THE ABC
CLINICAL GUIDE TO HERBS

The ABC
Clinical Guide to Herbs

Senior Editor
Mark Blumenthal

Founder and Executive Director
American Botanical Council

Managing Editor
Tara Hall

Editors
Alicia Goldberg
Tanja Kunz
Kara Dinda

Senior Writers
Josef Brinckmann
Bernd Wollschlaeger, M.D.

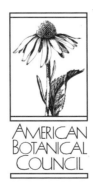

AMERICAN
BOTANICAL
COUNCIL

American Botanical Council
Austin, Texas
2003

Design and electronic production: Sean Barnes
Copyeditor and proofreader: Wendy Anderson
Indexer: Shirley Beckwith
Photography: Steven Foster
Illustrations: Peggy Duke
Printer: Sheridan Books, Inc.
Cover printer: Brady-Palmer Printing Corp.

American Botanical Council, Austin, Texas 78714-4345

First edition published 2003
Printed in the United States of America

ISBN for the Americas: 1-58890-157-2
ISBN for the Rest of the World: 3-13-132391-4

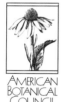

The American Botanical Council (ABC) is the nation's leading nonprofit education and research organization using science-based and traditional information to promote the responsible use of herbal medicine. The member-supported organization serves all populations interested in herbal medicine: consumers, healthcare professionals, researchers, educators, industry, and the media. American Botanical Council / P.O. Box 144345 / Austin, TX 78714-4345 / Phone: 512-926-4900 / Fax: 512-926-2345 / Toll free in the U.S.: 800-373-7105 / email: abc@herbalgram.org. This book may be ordered from the ABC website: www.herbalgram.org.

The exclusive distributor in the Americas is:

Thieme New York
333 Seventh Avenue
New York, NY 10001
United States of America
Phone: 1 800 782 3488 or +1 212 760 0888/Fax +1 212 947 1112
By email: customerservice@thieme.com

The exclusive distributor outside the Americas is:

Thieme International
Ruedigerstrasse 14
Stuttgart
D-70469 Germany
Phone: +49 (0) 711 8931 126/Fax +49 (0) 49 711 8931 410
By email: custserv@thieme.de

This book may also be ordered from www.thieme.com.

DEDICATION

This book is respectfully dedicated to the memory of the late Varro E. Tyler, Ph.D., Sc.D., Dean and Lilly Distinguished Professor Emeritus at the College of Pharmacy and Pharmacal Sciences at Purdue University.

Professor Tyler was a driving force behind "rational phytotherapy" in America—the concept that scientifically documented herbs and phytomedicinal products should be employed in popular self-care and modern clinical healthcare (in fact, he co-authored a book of that title). Through his articles, books, and lectures, he put forth the idea that there are many safe, appropriate, and scientifically justifiable applications for the chemically complex medicines made from herbs, whole plant extracts, and standardized medicinal plant preparations, often called phytomedicines.

As a member of the Board of Trustees of the American Botanical Council (ABC) Professor Tyler was the initial motivator of ABC's book, *The Complete German Commission E Monographs—Therapeutic Guide to Herbal Medicines*. He wrote the foreword in that book and its subsequent evolution, *Herbal Medicine: Expanded Commission E Monographs*.

Throughout his career, Professor Tyler promoted scientific education on the role of herbs and medicinal plants in modern medicine and pharmacy. He believed strongly that health professionals need to understand the actual and potential benefits and risks of herbs and phytomedicines. He also lamented the lack of inclusion of botanical medicine in the formal education of healthcare professionals. A committed proponent of quality control, clinical research, and rational, appropriate regulation of herbs and phytomedicinal products, he believed that both consumers and healthcare professionals could benefit from the judicious use of well-researched medicinal plant products.

ABC is grateful for Professor Tyler's involvement in the development of this book and for the significant and lasting contributions he made in the field of rational, science-based herbal medicine.

About the American Botanical Council

The American Botanical Council (ABC) is the nation's leading nonprofit education and research organization using science-based and traditional information to promote the responsible use of herbal medicine. The member-supported organization serves all populations interested in herbal medicine: consumers, healthcare professionals, researchers, educators, industry, and the media.

ABC's vision is that the public makes educated, responsible choices about herbal medicine as an accepted part of healthcare. Founded in 1988, ABC supports this vision through its mission to provide science-based and traditional information to promote the responsible use of herbal medicine.

ABC achieves its mission through:

- publication of its peer-reviewed journal *HerbalGram*
- the literature review service HerbClip™
- publication of books and literature
- continuing education materials for healthcare professionals
- information on its website, www.herbalgram.org
- internships for healthcare professionals
- safety guidelines for herbal products
- seminars, presentations and workshops
- serving as an information source to global print and electronic media

About Mark Blumenthal

Mark Blumenthal is the founder and executive director of ABC where he also serves as editor/publisher of *HerbalGram* and executive editor of HerbClip™. He is an adjunct associate professor of medicinal chemistry at the College of Pharmacy at the University of Texas at Austin. In addition, he is the senior editor of *The Complete German Commission E Monographs—Therapeutic Guide to Herbal Medicines* and *Herbal Medicine: Expanded Commission E Monographs*.

For information contact ABC at:

American Botanical Council
P.O. Box 144345
Austin, TX 78714-4345
Phone: 512-926-4900
Fax: 512-926-2345
Toll-free in the U.S.: 800-373-7105
Email: abc@herbalgram.org
Website: www.herbalgram.org

TABLE OF CONTENTS

List of Tables ix

Acknowledgements xi

Underwriters xiii

Disclaimers and Disclosures xiv

Author Disclosure of Commercial Affiliation xv

Learning Objectives and Accreditation xvi

Introduction xvii

    Part I: Background on Herbal Medicine xvii

        A Brief History of Medicinal Herbs in North America..xvii

        Recent Market and Consumer Use Information...xvii

        Herb Safety xviii

        Standardization xix

        Legal and Regulatory Status of Herbs and Phytomedicines in the U.S................xix

        Lack of Regulatory Assessment and Recognition of Benefits xxi

        Integrating Botanical Medicine into Modern Clinical Practice...........................xxi

        Rational Phytotherapy..xxiii

        Evidence-Based Medicine xxiii

        Interpreting Product Labels xxiv

    Part II: About This Book...xxv

        The Purpose of this Book xxv

        Potential Bias xxv

        Why the Herbs in this Book Were Selected xxv

        Description of the Herb Chapters xxvi

    References xxix

Herb Chapters: Clinical Overviews, Patient Sheets, and Single Herb Monographs 1

    Bilberry 3

    Black Cohosh 13

    Cat's Claw 23

    Cayenne 39

    Chamomile...51

    Chaste Tree 61

    Cranberry 73

    Echinacea 85

    Eleuthero 97

    Ephedra 107

    Evening Primrose Oil 123

    Feverfew 135

    Flax 143

    Garlic 153

    Ginger 171

    Ginkgo 185

    Ginseng, American 201

    Ginseng, Asian 211

    Goldenseal 227

    Hawthorn 235

    Horse Chestnut 247

    Kava 259

Licorice...273

Milk Thistle..285

Peppermint...297

Saw Palmetto..309

St. John's Wort...321

Tea, Black/Green..335

Valerian...351

Proprietary Herbal Product Monographs...365

Introduction 366

Monopreparations 369

Pycnogenol® (French Maritime Pine Bark Extract) 369

Multi-herb Propietary Product Monographs...374

Alluna™ 374

Esberitox® 375

Euvegal® forte 376

Hochu-ekki-to®..377

Hova® 378

Liv. 52® 379

Mastodynon®...381

Nutrilite® Saw Palmetto with Nettle Root 382

Padma® Basic/Padma® 28..383

Phytodolor®..385

Prostagutt® forte 387

Sinupret® 388

References 390

Appendix...393

Reviewers..394

General References 397

Commercial Products Used in Clinical Studies Listed in Single Herb Monographs..........398

Commercial Products Used in Clinical Studies Listed in Proprietary Herbal Product Monographs.....404

Company Contact Information for Commercial Products Used in Clinical Studies 405

Top-Selling Herbal Supplements in Food, Drug, and Mass Market Retail Outlets 409

Recent Studies 410

Abbreviations and Symbols...412

Glossary...416

Post Test...425

Applications For Receiving Credit...431

Index..441

LIST OF TABLES

Examples of Conventional Drugs Derived from Plants........xvii

Herbs and Herbal Materials Approved as Over-the-Counter (OTC) Drug Ingredients by the U.S. FDA.............xx

Reasons for Nondisclosure of Complementary and Alternative (CAM) Therapy Use With a Recognized Potential for Risk for Adverse Events xxii

Clinical Studies on Bilberry (*Vaccinium myrtillus* L.) 11

Clinical Studies on Black Cohosh (*Actaea racemosa* L.)..........21

Clinical Studies on Cat's Claw (*Uncaria guianensis* [Aubl.] Gmel.) 36

Clinical Studies on Cat's Claw (*Uncaria tomentosa* [Willd.] DC.)—Focusing on Preparations Standardized to Carboxy Alkyl Esters (CAEs) 36

Clinical Studies on Cat's Claw (*Uncaria tomentosa* [Willd.] DC.)—Focusing on Preparations Standardized to Pentacyclic Oxindole Alkaloids (POAs) with no Tetracyclic Oxindole Alkaloids (TOAs) 37

Clinical Studies on Cayenne (*Capsicum* spp.) 47

Clinical Studies on Capsaicin Preparations...........................48

Clinical Studies on Chamomile, German (*Matricaria recutita* L.) 59

Clinical Studies on Chaste Tree (*Vitex agnus-castus* L.) 69

Clinical Studies on Cranberry (*Vaccinium macrocarpon* Aiton)..81

Clinical Studies on Echinacea (*Echinacea* spp.) 94

Clinical Studies on Eleuthero (*Eleutherococcus senticosus* [Rupr. & Maxim.] Maxim.) 105

Clinical Studies on Ephedra (*Ephedra sinica* Stapf).............120

Clinical Studies on Ephedrine 121

Clinical Studies on Evening Primrose (*Oenothera biennis* L.)...131

Clinical Studies on Feverfew (*Tanacetum parthenium* [L.] Sch. Bip.)...142

Clinical Studies on Flax (*Linum usitatissimum* L.) 150

Clinical Studies on Garlic (*Allium sativum* L.) 167

Clinical Studies on Ginger (*Zingiber officinale* Roscoe)........179

Clinical Studies on Ginkgo (*Ginkgo biloba* L.) 195

Clinical Studies on Ginseng, American (*Panax quinquefolius* L.)..209

Clinical Studies on Ginseng, Asian (*Panax ginseng* C.A. Meyer) 222

Clinical Studies on Berberine 234

Clinical Studies on Hawthorn (*Crataegus* spp.) 244

Clinical Studies on Horse Chestnut (*Aesculus hippocastanum* L.) 255

Clinical Studies on Kava (*Piper methysticum* G. Forst.)........270

Clinical Studies on Licorice (*Glycyrrhiza* spp.) 282

Clinical Studies on Milk Thistle (*Silybum marianum* [L.] Gaertn.)..293

Clinical Studies on Peppermint (*Mentha* x *piperita* L.) 305

Clinical Studies on Saw Palmetto (*Serenoa repens* [W. Bartram] Small) 317

Clinical Studies on St. John's Wort (*Hypericum perforatum* L.) 331

Clinical Studies on Tea, Black/Green (*Camellia sinensis* [L.] Kuntze)...345

Clinical Studies on Valerian (*Valeriana officinalis* L.) 361

Clinical Studies on Pycnogenol®, French Maritime Pine Bark extract (*Pinus pinaster* Aiton subsp *atlantica*) 372

Clinical Studies on Alluna™ Sleep 374

Clinical Studies on Esberitox® 375

Clinical Studies on Euvegal® forte 376

Clinical Studies on Hochu-ekki-to®....................................377

Clinical Studies on Hova® 378

Clinical Studies on Liv.52® 380

Clinical Studies on Mastodynon® 381

Clinical Studies on Nutrilite® Saw Palmetto with Nettle Root 382

Clinical Studies on Padma® 28 384

Clinical Studies on Phytodolor® 386

Clinical Studies on Prostagutt® forte....................................387

Clinical Studies on Sinupret® 389

Commercial Products Used in Clinical Studies
Listed in Single Herb Monographs.....................................398

Commercial Products Used in Clinical Studies
Listed in Proprietary Herbal Product Monographs..............404

Top-Selling Herbal Supplements in Food, Drug,
and Mass Market Retail Outlets 409

ACKNOWLEDGEMENTS

This book is the product of a collaboration by many people and organizations, for which the editors and publisher are deeply grateful.

The person who deserves most credit for the idea and publication of this book is Wayne Silverman, Ph.D., Chief Administrative Officer at the American Botanical Council (ABC). Wayne originally envisioned a continuing medical education course for physicians, and spent months developing the idea with the Texas Medical Association (TMA). In his role as the chief development officer at ABC, he raised most of the funds necessary for the editorial development, publication, and distribution of this book and CME course.

There are two people at ABC who spent more time and energy on this project than almost any one else. Tara Hall, senior project manager, took over the role about midway during the editorial process and spent an incredible amount of time and focused energy coordinating literally hundreds of editorial and publication tasks. Sean Barnes, ABC's art director, designed the cover and layout of the entire book, entering additional changes into semi-final and final page proofs for months as the book came closer to publication. This book could not have been completed without their skillful, dedicated work.

During the writing and editorial process, two additional people served as project managers: Kara Dinda, M.S. and Alicia Goldberg. Each handled multiple tasks, dealing with writers, interns, libraries, peer reviewers, and others during the development of the monographs.

Our senior writers contributed immensely of their knowledge of herbs and herbal literature. Josef Brinckmann, former head of research and development at Traditional Medicinals in Sebastopol, California wrote the original drafts for some of the monographs, edited and revised some of the key sections in many others (e.g., Description, Regulatory), and provided translation of key German texts. Bernd Wollschlaeger, M.D., of the Aventura Family Health Center in Miami, Florida, provided translation of German papers, wrote the first drafts of the Clinical Overviews and the Clinical Review sections, and provided other valuable editorial input.

The staff of the American Botanical Council, past and present, deserve special mention. Of particular note is Tanja Kunz, former Education Coordinator, who provided extensive research while managing multiple tasks within the editorial process. Christina Allday-Bondy compiled and organized the extensive references and the brand cross-references. Judy Osburn and Kim West provided invaluable assistance in the development and fundraising efforts. Gayle Engels headed up much of the marketing and public relations efforts. The entire staff assisted in the final proofing of the Index. Special thanks are due to Stacy Elliott and Karen Robin, as well as Lori Glenn and Barbara Springer. Additional gratitude goes to Cecelia Thompson, Margaret Wright, George Solis, Kathleen Coyne, Cheryl Dipper, Jim Costello, and Roger Sleight. Former staff member Dawnelle Malone organized massive files for easier access to many of the references.

Julie Dennis contributed initial drafts of several sections of the Introduction. We also thank Candace Kiene for her copyediting; and extend appreciation to Wendy Anderson for her extensive editing and proofreading services, as well as for her work on certain sections, including the Glossary.

We are deeply grateful to Julie Bonifacio, of the Department of Health in Manila, the Phillipines. Julie came to ABC in 1999 as an intern under the aegis of the World Health Organization (WHO). During her three-month internship in 1999, Julie poured through ABC's library and began organizing the information that later developed into the monographs.

ABC is a preceptorship site for pharmacy students as well as students in nutrition and dietetics, as part of the fulfillment of their degree. From the College of Pharmacy at the University of Texas, we received assistance from Janice Ducoty, Pharm.D.; Lan Liu, Pharm.D.; Christine Formea, Pharm.D.; and Kathi Salerno–Faith, Pharm.D. From the University of Houston College of Pharmacy, we received assistance from Stan Eapen, Pharm.D; and Chelsea Tran, Pharm.D. From Southwest Texas State University, the following people assisted in the project: Hayley Dolezal, Jihyun Yoon, Patti Moody, Jill Ostendorf, Brady McConnell, Sara Davis, Sarah Harper-Becker, Angie Fiscus, Maggie Meyer, Diana Moyer, Tina Hammerschmidt, Jamie Stavinoha, and Nicholas Schnell. From Texas A&M University, the following interns assisted on the project: Amanda Scott, Erin Streiff, Mandy Clark, and Alicia Currado. Stacy Meyer, from Presbyterian Hospital, and Katherine Griffin, from Houston Veterans Administration Hospital, also assisted.

Like most nonprofit organizations, ABC depends on assistance from volunteers, who provide invaluable time and energy. The editors gratefully acknowledge Shirley Beckwith, ABC's volunteer librarian, who not only provided the indexing for the entire book, but assisted in accessing scientific studies from various libraries. Other volunteer contributions came from Erica Marchand, for her research on the Branded Products sections; Laurie Aroch, R.Ph., who created the first draft of the glossary; Karen Becker for her work on the Branded Products section; Susan Polasek, M.S.; Cynthia Warren; JoLyn Piercy; and Jeffrey Potts.

Significant assistance was provided by numerous reviewers from multiple academic disciplines, herbal industry, and related fields. These reviewers evaluated various drafts of the monographs offering expert advice and, in many cases, additional information, references, etc. The full list of reviewers can be found in the appendix on page 394; however, of particular importance are: Dennis V.C. Awang, Ph.D., of MediPlant Consulting Services in White Rock, British Columbia, who reviewed the Chemistry area of most of the monographs; Mary Chavez, Pharm.D., of Midwestern University, who provided detailed information on specific clinical trials summarized in the Clinical Tables; Jerry Cott, Ph.D., who reviewed much of the pharmacology of the monographs, and Thomas L. Kurt, M.D., M.P.H, Clinical Professor, Department of Internal Medicine, University of Texas Southwestern Medical School, who provided expert opinion and suggestions in many phases of the editorial process.

The editors and publisher acknowledge Donald R. Counts, M.D., a family practice physician in Austin, who integrates complementary and alternative treatments. Dr. Counts was a member of a the TMA planning committee organized in 1998 to discuss preliminary ideas for enduring material on therapeutic uses of herbs, and acted as this project's chief champion to TMA. He reviewed several drafts of the monographs and provided considerable constructive feedback, from a health professional's perspective, for improvement. Dr. Counts is a strong supporter of expanding the knowledge of physicians in the area of herbal medicine.

Invaluable support came from the Texas Medical Association Library, particularly Nancy Reynolds, Library Director, who provided access to TMA Library's extensive collection of clinical resources for research, document delivery services, and verification of references.

ABC is also most grateful to the Lloyd Library in Cincinatti, particularly to Erika Anderson, for supplying clinical trials and other scientific research articles from the Library's vast collection of journals and books.

ABC is also deeply grateful to the Council for Responsible Nutrition (CRN) in Washington, D.C., particularly John Cordaro, former President, and John Cardellina, Ph.D., former Vice-President for Botanical Sciences. CRN provided financial and administrative resources to convene a special expert panel of scientists and physicians who reviewed drafts of the major monographs. This process added an opportunity for additional review that greatly assisted in improving the material.

We are grateful to Alan Greenberg of the Greenberg Group who assisted with the marketing plan, as did Barbara Springer, Oliver Meek, Diane Graves, Denise Adams, and Jeffrey Potts.

Various attorneys in the natural products industry have provided review assistance and counsel. We are grateful to: Rakesh Amin of Weaver and Amin in Chicago; Loren D. Israelsen of LDI Group in Salt Lake City; A. Wesley Siegner of Hyman, Phelps and McNamara in Washington, D.C.; and Anthony L. Young of Piper Marbury in Washington, D.C. for their sage counsel and support.

We are also grateful to the members of the ABC Board of Trustees and ABC Advisory Board for their ongoing support of this project, many of whom acted as reviewers: Michael J. Balick, Ph.D., Director and Philecology Curator, Institute of Economic Botany, The New York Botanical Garden, Bronx, New York; James A. Duke, Ph.D., Economic Botanist (USDA, ret.) Author, Fulton, Maryland; Norman R. Farnsworth, Ph.D., Research Professor of Pharmacognosy, Program for Collaborative Research in the Pharmaceutical Sciences, University of Illinois at Chicago; Steven Foster, President, Steven Foster Group, Inc., Fayetteville, Arkansas; Fredi Kronenberg, Ph.D., Director, Rosenthal Center for Complementary and Alternative Medicine, Columbia University College of Physicians and Surgeons, New York; and Varro E. Tyler, Ph.D., Sc.D. (1926–2001), Dean and Distinguished Professor of Pharmacognosy Emeritus, School of Pharmacy and Pharmacal Sciences, Purdue University.

This book serves as both a reference book and a Continuing Medical Education course. In order to qualify for CME credit for physicians and CE credit for pharmacists, nurses and dieteticians (and other healthcare professionals) the accrediting organizations submitted drafts of the monographs to a committee of reviewers from each profession. Grateful thanks are due to many people at the various organizations listed below.

For accreditation for physicians, we are grateful to the staff at the Texas Medical Association (TMA), particularly Paige Miller, CME Program Manager, and Nancy Reynolds, Library Director. Also, as noted above, Donald R. Counts, M.D., and other TMA members for participating in the review process to provide continuing medical education credit for this book.

In the pharmacy profession, we offer grateful acknowledgement to the Texas Pharmacy Association (TPA), particularly Kim Roberson, R.Ph., Senior Director of Professional Affairs and Tanya Garde, R.Ph.

In the nursing profession, we offer grateful acknowledgement to the Texas Nurses Association (TNA), particularly, Wanda Douglas, M.S.N., R.N., Education Director, and Donna McCulloch, M.S., R.N., CNE Consultant.

We received assistance in the accreditation process from colleagues in the nutrition and dietetics profession. Our thanks go to B.J. Friedman, Ph.D., Professor of Nutrition, Chair of the Department of Family and Consumer Sciences at Southwest Texas State University, John Westerdahl, M.P.H., R.D., at the Castle Medical Center, Castle Center for Health Promotion; Cindy McClary, R.D., L.D., at St. Luke's Health Systems and Siouxland Regional Cancer Center in Sioux City, Iowa, and Susan Polasek, M.A., R.D., lecturer in nutrition at the University of Texas at Austin. We also gratefully acknowledge Gretchen Vannice, M.S., R.D., Continuing Professional Education Coordinator, and her colleagues at Nutrition in Complementary Care (NCC), Seattle, a dietetic practice group of the American Dietetics Association, for their financial support and for informing dietitians about this book.

There are probably other friends and colleagues who have contributed directly or indirectly, whom we have inadvertently overlooked. We sincerely apologize for any omissions. To all those listed above, and those whom we may have overlooked, the editors and publisher offer heartfelt gratitude and appreciation.

Mark Blumenthal
Austin, Texas
January 2003

UNDERWRITERS

As an independent nonprofit organization, the American Botanical Council depends on funding from the general public including its members and various companies, organizations, and foundations. We gratefully acknowledge the following underwriters for their generous support of *The ABC Clinical Guide to Herbs*.

VISIONARIES
Bionorica AG
Council for Responsible Nutrition
Horphag Research
Ricola USA

PARTNERS
ABKIT, Inc.
Campamed LLC
Enzymatic Therapy
GlaxoSmithKline
Metabolife International, Inc.
Pharmavite Corporation
PhytoPharmica
Rexall Sundown
Starlight International

SUPPORTERS
EcoNugenics, Inc.
Herbalife International, Inc.
Horst M. Rechelbacher Foundation
NBTY
Phoenix Laboratories, Inc.
Pierre Fabre
Schaper & Brümmer GmbH & Co. KG
Schwabe International

FRIENDS
American Health
Good 'N Natural
Holland & Barrett
The Jacob Teitelbaum Family Foundation
Nature's Bounty
Puritan's Pride
Renaissance Herbs, Inc.
Vitamin World

DISCLAIMERS AND DISCLOSURES

Medicine is an ever-changing art and science undergoing continual development. Research and clinical experience are constantly expanding our knowledge of proper treatment and therapy. The information contained in this book represents a compilation of authoritative scientific data. It is not an exhaustive listing of all possible uses, contraindications, adverse effects, interactions and other information. Insofar as this book mentions any use, dosage, contraindication, adverse effect, etc., readers may rest assured that the authors, editors, and publishers have consulted sources believed to be reliable in their efforts to provide information that is thorough and in accordance with the state of knowledge at the time of production of the book.

Nevertheless, in view of the possibility of human error by the authors, editors, or publisher of this work, or changes in the state of knowledge, this work does not involve, imply, or express any guarantee or responsibility on the part of the authors, editors, or publisher, nor any other party who has been involved in the preparation of this work, that the information contained herein is, in every respect, accurate or complete, and they are not responsible for any errors or omissions, or for the results obtained from use of such information. In addition, this book is not intended as a guide to self-medication by consumers. Every user is encouraged to carefully confirm this information with other sources. For example, readers are advised to consult their healthcare practitioner and to check the product information sheet included in the package of each product they plan to use to be certain that the information contained in this publication is accurate and that changes have not been made in the recommended dose or in the contraindications for administration. This recommendation is of particular importance in connection with new or infrequently used herbal preparations.

Some of the product names, patents, and registered designs referred to in this book are, in fact, registered trademarks or proprietary names even though specific reference to this fact is not always made in the text. Therefore, the appearance of a name without designation as proprietary is not to be construed as a representation by the publisher that it is in the public domain.

As a nonprofit organization, ABC serves the public by providing education and information on herbs and phytomedicines. In order to provide these services, ABC draws upon a multitude of sources for financial and research support. By disclosing the underwriters of this project (see page xiii), the commercial affiliations of the authors (see page xv), and the affiliations of the reviewers (see page 394), ABC is disclosing any conflict of interest on behalf of the authors, editors, reviewers, staff, and Trustees of ABC. The potential self-interest of any underwriter has not influenced the contents of this publication. ABC would like to assure the reader that its primary concern is to provide reliable information and education for the general public.

STATEMENTS OF NONENDORSEMENT

The inclusion of information on proprietary products is not an endorsement by the American Botanical Council of these products or the companies that produce them. Product brand names are listed for studies conducted using these preparations in order to acknowledge that these are the specific proprietary preparations on which particular trials were conducted.

The ABC Clinical Guide to Herbs was produced for educational purposes only; endorsement by Texas Medical Association of the use or efficacy of any treatments or methodologies included in this publication is not implied by their inclusion.

AUTHOR DISCLOSURE OF COMMERCIAL AFFILIATIONS

Texas Medical Association is accredited by the Accreditation Council for Continuing Medical Education to provide continuing education for physicians.

Policies and standards of the FDA, the American Medical Association, and the Accreditation Council for Continuing Medical Education require that authors for continuing medical education activities disclose any significant financial interests, relationships, or affiliations they may have with commercial entities whose products, devices, or services may be discussed in their book. They must also disclose discussion of investigational or unlabeled uses of a product.

The authors have asked that we advise readers that by law dietary supplement uses are not listed on product labels. Each monograph will discuss uses and clinical studies conducted using herbs and herbal products.

The following authors have asked that we advise participants in this activity that they have an affiliation with the following organization(s).

Mark Blumenthal	employee, American Botanical Council
	chairman, Board of Trustees, American Botanical Council
Tara Hall	employee, American Botanical Council
Alicia Goldberg	former contractor, American Botanical Council
Tanja Kunz	former employee, American Botanical Council
Kara Dinda, MS	former employee, American Botanical Council
Josef Brinckmann	former employee, Traditional Medicinals, Inc.
	consultant, Traditional Medicinals, Inc.
	(pertains to peppermint monograph only)
Bernd Wollschlaeger, MD	member, Advisory Board, American Botanical Council

LEARNING OBJECTIVES

The information is followed by a self-test. Upon completion of this course, health professionals should be able to:

1)   Identify the 29 most popular medicinal herbs available to consumers in the U.S. market.

2)   Explain the common therapeutic indications of the leading herbs.

3)   Provide an overview of the clinical study research of the leading herbs.

4)   Identify potential drug interactions and side effects.

5)   Evaluate the safety issues and contraindications.

6)   Interpret product labels for indications of clinical efficacy.

7)   Distinguish different types of brands on the marketplace which are backed by clinical research.

8)   Understand the implications of government regulations on the clinical use of herbs.

TARGET AUDIENCES
Dietitians, Naturopathic Physicians, Nurses, Pharmacists, and Physicians.

METHOD INSTRUCTION
Information is presented in monographs followed by test questions.

ACCREDITATION

DIETITIANS
A total of 12 CE hours will be awarded to Dietitians and Dietetic Technicians by the Commission on Dietetic Registration (CDR) of the American Dietetic Association, through Southwest Texas State University, for the successful completion of this program.

NATUROPATHIC PHYSICIANS
A total of 12 CE hours will be awarded by the American Botanical Council in collaboration with the Oregon Board of Naturopathic Examiners for the successful completion of this program.

NURSES
A total of 10 contact hours is provided by the Texas Nurses Association. Texas Nurses Association/Foundation is accredited as a provider of continuing nursing education by the American Nurses Credentialing Center's Commission on Accreditation (ANCC). This activity meets Type I criteria for mandatory continuing education requirements toward relicensure as established by the Board of Nurse Examiners for the State of Texas.

PHARMACISTS
A total of 1.2 CEU (12 contact hours) will be awarded to pharmacists for the successful completion of this program. The Texas Pharmacy Association is approved by the American Council on Pharmaceutical Education as a provider of continuing pharmaceutical education. The ACPE Program number is 154–999–03–700–H01 with an initial release date of March 2003. All requests for continuing education credit must be submitted to Texas Pharmacy Association prior to February 27, 2006.

PHYSICIANS
This activity has been planned and implemented in accordance with the Essential Areas and Policies of the Accreditation Council for Continuing Medical Education (ACCME) through the joint sponsorship of the Texas Medical Association and the American Botanical Council. Texas Medical Association is accredited by ACCME to provide continuing medical education for physicians.

Texas Medical Association designates this educational activity for a maximum of 13.5 category 1 credits toward the AMA Physician's Recognition Award. Each physician should claim only those credits he/she actually spent in the educational activity.

Expiration date: January 31, 2005

INTRODUCTION

by Mark Blumenthal
Founder and Executive Director, American Botanical Council

PART I: BACKGROUND ON HERBAL MEDICINE

A Brief History of Medicinal Herbs in North America

Herbs have enjoyed a long history of use as medicines in North America. Native Americans had medicinal uses for at least 2,582 species of plants, including such uses as analgesic, contraceptive, laxative, sedative, and remedies for colds, tuberculosis, and cancer (Moerman, 1998).

Until about 1930, herbs and herbal products constituted a significant proportion of the materia medica of North America during the 17th, 18th, 19th, and early 20th centuries. The first edition of the *United States Pharmacopeia* (USP) in 1820 contained 425 botanical substances (67% of all entries). Herb and herb product monographs reached their peak of 636 botanical substances (66%) in USP V in 1870, but by the time USP X was published in 1926, the total number of botanically-related monographs dropped to 203 botanical substances (36%) (Boyle, 1991). This reflected the trend that botanical medicine was widely used in the U.S. until about 1920 when herbs began to be replaced with pharmaceutical drugs, not because they were determined unsafe or ineffective, but because their actions were generally not as pharmacologically dramatic, and they were not as economically profitable as the newer synthetic drugs.

In 1888, the American Pharmaceutical Association published the *National Formulary* (NF), a compendium of formulae of primarily herb-based prepared medicines. In 1975 the publication of the NF was taken over by the USP and combined with the USP to create the USP-NF in 1980. In the 1990s, the USP renewed its efforts to address the issue of establishing quality standards for conventional dietary supplements (e.g., vitamins, minerals, etc.) and, in 1995, after the passage of the Dietary Supplement Health and Education Act of 1994 (DSHEA), USP began the development of monographs defining identity and purity standards for many of the best-selling herbs in the U.S. market. From 1995 to 2002, USP has published 86 standards monographs on 25 herbs (Blumenthal, 2003).

The recognition of the biological activity of herbs and medicinal plants is as old as medicine and pharmacy where many herbs have been used as medicines (so-called "crude drugs") and, in more recent times, as the sources of widely accepted pharmaceutical drugs. Table 1 contains a partial listing of modern plant-derived drugs.

Recent Market and Consumer Use Information

The need for professionally-oriented information and continuing education on the potential risks and benefits of herbal preparations is motivated by market factors in the past decade where consumers are using these products in larger numbers than ever before.

Consumers utilize herbs and other dietary supplements for a variety of purposes. A survey of 3,226 users of the ConsumerLab.com website stated they used supplements (herbal and non-herbal combined) for general health (67%), colds (53%), osteoarthritis (39%), energy enhancement (37%), cholesterol lowering (29%), cancer prevention (28%), allergy (27%), and weight management (25%). Fifty-four percent

Table 1: Examples of Conventional Drugs Derived from Plants*		
Drug	**Herb Common Name (Latin Name)**	**Action/Approved Use**
Colchicine	Autumn crocus (*Colchicum autumnale*)	Anti-inflammatory
Digoxin/Lanoxin	Digitalis/foxglove (*Digitalis* spp.)	Cardiotonic/Positive inotropic
Tubocurarine	Curare (*Chondrodendron tomentosum*)	Neuromuscular blocker
Ephedrine	Ephedra (*Ephedra sinica*)	Sympathomimetic
Etoposide	Mayapple (*Podophyllum peltatum*)	Antitumor
Physostigmine	Calabar bean (*Physostigma venenosum*)	Cholinesterase inhibitor (parasympathomimetic)
Reserpine	Rauwolfia (*Rauwolfia serpentina*)	Hypotensive
Scopolamine	Jimson weed (*Datura stramonium*) Duboisia (*Duboisia* spp.)	Antimuscarinic; antimotion sickness
Taxol®	Pacific yew (*Taxus brevifolia*)	Antitumor
Vincristine	Madagascar periwinkle (*Catharanthus roseus*)	Acute lymphocytic leukemia; non-Hodgkins lymphoma, etc.

* As of the mid 1980s, at least 119 plant-derived drugs were used in conventional medicine (Farnsworth *et al.*, 1985). Taxol® and several others have been added since then.

indicated that they used supplements for four or more conditions, with satisfaction with supplement brands being assessed as generally high, ranging from 97–63% of consumers being highly satisfied with their brands (ConsumerLab.com, 2002).

A recent survey of 2,590 respondents in the Slone Survey (Kaufman *et al.*, 2002) found the following 10 most common reasons for taking herbal and non-herbal dietary supplements (i.e., non vitamin and mineral supplements): "health/good for you (16%); arthritis (7%); memory improvement (6%); energy (5%); immune booster (5%); joints (4%); supplement the diet (45%); sleep aid (3%); prostate (3%); don't know/no reason specified (25%); all others (45%). There has been significant growth in other categories (e.g., menopause, weight loss, etc.) not noted specifically in this survey.

Over the past few years various surveys have reported differing statistics, but they tend to move in the same general direction. For example, in April and May 1999, *Prevention* magazine and Princeton Survey Research Associates conducted a survey of 2,000 adults indicating that 91 million consumers, about 49% of all the adult Americans, were estimated to have used an herbal product during the previous year. The survey also showed that about 24% (44.6 million) had used herbs frequently during the previous year, (Johnston, 2000), although another review and survey suggests that only 16–18% of adult Americans regularly use *dietary supplements* (which includes not only herbs, but also vitamins, minerals, amino acids, etc.) (Blendon *et al.*, 2001).

An earlier report estimated that 70 million Americans are using herbal supplements (Wasik, 1999). An often-cited study in the *Journal of the American Medical Association* (JAMA) (Eisenberg *et al.*, 1998) estimated that 46% of Americans saw an alternative practitioner in 1997, up from 36% in 1990, and spent $27.2 billion in 1998 on alternative care practitioners. Herb use reported in this survey grew from the baseline of 2.5% of the adult population measured in 1990 (Eisenberg *et al.*, 1993) to 12% of adults using herbs in a one-year period as measured in 1997, a growth factor of 380%.

In the 1990s, sales of herbal products became a phenomenon in mass market retail stores increasing from 1994 levels to their highest levels in 1998, then leveling off and subsequently dropping. Sales in this sector reached the high point of $688,352,192 (including Wal-Mart sales) in 1998 declining to $337,207,360 in 2001 (excluding Wal-Mart sales) (Blumenthal, 1999, 2002). (Recent market sales statistics are shown in the Appendix, page 409.) The decline of consumer demand in the mainstream market has been attributed to the following factors: negative media articles focusing on poor quality of some herbal products, adverse reaction reports and reports of interactions, the "myth" that the herb industry is unregulated—a message that lowers consumer confidence, unreasonable consumer expectations for the benefits of herbal products, and the cyclical nature of businesses (Blumenthal, 1999).

Meanwhile, sales in the natural/health food channels of trade continue to climb (albeit at a slower rate than previously.) This growth is explained by the fact that the more committed consumer shops for herbs and related supplements in health and natural food stores and appears to be less easily influenced by positive and negative publicity, rising 9% from $123,009,009 in 2000 to $134,086,587 in 2001 (Blumenthal, 2002).

Herb Safety

In general, it would appear that there are fewer adverse event reports (AERs) in the U.S. on a per capita basis for herbs than for conventional pharmaceutical drugs. On the other hand, it is also possible that the generally low incidents of AERs for herbs may be a result of poor reporting mechanisms and the possibility that many herb users simply may not report adverse events, because such events may be relatively minor (e.g., gastrointestinal upset, headache, etc.) and/or because many herb users may consider themselves outside the medical mainstream and may have a bias against making such a report. The truth of the situation in the U.S. is likely that both explanations are equally plausible; i.e, most commercially available herbs *are* generally gentler and safer than conventional drugs, *and* there needs to be better reporting mechanisms for herb-related adverse events.

The general safety of phytomedicines (advanced herbal preparations, often chemically standardized; see Standardization section on page xix) has been well documented in Western Europe, where the regulatory systems in many countries treat herbs and phytomedicines in the same way as they treat conventional drugs. That is, phytomedicines are made from raw materials and extracts that meet national or the European pharmacopeia standards for identity and purity, they are required to be manufactured by proper good manufacturing practices (GMPs: the body of federal requirements governing how food or drug manufacturers must operate their production facilities in order to ensure safe, properly labeled consumer foods and drugs), they are evaluated and approved by national governments for indications as nonprescription drugs and for safety parameters (e.g., the German Commission E), and any adverse effects are routinely reported within the same pharmacovigilance system designed for conventional drugs. In the European Union, the AERs for herbs and phytomedicinal preparations are lower than the AERs for conventional drugs, even when adjusted for total doses sold.

There are several voluntary reporting systems for herb and dietary supplement-related AERs in the U.S. One is the American Association of Poison Control Centers in Washington, D.C., the results from which are available on fee-for-service basis, usually for companies who check on reports on their specific products. Another is the Food and Drug Administration's (FDA) MedWatch system for drugs, used primarily by health professionals (sometimes considered controversial insofar as the reports are not always fully documented with adequate information). A new, improved system at FDA for reporting adverse events related to foods and dietary supplements is managed by the agency's Center for Food Safety and Applied Nutrition (CFSAN) and is called CAERS (CFSAN Adverse Event Reporting System). CAERS is replacing the older and much less reliable Special Nutritionals/Adverse Event Monitoring System (SN/AEMS) which was created in 1998. There were many problems associated with poor documentation of AERs associated with AEMS, as was eventually acknowledged on the AEMS website before it was removed in August, 2002: "There is no certainty that a reported adverse event can be attributed to a particular product or ingredient. The available information may not be complete enough to make this determination." (FDA, 2002a). The new CAERS system is expected to be pilot tested in 2003 and operational by 2004 (FDA, 2002b).

The FDA's 10-year work plan addresses the areas of safety, labeling, boundaries (related to appropriate definitions, etc.), enforcement activities, enhancement of the FDA's science/research capabilities, and outreach to consumers and manufacturers (Levitt, 2000). Included in the "Safety" section of the FDA's 10-year work plan, is the agency's commitment not only to publish regulations on GMPs, but also improve the AER system, as well as develop a database to enhance mechanisms for identifying potential health hazards related to foods and dietary supplements (Levitt, 2000). This is being implemented, as noted above.

The increasing use of herbs by consumers invariably suggests potential for interactions with conventional medications (Blumenthal, 2000; Fugh-Berman, 2000; Fugh-Berman and Ernst, 2001). Eisenberg *et al.* (1998) estimated that 15 million adults in 1997 used prescription drugs simultaneously with herbal remedies and/or high dose vitamin supplements, concluding that these persons were potentially at risk for adverse herb-drug or drug-supplement interactions. In a survey conducted by Princeton Survey Research Associates for *Prevention* magazine, researchers noted that 36% of herb users employ herbal remedies in place of prescription drugs; 31% *with* prescription drugs; 48% instead of over-the-counter (OTC) drugs; and 30% *with* OTC drugs (Johnston, 2000). In the Slone Survey (Kaufman *et al.*, 2002) of 2590 participants from about the same period of time, 81% stated that they used at least one medication (Rx or OTC), 50% took at least one prescription drug, and 7% took five or more drugs simultaneously. Fourteen percent said they used herbs and supplements during the previous week while 16% of the prescription drug users acknowledged also taking an herbal supplement. These authors conclude that one in seven adults consume at least one herbal supplement annually and that one in six patients taking a prescription drug is concurrently taking one or more herbal supplements, raising the potential for interactions.

A recent systematic review of herb-drug interactions (Fugh-Berman and Ernst, 2001) concluded that of the 108 interactions evaluated, 74 cases (68.5%) were considered unable to be evaluated due to the lack of adequate information, 14 (13%) were considered "well-documented" and thus likely, and 20 (18.5%) were considered "possible" interactions. The authors emphasize the need for better documentation of all relevant data in case studies of potential interactions. The most authoritative, evidence-based database of herb-drug interactions has been compiled by Brinker (2001).

Standardization

Many of the herbal preparations in this book upon which clinical trials were conducted are characterized as "standardized." This is one of the most misunderstood concepts in botanical medicine. While usually referring to the chemical process of "normalizing," "adjusting," or fixing a particular chemical or groups of chemicals, the concept of standardization has several meanings that warrant clarification.

There are numerous areas in which standardization occurs in the field of preparing botanical medicines and dietary supplements. First, there is nomenclature. The scientific terms (Latin binomials) are a standardized means used in botany and other sciences. In the U.S., there is also an initiative to standardize common names; the American Herbal Products Association (AHPA) has published a listing of about 1,650 herbs used in commerce in the U.S., with the "standardized common name" linked to the most recent Latin

binomial; "other common names" are also noted, although they are not preferred (McGuffin *et al.*, 2000). An earlier version of this self-regulatory initiative listing approximately 550 herbs was published in 1992 (Foster, 1992). In 1997, the U.S. Food and Drug Administration (FDA) adopted *Herbs of Commerce* as an official list for common names of herb products sold in the U.S. and thus federal regulations [21 C.F.R. Sec 101.4(h)(1)-(2)] require that common names used on herbal dietary supplement products be consistent with the names standardized in the 1992 edition of *Herbs of Commerce*. It is possible that the FDA will also similarly acknowledge the later publication.

The most frequently employed meaning of standardization refers to chemistry. *Standardization* often refers to the control of a particular marker compound or group of compounds (see discussion below). However, in a larger sense standardization can also refer to the entire process of controlling the supply chain of raw material quality and manufacturing process including, but not limited to, controlling various chemical components of the preparation (Eisner, 2001).

"Standardized" herbal products contain botanical ingredients that are chemically "standardized" to contain a consistent level of a major active constituent or marker compound or the botanical extract is defined by declaring the drug-to-extract ratio (e.g., 7–8:1), the extraction solvent (e.g., ethanol 60%), and the grade or quality of raw material that was used to make the extract (e.g., Senna Leaf USP). Chemical standardization has allowed manufacturers to offer greater consistency from batch to batch. In general, however, the term *standardization* encompasses far more than guaranteeing specific levels or ranges of certain constituents occurring in the final preparation. It involves the use of consistent, documented processes and standards throughout every step of production including adherence to Good Agricultural Practices (GAP), Good Manufacturing Practices (GMP) and Good Laboratory Practices (GLP), among others. AHPA has published its standardization guidance manual in 2001 (Eisner, 2001).

Standardizing herbal products does not necessarily guarantee potency because the medicinal activity is often not due to a single chemical but to a mixture of constituents (many still unidentified), and often to the additive, synergistic (or antagonistic) activity of several components (Robbers and Tyler, 1999). It is inherently difficult to control all the factors that affect a plant's chemical composition. For example, hypericins, a group of two naphthodianthrones, have long been held to be the active constituent of St. John's wort (*Hypericum perforatum*) (even though most commercial extracts incorrectly state that they are standardized to hypericin [singular] instead of hypericins). However, recent research suggests that the phloroglucinols hyperforin and adhyperforin, may be the prime active principles, and flavonoids such as amentoflavone have received consideration lately as possible active compounds (Awang, 1999). Other components may also be involved in biological activity.

Legal and Regulatory Status of Herbs and Phytomedicines in the U.S.

There appears to be considerable confusion about the regulation of herbs and other dietary supplements in the U.S. The herb and dietary supplement industries are characterized by a substantial level of laws, regulations, and proposed regulations on the federal level. Former FDA Commissioner Jane Henney, M.D.

testifying before the House Committee on Government Reform (March 25, 1999) stated, "The FDA has tools at its disposal to take enforcement actions against dietary supplements found to have safety, labeling, or other violations of the Food, Drug and Cosmetic (FD&C) Act, as amended by DSHEA." (Soller, 2000). As a result of DSHEA, dietary ingredients used in dietary supplements do not require pre-market documentation of safety for submission to the FDA unless they are *new dietary ingredients* (i.e., ingredients not sold before the passage of DSHEA in October 1994), subject to the notification requirement in Section 413(a)(2) of the FD&C Act. This has led critics of DSHEA to fear a potential "safety meltdown." Despite legitimate concerns about herb safety, the general lack of epidemiological evidence to the contrary suggests such a meltdown has not occurred since the passage of DSHEA, probably as a result of a combination of factors. These include the following considerations: (1) most dietary supplements have a very long history of relatively safe use; (2) consumers usually use self-care products, such as dietary supplements, in a responsible manner; (3) most companies are meeting the legal requirements of DSHEA; and, importantly, (4) the FDA and the FTC have sufficient enforcement authority in this area and have engaged in the development of the new regulatory framework for dietary supplements (Soller, 2000).

DSHEA places responsibility for ensuring herbal supplement safety on manufacturers, identifies how literature may be used in connection with sales, specifies types of statements of nutritional support that may be made on labels, specifies certain labeling requirements and provides for the establishment of regulations for GMPs. The FDA must model dietary supplement GMPs after food GMPs and may not impose standards for which there is no current and generally available analytical methodology. It is also important to point out that many dietary supplement companies have already been operating under GMPs that meet or exceed the proposed dietary supplement GMPs, particularly those companies who market their products outside of the U.S. or companies that also manufacture OTC drugs. Additionally, U.S. companies whose products are licensed as Traditional

Herbal Medicines (THMs) in Canada or as Therapeutic Goods in Australia must meet the GMP requirements of those countries, respectively. At press time (early 2003) the FDA had not yet published proposed rules for GMPs for dietary supplements, although such publication is considered imminent.

In passing DSHEA, Congress noted in the "findings" section of the Act that "consumers should be empowered to make choices about preventive health care programs based on data from scientific studies of health benefits related to particular dietary supplements." One of the purposes of passing DSHEA, therefore, was to provide consumer access to products and truthful information about those products, while maintaining authority for the FDA to take action against products that present safety problems or are improperly labeled (Soller, 2000).

Under DSHEA, dietary supplements are typically classified as foods, and defined as any product intended for ingestion as a supplement to the diet; but are not intended to replace food in the diet. They are specifically exempted from the definition of drugs (i.e. intended to diagnose, cure, mitigate, treat, or prevent diseases) and thus are not subjected to the same rigorous testing and approval processes required by the FDA for drugs. Manufacturers must label dietary supplements as such. Effective March 1999, supplement labels must carry a "Supplement Facts" panel, granting easier access to ingredients and suggested dosage.

One of the most misunderstood aspects of DSHEA is the issue of the FDA's ability to protect the public from unsafe dietary supplements. Once a supplement is on the market, the FDA must prove that it is unsafe before imposing restrictions on its use. The "burden of proof" has now shifted from the manufacturer proving safety to the FDA proving that a substance poses an "imminent health hazard" once that determination has been made by the Secretary of Health and Human Services. The issue of regulation, herb safety, and the impact on the general public can often be mischaracterized and exaggerated in the media to the extent that even FDA officials have misstated the agency's authority. According to Stephen H. McNamara, an attorney who specializes in food and drug law and formerly an attorney at the

Table 2: Herbs and Herbal Materials Approved as Over-the-Counter (OTC) Drug Ingredients by the U.S. FDA*

Herb Common Name	Latin Name	Approved Use
Capsicum fruit oleoresin	*Capsicum* spp.	Topical analgesic
Ipecac root	*Cephaelis ipecacuanha*	Emetic
Psyllium seed husk	*Plantago* spp.	Bulk laxative
Senna leaf and fruit	*Senna alexandrina*; *Cassia senna*	Stimulant laxative†
Slippery elm bark	*Ulmus rubra*	Demulcent
Witch hazel bark	*Hamamelis virginiana*	Astringent

* Herbs and herb materials refers to whole plants and/or plant parts, or their derived chemically complex products (e.g., oleoresin capsicum), but not single chemical entities (e.g., capsaicin, the primary active ingredient in capsicum oleoresin, approved as both an Rx and OTC drug, but not considered "herbal" although it is plant-derived). Further, pure compounds from herb-derived oils, although approved for OTC drug use, are not considered "herbal;" these include eucalyptol from eucalyptus leaf, menthol from peppermint leaf oil, and thymol from thyme leaf oil.

† In May 2002, the FDA issued a regulation effective November, 2002, deeming aloe (*Aloe ferox*, A. spp.) and cascara sagrada (*Rhamnus purshiana*) as laxative ingredients not generally recognized as safe for use as ingredients in OTC drug products. This regulation was based on the failure of members of the OTC drug and the herb industries to provide certain information requested by the FDA in June 1998 to help determine the safety of these ingredients. The FDA's request was based on previous research suggesting potential carcinogenicity associated with anthraquinone laxatives. Data on the potential safety of senna was submitted by members of the OTC drug industry, thereby allowing senna-based laxative preparations to stay on the market until the FDA's determination is issued (FDA, 2002c). The American Herbal Products Association and the International Aloe Science Council filed a petition with the FDA requesting a stay of this order until new safety data on aloe and cascara could be filed and considered (AHPA, 2002).

FDA, there are numerous provisions in the FDCA and DSHEA that give the FDA adequate authority to remove unsafe supplements from the market: "…it appears that the FDA has substantial and sufficient regulatory authority to protect the American public from any dangerous or otherwise unsafe herbs or other dietary supplement products despite statements to the contrary from FDA officials." (McNamara, 1996).

DSHEA also required the establishment of an Office of Dietary Supplements (ODS) within the National Institutes of Health (NIH) and a Commission on Dietary Supplement Labels. The ODS is responsible for conducting and coordinating research relating to dietary supplements (including botanicals) and collecting and compiling a database of scientific research on botanicals (ODS, 2002).

Consumer and professional confidence in herbal preparations and other dietary supplement products underwent a considerable degree of erosion during the late 1990s as various news organizations and independent groups reported that many of these products failed to meet a variety of labels claims related to content of certain ingredients, standardization markers, or other elements. While in some cases, these reports accurately reflected the wide variation in quality of herbal products, they sometimes were based upon improperly conducted analyses and/or inappropriate analytical methods (Raffman, 2000; Foreman, 2000).

For an extensive account of the legal and regulatory history of herbs in the U.S., see Blumenthal and Israelsen (1998).

Lack of Regulatory Assessment and Recognition of Benefits

One of the primary problems associated with the botanical products market in the U.S. is the lack of an official system to evaluate and recognize the benefits and risks of herbal preparations. While there is much attention focused on potential risks (for obvious reasons of concern for public safety and perhaps the less obvious reasons that many conventional health professionals are not adequately trained on the appropriate uses of these products), there is virtually no official recognition of the benefits of herbal products, except for the few herbs that are approved by the FDA for use as OTC drug ingredients (see Table 2). This lack of recognition of benefits fosters a situation in which safety problems become magnified and often disproportionately exaggerated relative to their actual public health implications. Thus, media reports of an adverse reaction to an herb or herbal product or an herb-drug interaction are viewed without any countervailing recognition of the benefits of the herb. This does not occur with OTC or prescription drugs as most of these ingredients have successfully undergone some form of formal risk-benefit assessment, i.e., the benefits outweigh the risks.

Some legislators and industry leaders are looking to countries with established herbal medicine regulatory systems. The Commission E in Germany is one such system frequently proposed as a potential model for consideration. There, herbal drugs are regulated in much the same way as conventional drugs, have to meet similar criteria of quality and safety that the country requires of all drugs (although herbal drugs are approved by a standard of "reasonable certainty" as compared to a stricter standard for pharmaceutical drugs), and are sometimes eligible for reimbursement by the national healthcare system (Blumenthal *et al.*, 1998). Commission E's findings on safety and efficacy have been called "the most accurate body of scientific knowledge on that subject available in the world today" (Robbers and Tyler, 1999). This statement is still probably true with respect to evaluations of herb safety and efficacy as sponsored by a Western industrialized nation. Commission E is a federally mandated panel of 24 experts from various disciplines associated with medicinal plants, including physicians and pharmacists. They met from 1978 to 1995 to assess the safety and efficacy of about 300 herbs and fixed herbal combinations to determine their approval as nonprescription drugs. Commission E conducted literature reviews as the primary method of determining safety and efficacy and did not employ the formal risk-benefit assessments used for conventional drugs. Nevertheless, of the 380 monographs published by Commission E, 254 were for herbs deemed positive (i.e., safe and effective—approved) while 126 were deemed either neutral (safe but insufficient data to approve use) or negative (unsafe and/or ineffective—unapproved) (Blumenthal *et al.*, 1998). Without a Commission E-like system or some other similar process for the rational and scientific evaluation of herb safety and benefits, and the eventual official recognition of these findings, it is highly likely that reports of adverse effects associated with herbs will continue to be viewed in an unbalanced manner without acknowledgement of their corresponding benefits.

Integrating Botanical Medicine into Modern Clinical Practice

Growing consumer use of herbs creates pressure on physicians and other healthcare providers to learn about their potential risks and benefits. Additionally, articles have begun to appear in medical journals urging conventionally trained physicians to become familiar with alternative medicine and to treat respectfully their patients who use such therapies (Eisenberg, 1997). Conferences and continuing medical education modules offer a variety of options, including information on medicinal herbs. For example, a week-long course on "Botanical Medicine in Modern Clinical Practice" has been offered by the Rosenthal Center for Complementary and Alternative Medicine at the Columbia University College of Physicians and Surgeons (www.rosenthal.hs.columbia.edu) since 1996.

Previous reports suggest that people who have used complementary medicine do not tell their physicians, as they are often concerned that the physician may either not understand or will criticize them; some of this is borne out in a recent survey summarized in Table 3 (Eisenberg *et al.*, 2001). As in all therapeutic relationships, communication and trust between doctor and patient are of primary importance (Zollman and Vickers, 1999). A University of Iowa study, however, suggests that herb users believe that herbs are generally safe, can improve their health, and that their physicians and their families share their positive perceptions about herbs. This same study noted the surprising finding that herb users tend to be heavier users of prescription drugs and to have more negative attitudes towards those medications than non-users (Klepser *et al.*, 2000).

Nearly two-thirds (64%) of the nation's medical schools now have courses on complementary and alternative medicine (CAM); many designed to help physicians answer patients' questions (Wetzel *et al.*, 1998; Stolberg, 2000). Of the 123 CAM courses reported in a survey, 68% were stand-alone electives and 31% were part of required curriculum (Wetzel *et al.*, 1998). Herbal medicine is usually included in the complementary medicine courses in these curricula, but the herb information is often relegated to cursory reviews and basic but incomplete information on only the most popular herbs in the market.

Nearly half of British medical schools offer some courses in complementary medicine and some postgraduate medical centers offer a basic introduction to complementary disciplines (Zollman and Vickers, 1999). In a survey of 550 European universities (141 having medical faculties), 43 (40%) universities of the 107 responding schools offer coursework in CAM; 8 teach herbal medicine/phytotherapy; 4 employ phytotherapy in university clinics; and 3 report clinical research on herbs (Barberis *et al.*, 2001).

The level of credibility in herbs and phytomedicines increased in the past decade among members of the conventional medical community in the U.S. after the publication of several papers in mainstream medical journals that support the safe and effective use of some of the more well-researched herbs. These papers include (in chronological order) the meta-analysis of clincal trials on St. John's wort for mild to moderate depression in the *British Medical Journal* (Linde *et al.*, 1996), the first American trial on ginkgo (*Ginkgo biloba*) leaf extract for early stage Alzheimer's dementia in the *Journal of the American Medical Association* (JAMA) (LeBars *et al.*, 1997), the meta-analysis of saw palmetto berry (*Serenoa repens*) extract for the treatment of symptoms of benign prostatic hyperplasia in JAMA (Wilt *et al.*, 1998), the meta-analysis of clinical trials on horse chestnut seed (*Aesculus hippocastanum*) extract for the treatment of chronic venous insufficiency in the *Archives of Dermatology* (Pittler and Ernst, 1998), and a clinical trial on a Chinese herbal combination formula demonstrating safety and efficacy in the treatment of irritable bowel syndrome in JAMA (Bensoussan *et al.*, 1998). Additional meta-analyses are being continually produced by the Cochrane Collaboration, an international group of reviewers from various medical centers who have been conducting evidence-based reviews on many of the more well-researched herbs and phytomedicines (as well as reviews on other modalities used in both conventional and complementary and alternative medicine <www.cochrane.org>). One example of such a review is the recent meta-analysis of trials on kava (*Piper methysticum*) for relief of symptoms of anxiety (Pittler and Ernst, 2002), based, in part, on an earlier meta-analysis of the same trials (Pittler and Ernst, 2000), and the meta-analysis of 33 clinical trials

conducted on ginkgo standardized extract showing "promising evidence" for the treatment of dementia in older patients (Birks *et al.*, 2002).

Healthcare providers should consider several important points when counseling patients on herbal treatments including: (1) herbal remedies are not usually as concentrated as conventional pharmaceuticals with some exceptions (i.e., some concentrated standardized extracts, e.g., milk thistle extract, ginkgo extract) and results may take longer; (2) like conventional pharmaceutical drugs, herbal remedies can produce unwanted side effects and adverse drug interactions; (3) many herbal remedies are not standardized like pharmaceutical drugs (which are almost always one single chemical entity), and different products may vary widely in chemistry, potency and activity; (4) although there is a growing body of data from controlled clinical trials on an increasing number of herbs, much of the data on herbs is based on empirical and/or anecdotal evidence. Reliable references for efficacy, dose, and safety should be consulted (D'Epiro, 1997).

In working with patients, healthcare professionals should ask about botanical medicine use when the patient has chronic or relapsing disease, is experiencing or concerned about adverse drug reactions, or there is unexplained poor compliance with treatment or follow-up. Useful questions when inquiring about use of botanical medicine include: "Have you tried other treatments for this problem?" "Have you changed your diet because you thought it might help this problem?" "Are you using or have you used any herbal remedies or other dietary supplements?"

Contrary to some publications suggesting that the relative high use of CAM therapy in the U.S. represents a large-scale rejection of orthodox and conventional medicine (Astin, 1998; Druss and Rosenheck, 1999), a recent survey by Eisenberg and colleagues (2001) found that "the use of CAM therapies cannot be attributed primarily to perceived dissatisfaction with conventional medical care or caregivers. Many adults seek, explore, and experience benefits from both conventional and CAM therapies....Only a minority of individuals seek the professional services of a CAM practitioner before seeking conventional medical care. As such, *conventional medical doctors and other conventional caregivers who are knowledgeable about CAM practices and the evidence to support or refute their application have a unique opportunity to advise patients on the use or avoidance of individual CAM therapies on a case-by-case basis.*" (emphasis added) (Eisenberg *et al.*, 2001).

The authors continue, "As evidence-based evaluation of CAM therapies materializes, let us be reminded that many adults currently choose to use CAM therapies to treat their most serious medical problems and appear to value both conventional and CAM approaches. Moreover, when patients choose not to tell their physicians that they use CAM therapies, *they appear to be less concerned about their physician's disapproval than their physician's perceived inability to understand or incorporate CAM therapies into their overall medical management.*" (emphasis added) (Eisenberg *et al.*, 2001).

Another recent survey reported that 44% of supplement consumers believe that physicians know "little" or "not much at all" about dietary supplements and 72% said they would continue using such products

Table 3: Reasons for Nondisclosure of Complementary and Alternative (CAM) Therapy Use With a Recognized Potential for Risk for Adverse Events*

Reason for nondisclosure	% responding
It wasn't important for your doctor to know	61
Your doctor never asked	60
It was none of your doctor's business	31
Your doctor would not understand	20
Your doctor would disapprove	14
Your doctor would discourage you	14

Based on Eisenberg *et al.*, 2001. Used with permission.

* Such therapies were listed as herbal remedies, chiropractic, naturopathy, megavitamins, and chelation therapy (n = 188 of total n = 726).

for their health even if a government-sponsored clinical trial resulted in negative findings (Blendon *et al.*, 2001).

Many users of herbs do not reveal this use to their primary physicians. Eisenberg *et al.* (2001) noted the main reasons that survey respondents gave for nondisclosure to their physicians of their use of CAM therapies with a "recognized potential for risk for adverse effects:" patients did not think it was important for the physician to know about the herb use and the physician did not inquire. (See Table 3 for more details.)

One of the biggest issues regarding herbal supplements facing conventional practitioners today is the question of trust. Many practitioners may be willing to recommend a particular herb for a patient, or counsel a patient who is already using an herbal remedy (e.g., the use of black cohosh to help treat symptoms of menopause, using saw palmetto to treat symptoms associated with BPH). However the clinician is often concerned about which *brand* of product to recommend, since there appears to be so much confusion about quality control among the many products that are available. One physician has proposed the following guidelines: In the absence of a clinical trial on a particular product, products manufactured or distributed by reputable herbal products manufacturers or major pharmaceutical firms, which have experience with and can ensure a high level of quality control, may be more safely recommended. Alternatively, standardized formulations, or those carrying a certified trade group seal, should be selected. Products with detailed labeling, including batch number, contact information, and expiration date, are also favored (Rotblatt, 1999).

However, these guidelines may not be adequate. Many manufacturers offer relatively detailed information on their product labels, including batch or lot numbers and expiration dates. These are required as part of federal regulations and good manufacturing practices (GMPs) and do not necessarily reflect the inherent quality of the herbal materials in the product, or the clinical reliability of the product. Many companies offer "standardized" herbal products, where the compound (or group of compounds) to which the product is standardized may or may not be based on activity-related parameters; products are often standardized to "marker" compounds simply for quality control purposes.

In the opinion of the editors of this publication, the first place to look for answers to the question "Which products should I recommend?" is the clinical literature. Although there may be numerous high quality, reliable herb products from which to choose, it seems reasonable to evaluate the clinical literature on each herb for which clinical trials have been conducted and determine which brand of commercial product was used in each study. While this may be only one criterion, the editors consider it a rational basis from which to consider making a product selection. Accordingly, such brand-related information is included in the monographs in this publication, intended as a guide for healthcare practitioners, although it should not be construed as a recommendation or endorsement by the editors or publishers of this volume. This information is found in the "Branded Products" section of each monograph (see description on page xxviii).

Rational Phytotherapy

Many people consider herbs and phytomedicines as CAM, which is the term that is now frequently employed in the U.S. However, in many modern European nations, the employment of herbs and phytomedicines in conventional medical practice is not considered alternative medicine but "rational phytotherapy," as these preparations are generally considered nonprescription medications and are regulated as such as far as their quality, safety, and efficacy are concerned.

According to the late Varro E. Tyler, the former Dean and Distinguished Professor of Pharmacognosy Emeritus at the School of Pharmacy and Pharmacal Sciences at Purdue University:

> Rational herbal medicine is conventional medicine. It is merely the application of diluted drugs to the prevention and cure of disease. The fact that the constituents and, sometimes, even the mode of action of these drugs are often incompletely understood and that instruction in their appropriate application is not a significant part of standard medical curricula does not in any way detract from their role in conventional medicine. If it did, we would be forced to discontinue the use of a number of popular products such as psyllium seed and senna laxatives, together with about 25% of our current materia medica that is derived from such sources. We would also have to conclude that some 62% of all German adults are unconventional because that is the percentage that turns first to a natural remedy (herbs or phytomedicines) to treat their illnesses….Although herbal therapy may not be mainstream American medicine, it certainly is conventional (Schulz *et al.*, 2001).

Evidence-Based Medicine

In the view of the editors, the term "evidence-based" presupposes a formal, systematic process in which clinical trials are ranked according to their size, design, and statistical power. This was *not* done in the preparation of *The ABC Clinical Guide to Herbs*, although such information *is* provided for most of the trials summarized in the clinical tables in each monograph. The editors have employed a relatively *informal evidence-based* approach in determining the "Primary Uses" of each herb in the herb's respective monograph, basing such uses on the availability of supporting clinical trials. However, in the view of the editors, this process did not meet the standards of a systematized process that is usually associated with the strict definition of "evidence-based." Therefore, the editors have chosen to use the phrase "science-based" rather than "evidence-based" when describing *The ABC Clinical Guide to Herbs*.

Interpreting Product Labels

1. Brand name

2. Product/herb name

3. Herbal products and other "dietary supplements" may make "statements of nutritional support," often referred to as "structure/function claims," as long as they are truthful and not misleading, are documentable by scientific data, and do not claim to diagnose, cure, treat, or prevent any disease, and carry a disclaimer on the product label to this effect. The disclaimer must also note that FDA has not evaluated the claim. The product manufacturer must also notify the FDA of the structure/function claim within 30 days of bringing the product to market. According to current FDA regulations, examples of acceptable structure/function claims include "supports the immune system" and "supports a healthy

Items 7-10 are part of the "Supplement Facts Panel"

7. "Serving Size" is the suggested number of tablets, capsules, softgels, tea bags, liquid extract, or tincture to take at one time.

8. "Amount per Serving" first indicates the nutrients present in the herb and then specifies the quantity. The following items must be declared if in excess of what can legally be declared as zero: calories, fat, carbohydrates, sodium, and protein. In addition, the following nutrients must also be declared if present in quantities exceeding what can legally be declared as zero: vitamins A, C, D, E, K, B-1, B-2, B-3, B-6, B-12, folic acid, biotin, calcium, iron, phosphorus, iodine, magnesium, zinc, selenium, copper, manganese, chromium, molybdenum, chloride, and potassium. Most herbal products contain negligible amounts of these nutrients.

9. "Percent Daily Value" (%DV) indicates the percentage of daily intake provided by the herb. An asterisk under the "Percent Daily Value" heading indicates that a Daily Value is not established for that dietary ingredient.

10. Herbs should be designated by their standardized common names as listed in the book *Herbs of Commerce*, published in 1992 by the American Herbal Products Association. If the common name is not listed in *Herbs of Commerce,* then the common name must be followed by the herb's Latin name. The plant part must be listed for each herb. The amount in milligrams of each herb must be listed unless the herbs are grouped as a proprietary blend—then only the total amount of the blend need be listed. For herbal extracts, the following information must be disclosed: 1. the ratio of the weight of the starting material to the volume of the solvent (even for dried extracts where the solvent has been removed, the solvent used to extract the herb must be listed); 2. whether the starting material is fresh or dry; and 3. the concentration of the botanical in the solvent.

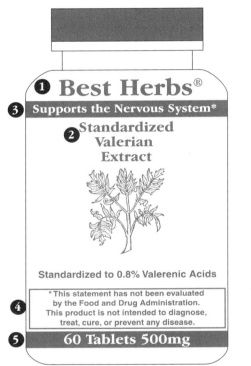

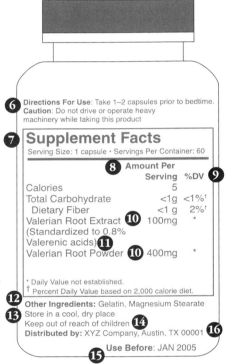

heart," while claims such as "helps treat the common cold" and "helps prevent heart disease" are considered unacceptable, as these are considered drug claims. Thus "helps maintain urinary tract health" is acceptable while "helps prevent urinary tract infections" is not.

4. A structure/function claim requires this disclaimer when it appears on the label of a dietary supplement, as well as in any brochures or advertising. The disclaimer must be in bold type and in a box.

5. Number of tablets, capsules, and net weight of each in package.

6. Directions for Use and Cautions.

11. Standardization. If a product is chemically standardized, the product label may list the component used to measure standardization (e.g., ginsenosides in Asian ginseng, valerenic acids in valerian, etc.) and the level to which the product is standardized (e.g. 4% ginsenosides). Therefore, if a product contained 100 mg of Asian ginseng extract per capsule and the extract was standardized to 4% ginsenosides, one capsule would contain 4 mg of ginsenosides. In most, but not all, cases, the component used to measure standardization is bioactive, although

the standardization component may not be responsible for the intended primary activity of the herbal supplement, other active compounds may be responsible. Products can also be standardized to "marker compounds" for purposes of quality control. Those markers may or may not be active.

12. A list of all other ingredients, in decreasing order by weight, must appear outside the Supplement Facts box. In herb formulas containing multiple herbal ingredients, the herbs must be listed in descending order of predominance.

13. The proper location for storage of herbal products is typically labeled as a cool, dry place.

14. All herbal products and other dietary supplements should be kept out of the reach of children.

15. The herb should be used before the expiration date for maximum potency and effectiveness. Expiration dates are often arbitrarily established by the manufacturer, regardless of the ingredients and their relative stability. Such dates are routinely set at two years from the date of manufacture of the finished dietary supplement, although this period may be longer or shorter depending on the manufacturer's policies, stability testing, dosage form, and other variables.

16. The product must list the manufacturer or distributor's name, city, state, and zip code.

PART II: ABOUT THIS BOOK

The Purpose of this Book

This book originally began on a significantly more modest scale as a continuing education (CE) module for medical doctors. It was to be patterned after the American Botanical Council's previous publication of brief monographs on 26 leading herbs, "Popular Herbs in the U.S. Marketplace," (Blumenthal and Riggins, 1997). Since the inception of this present publication in late 1998, *The ABC Clinical Guide to Herbs* has evolved into a comprehensive and up-to-date CE course on medicinal botanicals and is accredited for healthcare professionals including physicians, pharmacists, nurses, dieticians, and others.

This book provides a detailed review of relevant therapeutic and clinical data concerning some of the most frequently used medicinal herbs and their preparations that patients are likely to take. Therefore, *The ABC Clinical Guide to Herbs* (*The Guide*) can serve as a reference in clinical practice and in the curricula of medical, pharmacy, nursing, and dietician schools, among others. We have taken great care to provide clear differentiation between the specific products that have been the subject of clinical studies, the qualitative and quantitative standards that define them, along with corresponding pharmacopeial standards for herbs and herbal preparations, and correlations that can be made between specific product qualities and the results documented from published clinical trials.

The editors accessed a comprehensive range of authoritative data on the herbs and phytomedicines. However, the research has not been exhaustive, and it is possible that some clinically relevant research information was omitted. The editors anticipate the possibility of electronic versions of these monographs to be accessible on the American Botanical Council's website (www.herbalgram.org), and to be updated regularly as new clinically-relevant data is published.

Regardless of whether a healthcare professional chooses to incorporate an herb or phytomedicinal product in clinical practice—for treatment or prevention—the overwhelming fact is that many patients/consumers are using these natural products for their health in the belief that they provide some form of benefit. *It is thus essential that conventionally trained healthcare providers learn as much as possible about the clinical pharmacology of these products, their relative safety, and their potential applications, as suggested by the published literature. This is the primary purpose of this book and continuing education course.*

Potential Bias

It is understandable that some healthcare providers may hold a negative bias against herbs and herbal medicines. Most health professionals have not been taught about the potential benefits and relative risks of these therapeutic agents. They may also believe that herbs are not routinely screened by scientific evaluation of their safety and efficacy, and/or that they are not regulated as stringently as pharmaceutical drugs, etc. Thus, many healthcare professionals are quick to dismiss the validity of what others may consider a "reasonable" level of evidence in the form of clinical trials of various sizes and designs suggesting that an herb may provide some effective benefits. Such dismissal is frequently the result of *a priori* biases. This epistemological process occurs in both alternative and conventional medicine. According to a review by Vandenbroucke and de Craen (2001), physicians do reject seemingly solid evidence because it is not compatible with a pre-existing theory. They may be willing to discard a theory in the light of new data, but at other times they might also cling to an outmoded theory despite the compelling data suggesting otherwise. The authors write, "We propose that rational science is compatible with physicians' behavior, provided that physicians acknowledge the subjective element in the evaluation of science…" The editors of this publication are aware of these biases and have attempted to present evidence on the potential benefits and/or risks of these products in an open and straightforward manner.

Why the Herbs in this Book Were Selected

Most of the herbs in this book were selected because they consistently rank high in retail sales, in most channels of trade, particularly in 1999 when this project was initiated. A table of the top-selling herbal supplements in food, drug, and mass market retail outlets for the 52 weeks ending October 13, 2002, can be found in the Appendix on page 409.

Several herbs in this book are *not* listed among the top-selling herbs in mass markets, but were selected because they still are considered to be among the most popular herbs. Neither chamomile (*Matricaria recutita*) nor peppermint (*Mentha x piperita*) are highly popular as dietary supplements, however they are two of the most popular herbs sold as herbal tea ingredients. American ginseng (*Panax quinquefolius*) and eleuthero (*Eleutherococcus senticosus*) sales are high, but their sales data is usually subsumed under the generic term "ginseng" with Asian ginseng (*P. ginseng*). Chaste tree (*Vitex agnus-castus*), ephedra (*Ephedra sinica*), goldenseal (*Hydrastis canadensis*), and horse chestnut (*Aesculus hippocastanum*) are not top sellers in mainstream outlets. However, they are among the 35 top-sellers in the natural foods outlets (NBJ, 2002) and, with the exception of goldenseal, varying amounts of clinical research have been performed on each of these herbs.

Description of Herb Chapters

Each herb chapter contains a 2-page clinical overview, a 1-page patient information sheet, and a comprehensive monograph. The monographs include the following sections.

Overview. This section includes a brief background on the herb, geographical origin, brief historical data, market status, and other relevant background information. In the case of the relatively controversial herb ephedra (a.k.a. ma huang, *Ephedra sinica*), the Overview section has been expanded intentionally in order to provide the reader some detailed background on the legal and regulatory issues related to this herb over the past decade or so.

Description. This section provides a description of the crude herb material used in commerce and/or parameters for powdered crude material and/or extracts. This section is not intended to offer a detailed botanical description, since this book deals with materials of commerce and is not intended as a field guide or other type of reference where detailed botanical descriptions are needed.

Uses. The Uses section is divided into two parts: "Primary Uses" and "Other Potential Uses." By listing these as uses instead of indications, the editors are emphasizing that the herbs generally are not approved by the U.S. FDA (there are a few exceptions, e.g., the use of capsaicin, a primary active compound from cayenne or red pepper [*Capsicum* spp.]). Instead, Primary Uses refers usually to the most common use(s) of the herb or phytomedicine, especially as documented by published clinical trials. Other Potential Uses refers to the fact that there may be one or more trials suggesting possible use, that these trials may be small-scale pilot studies, that the design of the trial may be wanting for controls, and/or the trial's outcome may be equivocal. Uses documented in authoritative monographs (e.g., the German Commission E monographs, World Health Organization, or ESCOP [European Scientific Cooperative on Phytotherapy]), or uses that are acknowledged from long-standing empirical use in European or other forms of traditional medicine, may also qualify for mention as "potential or, in some cases, as Primary." Thus, the editors employed a type of evidence basis in qualifying the levels of use for an herb. By including potential uses, the editors are ensuring that healthcare professionals are aware that, as is often true with conventional pharmaceutical drugs, botanical medicines may have numerous possible applications beyond those documented by published clinical trials, or uses suggested by one or more trials.

It is not the intention of this book to determine the efficacy of particular herbs to a degree equivalent to those required for new drugs in a new drug application (NDA). Nor have the herbs been evaluated by a formal systematic review for the purposes of determination of their efficacy. However, an expert panel reviewed much of the literature upon which these monographs are based to assess the relative safety and potential efficacy for various uses.

Thus, the "Uses" are not meant to be considered in the same way as officially approved uses or indications for conventional drugs. The editors have based these uses on a variety of factors and the practitioner will have the opportunity to review the evidence presented in a variety of ways in the monographs and thus determine for him- or herself the appropriateness of using the herb or phytomedicine in a clinical setting. Thus, the primary or potential uses are proposed as a result of the totality of the evidence presented in the monograph and the appropriateness of their use is left to the judgment of the practitioner. In this sense, the uses are meant to be considered as guides, but are not necessarily presented as definitive uses as would be the case for approved conventional drugs.

Dosage. This section provides the recommended amount for effectiveness based on clinical research, authoritative monographs, or other sources. Unlike many herb publications currently available, the editors have gone to considerable length to provide various doses correlated to different types of preparations. Although authoritative monographs like those produced by the Commission E often refer to one or two types of preparations (e.g., dried herb ["crude drug"], liquid extracts, or solid extracts, etc.), they usually also add, "or equivalent preparations" to denote that other dosage forms of the herb (teas, concentrated extracts, etc.) might be substituted as long as their dosage is appropriately calculated. The challenge with this type of information is that it is often difficult to calculate such doses. When appropriate, the editors provide this information as a convenience to the practitioner. The doses are usually referenced from various authoritative sources, official monographs, clinical trials, and related sources. The reader may notice that there is often a range of dosage on any particular form of an herb, depending on either the intended use and/or the source of the information. This is a result of differences in the various sources and is indicative of the relative safety of many of these herbal preparations; i.e., precise dosing is often not as critical as it is with many pharmaceutical drugs.

Duration of Administration. This usually refers to periods of minimum or maximum use to ensure efficacy and/or reduce potential adverse reactions. However, in some monographs, the duration limit may also reflect the advisability of the patient's revisiting the physician, as is the case with the maximum of six months duration for preparations made from black cohosh rhizome (*Actaea racemosa*, syn. *Cimicifuga racemosa*). In this example, there is no evidence that use of black cohosh preparations for more than six months creates any risk; the six-month limit is based on the preference in Germany that women on hormone replacement therapy for the treatment of menopausal symptoms see their gynecologists every six months for a checkup. This duration was initially prescribed by the Commission E.

Chemistry. The chemistry of herbs and herbal preparations (phytomedicines) is by its nature very complex—a consideration that is especially important to maintain in relation to conventional pharmaceutical drugs, which are usually single chemical entities, whether they are naturally derived or synthetic. Medicinal plants contain hundreds of chemical compounds, most of them being relatively dilute. This section provides a brief listing of primary chemical constituents, particularly those believed to be related to the herb's known pharmacological activity.

Pharmacological Actions. This section provides information on activity of the herb and/or some of its isolated constituents. Many books on botanical medicine simply list all published actions as derived from the literature. This can be misleading, as animal data are not always clinically relevant to humans, especially when an isolated compound is given via injection. Additionally, much pharmacological data is published from *in vitro* studies (laboratory experiments in glass dishes on isolated cells or organs from animals or humans). While potentially insightful, *in vitro* studies suffer from the inability to fully recreate the environment of a living organism. Thus, their results are limited in scope and relevance to clinical considerations. The editors have separated pharmacological studies into three sections (human, animal, and *in vitro*) in order to put this information into clearer perspective. With most herbs (for example garlic [*Allium sativum*], Asian ginseng [*Panax ginseng*], ginkgo [*Ginkgo biloba*]), there are literally hundreds, in some cases thousands, of animal and *in vitro* studies in the literature, requiring the editors to limit the number of these studies referenced. While the editors have tried to include many that are representative of the actions of the herb, these sections are by no means exhaustive.

Mechanisms of Action. Mechanistic information regarding biochemical processes induced by an herbal preparation, studies showing where certain key compounds bind at receptor sites, and related data can be considered a subset of pharmacology. However, the editors have included some of this information in a separate section for the benefit of those researchers and clinicians having a special interest in such matters. Again, as with pharmacological actions, the editors have provided some data that provides insights into these areas, but did not embark on a quest to collect exhaustive data.

Contraindications. Safety data are clearly a matter of primary concern for clinicians, consumers, regulators, and manufacturers. The editors have attempted to provide as much data as they considered clinically relevant, although recent developments in herbal science and pharmacovigilance continue to provide new data that may require revision of these sections at any time. A case in point is the monograph on kava (*Piper methysticum*). After several drafts of the kava monograph were completed in late 2001, new data became available regarding potential hepatotoxicity associated with kava use (as suggested by AERs from Switzerland and Germany), and the subsequent regulatory concern in those and other countries. This situation required a significant revision of the kava monograph sections on contraindications and adverse events, even though several published reports by qualified pharmacologists and toxicologists who evaluated the kava AERs did not find adequate evidence of a causal relationship between kava use and most of the cases of hepatotoxicity (many of which were the result of pre-existing liver disease, concomitant use of hepatotoxic drugs, combination with alcohol, excessive dosage, etc.) (Waller, 2002).

The contraindications mentioned in this section are derived from various published reviews, official and unofficial monographs, etc. It should be noted that DSHEA allows for the disclosure of risk on the labels of herbs and other dietary supplements, but does not require such disclosure. However, the increased litigiousness in the American healthcare marketplace has created a deep concern from a product liability perspective to the extent that most companies will be compelled to publish more safety information on herbal products, although not currently required by law (Rubin, 2002).

In some monographs there are "no known" contraindications This usually means that the herb is generally safe to use with no known condition or known subset of individuals being precluded from use. However, this does not necessarily preclude pregnant or lactating women. A special subsection is provided in which specific information is given on pregnancy and lactation.

Adverse Effects. Adverse effects from herbs and herbal products are a reasonable expectation as is the case with any pharmacologically active agent. Historically, adverse effects from herbs and herbal products have been reported infrequently in the U.S. literature in comparison to the levels of use of these products. The argument has often been proffered that with the rise in widespread use of herbs in the U.S. there has not been a corresponding rise in herb-related AERs. This situation has been used as an indicator of the relative safety of the most popular herbs, which are generally known to exert more gentle, less dramatic physiological effects than conventional drugs. While this assertion is generally accurate, it is also true that adverse effects of herbs have not been collected in the same systems established for AERs for conventional medicines in the U.S., thereby suggesting that many may go unreported. However, in some leading western European countries (e.g., Germany, Switzerland), where herbs are routinely reported in the same systems of pharmacovigilance as conventional medications, herbs and phytomedicines have shown a remarkable record of relative safety. The monograph on St. John's wort provides an example: Between October 1991 and December 1999, over 8 million patients are estimated to have been treated with Germany's leading St. John's wort preparation (Jarsin® or Jarsin®300, manufactured by Lichtwer Pharma, Berlin); during this period only 95 reports of side effects were received by the German Adverse Drug Reaction Recording System. While it is possible that additional adverse reactions may have occurred and that there are additional reports relating to other St. John's wort products, this data strongly suggests a reasonable degree of safety relative to the levels of use.

One problem that arises in the reporting of herb adverse effects is the high degree of acceptance of poorly substantiated case reports and uncontrolled studies as evidence of risk. This stands in high contrast to the levels of evidence that health professionals normally require to document efficacy of a therapeutic agent. Another persistent problem plaguing the accurate reporting of adverse effects of herbs in the medical literature is the lack of adequate documentation of the botanical identity of the putatively offending herb.

The monographs in this publication contain adverse effects documented from the literature, including case reports, clinical studies, and authoritative monographs, often with explanatory data to help frame the clinical significance of the reports. In many cases, clinical trials suggest that a low percentage of subjects experienced gastric distress and/or nausea or headache—symptoms that are common in most clinical trials on pharmacological substances. In numerous trials, the adverse effects reported for an herb were consistent with those in the placebo group.

Drug Interactions. One of the biggest areas of concern in conventional medicine and the media is the issue of the potential interactions of herbal dietary supplements with prescription and/or OTC drugs. The April and May 1999 *Prevention* magazine survey reported that of patients taking prescription medications, 18.4% were also ingesting an herbal dietary supplement or a high-potency multivitamin and mineral supplement, which suggests the possibility of herb-drug interactions. The *Prevention* study indicates that many consumers use herbal supplements *with* drugs: 31% with prescription drugs, and 48% with OTC drugs (Johnston, 2000). Many of these patients acknowledge that they do not regularly report the use of dietary supplements to their physicians, so the need for physicians and pharmacists to request such information is increasingly compelling (Eisenberg *et al.*, 2001).

The recent revelations regarding the interaction of St. John's wort with drugs that are metabolized by the P450 system are examples of the developing body of knowledge being accumulated on the potential for herbs to interact with conventional medications. Only recently has systematic documentation of herb-drug interactions been published in the professional literature. The leading example of this trend is Francis Brinker's *Herb Contraindications and Drug Interactions,* 3rd edition (Brinker, 2001). Following the guidance of Brinker, the interactions noted in these monographs are based on a rational hierarchy of evidence, with usually only those reported in humans being listed. If other interactions are listed that are based on animal or *in vitro* data, or merely speculation, such levels of evidence are noted.

AHPA Safety Rating. The safety rating as assigned by the *American Herbal Products Association's Botanical Safety Handbook* (BSH) (McGuffin *et al.*, 1997) is noted, and in some other cases, some European organizations' assessments are also included. The AHPA safety classifications were based on data from more than 30 primary references (including the German Commission E) plus clinical trials, case reports and other forms of evidence. The BSH was developed as a voluntary form of self-regulation by the leading herb industry trade group in order to provide guidelines on the uniform disclosure of potential risk of approximately 550 of the most popular herbs sold in the U.S. The evaluation followed the passage of DSHEA in 1994 in which disclosure of potential risk on herb product labels was allowed for the first time.

The ratings are as follows:

Class 1: Herbs that can be safely consumed when used appropriately.

Class 2: Herbs for which the following use restrictions apply, unless otherwise directed by an expert qualified in the use of the described substance:

> 2a: For external use only.
>
> 2b: Not to be used during pregnancy.
>
> 2c: Not to be used while nursing.
>
> 2d: Other specific use restrictions as noted.

Class 3: Herbs for which significant data exists to recommend the following labeling: "To be used only under the supervision of an expert qualified in the appropriate use of this substance." Labeling must include proper use information: dosage, contraindications, potential adverse effects and drug interactions, and any other relevant information related to the safe use of this substance. [None of the herbs in the monographs in this book are designated as Class 3.]

Class 4: Herbs for which insufficient data is available for classification.

Regulatory Status in U.S. and Other Industrialized Nations. Although it may not be deemed directly relevant to the self-care or clinical applications of an herb, the editors considered it potentially constructive to include information on how the herbs are regulated in other industrialized nations. The status of these herbs ranges from food to dietary supplement, traditional medicine, nonprescription drug, etc.

Clinical Review. This section provides an overview of various clinical studies that are summarized in the table of clinical studies. Comments about specific studies, systematic reviews and meta-analyses, as well as other relevant observations on clinical trials are included. With a few exceptions, the editors have not devoted much space to discussing specific studies, since many of the most prominent trials are summarized in the Table of Clinical Studies on each herb.

Table of Clinical Studies. The purpose of the tables is to give the reader an at-a-glance view of summaries of many of the published clinical trials on a particular herb. In the case of herbs in which a significant number of trials have been published (e.g., garlic, ginkgo, Asian ginseng, saw palmetto, St. John's wort, etc.), it is not feasible to include all the studies in the literature. In these cases, many of the primary and most recent trials are included. In the case of other herbs (e.g., ginger [*Zingiber officinale*] and valerian [*Valeriana officinalis*]), as many of the clinical trials as the editors could locate are included. In the case of goldenseal root *(Hydrastis canadensis)*, no clinical trials have been published in the literature, so the table instead summarizes clinical trials on the alkaloid berberine, generally considered goldenseal's primary active compound. In the case of cayenne pepper (*Capsicum* spp.), clinical trials are summarized on the herb as well as the isolated primary active compound capsaicin, which is approved as a nonprescription drug ingredient.

Most tables are divided into various subsections dealing with the primary research parameter of the studies in each section (e.g., cardiovascular, chemoprevention, cognitive, diabetes, immunology, psychomotor response, etc.). The columns of the tables include the author and year, subject, design (including number of subjects, randomization, controls, etc.), duration, dose, preparation used (including brand name, if given), and results/conclusion. A key is provided in each table to clarify abbreviations.

An innovative feature of this book is the inclusion of the names of specific commercial brands of herbs and phytomedicinal products which are included in the Table of Clinical Studies. This is provided to give the clinician as much information as possible to make informed decisions and to underscore the issue of phytoequivalence. Phytoequivalence is the herbal counterpart to bioequivalence, an issue of concern in the prescription and generic drug industries. The concept refers to the fact that many of the clinical trials documenting the safety and the (actual or potential) efficacy of a particular herb are often conducted with one or a few leading proprietary phytomedicinal products. This is particularly true in studies on black cohosh, chaste tree, garlic, ginkgo, Asian ginseng, horse chestnut seed extract, milk thistle, and St. John's wort, among others.

Branded Products. This is a listing of the commercial products found in the Preparation column of the Table of Clinical Studies. It lists the brand name, manufacturer name, city and country, and a brief description of the product or parameters of the herbal extract. *The reader should note that the listing of a brand in these monographs is not to be construed as an endorsement of the particular product by the editors or publisher (the American Botanical Council). Mention of specific brands in each monograph and elsewhere in this publication is done solely as an acknowledgement of the research that has been conducted on the specific phytomedicinal product.* This has been done in response to numerous requests for such information from healthcare professionals, members of the media, and others. A table in the Appendix (see page 398) provides a cross-reference of the foreign brands and their U.S. counterparts if they are imported and marketed in this country. This is a unique feature of this publication and may become a valuable tool for clinicians to determine which specific herb products sold in the U.S. have been investigated in published clinical trials.

References. As with all publications of this type, complete references of all citations are included. These can be broken down into the following general categories: clinical trials, pharmacological studies, toxicological studies, epidemiological studies, chemical analyses, and profiles, monographs (official and nonofficial), general botanical and herbal reference books, government reports, review articles, meta-analyses and systematic reviews, historical accounts, national and international pharmacopeias, etc. For more information on General References, please see the listing on page 397. The editors have attempted to cite authoritative sources whenever possible, including secondary sources.

Clinical Overview

Clinical Overviews are intended to provide health professionals with quick, at-a-glance information on the most widely used product forms, their primary and other potential uses, and their key safety information. In order to give the clinician and general reader this quick look at the basic, clinically-relevant aspects of each herb, the essential elements of the monographs have been distilled into the two-page Clinical Overview that precedes each monograph. The editors anticipate that readers may refer to this section frequently for the sake of convenience. The editors suggest that readers refer to the monographs for in-depth guidance and to review the basis of the information in the Clinical Overviews.

An example of the type of "filtration" of the information from the monographs to the Clinical Overview, and subsequently, to Patient Information Sheets, can be seen in the monograph on horse chestnut seed extract (*Aesculus hippocastanum*). In this monograph, information on dosage and use of purified escin (a.k.a. aescin) preparations was removed from the Clinical Overview since to the editors' knowledge these preparations are not marketed in the United States. While the presence of such products in the European market warrants their inclusion in the monograph, since they are not available in North America, the editors did not consider this information relevant to the Clinical Overviews.

Patient Information Sheet

In order to assist both the practitioner and the patient, the Clinical Overviews have been further distilled into one-page Patient Information Sheets that are meant for photocopying and distribution to the patient. The editors have attempted to accurately and responsibly convey the essence of the information provided in the monographs; however, as is always the case in a process of simplification, important detailed information and nuance has been omitted. Although every effort has been made to ensure the accuracy of the data in the Patient Information Sheets, the clinician is advised to carefully evaluate them and provide to the patient whatever additional information the clinician deems appropriate.

Proprietary Products

This section reviews the clinical research on proprietary products including one monopreparation (i.e., containing one herb or herbal extract), Pycnogenol®, and 12 multi-herb products representing various herbal medicine traditions. The review of each product includes a table of clinical studies. The editors have included these proprietary products because monopreparations are the exception rather than the rule in most systems of traditional and indigenous medicine. Additional information is provided in the introduction to the proprietary products section on page 366.

REFERENCES

AHPA. See: American Herbal Products Association.

American Herbal Products Association (AHPA). AHPA & IASC Submit Petition to the FDA Regarding OTC Laxative Ingredients: Aloe and Cascara Sagrada [AHPA Update]. June 13, 2002.

Astin JA. Why patients use alternative medicine: results of a national study. *JAMA* 1998;279:1548–53.

Awang DVC. Standardization of Herbal Medicines. *Alternative Therapies in Women's Health* 1999;July:57–9.

Barberis L, De Toni E, Schiavone M, Zicca A, Ghio R. Unconventional medicine teaching at the universities of the European Union. *J Alt Compl Med* 2001;7(4):337–43.

Bensoussan A, Talley NJ, Hing, M, Menzies R, Guo A, Ngu M. Treatment of irritable bowel syndrome with Chinese herbal medicine: a randomized controlled trial. *J Amer Med Assn* 1998;280:1585–9.

Bent S, Tsourinas C, Romoli M, Linde K. Kava for anxiety disorder. In: *The Cochrane Library* 2001:1.

Birks J, Grimley Evans J, Van Dongen M. Ginkgo Biloba for Cognitive Impairment and Dementia (Cochrane Review). In: *The Cochrane Library*, Issue 4, 2002. Oxford: Update Software.

Blendon RJ, DesRoches CM, Benson JM, Brodie M, Altman DE. Americans' views on the use and regulation of dietary supplements. *Arch Int Med* 2001;161:805-810.

Blumenthal M. USP establishes botanical advisory panel. *HerbalGram* 2003;57:13.

Blumenthal M. Herb Sales Down in Mainstream Market, Up in Natural Food Supermarkets. *HerbalGram* 2002;55:60.

Blumenthal M. Interactions between herbs and conventional drugs: introductory considerations, *HerbalGram* 2000;49:52–63.

Blumenthal M. Herb market levels after five years of boom: 1999 sales in mainstream market up only 11% in first half of 1999 after 55% increase in 1998. *HerbalGram* 1999;47:64–65.

Blumenthal M, Busse WR, Goldberg A, Gruenwald J, Hall T, Riggins CW. et al. (editors). Klein S, Rister RS (trans). *The Complete German Commision E Monographs: Therapeutic Guide to Herbal Medicines*. Austin (TX): American Botanical Council; 1998.

Blumenthal M, Israelsen LD. The History of Herbs in the United States: Legal and Regulatory Perspectives. In: Miller LG, Murray WJ. *Herbal Medicinals: A Clinicians Guide*. Haworth Herbal Press: 1998;325–353.

Blumenthal M, Riggins CW. *Popular Herbs in the U.S. Marketplace*. Austin (TX): American Botanical Council; 1997.

Boyle W. *Official Herbs: Botanical Substances in the United States Pharmacopoeias 1820–1990*. East Palestine (OH): Buckeye Naturopathic Press; 1991.

Brinker F. *Herb Contraindications and Drug Interactions* 3d ed. Sandy (OR): Eclectic Medical Publications; 2001.

ConsumerLab.com. Supplement use in health conditions. March 2002 [Accessed 18 Dec 2002]. Available at: www.consumerlab.com/reports/otherreports.asp.

D'Epiro NW. Herbal medicine: what works, what's safe. *Patient Care* Oct 15, 1997;49–68, 77.

Dietary Supplement Health and Education Act of 1994 (DSHEA), Public Law 103-417, 21 USC § 3419.

Druss BG, Rosenheck RA. Association between use of unconventional therapies and conventional medical services. *JAMA* 1999;282:651–6.

DSHEA. See: Dietary Supplement Health and Education Act of 1994.

Eisenberg DM. Advising patients who seek alternative medical therapies. *Ann Intern Med* 1997;127(1):61–9.

Eisenberg DM, Kessler RC, Van Rompay MI, Kaptchuk TJ, Wilkey SA, Appel, S, Davis RB. Perceptions about complementary therapies relative to conventional therapies among adults who use both: results from national survey. *Ann Int Med.* 2001;135:344–51.

Eisenberg DM, Davis RB, Ettner SL, et al. Trends in alternative medicine use in the United States, 1990–1997: results of a follow-up national survey. *JAMA* 1998;280:1569–1575.

Eisenberg DM, Kessler RC, Foster C, Norlock FE, Calkins DR, Delbanco TL. Unconventional medicine in the United States. prevalence, costs, and patterns of use. *N Engl J Med* 1993;328:246–52.

Eisner S, managing editor. *Guidance for manufacture and sale of bulk botanical extracts.* Silver Spring (MD): American Herbal Products Assn;2001.

Farnsworth NR, Akerele O, Bingel AS, Soejarto DD, Guo ZG. Medicinal plants in therapy. *Bull WHO* 1985;965–81.

FDA. See: Food and Drug Administration.

Food and Drug Administration (FDA) SN/AEMS Web page. FDA Website. July 24, 2002a. This web page has since been removed as noted at URL: http://vm.cfsan.fda.gov/~dms/aems.html. Accessed 18 Dec 2002.

Food and Drug Administration (FDA). Letter to stakeholders: Announcing CAERS—the CFSAN adverse event reporting system [letter]. 29 Aug 2002b [Accessed 18 Dec 2002]. Available at URL: www.cfsan.fda.gov/~caersltr.html.

Food and Drug Administration (FDA). Status of Certain Additional Over-the-Counter Drug Category II and III Active Ingredients. *Federal Register* (codified at 21 CFR Part 310. Docket No. 78N-O36L. RIN 091 O-AA01). May 9, 2002c.

Food and Drug Administration (FDA). FDA Finalizes Rules for Claims on Dietary Supplements. *Press Office, Food and Drug Administration, U.S. Department of Health and Human Services, Public Health Service.* Jan. 5, 2000.

Foreman J. St. John's wort: Less than meets the eye. *Boston Globe.* Jan. 6, 2000.

Foster S. *Herbs of Commerce.* Austin (TX): American Herbal Products Assn;1992.

Fugh-Berman A. Herb-drug interactions. *Lancet* 2000;355, Jan. 8:134–138.

Fugh-Berman A, Ernst E. Herb-drug interactions: review and assessment of report reliability. *Br J Clin Pharmacol* 2001;52:587–95.

Johnston BA. *Prevention* Magazine Assesses Use of Dietary Supplements. *HerbalGram* 2000;48:65.

Kaufman DW, Kelly JP, Rosenberg L, Anderson TE, Mitchell AA. Recent patterns of medication use in the ambulatory adult population of the United States. The Slone Survey. *JAMA* 2002;287(3):337–344.

Klepser TB, Doucette WR, Horton MR, Buys LM, Ernst ME, Ford JK, et al. Assessment of patients' perceptions and beliefs regarding herbal therapies. *Pharmacotherapy* 2000;20(1):83–7.

Le Bars PL, Katz MM, Berman N, Itil TM, Freedman AM, Schatzberg AF. A placebo-controlled, double-blind, randomized trial of an extract of *Ginkgo biloba* for dementia. North American EGb Study Group [see comments]. *JAMA* 1997;278(16):1327–1332.

Levitt J. Letter and Outline on Dietary Supplement Strategy, Ten Year Plan. Center for Food Safety and Applied Nutrition, *Food and Drug Administration,* January 2000.

Linde K, Ramirez G, Mulrow C, Pauls A, Weidenhammer W, Melchart D. St. John's wort for depression—an overview and meta-analysis of randomized clinical trials. *BMJ* 1996;313(7052):253–8.

McGuffin M, Hobbs C, Upton R, Goldberg A, editors. *American Herbal Products Association's Botanical Safety Handbook.* Boca Raton (FL):CRC Press; 1997.

McGuffin M, Kartesz JT, Leung AY, Tucker AO. *Herbs of Commerce* 2d ed. Silver Spring (MD): American Herbal Products Assn; 2000.

McNamara S. FDA has adequate power and authority to protect the public from unsafe dietary supplements. *HerbalGram* 1996;25–7.

Moerman DE. *Native American Ethnobotany.* Portland (OR): Timber Press; 1998. p. 12, 19–21.

NBJ. See: *Nutrition Business Journal.*

Nutrition Business Journal (NBJ). Top selling U.S. herbs in 1999–2001 ($ millions, all channels). San Diego (CA): NBJ; 2002.

ODS. See: Office of Dietary Supplements.

Office of Dietary Supplements (ODS). About ODS. National Institutes of Health, Office of Dietary Supplements Web site. Available at: http://ods.od.nih.gov/about/law.html. Accessed 18 Dec 2002.

Pittler MH, Ernst E. Kava extract for treating anxiety [Cochrane Review]. In: The Cochrane Library; 2002;(2):CD00383.

Pittler M, Ernst E. Efficacy of kava extract for treating anxiety: systematic review and meta-analysis. *J Clin Psychopharmacol* 2000;20(1):84–9.

Pittler MH, Ernst E. Horse-chestnut seed extract for chronic venous insufficiency. a criteria-based systematic review. *Arch Dermatol* 1998;134(11):1356–1360.

Raffman G. Herbal remedy ripoffs. *D Magazine* 2000 (April);39–45.

Robbers JE, Tyler VE. *Tyler's Herbs of Choice: The Therapeutic Use of Phytomedicinals.* New York (NY): Haworth Herbal Press;1999.

Rotblatt MD. Herbal medicines: a practical guide to safety and quality assurance. *Western Journal of Medicine.* Sept 1999;171:172–175.

Rotblatt M, Ziment I. *Evidence-Based Herbal Medicine.* Philadelphia (PA): Hanley & Belfus, Inc.; 2002.

Rubin P. Herbal dietary supplements and foods: product liability analysis for a "failure to warn" of herb/drug interactions and guidelines to develop appropriate Warnings. *HerbalGram* 2002;55:56–59,71.

Schulz V, Hänsel R, Tyler VE. *Rational Phytohterapy: A Physician's Guide to Herbal Medicine.* New York (NY): Springer Verlag; 2001.

Soller, RW. Regulation in the herb market: The myth of the "Unregulated Industy." *HerbalGram* 2000;49:64–67.

Stolberg SG. Folk Cures on Trial: Alternative Care Gains a Foothold. *New York Times.* Jan. 31, 2000. 7 pp. A1, A16.

Vandenbroucke JP, de Craen AJ. Alternative medicine: a "mirror image" for scientific reasoning in conventional medicine. *Ann Intern Med.* 2001 Oct 2;135(7):507–13.

Waller DP. Report on Kava and Liver Damage. Silver Spring (MD): American Herbal Products Assn; 2002.

Wasik J. The truth about herbal supplements. *Consumers' Digest* July/August 1999:75–76,78–79.

Wetzel MS, Eisenberg DM, Kaptchuk TJ.Courses involving complementary and alternative medicine at U.S. medical schools. *JAMA* 1998;240:784–787.

Wilt J, et al. Saw palmetto extracts for treatment of benign prostatic hyperplasia: a systematic review. *JAMA* 1998;280(18):1604–9.

Zollman C, Vickers A. Complementary medicine and the doctor. *British Medical Journal* 1999;319:1558–1561.

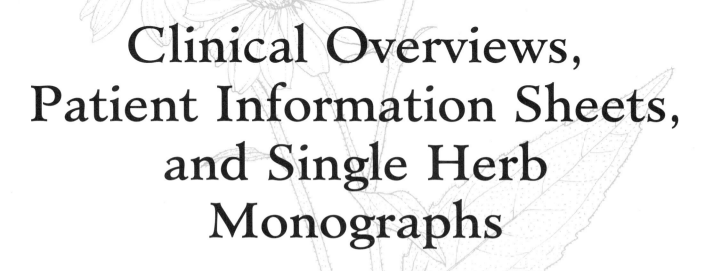

Clinical Overviews, Patient Information Sheets, and Single Herb Monographs

(This page intentionally left blank.)

Bilberry

Vaccinium myrtillus L.

[Fam. *Ericaceae*]

OVERVIEW

Bilberry is the name of a small European blueberry. Dietary supplements made from the standardized extract of bilberry have become popular in the U.S. over the past decade. Sales in the mainstream retail markets ranked 13th of all herbs in 2000. The standardized, concentrated extract of bilberry fruit is used by consumers primarily for ocular, microcirculatory and vascular-related disorders.

PRIMARY USES

- Retinopathy, hypertensive
- Retinopathy, diabetic
- Peripheral vascular disorders, blood purpuras
- Venous insufficiencies, varicose veins, capillary fragility, kidney capillary fragility
- Diarrhea (the bilberry fruits, not the standardized extracts)

OTHER POTENTIAL USES

- Blindness, night and day
- Cataracts
- Macular degeneration
- Retinitis pigmentosa
- Retinopathy, hemorrhagic
- Dysmenorrhea
- Reduction of surgical bleeding

PHARMACOLOGICAL ACTIONS

Astringent; antiplatelet aggregation; collagen-stabilizing activity; decreased vascular permeability associated with injury.

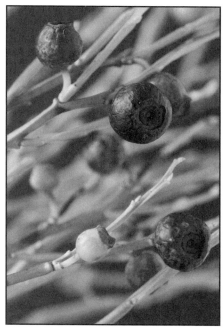

Photo © 2002 stevenfoster.com

DOSAGE AND ADMINISTRATION

Ranges from 160–480 mg daily depending on the conditions being treated. Therapeutic benefits appear to take effect in 4–8 weeks.

DRIED, RIPE FRUIT: 20–60 g daily (4–8 g with water, several times daily).

INFUSION/DECOCTION: 20–60 g daily.

COLD MACERATE: 20–60 g daily.

GARGLE: Mouthwash containing 10% decoction.

FLUID EXTRACT: 2–4 ml, 3 times daily [1:1 (*g/ml*)].

FOR DIARRHEA: Crude preparations (non-standardized) for no more than 3–4 days.

DRY STANDARDIZED EXTRACT: (25% anthocyanidins) 80–160 mg, 3 times daily.

CONTRAINDICATIONS

None known.

PREGNANCY AND LACTATION: No known restrictions.

ADVERSE EFFECTS

None known (at therapeutic dosages).

DRUG INTERACTIONS

Pharmacological studies suggest that very high doses (>170 mg anthocyanins per day for 30–60 days) may interact with warfarin or other antiplatelet drugs. Bilberry (form unstated) reportedly may reduce insulin requirements; therefore, conventional antidiabetic therapy would need close monitoring or dosage adjustment.

CLINICAL REVIEW

Fifteen clinical studies on bilberry that included a total of 694 participants were reviewed. All but one of the studies demonstrated positive effects for indications, including various ocular conditions (night/day vision and retinopathy), and vascular conditions, including venous insufficiencies and micro- and macro-peripheral circulation. Two double-blind, placebo-controlled (DB, PC) studies focused on retinopathy and confirmed results of two earlier open studies. One DB, PC study on nighttime vision confirmed preliminary findings of five previous open studies. A recent DB, PC, crossover study failed to find that bilberry extract (25% anthocyanosides) had an effect on night vision or night contrast sensitivity. One DB, PC study conducted on peripheral vascular disorder concluded positive results for Raynaud's sufferers. Another DB, PC study on chronic dysmenorrhea was positive and further supports pharmacological findings. One single-blind (SB), PC study on venous insufficiencies in 60 participants further supported the findings of four similar studies, including two open studies and two using pregnant subjects. Bleeding was investigated in a SB, PC study finding bilberry reduced intra- and postoperative bleeding and prevented subsequent hemorrhaging. Another study focused on bleeding associated with intrauterine devices.

Bilberry

Vaccinium myrtillus L.
[Fam. *Ericaceae*]

OVERVIEW

Bilberry is the name of a small, European blueberry. The standardized, concentrated extract of bilberry fruit is used by consumers mainly for disorders of the eyes and circulatory system. Sales in the mainstream retail markets ranked 13th of all herbs in 2000. Some concentrated extracts of the berry are standardized for an exact amount of water-soluble substances called anthocyanidins.

USES

Visual problems such as circulatory disorders of the retina; vein and circulatory disorders, including varicose veins, inadequate vein strength, and fragile capillaries.

DOSAGE

Ranges from 160–480 mg daily depending on the conditions being treated. Therapeutic benefits appear to take effect in 4–8 weeks.

FOR DIARRHEA: Non-standardized preparations for no more than 3–4 days.

DRIED, RIPE FRUIT: 20–60 g daily (4–8 g with water, several times daily).

INFUSION/DECOCTION: 20–60 g daily.

COLD MACERATE: 20–60 g daily.

GARGLE: Mouthwash containing 10% decoction.

FLUID EXTRACT: 2–4 ml, 3 times daily [1:1 (*g/ml*)].

DRY STANDARDIZED EXTRACT: 80–160 mg, 3 times daily [25% anthocyanidins].

CONTRAINDICATIONS

None known.

PREGNANCY AND LACTATION: None known.

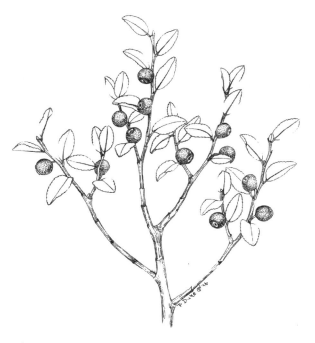

ADVERSE EFFECTS

Bilberry is not known to cause adverse effects in normally recommended therapeutic doses.

DRUG INTERACTIONS

There are no known drug interactions in therapeutic doses. However, very high doses (more than 170 mg anthocyanins daily for 30–60 days) may interact with anticoagulating drugs such as warfarin (Coumadin, Sofarin). Bilberry reportedly may reduce daily insulin requirements. Patients who are simultaneously taking antidiabetic medications and bilberry may need to be monitored or have the dosage of their antidiabetic drugs adjusted.

Comments

When using a dietary supplement, purchase it from a reliable source. For best results, use the same brand of product throughout the period of use. As with all medications and dietary supplements, please inform your healthcare provider of all herbs and medications you are taking. Interactions may occur between medications and herbs or even among different herbs when taken at the same time. Treat your herbal supplement with care by taking it as directed, storing it as advised on the label, and keeping it out of the reach of children and pets. Consult your healthcare provider with any questions.

AMERICAN
BOTANICAL
COUNCIL

The information contained on this sheet has been excerpted from *The ABC Clinical Guide to Herbs* © 2003 by the American Botanical Council (ABC). ABC is an independent member-based educational organization focusing on the medicinal use of herbs. For more detailed information about this herb please consult the healthcare provider who gave you this sheet. To order *The ABC Clinical Guide to Herbs* or become a member of ABC, visit their website at www.herbalgram.org.

Bilberry

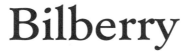

Vaccinium myrtillus L.

[Fam. *Ericaceae*]

OVERVIEW

Bilberry is the name of a small European blueberry. Dietary supplements made from the standardized extract of bilberry have become popular in the United States over the past decade. Sales in the mainstream retail markets ranked 13th of all herbs in 2000 (Blumenthal, 2001). The standardized, concentrated extract of bilberry is used by consumers to help treat or prevent ocular, microcirculatory, and vascular-related disorders. Bilberry *leaf* extract (not the fruit that is covered in this monograph) was used as a treatment for diabetes before the availability of insulin. It was found effective in adult onset diabetes as a method of reducing glycosuria and postprandial hyperglycemia (Allen, 1927). For that reason, the *leaf* extract is contraindicated for diabetes patients taking insulin (Bailey and Day, 1989).

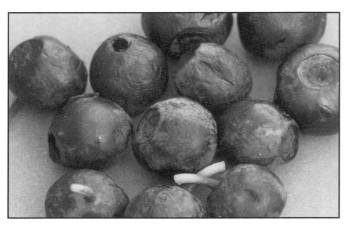

Photo © 2002 stevenfoster.com

DESCRIPTION

Bilberry preparations consist of the whole, dried, ripe, black or bluish-black fruit of *Vaccinium myrtillus* L. [Fam. *Ericaceae*]. Some concentrated extracts are standardized to anthocyanosides, calculated as 25% anthocyanidins, but may actually contain about 37% by weight (Pizzorno and Murray, 1999).

PRIMARY USES

Gastrointestinal
- Diarrhea: The German Commission E approved crude (i.e. non-concentrated) fruit preparations for acute diarrhea (Blumenthal *et al.*, 1998), particularly in children (Blumenthal *et al.*, 1998; Ofek *et al.*, 1996)

Ophthalmic
- Retinopathy, hypertensive (Repossi *et al.*, 1987), and diabetic (Ghiringhelli *et al.*, 1978; Treviso *et al.*, 1979; Scharrer *et al.*, 1981; Grismondi *et al.*, 1981; Orsucci *et al.*, 1983; Perossini *et al.*, 1987; Repossi *et al.*, 1987)

Vascular
- Peripheral vascular disorders and blood purpuras (Allegra *et al.*, 1982)
- Venous insufficiencies (Gatta *et al.*, 1988; Teglio *et al.*, 1987), varicose veins (Ghiringhelli *et al.*, 1978), capillary fragility (Coget and Merlen, 1980; Grismondi *et al.*, 1980; Mian *et al.*, 1977; Neumann, 1973; Treviso *et al.*, 1979), and kidney capillary fragility (Pennarola *et al.*, 1980)

OTHER POTENTIAL USES
- Blindness, night and day (Jayle *et al.*, 1965; Gloria and Peria, 1966; Sala *et al.*, 1979; Caselli, 1985; Vannini *et al.*, 1986; Zavarise *et al.*, 1987)
- Cataracts (Bravetti *et al.*, 1989)
- Gargle for inflamed oral and pharyngeal mucous membranes (Blumenthal *et al.*, 1998)
- Macular degeneration, retinitis pigmentosa, hemorrhagic retinopathy (Scharrer and Ober, 1981)
- Dysmenorrhea (Colombo and Vescovini, 1985)
- Reduction of intra- and post-operative bleeding (Gentile *et al.*, 1987; Cerutti *et al.*, 1984)

DOSAGE

Crude Preparations

DRIED, RIPE FRUIT: 20–60 g daily (4–8 g with water, several times daily) (Braun *et al.*, 1993; Meyer-Buchtela, 1999; Wichtl and Bisset, 1994).

INFUSION/DECOCTION: 20–60 g daily. The berries are prepared by placing 5–10 g crushed, dried fruit in 150 ml cold water. This mixture is boiled for approximately 10 minutes; then strained while hot. The preparation is drunk cold several times daily until the diarrhea subsides (Braun *et al.*, 1993; Meyer-Buchtela, 1999; Wichtl and Bisset, 1994).

COLD MACERATE: 20–60 g daily. The berries are prepared by soaking 5–10 g crushed dried fruit in 150 ml cold water for 2 hours, allowing the fruit to swell. The preparation is drunk cold several times daily (Braun *et al.*, 1993; Meyer-Buchtela, 1999; Wichtl and Bisset, 1994).

GARGLE: Mouthwash containing 10% decoction (prepared as described above) for local application in the treatment of mild inflammation of oral and pharyngeal mucous membranes (Blumenthal *et al.*, 2000).

FLUID EXTRACT: 1:1 (*g/ml*), 2–4 ml, 3 times daily (Anderhuber, 1991; Cunio, 1993).

Standardized Preparations

DRY STANDARDIZED EXTRACT: (25% anthocyanidins) 80–160 mg, 3 times daily (Pizzorno and Murray, 1999).

NOTE: Doses may range from 160–480 mg daily depending on the conditions being treated (see the following table, "Clinical

Studies on Bilberry"). Therapeutic benefits appear to take effect in 4–8 weeks.

DURATION OF ADMINISTRATION

Crude Preparations
DIARRHEA: Not more than 3–4 days.

Standardized Preparations
VASCULAR AND OCULAR-RELATED DISORDERS: 2–6 months depending on the condition.

CHEMISTRY

Dried bilberries contain 5–10% catechins (tannins), ca. 30% invertose (invert sugar) (Schulz *et al.*, 2001), and flavonoids. Bilberry contains a small amount of anthocyanosides (0.1–0.25% in fresh fruit) consisting of 3-O-glycosides of cyanidin, delphinidin, malvidin, peonidin, and petunidin (Baj *et al.*, 1983), and proanthocyanidins B1-B4 (Bruneton, 1999).

PHARMACOLOGICAL ACTIONS

Crude Preparations
Astringent (Blumenthal *et. al.*, 2000).

Standardized Preparations

Human
Anti-platelet aggregation (Pulliero *et al.*, 1989) (*ex vivo*); collagen-stabilizing activity (Mian *et al.*, 1977); decreased vascular permeability associated with injury (Mian *et al.*, 1977).

Animal
Antiplatelet aggregation (Morazzoni and Magistretti, 1990; Zaragoza *et al.*, 1985; Bottecchia *et al.*, 1987); anti-ulcer (Cristoni and Magistretti, 1987); decreased capillary fragility (anti-inflammatory activity) (Detre *et al.*, 1986; Lietti *et al.*, 1976); collagen-stabilizing (Detre *et al.*, 1986); vascular smooth muscle relaxant (Bettini *et al.*, 1984a; Bettini *et al.*, 1984b); vascular permeability regulator (Detre *et al.*, 1986; Lietti and Forni, 1976); increased regeneration of rhodopsin (a light-sensitive pigment found in rods and retina) (Alfieri *et al.*, 1966; Cluzel *et al.*, 1969).

In vitro
Antioxidant (Meunier *et al.*, 1989); free radical scavenger (Pietta *et al.*, 1998; Martin-Aragon *et al.*, 1998); inhibits cAMP phosphodiesterases (Ferretti *et al.*, 1988); chemopreventative (Bomser *et al.*, 1996); inhibits lipid peroxidation (Meunier *et al.*, 1989).

NOTE: The pharmacological actions — antioxidant, anti-inflammatory, decreases in capillary permeability, and stabilization of collagen — are further supported by research conducted on flavonoids in general (Gabor, 1972; Kuhnau, 1976; Havsteen, 1983; Monboisse *et al.*, 1983).

MECHANISM OF ACTION

- Inhibits enzymatic cleavage of collagen by enzymes secreted by leukocytes during inflammation (Mian *et al.*, 1977)
- Increases the endothelium barrier effect through stabilizing the membrane phospholipids and increasing the biosynthesis of the acid mucopolysaccharides of the connective ground substance, thus restoring the altered mucopolysaccharide pericapillary sheath (Mian *et al.*, 1977)
- Decreases basement membrane collagen hydrolysis by significantly reducing permeability of the blood-brain barrier (BBB), and increases recovery rate of the BBB caused by permeability-increasing agents (Robert *et al.*, 1977)
- Prevents the liberation of lactate dehydrogenase in heart,

plasma, and cardiac isoenzymes (Marcollet *et al.*, 1970)
- May result in retinal protection due to the inhibition of retinal phosphoglucomutase and glucose-6-phosphatase (Cluzel *et al.*, 1969)
- Reduces microvascular impairments due to ischemia reperfusion injury, with preservation of endothelium, attenuation of leukocyte adhesion, and improvement of capillary perfusion (Bertuglia *et al.*, 1995)
- Produces dose-dependent inhibition of platelet aggregation and clot retraction (Bottecchia, 1987)

CONTRAINDICATIONS
None known.

PREGNANCY AND LACTATION: No known restrictions.

ADVERSE EFFECTS
None known (at therapeutic doses).

DRUG INTERACTIONS
None known. It has been inferred, based on pharmacological studies, that very high doses (>170 mg anthocyanins per day for 30–60 days) may interact with warfarin or other antiplatelet drugs (Bone and Morgan, 1997). *Leaf only*: There have also been claims that bilberry *leaf*, as mentioned in the overview, may reduce insulin requirements. Therefore, conventional antidiabetic therapy would require close monitoring or adjustment (De Smet *et al.*, 1993; Bailey and Day, 1989).

AMERICAN HERBAL PRODUCTS ASSOCIATION (AHPA) SAFETY RATING
CLASS 1: Can be safely consumed when used appropriately (McGuffin *et al.*, 1997).

REGULATORY STATUS
AUSTRIA: Dried fruit official in the 1990 *Austrian Pharmacopoeia*, 1991 Addendum II (Meyer-Buchtela, 1999; ÖAB, 1991; Wichtl and Bisset, 1994).

CANADA: Multiple-ingredient Traditional Herbal Medicines (THMs) containing bilberry, in tea infusion form, and homeopathic mono-preparations of bilberry are scheduled OTC drugs requiring premarket registration and assignment of a drug identification number (DIN) (Health Canada, 2001).

FRANCE: Fresh or dried fruits are permitted for oral or topical use (Bruneton, 1999).

GERMANY: Dried fruit, for tea infusions and other equivalent galenical dosage forms, is an approved nonprescription drug of the German Commission E monographs (Blumenthal *et al.*, 1998). Dried fruit is official in the *German Drug Codex* supplement to the *German Pharmacopoeia* (DAC, 1998). Bilberry dried-fruit tea is an approved nonprescription drug listed in the *German Standard License* (St. Zul.) monographs (Braun *et al.*, 1993). The fresh, ripe fruit for preparation of hydro-alcoholic mother tincture and liquid dilutions is an official drug of the *German Homeopathic Pharmacopoeia* (GHP, 1993).

ITALY: Dried hydro-alcoholic extract is listed in the *Italian Pharmacopoeia* (Morazzoni and Bombardelli, 1996).

SWEDEN: Classified as foodstuff (De Smet *et al.*, 1993). As of January 2001, no bilberry products are listed in the Medical Products Agency (MPA) "Authorised Natural Remedies" (MPA, 2001).

SWITZERLAND: Dried fruit is official in the *Swiss Pharmacopoeia* (Meyer-Buchtela, 1999; Ph.Helv.VII, 1987–1997; Wichtl and Bisset, 1994). A semipurified extract (Myrtaven®), standardized to 58 mg anthocyanosides per capsule, is a Category C nonprescription drug with sale limited to pharmacies (Morant and Ruppanner, 2001).

U.K.: Not listed in *General Sale List* (GSL). No monograph in the *British Pharmacopoeia*.

U.S.: Dietary Supplement (USC, 1994). Tincture of the ripe berries is a Class D over-the-counter drug of the *Homeopathic Pharmacopoeia of the United States* (HPUS, 1993).

CLINICAL REVIEW

Fifteen studies are outlined in the following table, "Clinical Studies on Bilberry," including a total of 694 participants. All but one of the studies (Muth *et al.*, 2000) demonstrate positive effects for indications, including various ocular conditions (night/day vision and retinopathy), and vascular conditions, including venous insufficiencies and micro- and macroperipheral circulation. Two double-blind, placebo-controlled (DB, PC) studies (Perossini *et al.*, 1987; Repossi *et al.*, 1987) focused on retinopathy and confirmed results of two earlier open studies (Orsucci *et al.*, 1983; Scharrer and Ober, 1981). One DB, PC study (Vannini *et al.*, 1986) on nighttime vision confirmed preliminary findings of five previous open studies (Jayle and Auber, 1964; Jayle *et al.*, 1965; Gloria and Peria, 1966; Sala *et al.*, 1979; Terrasse *et al.*, 1966). A recent DB, PC, crossover study (Muth *et al.*, 2000) failed to find an effect of a bilberry extract (25% anthocyanosides) on night vision or night contrast sensitivity. One DB, PC study conducted on peripheral vascular disorder (Allegra *et al.*, 1982) concluded positive results for Raynaud's sufferers. Another DB, PC study (Colombo and Vescovini, 1985) on chronic dysmenorrhea was positive and further supports pharmacological findings (Bettini *et al.*, 1984a, Bettini *et al.*, 1984b). One single-blind, PC study on venous insufficiencies in 60 participants (Gatta *et al.*, 1988) further supported the findings of four similar studies, including two open studies (Ghiringhelli *et al.*, 1977; Mian *et al.*, 1977), and two using pregnant subjects (Teglio *et al.*, 1987; Grismondi *et al.*, 1980). Bleeding was investigated in a SB, PC study (Gentile *et al.*, 1987), finding bilberry reduced intra- and postoperative bleeding and prevented subsequent hemorrhaging. Another study (Cerutti *et al.*, 1984) focused on bleeding associated with intrauterine devices. The most comprehensive review of research and clinical information on bilberry was compiled by Morazzoni and Bombardelli (1996).

BRANDED PRODUCTS*

Difrarel 100™: Laboratoires Chibret / c/o Societe Anonyme Corporation / 200 Boulevard Etienne-Clementel Clermont-Ferrand / Puy-de-Dome / France. No product information available; no longer manufactured.

Myrtocyan®: Indena S.p.A. / Viale Ortles 12 / 20139 Milano / Italy / Tel: +39-02-57-4961 / Fax: +39-02-57-4046-20 / Email: indenami@tin.it. Extract standardized to 25% anthocyanidins containing 36% anthocyanosides.

Tegens™: Synthelabo-Pharma SA of France / 11 Rue de Veyrot, 1217 Meyrin / France / Tel: +33-02-29-89-0147 / Fax: +33-02-29-89-0188. The product is standardized to 25% anthocyanidins containing 36% anthocyanosides by the extract Myrtocyan®.

American equivalents, if any, are found in the Product Table beginning on page 398.

REFERENCES

Alfieri R, Sole P. Influence of anthocyanosides, in oral-perlingual administration, on the adapto-electroretinogram (AERG) in red light in humans. [in Italian]. *C R Seances Soc Biol Fil* 1966;160:1590–3.

Allegra C, Pollari G, Criscuolo A, Bonifacio M. Antocianosidi e sistema microvascolotessutale. *Minerva Angiol* 1982;7:39–44.

Allen FM. Blueberry leaf extract: physiologic and clinical properties in relation to carbohydrate metabolism. *JAMA* 1927;89:1577–81.

Bailey CJ, Day C. Traditional Plant Medicine as Treatment for Diabetes. *Diabetes Care* 1989;12(8):553–64.

Baj A, Bombardelli E, Gabetta B, Martinelli EM. Qualitative and quantitative evaluation of *Vaccinium myrtillus* anthocyanins by high-resolution gas chromatography and high-performance liquid chromatography. *J Chromatogr* 1983;279:365–72.

Belleoud L, Leluan D, Boyer Y. A study on the effect of anthocyanosides on nocturnal vision in air traffic controllers. [in' French]. *Rev Med Aeronaut Spat* 1966;18:3–7.

Belleoud L, Leluan D, Boyer Y. A study on the effect of anthocyanosides on nocturnal vision in ship personnel. [in French]. *Soc Franc Physiol Med Aeronaut Cosmonaut* 1967; May.

Bertuglia S, Malandrino S, Colantuoni A. Effect of *Vaccinium myrtillus* anthocyanosides on ischaemia reperfusion injury in hamster cheek pouch microcirculation. *Pharmacol Res* 1995;31:183–7.

Bettini V, Aragno R, Bettini M, *et al*. Vasodilator and inhibitory effects of *Vaccinium myrtillus* anthocyanosides on the contractile responses of coronary artery segments to acetylcholine: role of the prostacyclins and of the endothelium-derived relaxing factor. *Fitoterapia* 1991;62:15–28.

Bettini V, Aragno R, Bettini MB, *et al*. Facilitating influence of *Vaccinium myrtillus* anthocyanosides on the acetylcholine-induced relaxation of isolated coronary arteries: role of the endothelium-derived relaxing factor. *Fitoterapia* 1993;64:45–57.

Bettini V, Guerra B, Martino R, *et al*. Contractile responses of isolated rat stomach to stimulation of postganglionic cholinergic fibers in the presence of *Vaccinium myrtillus* anthocyanosides. *Fitoterapia* 1986;57:211–6.

Bettini V, Mayellaro F, Pilla I, Terribile Weil Marin V. Mechanical responses of isolated coronary arteries to barium in the presence of *Vaccinium myrtillus* anthocyanosides. *Fitoterapia* 1985;56:3–10.

Bettini V, Mayellaro F, Ton P, Zanella P. Effects of *Vaccinium myrtillus* anthocyanosides on vascular smooth muscle. *Fitoterapia* 1984a;55:265–72.

Bettini V, Mayellaro F, Ton P, Zogno M. Interactions between *Vaccinium myrtillus* anthocyanosides and serotonin on splenic artery smooth muscle. *Fitoterapia* 1984b;55:201–8.

Bever B, Zahnd G. Plants with oral hypoglycemic action. *Quart J Crude Drug Res* 1979;17:139–96.

Bilyk A, Sapers GM. Varietal differences in the quercetin, kaempferol, and myricetin contents of highbush blueberry, cranberry, and thornless blackberry fruits. *J Agric Food Chem* 1986;34:585–8.

Blumenthal M. Herb sales down 15% in mainstream market. *HerbalGram* 2001;51:69.

Blumenthal M, Busse WR, Goldberg A, Gruenwald J, Hall T, Riggins CW, Rister RS (eds.). Klein S, Rister RS (trans.). *The Complete German Commission E Monographs—Therapeutic Guide to Herbal Medicines*. Austin, TX: American Botanical Council; Boston: Integrative Medicine Communication; 1998: 88.

Blumenthal M, Goldberg A, Brinckmann J. (eds.) *Herbal Medicine: Expanded Commission E Monographs*. Newton, MA: Integrative Medicine Communications; 2000: 16–21.

Bomser J, Madhavi DL, Singletary K, Smith MA. *In vitro* anticancer activity of fruit extracts from *Vaccinium* species. *Planta Med* 1996;62:212–6.

Bone K, Morgan M. Bilberry: the vision herb. *MediHerb Prof Rev* 1997;59:1–4.

Boniface R, Robert AM. Effect of Anthocyanosides on Human Connective Tissue Metabolism. *Klin Monatsbl Augenheilkd* 1996;209:368–72.

Bottecchia D, Bettini V, Martino R, Camerra G. Preliminary report on the inhibitory effect of *Vaccinium myrtillus* anthocyanosides on platelet aggregation and clot retraction. *Fitoterapia* 1987;58:3–8.

Braun R, Surmann R, Wendt R, Wichtl M, Ziegenmeyer J (eds.). *Standardzulassungen für Fertigarzneimittel: Text und Kommentar* – 8. Ergänzungslieferung. Stuttgart, Germany: Deutscher Apotheker Verlag; Oct 1993;Nr.:1009.99.99.

Bravetti G, Fraboni E, Maccolini E. Preventive medical treatment of senile cataract with vitamin E and *Vaccinium myrtillus* anthocyanosides: clinical evaluation. [in Italian]. *Ann Ottalmol Clin Ocul* 1989;115:109–16.

Bruneton J. *Pharmacognosy Phytochemistry Medicinal Plants*, 2nd ed. Paris, France: Lavoisier Publishing; 1999:361–3.

Caselli L. Clinic, electroretinographic trial on the action of of anthocyanosides. *Arch Med Interna* 1985;37:29–35.

Cerutti R *et al*. Value of *Vaccinium myrtillus* anthocyanosides in the prophylaxis of minor side effects with copper intrauterine device contraception. *Ginecol Clin* 1984;(3-4):244–9.

Cluzel C, Bastide P, Tronche P. Phosphoglucomutase and glucose-6-phosphatase activities of the retina and anthocyanoside extracts from *Vaccinium myrtillus* (study *in vitro* and *vivo*). [in Italian]. *C R Seances Soc Biol Fil* 1969;163:147–50.

Coget J, Merlen J. Anthocyanosides and microcirculation. [in Italian]. *J Mal Vasc* 1980;5:43–6.

Coget J, Merlen J. Clinical study of a new chemical agent for vascular protection, Difrarel 20, compound of anthocyanosides extracted from *Vaccinum myrtillus*. [in Italian]. *Phlebologie* 1968;21:221–8.

Colombo D, Vescovini R. Controlled clinical trial of anthocyanosides from *Vaccinium myrtillus* in primary dysmenorrhea. *G Ital Obstet Ginecol* 1985;7:1033–8.

Cristoni A, Magistretti MJ. Antiulcer and healing activity of *Vaccinium myrtillus* anthocyanosides. *Farmaco [Prat]* 1987;42:29–43.

DAC. See: *Deutscher Arzneimittel-Codex*.

De Smet P, Keller K, Hänsel R, Chandler R. *Adverse Effects of Herbal Drugs*, Vol. 2. Berlin: Germany. Springer-Verlag; 1993;85:307–14.

Detre Z, Jellinek H, Miskulin M, Robert A. Studies on vascular permeability in hypertension: action of anthocyanosides. *Clin Physiol Biochem* 1986;4:143–9.

Deutscher Arzneimittel-Codex (DAC 1998 *Ergänzungsbuch zum Arzneibuch* – Band II). Stuttgart, Germany: Deutscher Apotheker Verlag. 1998;H-060:1–4.

Ferretti C, Magistretti M, Robotti A, Ghi P, Genazzani E. *Vaccinium myrtillus* anthocyanosides are inhibitors of cAMP and cGMP phosphodiesterases. *Pharmacol Res Comm* 1988;20:150.

Gabor M. Pharmacologic effects of flavonoids on blood vessels. *Angiologica* 1972;9:355–74.

Gatta L et al. *Vaccinium myrtillus* anthocyanosides in the treatment of venous stasis: controlled clinical study on sixty patients. *Fitoterapia* 1988;59:19–26.

General Sale List (GSL). Statutory Instrument 1994 No. 2410 – The Medicines (Products Other Than Veterinary Drugs). Amendment Order 1994. London, U.K.: Her Majesty's Stationery Office (HMSO). 1994.

Gentile A. The use of anthocyanidins in bilberry (Tegens™-Inverni della Beffa) to prevent hemorrhaging. [in Italian]. 1987. Unpublished, cited in Morazzoni P, Bombardelli E. *Vaccinium myrtillus* L. *Fitoterapia* 1996;67(1):3–29.

German Homeopathic Pharmacopoeia (GHP) 5th Supplement 1991 to the 1st ed. 1978. Translation of the German "Homöopathisches Arzneibuch (HAB 1), 5. Nachtrag 1991, Amtliche Ausgabe." Stuttgart, Germany: Deutscher Apotheker Verlag; 1993;383–4.

Ghiringhelli C, Gregoratti L, Marastoni F. Capillarotropic action of anthocyanosides in high dosage in phlebopathic stasis. [in Italian]. *Minerva Cardioangiol* 1978;26(4):255–76.

GHP. See: *German Homeopathic Pharmacopoeia*.

Gloria E, Peria A. Effect of anthocyanosides on the absolute visual threshold. [in Italian]. *Ann Oftalmol Clin Ocul* 1966;92:595–607.

Grismondi G. Treatment of phlebopathies caused by stasis in pregnancy. [in Italian]. *Minerva Ginecol* 1980;32:221–30.

GSL. See: *General Sale List*.

Havsteen B. Flavonoids, a class of natural products of high pharmacological potency. *Biochem Pharmacol* 1983;32:1141–8.

Health Canada. *Drug Product Database (DPD) Product Information*. Ottawa, Ontario: Health Canada; 2001.

Homeopathic Pharmacopoeia of the United States (HPUS) — Revision Service Official Compendium from July 1, 1992. Falls Church, VA: American Institute of Homeopathy; 1993 Dec;9412:VACM.

HPUS. See: *Homeopathic Pharmacopoeia of the United States*.

Jayle G, Aubert L. The action of anthocyanin glucosides on the scotopic and mesopic vision of a normal subject [in French]. *Thérapie* 1964;19:171–85.

Jayle G, Aubry M, Gavini H, et al. Study concerning the action of anthocyanoside extracts of *Vaccinium myrtillus* on night vision. [in French] *Ann Ocul (Paris)* 1965;198:556–62.

Kadar A, Robert L, Miskulin M, et al. Influence of anthocyanoside treatment on the cholesterol-induced atherosclerosis in the rabbit. *Paroi Arterielle* 1979;5:187–205.

Kuhnau J. The flavonoids. A class of semi-essential food components: their role in human nutrition. *World Rev Nutr Diet* 1976;24:117–91.

Leung A, Foster S. *Encyclopedia of Common Ingredients Used in Foods, Drugs, and Cosmetics*, 2d ed. New York: Wiley & Sons; 1996.

Lietti A, Cristoni A, Picci M. Studies on *Vaccinium myrtillus* anthocyanosides. I. Vasoprotective and antiinflammatory activity. *Arzneimittelforschung* 1976;26:829–32.

Lietti A, Forni G. Studies on *Vaccinium myrtillus* anthocyanosides. II. Aspects of anthocyanins pharmacokinetics in the rat. *Arzneimittelforschung* 1976;26:832–35.

Magistretti M, Conti M, Cristoni A. Antiulcer activity of an anthocyanidin from *Vaccinium myrtillus*. *Arzneimittelforschung* 1988;38:686–90.

Marcollet M, Bastide P, Tronche P. Angina protecting effect of *Vaccinium myrtillus* anthocyanosides aimed at the release of lactate dehydrogenase (LDH) and of its cardiac isoenzymes in the rat subjected to a swimming test. *C R Seances Soc Biol Fil* 1970;163:1786–9.

Martin-Aragon S, Basabe B, *et al*. Antioxidant action of *Vaccinium myrtillus* L. *Phytother Res* 1998;12:S104–6.

Martinelli E, Scilingo A, Pifferi G. Computer-aided evaluation of the relative stability of *Vaccinium myrtillus* anthocyanins. *Anal Chim Acta* 1992;259:109.

McGuffin M, Hobbs C, Upton R, Goldberg A. *American Herbal Product Association's Botanical Safety Handbook*. Boca Raton, FL: CRC Press; 1997.

Medical Products Agency (MPA). *Naturläkemedel: Authorised Natural Remedies* (as of January 24, 2001). Uppsala, Sweden: Medical Products Agency; 2001.

Meunier M, Duroux E, Bastide P. Antioxidizing action of procyanidolic oligomers and anthocyanosides. *Plant Médicin Phytothér* 1989;23(4):267–74.

Meyer-Buchtela E. *Tee-Rezepturen — Ein Handbuch für Apotheker und Ärzte*. Stuttgart, Germany: Deutscher Apotheker Verlag; 1999;Heidelbeeren.

Mian E, Curri S, Lietti A, Bombardelli E. Anthocyanosides and the walls of the microvessels: further aspects of the mechanism of action of their protective effect in syndromes due to abnormal capillary fragility. [in Italian]. *Minerva Med* 1977;68:3565–81.

Monboisse J, Braquet P, Borel J. Oxygen-free radicals as mediators of collagen breakage. *Agents Actions* 1984;15:49–50.

Monboisse J, Braquet P, Randoux A, Borel J. Non-enzymatic degradation of acid-soluble calf skin collagen by superoxide ion: protective effect of flavonoids. *Biochem Pharmacol* 1983;32:53–8.

Morant J, Ruppanner H (eds.). Fachinformation und Patientinformation: Myrtaven®. In: *Arzneimittel-Kompendium der Schweiz®* 2001. Basel, Switzerland: Documed AG. 2001.

Morazzoni P, Bombardelli E. Review: *Vaccinium myrtillus* L. *Fitoterapia* 1996;LXVII(1):3–29.

Morazzoni P, Magistretti M. Activity of Myrtocyan®, an anthocyanoside complex from *Vaccinium myrtillus* (VMA), on platelet aggregation and adhesiveness. *Fitoterapia* 1990;61:13–22.

MPA. See: Medical Products Agency.

Muth ER, Laurent JM, Jasper P. The effect of bilberry nutritional supplementation on night visual acuity and contrast sensitivity. *Altern Med Rev* 2000; 5(2):164–73.

Neumann L. Long-term therapy of vascular permeability disorders using anthocyanosides. [German]. *Munch Med Wochenschr* 1973;115:952–4.

ÖAB. See: *Österreichisches Arzneibuch*.

Ofek I, Goldhar J, Sharon N. Anti-*Escherichia coli* adhesin of cranberry and bilberry juices. *Adv Exp Med Biol* 1996;408:179–83.

Orsucci P, Rossi M, Sabbatini G, *et al*. Treatment of diabetic retinopathy with anthocyanosides: a preliminary report. *Clin Ocul* 1983;4:377.

Österreichisches Arzneibuch. (ÖAB 1991). Vienna, Austria: Verlag der Österreichischen Staatsdruckerei. 1991;Heidelbeeren.

Pennarola R, Roco P, Matarazzo G, *et al*. The therapeutic action of the anthocyanosides in microcirculatory changes due to adhesive-induced polyneuritis. [in Italian]. *Gazz Med Ital* 1980;139:485–91.

Perossini M, Guidi G, Chiellini S, Siravo D. Diabetic and hypertensive retinopathy therapy with *Vaccinium myrtillus* anthocyanosides (Tegens™). Double-blind placebo-controlled trial. *Ann Oftalmol Clin Ocul* 1987;113:1173–90.

Pharmacopoea Helvetica (Ph.Helv VII 1987 with supplements through 1997). Bern, Switzerland: Verlag Eidgenössische Drucksachen und Materialzentrale; 1987-1997.

Ph.Helv. See: *Pharmacopoea Helvetica*.

Pietta P, Simonetti P, Mauri P. Antioxidant activity of selected medicinal plants. *J Agric Food Chem* 1998;46:4487–90.

Pizzorno JE, Murray MT, editors. *Textbook of Natural Medicine*, Vol. 1., 2nd ed. New York: Churchill Livingstone;1999;991–6.

Pulliero G, Montin S, *et al*. Ex vivo study of the inhibitory effects of *Vaccinium myrtillus* anthocyanosides on human platelet aggregation. *Fitoterapia* 1989;60:69–75.

Repossi P, Malagola R, De Cadilhac C. The role of anthocyanosides on vascular permeability in diabetic retinopathy. *Ann Oftalmol Clin Ocul* 1987;113(4):357–361.

Robert A, Godeau G, Moati F, Miskulin M. Action of anthocyanosides of *Vaccinium myrtillus* on the permeability of the blood brain barrier. *J Med* 1977;8:321–2.

Sala D, Rolando M, Rossi P, Pissarello L. Effect of anthocyanosides on visual performances at low illumination. [in Italian]. *Minerva Oftalmol* 1979;21:283–5.

Scharrer A, Ober M. Anthocyanosides in the treatment of retinopathies. [in German]. *Klin Monatsbl Augenheilkd* 1981;178:386–9.

Schulz V, Hänsel R, Tyler V. *Rational Phytotherapy: A Physician's Guide to Herbal Medicine* 4th ed. Berlin Heidelberg: Germany. Springer-Verlag; 2001; 234.

Teglio L, Mazzanti C, Tronconi R, Guerresi E. *Vaccinium myrtillus* anthocyanosides (Tegens™) in the treatment of venous insufficiency of lower limbs and acute piles in pregnancy. *Quad Clin Ostet Ginecol* 1987;42:221–31.

Terrasse J, Moinade S. Initial results with a new vitamin P factor "the anthocyanosides" extracts of *Vaccinium myrtillus*. [in French]. *La Presse Med* 1964;72:397–400.

Tolan L, Barna V, Szigeti I, *et al*. [The use of bilberry powder in dyspepsia in infants]. *Pediatria (Bucur)* 1969;18:375–9.

Treviso A. Therapeutic value of the association of anthocyanin glucosides with gluta- mine and phosphorylserine in the treatment of learning disturbances at different ages. *Gazz Med Ital* 1979;138:217–32.

United States Congress (USC). Public Law 103-417: Dietary Supplement Health and Education Act of 1994. Washington, DC: 103rd Congress of the United States;1994.

USC. See: United States Congress.

Vannini L, Samuelly R, Coffano M, Tibaldi L. Study of the pupillary reflex after anthocyanoside administration. *Boll Ocul* 1986;65:11–2.

Wang H, Cao G, Prior R. Oxygen radical absorbing capacity of anthocyanins. *J Agric Food Chem* 1997;45:304–309.

Wichtl M, Bisset NG (eds.). *Herbal Drugs and Phytopharmaceuticals: A Handbook for Practice on a Scientific Basis.* Stuttgart, Germany: Medpharm Scientific Publishers; 1994;351–2.

Zaragoza F, Iglesias I, Benedi J. [Comparative study of the anti-aggregation effects of anthocyanosides and other agents]. *Arch Farmacol Toxicol* 1985;72:397–400.

Zavarise G. Effect of prolonged treatment with anthocyanosides on light sensitivity. [in Italian]. *Ann Oftalmol Clin Ocul* 1987;94:209–14.

Clinical Studies on Bilberry (Vaccinium myrtillus)

Ocular (night/day vision, retinopathy, etc.)

Author/Year	Subject	Design	Duration	Dosage	Preparation	Results/Conclusion
Muth et al., 2000	Night vision and contrast sensitivity	DB, PC n=15 males, all except 2 with good vision (ages 25–47 years)	90 days	160 mg, 3x/day (25% anthocyanosides)	Not specified	Study failed to find an effect of bilberry on night visual acuity (VA) (p>0.15) or night contrast sensitivity (CS) (p>0.35) for a high dose of bilberry taken for a significant duration. Hence, this study casts doubt on the proposition that bilberry supplementation, in forms currently available and in doses recommended, improves night VA or night CS.
Perossini et al., 1987	Retinopathy (patients with diabetic retinopathy, n=35; hypertensive vascular retinopathy n=5) (stage IV excluded)	DB, PC n=40	30 days	160 mg 2x/day	Tegens™ 160 mg capsule	Improved opthalmoscopic and angiographic patterns were demonstrated in 77–90% of the patients. Concluded to be an effective and safe treatment of diabetic and hypertensive retinopathy. (No statistics reported.)
Repossi et al., 1987	Early diabetic or hypertensive retinopathy	DB, PC n=40	1 year	160 mg 2x/day	Tegens™ 160 mg capsule	Improvements were observed in 50% (vs. 20% in control group). Patients with exudate deposits improved in 15% of the cases (vs. 10% control group). A lower percentage of patients (10% vs.15%) with hard exudates worsened.
Vannini et al., 1986	Nighttime vision in healthy subjects	DB, PC n=40 (mean age 25.5 years)	2 hours	240 mg/single dose	Myrtocyan®	Improved pupillary photomotor response, most evident 2 hours after administration; decreased total pupillary contraction time (p<0.05); increased pupillary contraction (p<0.05).
Orsucci et al., 1983	Diabetic retinopathy in Type II diabetes mellitus	O n=10	6 months	80 mg 3x/day	Tegens™ 80 mg capsule	Improvement in retinal picture; reduction or disappearance of hemorrhages.
Scharrer and Ober, 1981	Diabetic retinopathy	O n=31: 2 with hemorrhages due to anticoagulants, 4 with arterial sclerosis with hemorrhages of the retina, 20 with diabetic retinopathy (Keith Wagner Stages II and III)	4 weeks	Two, 80 mg capsules 3x/day	Difrarel 100™ capsule	Reduced vascular permeability during treatment. Mitigated changes of retinal vessels and prevented alterations in the visual field. (No statistics reported.)

KEY: **C** – controlled, **CC** – case-control, **CH** – cohort, **CI** – confidence interval, **Cm** – comparison, **CO** – crossover, **CS** – cross-sectional, **DB** – double-blind, **E** – epidemiological, **LC** – longitudinal cohort, **MA** – meta-analysis, **MC** – multi-center, **n** – number of patients, **O** – open, **OB** – observational, **OL** – open label, **OR** – odds ratio, **P** – prospective, **PB** – patient-blind, **PC** – placebo-controlled, **PG** – parallel group, **PS** – pilot study, **R** – randomized, **RC** – reference-controlled, **RCS** – retrospective cross-sectional, **RS** - retrospective, **S** – surveillance, **SB** – single-blind, **SC** – single-center, **U** – uncontrolled, **UP** – unpublished, **VC** – vehicle-controlled.

Clinical Studies on Bilberry (Vaccinium myrtillus) (cont.)

Vascular (micro and peripheral circulation, venous disorders/insufficiencies, etc.)

Author/Year	Subject	Design	Duration	Dosage	Preparation	Results/Conclusion
Gatta et al., 1988	Venous insufficiency (various causes)	SB, PC n=60 (mean age 44 years)	30 days	160 mg 3x/day	Tegens™ 160	Decreased severity of edema, sensations of pressure, paresthesia, and cramp-like pain were observed in the bilberry group (p<0.01 for all outcomes).
Gentile et al., 1987, unpublished	Preventive bleeding due to otorhinolaryngological surgery	SB, PC n=181 (ages 3–76 years)	10 days prior to surgery	160–320 mg/day dosed according to clinical symptoms	Myrtocyan®	Reduced intra- and postoperative bleeding and prevented subsequent hemorrhaging when treated with bilberry before surgery. (No statistics reported.)
Teglio, 1987	Venous insufficiency symptoms in pregnant women	n=51 (mean period of pregnancy 27 weeks) (mean age 30 years)	3 months	160, 240, 360 mg/day dosed according to symptom severity	Tegens™	Reduction in symptoms of pruritus (94.6%), paresthesia (87.5%), cramps (80.1%), pain (78.5%), exhaustion and heaviness (60%), and hemorrhoidal symptoms (75.5–83%).
Allegra et al., 1982	Peripheral vascular disorder	DB, PC n=47	30 days	480 mg/day	Myrtocyan®	Decreased edema, paresthesia, and pain while increasing joint mobility in patients with Raynaud's disease.
Grismondi et al., 1981	Phlebopathies induced by pregnancy	n=54 (ages 24–37 years)	60–90 days	320 mg/day started in 6th month of pregnancy	Myrtocyan®	Improvements in burning and itching (p<0.001), heaviness (p<0.001), and pain (p<0.001) were observed in bilberry users, as well as in diurnal and nocturnal cramps (p<0.01), and a reduction in edema and in capillary fragility (p<0.001).
Ghiringhelli et al., 1977	Varicose veins of lower limbs	O n=47 (mean age 45 years)	30 days	480 mg/day	Myrtocyan®	Bilberry significantly improved symptoms such as limb edema and dyschromic skin phenomena as well as heaviness, paresthesia, and pain.
Mian et al., 1977	Ulcerative dermatitis due to post thrombophlebitis	O n=15	10 days	240 mg/day	Myrtocyan®	Bilberry reduced the protein content of the exudate produced by venous occlusion and stasis, a symptom of post-thrombotic and varicose veins stasis. (No statistics reported.)

Other

Author/Year	Subject	Design	Duration	Dosage	Preparation	Results/Conclusion
Colombo, 1985	Chronic dysmenorrhea	DB, PC n=30	3 days prior to and during the cycle	320 mg/day	Myrtocyan® capsule	Bilberry significantly reduced dysmenorrhea symptoms including headache, heaviness of lower limbs, mammary tension, sickness and emesis, and pelvic and lumbosacral pain by the second month.
Cerutti et al., 1984	Side effects of copper IUD's	n=48	6 months	Two, 160 mg capsules 2x/day	Myrtocyan®	Decreased incidents of spotting and hyperpoly-menorrhea were observed in bilberry users.

KEY: C – controlled, **CC** – case-control, **CH** – cohort, **CI** – confidence interval, **Cm** – comparison, **CO** – crossover, **CS** – cross-sectional, **DB** – double-blind, **E** – epidemiological, **LC** – longitudinal cohort, **MA** – meta-analysis, **MC** – multi-center, **n** – number of patients, **O** – open, **OB** – observational, **OL** – open label, **OR** – odds ratio, **P** – prospective, **PB** – patient-blind, **PC** – placebo-controlled, **PG** – parallel group, **PS** – pilot study, **R** – randomized, **RC** – reference-controlled, **RCS** – retrospective cross-sectional, **RS** - retrospective, **S** – surveillance, **SB** – single-blind, **SC** – single-center, **U** – uncontrolled, **UP** – unpublished, **VC** – vehicle-controlled.

Black Cohosh

Actaea racemosa L. (syn. *Cimicifuga racemosa* [L.] Nutt.)

[Fam. *Ranunculaceae*]

OVERVIEW

Black cohosh is indigenous to the Eastern U.S. and Canada and has a long and widely recognized medicinal tradition. Native Americans and early colonists used black cohosh root to treat conditions including general malaise, malaria, rheumatism, abnormalities in kidney function, sore throat, menstrual irregularities, and childbirth. In Chinese medicine, rhizomes of many different species of *Actaea* have been traditionally used to treat inflammation, fever, headache, pain, sore throat, and chills. Black cohosh has been used in Europe for more than 40 years to treat symptoms associated with menopause. In 1996, nearly 10 million retail units of a standardized ethanolic and isopropanolic extract were sold monthly in Germany, Australia, and the U.S. The herb has become increasingly popular as a dietary supplement in the U.S., with retail sales in mainstream markets in 2000 ranking 14th among all herbals. Currently, black cohosh root is approved by the German Commission E to treat premenstrual discomfort, dysmennorhea, and neurovegetative complaints associated with menopause.

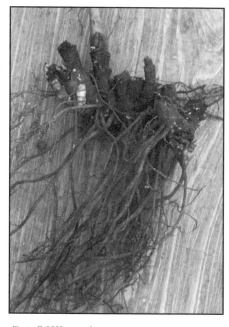

Photo © 2002 stevenfoster.com

PRIMARY USES

- Neurovegetative complaints associated with menopause, including hot flashes, heart palpitations, nervousness, irritability, sleep disturbances, tinnitus, vertigo, perspiration, depression
- Premenstrual discomfort
- Dysmenorrhea

OTHER POTENTIAL USES

- Surgical ovarian deficiencies

PHARMACOLOGICAL ACTIONS

Early research suggested estrogenic activity (with alcoholic fractions) inhibiting LH secretion, but not FSH secretion, in menopausal women and proliferating vaginal epithelium. However, other more recent studies have refuted estrogen-like activity. Further research needs to be conducted to determine the herb's mechanism of action.

DOSAGE AND ADMINISTRATION

The German Commission E monograph recommends a maximum treatment duration of six months. In Germany, prescriptions for hormone replacement therapy (HRT) are limited to a six-month duration in order to ensure that women return to their healthcare providers for general checkups. In the case of black cohosh, the Commission E has based its limitations of therapy with black cohosh on the same criteria as used for HRT.

DRIED RHIZOME AND ROOT: 40–200 mg daily.

DECOCTION: Daily dose, 240 ml boiling water poured onto 40–200 mg black cohosh (crude drug), simmered for 10–15 minutes.

FLUID EXTRACT: 0.3–1.0 ml, or 0.3–2.0 ml, or 5–30 drops [1:1 (*g/ml*) 90% alcohol].

TINCTURE: 0.4–2.0 ml daily, or 2–4 ml, or 40 drops twice daily [1:10 (*g/ml*) 40–60% alcohol].

STANDARDIZED DRY EXTRACT: 40%–60% ethanolic or isopropyl alcohol extracts of the rhizome with monitoring of active compounds (triterpene glycosides) corresponding to 40 mg of black cohosh daily.

CONTRAINDICATIONS

None known.

PREGNANCY AND LACTATION: Not recommended during pregnancy due to emmenagogue and uterine-stimulant effects (based on empirical observations). Not recommended during lactation (based on empirical observations).

ADVERSE EFFECTS

Occasional gastrointestinal discomfort has been reported. Vertigo, headache, nausea, vomiting, impaired vision, and impaired circulation have been reported in cases of overdose.

DRUG INTERACTIONS

None known.

CLINICAL REVIEW

Nine of 10 clinical studies (1,371 total participants) demonstrated positive effects for menopausal symptoms. Numerous clinical trials with varied methods and designs have been conducted on the standardized isopropanolic/ethanolic extract of black cohosh root, Remifemin®, from 1981 to the present. Five of the studies were open-label, and evaluated the effectiveness of the extract as a monotherapy for the treatment of menopausal complaints. Two studies compared black cohosh extract to conventional hormonal therapy in the treatment of complaints associated with menopause or hormonal deficiencies in ovariectomized/hysterectomized patients. One open-label, randomized (R), controlled study compared the efficacy of three different black cohosh therapies to conjugated estrogens and diazepam for menopausal problems. One R, double-blind study compared two dosages of Remifemin® for the treatment of menopausal symptoms. A decrease in the Kupperman-Menopause Index (KPI) was reported in five clinical studies on black cohosh extract.

Black Cohosh

Actaea racemosa L. (syn. *Cimicifuga racemosa* [L.] Nutt.)
[Fam. *Ranunculaceae*]

OVERVIEW

Black cohosh, a plant commonly found in the Eastern U.S. and Canada, was a botanical remedy of Native Americans. It has been used in Europe for over 40 years. Today, black cohosh root is approved by the German government as a treatment for premenstrual discomfort, painful menstruation, and menopausal symptoms.

USES

Menopausal complaints including hot flashes, heart palpitations, nervousness, irritability, sleep disturbances, ringing in the ears (tinnitus), whirling sense or dizziness (vertigo), perspiration, and depression; premenstrual discomfort; painful menstruation.

DOSAGE

The German Commission E monograph recommends taking black cohosh for a period of six months, after which a check-up with your healthcare practitioner is advised before resuming further use.

AVERAGE RECOMMENDED DOSE: 40mg–80mg (or oral dose equivalent) of black cohosh per day (available in tablet and liquid form).

DRIED RHIZOME AND ROOT: 40–200 mg.

DECOCTION: Pour 240 ml boiling water onto 40–200 mg black cohosh root, simmer for 10–15 minutes.

FLUID EXTRACT: 0.3–1.0 ml, 0.3–2.0 ml, 5–30 drops [1:1 (*g/ml*), 90% alcohol].

TINCTURE: 0.4–2.0 ml, 2-4 ml, 40 drops twice daily [1:10 (*g/ml*), 40–60% alcohol].

CONTRAINDICATIONS

None known.

PREGNANCY AND LACTATION: Patients who are pregnant and/or lactating should not use black cohosh. It is not recommended during pregnancy because it may promote menstrual flow or stimulate the uterus. Black cohosh is not recommended during breast-feeding.

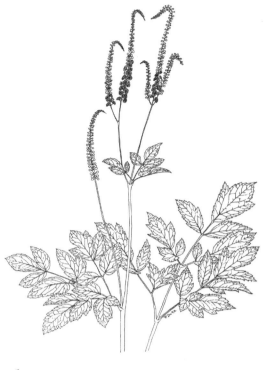

ADVERSE EFFECTS

Occasional gastrointestinal discomfort has been reported. Overdose may cause vertigo, headache, nausea, vomiting, impaired vision, and impaired circulation.

DRUG INTERACTIONS

None known. Minimal side effects were noted when standardized black cohosh extracts and estrogen-replacement therapy (hormone-replacement therapy, HRT) were taken at the same time.

Comments

When using a dietary supplement, purchase it from a reliable source. For best results, use the same brand of product throughout the period of use. As with all medications and dietary supplements, please inform your healthcare provider of all herbs and medications you are taking. Interactions may occur between medications and herbs or even among different herbs when taken at the same time. Treat your herbal supplement with care by taking it as directed, storing it as advised on the label, and keeping it out of the reach of children and pets. Consult your healthcare provider with any questions.

AMERICAN
BOTANICAL
COUNCIL

The information contained on this sheet has been excerpted from *The ABC Clinical Guide to Herbs* © 2003 by the American Botanical Council (ABC). ABC is an independent member-based educational organization focusing on the medicinal use of herbs. For more detailed information about this herb please consult the healthcare provider who gave you this sheet. To order *The ABC Clinical Guide to Herbs* or become a member of ABC, visit their website at www.herbalgram.org.

Black Cohosh

Actaea racemosa L. (syn. *Cimicifuga racemosa* [L.] Nutt.)

[Fam. *Ranunculaceae*]

OVERVIEW

Black cohosh is indigenous to the Eastern United States and Canada, and has a long and widely recognized medicinal tradition (Blumenthal *et al.*, 2000; Liske, 1998). Native Americans and early colonists used black cohosh root to treat conditions including general malaise, malaria, rheumatism, abnormalities in kidney function, sore throat, menstrual irregularities, and childbirth (Blumenthal *et al.*, 2000; Boon and Smith, 1999; Liske, 1998). In Chinese medicine, rhizomes of many different species of *Actaea* have been traditionally used to treat inflammation, fever, headache, pain, sore throat, and chills (Foster, 1999; Liske, 1998). Black cohosh has been used in Europe for more than 40 years to treat symptoms associated with menopause (Foster, 1999). In 1996, nearly 10 million retail units of a standardized ethanolic and isopropanolic extract were sold monthly in Germany, Australia, and the U.S. (Blumenthal *et al.*, 2000; Pizzorno and Murray, 1999). The herb has become increasingly popular as a dietary supplement in the U.S., with retail sales in mainstream markets in 2000 ranking 14th of all herbals (Blumenthal, 2001). Currently, black cohosh root is approved as a nonprescription drug to treat premenstrual discomfort, dysmennorhea, and neurovegetative complaints associated with menopause by the German Commission E (Blumenthal *et al* 1998; Liske, 1998).

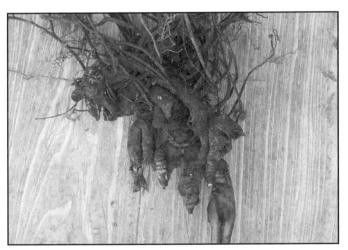

Photo © 2002 stevenfoster.com

DESCRIPTION

Crude preparations of black cohosh consist of the dried rhizome and roots of *Actaea racemosa* L. (syn. *Cimicifuga racemosa* [L.]) (Foster, 1999; McGuffin *et al.*, 2000) [Fam. *Ranunculaceae*], harvested in the fall (Blumenthal *et al.*, 2000; Bradley, 1992). Some commercial extracts have been standardized based upon triterpene glycoside content (Liske, 1998; McKenna, 1998). Remifemin®, a German standardized oral formulation used in all of the black cohosh clinical studies published through 2000, contains 20 mg of black cohosh extract standardized to 1 mg triterpene glycosides (calculated as 27-deoxyactein) per tablet or twenty drops (Blumenthal *et al.*, 2000; Liske, 1998; McKenna, 1998).

PRIMARY USES

Gynecology

* Menopause: Neurovegetative complaints associated with menopause, including hot flashes, heart palpitations, nervousness, irritability, sleep disturbances, tinnitus, vertigo, perspiration, and depression (Liske *et al.*, 2002; Düker *et al.*, 1991; Lehmann-Willenbrock and Riedel, 1988; Blumenthal *et al.*, 1998; Bratman and Kroll, 1999; Pethö, 1987; Stoll, 1987; Warnecke, 1985; Vorberg, 1984; Daiber 1983; Stolze 1982)

* Premenstrual discomfort (Blumenthal *et al.*, 1998; Bratman and Kroll, 1999)

* Dysmenorrhea (Blumenthal *et al.*, 1998; Bratman and Kroll, 1999)

OTHER POTENTIAL USES

* Treatment of surgical ovarian deficiencies (Lehmann-Willenbrock and Riedel, 1988; Liske, 1998)

DOSAGE

In clinical studies before 1996, the dose was 2x2 tablets/day, or 2x40 drops/day, which is equivalent to 48–140 mg of black cohosh extract per day (Foster, 1999; Liske, 1998). A recent clinical trial comparing two different dosages of Remifemin® (40 mg vs. 127 mg daily), for six months, in 116 women with menopausal complaints, found similar safety and efficacy profiles for both doses (Liske *et al.*, 2002). Based upon the results of this trial, a recommended dose equivalent to 40 mg of black cohosh (dried root) daily is currently recommended (Liske, 1998). Nevertheless, the dosage in most of the clinical trials shown in the table below is 80 mg daily of the extract (the doses in the studies using liquid preparation form at 40 drops twice daily are equivalent to 80 mg daily).

Internal

Crude Preparations

DRIED RHIZOME AND ROOT: 40–200 mg daily (Bradley, 1992).

DECOCTION: Daily dose 240 ml boiling water poured onto 40–200 mg black cohosh (cut, dried root) and simmered for 10–15 minutes (Bradley, 1992).

FLUID EXTRACT: 1:1 (*g/ml*) 90% alcohol, 0.3–1.0 ml (Karnick, 1994); 0.3–2.0 ml (Newall *et al.*, 1996).

TINCTURE: 1:10 (*g/ml*) 40–60% alcohol, 0.4–2.0 ml (Bradley, 1992); 2–4 ml (Newall *et al.*, 1996; Wren, 1988), 40 drops are taken twice daily (Hunter, 1999; Warnecke, 1985).

Standardized Preparations

EXTRACT: 40%–60% ethanolic or isopropyl alcohol extracts of the rhizome with monitoring of active compounds (triterpene glycosides) (Liske, 1998; Liske et al., 2002), corresponding to 40 mg of black cohosh daily (Blumenthal et al., 1998).

DURATION OF ADMINISTRATION

The German Commission E monograph recommends a maximum treatment duration of six months (Blumenthal et al., 1998). Some authors have suggested that this is due to a lack of clinical trials longer than six months published at the time the monograph was compiled (Bratman and Kroll, 1999; McKenna, 1998). According to Professor H. Schilcher, vice-president of the Commission E, the reason for this limitation is predicated on the Commission's desire to ensure that women return to their healthcare provider for periodic examinations at six-month intervals. The limitation is not based on any concerns about the long-term safety of black cohosh. Based on a long history (33 years) of black cohosh use in Germany at the time the monograph was written in 1989, and on the herb's general safety in long-term use (including data from clinical experience, post-marketing studies, and market data on daily doses prescribed, adverse events reports, etc.), the Commission E considered allowing unlimited duration of use of black cohosh without concern for safety. However, in Germany, prescriptions for hormone replacement therapy (HRT) are limited to a six-month duration in order to ensure that women return to their healthcare provider for general checkups; in the case of black cohosh, the Commission E treated it with the same limitations as HRT (Schilcher, 2001). The relative safety of black cohosh in long-term use is also supported by pharmacological and clinical research. In a six-month chronic toxicity study, followed by an eight-week recovery period, up to 1,800 mg/kg body weight, or roughly 90 times the therapeutic dose, of black cohosh granulate was administered to rats, and no detectable anomalies or toxic effects were observed (Korn, 1991). Although this study may support long-term use of black cohosh (Pizzorno and Murray, 1999), studies of carcinogens in rats must typically be two years long to equate to long-term use in humans (Cott, 2000). Ames tests (in vitro Salmonella microsomal assays) performed on isopropanolic extracts showed no evidence of mutagenicity (Bratman and Kroll, 1999; Liske, 1998). Although long-term studies may be warranted to satisfy current standards in toxicology, these findings suggest that black cohosh may be considered relatively safe for long-term therapy (Liske, 1998; Pizzorno and Murray, 1999).

CHEMISTRY

Constituents of black cohosh root and rhizome include triterpene glycosides: actein, cimicifugoside, cimigoside, 27-deoxyactein, deoxyacetylacteol, and racemoside (Bradley, 1992; Bratman and Kroll, 1999; McKenna, 1998; Newall et al., 1996). Eight new triterpene glycosides named cimiracemosides A-H have been identified (Shao et al., 2000). Some references state that it also contains isoflavones including formononetin (Bradley, 1992; Jarry et al., 1985; Pizzorno and Murray, 1999). NOTE: Although Jarry and coworkers reported the isolation of formononetin from a methanolic extract in 1985, more recent studies of Remifemin® (an isopropyl/ethanolic extract) along with five other commercial preparations failed to identify appreciable levels of the flavonoids (Liske, 1998; Foster, 1999; Stuck et al., 1997). An analysis of wild black cohosh from 13 different locations and two leading commercial extracts resulted in no detectable levels of formononetin

(Kennelly et al., 2002). A recent review suggests black cohosh does not contain isoflavones (Hagels et al., 2000). Constituents of black cohosh root and rhizomes also include the aromatic acids, isoferulic acid and salicylic acid (Bradley, 1992; Newall et al., 1996; Pizzorno and Murray, 1999) and other constituents including tannins, resin, phytosterols, fatty acids, starch, and sugars (Bradley, 1992; Foster, 1999; Newall et al., 1996).

PHARMACOLOGICAL ACTIONS

Studies refuting the estrogenic activity of black cohosh:

Human

A good-clinical-practices-compliance study (40 mg vs. 127 mg daily) in postmenopausal women yielded no estrogen-like lutenizing hormone (LH) or follicle-stimulating hormone (FSH) suppression. In addition, endogenous estradiol, sex hormone-binding globulin (SHBG), and prolactin levels remain unaffected (Liske et al., 1998; Liske et al., 2002). Estrogenic changes in vaginal cytological parameters (e.g., degree of vaginal proliferation) were not observed (Liske et al., 1998; Liske et al., 2002). No increase in thickness of the endometrium, no changes in vaginal cell status, and no changes in the hormone values of LH, FSH, prolactin, estradiol were observed before and after a black cohosh treatment (Nesselhut and Liske, 1999).

Animal

No estrogen-like uterine effects or changes in vaginal cytology were detected in animal experiments using an ethanolic extract (Einer-Jensen et al., 1996). In rats with artificially (DMBA) induced breast tumors, it was demonstrated that different doses of an isopropanolic black cohosh extract (1x, 10x, 100x human therapeutic dose) did not cause stimulation of mammary tumors compared to the placebo group. Estrogen substitution with mestranol resulted in a progression of the tumors. No estrogenic-agonistic effects on prolactin, LH, FSH, or on the uterine tissue were seen (Freudenstein et al., 2000). Pyridinoline and deoxypyridinoline as markers of bone metabolism in rats declined significantly under black cohosh administration (isopropanolic extract) compared to the control, suggesting potential benefits in retarding bone loss (Nisslein and Freudenstein, 2000).

In vitro

Formononetin, the isoflavone thought to be an active estrogenic component of black cohosh in earlier studies (Jarry et al., 1985; Jarry and Harnischfeger, 1985), is not detected in the commercially available isopropanolic and ethanolic extract (Struck et al., 1997) and is not a constituent of the dried root (Hagels et al., 2000). An isopropanolic/alcoholic extract inhibits the proliferation of estrogen-receptor positive (ER+) human breast cancer cell lines (MDA MB 435S) (Nesselhut et al., 1993). Investigations show that an isopropanolic-aqueous extract does not stimulate the proliferation of ER+ human breast cancer cell lines (MCF-7), but the extract does produce a dose-dependent inhibition of DNA synthesis, an antagonization of estradiol activity, and a synergistic increase in the anti-proliferative effect of tamoxifen (Freudenstein and Bodinet, 1999). An ethanolic black cohosh extract inhibited growth of T-47D human breast cancer cells (Dixon-Shanies and Shaikh, 1999).

Studies supporting the estrogenic activity of black cohosh:

Human

Earlier research showed that black cohosh improves neurovegetative symptoms (hot flashes, increased perspiration, headache, vertigo, heart palpitations, tinnitus) and psychological complaints (nervousness, irritability, sleep disturbances, depressive mood) associated with menopause or hormonal deficiencies experienced by hysterectomized/ovariectomized patients (Stolze, 1982; Daiber, 1983; Vorberg, 1984; Warnecke, 1985; Stoll, 1987; Pethö, 1987; Lehmann-Willenbrock and Reidel, 1988; Lieberman, 1998; Liske, 1998); proliferation of vaginal epithelium (Stoll, 1987). Three alcoholic fractions produced endocrine effects that inhibit LH secretion, but not FSH secretion, in menopausal women. The authors hypothesize that this is an estrogen-like effect (Düker *et al.*, 1991).

In vitro

A methanolic extract demonstrated endocrine activity in an *in vitro* estrogen-receptor assay. The three fractions identified were believed to compete with estradiol for binding sites on estrogen receptors (Jarry *et al.*, 1985).

MECHANISM OF ACTION

Although estrogen-like effects, such as LH suppression, have been proposed as the primary mechanism of action in alleviating the symptoms of menopause, results of recent animal investigations and clinical studies indicate that the mode of action is not identical with estrogen. On the contrary, estrogen-agonistic and estrogen-antagonistic effects on different target organs indicate a tissue selectivity for black cohosh ingredients (Boblitz *et al.*, 2000). Although some studies suggest black cohosh has an estrogen-like effect based on its observed LH-suppressive activity, a definite mechanism of action has not been established (Düker *et al.*, 1991). A recent animal study failed to detect estrogen-like uterine effects or changes in vaginal cytology with black cohosh administration. Thus, the authors concluded that LH suppression was associated with neurotransmitter interference instead of estrogenic activity (Einer-Jensen *et al.*, 1996). Similarly, another study comparing two different dosages of Remifemin® (40 mg vs. 127 mg daily) showed no effect on hormonal levels of LH, FSH, SHBG, prolactin, or estradiol, or on vaginal cytological parameters; however, menopausal symptoms were clearly alleviated (Liske *et al.*, 2002, 1998). Although the authors cannot definitively explain the mechanism responsible for the efficacy of black cohosh in the treatment of menopausal complaints, they agree that Remifemin® does not exert a hormonal (estrogenic) effect (Liske *et al.*, 2002, 1998).

CONTRAINDICATIONS

None known (Blumenthal *et al.*, 1998; Pizzorno and Murray, 1999).

NOTE: Despite earlier concerns about the possible estrogenicity of black cohosh, and thus a possible contraindication for women with estrogen-positive breast cancer, as explained in the Pharmacology and Mechanism of Action sections above and in the discussion below, it is clearly established that black cohosh is not estrogenic. Thus, no such contraindication is warranted.

According to an *in vitro* study, the use of an isopropanolic aqueous extract of black cohosh reportedly inhibited the proliferation of estrogen-receptor positive (ER+) human breast cancer cells and, although still debated, the present data indicate that black cohosh does not increase the risk of developing breast cancer (Nesselhut *et al.*, 1993). Another *in vitro* study reported that Remifemin® extract did not stimulate the proliferation of ER+ human breast cancer cells (Freudenstein and Bodinet, 1999). In addition, the extract inhibited DNA synthesis in a dose-dependent manner, antagonized the estrogenic activity of estradiol, and enhanced the anti-proliferative effect of tamoxifen (Freudenstein and Bodinet, 1999). In rats with artificially (DMBA) induced breast tumors, it could be demonstrated that different doses of an isopropanolic black cohosh extract (1x, 10x, 100x human therapeutic dose) did not cause any stimulation of mammary tumors compared to the placebo group. Estrogen substitution with mestranol resulted in a progression of the tumors. No estrogenic-agonistic effects on prolactin, LH, or FSH, or on uterine tissue were seen (Freudenstein *et al.*, 2000).

PREGNANCY AND LACTATION: Not recommended during pregnancy due to its emmenagogue and uterine-stimulant effect (based on empirical observations) (Brinker, 2001; McGuffin *et al.*, 1997). Not recommended during lactation (based on empirical observations) (Brinker, 2001; McGuffin *et al.*, 1997).

ADVERSE EFFECTS

Occasional gastrointestinal discomfort has been reported (Blumenthal *et al.*, 1998; Foster, 1999; McGuffin *et al.*, 1997). Vertigo, headache, nausea, vomiting, impaired vision, and impaired circulation have been reported with overdose (Foster, 1999; McGuffin *et al.*, 1997).

DRUG INTERACTIONS

None known (Blumenthal *et al.*, 1998; Brinker, 2001), including in cases of simultaneous administration of standardized black cohosh extracts and estrogen-replacement therapy (McKenna, 1998; Pethö, 1987; Warnecke, 1985).

AMERICAN HERBAL PRODUCTS ASSOCIATION (AHPA) SAFETY RATING

CLASS 2B: Not to be used during pregnancy.

CLASS 2C: Not to be used while nursing (McGuffin *et al.*, 1997).

REGULATORY STATUS

CANADA: Regulated as a drug if single dose is sufficiently high or as a potential "New Drug" for specific nontraditional use claims (HPB, 1993). Included in the Drugs Directorate "List of Herbs Unacceptable as Non-medicinal Ingredients in Oral Use Products" (Health Canada 1995a). When identified as a Traditional Herbal Medicine (THM) or as a homeopathic drug, black cohosh is regulated as a nonprescription over-the-counter (OTC) drug requiring premarket authorization and assignment of a drug identification number (DIN) (Health Canada, 1995b; Health Canada, 2001; WHO, 1998).

FRANCE: Traditional medicine.

GERMANY: Fresh or dried rhizome with attached roots is an approved nonprescription drug for oral use in the German Commission E Monographs (Blumenthal *et al.*, 1998). The fresh rhizome and roots for preparation of hydro-alcoholic mother tincture and liquid dilutions are an official drug of the *German Homeopathic Pharmacopoeia* (GHP, 1993). No monograph in the *German Pharmacopoeia* (DAB).

SWEDEN: Classified as a natural remedy; intended for self-medication; require advance application for marketing authorization. A monograph for the product Remifemin® is published in the Medical Products Agency (MPA) "Authorised Natural Remedies" (MPA, 1999, 2001; WHO, 1998).

SWITZERLAND: Approved as single-ingredient Herbal Medicine and as a component of multiple-ingredient Homeopathic Medicines, both classified by the *Interkantonale Kontrollstelle für*

Heilmittel (IKS) as List D medicinal products with sales limited to pharmacies and drugstores, without prescription (Morant and Ruppanner, 2001; WHO, 1998).

U.K.: OTC herbal medicine specified in the *General Sale List*, Schedule 1 (medicinal products requiring a full product license), Table A (for internal or external use); 200 mg maximum single dose and maximum daily dose (GSL, 1990).

U.S.: Dietary supplement (USC, 1994). The homeopathic mother tincture 1:10 (*w/v*), 55% (*v/v*), of fresh or dried black cohosh root, is a Class C OTC drug of the *Homeopathic Pharmacopoeia of the United States* (HPUS, 1990).

CLINICAL REVIEW

Ten clinical studies are outlined in the following table, "Clinical Studies on Black Cohosh," including a total of 1,371 participants. Nine of these studies demonstrated positive effects for menopausal symptoms. Numerous clinical trials with varied methods and designs have been conducted on the standardized isopropanolic/ethanolic extract of black cohosh root, Remifemin®, from 1981 to the present. Five of the studies were open-label, and evaluated the effectiveness of the extract as a monotherapy for the treatment of menopausal complaints (Pethö, 1987; Warnecke, 1985; Vorberg, 1984; Daiber, 1983; Stolze, 1982). Two studies, a randomized, double-blind (R, DB) study (Liske *et al.*, 1998), and a randomized study (Lehmann-Willenbrock and Reidel, 1988) compared black cohosh extract to conventional hormonal therapy in the treatment of complaints associated with menopause or hormonal deficiencies in ovariectomized/hysterectomized patients. One open-label, randomized, controlled study compared the efficacy of three different black cohosh therapies to conjugated estrogens and diazepam for menopausal problems (Warnecke, 1985). One R, DB study compared two dosages of Remifemin® for the treatment of menopausal symptoms (Liske *et al.*, 1998). A decrease in the Kupperman-Menopause Index (KPI) was reported in five clinical studies on black cohosh extract (Liske *et al.*, 1998; Lehmann-Willenbrock and Reidel, 1988; Stoll, 1987; Vorberg, 1984; Daiber, 1983).

BRANDED PRODUCTS

Remifemin®: GlaxoSmithKline / One Franklin Plaza / Philadelphia, PA 19102 / U.S.A. / Tel: (800) 366-8900. One tablet contains black cohosh extract corresponding to 20 mg of crude drug standardized to 1% 27-deoxyacteine.

Remifemin® drops: Schaper & Brümmer GmbH & Co. KG. / Bahnhofstrasse 35 / 38259 Salzgitter / Ringelheim / Germany / Tel: +49-5341-30-70 / Fax: +49-5341-30-71-24 / Email: info@schaperbruemmer.de / www.schaper-bruemmer.com/. Twenty drops correspond to 20 mg of crude drug. This product is no longer available.

REFERENCES

Anon. Black Cohosh. *Integrative Medicine Access*. Professional Reference to Conditions, Herbs and Supplements. Newton, MA: Integrative Medicine Communications; 2000.

Blumenthal M. Herb sales down 15% in mainstream market. *HerbalGram* 2001;51:69.

Blumenthal M, Busse WR, Goldberg A, Gruenwald J, Hall T, Riggins CW, Rister RS (eds.). Klein S, Rister RS (trans.). *The Complete German Commission E Monographs—Therapeutic Guide to Herbal Medicines*. Austin, TX: American Botanical Council; Boston: Integrative Medicine Communication; 1998.

Blumenthal M, Goldberg A, Brinckmann J. (eds.) *Herbal Medicine: Expanded Commission E Monographs*. Newton, MA: Integrative Medicine Communications; 2000:22–7.

Boblitz N, Liske E, Wüstenberg P. Black Cohosh–Efficacy, Effect and Safety of *Cimicifuga racemosa* in Gynecology. *Deutsche Apotheker Zeitung (DAZ)* 2000; 24:107–114.

Boon H, Smith M. *The Botanical Pharmacy: The Pharmacology of 47 Common Herbs*. Kingston, Ontario, Canada: Quarry Health Books; 1999:41–5.

Bradley P (ed.). *British Herbal Compendium* Vol. 1. Exeter, UK: British Herbal Medicine Association; 1992:34–6.

Bratman S, Kroll D. *The Healing Power of Herbs and Other Therapeutic Natural Products*. Rocklin, CA: Prima Publishing; 1999;1–5.

Brinker F. *Herb Contraindications and Drug Interactions*. 3rd ed. Sandy, OR: Eclectic Medical Publications. 2001:40-1.

Bruneton, J. *Pharmacognosy, Phytochemistry, Medicinal Plants*. Paris: Lavoisier Publishing; 1995.

Cott J. Personal Communication to M. Blumenthal. December 17, 2000.

Daiber W. Climacteric complaints: success without hormones – a phytotherapeutic agent lessens hot flushes, sweating and insomnia. [in German]. *Arztliche Praxis* 1983; 35(65):1946–7.

Dixon-Shanies D, Shaikh N. Growth inhibition of human breast cancer cells by herbs and phytoestrogens. *Oncol Rep* 1999;6:1383–7.

Düker E, Kopanski L, Jarry H, Wuttke W. Effects of extracts from *Cimicifuga racemosa* on gonadotropin release in menopausal women and ovariectomized rats. *Planta Med* 1991;57:420–4.

Einer-Jensen N, Zhao J, Andersen K, Kristoffersen K. *Cimicifuga* and *Melbrosia* lack oestrogenic effects in mice and rats. *Maturitas* 1996;25:149–53.

Farnsworth NR. Personal communication to M. Blumenthal. May 24, 1999.

Foster S. Black Cohosh: *Cimicifuga racemosa* – A Literature Review. *HerbalGram* 1999;45:35–50.

Freudenstein J, Bodinet C. Influence of an isopranolic aqueous extract of *Cimicifuga racemosa* rhizoma on the proliferation of MCF-7 cells. In abstracts of *23rd International LOF-Symposium on Phyto-estrogens*. University of Gent, Belgium; 15 January 1999.

Freudenstein J, Dasenbrock C, Nisslein T. Lack of promotion of estrogen dependent mammary tumors *in vivo* by an isopropanolic black cohosh extract. *Phytomedicine* 2000. 7(Supplement II 13), "3rd International Congress on Phytomedicine", Oct. 11–13, 2000, Munich, Germany.

GHP. See: *German Homeopathic Pharmacopoeia*.

GSL See: *General Sale List*.

General Sale List (GSL). Statutory Instrument 1990 No. 1129 The Medicines (Products Other Than Veterinary Drugs) Amendment Order 1990. London, U.K.: Her Majesty's Stationery Office (HMSO); 1990.

German Homeopathic Pharmacopoeia (GHP) 1st edition 1978 with 5 supplements through 1991. Translation of the German "*Homöopathisches Arzneibuch* (HAB 1) Amtliche Ausgabe." Stuttgart, Germany: Deutscher Apotheker Verlag; 1993;323–4.

HPB. See: Health Protection Branch.

HPUS. See: *Homeopathic Pharmacopoeia of the United States*.

Hagels H, Baumert-Krauss J, Freudenstein J. Composition of Phenolic Constituents in *Cimicifuga racemosa*. International Congress and 48th annual meeting of the Society of Medicinal Plant Research (GA), 6th International Congress on Ethnopharmacology of the International Society for Ethnopharmacology (ISE), Zürich, Switzerland, 2000.

Health Canada. *Drugs Directorate Guidelines: Traditional Herbal Medicines*. Ottawa, Ontario: Minister of National Health and Welfare; 1995b Oct.

Health Canada. Drugs Directorate Policy on Herbals Used as Non-medicinal Ingredients in Nonprescription Drugs in Human Use — Appendix II: List of Herbs Unacceptable as Non-medicinal Ingredients in Oral Use Products Subject to Part B. Ottawa, Ontario: Health Canada Drugs Directorate Bureau of Nonprescription Drugs; 1995a.

Health Canada. *Drug Product Database* (DPD) *Product Information*. Ottawa, Ontario: Health Canada Therapeutic Products Programme; 2001.

Health Protection Branch. *HPB Status Manual*. Ottawa, Ontario: Health Protection Branch. February 19, 1993;22.

Homeopathic Pharmacopoeia of the United States (HPUS) — Revision Service Official Compendium from July 1, 1992. Falls Church, VA: American Institute of Homeopathy. 1990 Dec;2175:CMCF.

Hunter A. *Cimicifuga racemosa*: pharmacology, clinical trials and clinical use. *Eur J Herbal Med* 1999; 5(1):19–25.

Jacobson JS, Traxel AB, Evans J, Klasus L, Vahdat L, Kinne D, *et al*. Randomized trial of black cohosh for the treatment of hot flashes among women with a history of breast cancer. *J Clin Oncol* 2001;19(10):2739-45.

Jarry H, Harnischfeger G, Düker E. Studies on the endocrine efficacy of the constituents of *Cimicifuga racemosa*: 2. *In vitro* binding of constituents to estrogen receptors. *Planta Med* 1985;51(4):316–9.

Jarry H, Harnischfeger G. Studies on the endocrine effects of the contents of *Cimicifuga racemosa*. Influence on the serum concentration of pituitary hormones in ovariectomized rats. *Planta Med* 1985;51(4):46–9.

Karnick C. *Pharmacopoeial Standards of Herbal Plants*. Delhi, India: Srit Satguru Publications; 1994; 1,2:61–2, 13.

Kennelly EF, Baggett S, Nuntanakorn P, Ososki AL, Mori SA, Duke J, et al. Analysis of thirteen populations of black cohosh for formononetin. *Phytomed* 2000;9(5):461–5.

Korn WD. Six–month oral toxicity study with Remifemin®-granulate in rats followed by an 8-week recovery period. Hannover: International Bioresearch. 1991.

Lehmann-Willenbrock E, Riedel H. Clinical and endocrinologic examinations concerning therapy of climacteric symptoms following hysterectomy with remaining ovaries. [in German]. *Zentralblatt Gynäkologie* 1988;110(10):611–8.

Lieberman S. A review of the effectiveness of *Cimicifuga racemosa* (black cohosh) for the symptoms of menopause. *J Womens Health* 1998 Jun;7(5):525–9.

Liske E. Therapeutic efficacy and safety of *Cimicifuga racemosa* for gynecological disorders. *Advances in Ther* 1998;15(1): 45–53.

Liske E, Hänggi W, Henneicke-von Zepelin HH, Boblitz N, Wüstenberg P, Rahlfs VW. Physiological investigation of a unique extract of black cohosh (*Cimicifugae racemosae rhizoma*): a 6-month clinical study demonstrates no systemic estrogenic effect. *J Womens Health Gend Based Med* 2002;11(2):163–74.

Liske E, Wüstenberg P. Therapy of climacteric complaints with *Cimicifuga racemosa*: a herbal medicine with clinically proven evidence. *Menopause* 1998;5(4):250.

Liske E, Wüstenberg P, Boblitz N. Human-pharmacological investigations during treatment of climacteric complaints with *Cimicifuga racemosa* (Remifemin®): No estrogen-like effects. *ESCOP. The European Phytojournal* 1998.

Lust J. *The Herb Book*. New York, NY: Bantam Books;1974;124–5.

MPA. See: Medical Products Agency.

McGuffin M, Hobbs C, Upton R, Goldberg A. *American Herbal Products Association's Botanical Safety Handbook: Guidelines for the Safe Use and Labeling for Herbs of Commerce*. Boca Raton, FL: CRC Press:1997;29-30.

McGuffin M, Kartesz J, Leung A, Tucker A (eds.). *American Herbal Products Association's Herbs of Commerce*, 2nd ed. Silver Spring (MD):American Herbal Products Association; 2000.

McKenna D (ed.). *Natural Dietary Supplements: A Desk Top Reference*. St. Croix, MN: Institute for Natural Products Research; 1998.

Medical Products Agency (MPA). *Naturläkemedelsmonografi: Remifemin®*. Uppsala, Sweden: Medical Products Agency. 1999.

Medical Products Agency (MPA). *Naturläkemedel: Authorised Natural Remedies* (as of January 24, 2001). Uppsala, Sweden: Medical Products Agency. 2001.

Morant J, Ruppanner H (eds.). Fachinformation und Patienteninformation: Zeller Cimifemin®; Omida Klimaktoplant®; Bioforce Menosan. In: *Arzneimittel-Kompendium der Schweiz®* 2001. Basel, Switzerland: Documed AG. 2001.

Murray M. *The Healing Power of Herbs*, 2nd ed. Rocklin, CA: Prima Publishing; 1992:376.

Nesselhut T, Liske E. Pharmacological measures in postmenopausal women with an isopropanolic aqueous extract of *Cimicifuga racemosa* rhizoma. *Menopause* 1999; 6(4):331.

Nesselhut T, Schellhase C, Dietrich R, Kuhn W. Assessment of the proliferative potency of phytopharmaceuticals with estrogen-like effect on breast cancer cells. [in German]. *Arch Gynecol Obstet* 1993;254:817–8.

Newall C, Anderson L, Phillipson J. *Herbal Medicines: A Guide for Health-Care Professionals*. London: The Pharmaceutical Press; 1996.

Nisslein T, Freudenstein J. Effects of black cohosh on urinary bone markers and femoral density in an OVX-rat model. Osteoporosis International 2000; 11 (Supplement 2); World Congress on Osteoporosis 2000, June 15–18, Chicago, USA.

Pethö A. Climacteric complaints are often helped with black cohosh. [in German]. *Arztliche Praxis* 1987;47:1551–3.

Pizzorno JE, Murray MT, editors. *Textbook of Natural Medicine*. Vol. 1, 2nd ed. New York: Churchill Livingston;1999. p. 657–61.

Schilcher H. Personal communication to Uwe Koetter. October 2000.

Schulz V, Hänsel R, Tyler V. *Rational Phytotherapy: A Physicians' Guide to Herbal Medicine*. 3rd ed. Berlin: Springer; 2000.

Shao Y, Harris A, Wang M *et al.* Triterpene glycosides from *Cimicifuga racemosa*. *J Nat Prod* 2000;63:905–910.

Stoll W. Phytopharmacon influences atrophic vaginal epithelium: double-blind study – *Cimicifuga* vs. estrogenic substances. [in German]. *Therapeutikon* 1987;1:23–31.

Stolze H. An alternative to treat menopausal complaints. *Gynecology* 1982;1:14–6.

Struck D, Tegtmeier M, Harnischfeger G. Flavones in extracts of *Cimicifuga racemosa*. *Planta Med* 1997;63(3):289.

United States Congress (USC). Public Law 103–417: Dietary Supplement Health and Education Act of 1994. Washington, DC: 103rd Congress of the United States; 1994.

USC. See: United States Congress.

Vorberg G. Therapy of climacteric complaints. *Z Allgemeinmed* 1984; 60:626–9.

Warnecke G. Influencing menopausal symptoms with a phytotherapeutic agent. Successful therapy with *Cimicifuga* mono-extract. *Med Welt* 1985;36(2):871–4.

WHO. See: World Health Organization.

World Health Organization. *Regulatory Status of Herbal Medicines: A Worldwide Review*. Geneva, Switzerland: World Health Organization Traditional Medicine Programme; 1998;8–9, 26–7.

Wren R. *Potter's New Cyclopaedia of Botanical Drugs and Preparations*, 8th ed. Essex, UK: CW Daniel Co. 1988;83.

Clinical Studies on Black Cohosh (*Actaea racemosa* L., syn. *Cimicifuga racemosa*)

Gynecology

Author/Year	Subject	Design	Duration	Dosage	Preparation	Results/Conclusion
Jacobson *et al.*, 2001	Menopausal symptoms: Hot flashes in women with history of breast cancer	R, DB, PC n=69 (randomized based on current tamoxifen use)	2 months	One, 20 mg tablet, 2 x daily with meals	Remifemin®	Although both treatment and placebo groups self-reported declines in number and intensity of hot flashes, black cohosh was not found to be statistically more harmful or beneficial than placebo in treating menopausal symptoms. Sweating was the only symptom that did show significantly greater improvement over placebo in the black cohosh group (p=0.4). Subset analysis showing effects on patients taking tamoxifen was not reported.
Liske *et al.*, 2002	Menopause complaints; comparison of standard safety and efficacy and high dose	R, DB, C, PG n=116 (women ages 42–60 with climacteric complaints)	6 months	40 mg/day (crude drug) vs. 127 mg/day (crude drug)	Remifemin®	Decrease in the Kupperman-Menopause Index (KPI) (values ~31 at the beginning) was observable after 2 weeks of Remifemin® therapy. Median scores dropped to 8 (standard dosage) and 7 (high dosage) after 12 weeks. Similar results in safety and efficacy were observed for both dosages. After 6 months, a positive response (KPI<15) was seen in ~90% of patients. No detectable changes were seen in hormone levels of LH, FSH, SHBG, prolactin, or estradiol. Remifemin® did not influence vaginal cytological parameters (degree of proliferation). The authors concluded that Remifemin may act as a selective estrogen receptor modulator ("Phyto-SERM").
Düker *et al.*, 1991	FSH and LH levels during menopause	PC n=110 female patients with menopausal-complaints who have received no hormonal therapy for at least 6 months (mean age=52)	2 months	8 mg/day extract vs. placebo	Remifemin® tablet vs. placebo	Remifemin® showed an estrogen-like mode of action with selective LH suppression in menopausal women. No significant change in FSH was observed. Mean LH levels significantly reduced compared to placebo (p<0.05).
Lehmann-Willenbrock and Riedel, 1988	Menopause complaints	R, Cm n=60 randomized into 4 treatment groups (Estriol, conjugated estrogen, estrogen gestation, black cohosh)	6 months	1 mg tablet/day Ovestin® or 1.25 mg tablet/day Presomen® or 1 tablet/day Trisequens® or 48–140 mg/day Remi-femin®	Ovestin®, Estriol alone; Presomen®, conjugated estrogens; Trisequens®, combined estrogen-gestagen theapy; Remifemin® tablet	Remifemin® extract was shown to produce a decline in modified KPI and improvement of complaints associated with postoperative ovarian function deficiencies. No significant differences were noted among treatment groups. No differences in LH or FSH levels were observed.
Pethö, 1987	Menopause complaints	O n=50 (female patients converting from hormone injections to black cohosh over 6 months)	6 months	48–140 mg/day	Remifemin® tablet	Hormone replacement therapy (Gynodian, injection) may be switched to black cohosh extract with equivalent success. Of the patients, 82% reported black cohosh preparation good or very good; 56% of patients did not require additional hormone injections. No side effects were noted. Significant improvement in mean menopausal index after 2 months (p<0.001).

KEY: C – controlled, **CC** – case-control, **CH** – cohort, **CI** – confidence interval, **Cm** – comparison, **CO** – crossover, **CS** – cross-sectional, **DB** – double-blind, **E** – epidemiological, **LC** – longitudinal cohort, **MA** – meta-analysis, **MC** – multi-center, **n** – number of patients, **O** – open, **OB** – observational, **OL** – open label, **OR** – odds ratio, **P** – prospective, **PB** – patient-blind, **PC** – placebo-controlled, **PG** – parallel group, **PS** – pilot study, **R** – randomized, **RC** – reference-controlled, **RCS** – retrospective cross-sectional, **RS** - retrospective, **S** – surveillance, **SB** – single-blind, **SC** – single-center, **U** – uncontrolled, **UP** – unpublished, **VC** – vehicle-controlled.

Gynecology (cont.)

Author/Year	Subject	Design	Duration	Dosage	Preparation	Results/Conclusion
Stoll, 1987	Menopause complaints	R, DB, PC, Cm n=80 female patients (ages 46 to 56)	12 weeks	48–140 mg/day or 0.625 mg CE/day plus 3 placebo tablets/day on days 1–21, then 2 place- bo tablets 2x/day on days 22–28 or 2 placebo tablets 2x/day	Remifemin® tablet or conjugated estrogens (CE) or placebo	Patients treated with Remifemin® showed significant increase in proliferation status of vaginal epithelium compared to those patients treated with estrogens or placebo (p<0.001) and significant improvements in somatic and psychological parameters (p<0.001) (meas- ured by KPI and Hamilton Anxiety (HAMA) scales). The number of hot flashes dropped from average of 4.9 daily to < 1 in black cohosh group; estrogen group, dropped from 5.2 to 3.2 average daily; and placebo dropped from 5.1 to 3.1 average daily occurrences. Improvements in vaginal lining were so significant, author suggests that black cohosh extract is suited as a remedy of first choice to treat menopausal symptoms, particularly if HRT is contraindicated or not desired by patient. Significant improvement of proliferation of vaginal epithelium with Remifemin®, compared to other groups (p<0.001).
Warnecke, 1985	Menopause complaints	O, C, Cm n=60 female patients with menopausal complaints (average age 54 years)	12 weeks	48–140 mg/day or 0.6 mg/day or 2 mg/day	Remifemin® drops or Conjugated estrogens or diazepam	Patients showed similar cytological responses (meas- ured by proliferation and maturation of vaginal epithelial cells) to Remifemin® and estrogens. Patients receiving diazepam had no observable cytological changes. Comparable improvements in neurovegetative and psy- chological symptoms (measured by Self-Assessment Depression scale, HAMA, and Clinical Global Impressions (CGI) scale) were seen in all 3 treatment groups.
Vorberg, 1984	Menopause complaints	O n=50 menopausal women (39 patients showed con- traindications to HRT, and 11 refused hormone treatment)	12 weeks	48–140 mg/day	Remifemin® drops	Improvements in psychological symptoms, KPI (p<0.001), Profile of Mood States (POMS) (p<0.001), and CGI (p<0.001) were all significant to highly signifi- cant in treatment group. No serious side effects were observed. Only mild gastrointestinal disturbances, which did not require discontinuation of treatment, were observed.
Daiber, 1983	Menopause complaints	O n=36 menopausal women; hor- mone replace- ment therapy was refused or contraindi- cated for these subjects (ages 45–62 years)	12 weeks	48–140 mg/day	Remifemin® drops	Highly significant decreases in KPI were observed, as was improvement in psychological symptoms including decreases in weariness and despondency, and increases in motivation and positive mood. A positive response in the CGI scale was also observed. No side effects or incompatibility reactions were observed during the 12 weeks of administration. Reduction of hot flashes (p<0.001), nervousness (p<0.001), depressive psychosis (p<0.01).
Stolze, 1982	Menopause complaints	O, MC n=704 female patients, 629 evaluated (mean age 51 years)	6 to 8 weeks	48–140 mg/day	Remifemin® drops	Significant improvements in neurovegetative complaints and psychological disturbances were experienced by 3 of 4 patients after 4 weeks of Remifemin® therapy. After 6 to 8 weeks, 40–50% of patients experienced complete relief from symptoms and another 30–40% of patients reported marked improvement in symptoms. The Remifemin® was well-tolerated, with no discontin- uation of therapy. Only 7% of patients reported mild, transitory nonspecific complaints. In 72% of cases, physicians observed advantages of Remifemin® over previous hormonal treatment. In 54.3% of the cases, physicians stated advantages of Remifemin® compared to previous treatment with psychoactive drugs. No sta- tistics provided.

KEY: C – controlled, **CC** – case-control, **CH** – cohort, **CI** – confidence interval, **Cm** – comparison, **CO** – crossover, **CS** – cross-sectional, **DB** – double-blind, **E** – epidemiological, **LC** – longitudinal cohort, **MA** – meta-analysis, **MC** – multi-center, **n** – number of patients, **O** – open, **OB** – observational, **OL** – open label, **OR** – odds ratio, **P** – prospective, **PB** – patient-blind, **PC** – placebo-controlled, **PG** – parallel group, **PS** – pilot study, **R** – randomized, **RC** – reference-controlled, **RCS** – retrospective cross-sectional, **RS** - retrospective, **S** – surveillance, **SB** – single-blind, **SC** – single-center, **U** – uncontrolled, **UP** – unpublished, **VC** – vehicle-controlled.

Cat's Claw

Uncaria tomentosa (Willd.) DC.; *Uncaria guianensis* (Aubl.) Gmel.

[Fam. *Rubiaceae*]

OVERVIEW

Cat's claw (*uña de gato* in Spanish) is the common name for at least 20 plants (from 12 families) with sharp, curved thorns. Among them are the two climbing, woody vine discussed in this clinical overview: *Uncaria tomentosa* and *U. guianensis,* both native to the South and Central American tropical rain forests. [EDITORS' NOTE: In this clinical overview, *U. tomentosa* will be abbreviated as "UT" and *U. guianensis* as "UG".] Both UT and UG are said to have a long history of use by indigenous people to treat health problems including rheumatism, arthritis, and other chronic inflammatory disorders, gastric ulcers and gastrointestinal disorders, tumors, and as a contraceptive.

UT plants occur naturally as two chemotypes that appear botanically identical, but are chemically different. One chemotype contains predominantly pentacyclic oxindole alkaloids (POAs) with little or no tetracyclic oxindole alkaloids (TOAs), and the other contains TOAs with either no POAs or up to a considerable amount of POAs. TOAs are reported to act antagonistically to some POA activity. While early studies focused on POAs as the primary active components, more recent studies report that activity is well spread over a range of polar constituents.

Cat's claw has gained recent popularity in the U.S. herb market, but not yet in mainstream retail markets, being sold primarily in health food stores, mail order, and ethnic markets. The cat's claw market is defined by the following five types of products offered mainly by three manufacturers: (1) an aqueous-acid or hydroalcoholic extract of UT root standardized to POAs with no TOAs [herein referred to as UT-POA], (2) an aqueous UT extract standardized to carboxy alkyl esters (CAEs) [herein referred to as UT-CAE], (3) and an aqueous UG extract [herein referred to as UG]. Two additional types of cat's claw products are relatively generic and usually labeled as UT: extracts not standardized to any particular constituent [herein referred to as UT-unspecified] and raw root bark products powdered in capsules or tablets, or finely cut for teas (decoction, the traditional form of use). Little scientific research has been performed on this fifth class of crude products. Because there are numerous plants in Central and South America commonly referred to "uña de gato," there have been reports of inappropriately labeled products in ethnic markets. [Editor's NOTE: Because the information on each species and preparation type may be specific to that particular species or preparation type, the actions and uses of 1 may not apply to another.]

PRIMARY USES

Anti-Inflammatory

- Osteoarthritis (of the knee); reduces pain (UG)
- Rheumatoid arthritis, adjunct therapy to conventional treatment: reduces number of painful and swollen joints (UT-POA)

OTHER POTENTIAL USES

- UT-CAE: enhanced DNA repair; extends immunity from pheumonia vaccine
- UT-POA: ulcers and gastritis; in cancer patients as an adjunctive to chemotherapy and radiation increases vitality and reduces side effects; in HIV patients as an adjunctive to antiretroviral therapy stablizes and/or reduces CD4-cell count, increases vitality and mobility, and reduces HIV-related symptoms; externally, active against *Herpes simplex* and *Varicella-zoster*
- UT-UNSPECIFIED: decreased mutagenicity of one smoker's urine

PHARMACOLOGICAL ACTIONS

UG: Anti-inflammatory. In *in vitro* studies: antioxidant.

UT-UNSPECIFIED: Antimutagenic. In animal studies: anti-inflammatory. In *in vitro* studies: antioxidant.

UT-CAE: Immunomodulation/immune support; antimutagenic.

UT-POA: Anti-inflammatory; immunomodulation/immune support.

DOSAGE AND ADMINISTRATION

At this time, there is little scientific information on how long cat's claw can be consumed safely. Published clinical trials have been conducted from 4 weeks to 1 year of continuous internal use, while unpublished treatment observations report continuous (uncontrolled) use for up to 10 years. There are no known reports of adverse effects associated with use of cat's claw preparations for extended periods.

Crude Preparations

UG

- CAPSULES: aqueous extract of bark powder, freeze-dried: 100 mg 1–3x/day.

UT-unspecified

- CAPSULES: 350–500 mg, 1–2x/day.
- DECOCTION: 1 g root bark boiled for 15 min. in 250 ml water, 1–3x/day.
- TINCTURE: 1–2 ml, 2–3x/day.

Standardized Preparations
UT-CAE
- TABLETS: 350 mg/day.

UT-POA
- CAPSULES: One, 3x/day for the 1st 10 days, and 1/day thereafter.

CONTRAINDICATIONS
None reported for UG, UT-unspecified, and UT-CAE.

UT-POA: Based on the belief that cat's claw is an immunostimulant, the herb has been contraindicated for leukemia patients awaiting bone marrow or organ transplant and persons with iatrically-induced immunosuppression (e.g., organ transplants), autoimmune disease, multiple sclerosis, or tuberculosis. However, some researchers disagree with this view and suggest that cat's claw may be helpful for transplant patients. Elevated production of TNFα is characteristic of numerous autoimmune disorders, including those in which cat's claw offers benefits (arthritis, gut inflammation); and lowering TNFα levels, as has been documented with cat's claw, may be desirable rather than contraindicated for these patients. HIV/AIDS patients should proceed with caution when introducing any new therapeutic agent. Cat's claw is not for use in children under 3 years due to lack of data regarding its effects on the immature immune system.

PREGNANCY AND LACTATION: Not recommended due to lack of data regarding the effects of cat's claw during pregnancy and on the immature immune system.

ADVERSE EFFECTS
Recent human trials conclude that various cat's claw preparations tested are safe, with no adverse effects reported in hepatic, renal, central nervous system, or hematological functions. Cat's claw teas or crude extracts may cause mild nausea, due to bitter taste; however, this appears speculative as nausea is not a frequently reported effect.

UG: One study reports infrequent headache, dizziness, and vomiting, but the incidence and frequency were the same as with placebo.

UT-CAE: None reported.

UT-POA: In AIDS patients and patients receiving large doses of chemotherapy, individual cases of a mild erythrocytosis have been reported. During the first 1–2 weeks of cat's claw tea use, temporary constipation or mild diarrhea was sometimes observed. Increased occurrence of acne symptoms has been reported in HIV patients with prior symptoms. In rare cases, elevated uric acid values were observed in HIV and cancer patients; extensive cell die-off in tumor patients may cause lytic fever lasting 1–2 weeks.

DRUG INTERACTIONS
UG: None reported.

UT-UNSPECIFIED: May potentially reduce the metabolism rate, increasing serum levels of drugs taken orally as observed in an *in vitro* assay where the CYP3A4 isozyme production was inhibited.

UT-CAE: None reported.

UT-POA: According to a communication to physicians and pharmacists from the leading Austrian research and manufacturing company on cat's claw, the following advice should be given to patients, based on the product's proposed immunomodulatory effects:

Take between chemotherapy treatments and after completion, but not with chemotherapy treatments; Do not take in conjunction with passive animal vaccines, intravenous hyperimmunoglobulin therapy; intravenous thymic extracts, drugs using animal protein or peptide hormones (e.g., bovine or porcine insulin), cryoprecipitates, or fresh blood plasma.

CLINICAL REVIEW
Fourteen clinical trials on various cat's claw preparations are summarized in the monograph. In general, the studies are small, most are uncontrolled (U), and some unpublished (UP). One prospective, randomized, double-blind, placebo-controlled, parallel group, multi-center (P, R, DB, PC, PG, MC) trial was conducted on UG for osteoarthritis of the knee. The study reports a significant improvement in pain associated with activity and in medical and patient assessment scores, but no significant improvement in knee circumference or pain at rest or at night. There were no significant adverse side effects in UG and placebo groups.

The UT-CAE preparation was tested in 3 trials. One small R, PC trial resulted in no loss of immunity after 5 months in patients given a pneumonia vaccine after 2 months of treatment with the UT-CAE extract compared to loss with placebo. Another small trial reported an increase in DNA repair with no adverse effects. One U trial on healthy volunteers resulted in an increase in white blood cells.

UT-POA extract was tested for anti-inflammatory effects in 3 trials. One 52-week trial tested cat's claw for rheumatoid arthritis (RA). The first phase was R, DB, PC; in the second phase all patients received the treatment. There was a significant decrease in pain and a shorter period of morning stiffness for the treatment group compared to placebo after the first phase and a further reduction after the second phase. The placebo-cat's claw treatment group experienced some reduction of symptoms in the second phase. Two small uncontrolled, unpublished trials tested the UT-POA extract on patients with RA, and on ulcers and gastritis.

The UT-POA extract was tested for immune function effects in 5 trials. All 5 trials are U, UP, thereby raising questions as to the significance of the results. Two trials tested the UT-POAs extract as an adjuvant therapy for cancer patients undergoing chemotherapy, radiation, and/or surgery with generally favorable results, 3 trials testing UT-POA extract as an adjuvant therapy for HIV-positive patients reported stabilized or increased CD-4 cell counts, increased vitality and no adverse effects.

Two U, UP trials using the UT-POA extract in topical preparations for *Herpes simplex* and *Varicella zoster* lesions, showed improvement and no adverse effects.

Cat's Claw

Uncaria tomentosa (Willd.) DC.; *Uncaria guianensis* (Aubl.) Gmel.
[Fam. *Rubiaceae*]

OVERVIEW

Cat's claw (*uña de gato* in Spanish), refers to at least 20 plants with sharp, curved thorns, two of which are discussed in this sheet: *Uncaria tomentosa* (UT) and *U. guianensis* (UG), both native to the South and Central American tropical rain forests. UT and UG have a long history of use by indigenous people of these areas to treat health problems including rheumatism, arthritis, other chronic inflammatory disorders, gastric ulcers, gastrointestinal disorders, tumors, and as a contraceptive.

There are five types of products offered mainly by three manufacturers: (1) an aqueous-acid or hydroalcoholic extract of UT root standardized to pentacyclic onxindole acids (POAs) with no tetracyclic oxindole acids (TOAs) [herein referred to as UT-POA]; (2) an aqueous UT extract standardized to carboxy alkyl esters (CAEs) [UT-CAEs]; (3) and an aqueous UG extract [UG]. Two additional types of cat's claw products are relatively generic and usually labeled as UT: extracts not standardized to any particular constituent [UT-unspecified] and raw root bark products powdered in capsules or tablets, or finely cut for teas (the traditional form of use). [EDITORS' NOTE: Because each cat's claw species and preparation-type has a different chemical profile, the biological actions and uses for one may not apply to another.]

PRIMARY USES

Osteoarthritis (of the knee); rheumatoid arthritis along with conventional treatment. Other potential uses: anti-inflammatory; immune system modulator.

DOSAGE

Crude Preparations

UG CAPSULES: 100 mg 1–3x/day.

UT-unspecified:

CAPSULES: 350–500 mg, 1–2x/day.

TEA: 1 g root bark boiled for 15 min. in 250 ml water, 1–3x/day.

TINCTURE: 1–2 ml, 2–3x/day.

Standardized Preparations

UT-CAE TABLETS: 350 mg/day.

UT-POA CAPSULES: One capsule 3x/day for the 1st 10 days, and one capsule/day thereafter.

CONTRAINDICATIONS

None reported for UG, UT-unspecified, and UT-CAE.

UT-POA: Based on the belief that cat's claw is an immunostimulant, it is not advised for patients awaiting bone marrow or organ transplant, persons with medically-induced immunosuppression (e.g., patients with organ transplants), autoimmune disease, multiple sclerosis, or tuberculosis. HIV/AIDS patients should proceed with caution when introducing any new therapeutic agent. Cat's claw is not for use in children under 3 years.

PREGNANCY AND LACTATION: Not recommended due to lack of data.

ADVERSE EFFECTS

Recent human trials conclude that various cat's claw preparations are safe, with no adverse effects reported in liver, kidney, central nervous system, cardiovascular or blood functions. Cat's claw teas or crude extracts may cause mild nausea, due to bitter taste; however, this appears speculative as nausea is not frequently reported.

UT-POA: In AIDS patients and patients receiving large doses of chemotherapy, individual mild cases of red blood cell elevation were reported. During the first 1–2 weeks of cat's claw tea use constipation or mild diarrhea was sometimes observed. Increased occurrence of acne symptoms was reported in HIV patients with prior acne symptoms. In rare cases, elevated uric acid values were observed in HIV and cancer patients; extensive cell die-off in cancer patients may cause a fever lasting 1–2 weeks.

DRUG INTERACTIONS

None reported for UG, UT-unspecified, and UT-CAE.

UT-POA: The leading Austrian cat's claw manufacturer advises: Take between and after chemotherapy treatment, but not during; do not take with passive animal vaccines, intravenous hyperimmunoglobulin therapy; intravenous thymic extracts, drugs using animal protein or peptide hormones (e.g., bovine or porcine insulin), or precipitate from frozen or fresh blood plasma.

Comments

When using a dietary supplement, purchase it from a reliable source. For best results, use the same brand of product throughout the period of use. As with all medications and dietary supplements, please inform your healthcare provider of all herbs and medications you are taking. Interactions may occur between medications and herbs or even among different herbs when taken at the same time. Treat your herbal supplement with care by taking it as directed, storing it as advised on the label, and keeping it out of the reach of children and pets. Consult your healthcare provider with any questions.

AMERICAN BOTANICAL COUNCIL

The information contained on this sheet has been excerpted from *The ABC Clinical Guide to Herbs* © 2003 by the American Botanical Council (ABC). ABC is an independent member-based educational organization focusing on the medicinal use of herbs. For more detailed information about this herb please consult the healthcare provider who gave you this sheet. To order *The ABC Clinical Guide to Herbs* or become a member of ABC, visit their website at www.herbalgram.org.

Cat's Claw

Uncaria tomentosa (Willd.) DC.; *Uncaria guianensis* (Aubl.) Gmel.

[Fam. *Rubiaceae*]

OVERVIEW

Cat's claw, also known by its Spanish name, *uña de gato*, is an herb that has gained recent popularity in the U.S. herb market. *Uña de gato* is the common name for at least 20 plants (from 12 different families) with sharp, curved thorns (Obregon, 1995; Cabieses, 1994). Among them are two climbing, woody vines: *Uncaria tomentosa* and *U. guianensis*, the two species of *Uncaria* (there are approximately 60 species) (Obregon, 1995; Cabieses, 1994) native to the South and Central American tropical rain forests that are the subject of this monograph. According to U.S. herb industry policy, the standardized common name "cat's claw" refers to only *U. tomentosa* (McGuffin *et al.*, 2000), presumably because products containing *U. guianensis* were not generally available in the U.S. market during most of the 1990s, having been introduced in the past several years. [EDITORS' NOTE: For the purposes of this monograph, *U. tomentosa* will be abbreviated as "UT" and *U. guianensis* will be abbreviated as "UG." Because the information on each species and preparation type may be specific to that particular species or preparation type, it may have been preferable to write two or three separate monographs instead of one. However, the editors chose to include all the relevant information on "cat's claw" in this single monograph, with subheadings designating species and preparation type, where applicable. In doing so, the editors acknowledge that actions and uses based on one species or preparation type may not be transferable to another.]

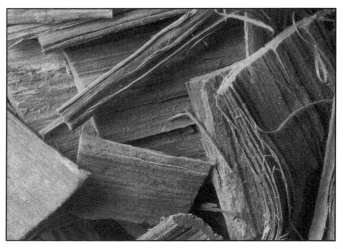

Photo © 2003 stevenfoster.com

Both UT and UG are said to have a long history of use by indigenous people to treat a diverse set of health problems, particularly rheumatism, arthritis, and other chronic inflammatory disorders, gastric ulcers and gastrointestinal disorders, tumors, and as a contraceptive (Cabieses, 1994; Jones, 1995; Obregon, 1995; Anon.,1996; Miller, 2001a). Although no written records are available describing their traditional use (Cabieses, 1994), a study of the medicinal system of the Ashaninca (also spelled Asháninka) tribe in Peru has been published. To the priests of this tribe, cat's claw (UT) is a sacred plant used to eliminate disturbance in the communication between body and spirit (Keplinger *et al.*, 1999). One account of the Asháninka Indians states that the priests differentiate between the two UT chemotypes and use only the pentacyclic oxindole alkaloid (POA) chemotype (Keplinger *et al.*, 1999), but how the priests can distinguish between chemotypes without the scientific tools of chemical analysis is not described. Despite some recent interest in this herb's potential immunomodulating activity, ethnomedical evidence of such use is lacking.

Several types of cat's claw preparations have grown in popularity in the U.S. with the market defined by the following five types of products offered mainly by three manufacturers, each with their own distinct focus: (1) an aqueous-acid or hydroalcoholic extract of UT root standardized to pentacyclic oxindole alkaloids (POAs) with no tetracyclic oxindole alkaloids (TOAs) [herein referred to as UT-POA], (2) an aqueous UT extract standardized to carboxy alkyl esters (CAEs) [herein referred to as UT-CAE], (3) and an aqueous UG extract [herein referred to as UG]. Two additional types of cat's claw products are relatively generic and usually labeled as UT: extracts not standardized to any particular constituent [herein referred to as UT-unspecified] and raw root bark products powdered in capsules or tablets, or finely cut for teas (decoctions, the traditional form of use). Little scientific research has been performed on this fifth class of crude products. Occasionally, products labeled as "cat's claw" in ethnic markets have been shown to be mislabeled due to the vast number of plants known by the common name cat's claw, and the lack of adequate quality control with some small importers and distributors.

Fourteen clinical trials on various preparations are summarized herein. One controlled clinical trial with UG suggests efficacy in the treatment of osteoarthritis of the knee (Piscoya *et al.*, 2001). While cat's claw's popularity is partly due to European reports of its clinical effectiveness in combination with AZT (zidovudine) for AIDS treatment, these findings lack confirmation by well-controlled clinical studies. Other current studies report on cat's claw's anti-inflammatory and antioxidant properties, and its ability to affect gene expression and thereby modulate the immune system.

Cat's claw is not yet popular in mainstream retail markets, being sold primarily in health food stores where it ranked 25th in total herb sales in 2000 (Richman and Witkowski, 2001), mail order, and in the ethnic Hispanic market.

DESCRIPTION

Cat's claw preparations are made from extracts of the dried stalk, stalk bark (commonly called "root" bark), or actual root of *U. tomentosa* (Willd.) DC. or *U. guianensis* (Aubl.) Gmel. [Fam. *Rubiaceae*]. Products standardized to POAs will often use the root rather than the root (stalk) bark, as it contains a higher concentration of POAs. However, this practice destroys the plant, whereas use of the stalk or root bark allows the vine to regenerate. Given that a considerable portion of cat's claw is still wild harvested, from an environmental/sustainability perspective it may be more prudent long-term to utilize the stalk and root bark rather than the actual root, or cultivate the plants if the actual root is desired. *Uncaria tomentosa* and *U. guianensis* are distinguished by flower color, thorn shape, and leaf characteristics (Jones, 1995; Cabrieses, 1994). In addition, *U. guianensis* contains lower levels of alkaloids (35 times less) and flavanols than *U. tomentosa* (Sandoval *et al.*, 2002, 2000; Miller *et al.*, 2001). The *U. tomentosa* plants occur naturally as two chemotypes that appear botanically identical, but are chemically different in their alkaloid content (Laus *et al.*, 1997). One chemotype contains predominantly POAs with little or no TOAs, and the other contains TOAs with either no POAs or up to a considerable amount. TOAs are reported to act antagonistically to some POA activity (Wurm *et al.*, 1998). While early studies focused on POAs as the active components, more recent studies report that activity is well spread over a range of polar materials. Several commercial preparations of *U. tomentosa* are available: aqueous-acid and hydroalcoholic extracts standardized to POAs (containing no TOAs); a nonstandardized mixture of both chemotypes; and an aqueous extract, ultrafiltrated, containing a negligible level of oxindole alkaloids, and standardized to CAEs. One *U. guianensis* preparation is composed of a freeze-dried aqueous extract. No monographs on any cat's claw preparation have been published to date in any official pharmacopeias.

PRIMARY USES
Anti-inflammatory
- **Osteoarthritis (of the knee)**
  UG: reduces pain (Piscoya *et al.*, 2001)

- **Rheumatoid arthritis–adjunct therapy to conventional treatment**
  UT-POA: reduces number of painful and swollen joints (Mur *et al.*, 2002; Immodal, 1995, 2002)

OTHER POTENTIAL USES
[EDITORS' NOTE: the following potential uses are based on clinical trials unless otherwise noted.]

- **Anti-inflammatory/Gastrointestinal**
  UG: protects gastric epithelial cells against NSAID-induced gastritis and apoptosis in *in vitro* tests (Sandoval *et al.*, 2002)

  UT-UNSPECIFIED: protects gastric epithelial cells against NSAID-induced gastritis and apoptosis in animal and *in vitro* tests (Sandoval *et al.*, 2002; Sandoval-Chacón *et al.*, 1998)

  UT-POA: ulcers and gastritis (Immodal 1995, 1999a)

- **Antioxidant**
  UG: effectively scavenges DPPH (α, α-diphenyl-β-picryl-hydrazyl), protects against deoxyribose degradation, and inhibits ABTS (2,2'-azinobis [3-ethyl-benzthiazoline-6-sulfonic acid]) radicals in *in vitro* tests (Sandoval *et al.*, 2002); limits gastric epithelial cell death in response to oxidative stress *in vitro* (Miller *et al.*, 2001)

  UT-UNSPECIFIED: effectively scavenges DPPH, protects against deoxyribose degradation, and inhibits ABTS radicals in *in vitro* tests (Sandoval *et al.*, 2002); cytoprotective

against oxidative stress *in vitro* (Sandoval-Chacón *et al.*, 1998)

- **Cancer–adjunctive to chemotherapy & radiation**
  UT-POA: increases vitality and reduces side effects (Immodal, 1995, 1999a, 2002)

- **DNA-Repair/Antimutagenic**
  UT-UNSPECIFIED: decreased mutagenicity of one smoker's urine (Rizzi *et al.*, 1993)

  UT-CAE: enhanced DNA repair (Sheng *et al.*, 2001)

- **External Use**
  UT-POA: *Herpes simplex* and *Varicella-zoster* (Immodal 1995, 1999a, 2002)

- **HIV–adjunctive to antiretroviral therapy**
  UT-POA: stabilizes and/or reduces CD4-cell count, increases vitality and mobility, reduced HIV-related symptoms (Immodal, 1995, 1999a, 2002)

- **Immune system support**
  UT-CAE: extends immunity from pneumonia vaccine (Lamm *et al.*, 2001); increases white blood cells (Sheng *et al.*, 2001, 2000a) in animal study (Sheng *et al*, 2000b)

- **Protection against UV radiation**
  UT-UNSPECIFIED: cytoprotective against UV radiation *in vitro* (Sandoval *et al.*, 2000; Rizzi *et al.*, 1993)

DOSAGES
Crude Preparations
[EDITOR'S NOTE: There is little scientific or clinical documentation supporting the use of crude cat's claw products. Most clinical research has been conducted on special standardized preparations of various types.]

- ***Uncaria guianensis***
  CAPSULES: aqueous extract of bark powder, freeze-dried: 100 mg 1–3 times daily (Piscoya *et al.*, 2001; Miller, 2001a).

- ***Uncaria tomentosa*–chemotype and active component unspecified**
  CAPSULES: 350–500 mg, 1–2 times daily (CAMR, 1999).

  DECOCTION: 1 g root bark boiled for 15 minutes in 250 ml water, 1–3 times daily (Access, 2000; CAMR, 1999).

  TINCTURE: 1–2 ml, 2–3 times daily (CAMR, 1999).

Standardized Preparations
- ***Uncaria tomentosa*–standardized to CAEs**
  TABLETS: 350 mg daily (Lamm *et al.*, 2001; Sheng *et al.*, 2001, 2000a).

- ***Uncaria tomentosa*–standardized to POAs**
  CAPSULES: 20 mg (0.26 mg POAs), 3 times daily for the first 10 days, and one capsule daily thereafter (Enzymatic Therapy, 2002).

  CAPSULES: 1–3 capsules/day (in acute cases, triple dose for 1st wk) (Immodal, 1995).

  DROPS (d): Adults: 3x20 d/day; 3–6 yrs: 3x7 d/day; 7–9 yrs: 3x10 d/day; 10–12 yrs: 3x15 d/day; 12+ yrs: 3x20 d/day (Immodal, 1995).

  TEA: 20 g ground root bark in 1 L water, boiled 45 min, cooled 10 min, filtered water added to make 1 L. Adults: 60 ml decoction in 60 ml hot water before breakfast; Children: decoction in hot water before breakfast according to the following amounts: 3–6 yrs: 20 ml in 20 ml;

7–9 yrs: 30 ml in 30 ml; 10–12 yrs: 50 ml in 50 ml; 12+ yrs: same as adult (Immodal, 1995).

OINTMENT: applied externally several times daily (Immodal, 1995).

SPRAY: applied externally several times daily (Immodal, 1995).

DURATION OF ADMINISTRATION

At this time, there is little scientific information other than ethnobotanical observations and 14 clinical trials (including case reports and treatment observations) on how long cat's claw can be consumed. Published clinical trials have been conducted from as short as 4 weeks to 1 year of continuous internal use, while unpublished treatment observations using Krallendorn® (Immodal Pharmaka GmbH) products report on continuous (uncontrolled) use for up to 10 years. There are no known reports of adverse effects associated with the use of cat's claw preparations for extended periods.

CHEMISTRY

Although chemical research on cat's claw began with UG in 1952 (Cabieses, 1994), most of the chemical research since then has focussed on UT and its alkaloids, particularly the oxindole alkaloids. However, these alkaloids are a small component of cat's claw (approximately 0.9% in UT and 0.03% in UG [Sandoval et al., 2002]), which is rich in flavonoids, quinovic glycosides, polyhydroxylated triterpenes, and tannins. While earlier studies reported alkaloids as the active components of cat's claw (Aguilar et al., 2000; Laus et al., 1998; Stuppner et al., 1993; Kreutzkamp, 1984; Wagner et al., 1985a, 1985b), more recent studies report that bioactivity is spread over a wide range of components (Aguilar et al., 2002; Sandoval et al., 2002; Kitajima et al., 2000; Lee et al., 1999; Sheng et al., 1998; Wirth and Wagner, 1997; Aquino et al., 1991, 1989; Cerri et al., 1988), and one study suggests that the anti-inflammatory and antioxidant activities of cat's claw are not affected by the presence or relative level of alkaloids (Sandoval et al., 2002).

Uncaria guianensis

The little chemical research performed on UG has been limited to its alkaloid, quinovic acid glycoside, and flavanol content. UG contains very low levels of alkaloids—35 times less than UT (Sandoval et al., 2002; Miller et al., 2001)—including speciophylline, mitraphylline, isomitraphylline, uncarine E, and uncarine C (Sandoval et al., 2002; Miller et al., 2001; Lee et al., 1999). UG also contains quinovic acid glycosides (Yépez et al., 1991), flavanols (catechin, epigallocatechin, epicatechin, and epigallocatechin) (Sandoval et al., 2002; Miller et al., 2001), and polyphenols (Miller et al., 2001). UG has lower concentrations of the flavanols (except for epigallocatechin) than does UT (Sandoval et al., 2002).

Uncaria tomentosa

UT has two chemotypes: the pentacyclic alkaloid type and tetracyclic alkaloid type. The first contains POAs, which some consider to be the main active component of cat's claw (Immodal 1995, 1999a, 1999b), with little or no TOAs. The second chemotype contains predominantly TOAs with either no POAs or up to a considerable amount of POAs (Laus et al., 1997). TOAs are considered antagonistic to the purported beneficial effects of the POAs (Wurm et al., 1998) and thus, the significance in distinguishing between the two chemotypes. As in any determination of the source of bioactivity in an unknown natural product any proposed active constituent must mimic the actions of the extract from which it was derived, and exert these actions at a concentration that reflects its relative amount within that botanical or botanical extract. Studies demonstrating that purified POAs or TOAs share the same bioactivity of cat's claw preparations but enhanced for the relative concentrations in these extracts are lacking. Therefore, these chemical constituents may be more useful as marker compounds rather than mediating the bioactivity of the botanical.

POAs in UT include pteropodine (uncarine C), isopteropodine (uncarine E), speciophylline (uncarine D), uncarine F, mitraphylline, and isomitraphylline (Muhammad et al., 2001a; Laus et al., 1997; Stuppner et al., 1992; Wagner et al., 1985b). The TOAs present in UT include rhynchophylline, isorhynchophylline, corynoxeine, isocorynoxeine (Keplinger et al., 1999; Laus et al., 1997; Wagner et al., 1985b). Other alkaloids in UT include pentacyclic indol alkaloids (akuammigine, tetrahydroalstonine, isoajmalicin) (Laus et al., 1997), tetracyclic indol alkaloids (hirsutine, dihydrocorynantheine, hirsuteine, corynantheine) (Keplinger et al., 1999; Laus et al., 1997), and precursor alkaloids (5α-carboxystrictosidine, lyaloside) (Aquino et al., 1991).

In addition to alkaloids, UT contains triterpenes (ursolic acid derivatives, quinovic acid glycosides, oleanolic acid derivatives) (Laus et al., 1997; Aquino et al., 1991, 1990, 1989; Cerri et al. 1988), polyhydroxylated triterpenes (Aquino et al., 1991, 1990, 1989; Cerri et al. 1988), procyanidins ([-]-epicatechin, cinchonain 1a, cinchonain 1b) (Wirth and Wagner, 1997), sterols (β-sitosterol, stigmasterol, campesterol) (Senatore et al., 1989), flavanols (catechin, epigallocatechin, epicatechin and epigallocatechin) (Sandoval et al., 2002), tannins (Wagner et al., 1985b) and CAEs (Sheng et al., 2001).

PHARMACOLOGICAL ACTIONS
Human
- **Uncaria guianensis**
  ANTI-INFLAMMATORY: significantly reduced pain associated with activity in patients with osteoarthritis of the knee (Piscoya et al., 2001).

- **Uncaria tomentosa–unspecified preparations**
  ANTIMUTAGENIC: ingestion for 15 days decreased mutagenicity of one smoker's urine (Rizzi et al., 1993).

- **Uncaria tomentosa–standardized to CAEs**
  IMMUNOMODULATION/IMMUNE SUPPORT: enhanced response to pneumococcal vaccine by reducing decay of antibody titers and elevating lymphocyte/neutrophil (Lamm et al., 2001); decreased DNA damage (measured as single strand breaks in DNA) from single dose of hydrogen peroxide and increased DNA repair (Sheng et al., 2001); increased white blood cell levels in healthy males (Sheng et al., 2000a).

  ANTIMUTAGENIC: decreased DNA damage (measured as single strand breaks in DNA) from single dose of hydrogen peroxide and increased DNA repair (Sheng et al., 2001); enhances DNA repair (Sheng et al., 2000a).

- **Uncaria tomentosa–POA chemotype**
  ANTI-INFLAMMATORY: reduced number of painful and tender joints and decreased duration of morning stiffness in rheumatoid arthritis patients (Mur et al., 2002; Immodal, 1995, 2002); eliminated symptoms and need for antacids in ulcer and gastritis patients (Immodal 1995, 1999a).

IMMUNOMODULATION/IMMUNE SUPPORT: increased vitality and reduced side effects in cancer patients undergoing chemotherapy, radiation, or surgery (Immodal 1995, 1999a, 2002); reduced HIV-related symptoms and increased vitality of HIV patients receiving antiretroviral treatment, increased lymphocyte numbers in HIV patients although total leukocyte numbers remained unchanged, stabilized or increased CD4 cell count in HIV patients (Immodal 1995, 1999a, 2002).

Animal

- *Uncaria tomentosa*–**unspecified preparations**

    ANTI-INFLAMMATORY: significantly reduced paw volume in carrageen-induced rat paw edema (Aguilar *et al.*, 2002, 2000; Aquino *et al.*, 1991); protected against NSAID-induced gastritis by reducing lesions and apoptosis of the mucosal epithelial cells (Sandoval *et al.*, 2002); prevention of NSAID-induced enteropathy in rats (Sandoval-Chacón *et al.*, 1998).

- *Uncaria tomentosa*–**standardized to CAEs**

    IMMUNOMODULATION/IMMUNE SUPPORT: increased DNA repair of single and double strand breaks from whole body irradiation in rats (Sheng *et al.*, 2000a); increased white blood cell count sooner, and all fractions proportionally, compared with control in rat model of chemotherapy-induced leukopenia (Sheng *et al*, 2000b); prolonged leukocyte survival in rats at daily doses of 125–500 mg/kg body weight (Åkesson *et al.*, 2003).

- *Uncaria tomentosa*–**POA chemotype**

    ANTI-INFLAMMATORY: significantly reduced paw volume in carrageen-induced rat paw edema (Aguilar *et al.*, 2002, 2000).

- **Isolated components of *Uncaria* species**

    [EDITORS' NOTE: The studies referenced in this subsection were performed with compounds isolated from *U. rhynchophylla* or *U. sinensis*. While these compounds are also found in *U. guianensis* and/or *U. tomentosa*, no studies have been performed on extracts or fractions derived from UG or UT to verify that these actions apply to them as well; thus their clinical significance is undetermined. These studies have been included because some proponents of the UT products standardized to POAs and no TOAs, cite them in support of the need for removal of TOAs from cat's claw products.]

    Isorhynchophylline reduced blood pressure and heart rate in rats and dogs (Shi *et al.*, 1989); rhynchophylline and isorhynchophylline reduced blood pressure and heart rate in dogs, with isorhychophylline demonostrating a stronger effect (Shi *et al.*, 1992).

In vitro

- *Uncaria guianensis*

    ANTI-INFLAMMATORY: reduces excessive production of cytokines and inflammatory mediators at the genetic level (Sandoval *et al.*, 2002; Piscoya *et al.*, 2001) with UG being more potent than UT (Sandoval *et al.*, 2002), and at extract concentrations far lower than required for antioxidant activity (Piscoya *et al.*, 2001); prevents and eliminates gastrointestinal injury and inflammation in NSAID-induced gastritis (Sandoval *et al.*, 2002).

    ANTIOXIDANT: scavenges DPPH (UG more potent than UT despite lower concentrations of alkaloids and flavanols), protects against deoxyribose degradation in a dose-dependent

manner, and inhibits ABTS-radicals (Sandoval *et al.*, 2002); effectively scavenges free radicals and inhibits lipid peroxidation (Piscoya *et al.*, 2001); protects human gastric epithelial cells from apoptosis induced by DPPH, peroxynitrite and H_2O_2 (Miller *et al.*, 2001).

- *Uncaria tomentosa*–**unspecified preparations**

    ANTI-INFLAMMATORY: reduces excessive production of cytokines and inflammatory mediators at the genetic level with UG being more potent than UT, and at extract concentrations far lower than required for antioxidant activity (Sandoval *et al.*, 2002; Piscoya *et al.*, 2001); suppressed tumor necrosis factor alpha (TNFα) production by 65–85% (Sandoval *et al.*, 2000); prevents and eliminates gastrointestinal injury and inflammation in NSAID-induced gastritis (Piscoya *et al.*, 2001; Sandoval *et al.*, 2000; Sandoval-Chacón *et al.*, 1998); reduces cyclo-oxygenase-2 (COX-2) expression (Piscoya *et al.*, 2001).

    ANTIOXIDANT: scavenges DPPH (UG more potent than UT reflected as lower IC50 value despite lower concentrations of alkaloids and flavanols), protects against deoxyribose degradation in a dose-dependent manner, and inhibits ABTS-radicals (Sandoval *et al.*, 2002, 2000); effectively scavenges free radicals and inhibits lipid peroxidation (Piscoya *et al.*, 2001); protects human gastric epithelial cells from apoptosis induced by DPPH, peroxynitrite and hydrogen peroxide (Miller *et al.*, 2001); reduces peroxynitrite-induced apoptosis in human gastric epithelial cells and in macrophages (Sandoval-Chacón *et al.*, 1998); protective against UV irradiation-induced cytotoxicity (Sandoval *et al.*, 2000).

    IMMUNOMODULATION/IMMUNE SUPPORT: Increased cytokine (IL-1 and IL-6) production in alveolar macrophages (Lemaire *et al.*, 1999) although high concentrations were used that might reflect a toxicologic response and may be incompatible with *in vivo* efficacy (Sandoval *et al.*, 2002).

    ANTIMUTAGENIC: protective against photomutagenesis, (Rizzi *et al.*, 1993).

- *Uncaria tomentosa*–**standardized to CAEs**

    IMMUNOMODULATION/IMMUNE SUPPORT: CAE: significantly increased PHA (phytohemagglutinin)-stimulated lymphocyte proliferation in splenocytes and significantly elevated white blood cell (WBC) count (Sheng *et al.*, 2000a).

    ANTIPROLIFERATIVE: inhibited proliferation and induced apoptosis in some tumor cell lines (Sheng *et al.*, 1998) at high concentrations that might reflect a toxicologic response (Sandoval *et al.*, 2000).

- *Uncaria tomentosa*–**POA chemotype**

    ANTI-INFLAMMATORY: moderate to weak activity against cyclo-oxygenase-1 and -2 (COX-1 and COX-2) (Aguilar *et al.*, 2002).

    ANTIPROLIFERATIVE: Inhibited proliferation of some human tumor cell lines (Immodal, 1999b).

- **Isolated Chemical Components from Cat's Claw**

    [EDITORS' NOTE: As in any determination of the source of bioactivity in an unknown natural product, any proposed active constituent must mimic the actions of the extract from which it was derived, and exert these actions at a concentration that reflects its relative amount within that botanical or botanical extract. Studies demonstrating that purified POAs or TOAs share the same bioactivity of cat's claw preparations but enhanced for the relative concentrations in these extracts are lacking. Therefore, these chemical constituents may be more useful as marker compounds rather than mediating the bioactivity of the botanical.]

IMMUNOMODULATION/IMMUNE SUPPORT: Phagocytosis was enhanced *in vitro* by pteropodine, isomitraphylline, and isorhynchophylline (two POAs and one TOA, isolated from UT), but phagocytosis was enhanced *in vivo* only after addition of catechin to POAs (Wagner *et al.*, 1985a, 1985b; Kreutzkamp, 1984); POAs isolated from UT induced endothelial cells to release a factor that inhibited proliferation of normal human lymphoblasts and stimulated proliferation of normal human resting lymphocytes, while TOAs dose-dependently reduced these effects (Wurm *et al.*, 1998); POAs isolated from UT inhibited growth of HL60 and U-937 leukemic cells, with uncarine F demonstrating the strongest effect; (Stuppner *et al.*, 1993 cited in Keplinger *et al.*, 1999); isopteropodine (POA isolated from UT) increases the phagocytosis of granulocytes and reticuloendothelial system (RES) cells (Kreutzkamp, 1984; Wagner *et al.*, 1985a, 1985b).

ANTI-INFLAMMATORY: 17 non-alkaloid HPLC fractions from UT reduced TNFα and nitrite production induced by lipopolysaccharide (LPS) in RAW 264.7 cells (Sandoval *et al.*, 2002); one quinovic acid glycoside isolated from UT demonostrated anti-inflammatory effects, but it appears that the strong anti-inflammatory effects of cat's claw extracts and fractions may be the result of the synergistic activity of a combination of compounds (Aquino *et al.*, 1991); moderate anti-inflammatory activity has been demonstrated for β-sitosterol, stigmasterol and campesterol isolated from UT (Senatore *et al.*, 1989); one procyanidine (cinchonain Ib) isolated from UT inhibited 5-lipoxygenase, demonstrating anti-inflammatory activity (Wirth and Wagner, 1997).

ANTIVIRAL: 9 quinovic acid glycosides isolated from UT showed moderate antiviral activity against vesicular stomatitis virus, but at concentrations approaching cellular toxicity (Aquino *et al.*, 1989); two quinovic acid glycocides isolated from UT (those with free carboxyl groups) reduced by 50% the viral cytopathic effect of rhinovirus type 1b infection (Aquino *et al.*, 1989).

ANTIPROLIFERATIVE: Uncarine D showed weak cytotoxic activity against SK-MEL, KB, BT-549 and SK-OV-3 cell lines with IC50 values between 30 and 40 µg/ml, while uncarine C exhibited weak cytocoxicity only against ovarian carcinoma (IC50 at 37 µg/ml) (Muhammad *et al.*, 2001b). However, given the concentration of uncarine C in cat's claw, the amount of cat's claw that would have to be consumed to achieve these concentrations *in vivo* may be unrealistic. In addition to the antimutagenic activity, UT extracts and factions exert a direct antiproliferative activity on the MCF7 human breast cancer cell line. The bioassay-directed fraction from barks and leaves resulted in the isolation of 2 active fractions, displaying an IC50 of 10 mg/ml and 20 mg/ml, respectively and an antiproliferative effect, with about 90% of inhibition at a concentration of 100 mg/ml (Riva *et al.*, 2001). As noted above, for the alkaloids uncarine D and C, these fractions would require an unrealistic consumption of kilogram quantities of cat's claw to achieve these actions.

- **Isolated Chemical Components from other *Uncaria* species**
[EDITORS' NOTE: The studies referenced in this subsection were performed with compounds isolated from *U. rhynchophylla* or *U. sinensis*. While these compounds are also found in *U. guianensis* and/or *U. tomentosa*, no studies have been performed on extracts or fractions derived from UG or UT to verify that these actions apply to them as well; thus their clinical significance is undetermined. These studies have been included because some proponents of the UT products standardized to POAs and no TOAs, cite them in support of the need for removal of TOAs from cat's claw products.]

Rhynchophylline and isorhynchophylline produced negative chronotropic and inotropic effects (Zhu and Guozing, 1993); rhynchophylline inhibits platelet aggregation (Chen *et al.*, 1992; Jin *et al.*, 1991); rhynchophylline may be a calcium antagonist (Sun *et al.*, 1988; Zhang *et al.*, 1987); rhynchophylline, corynoxeine, isorhynchophylline, isocorynoxeine, and indole alkaloids such as hirsuteine and hirsutine inhibit Ca2+ influx which protects against glutamate-induced neuronal death (Shimada *et al*, 1999; Yano *et al.*, 1991); corynantheine and dihydrocorynantheine have sedative action which in toxic dosages may lead to respiratory paralysis and ataxia (Kanatani, 1985); corynantheine and dihydrocorynantheine reduced specific [3H]5-HT binding and were found to be partial agonists for 5-HT receptors (Kanatani, 1985).

MECHANISMS OF ACTION
Uncaria guianensis
ANTI-INFLAMMATORY

- Modifies gene expression by inhibiting redox-sensitive transcription factors (Piscoya *et al.*, 2001; Sandoval *et al.*, 2002).

- Inhibits transcription factor NF-kB thereby modifying expression of genes involved in the inflammatory process including TNFα, inducible nitric oxide synthase (iNOS), and COX-2 (Sandoval *et al.*, 2002; Piscoya *et al.*, 2001).

- Inhibits production of TNFα (Sandoval *et al.*, 2002; Piscoya *et al.*, 2001) with UG being more potent than UT (Sandoval *et al.*, 2002).

- Decreases production of lipopolysaccharide-induced prostaglandin E-2 (Piscoya *et al.*, 2001).

ANTIOXIDANT

- Scavenges DPPH (UG more potent than UT despite lower concentrations of alkaloids and flavanols), protects against deoxyribose degradation in a dose-dependent manner, and inhibits ABTS-radicals (Sandoval *et al.*, 2002).

- Effectively scavenges free radicals and inhibits lipid peroxidation (Piscoya *et al.*, 2001; Miller *et al.*, 2001).

- Protects human gastric epithelial cells from apoptosis induced by DPPH, peroxynitrite and hydrogen peroxide (Miller *et al.*, 2001).

- More effective in limiting the cellular response to oxidants than degrading the oxidant itself (Miller *et al.*, 2001; Piscoya *et al.*, 2001).

Uncaria tomentosa–unspecified

ANTI-INFLAMMATORY

- Modifies gene expression by inhibiting redox-sensitive transcription factors (Piscoya *et al.*, 2001; Sandoval *et al.*, 2000; Sandoval-Chacón *et al.*, 1998).
- Inhibits transcription factor NF-kB thereby modifying expression of more than 28 genes involved in the inflammatory process including TNFα, iNOS, and COX-2 (Aguilar *et al.*, 2002; Sandoval *et al.*, 2002; Piscoya *et al.*, 2001; Sandoval-Chacón *et al.*, 1998).
- Inhibits lipopolysaccharide-induced iNOS gene expression, nitrite formation, and cell death (Sandoval-Chacón *et al.*, 1998).
- Inhibits production of TNFα, iNOS, and COX-2 (Sandoval *et al.*, 2002; Piscoya *et al.*, 2001; Sandoval-Chacón *et al.*, 1998).
- Moderate to weak activity against COX-1 and COX-2 (Aguilar *et al.*, 2002).
- Decreased production of lipopolysaccharide-induced prostaglandin E-2 (Piscoya *et al.*, 2001).
- Suppressed TNFα production (Sandoval *et al.*, 2002; Piscoya *et al.*, 2001; Sandoval-Chacón *et al.*, 1998) by 65–85% (Sandoval *et al.*, 2000).

ANTIOXIDANT

- Scavenges DPPH (UG more potent than UT despite lower concentrations of alkaloids and flavanols), protects against deoxyribose degradation in a dose-dependent manner, and inhibits ABTS-radicals (Sandoval *et al.*, 2002; 2000).
- Effectively scavenges free radicals and inhibits lipid peroxidation (Piscoya *et al.*, 2001).
- Protects human gastric epithelial cells from apoptosis induced by DPPH, peroxynitrite and H_2O_2 (Miller *et al.*, 2001).
- Reduces peroxynitrite-induced apoptosis in human gastric epithelial cells and in macrophages (Sandoval-Chacón *et al.*, 1998).
- Cytoprotective against UV irradiation (Sandoval *et al.*, 2000).

IMMUNOMODULATION/IMMUNE SUPPORT

- Increased cytokine (IL-1 and IL-6) production in alveolar macrophages (Lemaire *et al.*, 1999) although high concentrations were used suggesting that this action could only be observed *in vivo* with ingestion of kilogram quantities; a dosing regimen that might reflect a toxicologic response (Sandoval *et al.*, 2002).
- Stimulates interleukin-1 (IL-1) and interleukin-6 (IL-6) production at a rate of 10.0x and 7.5x control levels, respectively. The effect is dose-dependent and diminishes when the dose exceeds the range of 0.025–0.1 mg/ml (Lemaire *et al.*, 1999).

Uncaria tomentosa–standardized to CAEs

ANTIMUTAGENIC

- Stimulation of DNA repair mechanisms (Sheng *et al.*, 2000a, 2001).

IMMUNOMODULATION/IMMUNE SUPPORT

- Stimulates lymphocyte proliferation and elevates white blood cells (Sheng *et al.*, 2000a, 2000b; Lamm *et al.*, 2001).

ANTI-TUMOR

- Suppresses tumor growth through selective induction of apoptosis in two human leukemic cell lines (K562 and HL60) and one human EBV-transformed B-lymphoma cell line (Raji) (Sheng *et al.*, 1998); however, some authors have reported apoptosis in these same cell lines due to inhibition of NF-kB (Sandoval *et al.*, 2002; Mannick *et al.*, 1997; Beg and Baltimore, 1996).

Uncaria tomentosa–POA chemotype

ANTI-INFLAMMATORY

- Moderate to weak activity against COX-1 and COX-2 (Aguilar *et al.*, 2002).
- Inhibits synthesis of NF-kB (Aguilar *et al.*, 2002; 2000).

IMMUNOMODULATION/IMMUNE SUPPORT

- POAs induce the release of a lymphocyte-growth factor from endothelial cells that regulates lymphocyte proliferation (Wurm *et al.*, 1998), but does not change total leukocyte numbers (Keplinger *et al.*, 1999). TOAs act antagonistically to this effect of POAs (Wurm *et al.*, 1998; Keplinger *et al.*, 1999).

CONTRAINDICATIONS

Cat's claw has been contraindicated for leukemia patients awaiting bone marrow transplant, any patient awaiting organ transplant, persons with iatrically-induced immunosuppression (e.g., organ transplants), autoimmune disease, multiple sclerosis, or tuberculosis (CAMR, 1999). These contraindications are based on the belief that cat's claw is an immunostimulant. However, some researchers disagree with this view (Miller, 2001b; Sandoval-Chacón *et al.*, 1998; Sandoval *et al.*, 2000, 2002) and suggest that cat's claw may be helpful for transplant patients (Miller, 2001a). The elevated production of TNFα is a characteristic of numerous autoimmune disorders, including those in which cat's claw offers benefits (arthritis, gut inflammation) and lowering TNFα levels, as with cat's claw, may be desirable rather than contraindicated for these patients. HIV/AIDS patients should proceed with caution when introducing any new therapeutic agent (Miller, 2001b). Cat's claw is not for use in children under 3 years due to lack of data regarding its effects on the immature immune system (Immodal, 1995).

PREGNANCY AND LACTATION: Not recommended (Jones, 1995) due to lack of data regarding the effects of cat's claw on the immature immune system (Immodal, 1995).

ADVERSE EFFECTS

Recent human trials have concluded that the various cat's claw preparations tested are safe, with no adverse effects reported in liver, renal, central nervous system, or hematological function (Piscoya *et al.*, 2001; Sheng *et al.*, 2001, 2000a; Lamm *et al.*, 2001). Cat's claw teas or crude extracts may cause mild nausea, due to the bitter taste (Williams, 2001); however, this appears speculative as nausea is not a frequently reported effect. In one case report, a patient with systemic lupus erythematosus (SLE) experienced acute renal failure, which the authors attributed to an idiosyncratic adverse reaction to the purported cat's claw preparation which was not adequately documented (Hilepo *et al.*, 1997).

Uncaria guianensis

In one study infrequent reports of headache, dizziness, and vomiting were reported but the incidence and frequency were the same as with placebo (Piscoya *et al.*, 2001).

Uncaria tomentosa–standardized to CAEs
None reported.

Uncaria tomentosa–POA chemotype
In AIDS patients and patients receiving large doses of chemotherapy, individual cases of a mild erythrocytosis have been reported. During the first 1–2 weeks of ingesting cat's claw tea (Krallendorn®) temporary constipation or mild diarrhea was sometimes observed. Increased occurrence of acne symptoms has been reported in HIV patients with prior symptoms. In rare cases, elevated uric acid values were observed in HIV and cancer patients; extensive cell die-off in tumor patients may cause lytic fever lasting 1–2 weeks (Immodal, 1999a, 1995).

Components from Other Species of *Uncaria*
Cat's claw products containing larger amounts of TOAs could possibly result in sedative effects and circulatory complaints (e.g., reduced blood pressure, coronary blood flow, and heart rate; inhibited platelet aggregation) (Reinhard, 1999), due to the reported effects of TOAs in *Uncaria* species other than UT or UG (Shi *et al.*, 1992, 1989; Jin *et al.*, 1991). However, no such effects have been reported in studies using products made with UT or UG.

DRUG INTERACTIONS

Uncaria guianensis
None reported.

Uncaria tomentosa–unspecified preparations
UT may potentially reduce the rate of metabolism and thus increase serum levels of drugs taken orally as observed in an *in vitro* assay on an unspecified UT tincture where the CYP3A4 isozyme production was inhibited (Budzinski *et al.*, 2000).

Some authors warn that some unspecified forms of cat's claw may increase the effects of anticoagulants and antihypertensives (Fetrow and Avila, 2000; CAMR, 1999; Spaulding-Albright, 1997; INPR, 1999). However, this is based on research on TOA components isolated from *Uncaria* species other than UG or UT. While it is possible that cat's claw products rich in TOAs may interact with these classes of drugs, there are no reliable data to support this conclusion. Further, there is little evidence to support this interaction with cat's claw products that contain little or no TOAs such as UG products or the UT product Krallendorn®, or C-Med-100® (AF Nutraceutical Group).

Uncaria tomentosa–standardized to CAEs
None reported.

Uncaria tomentosa–POA chemotype
According to a communication to physicians and pharmacists from the leading Austrian research and manufacturing company of cat's claw, the following advice should be given to patients, based on the products proposed immunomodulatory effects:

Take between chemotherapy treatments and after completion, but not with chemotherapy treatments; do not take in conjunction with passive animal vaccines, intravenous hyperimmunoglobulin therapy; intravenous thymic extracts, drugs using animal protein or peptide hormones (e.g., bovine or porcine insulin), cryoprecipitates, or fresh blood plasma (Immodal, 1995).

AMERICAN HERBAL PRODUCTS ASSOCIATION (AHPA) SAFETY RATING
CLASS 4: Insufficient data available for classification (McGuffin *et al.*, 1997).

[EDITORS' NOTE: Cat's claw was not widely marketed during the time that the literature upon which this book is based was published, mainly 1980s and early to mid-1990s. Of potential relevance is the fact that numerous studies show cat's claw to be safe. Human, animal, and *in vitro* studies demonstrate the antimutagenic activity of cat's claw (Sheng *et al.*, 2001, 2000a, 1998; Immodal, 1999b; Leon *et al.*, 1996; Rizzi *et al.*, 1993). One human trial found no toxic effects at a dose of 350 mg/day of C-Med-100® for 6 consecutive weeks (Sheng *et al.*, 2000a). One animal study reports an LD50 of greater than 16 g/kg of body weight using a freeze-dried aqueous extract of POA type UT (Kynoch and Lloyd, 1975), while a second reports an LD50 of greater than 8 g/kg for C-Med-100. Another study found daily oral administration of an aqueous-acid extract of UT at 1,000 mg/kg body weight for 28 days to be atoxic in rats (Svendson and Skydsgaard, 1986). In an additional test, an aqueous extract of UT was atoxic up to the maximum dosage of 5 g/kg body weight administered orally, and up to a concentration of 2 g/kg body weight administered intraperitoneally (Kreutzkamp, 1984). The alkaloid fraction of UT was found to be atoxic up to the maximum dosage of 2 g/kg body weight orally, and 1 g/kg body weight intraperitoneally (Kreutzkamp, 1984).]

REGULATORY STATUS
AUSTRIA: Prescription drug Krallendorn® (pentacyclic chemotype).

CANADA: Status undetermined. No products containing cat's claw are listed in the Health Canada Drugs Product Database (Health Canada, 2001).

GERMANY: No German Commission E monograph (Blumenthal *et al.*, 1998). No monograph in the *German Pharmacopoeia* (DAB, 1999).

SWEDEN: No products containing cat's claw are listed in the Medical Products Agency (MPA) "Authorised Natural Remedies" (MPA, 2001).

SWITZERLAND: No products containing cat's claw are listed in the *Swiss Drug Compendium* (Morant and Ruppanner, 2001). No monograph in the *Swiss Pharmacopoeia*.

U.K.: Not listed in the *General Sale List* (GSL, 1994). No monograph in the *British Pharmacopoeia*.

U.S.: Dietary supplement (USC, 1994). No monograph in the USP-NF.

CLINICAL REVIEW
There are 14 clinical trials on various preparations made from the two species of *Uncaria* summarized in the clinical studies Tables in this monograph. In general, the studies are relatively small, most are uncontrolled, and some have not been published. One prospective (P), randomized (R), double-blind (DB), placebo-controlled (PC), parallel group (PG), multi-center (MC) trial was conducted on 45 men who consumed 100 mg of a freeze-dried aqueous extract of UG for 4 weeks for osteoarthritis of the knee (Piscoya *et al.*, 2001). The study reports a significant improvement in pain associated with activity, and medical and patient assessment scores, but no significant improvement in pain at rest or at night, or knee circumference. There were no significant side effects in the UG and placebo groups.

Three trials tested the UT-CAE preparation (C-Med-100®) on immunomodulatory parameters. One small R, PC trial (n=23) resulted in no loss of immunity after 5 months in patients given a pneumonia vaccine after 2 months of treatment with 700 mg per day of the UT-CAE extract when compared to loss in the placebo group (Lamm *et al.*, 2001). Another small trial (n=12) reported an increase in DNA repair with no adverse effects (Sheng *et al.*, 2001). An uncontrolled trial on healthy volunteers resulted in an increase in white blood cells (Sheng *et al.*, 2000a).

Three trials tested a proprietary extract of UT standardized to POAs (Krallendorn®) for anti-inflammatory effects. One 52-week trial on 40 people with rheumatoid arthritis (RA) used 60 mg per day of the extract in capsules (Mur *et al.*, 2002). The first phase (24 weeks) was R, DB, PC; the second phase (28 weeks) was not blinded—all patients received the treatment. There was a significant decrease in pain and a shorter period of morning stiffness for the treatment group compared to placebo after the first phase and a further reduction after the second phase. The placebo-cat's claw treatment group experienced some reduction of symptoms in the second phase. Two small uncontrolled, unpublished trials test the UT-POA extract on patients with RA (Immodal, 1995, 2002) and on ulcers and gastritis (Immodal, 1995, 1999a).

Five trials tested the UT-POA extract for its effects on immune function. All five trials were uncontrolled and unpublished, thereby raising questions as to the significance of the results. Two trials tested the UT-POA extract as an adjuvant therapy for cancer patients undergoing chemotherapy, radiation, and/or surgery (Immodal 1995, 1999a, 2002) with generally favorable results, including patients' reports of a greater sense of vitality and fewer side effects; three additional trials tested UT-POA extract as an adjuvant therapy for HIV-positive patients (Immodal 1995, 1999a, 2002) and reported stabilized or increased CD-4 cell counts, increased vitality, and no adverse effects.

Two uncontrolled, unpublished trials were performed on the UT-POA extract in topical preparations for use on lesions caused by *Herpes simplex* (Immodal, 1995, 1999a, 2002) and *Varicella zoster* (Immodal, 1995, 1999a, 2002), showing improvement and no adverse effects.

BRANDED PRODUCTS

C-MED-100®: Campamed, LLC / 437 Madison Avenue / New York, NY 10022 / U.S.A. / Tel: 212-616-6814 / Fax: 212-838-8918. Patented extract of *Uncaria tomentosa*, standardized to 8% by carboxy alkyl esters. Ultrafiltrated, 100% water soluble extract spray-dried and compressed into 350 mg tablets.

Krallendorn® Capsules: Immodal Pharmaka GmbH / Bundesstrasse 44 / 6111 Volders / Austria / Tel: +43-05-22-45-7678 / Fax: +43-05-22-45-7646. Cat's claw root (pentacyclic chemotype) aqueous-acid extract standardized to contain 1.3% POAs, and undetectable TOAs.

Krallendorn® Drops: Immodal Pharmaka GmbH. Cat's claw root (pentacyclic chemotype) aqueous-acid extract standardized to contain 1.3% POAs, and undetectable TOAs; each 100 g of drop solution contains 600 mg cat's claw extract, water, ethanol (95% by volume).

Krallendorn® Ointment: Immodal Pharmaka GmbH. Cat's claw root (pentacyclic chemotype) aqueous-acid extract standardized to contain 1.3% POAs, and undetectable TOAs; each 75 g of ointment contains 300 mg cat's claw extract.

Krallendorn® Spray: Immodal Pharmaka GmbH. Cat's claw root (pentacyclic chemotype) aqueous-acid extract standardized to contain 1.3% POAs, and undetectable TOAs; each 100 g of spray solution contains 600 mg cat's claw extract.

Krallendorn® Tea: Immodal Pharmaka GmbH. Cat's claw root (pentacyclic chemotype), ground.

*American equivalents, if any, are found in the Product Table beginning on page 398.

REFERENCES

Access. *Professional Reference to Conditions, Herbs and Supplements*. Newton (MA): Integrative Medicine Communications; 2000.

Aguilar JL, Rojas PA, Capcha RC, Plaza A, Merfortl I. Anti-inflammatory and molecular activity of extracts of *Uña de gato* with different concentrations of pentacyclic and tetracyclic alkaloids and of a freeze-dried extract. Congreso Internacional FITO 2000; Lima, Peru.

Aguilar JL, Rojas P, Marcelo A, Plaza A, Bauer R, Reininger E, et al. Anti-inflammatory activity of two different extracts of *Uncaria tomentosa* (Rubiaceae). *J Ethnopharmacol* 2002;81(2):271–6.

Åkesson C, Pero RW, Ivars F. C-Med 100®, a hot water extract of *Uncaria tomentosa*, prolongs leukocyte survival in vivo. *Phytomedicine* 2003;30 [in press].

Anonymous. Cat's Claw. *The Lawrence Review of Natural Products* Apr 1996;1–3.

Aquino R, DeFeo V, DeSimone F, Pizza C, Cirino G. Plant metabolites. New compounds and anti-inflammatory activity of *Uncaria tomentosa*. *J Nat Prod* 1991;54(2):453–459.

Aquino R, DeSimone F, Vincieri FF, Pizza C, Gaes-Baitz E. New polyhydroxylated triterpenes from *Uncaria tomentosa*. *J Nat Prod* 1990 May-Jun:53(3):559–64.

Aquino R, DeSimone C, Pizza. Plant metabolites. Structure and in vitro antiviral activity of quinovic acid glycosides from *Uncaria tomentosa* and *Guettarda platypoda*. *J Nat Prod* 1989;52(4):679–685.

Beg AA, Baltimore D. An essential role for NF-kB in preventing TNFα-induced cell death. *Science* 1996;274:782–410. Cited in Sandoval M, Okuhama NN, Zhang X-J, Condezo LA, Lao J, Angeles FM, Bobrowski P, Miller MSJ. Anti-inflammatory and antioxidant activities of cat's claw (*Uncaria tomentosa* and *Uncaria guianensis*) are independent of their alkaloid content. *Phytomed* 2002;9(4):325–37.

Blumenthal M, Busse WR, Goldberg A, Gruenwald J, Hall T, Riggins CW, Rister RS, editors. Klein S, Rister RS (trans.). *The Complete German Commission E Monographs—Therapeutic Guide to Herbal Medicines*. Austin (TX): American Botanical Council; Boston: Integrative Medicine Communication; 1998.

Budzinski JW, Foster BC, Wandenhoek S, Arnason JT. An in vitro evaluation of human cytochrome P450 3A4 inhibition by selected commercial herbal extracts and tinctures. *Phytomedicine* 2000 Jul;7(4):273–82.

Cabieses F. *The saga of the cat's claw*. Lima, Peru: Via Lactea Editores; 1994.

CAMR. See: Center for Alternative Medicine Research.

Center for Alternative Medicine Research. Cat's Claw Summary [University of Texas, Health Science Center at Houston, School of Public Health web site]. 4 May 1999. Available at: http://www.sph.uth.tmc.edu/utcam/summary/cat.htm. Accessed 18 Oct 1999.

Cerri R, Aquino R, De Simone F, Pizza C. New quinovic acid glycosides from *Uncaria tomentosa*. *J Nat Prod* 1988;51:257–61. Cited in Sandoval M, Okuhama NN, Zhang X-J, Condezo LA, Lao J, Angeles FM, Bobrowski P, Miller MSJ. Anti-inflammatory and antioxidant activities of cat's claw (*Uncaria tomentosa* and *Uncaria guianensis*) are independent of their alkaloid content. *Phytomed* 2002;9(4):325–37.

Chen CX, Jin RM, Li YK, Zhong J, Yue L, Chen SC, Zhou JY. Inhibitory effect of rhynchophylline on platelet aggregation and thrombosis. *Acta Pharmacol Sin* 1992;13(2):126-130.

DAB. See: *Deutsches Arzneibuch*.

Deutsches Arzneibuch (DAB). Stuttgart, Germany: Deutscher Apotheker Verlag; 1999.

Enzymatic Therapy. Saventaro® [product information]. Accessed 26 Jul 2002. Available at URL: www.enzy.com/products.

Fetrow CW, Avila JR. *The Complete Guide to Herbal Medicines*. Springhouse(PA):Springhouse Corporation; 2000. p. 113–4.

General Sale List (GSL). Statutory Instrument 1994 No. 2410: The Medicines (Products Other than Veterinary Drugs). London, UK: Her Majesty's Stationery Office (HMSO); 1994.

GSL. See: *General Sale List*.

Health Canada. *Drug Product Database (DPD) Product Information*. Ottawa, Ontario: Health Canada Therapeutic Products Programme; 2001.

Hilepo J, Bellucci A, Mossey R. Acute renal failure caused by cat's claw herbal remedy in a patient with systemic lupus erythematosus [letter]. *Nephron* 1997;77:361.

Immodal Pharmaka. Krallendorn® *Uncaria tomentosa* (Willd.) DC Root Extract: Information for Physicians and Dispensing Chemists. 3rd revised ed. Volders, Austria: Immodal; 1995. Available on request from immodal@volders.netwing.at.

Immodal Pharmaka. Radix *Uncariae tomentosae* (Willd.) DC., pentacyclic chemotype (Krallendorn®): summarized research. Volders, Austria: Immodal; 2002.

Immodal Pharmaka. Summary and assessment of clinical examinations of Krallendorn® products. Volders, Austria: Immodal; 1999a. Available on request from immodal@volders.netwing.at.

Immodal Pharmaka. Summary and assessment of: Pharmacodynamical examinations of extracts of *Uncaria tomentosa* (Willd.) DC. mod. pent. Volders, Austria: Immodal; 1999b.

INPR. See: Institute for Natural Products Research.

Institute for Natural Products Research (INPR). The NPDR Quick Reference—Cat's Claw [INPR web site]. 1999. Available at URL: http://www.naturalproducts.org/public/qr/catsclaw.html. Accessed 4 Dec 2002.

Jin R, Chen C, Li Y, Xu, P. Effect of rhynchophylline on platelet aggregation and experimental thrombosis. *Acta Pharm Sinica* 1991;26(4):246–249.

Jones K. *Cat's Claw—Healing Vine of Peru*. Seattle (WA): Sylvan Press; 1995.

Kanatani H, Kohda H, Yamasaki K, Hotta I, Nakata Y, Segawa T. The active principles of the branchlet and hook of *Uncaria sinensis* Oliv. examined with a 5-hydroxytryptamine receptor binding assay. *J Pharm Pharmacol* 1985;37:401–404.

Keplinger K, Laus G, Wurm M, Dierich MP, Teppner H. *Uncaria tomentosa* (Willd.) DC–Ethnomedicinal use and new pharmacological, toxicological and botanical results. *J Ethnopharmacol* 1999;64:23–34.

Kitajima M, Hashimoto K, Yokoya M, Takayama H, Aimi N, Sakai LI. A new gluco indole alkaloid, 3, 4-dehydro-5-carboxystricosidine, from Peruvian *Una de Gato* (*Uncaria tomentosa*). *Chem Pharm Bull* (Tokyo) 2000;48(10):1410–2.

Kreutzkamp B. Niedermolekulare Inhaltsstoffe mit immunstimulierenden Eigenschaften aus *Uncaria tomentosa*, Okoubaka aubrevillei und anderen Drogen [dissertation]. Munich, Germany: University of Munich; 1984. Cited in Keplinger K, Laus G, Wurm M, et al. *Uncaria tomentosa* (Willd.) DC–Ethnomedicinal use and new pharmacological, toxicological and botanical results. *J Ethnopharmacol* 1999;64:23–34.

Kynoch SR, Lloyd GK. Acute oral toxicity to mice of substance E-2919. Huntingdon Research Centre. Huntingdon, Cambridgeshire, England: 1975. Cited in Reinhard K. *Uncaria tomentosa* (Willd.) D.C. Cat's claw, una de gato, or saventaro. *J Alternative Complement Med* 1999;5(2):143–51.

Lamm S, Sheng Y, Pero RW. Persistent response to pneumococcal vaccine in individuals supplemented with a novel water soluble extract of *Uncaria tomentosa*, C-Med-100®. *Phytomedicine* 2001;8(4):267–274.

Laus G, Brössner D, Keplinger K. Alkaloids of Peruvian *Uncaria tomentosa*. *Phytochemistry* 1997;45(4):855–860.

Laus G, Keplinger K, Wurm M, Dierich MP. Pharmacological activities of two chemotypes of *Uncaria tomentosa* (Willd.) DC. 46th Annual Congress of the Society for Medicinal Plant Research, Vienna, Austria, 1998.

Lee KK, Zhou BN, Lingston DG Vaisberg AJ, Hammond GB. Bioactive indole alkaloids from the bark of *Uncaria guianensis*. *Planta Med* 1999;65:759–60.

Lemaire I, Assinewe V, Cano P, Awang D, Arnason J. Stimulation of interleukin-1 and -6 production in alveolar macrophages by the neotropical liana, *Uncaria tomentosa* (Uña de Gato). *J Ethnopharmacol* 1999;64:109–115.

Leon FR, Ortiz N, Antunez de Mayolo A, Namisato T, Monge R. Antimutagnic activity of a freeze-dried aqueous extract of *Uncaria tomentosa* in smokers and non-smokers. Third European Colloquium on Ethnopharmacology, Genova, Italy 1996:255. Cited in Reinhard K. *Uncaria tomentosa* (Willd.) D.C. Cat's claw, una de gato, or saventaro. *J Alternative Complement Med* 1999;5(2):143–51.

Mannick EE, Mishra J, Marque J, Clavell M, Miller MJS, Oliver PD. Inhibitors of nuclear factor Kappa B cause apoptosis in cultured macrophages. *Mediators Inflammation* 1997;6:225–32. Cited in Sandoval et al., 2002 Sandoval M, Okuhama NN, Zhang X-J, Condezo LA, Lao J, Angeles FM, Bobrowski P, Miller MSJ. Anti-inflammatory and antioxidant activities of cat's claw (*Uncaria tomentosa* and *Uncaria guianensis*) are independent of their alkaloid content. *Phytomed* 2002;9(4):325–37.

McGuffin M, Kartesz JT, Leung AY, Tucker AO. *The American Herbal Product Association's Herbs of Commerce*, 2nd ed. Silver Spring (MD): American Herbal Products Association; 2000.

McGuffin M, Hobbs C, Upton R, Goldberg A. *American Herbal Products Association's Botanical Safety Handbook: Guidelines for the Safe Use and Labeling for Herbs of Commerce*. Boca Raton (FL): CRC Press; 1997.

Medical Products Agency (MPA). Naturläkemedel: Authorised Natural Remedies (as of January 24, 2001). Uppsala, Sweden: Medical Products Agency; 2001.

Miller MJS. Personal communication to M. Blumenthal. Jun 4, 2001a.

Miller MJS. Alternative focus: Amazonian medicinals for gastrointestinal health. *HIV Resource Review* 2001b;5:1–6.

Miller MJS, Angeles FM, Reuter BK, Bobrowski P, Sandoval M. Dietary antioxidants

protect gut epithelial cells from oxidant-induced apoptosis. *BMC Complement Altern Med* 2001;1:11.

Morant J, Ruppanner H (eds.). *Arzneimittel-Kompendium der Schweiz® 2001*. Basel, Switzerland: Documed AG; 2001.

MPA. See: Medical Products Agency.

Muhammad I, Khan IA, Fischer NH, Fronczek FR. Two stereoisomeric pentacyclic oxindole alkaloids from *Uncaria tomentosa*: uncarine C and uncarine E. *Acta Cryst* 2001a;C57:240–2.

Muhammad I, Dunbar DC, Khan RA, Ganzera M, Khan IA. Investigation of Una de Gato. 7-deoxyloganic acid and 15N NMR spectroscopic studies on pentacyclic oxindole alkaloids from *Uncaria tomentosa*. *Phytochemistry* 2001b;57(5):781–5.

Mur E, Hartig F, Eibl G, Schirmer M. Randomized double blind trial of an extract from the pentacyclic alkaloid-chemotype of *Uncaria tomentosa* for the treatment of rheumatoid arthritis. *J Rheumatol* 2002;29:678–81.

Obregon VL. Cat's Claw. Genus *Uncaria*. Botanical, Chemical and Pharmacological Studies of *Uncaria tomentosa* (Willd.) DC and *Uncaria guianensis* (Aubl.). 1995; Lima, Peru: Institute of American Phytotherapy. (English translation of work published in Spanish in 1994).

Piscoya J, Rodriguez Z, Bustamante SA, Okuhama NN, Miller MJS, Sandoval M. Efficacy and safety of freeze-dried cat's claw in osteoarthritis of the knee: mechanisms of action of the species *Uncaria guianensis*. *Inflamm Res* 2001;50:442–8.

Reinhard K. *Uncaria tomentosa* (Willd.) D.C. Cat's claw, una de gato, or saventaro. *J Alternative Complement Med* 1999;5(2):143–151.

Richman A, Witkowski JP. Annual herb sales survey. *Whole Foods* 2001 Oct:23–30.

Riva L, Coradini D, Di Fronzo G, De Feo V, De Tommasi N, De Simone F, Pizza C. The antiproliferative effects of *Uncaria tomentosa* extracts and fractions on the growth of breast cancer cell line. *Anticancer Res* 2001;21(4A):2457–61.

Rizzi R, Re F, Bianchi A, De Feo V, de Simone F, Bianchi L, Stivala L. Mutagenic and antimutagenic activities of *Uncaria tomentosa* and its extracts. *J Ethnopharmacol* 1993;38:63–77 .

Sandoval M, Charbonnet R, Okuhama N, Roberts J, Krenova Z, Trentacosti A, Miller M. Cat's claw inhibits TNFα production and scavenges free radicals: role in cytoprotection. *Free Radic Biol Med* 2000;29(1):71–78.

Sandoval M, Okuhama NN, Zhang X-J, Condezo LA, Lao J, Angeles FM, Bobrowski P, Miller MJS. Antiinflammatory and antioxidant activities of cat's claw (*Uncaria tomentosa* and *Uncaria guianensis*) are independent of their alkaloid content. *Phytomedicine* 2002;9(4):325–37.

Sandoval-Chacón M, Thompson JH, Lui X, Mannick E, Sadowska-Krowicka H, Charbonnet R, Clark D, Miller M. Anti-inflammatory actions of Cat's claw: the role of NF-kappaB. *Aliment Pharmacol Ther* 1998;12:1279–1289.

Senatore A, Cataldo A, Iaccarino FP, Elberti MG. Phytochemical and biological study of *Uncaria tomentosa*. *Bulletin de la Societe Italie Speriment* 1989;65:517–520.

Sheng Y, Pero R, Amiri A et al. Induction of apoptosis and inhibition of proliferation in human tumor cells treated with extracts of *Uncaria tomentosa*. *Anticancer Res* 1998;18:3363–3368.

Sheng Y, Li L, Holmgren C, Pero RW. DNA repair enhancement of aqueous extracts of *Uncaria tomentosa* in a human volunteer study. *Phytomedicine* 2001;8(4) 275–282.

Sheng Y, Bryngelsson C, Pero R. Enhanced DNA repair, immune function and reduced toxicity of C-Med-100®, a novel aqueous extract from *Uncaria tomentosa*. *J Ethnopharmacol* 2000a;69:115–126.

Sheng Y, Pero R, Wagner H. Treatment of chemotherapy-induced leukopenia in the rat model with aqueous extract from *Uncaria tomentosa*. *Phytomedicine* 2000b;7(2):137–143.

Shi JS, Huang B, Wu Q, Ren RX, Xie XL. Effects of rhynchophylline on motor activity of mice and serotonin and dopamine in rat brain. *Acta Pharm Sinico* 1992; 14(2):114–7.

Shi JS, Liu GX, Wu Q, Zhang W, Huang XN. Hypotensive and hemodynamic effects of isorhynchophylline in conscious rats and anesthetized dogs. *Chin J Pharmacol Toxicol.* 1989;3(3):205–10.

Shimada Y, Goto H, Itoh T, Sakakibara I, Kubo M, Sasaki H, Terasawa K. Evaluation of the protective effects of alkaloids isolated from the hooks and stems of *Uncaria sinensis* on glutamate-induced neuronal death in cultured cerebellar granule cells from rats. *J Pharm Pharmacol* 1999;51(6):715–22.

Spaulding-Albright N. A review of some herbal and related products commonly used in cancer patients. *J Am Diet Assoc* 1997;97:S208–15.

Stuppner H, Sturm S, Geisen G, Zillian U, Konwalinka G. A differential sensitivity of oxindole alkaloids to normal and leukemic cell lines. *Planta Medica*. 1993;59:Supplement,A583.

Stuppner H, Sturm S, Konwalinka G. HPLC analysis of the main oxindole alkaloids of *Uncaria tomentosa*. *Chromatographia* 1992;34:597–600.

Sun A-S, Liu G-X, Wang X-Y, Zhang W, Luang X-N. Effects of rhynchophylline on contraction of isolated rat uterus. [in Chinese]. *Ch J Pharm Tox* 1988;2(2):93–97.

Svendson O, Skydsgaard K. Test report, *Extratum Redicis Uncariae tomentosae*: 28-day oral rat toxicity study. Uppsala: Scantox; 1986. Cited in Reinhard K. *Uncaria tomentosa* (Willd.) D.C. Cat's claw, una de gato, or saventaro. *J Alternative Complement Med* 1999;5(2):143–51.

United States Congress (USC). Public Law 103–417: Dietary Supplement Health and Education Act of 1994. Washington, DC: 103rd Congress of the United States; 1994.

USC. See: United States Congress.

Wagner H, Proksch A, Vollmar A, Kreutzkamp B, Bauer J. In vitro phagocytosis stimulation by isolated plant materials in a chemoluminescence-phagocytosis model [in German]. *Planta Med* 1985a Apr;(2):139–44.

Wagner H, Kreutzkamp B, Jurcic K. The alkaloids of *Uncaria tomentosa* and their phagocytosis-stimulating action [in German]. *Planta Med* 1985b Oct;(5):419–23.

Williams JE. Review of antiviral and immunomodulating properties of plants of the Peruvian rainforest with a particular emphasis on Uña de gato and Sangre de grado. *Altern Med Rev* 2001 Dec;6(6):567–79.

Wirth C, Wagner H. Pharmacologically active procyanidines from the bark of *Uncaria tomentosa*. *Phytomedicine* 1997;4(3):265–266.

Wurm M, Kacani L, Laus G, Keplinger K, Dierich M. Pentacyclic oxindole alkaloids from *Uncaria tomentosa* induce human endothelial cells to release a lymphocyte-proliferation-regulating factor. *Planta Med* 1998;64:701–704.

Yano S, Horiuchi H, Horie S, Aimi N, Sakai S, Watanabe K. Ca2+ channel blocking effects of hirsutine, an indole alkaloid from *Uncaria* genus, in the isolated rat aorta. *Planta Med* 1991;57:403–5.

Yepez AM, de Ugaz OL, Alvarez CM, De Feo V, Aquino R, De Simone F, et al. Quinovic acid glycosides from *Uncaria guianensis*. *Phytochemistry* 1991;30(5):1635–7.

Zhang W, Liu GX, Huang XN. Effect of rhynchophylline on contraction of rabbit aorta. *Acta Pharmacol Sin* 1987;8(5):425–429.

Zhu Y, Guoxing HX. Negative chronotropic and inotropic effects of rhynchophylline and isorhynchophylline on isolated guinea pig arteria. *Chin J Pharmacol Toxicol* 1993;7(2):117–121.

Clinical Studies on Cat's Claw (*Uncaria guianensis* [Aubl.] Gmel.)

Anti-inflammatory

Author/Year	Subject	Design	Duration	Dosage	Preparation	Results/Conclusion
Piscoya *et al.*, 2001	Safety and efficacy for osteoarthritis (knee)	P, R, DB, PC, PG, MC n=45 men (30=cat's claw; 15=placebo); with symptomatic osteoarthritis (OA) of knee, experiencing pain for most of prior month and requiring NSAID therapy for 3 months prior to study, with knee pain on movement (45–75 years)	4 weeks 7-day washout for NSAIDs; 12 hours for analgesics	One, 100 mg capsule/day	Freeze-dried cat's claw water extract; material made for study	UG group had significant improvement in pain associated with activity and patient assessment scores determined after 1 week of trial (p<0.05). Further, UG group showed highly significant improvement of these indices and medical assessment scores at weeks 2 and 4 (p<0.001). There was significant improvement in all 3 indices with treatment at week 4, compared to baseline and week 1 (p<0.05). However, pain at rest or at night, and knee circumference, were not significantly altered in either placebo or UG group, and there was no significant difference in side effects in either group and no adverse effects in blood or liver function were observed. Authors conclude based on human trial and in vitro component of study that UG and UT are safe and effective antioxidants, and UG and UT are equally bioactive for treatment of OA.

Clinical Studies on Cat's Claw (*Uncaria tomentosa* [Willd.] DC.)—focusing on preparations standardized to carboxy alkyl esters (CAEs)

Immunomodulation

Author/Year	Subject	Design	Duration	Dosage	Preparation	Results/Conclusion
Lamm *et al.*, 2001	Immune system response to pneumonia vaccine	R, PC n=23 healthy caucasian males (40–60 years old)	2 months of treatment; evaluation at days 1, 30, 60, 180	700 mg/day (350 mg 2x/day) or placebo	C-Med-100® tablets (water soluble UT extract standardized to 8–10% CAEs)	UT group had elevated lymphocyte/neutrophil ratio at 2 months (p<0.05) and at 5 months showed no loss of immunity based on decay of 12 serotype pneumococcal antibody titers (p<0.01). Placebo group showed highly significant loss of immunity at 5 months. No toxic side effects were reported.
Sheng *et al.*, 2001	DNA repair, immune enhancement, and safety	R, PC n=12 healthy volunteers (mean age 44 years)	Baseline period of 3 weeks, then 8-week treatment	250 mg/day, or 350 mg/day, or placebo	C-Med-100® tablets	In both UT groups, there was 12–15% enhanced DNA repair (from 72–74% before treatment to 81–85% after treatment), as measured by alkaline elution, after 8 weeks of treatment (p<0.05). There was a tendency towards increased proliferation of phytohemagglutinin-induced lymphocyte proliferation, but results were not significant. No toxic responses were observed.
Sheng *et al.*, 2000a	Safety and immune enhancement	Volunteer supplement study n=4 apparently healthy adult males (32–58 years)	9 weeks Baseline then 6 weeks treatment	350 mg/day	C-Med-100® tablets	Subjects showed a significantly (p<0.05) increased level of white blood cells. No signs or symptoms of toxicity were observed.

KEY: C – controlled, **CAEs** – carboxy alkyl esters, **CC** – case-control, **CH** – cohort, **CI** – confidence interval, **Cm** – comparison, **CO** – crossover, **CS** - cross-sectional, **DB** – double-blind, **E** – epidemiological, **LC** – longitudinal cohort, **MA** – meta-analysis, **MC** – multi-center, **n** – number of patients, **O** – open, **OB** – observational, **OL** – open label, **OR** – odds ratio, **P** – prospective, **PB** – patient-blind, **PC** – placebo-controlled, **PG** – parallel group, **POAs** – pentacyclic oxindole alkaloids, **PS** – pilot study, **R** – randomized, **RC** – reference-controlled, **RCS** – retrospective cross-sectional, **RS** - retrospective, **S** – surveillance, **SB** – single-blind, **SC** – single-center, **TOAs** – tetracyclic oxindole alkaloids, **U** – uncontrolled, **UG** – *Uncaria guianensis*, **UP** – unpublished, **UT** – *Uncaria tomentosa*, **VC** – vehicle-controlled.

Clinical Studies on Cat's Claw (*Uncaria tomentosa* [Willd.] DC.)—focusing on preparations standardized to pentacyclic oxindole alkaloids (POAs) with no tetracyclic oxindole alkaloids (TOAs)

Anti-inflammatory

Author/Year	Subject	Design	Duration	Dosage	Preparation	Results/Conclusion
Mur et al., 2002	Safety and efficacy in active rhuematoid arthritis (RA)	Phase 1: R, DB, PC Phase 2: all participants received cat's claw extract n=40 patients with active RA (Steinbrocker functional class II or III) (> or = 20 years of age)	52 weeks total with assessment at weeks 4, 8, 16, 24, 36, 52: Phase 1: 24 weeks Phase 2: 28 weeks	One capsule 3x/day (total 60 mg/day)	Krallendorn® capsules (20 mg cat's claw extract per capsule, containing 14.7 mg/g POAs and no TOAs)	At 24 weeks UT group compared to placebo showed reduced number of painful joints (by 53.2% vs. 24.1%; p=0.044). UT group experienced fewer tender joints (p=0.001) decrease in Ritchie Index (p=0.002) and shorter period of morning stiffness (p=0.002), whereas placebo group experienced no significant change. At 52 weeks UT-UT group showed further reduction in number of tender joints and in Ritchie Index, while placebo-UT group had a decrease in the number of painful and swollen joints (p=0.003; p=0.007) and decrease in Ritchie Index (p=0.004) compared to values at end of Phase I (placebo).
Immodal, 1995, 2002	Rhuematoid arthritis (RA), adjuvant to conventional treatment	C, UP n=6 patients (2 in Steinbrocker class I/II, 4 in Steinbrocker class II/III)	24 months of cat's claw treatment with assessment at months 3, 6, 12, 18, 24, and 8 years after completion of cat's claw treatment	Months 1–24: 60 mL tea/day (3 mg alkaloids/day) 4 patients continued treatment on their own after 2 years controlled phase: 1–3 capsules daily	Krallendorn® tea and capsules	At 3 months 3 patients had an increase in pain, while the other 3 had reduced pain. At 6 months all patients experienced reduced pain and joint stiffness. At 12 months 3 were largely pain-free, 3 had reduced pain with some pain-free periods, and dosages of conventional medications were reduced. At 18 months all patients were pain free. The 2 patients in class I/II remained symptom-free for 5–7 years after cat's claw treatment, while class II/III patients remained symptom-free for 1–2 years after cat's claw treatment. No adverse effects were reported.
Immodal, 1995, 1999a	Ulcers and gastritis	C, OB, UP Case reports n=7 patients with stomach or duodenal ulcers (n=5) or gastritis (n=2)	4 months. Months 1–3: cat's claw treatment Month 4 observation only	Decoction of 1.5 g in 120 ml water taken on empty stomach in morning	Krallendorn® tea	All 5 ulcer patients were asymptomatic after an average of 10 days and discontinued antacid treatment. Both patients with recurrent gastritis were asymptomatic after an average of 3 days and also stopped antacid treatment. All patients remained asymptomatic 1 month after discontinuation of cat's claw.

Immunomodulation

Author/Year	Subject	Design	Duration	Dosage	Preparation	Results/Conclusion
Immodal, 1999a, 2002	Adjuvant to chemotherapy, radiation, and brain tumor resection	O, U, UP n=60	Varied: 12–31 months	60 mg/day	Krallendorn® drops	All patients reported greater vitality and fewer side effects from chemotherapy and radiation. Survival rates were not measurable since there were no controls.
Immodal, 1995, 2002	Adjuvant to chemotherapy, radiation, and surgery	U, UP n=22 patients with tumor diseases	12 months to 10 years	Tea: 60 ml/day Capsules: one capsule 1–3 x/day (20–60 mg/day)	Krallendorn® tea or Krallendorn® capsules	All patients showed increased vitality and fewer side effects. Partial remission in 5 patients, full remission in 13 patients, and prolonged survival time (>4 years in 7 patients). However, survival rates were not measurable, since there were no controls.
Immodal, 1995, 1999a, 2002	Adjuvant therapy for HIV patients	MC, O, U, UP n=44 patients in stages CDC A (n=16), CDC B (n=13), and CDC C (n=15)	12–60 months	1–6 capsules/day or equivalent amounts of drops or tea (20–120 mg/day capsules)	Krallendorn® capsules (n=41) or Drops (n=2) or Tea (n=1)	Cat's claw stabilized CD4-cell count in stage A patients and stabilized or increased it in stage B & C patients. A direct correlation was observed between CD4 cell count and total leukocyte and CD8 cell count. Symptoms decreased in stage B patients and disease progression was reduced in stage C patients. All patients experienced increased vitality and mobility. No adverse effects or drug interactions were observed.

KEY: **C** – controlled, **CAEs** – carboxy alkyl esters, **CC** – case-control, **CH** – cohort, **CI** – confidence interval, **Cm** – comparison, **CO** – crossover, **CS** - cross-sectional, **DB** – double-blind, **E** – epidemiological, **LC** – longitudinal cohort, **MA** – meta-analysis, **MC** – multi-center, **n** – number of patients, **O** – open, **OB** – observational, **OL** – open label, **OR** – odds ratio, **P** – prospective, **PB** – patient-blind, **PC** – placebo-controlled, **PG** – parallel group, **POAs** – pentacyclic oxindole alkaloids, **PS** – pilot study, **R** – randomized, **RC** – reference-controlled, **RCS** – retrospective cross-sectional, **RS** - retrospective, **S** – surveillance, **SB** – single-blind, **SC** – single-center, **TOAs** – tetracyclic oxindole alkaloids, **U** – uncontrolled, **UG** – *Uncaria guianensis*, **UP** – unpublished, **UT** – *Uncaria tomentosa*, **VC** – vehicle-controlled.

Immunomodulation (cont.)

Author/Year	Subject	Design	Duration	Dosage	Preparation	Results/Conclusion
Immodal, 1999a	Adjuvant therapy for HIV patients	O, U, UP n=14 patients with HIV or AIDS and a T4-cell count of 200–500 cells/mcL (6 also received AZT, 1 also received DDI)	1 year with assessments at months 0, 3, 6, 9, 12	2–3 capsules/day (40–60 mg/day)	Krallendorn® capsules	HIV-related symptoms were reduced. Slight increases were observed in heart beat, lymphocytes, uric acid, and in percent of T8 cells, as well as a decrease in granulocytes and a slight decrease in percent of T4 cells. Patients reported increased vitality.
Immodal, 1999a, 2002	Adjuvant therapy for HIV patients	RS, O, U, UP n=16 patients with HIV or AIDS	1–5.8 years	1–6 capsules/day (20–120 mg/day)	Krallendorn® capsules	Patients receiving antiretroviral therapy and cat's claw remained clinically stable and showed stable or increased CD4-cell counts. In those patients receiving cat's claw only, most remained clinically stable with stable CD4-cell counts. All patients reported increased vitality and mobility. No adverse effects or drug interactions were observed.

External Use

Author/Year	Subject	Design	Duration	Dosage	Preparation	Results/Conclusion
Immodal, 1995, 1999a, 2002	*Herpes simplex*	O, MC, U, UP n=17	17 days	Once daily	Krallendorn® topical preparations of root extract: spray, ointment, cream, or gel containing 8 mcg POA/mg	Pain was eliminated in 14 patients by day 3 and in all 17 patients by day 7. Lesions had healed completely in 9 patients by day 7 and in all 17 patients by day 17. No adverse effects were observed.
Immodal, 1995, 1999a, 2002	*Varicella zoster*	O, U, UP n=20	13 days	Low dose group (n=16): once daily; High dose group (n=4): every 2 hours during waking hours	Krallendorn® topical preparations of root extract: spray, ointment, or cream containing 8 mcg POA/mg	Low dose group: 15 of 16 were symptom free by day 7 and lesions had healed for 15 of 16 by day 13. High dose group: all had greatly reduced pain on day 2 and all were pain-free by day 4. Scabs had disappeared by day 5. No adverse effects were observed.

KEY: C – controlled, **CAEs** – carboxy alkyl esters, **CC** – case-control, **CH** – cohort, **CI** – confidence interval, **Cm** – comparison, **CO** – crossover, **CS** - cross-sectional, **DB** – double-blind, **E** – epidemiological, **LC** – longitudinal cohort, **MA** – meta-analysis, **MC** – multi-center, **n** – number of patients, **O** – open, **OB** – observational, **OL** – open label, **OR** – odds ratio, **P** – prospective, **PB** – patient-blind, **PC** – placebo-controlled, **PG** – parallel group, **POAs** – pentacyclic oxindole alkaloids, **PS** – pilot study, **R** – randomized, **RC** – reference-controlled, **RCS** – retrospective cross-sectional, **RS** - retrospective, **S** – surveillance, **SB** – single-blind, **SC** – single-center, **TOAs** – tetracyclic oxindole alkaloids, **U** – uncontrolled, **UG** – *Uncaria guianensis*, **UP** – unpublished, **UT** – *Uncaria tomentosa*, **VC** – vehicle-controlled.

Cayenne

Capsicum spp.

Capsicum annuum L. var. *annuum*; *C. annuum* L. var. *glabriusculum* (Dunal) Heiser & Pickersgill [syn. *C. frutescens* L.]; *C. baccatum* L.; *C. chinense* Jacq.
[Fam. *Solanaceae*]

OVERVIEW

Cayenne is marketed in the U.S. as a food, spice, and dietary supplement in tablets, capsules, and occasionally as a tincture. Common names for cayenne include cayenne pepper, chili pepper, paprika, red pepper, tabasco pepper, bird pepper, African bird pepper, piquin, aji pepper, Brown's pepper, Peruvian pepper, piris, habañero pepper, and bonnet pepper. Cayenne is one of the fastest growing botanical imports, accounting for approximately 12% of the total annual value of U.S. spice imports. New Mexico alone produces approximately 100 million pounds of dried peppers annually. Twenty-three percent of natural food store consumers purchased cayenne at least once during the first half of 1999. Preparations made from the oleoresin in cayenne, and the oleoresin's isolated constituent capsaicin, are used in topical, over-the-counter (OTC) drug products. Capsicum oleoresin topical analgesic lotions and creams, containing the pure compound capsaicin, are available OTC in three strengths (0.025%, 0.075%, and 0.25%) for the following uses: inflammation and pain due to shingles, pain associated with postherpetic neuralgia, rheumatoid arthritis, osteoarthritis, diabetic neuropathy, and post-surgical pain. Other off-label uses for these lotions and creams are to relieve pain associated with psoriasis, chronic neuralgia unresponsive to other forms of therapy, and intractable pruritus.

PRIMARY USES

External
Capsaicin preparations
- Neuralgia, postherpetic (acute and chronic pain)
- Neuropathy, diabetic
- Psoriasis
- Osteoarthritis

OTHER POTENTIAL USES

Internal
Cayenne preparations
- Peptic ulcer, prevention
- Gastrointestinal cytoprotective effect

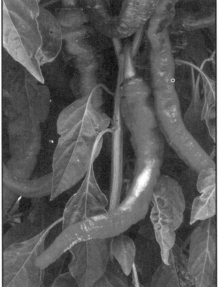

Photo © 2003 stevenfoster.com

External
Capsaicin preparations
- Fibromyalgia
- Cluster headache
- Chronic rhinopathy

PHARMACOLOGICAL ACTIONS

Protects stomach; protects against peptic ulcer; increases fibrinolytic activity; stimulates carbohydrate oxidation.

DOSAGE AND ADMINISTRATION

Internal

DRIED FRUIT: 30–120 mg, 3 times daily. As a digestive aid, 120–450 mg, 2–3 times daily with meals.

INFUSION: 240 ml boiling water poured over 0.5–1.0 teaspoon of cayenne, steeped for 10 minutes, 1 tablespoon drunk, diluted with hot water when needed.

TINCTURE: 0.3–1.0 ml, 3 times daily, or as needed [1:20 (*g/ml*), 60% ethanol].

OLEORESIN (STANDARDIZED): 1.2 mg.

External

Commission E recommends taking capsaicin for no longer than 2 days; 14 days must pass before a new application can be used on the same location. Longer use on the same area may cause damage to sensitive nerves. In a contradictory recommendation, the *Physicians Desk Reference* listing for Zostrix®, a cream that contains capsaicin, states that capsaicin-containing preparations must be used continuously for up to several weeks (i.e., 3 to 4 applications daily for 2–6 weeks may be required) to be effective.

LINIMENT: Hot oil emulsion containing dried cayenne powder or alcoholic tincture, applied locally by friction method.

OINTMENT OR CREAM (STANDARDIZED): Semiliquid preparation containing 0.02–0.05% capsaicinoids in an emulsion base, applied to affected area.

OLEORESIN (STANDARDIZED): 2.5% maximum strength.

POULTICE (STANDARDIZED): Semisolid paste or plaster which, when applied locally, produces 10–40 mcg capsaicinoids per cm^2.

Cayenne

Clinical Overview

TINCTURE (STANDARDIZED): 1:10 (*g/ml*), 90% ethanol, aqueous-alcoholic preparation containing 0.005–0.01% capsaicinoids, applied locally.

PURE CAPSAICIN CREAM OR OINTMENT: For diabetic neuropathy, 0.075% (pure) capsaicin cream or ointment is applied 4 times daily. For postherpetic neuralgia, 0.025% capsaicin cream or ointment is applied 4 times daily.

CONTRAINDICATIONS

Internal

Inhalation is contraindicated because capsaicin causes immediate bronchoconstriction. Ingestion is contraindicated in the following conditions: chronic irritable bowel (because capsaicin is a neural irritant and causes intestinal contractions), gastroduodenal ulcers (although there are conflicting results for duodenal ulcers), acute gastritis, pulmonary tuberculosis, and hemorrhoids.

External

Cayenne preparations are contraindicated for application on injured skin, for use near the eyes, and for individuals with allergies to cayenne preparations.

PREGNANCY AND LACTATION: No known restrictions.

ADVERSE EFFECTS

The German Commission E noted that in rare cases, a hypersensitivity rash (urticaria) could occur. Capsaicinoids are strongly irritating to mucosal membranes, and inhaling cayenne can produce a form of allergic alveolitis.

DRUG INTERACTIONS

External

Commission E reported no known drug interactions but warned: "No additional heat application." Angiotensin-converting enzyme (ACE) inhibitors can predispose patients to coughing with application of topical preparations containing capsaicin.

Internal

Dried powder can protect against aspirin-induced gastroduodenal mucosal injury when taken one-half hour before aspirin (although this is more of a pharmacological action, not a true interaction). Capsicum may interfere with monoamine oxidase inhibitors (MAOIs) and antihypertensive therapy due to its ability to increase catecholamine secretion. It also may increase hepatic metabolism of drugs (i.e., via elevated glucose-6-phosphate dehydrogenase and adipose lipoprotein lipase activity).

CLINICAL REVIEW

Internal

All but one of eight clinical studies involving a total of 1,405 participants demonstrated positive effects for indications including gastrointestinal and metabolic conditions. Five studies investigated gastrointestinal effects related to the regular dietary intake of cayenne powder vs. non-ingestion of cayenne. The gastrointestinal effects under examination included a protective effect against peptic ulcer, a gastroprotective effect following ingestion of aspirin, risk of gastric cancer, gastric or duodenal mucosal damage, and elevated metabolic rate. In addition, a hematology study investigated fibrinolytic activity.

External (Preparations Containing Pure Capsaicin)

Eighteen clinical studies on pure capsaicin preparations involving a total of 1,326 participants were reviewed. All but one of the studies demonstrated positive effects for indications including neuralgia, neuropathy, psoriasis, arthritis, and fibromyalgia. Of 14 double-blind, placebo-controlled (DB, PC) studies that included a total of 1,036 participants, two investigated topical capsaicin in painful diabetic neuropathy and showed statistically significant results related to pain status. Four DB, PC studies on osteoarthritis all yielded statistically significant results, thus confirming capsaicin's efficacy in pain reduction. Three DB, PC studies focused on the treatment of rheumatoid arthritis, with two studies reporting significant reduction in pain. One study reported a significant reduction in primary osteoarthritis pain, but no significant reduction in rheumatoid arthritis pain. Other conditions for which topical capsaicin was evaluated in DB, PC studies include notalgia paresthetica, fibromyalgia, psoriasis, and postherpetic neuralgia. Only one study, a 12-week, DB, PC study on chronic distal painful polyneuropathy, failed to demonstrate a trend in favor of treatment with capsaicin. In clinical trials, creams containing low concentrations (0.025–0.075%) of capsaicin have been shown to be effective in the treatment of postherpetic neuralgia and other pain syndromes, including cluster headache.

Cayenne

Capsicum spp.

Capsicum annuum L. var. *annuum*; *C. annuum* L. var. *glabriusculum* (Dunal) Heiser & Pickersgill [syn. *C. frutescens* L.]; *C. baccatum* L.; *C. chinense* Jacq.

[Fam. *Solanaceae*]

OVERVIEW

Cayenne consists of the dried fruits of various capsaicin-containing *Capsicum* species, including many cultivated peppers found in the home garden. Common names for cayenne include cayenne pepper, chili pepper, paprika, red pepper, tabasco pepper, bird pepper, African bird pepper, piquin, aji pepper, Brown's pepper, Peruvian pepper, piris, habañero pepper, and bonnet pepper. Preparations made from various parts of the pepper are used in creams and ointments, and are available in three strengths: 0.025%, 0.050%, and 0.075%. The dried fruits of cayenne are also used for treating various illnesses.

USES

External

Neuralgia (nerve pain) caused by herpes infections; diabetic neuropathy; psoriasis; osteoarthritis.

DOSAGE

Internal

DRIED FRUIT: 30–120 mg, 3 times daily. As a digestive aid, 120–450 mg, 2–3 times daily with meals.

TINCTURE: 0.3–1.0 ml, 3 times daily, or as needed [1:20 (*g/ml*), 60% ethanol].

External

Commercial creams that contain capsaicin (in dilutions of 0.025-0.75%), may require 3–4 applications daily for 2–6 weeks to be effective.

LINIMENT: Hot-oil emulsion containing dried cayenne powder or alcoholic tincture, applied locally by friction method.

OINTMENT OR CREAM (STANDARDIZED): Semiliquid preparation containing 0.02–0.05% capsaicinoids in an emulsion base, applied to affected area.

OLEORESIN (STANDARDIZED OIL-BASE PREPARATIONS): 2.5% maximum strength.

PURE CAPSAICIN CREAM OR OINTMENT: For diabetic neuropathy, apply 0.075% capsaicin cream or ointment, 4 times daily. For postherpetic neuralgia, apply 0.025% capsaicin cream or ointment, 4 times daily.

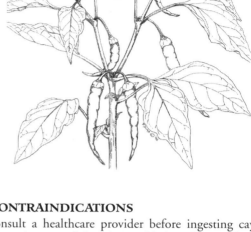

CONTRAINDICATIONS

Consult a healthcare provider before ingesting cayenne pepper in cases of chronic irritable bowel, gastroduodenal ulcer, acute gastritis, pulmonary tuberculosis, or hemorrhoids. Do not inhale cayenne-containing products because they are strongly irritating to mucous membranes. Cayenne preparations should not be applied to injured skin, used near the eyes, or taken by individuals allergic to cayenne preparations.

ADVERSE EFFECTS

In rare cases, a hypersensitivity rash (urticaria) can occur.

DRUG INTERACTIONS

Cayenne has been reported to interfere with monoamine oxidase (MAO) inhibitors and with blood pressure lowering medications (i.e., ACE inhibitors). It may increase the rate at which the liver metabolizes other drugs.

Comments

When using a dietary supplement, purchase it from a reliable source. For best results, use the same brand of product throughout the period of use. As with all medications and dietary supplements, please inform your healthcare provider of all herbs and medications you are taking. Interactions may occur between medications and herbs or even among different herbs when taken at the same time. Treat your herbal supplement with care by taking it as directed, storing it as advised on the label, and keeping it out of the reach of children and pets. Consult your healthcare provider with any questions.

AMERICAN BOTANICAL COUNCIL

The information contained on this sheet has been excerpted from *The ABC Clinical Guide to Herbs* © 2003 by the American Botanical Council (ABC). ABC is an independent member-based educational organization focusing on the medicinal use of herbs. For more detailed information about this herb please consult the healthcare provider who gave you this sheet. To order *The ABC Clinical Guide to Herbs* or become a member of ABC, visit their website at www.herbalgram.org.

Cayenne

Capsicum spp.

Capsicum annuum L. var. *annuum*; *C. annuum* L. var. *glabriusculum* (Dunal) Heiser & Pickersgill [syn. *C. frutescens* L.];
C. baccatum L.; *C. chinense* Jacq.
[Fam. *Solanaceae*]

OVERVIEW

Cayenne is marketed in the U.S. as a food, spice, and dietary supplement (in tablets, capsules, and occasionally, as a tincture). Common names for cayenne include cayenne pepper, chili pepper, paprika, red pepper, tabasco pepper, bird pepper, African bird pepper, piquin, aji pepper, Brown's pepper, Peruvian pepper, piris, habañero pepper, and bonnet pepper. Cayenne is one of the fastest growing botanical imports, accounting for approximately 12% of the total annual value of U.S. spice imports. New Mexico alone produces approximately 100 million pounds of dried peppers annually (Buzzanell and Gray, 1999). Twenty-three percent of natural food store consumers purchased cayenne at least once during the first half of 1999 (Richman and Witkowski, 1999). Preparations made from the oleoresin in cayenne and oleoresin's isolated constituent, capsaicin, are used in topical, over-the-counter (OTC) drug products. Capsicum oleoresin topical analgesic lotions and creams, containing the pure compound capsaicin, are available OTC in three strengths, 0.025%, 0.075%, and 0.25% (Palevitch and Craker, 1995; Rosenstein, 1999) for the following uses: inflammation and pain due to shingles, postherpetic neuralgia, rheumatoid arthritis, osteoarthritis, diabetic neuropathy, and post-surgical pain. Other uses for these lotions and creams that are not specified on the labels are to relieve pain associated with psoriasis, chronic neuralgia unresponsive to other forms of therapy, and intractable pruritus (Turkoski *et al.*, 1998).

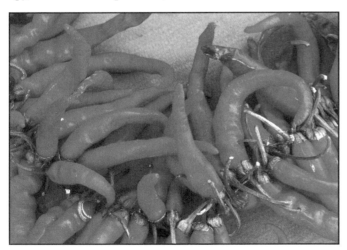

Photo © 2003 stevenfoster.com

DESCRIPTION

Cayenne preparations consist of the dried, ripe fruit, usually removed from the calyx, of various capsaicin-rich *Capsicum* species, such as *C. annuum* L. [Fam. *Solanaceae*], including a large number of varieties (Blumenthal, *et al.*, 2000). In Germany, pharmacopeial grade cayenne must contain no less than 0.4% total capsaicinoids, as determined by liquid chromatography (DAB, 1999). [NOTE: This herb was described under the monograph heading "Paprika (Cayenne)" in the German Commission E monographs (Blumenthal *et al.*, 1998).]

PRIMARY USES

External
Capsaicin preparations
Neuralgia
- Significant reduction of postherpetic neuralgia (Watson *et al.*, 1993; Peikert *et al.*, 1991; Bernstein *et al.*, 1989)

Neuropathy
- Improved pain relief for diabetic neuropathy (Capsaicin Study Group, 1991, 1992; Chad *et al.*, 1990)

Psoriasis
- Improvement in global evaluation, pruritus relief and combined psoriasis severity scores (Krogstad *et al.*, 1999; Ellis *et al.*, 1993)

Osteoarthritis
- Significant reduction in pain and joint tenderness (Altman *et al.*,1994; Schnitzer *et al.*, 1994; Weisman *et al.*, 1994; McCarthy and McCarty, 1992; Deal *et al.*, 1991)

OTHER POTENTIAL USES

Internal
Cayenne preparations
Gastrointestinal
- Cytoprotective effect (Yeoh *et al.*, 1995)
- Peptic ulcer, prevention (Kang *et al.*, 1995; Yeoh *et al.*, 1995)

External
Capsaicin preparations
- Fibromyalgia (McCarty *et al.*, 1994)
- Cluster headache (Marks *et al.*, 1993)
- Chronic rhinopathy (Eberle and Gluck, 1994)

DOSAGE

Internal
Crude Preparations
DRIED FRUIT: 30–120 mg, 3 times daily, (BHP, 1983). As a digestive aid, 120–450 mg, 2–3 times daily with meals (McKenna *et al.*, 1998). In a clinical study, 10 g powdered fruit was administered one time with meals to stimulate carbohydrate oxidation (Lim *et al.*, 1997). However, this dose is probably too high for regular consumption.

INFUSION: 240 ml boiling water is poured over 0.5–1.0 teaspoon of cayenne and steeped for 10 minutes; 1 tablespoon is drunk, diluted with hot water when needed (Hoffmann, 1992; Lust, 1974).

TINCTURE: 1:20 (*g/ml*), 60% ethanol: 0.3–1.0 ml, 3 times daily, or when needed (Boon and Smith, 1999; BPC, 1968; Hoffmann, 1992; Karnick, 1994).

Standardized Preparations
OLEORESIN: 1.2 mg (maximum dose) (MD), 1.8 mg (maximum daily dose) (MDD) (GSL, 1984–1994).

External
Crude Preparations
LINIMENT: Hot oil emulsion containing dried cayenne powder or alcoholic tincture is applied locally by friction method (Blumenthal *et al.*, 2000).

Standardized Preparations
OINTMENT OR CREAM: Semiliquid preparation containing 0.02–0.05% capsaicinoids in an emulsion base, is applied to affected area (Blumenthal *et al.*, 2000).

OLEORESIN: 2.5% maximum strength (GSL, 1984–1994 from Newall *et al.*, 1996) is applied locally.

POULTICE: Semisolid paste or plaster which, when applied locally, produces 10–40 mcg capsaicinoids per cm^2 (Blumenthal *et al.*, 2000).

TINCTURE: 1:10 (*g/ml*), 90% ethanol, aqueous-alcoholic preparation containing 0.005–0.01% capsaicinoids, is applied locally (Blumenthal *et al.*, 2000).

Pure Capsaicin Preparations
For diabetic neuropathy, 0.075% capsaicin cream or ointment is applied 4 times daily. For postherpetic neuralgia, 0.025% capsaicin cream or ointment is applied 4 times daily (Boon and Smith, 1999; Pizzorno and Murray, 1999).

DURATION OF ADMINISTRATION
External
Crude Preparations
Commission E recommends no longer than two days; 14 days must pass before a new application can be used in the same location. Longer use on the same area may cause damage to sensitive nerves (Blumenthal *et al.*, 1998).

Preparations Containing Pure Capsaicin
Three to four applications daily for 2–6 weeks may be required (Kruse and Eland, 1999).

WARNING: Preparations made from cayenne irritate the mucous membranes even in very low concentrations and cause a painful burning sensation. Patients should avoid the contact of cayenne preparations with mucous membranes, especially the eyes (Blumenthal *et al.*, 1998).

CHEMISTRY
Cayenne contains up to 1.5% pungent principles known as capsaicinoids (usually 0.1–1.0%), composed of 49–69% capsaicin, 22–36% dihydrocapsaicin, 7.0–7.4% nordihydrocapsaicin, 1–2% homodihydrocapsaicin, and 1–2% homocapsaicin (Bennet and Kirby, 1968; Duke, 1985; Wood, 1987). Other constituents of cayenne include carotenoids and ascorbic acid (vitamin C) (Bruneton, 1999).

PHARMACOLOGICAL ACTIONS
Internal
Human
Crude Preparations

Dried powder can protect against aspirin-induced gastroduodenal mucosal injury when taken 1/2 hour prior to aspirin (Brinker, 2001; Yeoh *et al.*, 1995); protects against peptic ulcer (Kang *et al.*, 1995); increases fibrinolytic activity (Visudhiphan *et al.*, 1982); stimulates carbohydrate oxidation (Lim *et al.*, 1997); gastrointestinal stimulant (Osol and Farrar, 1955).

Animal
Antigenotoxic and anticarcinogenic (Surh *et al.*, 1998).

External
Crude Preparations
Local hyperemic and local nerve-damaging activity (Blumenthal *et al.*, 1998); rubefacient and vasostimulant (BHP, 1996; Kapoor, 1990). Capsicum oleoresin does not uniformly induce neuropeptide activity as reliably as purified capsaicin. Clinical efficacy studies have shown purified capsaicin depletes the neuropeptide-active agent substance P, which is stored in sensory neurons, though no similar studies have been done on capsicum oleoresin. Capsascin also further blocks resynthesis of substance P (Cordell and Araujo, 1993).

Pure Capsaicin Preparations
Block pain neurotransmitter, substance P (Ellison *et al.*, 1997); dilate blood vessels, release histamine and reduce perfusion in lesional skin (Krogstad *et al.*, 1999); reduce and relieve pain; cause activation followed by desensitization of the sensory neurons on short- and long-term treatments (Ellison *et al.*, 1997; Munn *et al.*, 1997; Vickers *et al.*, 1998).

MECHANISM OF ACTION
Internal
- Intragastric capsaicin stimulates afferent nerve endings in animal tests, suggesting that its gastroprotective effects may be caused by increased mucosal blood flow rather than by prostaglandin production (Yeoh *et al.*, 1995).
- Cayenne affects the cardiovascular system, reducing triglyceride levels and platelet aggregation, and increasing fibrinolytic activity (Pizzorno and Murray, 1999).
- Reduces serum triglyceride levels without an alteration in serum cholesterol or pre-β-lipoproteins, and stimulates lipid mobilization from adipose tissue (Boon and Smith, 1999).
- Increases catecholamine (plasma epinephrine and norepinephrine concentration) levels (Barna and Sreter, 1986; Lim *et al.*, 1997).
- Inhibits lipid peroxidation and myeloperoxidase activity in ethanol-induced gastric mucosal lesions; thereby demonstrating gastroprotective activity, which may be useful in chemoprevention (Park *et al.*, 2000).
- Vanilloid (capsaicin) receptors act in nonspecific manner (not specifically as previously believed) to activate sensory neurons. Capsaicin and the protons lower the heat threshold of the receptor, while it is the heat (<48°C) that opens the channel pore of the vanilloid receptor neurons (Szallasi and Blumberg, 1999).

External
Capsaicin Preparations
- Activate nociceptive fibers, which induces the release of excitatory neurotransmitters (substance P, N-methyl-D-asparic acid), bind to specific vanilloid (capsaicin) receptors, and its effects are reversible (Szallasi and Blumberg, 1999; Fusco and Giacovazzo, 1997; Lotz, 1994).
- Induce a selective analgesic effect by depleting substance P, a neuropeptide of 11 amino acids that mediates the transmission and modulation of pain impulses from the peripheral nerves to the spinal column. Capsaicin initially stimulates substance P release from peripheral sensory, C-type nerve fibers, then prevents its reuptake, and also blocks its transport within the neuron, which causes its eventual depletion, resulting in analgesia. The depletion of substance P initially takes one to three days, though with continued use the analgesic effect may last for weeks (Boon and Smith, 1999; Fusco and Giacovazzo, 1997; Tyler, 1992).

CONTRAINDICATIONS
Internal
Crude Preparations
Inhalation is contraindicated due to immediate bronchoconstriction caused by capsaicin (Fuller *et al.,* 1985). Ingestion is contraindicated in cases of chronic irritable bowel due to neural irritant and intestinal contraction properties of capsaicin (Buck and Burks, 1986), gastroduodenal ulcers, acute gastritis, pulmonary tuberculosis, and hemorrhoids (But *et al.,* 1997). However, a randomized, comparison clinical study did not find gastric mucosal damage in patients with duodenal ulcers who consumed cayenne (Kumar *et al.,* 1984).

External
Cayenne preparations are contraindicated for application on injured skin, allergies to cayenne preparations (Blumenthal *et al.,* 1998), or use near the eyes (Brinker, 2001).

PREGNANCY AND LACTATION: No known restrictions (McGuffin *et al.,* 1997).

ADVERSE EFFECTS
Commission E noted that in rare cases, a hypersensitivity reaction (urticaria) can occur (Blumenthal *et al.,* 1998). Capsaicinoids are strongly irritating to mucosal membranes and inhalation of cayenne can produce a form of allergic alveolitis.

DRUG INTERACTIONS
External
Commission E reported no drug interactions are known, but included the following note: "No additional heat application" (Blumenthal *et al.,* 1998). Angiotensin-converting enzyme (ACE) inhibitors can predispose patients to coughing with application of topical preparations containing capsaicin according to human case reports (Brinker, 2001).

Internal
CRUDE HERB: Capsicum may interfere with monoamine oxidase inhibitors (MAOIs) and antihypertensive therapy (increased catecholamine secretion), and may increase the hepatic metabolism of drugs (glucose-6-phosphate dehydrogenase and adipose lipoprotein lipase activity elevated) (Newall *et al.,* 1996). In an animal study (rabbits), theophylline absorption was enhanced when administered before or simultaneously with cayenne (Bouraoui *et al.,* 1988).

AMERICAN HERBAL PRODUCTS ASSOCIATION (AHPA) SAFETY RATING
CLASS 2D: External: Contraindicated on injured skin or near eyes.

CLASS 1: Internal: Can be safely consumed when used appropriately. NOTE: Excessive doses may cause gastrointestinal irritation in sensitive individuals (McGuffin *et al.,* 1997).

REGULATORY STATUS
AUSTRIA: Official in the *Austrian Pharmacopoeia,* ÖAB 1991 (Wichtl, 1997).

CANADA: Topical liniments, lotions, and plasters containing capsicum oleoresin or purified capsaicin are schedule OTC (over-the-counter) drugs requiring pre-market authorization and assignment of a Drug Identification Number (DIN) (Health Canada, 2001).

FRANCE: Topical preparations are approved for relieving minor articular pain in *French Pharmacopoeia,* Ph.Fr. X (Bradley, 1992; Reynolds *et al.,* 1993).

GERMANY: Topical preparations are approved nonprescription drugs of the Commission E monographs (Blumenthal *et al.,* 1998). Dried ripe fruit is official in the *German Pharmacopoeia* (DAB, 1999). Dried ripe fruit for preparation of hydro-alcoholic mother tincture and liquid dilutions is an official drug of the *German Homoeopathic Pharmacopoeia* (GHP, 1993).

ITALY: Official in *Italian Pharmacopoeia* (Newall *et al.,* 1996).

JAPAN: Dried fruit and powdered dried fruit are both official in the *Pharmacopoeia of Japan* (JSHM, 1993).

SWEDEN: Topical capsaicin cream is an approved non-prescription drug (MPA, 1997). No capsicum products are listed in the Medical Products Agency (MPA) "Authorized Natural Remedies" (MPA, 2001).

SWITZERLAND: Official in *Swiss Pharmacopoeia,* Ph.Helv.VII (Wichtl, 1997). External-use plasters containing cayenne and cayenne extract are nonprescription drugs, with sale limited to pharmacies and drugstores (Morant and Ruppanner, 2001).

U.K.: Capsicum oleoresin and water-soluble capsicum oleoresin are herbal medicines specified in the *General Sale List,* Schedule 1 (medicinal products requiring a full product license), Table B (external use only) (GSL, 1995).

U.S.: Generally recognized as safe (GRAS) (US FDA, 1998). Dietary supplement (USC, 1994). Capsicum oleoresin and purified capsaicin are safe and effective for use as OTC external analgesics (US FDA, 1979; US FDA, 1983).

CLINICAL REVIEW
A total of 26 clinical trials conducted on cayenne and capsaicin are summarized in the following tables, "Clinical Studies on Cayenne" and "Clinical Studies on Capsaicin Preparations." All but one of these studies (López-Carrillo *et al.,* 1994), demonstrated positive effects for indications including gastrointestinal and metabolic conditions. Five studies investigated gastrointestinal effects related to the regular dietary intake of cayenne powder vs. non-ingestion of cayenne including a protective effect against peptic ulcer (Kang *et al.,* 1995), a gastroprotective effect following ingestion of aspirin (Yeoh *et al.,* 1995), risk of gastric cancer (Lopez-Carrillo *et al.,* 1994), gastric or duodenal mucosal damage (Graham *et al.,* 1988; Kumar *et al.,* 1984), and elevated metabolic rate (Henry and Emery, 1986). A hematology study found significantly higher fibrinolytic activity in Thai subjects who con-

sumed cayenne regulary, compared with American subjects (Visudhiphan *et al.*, 1982).

Table 2, "Clinical Studies on Capsaicin Preparations," summarizes 18 studies involving a total of 1,326 participants, evaluating the external use of preparations containing pure capsaicin. All but one of the studies (Low *et al.*, 1995) demonstrated positive effects for indications including neuralgia, neuropathy, psoriasis, arthritis, and fibromyalgia. The table includes 14 double-blind, placebo-controlled (DB, PC) studies involving a total of 1,036 participants. Two DB, PC studies investigated topical capsaicin in painful diabetic neuropathy, with statistically significant results related to pain status (Capsaicin Study Group, 1992; Chad *et al.*, 1990). Osteoarthritis was the subject of four DB, PC studies, all with statistically significant results confirming capsaicin's efficacy in pain reduction (Altman *et al.*, 1994; Deal *et al.*, 1991; McCarthy and McCarty, 1992; Schnitzer *et al.*, 1994). Three DB, PC studies focused on the treatment of rheumatoid arthritis, with two studies reporting significant reduction in pain (Deal *et al.*, 1991; Weisman *et al.*, 1994). One study reported a significant reduction in primary osteoarthritis pain, but no significant reduction in rheumatoid arthritis pain (McCarthy and McCarty, 1992). Other topics investigated with topical capsaicin in DB, PC studies include notalgia paresthetica (Wallengren and Klinker, 1995), fibromyalgia (McCarty *et al.*, 1994), psoriasis (Ellis *et al.*, 1993), and postherpetic neuralgia (Watson *et al.*, 1993). Only one study did not demonstrate a trend in favor of treatment with capsaicin. This was a 12-week, DB, PC study investigating chronic distal painful polyneuropathy (Low *et al.*, 1995). Creams containing low concentrations (0.025–0.075%) of capsaicin have been shown in clinical trials to be effective in the treatment of postherpetic neuralgia (Bernstein *et al.*, 1987; Bernstein *et al.*, 1989; Menke and Heins, 1999; Peikert *et al.*, 1991; Watson *et al.*, 1988; Watson *et al.*, 1993), diabetic neuropathy (Basha and Whitehouse, 1991; Tandan *et al.*, 1992), and other pain syndromes, including cluster headache (Marks *et al.*, 1993).

BRANDED PRODUCTS

Axsain®: GenDerm Corporation / 4343 East Camelback Road / Phoenix, Arizona 85012 / U.S.A. Cream product with 0.075% capsaicin. This product is no longer available.

Capsig®: Schering-Plough / 2000 Galloping Hill Road / Kenilworth, NJ 07033 / U.S.A. / Tel: (908) 298-4000 / www.sch-plough.com. Cream with 0.025% capsaicin. This product is no longer available.

Chili powder (no product name specified): KNP Trading Pte Ltd, 50 Senoko Drive / Singapore 758 232 / Tel: 65-257 6916 / Fax: 65-753 6916 / www.knp-housebrand.com. Chili powder containing 478 ppm capsaicin.

Saemaul Kongjang 1: No product information available.

Zostrix®-HP: GenDerm Corporation. Cream product with 0.075% capsaicin.

REFERENCES

Altman R, Aven A, Holmberg C *et al*. Capsaicin cream 0.025% as monotherapy for osteoarthritis: a double-blind study. *Semin Arthritis Rheum* 1994;23(No. 6 Suppl 3):25–33.

Barna J, Sreter F. Effect of chronically administered large amount of "sweet" paprika on some muscle characteristics. *Acta Aliment* 1986;15:299–305.

Basha K, Whitehouse F. Capsaicin: a therapeutic option for painful diabetic neuropathy. *Henry Ford Hosp Med J* 1991; 39(2):138–40.

Bennet D, Kirby G. Constitution and biosynthesis of capsaicin. *J Chem Soc C* 1968;442–6.

Berger A, Henderson M, Nadoolman W, *et al*. Oral capsaicin provides temporary relief for oral mucositis pain secondary to chemotherapy/radiation therapy. *J Pain Symptom Manage* 1995;10(3):243–8.

Bernstein J, Bickers D, Dahl M, Roshal J. Treatment of chronic postherpetic neuralgia with topical capsaicin. A preliminary study. *J Am Acad Dermatol* 1987; 17(1):93–6.

Bernstein J, Korman N, Bickers D, Dahl M, Millikan L. Topical capsaicin treatment of chronic postherpetic neuralgia. *J Am Acad Dermatol* 1989; 21(2 Pt 1):265–70.

BHP. See: *British Herbal Pharmacopoeia*.

Blumenthal M, Busse WR, Goldberg A, Gruenwald J, Hall T, Riggins CW, Rister RS (eds.). Klein S, Rister RS (trans.). *The Complete German Commission E Monographs—Therapeutic Guide to Herbal Medicines*. Austin, TX: American Botanical Council; Boston: Integrative Medicine Communication; 1998; 178.

Blumenthal M, Goldberg A, Brinckmann J (eds.). *Herbal Medicine: Expanded Commission E Monographs*. Newton, MA: Integrative Medicine Communications; 2000; 52–6.

Boon H, Smith M. *The Botanical Pharmacy: The Pharmacology of 47 Common Herbs*. Kingston, Ontario, Canada: Quarry Health Books; 1999;56–61.

Bouraoui A, Toumi A, Mustapha H, Brazier J. Effects of capsicum fruit on theophylline absorption and bioavailability in rabbits. *Drug-Nutrient Interact* 1988;5:345–50.

BPC. See: *British Pharmaceutical Codex*.

Bradley P (ed.). *British Herbal Compendium*, Vol. 1. Dorset, UK: British Herbal Medicine Association 1992;174–6.

Brinker F. *Herb Contraindications and Drug Interactions*, 3rd ed. Sandy, OR: Eclectic Medical Publications; 2001;57–59.

British Herbal Pharmacopoeia (BHP). Cayenne monograph. Exeter, U.K.: British Herbal Medicine Association; 1996;55–6.

British Herbal Pharmacopoeia (BHP). Cayenne monograph. Keighley, UK: British Herbal Medicine Association; 1983.

British Pharmaceutical Codex (BPC). London, UK: The Pharmaceutical Press; 1968.

Bruneton, J. *Pharmacogonosy, Phytochemistry, Medicinal Plants*, 2nd ed. Hatton, C.K (trans.). Paris: Intercept, Ltd.; 1999.

Buck S, Burks T. The neuropharmacology of capsaicin: review of some recent observations. *Pharmacol Rev* 1986;38(3):179–226.

But P, Kimura T, Guo J, Sung C (eds.). *International Collation of Traditional and Folk Medicine*, Vol. 2, Northeast Asia, Part II. River Edge, NJ: World Scientific Publishing, Co; 1997;138–9.

Buzzanell P, Gray F. The spice market in the United States: Recent developments and prospects. Economic Research Service, U.S. Department of Agriculture; Agricultural Information Bulletin No. 709. 1999.

Capsaicin Study Group. Effect of treatment with capsaicin on daily activities of patients with painful diabetic neuropathy. *Diabetes Care* 1992;15(2):159–65.

Capsaicin Study Group. Treatment of painful diabetic neuropathy with topical capsaicin. *Arch Intern Med* 1991;151:2225–9.

Chad D, Aronin N, Lundstrom R *et al*. Does capsaicin relieve the pain of diabetic neuropathy? *Pain* 1990;42:387–8.

Cordell G, Araujo O. Capsaicin: identification, nomenclature, and pharmacotherapy. *Ann Pharmacother* 1993;27:330–6.

DAB. See: *Deutsches Arzneibuch*.

Deal C, Schnitzer T, Lipstein E, *et al*. Treatment of arthritis with topical capsaicin: a double-blind trial. *Clin Therapeut* 1991;13(3):383–395.

Desai H *et al*. Effect of red chilli powder on DNA content of gastric aspirates. *Gut* 1973;14:974–6.

Deutsches Arzneibuch (DAB). Stuttgart, Germany: Deutscher Apotheker Verlag. 1999.

Duke J. *CRC Handbook of Medicinal Herbs*. Boca Raton, FL: CRC Press, Inc; 1985;98–9.

Eberle E, Gluck U. Clinical experiences with local capsaicin treatment of chronic rhinopathy. [in German]. *HNO* 1994;42(11):665–9.

Ellis C, Berberian B, Sulica V, *et al*. A double-blind evaluation of topical capsaicin in pruritic psoriasis. *J Am Acad Dermat* 1993;29:438–42.

Ellison N, Loprini C, Kugler J, *et al*. Phase III placebo-controlled trial of capsaicin cream in the management of surgical neuropathic pain in cancer patients. *J Clin Oncol* 1997;15(8):2974–80.

Fuller R, Dixon C, Barnes P. Bronchoconstrictor response to inhaled capsaicin in humans. *J Appl Physiol* 1985;58(4):1080–4.

Fusco B, Alessandri M. Analgesic effect of capsaicin in idiopathic trigeminal neuralgia. *Anest Analg* 1992;74:375–377.

Fusco BM Giacovazzo M. Peppers and pain: The promise of capsaicin. *Drugs* 1997;53(6):909–14.

General Sale List (GSL). Statutory Instrument 1995 No. 3216 The Medicines (Products Other Than Veterinary Drugs) Amendment Order 1995. London, U.K.: Her Majesty's Stationery Office (HMSO). 1995.

General Sale List (GSL). Statutory Instrument (S.I.). The Medicines (Products other than Veterinary Drugs). London, UK: Her Majesty's Stationery Office; 1984; S.I. No. 769, as amended 1985; S.I. No. 1540, 1990; S.I. No. 1129, 1994; S.I. No. 2410.

German Homeopathic Pharmacopoeia (GHP), 1st ed. 1978 with 5 supplements through 1991. Translation of the German "*Homöopathisches Arzneibuch* (HAB 1) Amtliche

Ausgabe." Stuttgart, Germany: Deutscher Apotheker Verlag; 1993;275–7.

GHP. See: *German Homeopathic Pharmacopoeia.*

Graham D, Smith J, Opekum A. Spicy food and the stomach: Evaluation by videoendoscopy. *JAMA* 1988;260(23):3473–5.

GSL. See: *General Sale List.*

Health Canada. *Drug Product Database (DPD) Product Information.* Ottawa, Ontario: Health Canada Therapeutic Products Programme; 2001.

Henry C, Emery B. Effect of spiced food on metabolic rate. *Human Nutr Clin Nutr* 1986;40(2):165–8.

Hoffmann D. *The New Holistic Herbal.* Rockport, MA: Element, Inc;. 1992;189.

Japanese Standards for Herbal Medicines (JSHM). Tokyo, Japan: Yakuji Nippo, Ltd; 1993;59–60.

JSHM. See: *Japanese Standards for Herbal Medicines.*

Kang J, Yeoh K, Chia H, *et al.* Chili – protective factor against peptic ulcer? *Dig Dis Sci* 1995;40(3)576–9.

Kapoor L. *CRC Handbook of Ayurvedic Medicinal Plants.* Boca Raton, FL: CRC Press; 1990; 98.

Karnick C. *Pharmacopoeial Standards of Herbal Plants,* Vol. 1. Delhi, India: Sri Satguru Publications; 1994;79–80.

Krogstad A, Lönnroth P, Larson G, Wallin B. Capsaicin treatment induces histamine release and perfusion changes in psoriatic skin. *Brit J Derm* 1999;141:87–93.

Kruse L, Eland J. *Capsaicin (Axsain®, Capsaicin-P, Zostrix® HP, Dolorac): Healthcare Professional Version.* Iowa City, IA: The University of Iowa College of Nursing; 1999 available at: <http://www.nursing.uiowa.edu/sites/PedsPain/Topicals/CAPSAIte.htm>.

Kumar N, Vij C, Sarin S, Anand B. Do chilies influence healing of duodenal ulcer? *Br Med J* 1984;288:1803–1804.

Lim K, Yoshioka M, Kikuzato S, *et al.* Dietary red pepper ingestion increases carbohydrate oxidation at rest and during exercise in runners. *Med Sci Sports Exerc* 1997 March;29(3):355–61.

Locock R. Capsicum. *Can Pharm J* 1985;118:517–9.

López-Carrillo L, Avila M, Dubrow R. Chili pepper consumption and gastric cancer in Mexico: A case-control study. *Am J Epidem* 1994;139(3):264–71.

Lotz M. 1994. Experimental models of arthritis: Identification of substance P as a therapeutic target and use of capsaicin to manage joint pain and inflammation. *Semin Arthritis Rheum* 1994; 23(6)Suppl 3:10–17.

Low P, Opfer-Gehrking T, Dyck P, Litchy W, O'Brien P. Double-blind, placebo-controlled study of the application of capsaicin cream in chronic distal painful polyneuropathy. *Pain* 1995;62:163–8.

Lust J. *The Herb Book.* New York, NY: Bantam Books; 1974;151–2.

Marks D, Rapoport A, Padla D, *et al.* A double-blind placebo-controlled trial of intranasal capsaicin for cluster headache. *Cephalalgia* 1993;13(2):114–6.

McCarthy G, McCarty D. Effect of topical capsaicin in the therapy of painful osteoarthritis of the hands. *J Rheumatol* 1992;19:604–7.

McCarty D, Csuka M, McCarthy G, Trotter D. Treatment of pain due to fibromyalgia with topical capsaicin: a pilot study. *Semin Arthritis Rheum* 1994;23(No. 6, Suppl 3):41–7.

McGuffin M, Hobbs C, Upton R, Goldberg A (eds.). *American Herbal Products Association's Botanical Safety Handbook.* Boca Raton, FL: CRC Press; 1997;23.

McKenna D, Hughes K, Jones K (eds.). *Natural Dietary Supplements: A Desktop Reference.* Marine on St. Croix, MN: Institute for Natural Products Research; 1998.

Medical Products Agency (MPA). *Läkemedelsmonografi: Capsina (kapsaicin).* Uppsala, Sweden: Medical Products Agency; 1997.

Medical Products Agency (MPA). *Naturläkemedel: Authorised Natural Remedies* (as of January 24, 2001). Uppsala, Sweden: Medical Products Agency; 2001.

Menke J, Heins J. Treatment of postherpetic neuralgia. *J Am Pharm Assoc (Wash)* 1999; 39(2):217–21.

Morant J, Ruppanner H (eds.). Patienteninformation: Democal Kreuz-Pflaster D. In: *Arzneimittel-Kompendium der Schweiz®* 2001. Basel, Switzerland: Documed AG. 2001.

MPA. See: Medical Products Agency.

Munn S, Burrows N, Abadia-Molina F. The effect of topical capsaicin on substance P immunoreactivity: a clinical trial and immunohistochemical analysis [letter]. *Acta Derm Venereol (Stockh)* 1997; 77(2):158–9.

Newall C, Anderson L, Phillipson J. *Herbal Medicines: A Guide for Health-care Professionals.* London, UK: The Pharmaceutical Press; 1996;60–61.

Osol A, Farrar G. *The Dispensatory of the United States of America,* 25th edition. Philadelphia, PA: Lippincott; 1955;239–42.

Paice J, Ferrans C, Lashley F, *et al.* Topical capsaicin in the management of HIV-associated peripheral neuropathy. *J Pain Symptom Manage* 2000;19(1):45–52.

Palevitch D, Craker L. Nutritional and medical importance of red peppers (*Capsicum* spp.). *J Herbs Spices Med Plants* 1995; 3(2):55–83.

Park JS, Choi MA, Kim BS, *et al.* Capsaicin protects against ethanol-induced oxidateive injury in the gastric mucosa of rats. *Life Sci* 2000;67: 3087–93.

Peikert A, Hentrich M, Ochs G. Topical 0.025% capsaicin in chronic post-herpetic neuralgia: efficacy, predictors of response and long-term course. *J Neurol* 1991; 238(8):452–6.

Pimparkar B *et al.* Effects of commonly used spices on human gastric secretion. *J Assoc Physicians India* 1972;20:901–10.

Pizzorno JE, Murray MT, editors. Capsicum frutescens. In: *Textbook of Natural Medicine,* Vol. 1, 2nd ed. New York: Churchill Livingstone; 1999;629–32.

Reynolds JEF, Pafitt K, Parsons AV, Sweetman SC (eds.). *Martindale: The Extra Pharmacopoeia,* 30th edition. London, U.K.: The Pharmaceutical Press. 1993;899.

Richman A, Witkowski J. 17th annual consumer survey. *Whole Foods* 1999 Aug;33–8.

Rosenstein E. Topical agents in the treatment of rheumatic disorders. *Complement Alternative Ther Rheum Dis I* 1999;25(4):899–918.

Schnitzer T, Morton C, Coker S. Topical capsaicin therapy for osteoarthritis pain: Achieving a maintenance regimen. *Semin Arthritis Rheum* 1994;23(No. 6 Suppl 3):34–40.

Surh Y, Lee E, Lee J. Chemoprotective properties of some pungent ingredients present in red pepper and ginger. *Mut Res* 1998;402:259–67.

Szallasi A, Blumberg, PM. Vanilloid (capsaicin) receptors and mechanisms. *Pharmacol Rev* 1999;51(2):159–95.

Tandan R, Lewis G, Krusinski PB, Badger GB, Fries TJ. Topical capsaicin in painful diabetic neuropathy. Controlled study with long-term follow-up. *Diabetes Care* 1992; 15(1):8–14.

Turkoski B, Lance B, Janosik J. *Drug Information Handbook for Nursing.* Hudson, Ohio: Lexi-Comp Inc. 1998;1475.

Tyler, VE. *The Honest Herbal: A Sensible Guide to the Use of Herbs and Related Remedies,* 3rd ed. New York: Pharmaceutical Products Press; 1992;79–80.

United States Congress (USC). Public Law 103–417: Dietary Supplement Health and Education Act of 1994. Washington, DC: 103rd Congress of the United States; 1994.

United States Food and Drug Administration (U.S. FDA). *Code of Federal Regulations,* Title 21, Part 182 – Substances Generally Recognized as Safe. Washington, DC: Office of the Federal Register National Archives and Records Administration; 1998;427–33.

United States Food and Drug Administration (U.S. FDA). *Code of Federal Regulations 21* (CFR 21). Proposed monographs on analgesic drug products for over-the-counter (OTC) human use. Washington, D.C.: Office of the Federal Register National Archives and Records Administration; 1979;44:69804–5; 1983;48:5852–69.

US FDA. See: United States Food and Drug Administration.

USC. See: United States Congress.

Vickers E, Cousins M, Walker S, Chisolm K. Analysis of 50 patients with atypical odontalgia. *Oral Surg Oral Med Oral Pathol Oral Radiol Endod* 1998;85:24–32.

Visudhiphan S, Poolsuppasit S, Piboonnukarintro S, *et al.* The relationship between high fibrinolytic activity and daily capscium ingestion in Thais. *Am J Clin Nutr* 1982;35:1452–58.

Wallengren J, Klinker M. Successful treatment of notalgia paresthetica with topical capsaicin: Vehicle-controlled, double-blind, crossover study. *J Am Academy Dermatol* 1995;32(No. 2, Part 1)287–9.

Watson C, Tyler K, Bickers D *et al.* A randomized vehicle-controlled trial of topical capsaicin in the treatment of postherpetic neuralgia. *Clin Ther* 1993; 15(3):510–26.

Watson C, Evans R, Watt V. Post-herpetic neuralgia and topical capsaicin. *Pain* 1988;33(3):333–40.

Watson C, Evans R. The postmastectomy pain syndrome and topical capsaicin: a randomized trial. *Pain* 1992;51(3):375–9.

Weisman M, Hagaman C, Yaksh T, Lotz M. Preliminary findings on the role of neuropeptide suppression by topical agents in the management of rheumatoid arthritis. *Semin Arthritis Rheum* 1994;23(No 6, Suppl 3):18-24.

Westerman R, Roberts R, Kotzmann R, *et al.* Effects of topical capsaicin on normal skin and affected dermatomes in *Herpes zoster. Clin Exp Neurol* 1988;25:71–84.

Wichtl M (ed.). *Tea Derived Drugs and Phytopharmaceuticals,* 3rd Edition: *A pocket reference for the evidence-based clinical practice.* [in German]. Stuttgart, Germany: Wissenschaftliche Verlagsgesellschaft GmbH; 1997;123–5.

Willard T. *The Wild Rose Scientific Herbal.* Calgary, Alberta: Wild Rose College of Natural Healing; 1991;68–73.

Wood A. Determination of the pungent principles of chilies and ginger by reversed-phase high-performance liquid chromatography with use of a single standard substance. *Flavour Fragrance J* 1987;2:1–12.

Yeoh K, Kang J, Yap I, *et al.* Chili protects against aspirin-induced gastroduodenal mucosal injury in humans. *Dig Dis Sci* 1995;40(3):580–3.

Clinical Studies on Cayenne (*Capsicum* spp.)

Internal Use of Cayenne Crude Herb Preparations

Author/Year	Subject	Design	Duration	Dosage	Preparation	Results/Conclusion
Lim et al., 1997	Metabolic elevation of plasma catecholamine levels and alteration of energy substrate utilization	R n=8 male middle- and long-distance runners (mean age 20.8 years)	1 dose on 2 occasions, separated by 1 week, or placebo	Experimental meal with or without 1 dose of 10 g pepper	Dried hot red pepper powder (Saemaul Kongjang 1) containing 0.3% capsaicin	Capsicum increased carbohydrate oxidation for energy substrate more than meal without capsicum, at rest and during exercise. Subjects had meal (2,720 kilojoules) with or without 10 g capsicum. During rest (2.5 hours after meal) and exercise (pedaling for 1 hour), expired gasses and venous blood were collected. Capsicum significantly elevated respiratory quotient (p<0.05) and blood lactate levels (p<0.05) at rest and during exercise. Capsicum group had significantly higher plasma epinephrine and norepinephrine levels 30 minutes after meal, compared to patients without capsicum-containing meal.
Kang et al., 1995	Gastrointestinal amount of chili in patients with peptic ulcer	Cm n=190: 103 peptic ulcer patients; 87 controls without peptic ulcer or dyspepsia	2 years prior to interviews with standard questionnaire	Peptic ulcer group, median amount 312 teaspoons per month; control group, median amount 834 teaspoons per month	Dietary intake of fresh chilis, dried chili powder, chili sauces and dips, curry powder, etc.	Compared to controls, ulcer patients ingested chili less frequently and in smaller portions during the 2 years before diagnosis. The odds ratio of having peptic ulcer disease was 0.47 (95% confidence intervals: 0.25–0.89) for subjects who ingested chili more frequently and in larger amounts. Chili use appears to have a protective effect against peptic ulcer disease.
Yeoh et al., 1995	Gastrointestinal (protective effect of chili against acute gastroduodenal mucosal injury induced by aspirin)	R, SB n=18 volunteers without a history of dyspeptic symptoms (ages 21–26 years)	2 days, 4 weeks apart	20 g chili powder (containing 9.5 mg capsaicin), mixed with 200 ml water followed by 600 mg aspirin with 200 ml water vs. aspirin without chili	Chili powder containing 478 ppm capsaicin (KNP Trading Pte Ltd., Singapore)	Chili powder demonstrated a gastroprotective effect in human subjects as determined by endoscopy. Median gastric injury score after chili was 1.5 compared to 4 in control group (p<0.05).
López-Carrillo et al., 1994	Gastric cancer risk	E n=972 (incident group n=220; control group n=752) (mean age 57.2 years)	286 days	Approximately 20 g peppers/day	Chili peppers	Chili pepper consumers had a 5.5-fold greater risk for gastric cancer than non-chili pepper consumers. Among consumers, there was a highly significant trend of increasing risk with increasing, self-rated level of consumption. The odds ratio for high-level consumers compared with non-consumers was 17.11 (95% CI 7.78–37.59). The authors could not conclude definite results because there was a lack of a dose-response relationship observed when chili pepper consumption was measured as a frequency of consumption per day.
Graham et al., 1988	Gastrointestinal (effect of spiced food on gastric mucosa)	SB, R, CO n=12 (ages 24–43 years)	4 days	30 g jalapeño peppers with spicy meal vs. bland meal	Jalapeño peppers	Ingestion of highly spiced meals by normal individuals did not cause endoscopically demonstrable gastric or duodenal mucosal damage.
Henry and Emery, 1986	Gastrointestinal (effect of spiced food on metabolic rate)	OL, Cm n=12	2 days, 180 minutes each day	3 g mustard and chili sauce	1 meal with 3 g mustard and chili sauce vs. 1 non-spicy meal	A statistically significant increase of 25% in the post-spicy meal resting metabolic rate (RMR) was measured, peaking at around 75–90 minutes post-meal. The peak increase in the non-spicy meal rate was smaller and came earlier, at 60–75 minutes. After 180 minutes, the metabolic rate after the spicy meal was still relatively elevated.
Kumar et al., 1984	Gastrointestinal (effect of chili on healing rate of duodenal ulcers)	Cm, R n=50 (mean age chili group 32.6 years; mean age control group 36.8 years)	1 month	1 g red chili powder 3x/day with meals vs. meals without chili powder	Capsicum powder added to food (both groups also took 15 ml liquid antacid 6x/day)	Red chilies were found not to influence the healing of duodenal ulcer. No gastric mucosal damage in the form of hyperemia or erosions was observed. The authors concluded that patients with duodenal ulcer may consume a normal diet and that bland food is unlikely to serve any useful purpose.

KEY: **C** – controlled, **CC** – case-control, **CH** – cohort, **CI** – confidence interval, **Cm** – comparison, **CO** – crossover, **CS** – cross-sectional, **DB** – double-blind, **E** – epidemiological, **LC** – longitudinal cohort, **MA** – meta-analysis, **MC** – multi-center, **n** – number of patients, **O** – open, **OB** – observational, **OL** – open label, **OR** – odds ratio, **P** – prospective, **PB** – patient-blind, **PC** – placebo-controlled, **PG** – parallel group, **PS** – pilot study, **R** – randomized, **RC** – reference-controlled, **RCS** – retrospective cross-sectional, **RS** - retrospective, **S** – surveillance, **SB** – single-blind, **SC** – single-center, **U** – uncontrolled, **UP** – unpublished, **VC** – vehicle-controlled.

Clinical Studies on Cayenne (*Capsicum* spp.) (cont.)

Internal Use of Cayenne Crude Herb Preparations (cont.)

Author/Year	Subject	Design	Duration	Dosage	Preparation	Results/Conclusion
Visudhiphan et al., 1982	Hematology (effect on fibrinolytic activity and blood coagulation)	Cm n=143: 88 Thai and 55 American subjects (ages 12–68 years)	1 day	Thai meals w/ capsicum vs. American meals without capsicum	Powder of *C. frutescens* added to food	Fibrinolytic activity measured in 88 Thai subjects (mean ± SD = 167 ± 66.84 minutes) was significantly higher than in 55 American whites (mean ± SD = 254 ± 126.70 minutes) residing in Thailand for a period of time (p<0.001), presumably due to Thai population's daily consumption of capsicum with their food compared to the absence of daily capsicum in the American diet. Additionally, the Thai population had lower plasma fibrinogen (p<0.01) and higher anti-thrombin III (statistics not reported) compared to Americans.

Clinical Studies on Capsaicin Preparations

Neuralgia

Author/Year	Subject	Design	Duration	Dosage	Preparation	Results/Conclusion
Watson et al., 1993	Postherpetic neuralgia	DB, PC, PG n=143 patients with chronic postherpetic neuralgia	6 weeks	0.075% capsaicin in cream base 4x/day	Zostrix®-HP	Statistically significant pain reduction. Average reduction in pain by visual analog scale (VAS) ~15% decrease for capsaicin and 5% increase for placebo.
Peikert et al., 1991	Postherpetic neuralgia	OL n=39 patients with chronic post-herpetic neuralgia	2 months with follow-up after 10–12 months	0.025% capsaicin in cream base	Brand not stated	Of the patients, 48% experienced substantial improvement. Of the 48% who responded, 72% were still improved after 10–12 months. Topically applied capsaicin may be effective in relieving pain of postherpetic neuralgia.
Bernstein et al., 1989	Chronic post-herpetic neuralgia	DB, PG n=32 elderly patients	6 weeks	0.075% capsaicin in cream base 4x/day	Zostrix®-HP	After 6 weeks, nearly 80% of capsaicin group experienced some pain relief. The investigators' global evaluation for symptom relief at end of treatment indicated capsaicin was better than placebo.

Neuropathy

Author/Year	Subject	Design	Duration	Dosage	Preparation	Results/Conclusion
Ellison et al., 1997	Surgical neuropathic pain for at least 3 months	R, PC n=99 (median age in first capsaicin group 66 years; median age in first placebo group 64 years)	2 months	Rubbing preparation in until it vanished 4x/day	Zostrix®-HP	Average pain reduction of 53% vs. 17% placebo (p=0.0005). Post-surgical neuropathic pain decreased significantly and, despite some toxicities, was preferred 3:1 over placebo.
Low et al., 1995	Chronic distal painful poly-neuropathy	DB, PC, R n=39 patients with bilateral symmetric painful peripheral neuropathy in distal lower extremities for at least 6 months (mean age 56 years)	3 months	0.075% capsaicin in cream base 4x/day	Brand not stated	This study did not demonstrate a trend in favor of capsaicin. No statistically significant difference was found.
Capsaicin Study Group, 1992, 1991	Diabetic neuropathy	R, DB, PC, MC n=277 patients with peripheral polyneuropathy or radiculopathy (ages 22–92 years)	8 weeks	0.075% capsaicin in cream base 4x/day	Axsain®	Of capsaicin group, 69.5% showed improvement in pain relief compared to 53.4% with vehicle cream (p=0.012); 18.3 vs. 9.2% showed improvement in working (p=0.019); 26.1 vs 14.6% showed improvement in walking (p=0.029); 29.5 vs. 20.3% showed improvement in sleeping (p=0.036). 22.8 vs. 12.1% had improved participation in recreational activities (p=0.037).

KEY: C – controlled, **CC** – case-control, **CH** – cohort, **CI** – confidence interval, **Cm** – comparison, **CO** – crossover, **CS** – cross-sectional, **DB** – double-blind, **E** – epidemiological, **LC** – longitudinal cohort, **MA** – meta-analysis, **MC** – multi-center, **n** – number of patients, **O** – open, **OB** – observational, **OL** – open label, **OR** – odds ratio, **P** – prospective, **PB** – patient-blind, **PC** – placebo-controlled, **PG** – parallel group, **PS** – pilot study, **R** – randomized, **RC** – reference-controlled, **RCS** – retrospective cross-sectional, **RS** – retrospective, **S** – surveillance, **SB** – single-blind, **SC** – single-center, **U** – uncontrolled, **UP** – unpublished, **VC** – vehicle-controlled.

Clinical Studies on Capsaicin Preparations (cont.)

Neuropathy (cont.)

Author/Year	Subject	Design	Duration	Dosage	Preparation	Results/Conclusion
Chad et al., 1990	Diabetic neuropathy	DB, R n=46 patients with painful distal, symmetrical polyneuropathy	1 month	0.075% capsaicin in cream base 4x/day	Axsain®	Assessed by physician's global evaluation scores, capsaicin group showed trend towards beneficial effect and greater improvement. However, a clear positive therapeutic conclusion was not determined in this study due to the difficulty in separating the salutary effects of capsaicin from vehicle.

Psoriasis

Author/Year	Subject	Design	Duration	Dosage	Preparation	Results/Conclusion
Krogstad et al., 1999	Psoriatic lesions	PC n=22 psoriatic patients (mean age 44 years)	24 hours	0.75–1.0%, 1x capsaicin epicutaneously to skin	Essex cream	Compared with placebo, 24-hour treatment caused 15% decrease in basal perfusion in lesional skin. After 50 minutes of capsaicin treatment, histamine release increased by 30% (p<0.05). After 50–60 minutes, capsaicin increased perfusion in lesional skin by 30% (p<0.001).
Ellis et al., 1993	Psoriasis	DB, PC, MC, PG n=197 patients with stable, plaque-type psoriasis with pruritis, involving >5% body surface (mean age capsaicin group 47 years; mean age placebo group 45 years)	6 weeks	0.025% cream 4x/day	Brand not stated (0.025% capsaicin cream)	Capsaicin-treated patients demonstrated significantly greater improvement in global evaluation (p=0.024 at 4 weeks; p=0.03 at 6 weeks), pruritus relief (p=0.002 at 4 weeks; p=0.06 at 6 weeks) and combined psoriasis severity scores (p=0.3 at 4 weeks; p=0.36 at 6 weeks). The most frequently reported side effect was transient burning sensation at application sites.

Osteoarthritis (OA)/Rheumatoid Arthritis (RA)

Author/Year	Subject	Design	Duration	Dosage	Preparation	Results/Conclusion
Altman et al., 1994	OA	DB, R, PC, MC n=113 (ages 18–86 years)	3 months	0.025% cream 4x/day	Zostrix®	Significantly better pain and tenderness relief with topical capsaicin than with placebo. Significant improvement of physicians' and patients' global evaluations with capsaicin (p=0.03). Capsaicin-treated patients reported great reduction of pain on the visual analog scale (VAS) (p=0.02 at 12 weeks) and on passive range of motion (p=0.03), and of joint swelling and tenderness (p=0.01). Results support use of capsaicin 0.025% as first-line therapy for OA pain.
Schnitzer et al., 1994	OA involving one or both hands	DB, R, PC, PG n=59 4x/day regimen vs. 2x/day regimen (mean age capsaicin 69.3 years; mean age placebo 66.8 years)	9 weeks	Phase I: 0.025% cream 4x/day, 3 weeks; Phase II: 0.025% cream 2x/day, 6 weeks	Zostrix®	Study confirmed that topical capsaicin 4 times per day is safe and effective adjunctive therapy for OA pain (p=0.018 at 3 weeks; p=0.13 capsaicin vs. placebo after 6 weeks) and once effective symptomatic relief is achieved, reducing dosage to 4 times per day appears to provide relief with continued application.
Weisman et al., 1994	RA (effect of capsaicin on synovial fluid of knee)	DB, PC, R n=10 (mean age capsaicin group 47.1 years; mean age placebo group 50.9 years)	6 weeks	0.075% cream 4x/day	Brand not stated	Analysis of synovial fluid showed that topical capsaicin caused greater reductions of inflammatory mediators than placebo. Study suggests that in addition to its effects on afferent neurons, capsaicin might also provide additional anti-inflammatory activity.

KEY: **C** – controlled, **CC** – case-control, **CH** – cohort, **CI** – confidence interval, **Cm** – comparison, **CO** – crossover, **CS** – cross-sectional, **DB** – double-blind, **E** – epidemiological, **LC** – longitudinal cohort, **MA** – meta-analysis, **MC** – multi-center, **n** – number of patients, **O** – open, **OB** – observational, **OL** – open label, **OR** – odds ratio, **P** – prospective, **PB** – patient-blind, **PC** – placebo-controlled, **PG** – parallel group, **PS** – pilot study, **R** – randomized, **RC** – reference-controlled, **RCS** – retrospective cross-sectional, **RS** - retrospective, **S** – surveillance, **SB** – single-blind, **SC** – single-center, **U** – uncontrolled, **UP** – unpublished, **VC** – vehicle-controlled.

Cayenne

Monograph

Osteoarthritis (OA)/Rheumatoid Arthritis (RA) (cont.)

Author/Year	Subject	Design	Duration	Dosage	Preparation	Results/Conclusion
McCarthy and McCarty, 1992	Primary OA and RA on the hand with at least moderate severity	DB, R, PC OA: n=14 RA: n=7 (mean age 61 years)	1 month	0.075% cream 4x/day vs. vehicle-only cream	Brand not stated	OA: Significant reduction in pain (p<0.02). RA: No significant reduction in pain. Capsaicin reduced tenderness and pain associated with osteoarthritis (p<0.02). Local burning sensation was only adverse effect noted.
Deal et al., 1991	Primary OA and RA with moderate to severe knee pain	DB, R, PC, MC OA: n=70 RA: n=31 patients with primary OA or RA of 1 or both knees (mean ages with OA: capsaicin 62 years, placebo 60 years; mean ages with RA: capsaicin 52 years, placebo 56 years)	1 month	0.025% cream 4x/day	Zostrix®	OA: mean reduction in pain of 33% (p=0.033). RA: mean reduction in pain of 57% (p=0.003). With global evaluation, 80% of the capsaicin-treated patients reported reduction in pain after 2 weeks of treatment. Both OA and RA patients had significant reduction of knee pain severity (categorical scale and visual analog scale [VAS]).

Other

Author/Year	Subject	Design	Duration	Dosage	Preparation	Results/Conclusion
Vickers et al., 1998	Atypical odontalgia (AO)	O n=50 duration of pain from 3 months to 32 months (ages 21–82 years)	1 month	Topical anesthetic mouthwash (benzocaine 15%), application for 3 minutes 2x/day, followup for at least 3 months	Capsig® (0.025% capsaicin)	Of 30 subjects, 19 responded positively, with pain reduction ranging from 10–100% (mean=58 ± 25 [SD]; p<0.01) using visual analog scale (VAS).
Wallengren and Klinker, 1995	Notalgia paresthetica	R, DB, PC, C n=20 duration of symptoms 3 years (mean age 59 years)	10 weeks	0.025% capsaicin in cream base 5x/day for 1 week, then 3x daily for 3 weeks, followed by 2-week washout, then crossover repeat application for 4 weeks	Zostrix®	Of capsaicin group, 70% showed improvement vs. 30% placebo. Improvement in capsaicin group was long-lasting in some cases for several months.
McCarty et al., 1994	Fibromyalgia	DB, PC n=45 (ages 18–70 years)	1 month	0.025% capsaicin in cream base 4x/day	Zostrix®	Capsaicin group reported significantly less tenderness in the tender points than placebo at week 4. No statistically significant differences between groups on visual analog scale (VAS). Significant increase (p = .02) in grip strength was noted at week 2 for capsaicin group.
Marks et al., 1993	Cluster headache	DB, PC, R n=13	7 days, then recorded severity of each headache for 15 days	0.025% capsaicin in cream base	Intranasal capsaicin ointment	Headaches were significantly less severe in capsaicin-treated group on days 8–15 and on days 1–7 compared to placebo. Results indicated that intranasal capsaicin may provide new therapeutic option for treatment of cluster headaches.

KEY: C – controlled, **CC** – case-control, **CH** – cohort, **CI** – confidence interval, **Cm** – comparison, **CO** – crossover, **CS** – cross-sectional, **DB** – double-blind, **E** – epidemiological, **LC** – longitudinal cohort, **MA** – meta-analysis, **MC** – multi-center, **n** – number of patients, **O** – open, **OB** – observational, **OL** – open label, **OR** – odds ratio, **P** – prospective, **PB** – patient-blind, **PC** – placebo-controlled, **PG** – parallel group, **PS** – pilot study, **R** – randomized, **RC** – reference-controlled, **RCS** – retrospective cross-sectional, **RS** - retrospective, **S** – surveillance, **SB** – single-blind, **SC** – single-center, **U** – uncontrolled, **UP** – unpublished, **VC** – vehicle-controlled.

Chamomile, German

Matricaria recutita L. (syn. *Chamomilla recutita* [L.] Rauschert;
M. chamomilla L.; *M. suaveolens* L.)
[Fam. *Asteraceae*]

OVERVIEW

Chamomile is one of the most widely used ingredients in herbal teas worldwide. The amount of chamomile imported into the U.S. each year is between 750,000 and one million pounds, with an estimated 90% used in teas. In the U.S. and Europe, chamomile is also a popular ingredient for external use in health and beauty aids. In commerce, chamomile is often called German chamomile or Hungarian chamomile, which should not be confused with the rarer, and more costly, Roman or English chamomile (*Anthemis nobilis* syn. *Chamaemelum nobile*).

PRIMARY USES

Internal
- Gastrointestinal spasms
- Inflammatory diseases of the gastrointestinal tract
- Indigestion, flatulence, and/or excess gas production, bloating

External
- Inflammatory dermatosis
- Neurodermatitis
- Wound treatment after dermabrasion for tattoo removal
- Ano-genital inflammation (baths and irrigation)

OTHER POTENTIAL USES
- Diarrhea in children
- Common cold symptoms
- Alleviation of mucositis induced by radiation and chemotherapy

PHARMACOLOGICAL ACTIONS

Anti-inflammatory; muscle relaxant; antispasmodic; promotes wound-healing; deodorant; antibacterial and bacteriostatic; stimulates skin metabolism; mild sedative; carminative.

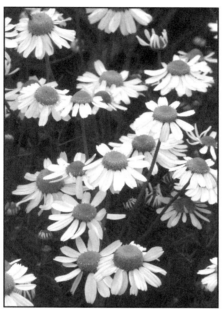

Photo © 2003 stevenfoster.com

DOSAGE AND ADMINISTRATION

Internal and External
Caution patients to report any acute complaints that last more than one week, or recur periodically.

Internal
DRIED FLOWER HEADS: 2–4 g, 3 times daily; 5 g single dose.

INFUSION: The German Commission E dosage: 150 ml boiling water poured over approximately 3 g dried flower and steeped, covered, for 5–10 minutes, 3–4 times daily between meals for gastrointestinal complaints. The official Swiss tea infusion dosage for the same indication is 900 mg, 3–5 times daily.

FLUID EXTRACT: 1:1 (*g/ml*), 38–53% ethanol (*v/v*), containing minimum 0.3% (*m/m*) blue volatile oil, 1–4 ml, 3 times daily.

TINCTURE: 1:5 (*g/ml*), 45% ethanol, 3–10 ml, 3 times daily. The Kamillosan® Konzentrat product has an approximately 1:4.0–4.5 (*w/v*) ratio in 42.8% ethanol; each 100 ml contains 150–300 mg essential oil, 150–300 mg apigenin-7-glucoside, and 50 mg (-)-α-bisabolol. Adults: 5 ml in 100 ml warm water, 4 times daily. Children: 2.5 ml, 4 times daily.

External
BATH ADDITIVE: 50 g dried flower added to 10 liters (about 2.5 gallons) water, as a bath for ano-genital inflammation.

GARGLE: 100 ml boiling water poured over 3–10 g dried flower and steeped, covered, for 5–10 minutes. The tea infusion used as a wash or gargle for inflammation of the mucous membranes of the mouth and throat. Or, 5 ml tincture poured into 100 ml warm water and gargled 3 or more times daily.

INHALATION: 100 ml boiling water poured over 3–10 g dried flower and steeped, covered, for 5–10 minutes. Or, 15 ml tincture poured into 0.5 liter boiled water, 1–3 times daily. Steam vapor inhaled for inflammation of the upper respiratory tract.

POULTICE: Semisolid paste or plaster containing 3–10% (*m/m*) of flower heads.

RINSE: Hot aqueous rinse containing 3–10% infusion.

NOTE: Do not apply the infusion near the eyes.

CONTRAINDICATIONS

Known hypersensitivity to plants of the *Asteraceae (Compositae)* family such as arnica flower (*Arnica* spp.), chamomile flower (*Matricaria* spp.), marigold flower (*Calendula officinalis*), and yarrow flower (*Achillea* spp.); ragweed (*Ambrosia* spp.); asters (*Aster tataricus*); and chrysanthemums (*Chrysanthemum* spp.).

PREGNANCY AND LACTATION: No known restrictions.

ADVERSE EFFECTS

Minor side effects have been recorded. In rare cases, a contact allergy may occur. Washing the eyes with chamomile tea may cause allergic conjunctivitis in rare cases. The highly concentrated hot tea has been reported to act as an emetic. The unprocessed, crude flower is free from any toxic effects. Rarely, anaphylactic reactions can occur. Case reports have documented contact dermatitis and urticaria as well as one fatal anaphylaxis after a chamomile-containing enema was given during labor.

DRUG INTERACTIONS

No known interactions. Fluid extract may prevent ethyl alcohol-induced ulcer formation. Potential interactions with warfarin have been cautioned.

CLINICAL REVIEW

Of 10 clinical studies on German chamomile extract (8,668 total participants), all but 1 demonstrated positive effects for indications including dermatological, neurological, and respiratory conditions. Three studies focused on the use of chamomile as a mouthwash for stomatitis and for its astringent and cooling effects. One stomatitis study did not notice significant improvement. Dermatological studies included a controlled, bilateral, comparative study investigating a chamomile cream against inflammatory dermatoses, and a double-blind (DB) study on use of a chamomile extract to promote wound-healing after dermabrasion. Other studies demonstrating positive results included inhalation of the steam vapor of chamomile extract to treat respiratory tract conditions related to the common cold, inhalation of the volatile oil to determine the effect of olfactory stimulation on mood, and oral ingestion of the aqueous infusion to investigate cardiac effects after ventricular catheterization. In a study of 8,058 mothers in childbirth conducted over a period of eight years, two essential oils, clary sage (*Salvia sclarea*) and chamomile, were shown to be effective in alleviating pain during labor. A recent DB, placebo-controlled study investigated the use of a chamomile fluid extract and apple pectin combination product for treating young children with acute, non-complicated diarrhea.

Chamomile, German

Matricaria recutita L. (syn. *M. recutita* L. Rauschert; *M. chamomilla* L.; *M. suaveolens* L.)
[Fam. *Asteraceae*]

OVERVIEW

In the U.S., chamomile is one of the most widely used herbal ingredients in teas as well as in cosmetic, health, and beauty aid products. The amount of chamomile imported into the U.S. each year is between 750,000 and one million pounds, with an estimated 90% used in teas. In commerce, chamomile is often called German chamomile or Hungarian chamomile, which should not be confused with the rare, and more costly, Roman or English chamomile (*Anthemis nobilis* syn. *Chamaemelum nobile*).

USES

Internal

Indigestion; flatulence (gas); bloating; gastrointestinal spasms; inflammatory diseases of the gastrointestinal tract.

External

Inflammatory skin conditions; scaly patches of skin resulting from an itch that is irritated when scratched; wound treatment after dermabrasion for tattoo removal; inflamed anal and genital areas (baths and irrigation).

DOSAGE

For acute complaints that last more than one week, or recur periodically, consult your healthcare provider.

Internal

FLUID EXTRACT: 1–4 ml, 3 times daily.

TINCTURE: Adults: 5 ml in 100 ml warm water, 4 times daily. Children: 2.5 ml, 4 times daily.

External

BATH ADDITIVE: Add 50 g dried flower per 10 liters (approximately 2.5 gallons) water. Bathe in the infusion for ano-genital inflammation.

GARGLE: Pour 100 ml boiling water over 3–10 g dried flower and steep, covered, for 5–10 minutes. Use the tea infusion as a wash or gargle for inflammation of the mucous membranes of the mouth and throat, or pour 5 ml tincture into 100 ml warm water, and gargle 3 or more times daily.

INHALATION: Pour 100 ml boiling water over 3–10 g dried flower and steep, covered, for 5–10 minutes, or pour

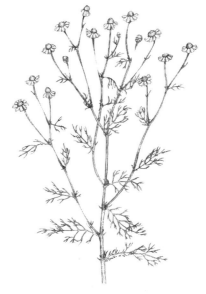

15 ml tincture into approximately 2 cups boiled water, 1–3 times daily. Inhale steam vapor for inflammation of the upper respiratory tract.

CONTRAINDICATIONS

Individuals allergic to plants in the same family (including arnica, marigold, yarrow, chrysanthemum, and ragweed, for example) may experience a similar reaction to chamomile.

PREGNANCY AND LACTATION: There are no known restrictions for usage during pregnancy or while breast-feeding.

ADVERSE EFFECTS

Rare cases of allergic reactions to chamomile used as an eyewash have been reported. A fatal, possibly allergic, reaction occurred during labor after a chamomile enema was used. Highly concentrated hot tea may cause vomiting. Other adverse effects include dermatitis and urticaria.

DRUG INTERACTIONS

The fluid extract may prevent ulcers caused by alcohol consumption. Potential interactions with the anticoagulating drug warfarin have been speculated.

Comments

When using a dietary supplement, purchase it from a reliable source. For best results, use the same brand of product throughout the period of use. As with all medications and dietary supplements, please inform your healthcare provider of all herbs and medications you are taking. Interactions may occur between medications and herbs or even among different herbs when taken at the same time. Treat your herbal supplement with care by taking it as directed, storing it as advised on the label, and keeping it out of the reach of children and pets. Consult your healthcare provider with any questions.

The information contained on this sheet has been excerpted from *The ABC Clinical Guide to Herbs* © 2003 by the American Botanical Council (ABC). ABC is an independent member-based educational organization focusing on the medicinal use of herbs. For more detailed information about this herb please consult the healthcare provider who gave you this sheet. To order *The ABC Clinical Guide to Herbs* or become a member of ABC, visit their website at www.herbalgram.org.

Chamomile, German

Matricaria recutita L. (syn. *Chamomilla recutita* [L.] Rauschert; *M. chamomilla* L.; *M. suaveolens* L.)

[Fam. *Asteraceae*]

OVERVIEW

Chamomile is one of the most widely used ingredients in herbal teas worldwide. The amount of chamomile imported into the U.S. each year is between 750,000 and one million pounds, with an estimated 90% used in teas (Keating, 2001). In the U.S. and Europe, chamomile is also a popular ingredient for external use in health and beauty aids. In commerce, chamomile is often called German chamomile or Hungarian chamomile, which should not be confused with the rarer, and more costly, Roman or English chamomile (*Anthemis nobilis* syn. *Chamaemelum nobile*).

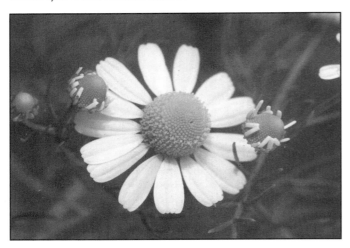

Photo © 2003 stevenfoster.com

DESCRIPTION

Chamomile preparations consist of the fresh or dried flower heads of *Matricaria recutita* L. (syn. *Chamomilla recutita* [L.] Rauschert; *M. chamomilla* L.; *M. suaveolens* L.) [Fam. *Asteraceae*]. Pharmacopeial grade chamomile must contain no less than 0.4% of blue volatile oil, and no less than 0.3% of apigenin-7-glucoside (USP, 2002). Pharmacopeial grade chamomile fluid extract contains not less than 0.3% of blue residual oil with an ethanol content of 38%–53% (*v/v*) (Ph.Eur., 2001).

PRIMARY USES

Internal
- Gastrointestinal spasms, inflammatory diseases of the gastrointestinal tract (Morant and Ruppanner, 2001; Blumenthal *et al.*, 1998; Bradley, 1992; Braun *et al.*, 1996)
- Indigestion, flatulence and/or excess gas production, bloating (Health Canada, 1996)

External
Dermatology
- Inflammatory dermatosis and neurodermatitis (Aertgeerts *et al.*, 1985)

- Wound treatment after dermabrasion for tattoo removal (Glowania *et al.*, 1987)
- Ano-genital inflammation (baths and irrigation) (Blumenthal *et al.*, 1998; Braun *et al.*, 1996)

OTHER POTENTIAL USES
- Diarrhea in children (de la Motte *et al.*, 1997)
- Common cold symptoms (Saller *et al.*, 1990)

Oncology
- Alleviation of radiation and chemotherapy induced mucositis (Carl and Emrich, 1991)

DOSAGE

Internal
Crude Preparations
DRIED FLOWER HEADS: 2–4 g, 3 times daily (Bradley, 1992), 5 g single dose (CCRUM, 1992).

INFUSION: The German Commission E dosage is 150 ml boiling water poured over approximately 3 g dried flower and steeped, covered, for 5–10 minutes, 3–4 times daily between meals for gastrointestinal complaints (Blumenthal *et al.*, 1998; Braun *et al.*, 1996). The official Swiss tea infusion dosage for the same indication is 900 mg, 3–5 times daily (Morant and Ruppanner, 2001).

FLUID EXTRACT: 1:1 (*g/ml*), 38–53% ethanol (*v/v*), containing minimum 0.3% (*w/w*) blue volatile oil, 1–4 ml, 3 times daily (Bradley, 1992).

TINCTURE: 1:5 (*g/ml*), 45% ethanol, 3–10 ml, 3 times daily (Bradley, 1992).

TINCTURE: 1:4.0–4.5 (*w/v*) ratio in 42.8% ethanol. Adults: 5 ml in 100 ml warm water, 4 times daily. Children: 2.5 ml, 4 times daily (Asta Medica, 1998; Gelbe Liste Pharmindex, 2000).

External
Crude Preparations
BATH ADDITIVE: 50g dried flower added per 10 liters (ca. 2.5 gallons) water as a bath for ano-genital inflammation (Blumenthal *et al.*, 1998; Braun *et al.*, 1996).

GARGLE: 100 ml boiling water poured over 3–10 g dried flower and steeped, covered, for 5–10 minutes (Braun *et al.*, 1996). The tea infusion is used as a wash or gargle for inflammation of the mucous membranes of the mouth and throat (Blumenthal *et al.*, 1998; Braun *et al.*, 1996). Or 5 ml tincture poured into 100 ml warm water and gargled 3 or more times daily (Asta Medica, 1998).

INHALATION: 100 ml boiling water poured over 3–10 g dried flower and steeped, covered, for 5–10 min. (Braun *et al.*, 1996). Or 15 ml tincture poured into 0.5 liter boiled water, 1–3 times daily (Asta Medica, 1998). Steam vapor inhaled for inflammation of the upper respiratory tract.

POULTICE: Semisolid paste or plaster containing 3–10% (*m/m*) of flower heads (Blumenthal *et al.*, 1998).

RINSE: Hot aqueous rinse containing 3–10% infusion (Blumenthal *et al.*, 1998).

NOTE: Do not apply infusion near eyes (Braun *et al.*, 1996).

DURATION OF ADMINISTRATION
Internal and external
For acute complaints that last more than one week, or recur periodically, consult a healthcare provider (Braun *et al.*, 1996).

CHEMISTRY
Chamomile contains from 6–8% flavonoids (Hänsel *et al.*, 1999; Bruneton, 1999; Dölle *et al.*, 1985), composed of flavone glycosides including apigenin 7-glucoside and its 6'-acetylated derivative and flavonols including luteolin glucosides, quercetin glycosides, and isorhamnetin (Bruneton, 1999); up to 10% mucilage polysaccharides (Carle and Isaac, 1985; Meyer-Buchtela, 1999); 0.4–2.0% volatile oil, composed of bisabolane sesquiterpenes (up to 50%) and chamazulene (1–15%); sesquiterpene lactones (matricin and matricarin) (Bruneton, 1999; Carle and Isaac, 1985); and up to 0.3% choline (Schilcher, 1987).

PHARMACOLOGICAL ACTIONS
According to the German Commission E, chamomile is anti-inflammatory; muscle relaxant; antispasmodic; promotes wound-healing; deodorant; antibacterial; bacteriostatic; stimulates skin metabolism (Blumenthal *et al.*, 1998).

Internal
Human
Sedative (Bradley, 1992; Gould *et al.*, 1973; Mann and Staba, 1986); carminative (CCRUM, 1992).

Animal
Inhibits ulceration (Szelenyi *et al.*, 1979); relaxes smooth muscle (Carle and Gomaa, 1991,92); depresses central nervous system (CNS) (Della Loggia *et al.*, 1982). Apigenin binds to central benzodiazepine receptors, producing anxiolytic effects in mice but without any sedative or myorelaxant effects (Viola *et al.*, 1995). A subsequent study reports, in contrast, that apigenin has sedative action without anxiolytic and/or myorelaxant effect. The study links the sedative action of chamomile extracts not to an activation of GABA$_A$ receptors by apigenin, but to other compounds with benzodiazepine-like activity (Avallone *et al.*, 2000).

In vitro
Antipeptic (reduces proteolytic activity of pepsin by 50%) (Thiemer *et al.*, 1972; Isaac and Thiemer, 1975); prevents and relieves inflammation (Ammon and Sabieraj, 1996).

External
Human
Anti-inflammatory (Aertgeerts *et al.*, 1985); astringent; cooling (Nasemann, 1975); promotes wound-healing (Glowania *et al.*, 1987).

Animal
Anti-inflammatory (Carle and Gomaa, 1991,92; Tubaro *et al.*, 1984; WHO, 1999).

MECHANISM OF ACTION
- Whole plant extracts of chamomile have demonstrated antispasmodic action, though the mechanism of action was unclear (Forster *et al.*, 1980). Antispasmodic effects are due mainly to chamomile's water-soluble constituents (Carle and Gomaa, 1991,92) such as the flavonoids apigenin and apigenin-7-O-glucoside and the volatile oil (–)-α-bisabolol, which act similarly to papaverine (Bruneton, 1999; WHO, 1999).
- Sedative effects are attributed to the flavonoids, including apigenin, which acts as a ligand for the central benzodiazepine receptors. Apigenin competitively inhibits the binding of flunitrazepam, thus providing a molecular basis for possible weak CNS-depressing activity of water-based preparations (e.g., teas) (Viola *et al.*, 1995).
- Apigenin may be an anti-inflammatory constituent (Hadley and Petry, 1999), due to the water-soluble and lipophilic components. The flavones block the arachidonic acid pathway by inhibiting phospholipase A, cyclo-oxygenase, and lipoxygenase pathways. The volatile oil components, chamazulene and α-bisabolol, have also demonstrated anti-inflammatory action by interfering with 5-lipoxygenase and cyclo-oxygenase production (Carle and Gomaa, 1991,92).
- The azulene components of the volatile oil have anti-allergenic and anti-inflammatory actions, though the mechanism of action was unclear (Farnsworth and Morgan, 1972).
- Azulene may prevent histamine discharge from tissue by activating the pituitary-adrenal system, causing the release of cortisone (Stern and Milin, 1956); or azulene may prevent allergic seizures caused by histamine release, activating cellular resistance and speeding the process of healing (Meer and Meer, 1960).
- Chamomile extract accelerates wound-healing, reportedly by reducing inflammation and promoting tissue granulation and regeneration on topical application (Carle and Isaac, 1987).

CONTRAINDICATIONS
Known hypersensitivity to plants of the *Asteraceae (Compositae)* family such as arnica flower (*Arnica* spp.), chamomile flower (*Matricaria* spp.), marigold flower (*Calendula officinalis* L.), and yarrow flower (*Achillea* spp.) (Braun *et al.*, 1996); ragweed (*Ambrosia* spp.); asters (*Aster tataricus* L. f.); and chrysanthemums (*Chrysanthemum* spp.) (WHO, 1999).

PREGNANCY AND LACTATION: No known restrictions in pregnancy or lactation (De Smet *et al.*, 1992; McGuffin *et al.*, 1997). No adverse teratogenic effects have been reported *in vivo* (WHO, 1999).

ADVERSE EFFECTS
Minor side effects are recorded by several references (McGuffin *et al.*, 1997). There is empirical evidence of extremely rare contact allergy (Bradley, 1992; Brinker, 2001). Eye washing with chamomile tea may induce allergic conjunctivitis in rare cases (Subiza *et al.*, 1990). Highly concentrated hot tea has been reported to act as an emetic (Chadha, 1952–1988). The unprocessed crude flower is free from any toxic effects (CCRUM, 1992). Case reports describing contact dermatitis and urticaria have been documented (Foti *et al.*, 2000; Giordano-Labadie, 2000; Rodriguez-Serna *et al.*, 1998; Pereira, 1997; McGeorge and Steele, 1991; van Ketel, 1982). A case report regarding a fatal outcome of anaphylaxis when a chamomile-containing enema was given during labor has been documented (Jensen-Jarolim *et al.*, 1998). Rarely, anaphylactic reactions can occur (Casterline, 1980; Subiza *et al.*, 1989).

There have been several reports in the literature of suspected anaphylaxis associated with the use of chamomile. One authoritative source, reviewing the available literature from over almost 100 years, concluded, "This rather remote possibility may have been greatly overemphasized in the nonmedical literature. Only five cases of allergy specifically attributed to German chamomile were identified worldwide between 1887 and 1982; however, a recent report indicates that a German chamomile ether extract used in allergic patch testing from 1985 to 1990 in 3,851 tested individuals produced an allergic reaction in sixty-six patients or 1.7%." (Robbers and Tyler, 1999). One of the reports receiving widespread attention in the medical press was based on a misinterpretation of the taxonomic identity of the so-called "chamomile" (Anon., 1979). This article warned readers to avoid teas made from the Composite family, including chamomile, goldenrod (*Solidago virgaurea*), marigold, and yarrow. The article cited a paper titled "Anaphylactic reaction to chamomile tea" (Benner and Lee, 1973), which does not specify the genus or species of the purported chamomile material implicated in the single case described, a 35-year old woman who suffered from ragweed hay fever and who developed anaphylaxis following ingestion of one cup of the purported "chamomile tea" (Awang, 1990). The incident was incorrectly inferred to be the popular German or Hungarian chamomile (*M. recutita*). The actual case was based on ingestion of dog fennel (*Anthemis cotula*), a plant not widely used in commercial products, and generally unavailable in the U.S. Dog fennel is a member of the genus *Anthemis*, the same as Roman or English chamomile (*A. nobilis*, syn. *Chamaemelum nobile*) — hence the erroneous appellation "chamomile" by the authors of the case reports (Lewis, 1992). Dog fennel contains a higher level of anthecotulid, a sesquiterpene lactone that has demonstrated activity in primary irritant contact dermatitis (Hausen *et al.*, 1984).

However, there have been some recent reports of anaphylaxis to German chamomile (*M. recutita*). In one study, 10 out of 14 patients with a history of allergy to chamomile, spices, or "weeds" tested positive to chamomile in a skin prick/RAST test (Reider *et al.*, 2000). Curiously, chamazulene in German chamomile has anti-allergenic and anti-inflammatory activity, and another constituent, an EN-IN-dicycloether, has demonstrated anti-inflammatory, anti-anaphylactic, spasmolytic, and bacteriostatic activity (Farnsworth and Morgan, 1972).

DRUG INTERACTIONS

According to the German Commission E, no interactions are known (Blumenthal *et al.*, 1998). The fluid extract may prevent ethyl alcohol-induced ulcer formation (Brinker, 2001). *In vitro* studies of the inhibitory effect of ethanolic herbal extracts and tinctures on the cytochrome P450 3A4 (CYP3A4) system revealed a median inhibitory concentration (IC50) of a chamomile extract ranging from 1–2%. This might have implications for predicting the likelihood of potential herb-drug interactions (Budzinski *et al.*, 2000), although such reactions have not been reported. Potential interactions with warfarin have been reported, and caution regarding their concomitant use has been suggested (Heck *et al.*, 2000), although this remains speculative.

AMERICAN HERBAL PRODUCTS ASSOCIATION (AHPA) SAFETY RATING

CLASS 1: Herbs that can be safely consumed when used appropriately (McGuffin *et al.*, 1997).

REGULATORY STATUS

AUSTRIA: Official in the *Austrian Pharmacopoeia* (ÖAB) (Wichtl, 1997).

BELGIUM: Herbal medicine for oral or external use for specific indication (Bradley, 1992; Van Hellemont, 1986; WHO, 1998).

CANADA: Permitted as a Traditional Herbal Medicine (THM) or homeopathic drug for oral use. Requires premarket authorization and assignment of a Drug Identification Number (DIN) if labeled as a THM or homeopathic drug (Health Canada, 1996). Food, if no claim statement is made.

COUNCIL OF EUROPE: Dried flower, essential oil and fluid extract official in *European Pharmacopoeia*, 3rd edition (Ph.Eur., 2001).

FRANCE: Traditional Herbal Medicine (THM) for oral and external use for specific indications (Bradley, 1992; Bruneton, 1999). Official in the *French Pharmacopoeia*, 10th edition (Ph.Fr.X) (WHO, 1999).

GERMANY: Approved nonprescription drug of the German Commission E for oral and external use (Blumenthal *et al.*, 1998). Tea infusion form is an approved nonprescription drug in the *German Standard License* monographs (Braun *et al.*, 1996). The alcoholic fluid extract and the volatile oil forms are official in the *German Pharmacopoeia* (DAB, 1999).

INDIA: Licensed single drug in Unani system of medicine (CCRUM, 1992). Also listed in compound formulations official in the *National Formulary of Unani Medicine* (NFUM I) with standards approved by the Unani Pharmacopoeia Committee (UPC) (NFUM, 1983).

ITALY: Listed in the *Italian Pharmacopoeia* (Newall *et al.*, 1996).

RUSSIAN FEDERATION: Official in the USSR X (Bradley, 1992; Newall *et al.*, 1996).

SWEDEN: Natural remedy for self-medication. Requires marketing authorization by the Medical Products Agency (WHO, 1998).

SWITZERLAND: Official in the *Swiss Pharmacopoeia* (Ph.Helv.) (Wichtl, 1997). Creams, fluid extracts, powders, sprays, and tea infusions are Category D non-prescription drugs with sale limited to pharmacies and drugstores (Morant and Ruppanner, 2001; Asta Medica, 2000; WHO, 1998).

U.K.: Herbal medicine specified in the *General Sale List*, Schedule 1 (medicinal products requiring a full product license), Table A (internal or external use) (GSL, 1990).

U.S.: Generally recognized as safe (GRAS) (US FDA, 1998). Food or dietary supplement, depending on the claim statement (USC, 1994). Listed in the Official Monographs of the U.S. *National Formulary*, 19th edition (USP, 2002). Tincture of the whole flower plant, 1:10 (*w/v*) in 45% alcohol (*v/v*), is a Class C over-the-counter (OTC) drug of the *Homeopathic Pharmacopoeia of the United States* (HPUS, 1990).

CLINICAL REVIEW

Ten studies are outlined in the following table, "Clinical Studies on German Chamomile," including a total of 8,668 participants. All but one of the studies (Fidler *et al.*, 1996) demonstrated positive effects for indications including dermatological, neurological, and respiratory conditions. Three studies (Fidler *et al.*, 1996; Carl and Emrich, 1991; Nasemann, 1975) focused on the the use of chamomile as a mouthwash for its astringent and cooling effects, stomatitis, and mucositis (Fidler *et al.*, 1996; Carl and Emrich, 1991; Nasemann, 1975). One stomatitis study did not notice significant improvement (Fidler *et al.*, 1996). Other dermatological studies included one controlled, bilateral, comparative study investigating a chamomile cream against inflammatory dermatoses (Aertgeerts *et al.*, 1985), and a DB study on using a chamomile extract to promote wound-healing after dermabrasion (Glowania *et al.*, 1987). Other studies demonstrating positive results included inhalation of the steam vapor of chamomile extract to treat respiratory tract conditions related to the common cold (Saller *et al.*, 1990); inhalation of volatile oil to determine the effect of olfactory stimulation on mood (Roberts and Williams, 1992); and oral ingestion of the aqueous infusion to investigate cardiac effects after ventricular catheterization (Gould *et al.*, 1973). In a study of 8,058 mothers in childbirth conducted over a period of eight years, two essential oils, clary sage (*Salvia sclarea* L.) and chamomile were shown to be effective in alleviating pain during labor (Burns *et al.*, 2000). A recent DB,PC study investigated the use of a chamomile fluid extract and apple pectin combination product for treating young children with acute, non-complicated diarrhea (de la Motte *et al.*, 1997).

BRANDED PRODUCTS

Diarrhoesan® Chamomile fluidextract: Dr. Loges & Co. GmbH / Postfach 1262 / Schützenstrasse 5 / 21423 Winsen / Germany / Tel.: +49-041-71-7070 / Fax: +49-041-71-7071-00 / Email: info@loges.com. Each 100 ml of solution contains 2.5 ml of chamomile fluidextract (1:1),eluent: ethanol 55% and 3.2 g of apple pectin.

Kamillosan® Creme: VIATRIS GmbH & Co. KG / Weismüllerstrasse., 45 / D-60314 Frankfurt/Main / Germany / Tel: +49-69-4001 2811 / Fax: +49-69-4001 2951 / Email: info@viatris.com / www.viatris.com (formerly known as ASTA Medica AG). One gram cream contains 20 mg ethanolic dry extract (2.75:1) in a fatty ointment base. The extract contains no less than 0.2 mg volatile oil and a minimum of 0.07 mg (-)-α-bis-abolol.

Kamillosan® Konzentrat: VIATRIS GmbH & Co. KG. Hydroalcoholic tincture extracted with 38.5% (*m/m*) ethanol; drug-to-extract ratio of approximately 1:4.0–4.5 (*w/v*), in 42.8% ethanol. Each 100 ml of tincture contains 150–300 mg essential oil; 150–300 mg apigenin-7-glucoside and 50 mg (-)-α-bis-abolol.

Kamillosan® Liquidum: VIATRIS GmbH & Co. KG. Standardized hydroalcoholic fluid extract; 150 mg of essential oil per 100 ml fluid extract containing a minimum of 3 mg chamazulene and 50 mg α-bisabolol.

Kneipp® Kamillen-Konzentrat: Kneipp Werke /105-107 Stonehurst Court / Northvale, NJ 07647 / U.S.A. / Tel: (201) 750-0600 / Fax: (201) 750-2070 / www.kneipp.com. Hydroalcoholic fluid extract.

American equivalents, if any, are found in the Product Table beginning on page 398.

REFERENCES

Aertgeerts P, Albring M, Klaschka F, *et al.* Comparative testing of Kamillosan® cream and steroidal (0.25% hydrocortisone, 0.75% fluocortin butyl ester) and non-steroidal (5% bufexamac) dermatologic agents in maintenance therapy of eczematous diseases. [in German]. *Z Hautkr* 1985;60(3):270–7.

Ammon HPT, Sabieraj J. Kamille: Mechanismus der antiphlogistischen Wirkung von Kamillenextrakten und –inhaltsstoffen. *Deutsche Apotheker Zeitung* 1996;136(22):17.

Anon. Toxic reactions to plant products sold in health food stores. Abromowicz M (ed.). *Medical Letter on Drugs and Therapeutics* 1979;21(7):29–32.

Asta Medica. *Fachinformation: Kamillosan® Konzentrat.* Frankfurt, Germany: Asta Medica AG; March 1998.

Asta Medica. *Kamillosan® Produkteübersicht.* Frankfurt, Germany: Asta Medica, Division of Degussa-Hüls Group; 2000.

Avallone R, Zanoli P, Puia G, *et al.* Pharmacological profile of apigenin, a flavonoid isolated from *Matricaria chamomilla.* *Biochem Pharmacol* 2000; 59:1387–94.

Awang DVC. Chamomile, allergy and anaphylactic shock. [unpublished] Feb. 1, 1990.

Benner MH, Lee HJ. Anaphylactic reaction to chamomile tea. *J Allergy Clin Immunol* 1973 Nov;52(5):307–8.

Blumenthal M, Busse WR, Goldberg A, Gruenwald J, Hall T, Riggins CW, Rister RS (eds.). Klein S, Rister RS (trans.). *The Complete German Commission E Monographs—Therapeutic Guide to Herbal Medicines.* Austin, TX: American Botanical Council; Boston: Integrative Medicine Communication; 1998; 108.

Bradley P (ed.). *British Herbal Compendium,* Vol. 1. Bournemouth, UK: British Herbal Medicine Association; 1992;154–7.

Braun R, Surmann P, Wendt R, *et al* (eds.). *Standardzulassungen für Fertigarzneimittel—Text und Kommentar.* Stuttgart, Germany: Deutscher Apotheker Verlag; 1996.

Brinker F. *Herb Contraindications and Drug Interactions,* 3rd ed. Sandy, OR: Eclectic Medical Publications; 2001;62.

Bruneton J. *Pharmacognosy, Phytochemistry, Medicinal Plants,* 2nd ed. Paris: Lavoisier Publishing; 1999;520–3.

Budzinski J, Foster B, Vandenhoek S, Arnason J. An *in vitro* evaluation of human cytochrome P450 3A4 inhibition by selected commercial herbal extracts and tinctures. *Phytomed* 2000 Jul;7(4):273–82.

Burns E, Blamey C, Ersser S, Barnetson L, Lloyd A. The use of aromatherapy in intrapartum midwifery practice an observational study. *J Altern Complement Med* 2000 Apr;6(2):141–7.

Carl W, Emrich L. Management of oral mucositis during local radiation and systemic chemotherapy: a study of 98 patients. *J Prosthet Dent* 1991;66(3):361–9.

Carle R, Gomaa K. Chamomile: a pharmacological and clinical profile. *Drugs of Today* 1992;28:559–65.

Carle R, Gomaa K. The medicinal use of Matricariae flos. *Br J Phytother* 1991/92;2(4):147–53.

Carle R, Isaac O. Chamomile—Effect and Efficacy: Comments to the monograph. Matricariae flos (Chamomile flowers). [in German]. *Z Phytother* 1987;8:67–77.

Carle R, Isaac O. Advances in chamomile research between 1974-1984. [in German]. *Dtsch Apoth Ztg* 1985;125(43, Suppl I):2–8.

Casterline C. Allergy to chamomile tea [letter]. *JAMA* 1980 July;244(4):330–1.

CCRUM. See: Central Council for Research in Unani Medicine.

Central Council for Research in Unani Medicine (CCRUM). *Standardisation of Single Drugs in Unani Medicine,* Part II. New Delhi, India: CCCRUM Ministry of Health & Family Welfare Government of India; 1992;141–7.

Chadha Y *et al.* (eds.). *The Wealth of India* (Raw Materials), 11 vols. New Delhi, India: Publications and Information Directorate, CSIR; 1952–1988.

DAB. See: *Deutsches Arzneibuch.*

de la Motte S, Bose-O'Reillly S, Heinisch M, Harrison F. Doppelblind-Vergleich zwischen einem Apfelpektin/Kamillenextrakt-Präparat und Plazebo bei Kindern mit Diarrhoe. *Arzneimittelforschung* 1997;47(11):1247–9.

De Smet P, Keller K, Hänsel R, Chandler R (eds.). *Adverse Effects of Herbal Drugs 1.* New York, NY: Springer Verlag; 1992;243–7.

De Smet P, Keller K, Hänsel R, Chandler R (eds.). *Adverse Effects of Herbal Drugs 2.* New York, NY: Springer Verlag; 1993;55.

Della Loggia R, Traversa U, Scarcia V, Tubaro A. Depressive effects of *Chamomilla recutita* (L.) Rausch, tubular flowers, on central nervous system in mice. *Pharmacol Res Commun* 1982;14(2):153–62.

Della Loggia R. Evaluation of the anti-inflammatory activity of chamomile preparations. *Planta Medica* 1990;56:657–8.

Deutsches Arzneibuch. (DAB). Stuttgart, Germany: Deutscher Apotheker Verlag; 1999.

Dölle B, Carle R, Müller W. Flavonoidbestimmung in Kamillenextraktpräparaten. *Dtsch Apoth Ztg* 1985; 125(Suppl. I):14–9.

European Pharmacopoeia (Ph.Eur. 3rd edition, Supplement 2001). Strasbourg: Council of Europe; 2001;1102–3.

Farnsworth N, Morgan B. Herb drinks: Camomile tea [letter]. *JAMA* 1972;221(4):410.

Fidler P, Loprinzi C, O'Fallon J, *et al.* Prospective evaluation of a chamomile mouthwash for prevention of 5-FU- induced oral mucositis. *Cancer* 1996;77(3):522–5.

Forster H, Niklas H, Lutz S. Antispasmodic effects of some medicinal plants. *Planta Med* 1980;40(4):309–19.

Foti C, Nettis E, Panebianco R, Cassano N, Diaferio A, Pia D. Contact urticaria from *Matricaria chamomilla.* *Contact Dermatitis* 2000 Jun;42(6):360–1.

Gelbe Liste Pharmindex. 3. Quartal 2000. Germany: Available at: http://www.gelbe-liste.de.

General Sale List (GSL). Statutory Instrument (S.I.) The Medicines (Products Other Than Veterinary Drugs) Amendment Order 1990; No. 1129. London, U.K.: Her Majesty's Stationery Office (HMSO). 1990.

Giordano-Labadie F, Schwarze H, Bazex J. Allergic contact dermatitis from chamomile used in phytotherapy. Contact Dermatitis 2000 Apr;42(4):247.

Glowania H, Raulin C, Swoboda M. The effect of chamomile on wound healing— a controlled clinical-experimental double-blind study. [in German]. Z Hautkr 1987;62(17):1262, 1267–71.

Gould L, Reddy C, Gomprecht R. Cardiac effects of chamomile tea. J Clin Pharmacol 1973;13(11):475–9.

GSL. See: General Sale List.

Hadley S, Petry J. Medicinal herbs: A primer for primary care. Hosp Pract 1999;34(6):109–12, 115–6.

Hänsel R, Sticher O, Steinegger E. Pharmakognosie–Phytopharmazie, 6th ed. Berlin, Germany: Springer Verlag; 1999;699.

Hausen BM, Busker E, Carle R. The sensitizing capacity of Compositae Plants VII. Experimental Investigations, with extracts and Compounds of Chamomilla recutita (L.) Rauschert and Anthemis cotula L. Planta Medica 1984;34:229–34.

Health Canada. Chamomile Labeling Standard. Ottawa, Canada: Health Canada Therapeutic Products Programme. 1996.

Heck A, DeWitt B, Lukes A. Potential interactions between alternative therapies and warfarin. Am J Health-Syst Pharm 2000;57(13):1221–7.

Homeopathic Pharmacopoeia of the United States (HPUS) — Revision Service Official Compendium from July 1, 1992. Falls Church, VA: American Institute of Homeopathy; 1990 June;2127:CHAM.

HPUS. See: Homeopathic Pharmacopoeia of the United States.

Isaac O, Thiemer K. Biochemical Assessments of Chamomile extracts. Arzneimittelforschung 1975;25(9):1352-4.

Jensen-Jarolim E, Reider N, Fritsch R, Breiteneder H. Fatal outcome of anaphylaxis to chamomile-containing enema during labor: a case study. J Allergy Clin Immunol 1998 Dec;102(6 Pt 1):1041–2.

Keating B. Sage Group, Seattle WA. Personal communication to T. Kunz. April 19, 2001.

Lang W, Schwandt K. Assessment of the glycoside content of chamomile. [in German]. Deutsche Apotheker Zeitung 1957;97:149–51.

Leslie G, Salmon G. Repeated dose toxicity studies and reproductive studies on nine Bio-Strath herbal remedies. Swiss Medicine 1979;1:1–3.

Lewis WH. Notes on economic plants. Econ Botany 1992;46(4):426–30.

Mann C, Staba EJ. The Chemistry, Pharmacology, and Commercial Formulations of Chamomile. In: Craker L, Simon J (eds.). Herbs, Spices, and Medicinal Plants— Recent Advances in Botany, Horticulture, and Pharmacology. Phoenix, AZ: Oryx Press; 1986;235–80.

McGeorge B, Steele M. Allergic contact dermatitis of the nipple from Roman chamomile ointment. Contact Dermatitis 1991 Feb;24(2):139–40.

McGuffin M., Hobbs C, Upton R, Goldberg A (eds.). American Herbal Product Association's Botanical Safety Handbook. Boca Raton, FLA: CRC Press; 1997;74.

Meer G, Meer W. Chamomile flowers. Am Perfum 1960;November.

Meyer-Buchtela E. Tee-Rezepturen: Ein Handbuch für Apotheker und Ärzte. Stuttgart, Germany: Deutscher Apotheker Verlag; 1999.

Morant J, Ruppanner H (eds.). Asta Medica Kamillosan®; Sidroga® Kamillenblütentee. In Arzneimittel-Kompendium der Schweiz® 2001. Basel, Switzerland: Documed AG. 2001.

Nasemann T. Kamillosan®-(Chamomile) Applications in dermatology. [in German]. Z Allgemeinmed 1975;51(25):1105–6.

National Formulary of Unani Medicine (NFUM I) Part I (English Edition). New Delhi, India. Government of India Department of Indian Systems of Medicine & Homeopathy, Ministry of Health & Family Welfare; 1983.

Newall CA, Anderson LA, Phillipson JD. Herbal Medicines: A Guide for Health-care Professionals. London, UK: The Pharmaceutical Press; 1996;69–71.

NFUM. See: National Formulary of Unani Medicine.

Pereira F, Santos R, Pereira A. Contact dermatitis from chamomile tea. Contact Dermatitis 1997;36(6):307.

Ph.Eur. See: European Pharmacopoeia.

Ph.Fr.X. See: Pharmacopée Française.

Pharmacopée Française, Xe Édition (Ph.Fr.X.). Paris, France: Adrapharm; 1982–1996.

Reider N, Sepp N, Fritsch P. Anaphylaxis to chamomile: clinical features and allergen cross-reactivity. Clin & Exp Allergy 2000;30:1436–43.

Robbers JE, Tyler VE. Tyler's Herbs of Choice: The Therapeutic Use of Phytomedicinals. New York: Haworth Herbal Press, 1999;70.

Roberts A, Williams J. The effect of olfactory stimulation on fluency, vividness of imagery and associated mood: a preliminary study. Br J Med Psychol 1992;65(Pt2):197–9.

Rodriguez-Serna M, Sanchez-Motilla J, Ramon R, Aliaga A. Allergic and systemic contact dermatitis from Matricaria chamomilla tea. Contact Dermatitis 1998;39(4):192–3.

Saller R, Beschorner M, Hellenbrecht D, Bühring M. Dose-dependency of symptomatic relief of complaints by chamomile steam inhalation in patients with common cold [Abstract]. Eur J Pharmacol 1990;183:728–9.

Schilcher H. Die Kamille. In: Handbuch für Ärzte, Apotheker und andere Naturwissenschafter. Stuttgart, Germany: Wissenschaftliche Verlagsgesellschaft; 1987.

Stern P, Milin R. Anti-allergic and anti-inflammatory effect of azulenes. [in German]. Arzneimittelforschung 1956;6:445–50.

Subiza J, Subiza JL, Alonso M, et al. Allergic conjunctivitis to chamomile tea. Ann Allergy 1990;65(2):127–32.

Subiza J, Subiza J, Hinojosa M, et al. Anaphylactic reaction after the ingestion of chamomile tea: A study of cross-reactivity with other composite pollens. J Allergy Clin Immunol 1989;84(3):353–8.

Szelenyi I, Isaac O, Thiemer K. Pharmacological assessment of chamomile extracts. [in German]. Planta Med 1979;35:218–27.

Thiemer K, Stadler R, Isaac O. Assessment of chamomile extracts. [in German]. Arzneimittelforschung 1972;22(6):1086–7.

Tubaro A, Zilli C, Della Loggia R. Evaluation of anti-inflammatory activity of a chamomile extract after topical application. Planta Med 1984;51:359.

United States Congress (USC). Public Law 103–417: Dietary Supplement Health and Education Act of 1994. Washington, DC: 103rd Congress of the United States; 1994.

United States Food and Drug Administration (US FDA). Code of Federal Regulations, Title 21, Part 182 – Substances Generally Recognized as Safe. Washington, DC: Office of the Federal Register National Archives and Records Administration. 1998;427–33.

United States Pharmacopeia, (USP 25th revision) – National Formulary (NF 20th Edition). Rockville, MD: United States Pharmacopeial Convention, Inc. 2002.

US FDA. See: United States Food and Drug Administration.

USC. See: United States Congress.

USP. See: United States Pharmacopeia.

Van Hellemont J. Compendium de phytotherapie. Bruxelles, Belgique: Association Pharmaceutique Belge, 1986.

van Ketel W. Allergy to Matricaria chamomilla. Contact Dermatitis 1982 Mar;8(2):143.

Viola H, Wasowski C, Levi de Stein M, et al. Apigenin, a component of Matricaria recutita flowers, is a central benzodiazepine receptors-ligand with anxiolytic effects. Planta Med 1995;61(3):213–6.

WHO. See: World Health Organization.

Wichtl M (ed.). Teedrogen und Phytopharmaka, 3. Auflage: Ein Handbuch für die Praxis auf wissenschaftlicher Grundlage. Stuttgart, Germany: Wissenschaftliche Verlagsgesellschaft GmbH; 1997;375–95.

World Health Organization (WHO). Regulatory Status of Herbal Medicines: A Worldwide Review. Geneva, Switzerland: World Health Organization Traditional Medicine Programme; 1998.

World Health Organization (WHO). WHO Monographs on Selected Medicinal Plants, Vol. 1. Geneva, Switzerland: World Health Organization; 1999;86–94.

Clinical Studies on Chamomile (*Matricaria recutita* L.)

Oral/Gastrointestinal

Author/Year	Subject	Design	Duration	Dosage	Preparation	Results/Conclusion
Fidler *et al.*, 1996	Stomatitis	Phase III, DB, PC, R n=164	2 weeks	30 drops extract in 100 ml water as mouthwash 3x/day vs. placebo	Kamillosan® Konzentrat, diluted in water	Chamomile mouthwash administered in addition to cryotherapy did not significantly alleviate 5 flourouracil (5-FU)-induced stomatitis (p=0.32). However, subset analysis based on gender did reveal unexpected differential effects, suggesting that chamomile might be beneficial for males but detrimental for females. This could not be explained by reasons other than chance.
Carl and Emrich, 1991	Stomatitis and mucositis	U n=98	Varying durations for different treatment groups	Oral rinse during repeated cycles	Kamillosan® Liquidum	Chamomile oral rinse decreased stomatitis and was found to be beneficial in the treatment of mucositis resulting from radiation and cancer chemotherapeutic agents. The resolution of mucositis appeared to be accelerated by the chamomile rinse. Prophylactic oral care appeared to modify oral environment favorably and maintain tissue integrity.
Nasemann, 1975	Astringent and cooling effect	DB n=36	18 months	Mouth wash, 5–6x/day	Kamillosan®	With exception of patients with glossodynia, extract showed astringent and cooling action.

Dermatological

Author/Year	Subject	Design	Duration	Dosage	Preparation	Results/Conclusion
Glowania *et al.*, 1987	Dermabrasion	R, PC, DB n=14 healthy males with abrasions of tattoos on the arms with Derma III equipment (1.5 mm depth)	14 days	Chamomile extract compresses for 1 hour, 3x/day until wounds are completely dry	Chamomile extract standardized to 3 mg chamazulene and 50 mg levomenol	Objective parameters were used to evaluate epithelial and drying effect of chamomile preparation applied topically to weeping wound area after dermabrasion from tattoo removal. Chamomile extract significantly decreased weeping wound size, and sped up healing time by enhancing drying of oozing wounds.
Aertgeerts *et al.*, 1985	Inflammatory dermatoses	Cn, Cm, MC n=161	3–4 weeks	Chamomile cream vs. 0.25% hydrocortisone, 0.75% fluocortin butyl ester, 5% bufexamac	Kamillosan® Crème	Chamomile cream showed more or less equally effective therapeutic results as hydrocortisone for treatment of inflammatory dermatoses. It proved superior to the nonsteroidal, anti-inflammatory agent 5% bufexamac as well as to 0.75% fluocortin butyl ester. For treatment of neurodermatitis, chamomile cream was therapeutically comparable to hydrocortisone and superior to other tested products.

KEY: C – controlled, **CC** – case-control, **CH** – cohort, **CI** – confidence interval, **Cm** – comparison, **CO** – crossover, **CS** – cross-sectional, **DB** – double-blind, **E** – epidemiological, **LC** – longitudinal cohort, **MA** – meta-analysis, **MC** – multi-center, **n** – number of patients, **O** – open, **OB** – observational, **OL** – open label, **OR** – odds ratio, **P** – prospective, **PB** – patient-blind, **PC** – placebo-controlled, **PG** – parallel group, **PS** – pilot study, **R** – randomized, **RC** – reference-controlled, **RCS** – retrospective cross-sectional, **RS** - retrospective, **S** – surveillance, **SB** – single-blind, **SC** – single-center, **U** – uncontrolled, **UP** – unpublished, **VC** – vehicle-controlled.

Other

Author/Year	Subject	Design	Duration	Dosage	Preparation	Results/Conclusion
de la Motte et al., 1997	Acute diarrhea in children	P, DB, R, MC, PG, PC n=79 children, 6 months to 5.5 years	3 days	1st dose 10 ml, followed by 5 ml/hour, up to 60 ml/day	Diarrhoesan® Chamomile fluid extract (0.035 mg/g chamazulene and 0.5 mg/g (-)-α-bis-abolol) combined with apple pectin	After 3 days of treatment, diarrhea in the pectin/chamomile group had ended significantly (p<0.05) more frequently than placebo. Pectin/chamomile reduced duration of diarrhea significantly (p<0.05) by at least 5.2 hours. Parents documented subjects' well-being in a diary twice daily and, compared to placebo, a trend of continuous improvement was observed in the pectin/chamomile group.
Roberts and Williams, 1992	Neurology, psychiatry	PC n=22	1 day	1x exposure vs. placebo	Chamomile flower volatile oil	Patients were asked to visualize positive and negative phrases following olfactory stimulation by chamomile oil or placebo. Chamomile oil significantly increased latency for all images, and shifted mood ratings and frequency judgments in a more positive direction, suggesting a possible mode of action.
Saller et al., 1990	Respiratory	PC, R n=60	1 day	Steam inhalation, 1x/5 hours	Kneipp® Kamillen-Konzentrat, alcoholic flu-idextract diluted in boiled water	Steam inhalation, below a towel, with chamomile extract in hot water reduced the severity of common cold symptoms in a pronounced and dose-dependent manner. Onset of action occurred within 15 minutes and reached maximum effect between 30–120 minutes; then efficacy declined after 2–3 hours.
Gould et al., 1973	Cardio-vascular effects	U n=12 hospitalized patients	1 day	2 tea bags in 6 ounces boiled water, 1x	Chamomile flower tea infusion (brand not stated)	Significant increase in mean brachial artery pressure from 91 to 98 mmHg (p<0.05). No other significant hemodynamic changes were observed. Blood pressure and cardiac output were measured prior to drinking tea and 30 minutes later. Average cardiac index showed only slight decrease, and average stroke index was essentially unchanged. 10 of the 12 patients fell into deep sleep 10 minutes after ingestion, lasting until end of cardiac catheterization approximately 90 minutes.

Combination Product with Chamomile (Essential Oil)

Author/Year	Subject	Design	Duration	Dosage	Preparation	Results/Conclusion
Burns et al., 2000	Pain during childbirth	O n=8,058	8 years	Not stated	10 essential oils, including chamomile	The study found that aromatherapy with 2 of the tested essential oils, clary sage and chamomile, reduced maternal anxiety, fear, and/or pain during labor. The use of aromatherapy was found to reduce the use of systemic opioids in the study center, from 6% in 1990 per woman to 0.4% in 1997.

KEY: **C** – controlled, **CC** – case-control, **CH** – cohort, **CI** – confidence interval, **Cm** – comparison, **CO** – crossover, **CS** – cross-sectional, **DB** – double-blind, **E** – epidemiological, **LC** – longitudinal cohort, **MA** – meta-analysis, **MC** – multi-center, **n** – number of patients, **O** – open, **OB** – observational, **OL** – open label, **OR** – odds ratio, **P** – prospective, **PB** – patient-blind, **PC** – placebo-controlled, **PG** – parallel group, **PS** – pilot study, **R** – randomized, **RC** – reference-controlled, **RCS** – retrospective cross-sectional, **RS** - retrospective, **S** – surveillance, **SB** – single-blind, **SC** – single-center, **U** – uncontrolled, **UP** – unpublished, **VC** – vehicle-controlled.

Chaste Tree

Vitex agnus-castus L.

[Fam. *Verbenaceae*]

OVERVIEW

Chaste tree derived its common name from the traditional belief that the plant promoted chastity. The fruit of *Vitex agnus-castus* (hereafter referred to as chaste tree) was used to suppress sexual desire by both the men and women of ancient Greece and Rome. During the Middle Ages, monks used chaste tree as a "functional" food flavoring for the same purpose. In Germany, chaste tree is a common treatment for gynecological disorders including corpus luteum insufficiency, premenstrual syndrome (PMS), and hormonally-induced acne. Although chaste tree is widely used in Germany, it has not been used extensively in the U.S. until recently.

PRIMARY USES

- Dysmenorrhea
- Hyperprolactinemia and corpus luteum insufficiency
- Premenstrual syndrome (PMS)

NOTE: The German Commission E recommended that women who experience tension or swelling of the breasts, or menstrual disturbances should consult a healthcare provider for proper diagnosis (Blumenthal, *et al.,* 1998).

OTHER POTENTIAL USES

- Acne vulgaris
- Prevention of miscarriage in the first trimester of pregnancy in cases of progesterone insufficiency
- Mastodynia
- Insufficient lactation

PHARMACOLOGICAL ACTIONS

Hormonal modulator; increases progesterone levels with corresponding reduction in estrogen levels via corpus luteum hormone effect (i.e, central action at pituitary level that inhibits release of follicle-stimulating hormone (FSH) and promotes release of luteinizing hormone (LH)); decreases prolactin secretion by the pituitary gland via dopamine antagonistic effect.

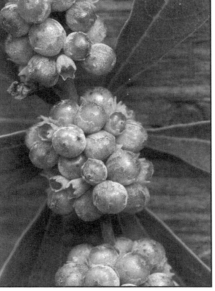

Photo © 2003 stevenfoster.com

DOSAGE AND ADMINISTRATION

Chaste tree does not have an immediate effect. The following are recommendations for minimum treatment duration: 3 months for PMS; 5–7 months for anovulation and infertility; up to 18 months for amenorrhea lasting longer than 2 years; 4–6 months for complete relief from symptoms of most conditions.

Internal

The German Commission E recommended the following daily dosage: 30–40 mg dried fruit [aqueous-alcoholic extract (50–70% *v/v*)].

DRY NATIVE EXTRACT: 1 tablet swallowed with some liquid each morning [2.6–4.2 mg, depending on concentration ratio, standardized to contain approximately 0.6–1.0% casticin].

FLUID EXTRACT: 0.5–1.0 ml [1:1 (*g/ml*), 70% alcohol (*v/v*)].

FLUID EXTRACT: 1.2–4.0 ml [1:2 (*g/ml*)].

TINCTURE: 40 drops, once daily with some liquid each morning [alcohol 58% volume, 100 g of aqueous-alcoholic solution contains 9 g of 1:5 tincture].

CONTRAINDICATIONS

None known. In theory, chaste tree should not be given with dopamine antagonists.

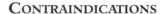

PREGNANCY AND LACTATION: Not recommended for use during pregnancy. No known restrictions during lactation. There is insufficient information regarding chaste tree's influence on prolactin levels in lactating women to reliably predict the lactogenic response. Clinical information and traditional use suggest a galactogogue effect, while *in vitro* and animal studies using a high dosage range suggest an anti-galactogogue effect. Long-term use of chaste tree (more than two weeks) during lactation may lead to disruption of the lactation amenorrhea state and an early return to fertility, which may or may not be desired.

Chaste Tree

Clinical Overview

ADVERSE EFFECTS

Side effects are rare, occurring in 1–2% of all patients treated (in clinical trials), and may include rash, headache, hair loss, fatigue, agitation, dry mouth, tachycardia, nausea, and increased menstrual flow. Itching and urticarial exanthemas occasionally occur. Caution patients to report tension, swollen breasts, or menstrual disturbances.

DRUG INTERACTIONS

None known. Evidence of a dopaminergic effect in animals suggests that a reciprocal weakening effect may occur with ingestion of dopamine-receptor antagonists such as haloperidol and potentially with dopamine-receptor blocking agents, such as metoclopramide, widely used as an antiemetic. Because of its apparent hormonal activity, chaste tree may interfere with the effectiveness of oral contraceptives and hormone-replacement therapy, although this is speculative and has not been substantiated in clinical case reports.

CLINICAL REVIEW

Eighteen clinical studies on chaste tree that included 8,336 participants all demonstrated positive effects for indications including corpus luteum abnormalities, menstrual cycle abnormalities, and PMS. Most of the studies were open, uncontrolled studies. One double-blind, placebo-controlled (DB, PC) study investigated a native dry extract of chaste tree in the treatment of luteal phase defects due to hyperprolactinemia. Two other DB, PC studies investigated native dry extracts in the treatment of PMS. A randomized (R), DB, PC, parallel study on a commercial chaste tree preparation (Ze440) on 170 women with PMS concluded that the fruit extract is safe and effective in reducing PMS symptoms. Another recent, multi-center trial on the efficacy of a chaste tree extract (Ze440) investigated 50 patients with PMS, concluding that PMS can be treated successfully as indicated by clear improvement in the main-effect parameter during treatment and the gradual return of that symptom after cessation of treatment. The main effect of treatment seems related to symptomatic relief rather than to the duration of the syndrome. From 1943 to 1997, approximately 32 clinical studies were conducted on a proprietary chaste berry product (Agnolyt®, Madaus, Germany). Eight studies focused on the product's effect on PMS, 4 on mastitis and fibrocystic disease, 3 on menopausal symptoms, 3 on increasing lactation, 4 on hyperprolactinemia, 7 on uterine bleeding disorders, 3 on acne, and 4 on miscellaneous menstrual irregularities.

Chaste Tree

Vitex agnus-castus L.
[Fam. *Verbenaceae*]

OVERVIEW

Chaste tree, also called chaste berry or vitex, derives its common name from the traditional belief that the plant promoted chastity. The fruit was used by both men and women in ancient Greece and Rome, and by monks during the Middle Ages, to suppress sexual desire. In Germany, chaste tree is a common treatment for gynecological disorders and it has recently become popular in the U.S.

USES

Premenstrual syndrome (PMS); painful menstruation; hyperprolactinemia and corpus luteum insufficiency.

NOTE: The German Commission E recommended that women who experience tension or swelling of the breasts or menstrual disturbances should consult a healthcare provider for proper diagnosis.

OTHER POTENTIAL USES

Breast pain.

DOSAGE

DRY NATIVE EXTRACT: One 2.6–4.2 mg tablet, standardized to contain approximately 0.6–1.0% casticin, swallowed with some liquid each morning.

FLUID EXTRACT: 0.5–4.0 ml, daily.

TINCTURE: 40 drops, daily.

CONTRAINDICATIONS

No known contraindications.

PREGNANCY AND LACTATION: Not for use during pregnancy. No restrictions known during breast-feeding. There is insufficient information on chaste tree's effect on breast-feeding. Long-term use of chaste tree (more than 2 weeks) may lead to disruption of the cessation of the menstrual cycle that normally accompanies breast-feeding and an early return to fertility which may or may not be desired. Consult a healthcare provider prior to use while breast-feeding.

ADVERSE EFFECTS

Itching, rash, headache, hair loss, fatigue, agitation, dry

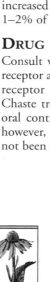

mouth, rapid heartbeat (tachycardia), nausea, and increased menstrual flow may occur rarely (noted in 1–2% of patients in clinical studies).

DRUG INTERACTIONS

Consult with a healthcare provider if using dopamine-receptor antagonists such as haloperidol, and dopamine-receptor blocking agents such as metoclopramide. Chaste tree may also interfere with the effectiveness of oral contraceptives and hormone-replacement therapy; however, this potential interaction is theoretical and has not been documented in case reports.

Comments

When using a dietary supplement, purchase it from a reliable source. For best results, use the same brand of product throughout the period of use. As with all medications and dietary supplements, please inform your healthcare provider of all herbs and medications you are taking. Interactions may occur between medications and herbs or even among different herbs when taken at the same time. Treat your herbal supplement with care by taking it as directed, storing it as advised on the label, and keeping it out of the reach of children and pets. Consult your healthcare provider with any questions.

AMERICAN BOTANICAL COUNCIL

The information contained on this sheet has been excerpted from *The ABC Clinical Guide to Herbs* © 2003 by the American Botanical Council (ABC). ABC is an independent member-based educational organization focusing on the medicinal use of herbs. For more detailed information about this herb please consult the healthcare provider who gave you this sheet. To order *The ABC Clinical Guide to Herbs* or become a member of ABC, visit their website at www.herbalgram.org.

Chaste Tree

Vitex agnus-castus L.
[Fam. Verbenaceae]

OVERVIEW

Chaste tree, sometimes called chaste berry or vitex, derived its common name from the traditional belief that the plant promoted chastity (Winterhoff, 1998; Christie and Walker, 1997). The fruit of *Vitex agnus-castus* (hereafter referred to as chaste tree) was used in ancient Greece and Rome by males and females, including the monks of the Middle Ages (as a "functional" food flavoring), to suppress sexual desire (Winterhoff, 1998; Upton, 2001). Chaste tree is a widely used and popular treatment for gynecological disorders, including corpus luteum insufficiency (Merz *et al.*, 1996; Milewicz *et al.*, 1993); premenstrual syndrome (PMS) (Schellenberg *et al.*, 2001, Loch *et al.*, 2000; Dittmar and Böhnert, 1992; Coeugniet *et al.*, 1986; Wuttke *et al.*, 1995); menstrual problems (Loch *et al.*, 1991; Loch and Kaiser, 1990); and cyclic mastalgia (Halaska *et al.*, 1998; Kress and Thanner, 1981; Kubista *et al.*, 1983). It has also been used to treat hormonally induced acne (Amann, 1967). Chaste tree has been traditionally used to treat fibroid cysts and infertility, to stop miscarriages caused by progesterone insufficiency, to flush out the placenta after birth (McGuffin *et al.*, 1997; Peirce, 1999), and as a digestive aid, sedative, and anti-infective (Christie and Walker, 1997). Although chaste tree is widely used in Germany, it has not been used in the U.S. much until relatively recently. It has not yet achieved significant popularity in mainstream retail outlets but ranked 54th in natural food store sales in 2001 (Richman and Witkowski, 2001).

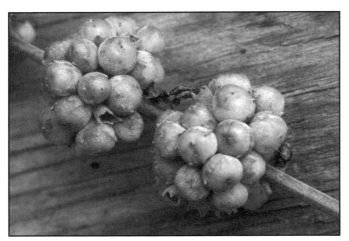

Photo © 2003 stevenfoster.com

DESCRIPTION

Chaste tree is the ripe, dried fruit of *Vitex agnus-castus* L. [Fam. Verbenaceae], containing no less than 0.4% (*v/w*) of volatile oil (GHP, 1993), and no less than 8% water-soluble extractive (BHP, 1996). The average water- and ethanol-soluble extractive content is approximately 10% (Abel, 1999). It is unknown which constituents are responsible for chaste tree's activity, and up to this point there are no official published guidelines for the standardization of chaste tree preparations (Meier, 1999). However, two compounds are presently used as marker compounds for quality control: the iridoid glycoside *agnuside* and the flavonol *casticin* (Abel, 1999). Most chaste tree preparations used in European medicine are nonstandardized fluid extracts, tinctures, and/or native dry extracts. The "native" or "total" extract has an approximate 10:1 (*w/w*) drug-to-extract ratio containing 0.6–1.0% casticin (Abel, 1999; Morant and Ruppanner, 2001). It has been suggested in the future, pharmaceutical-grade chaste tree preparations should be characterized qualitatively and quantitatively, based on hydrophilic flavonoids, lipophilic compounds, and iridoid glycosides (Hoberg *et al.*, 1999; Upton, 2001).

PRIMARY USES
Gynecology

- Dysmenorrhea (Bubenzer, 1993; Loch *et al.*, 1991; Loch and Kaiser, 1990; Bleier, 1959; Probst and Roth, 1954)
- Hyperprolactinemia and corpus luteum insufficiency (Merz *et al.*, 1996; Milewicz *et al.*, 1993; Propping *et al.*, 1991; Propping and Katzorke, 1987)
- Premenstrual syndrome (PMS) (Schellenberg *et al.*, 2001; Loch *et al.*, 2000; Berger *et al*, 2000; Berger *et al.*, 1999; Lauritzen *et al.*, 1997; Turner and Mills, 1993; Dittmar and Böhnert, 1992; Coeugniet *et al.*, 1986)

NOTE: The German Commission E recommended that women who experience tension or swelling of the breasts, or menstrual disturbances should consult a healthcare provider for proper diagnosis (Blumenthal, *et al.*, 1998)

OTHER POTENTIAL USES
Dermatology
- Acne vulgaris (Giss and Rothenburg, 1968; Amann, 1967; Bleier, 1959)

Gynecology
- Prevention of miscarriage in the first trimester of pregnancy in cases of progesterone insufficiency (McGuffin *et al.*, 1997)
- Mastodynia (Halaske *et al.*, 1999; Blumenthal *et al.*, 1998; Kubista *et al.*, 1986)
- Insufficient lactation (Bruckner, 1989)

DOSAGE
Internal
The German Commission E recommended the following daily dosage: Aqueous-alcoholic extract (50–70% *v/v*), corresponding to 30–40 mg dried fruit (Blumenthal *et al.*, 1998).

DRY NATIVE EXTRACT [2.6–4.2 mg, depending on concentration ratio, standardized to contain approximately 0.6–1.0% casticin]: 1 tablet swallowed with some liquid each morning (Abel, 1999; Bionorica, 1998; Lauritzen *et al.*, 1997; Madaus, 1996). NOTE: Some products (Zeller PreMens® Ze440) recommend up to 20 mg native extract daily (Morant and Ruppanner, 2001; Berger *et al.*, 1999).

FLUID EXTRACT [1:1 (*g/ml*), 70% alcohol (*v/v*)]: 0.5–1.0 ml (Karnick, 1994).

FLUID EXTRACT [1:2 (*g/ml*)]: 1.2–4.0 ml (Bone, 1989).

TINCTURE [Alcohol 58% volume, 100 g of aqueous-alcoholic solution contains 9 g of 1:5 tincture]: 40 drops, once daily with some liquid each morning (Madaus, 1996).

DURATION OF ADMINISTRATION

Chaste tree does not have an immediate effect. For treatment of PMS, a minimum treatment duration of three months is recommended (Morant and Ruppanner, 2001). A survey of medical herbalists in the U.K. reported a mean average of 4.8 months of treatment is necessary before patients with PMS symptoms respond to chaste tree (Christie and Walker, 1997). For anovulation and infertility, a treatment duration of five to seven months may be necessary. For amenorrhea lasting longer than two years, a treatment period of up to 18 months may be required (Pizzorno and Murray, 1999; Boon and Smith, 1999; Brown, 1994). For most other conditions, symptoms usually start to diminish within one to two months. After four to six months, extensive or complete relief from symptoms may be seen (Pizzorno and Murray, 1999; Brown, 1994).

CHEMISTRY

Mature chaste tree fruit yields 0.4–0.7% (% *v/w*) essential oil, depending on distillation time and size of comminuted particles (Sørensen and Katsiotis, 2000), and is composed mainly of bornyl acetate, 1,8-cineole, limonene, α- and β-pinene, β-caryophyllene, and α-terpinyl acetate (Meier and Hoberg, 1999). It also contains labdane diterpenoids: 0.04–0.3% rotundifuran, 0.04–0.17% vitexilactone, 0.02–0.1% 6β, 7β-diacetoxy-13-hydroxy-labda-8,14-diene (Hoberg et al., 1999); flavonoids: 0.10–0.16% casticin (Abel, 1999); iridoid glycosides: 0.2–0.4% agnuside (Abel, 1999); and 0.3% aucubin (Newall *et al.*, 1996). NOTE: For optimal yield of isoorientin, agnuside, and casticin in extraction, tincture maceration with a drug-to-extract ratio of 1:5 (*w/v*) in 52% ethanol (*v/v*) is most effective and will also extract a significant amount of the diterpenes (Meier, 1999).

PHARMACOLOGICAL ACTIONS

Human

Hormonal modulator (BHP, 1996). Early research suggested that chaste tree acts centrally, at the pituitary level, to inhibit release of follicle-stimulating hormone (FSH) and promote the release of luteinizing hormone (LH) (Boon and Smith, 1999; Weiss and Fintelmann, 2000). This action, referred to as a "corpus luteum hormone effect" (Weiss, 1988), was previously thought to lead to an increase in progesterone levels and a corresponding reduction in estrogen levels (Boon and Smith, 1999; Weiss, 1988). However, more recent research indicates that chaste tree appears to exert its medicinal actions through the reduction of prolactin secretion by the pituitary gland (Upton, 2001; Boon and Smith, 1999; Winterhoff, 1998; Newall *et al.*, 1996), through a mechanism involving dopamine antagonism.

Animal

Chaste tree significantly inhibits the stress-induced secretion of prolactin in male rats via its activity on the pituitary gland (Jarry *et al.*, 1991; Winterhoff, 1993; Wuttke *et al.*, 1995). In healthy lactating rats, high doses of chaste tree significantly reduced milk production compared to controls (Winterhoff, 1993, 1998).

In vitro

Chaste tree extract displaces ligands of human opioid-receptor-binding (Brugisser *et al.*, 1999), inhibits prolactin release from rat pituitary cells and exerts a dopamine-agonistic effect through direct dopamine receptor-binding (Jarry *et al.*, 1994; Sluitz *et al.*, 1993; Winterhoff, 1993; Wuttke *et al*, 1995). It does not appear to modulate rat pituitary cell production of FSH or LH (Jarry *et al.*, 1994) or inhibit spontaneous activity of the isolated rat uterus (Lal *et al.*, 1985). It has antimicrobial activity (Pepeljnjak, *et al.*, 1996).

MECHANISM OF ACTION

The exact mechanism of action of chaste tree has not been established (Upton, 2001). However, *in vitro* and *in vivo* studies have shown a dopaminergic action resulting in a reduction in elevated prolactin levels (Jarry *et al.*, 1994, 1991; Milewicz *et al.*, 1993; Sluitz *et al.*, 1993; Upton, 2001; Winterhoff, 1998; Wuttke *et al.*, 1995) and a cholinergic mechanism of action (Berger *et al.*, 1999). Isolated diterpenoids, rotundifuran, and 6β,7β-diacetoxy-13-hydroxy-labda-8,14-diene have shown dopaminergic activity in studies on receptor-binding (Hoberg *et al.*, 1999). Chaste tree extract inhibit release of FSH, and promote the release of LH (Boon and Smith, 1999; Weiss and Fintelmann, 2000). This action, referred to as a "corpus luteum hormone effect" (Weiss, 1988), leads to an increase in progesterone levels and a corresponding reduction in estrogen levels (Boon and Smith, 1999; Weiss, 1988). Furthermore, new research indicates that chaste tree appears to exert its medicinal actions through the reduction of prolactin secretion from the pituitary gland (Boon and Smith, 1999; Winterhoff, 1998; Newall *et al.*, 1996).

Animal

• Healthy male rats have been involved in studies in which plasma levels of prolactin were measured before and after exposure to chaste tree. Post-treatment prolactin levels were significantly reduced in the chaste tree treatment groups compared to control groups, which indicates inhibition of prolactin secretion *in vivo* (Winterhoff, 1998; Wuttke *et al.*, 1995).

In vitro

• Studies using a test system consisting of rat pituitary cultures revealed a dose-dependent decrease in prolactin secretion (Jarry *et al.*, 1994, 1991; Sluitz *et al.*, 1993; Winterhoff, 1998; Wuttke *et al.*, 1995). Since the prolactin inhibitory effects could be blocked by haloperidol, a dopamine receptor antagonist, chaste tree appears to exert its prolactin-lowering action via dopamine agonism (Merz *et al.*, 1996; Winterhoff, 1998).

CONTRAINDICATIONS

According to the German Commission E, no contradictions are known (Blumenthal *et al.*, 1998).

PREGNANCY AND LACTATION: Not recommended for use during pregnancy, according to the Commission E (Blumenthal *et al.*, 1998). The corpus luteum hormone effect of chaste tree can adversely effect the fetal sexual development and therefore chaste tree extract should not be taken during pregnancy. However, in cases of progesterone insufficiency, the increase in progesterone levels can prevent miscarriage in the first trimester of pregnancy (McGuffin *et al.*, 1997), but this exceptional indication during pregnancy should be discussed with the healthcare provider prior to use. Progesterone levels should be closely monitored in the early weeks of pregnancy if a decision is made to withdraw chaste tree before four months.

No known restrictions during lactation (McGuffin *et al.*, 1997). There is insufficient information regarding chaste tree's influence on prolactin levels in lactating women to reliably predict the lactogenic response. Clinical information and traditional use suggest a galactogogue effect, while *in vitro* and animal studies using a high dosage range suggest an anti-galactogogue effect. Long-term use of chaste tree (more than two weeks) during lactation may lead to disruption of the lactation amenorrhea state and an early return to fertility, which may or may not be desired.

ADVERSE EFFECTS

Commission E noted occasional occurrence of itching and urticarial exanthemas. If feelings of breast tension, breast swelling, or menstrual disturbances occur, a healthcare provider should be consulted for diagnosis (Blumenthal *et al.*, 1998). Side effects are rare, occurring in 1–2% of all patients treated (Loch *et al.*, 2000), and may include itching, rash, headache, hair loss, fatigue, agitation, dry mouth, tachycardia, nausea, and increased menstrual flow (Anon., 1998; Dittmar and Böhnert, 1992; Loch *et al.*, 1991; Newall, *et al.*, 1996). The usual percentage of side effects reported in clinical trials is 1–2% of subjects, or 246 side effects in 30 studies, with some subjects reporting multiple effects (total subjects=11,506) (Upton, 2001). The most frequent side effects reported were gastrointestinal distress/nausea (75), acne, skin reactions, urticaria (58), cycle changes (24), headache (10). There is one case report of mild ovarian hyperstimulation in a woman who self-prescribed chaste tree (Cahill, *et al.*, 1994).

DRUG INTERACTIONS

None known. There is evidence of a dopaminergic effect in animals, which suggests a reciprocal weakening effect can occur with ingestion of dopamine-receptor antagonists such as haloperidol and potentially with dopamine-receptor blocking agents, such as metoclopramide, widely used as an antiemetic (Blumenthal *et al.*, 1998). Due to its apparent hormonal activity, chaste tree may interfere with the effectiveness of oral contraceptives and hormone-replacement therapy (McGuffin *et al.*, 1997; Boon and Smith, 1999); however, this speculative interaction has not been substantiated in clinical case reports (Upton, 2001).

AMERICAN HERBAL PRODUCTS ASSOCIATION (AHPA) SAFETY RATING

CLASS 2B: Should not be used during pregnancy (McGuffin *et al.*, 1997).

CLASS 2D: May counteract the effectiveness of birth control pills (McGuffin *et al.*, 1997). However, a subsequent in-depth review of chaste tree pharmacology and clinical trials by a co-editor of the AHPA rating writes that this precaution "lacks substantiation" (Upton, 2001).

REGULATORY STATUS

CANADA: 32 chaste tree-containing homeopathic drugs have marketing authorization with Drug Identification Numbers (DIN) assigned (Health Canada, 2001). No chaste tree-containing

Traditional Herbal Medicines (THM) are presently authorized, though there are no known restrictions.

FRANCE: Chaste tree fruit for homeopathic preparations is official in the Pharmacopée Française (Ph.Fr. X, 1989).

GERMANY: Approved nonprescription drug by the Commission E (Blumenthal *et al.*, 1998). Dried ripe fruit, containing no less than 0.4% (*v/w*) volatile oil, for preparation of mother tincture and liquid dilutions is official in the *German Homeopathic Pharmacopoeia* (GHP, 1993). Chaste tree is the subject of a botanical monograph in development for the DAB by the German pharmacopeial commission (Meier, 1999).

ITALY: No monograph in the *Italian Pharmacopoeia* (Meier, 1999).

SWEDEN: Classified as a drug which must be registered as a pharmaceutical specialty (De Smet *et al.*, 1993). No chaste tree-containing products are presently registered in the Medical Products Agency's (MPA) "Authorised Natural Remedies" (MPA, 2001a), but chaste tree homeopathic drugs in tablets (D6, D12, and D30) have been registered (MPA, 2001b).

SWITZERLAND: Category D nonprescription drug with sale limited to pharmacies and drugstores (Meier and Hoberg, 1999; Morant and Ruppanner, 2001). Two chaste tree phytomedicines and two chaste tree-containing homeopathic drugs are listed in the *Swiss Codex* 2000/01 (Ruppanner and Schaefer, 2000). Chaste tree is the subject of a botanical monograph in development by the Swiss pharmacopeial commission (Meier, 1999).

U.K.: Herbal medicine on *General Sale List* (GSL), Table A (internal or external use), Schedule 1 (requires full Product License) (GSL, 1994). No monograph in the *British Pharmacopoeia* (Meier, 1999), but one is found in *British Herbal Pharmacopoeia*.

U.S.: Dietary supplement (USC, 1994). Tincture of the dried or fresh berries, 1:10 (*w/v*) in 65% alcohol (*v/v*), is official in the *Homeopathic Pharmacopoeia of the United States* (HPUS, 1989). No monograph in the USP-NF.

CLINICAL REVIEW

Eighteen studies are outlined in the table, "Clinical Studies on Chaste Tree," including 8,336 participants. All of these studies demonstrate positive effects for indications including corpus luteum abnormalities, menstrual cycle abnormalities, and PMS. Most of the studies are open, uncontrolled studies. One double-blind, placebo-controlled (DB, PC) study investigated a native dry extract of chaste tree in the treatment of luteal phase defects due to hyperprolactinemia (Milewicz *et al.*, 1993). Two other studies investigated native dry extracts in the treatment of PMS (Lauritzen *et al.*, 1997; Turner and Mills, 1993). A randomized, DB, PC, parallel study on a commercial chaste tree preparation (Ze440) on 170 women with PMS concluded that the fruit extract is safe and effective in reducing PMS symptoms (Schellenberger *et al.*, 2001). Another recent, multi-center trial on the efficacy of a chaste tree extract (Ze440) investigated 50 patients with PMS, concluding that PMS can be treated successfully as indicated by clear improvement in the main-effect parameter during treatment and the gradual return of that symptom after cessation of treatment. The main effect of treatment seems related to symptomatic relief rather than to the duration of the syndrome (Berger *et al.*, 2000). From 1943 to 1997, approximately 32 clinical studies were conducted on a proprietary chaste berry product (Agnolyt®, Madaus, Germany). Eight studies were on the product's effect on PMS, 4 on mastitis and fibrocystic disease, 3 on menopausal symptoms, 3 on increasing lactation, 4 on hyperprolactinemia, 7 on uterine bleeding disorders, 3 on acne, and 4 on miscellaneous menstrual irregularities.

BRANDED PRODUCTS*

Agnolyt® Capsules: Madaus AG / Ostermerheimer Strasse 198 / Köln / Germany / Tel: +49-22-18-9984-76 / Fax: +49-22-18-9987-21 / Email: b.lindener@madaus.de. Chaste tree fruit, hydro-alcoholic, native dry extract 9.58–11.5:1 (*w/w*), 60% ethanol volume. This product is no longer available.

Agnolyt® Solution: Madaus AG Chaste tree fruit tincture, ethanol 68% volume. Each 100 g of aqueous-alcoholic solution contains 9 g of a 1:5 tincture.

Alyt® Solution: Ciba-Geigy AG / Contact: Novartis Consumer Health AG / Route de l'Etraz / CH 1260 Nyon 1 / Switzerland / www.consumer-health.novartis.com. Chaste tree fruit tincture, ethanol 68% volume. Each 100 g of aqueous-alcoholic solution contains 9 g of a 1:5 tincture. Unable to verify manufacturer and availability.

BNO 1095 capsules (Bionorica Agnus castus extract), Bionorica AG / P.O. Box 1851 / D-92308 Neumarkt / Germany / Tel: +49(0)9181-231-90 / Email: international@bionorica.de / www.bionorica.de. Capsules contain 40 mg BP1095E1 [6–12:1 extract (spissum) (70% ethanol)]. This product is not distributed; Bionorica does distribute a tablet product containing BP1095 extract (6–12:1) equivalent to 40 mg crude drug.

Femicur® N Kapseln: Schaper & Brümmer GmbH & Co. KG/ Bahnhofstrasse 35 / 38259 Salzgitter / Ringelheim / Germany / Tel: +49-5341-30-70 / Fax: +49-5341-30-71-24 / Email: info@schaperbruemmer.de / www.schaper-bruemmer.com. 1 capsule contains dry extract of fruits of Vitex agnus-castus (7–13:1) 4 mg, extractant: ethanol 60% (m/m).

PreMens® Ze440: Zeller AG / Seeblickstrasse 4 / CH-8590 Romanshorn 1 / Switzerland / www.zellerag.ch. One coated tablet contains 40 mg chaste tree fruit hydro-alcoholic extract of which 20 mg is native dry extract, 6.0–12.0:1 (*w/w*) and 20 mg is lactose as excipient, 60% ethanol by weight. Normalized to contain a minimum of 0.6% casticin.

Strotan® Kapseln: Strathmann AG & Co. / Sellhopsweg 1 / 22459 Hamburg / Germany / Tel: +49-40-55-9050 / Fax: +49-40-55-9051-00 / Email: info@strathmann.de / www.strathmann.de. Soft-gel capsule contains 20 mg chaste tree fruit, hydro-alcoholic (50–70% *v/v*), native dry extract. Chemically defined constituents include the iridoids aucubin and agnuside, flavonoids, essential and fatty oils, and the bitter principle castin.

*American equivalents are found in the Product Table beginning on page 398.

REFERENCES

Abel G. Experience with the analytical methods from raw extract to drug product. [in German]. *Z Phytother* 1999;20:147–8.

Amann W. Improvement of acne vulgaris following therapy with agnus-castus (Agnolyt®). [in German]. *Ther Ggw* 1967;106:124–6.

Anon. Chaste Tree. In: Dombek C (ed.). *Lawrence Review of Natural Products*. St. Louis: Facts and Comparisons; 1998.

BHP. See: *British Herbal Pharmacopoeia*.

Berger D, *et al*. Efficacy of *Vitex agnus-castus* L. extract Ze 440 in patients with premenstrual syndrome (PMS). *Arch Gynecol Obstet* 2000 Nov;264(3):150–3.

Berger D, Aebi S, Samochowiec E, Schaffner W. Clinical Applications in premenstrual syndrome. [in German]. *Z Phytother* 1999;20:155–7.

Berger D, Burkard W, Schaffner W, Meier B. Receptorligation studies with extracts

and their isolated substances. [in German]. *Z Phytother* 1999;20:153–4.

Bionorica. Agnucaston®. In: *Präparateverzeichnis*. Neumarkt/Opf., Germany: Bionorica Arzneimittel GmbH; 1998;70.

Bleier W. Phytotherapy in irregular menstrual cycles or bleeding periods and the gynecological disorders of endocrine origin. [in German]. *Zentralbl Gynäkol* 1959;18:701–9.

Blumenthal M, Busse WR, Goldberg A, Gruenwald J, Hall T, Riggins CW, Rister RS (eds.). Klein S, Rister RS (trans.). *The Complete German Commission E Monographs—Therapeutic Guide to Herbal Medicines*. Austin, TX: American Botanical Council; Boston: Integrative Medicine Communication; 1998;108.

Blumenthal M, Goldberg A, Brinckmann J (eds.). *Herbal Medicine: Expanded Commission E Monographs*. Austin: American Botanical Council; Newton, MA: Integrative Medicine Communications; 2000;62–3.

Böhnert K. The use of *Vitex agnus-castus* for hyperprolactinemia. *Q Rev Nat Med* 1997 Spring;19–21.

Bone K. *Vitex agnus-castus* — scientific studies. *MediHerb Newsletter* February 1989.

Boon H, Smith M. *The Botanical Pharmacy*. Quarry Health Books; 1999;76-81.

British Herbal Pharmacopoeia (BHP 1996), 4th edition. Exeter, UK: British Herbal Medicine Association; 1996;19–20.

Brown D. *Vitex agnus-castus*: clinical monographs. *Q Rev Nat Med* 1994 Summer; 111–21.

Bruckner C. The application of phytopharmaceuticals in central Europe and their stimulating effect on lactation. [in German]. *Gleditschia* 1989;17:189–201.

Brugisser R, Burkard W, Simmen U, Schaffner W. Assessment of opioid receptor activity with *Vitex agnus-castus*. [in German]. *Z Phytother* 1999;20:154.

Bubenzer R. Therapy with Agnus-castus extract (Strotan®). [in German]. *Therapiewoche* 1993;43:32–3, 1705–6.

Cahill D, Fox R, Wardle P, Harlow C. Multiple follicular development associated with herbal medicine. *Hum Reprod* 1994;9:1469–70.

Christie S, Walker A. *Vitex agnus-castus*, A review of its traditional and modern therapeutic use, current use from a survey of practitioners. *Euro J Herbal Med* 1997;3:29–45.

Coeugniet E, Elek E, Kühnast R. Premenstrual syndrome and its treatment. [in German]. *Arztezeitchr Naturheilverf* 1986;27:619–22.

De Smet, P, Keller K, Hänsel R, Chandler R. *Adverse Effects of Herbal Drugs*, Vol. 2. Berlin, Heidelberg: Springer-Verlag; 1993;1–17, 87.

Dittmar F, Böhnert K. Premenstrual Syndrome: Treatment with a phytopharmceutical. [in German]. *TW Gynakol* 1992;5:60–8.

Du Mee C. *Vitex agnus-castus*. *Aust J Med Herbalism* 1993;5:63–5.

Fleming T (ed.). *PDR for Herbal Medicines*. Montvale, NJ: Medical Economics Company, Inc.; 1998.

Gerhard I, Patek A, Monga B, Blank A, Gorkow C. Mastodynon® for female sterility. [in German]. *Forsch Komplementarmed* 1998;5:272–8.

General Sale List (GSL). Statutory Instrument 1994 No. 2410 — The Medicines (Products Other Than Veterinary Drugs) Amendment Order 1994. London, U.K.: Her Majesty's Stationery Office (HMSO); 1994.

German Homeopathic Pharmacopoeia (GHP), 1st edition 1978 with supplements through 1991. Translation of the German "*Homöpathisches Arzneibuch* (HAB 1), Amtliche Ausgabe." Stuttgart, Germany: Deutscher Apotheker Verlag; 1993;907–8.

GHP. See: *German Homoeopathic Pharmacopoeia*.

GSL. See: *General Sale List*.

Giss G, Rothenburg W. Treatment of acne with phytopharmaceuticals. [in German]. *Z Haut und Geschlechtskrankheiten* 1968;43(15):645–7.

Halaska M, Raus K, Beles P, Martan A, Paithner K. Treatment of cyclical mastodynia using an extract of *Vitex agnus-castus*: results of a double-blind comparison with a placebo. [in Czech.]. *Ceska Gynekol* 1998;63:388–92.

Health Canada. Agnus-castus. In: Drug Product Database (DPD). Ottawa, Ontario: Health Canada Therapeutic Products Programme; 2001.

Hobbs C, Blumenthal M. Chaste Tree: *Vitex agnus-castus*—A Literature Review [unpublished].

Homeopathic Pharmacopoeia of the United States — HPUS Revision Service Official Compendium from July 1, 1992. Falls Church, VA: American Institute of Homeopathy. June 1989;0066;AGNS.

HPUS. See: *Homeopathic Pharmacopoeia of the United States*.

Hoberg E, Sticher O, Orjala J, Meier B. The analysis of diterpne from agni casti fructus extract. [in German]. *Z Phytother* 1999;s0:149–150.

IKS. See: *Interkantonale Kontrollstelle für Heilmittel*.

Interkantonale Kontrollstelle für Heilmittel (IKS). Liste D: Richtlinien der IKS für die Verkaufsabgrenzung der Arzneimittel für Drogerien. Bern, Switzerland: IKS; 1988, Nov 25.

Jarry H, Leonhardt S, Wuttke W, Behr B, Gorkow C. Principal dopaminergic action of an agnus-castus extract (Mastodynon®). [in Geman]. *Z Phytother* 1991;12:77–82.

Jarry H, Leonhardt S, Gorkow C, Wuttke W. *In vitro* prolactin but not LH and FSH release is inhibited by compounds in extracts of *Agnus-castus*: direct evidence for a dopaminergic principle by the dopamine receptor assay. *Exp Clin Endocrinol* 1994;102:448–54.

Jarry H, Leonhardt S, Wuttke W, *et al.* In search of dopaminergic substances in agni-casti-fructus extracts. Why actually? [in German]. *Z Phytother* 1999;20:150–2.

Karnick C. *Pharmacopoeial Standards of Herbal Plants*, Vol. II. Delhi, India: Sri Satguru Publications; 1994;32.

Kress D, Thanner E. Treatment of mastitis. [in German]. *Med Klinik* 1981;76:566.

Kubista E, *et al.* Conservative treatment of mastitis. [in German]. *Z Gynakologie* 1983;105:1153–62.

Kubista E, *et al.* Treatment of mastopathy with cyclic mastodynia. Clinical results and hormone profiles. *Gynak Rdsch* 1986;26:65–79.

Lal R, Sankaranarayanan A, Mathur V, Sharma P. Antifertility and oxytocic activity of *Vitex agnus-castus* seeds in female albino rats. *Bulletin of Postgraduate Institute of Medical Education and Research Chandigarh* 1985;19:44-7.

Lauritzen C, Reuter H, Repges R. Böhnert K, Schmidt U. Treatment of premenstrual tension syndrome with *Vitex agnus-castus*: controlled double-blind study versus pyridoxine. *Phytomedicine* 1997;4(3):183–9.

Leung A, Foster S. *Encyclopedia of Common Natural Ingredients Used in Food, Drugs and Cosmetics*, 2nd ed. New York, NY: John Wiley & Sons, Inc.; 1996.

Loch E, Selle H, Boblitz N. Treatment of premenstrual syndrome with a phytopharmaceutical formulation containing *Vitex agnus-castus*. *J Women's Health and Gender-Based Med* 2000;9(3):315–20.

Loch E, *et al.* The treatment of menstrual disorders with *Vitex agnus-castus* tincture. [in German]. *Der Frauenarzt* 1991;32:867–70.

Loch E, Kaiser E. Diagnosis and treatment of dyshormonal menstrual periods in the general practice. [in German]. *Gynakol Praxis* 1990;14:489–95.

Madaus GmbH. Product Information: Agnolyt® Solution; Agnolyt® Capsules. Köln, Germany: Dr. Madaus GmbH & Co.; 1996.

McGuffin M, Hobbs C, Upton R, Goldberg A (eds.). *American Herbal Products Association's Botanical Safety Handbook*. Boca Raton, FL: CRC Press; 1997:123–4.

Medical Products Agency (MPA). *Naturläkemedel: Authorised Natural Remedies* (as of Jan 24, 2001). Uppsala, Sweden: Medical Products Agency; 2001a.

Medical Products Agency (MPA). *Läkemedelsnära Produkter; Homeopatika: Företag med registrerade homeopatika*. Uppsala, Sweden: Medical Products Agency; 2001b.

Meier B. Standardization problems of pharmaceutical preparations. [in German]. *Z Phytother* 1999;20(3):145–7.

Meier B, Hoberg E. *Agni-casti fructus*: New insights in quality and efficacy. [in German]. *Z Phytother* 1999;20:140–1.

Merz P, Gorkow C, Schrödter A, *et al.* The effects of a special Agnus-castus extract (BP1095E1) on prolactin secretion in healthy male subjects. *J Exp Clin Endocrinol Diabetes* 1996;104:447–53.

Milewicz A, Gejdel E, Sworen H, *et al. Vitex agnus-castus* extract in the treatment of luteal phase defects due to latent hyperprolactinemia. Results of a randomized placebo-scontrolled double-blind study. [in German]. *Arzneimittelforschung* 1993;43(7):752–6.

Morant J, Ruppanner H (eds.). Zeller Medical Prefemin®; PreMens®. In: *Arzneimittel Kompendium der Schweiz® 2001*. Basel, Switzerland: Documed AG. 2001.

MPA. See: Medical Products Agency.

Newall C, Anderson L, Phillipson J. *Herbal medicines: a guide for health-care professionals*. London, UK: Pharmaceutical Press; 1996;296.

Peirce A. *The American Pharmaceutical Association Practical Guide to Natural Medicines*. New York: William Morrow and Company, Inc.; 1999.

Pepeljnjak S, Antolic A, Kustrak D. Antibacterial and antifungal activities of the *Vitex agnus-castus* L. extracts. *Acta Pharmaceutica Zagreb* 1996;46:201–6.

Ph.Fr. X. See: Pharmacopée Française.

Pharmacopée Française (Ph.Fr. X). Paris, France: Adrapharm. 1982–1996; Supplement January 1989.

Pizzorno JE, Murray MT, editors. *Textbook of Natural Medicine*. Vol.1, 2nd ed. New York: Churchill Livingston; 1999;1:1020–3, 1395,1510.

Probst V, Roth O. A plant extract with a hormone like effect. [in German]. *Dtsch Med Wschr* 1954;79(35):1271– 4.

Propping D, Katzorke T. Treatment of corpus luteum insufficiency. [in German]. *Z Allgemeinmed* 1987;63(31):932–3.

Propping D, Böhnert K, Peeters M, *et al. Vitex agnus-castus* treatment of gynecological syndromes. [in German]. *Therapeutikon* 1991;5:581–5.

Reuter H, *et al.* The management of the premenstrual syndrome with *Vitex agnus-castus*. Double-blind controlled study with pyridoxin. [in German]. *Z Pyhtother Abstractband* 1995;7.

Richman A, Witkowski P. 7th annual herb sales survey. *Whole Foods* 2001;24(11):23–30.

Ruppanner H, Schaefer U (eds.). *Codex 2000/01 — Die Schweizer Arzneimittel in einem Griff*. Basel, Switzerland: Documed AG. 2000; 256, 684, 688.

Schellenberg R. Kunze G, Pfaff E, *et al.* Treatment for the premenstrual syndrome with agnus-castus fruit extract: prospective, randomized, placebo controlled study. *BMJ* 2001 Jan;322:134–7.

Sliutz G, Speiser P, Schultz AM, Spona J, Zeillinger R. Agnus-castus extracts inhibit prolactin secretion of rat pituitary cells. *Horm Metab Res* 1993;25:253–5

Sørensen J, Katsiotis S. Parameters influencing the yield and composition of the essential oil from Cretan *Vitex agnus-castus* fruits. *Planta Med* 2000;66:245–50.

Turner S, Mills S. A double-blind clinical trial on a herbal remedy for premenstrual syndrome; a case study. *Comp Ther Med* 1993;1:73–7.

United States Congress (USC). Public Law 103–417: Dietary Supplement Health and Education Act of 1994. Washington, DC: 103rd Congress of the United States; 1994.

Upton R (ed.). Chaste Tree Fruit. Santa Cruz, CA: American Herbal Pharmacopoeia; 2001.

USC. See: United States Congress.

Weiss R. *Herbal Medicine*. Beaconsfield, England: Beaconsfield Publishers, 1988;318.

Weiss R, Fintelmann V. *Herbal Medicine*. 2nd ed. New York: Thieme; 2000;331.

Winterhoff H. Phytobotanicals and their endocrine effect. [in German.] *A Phytother* 1993;14:83–94.

Winterhoff H. *Vitex agnus-castus* (chaste tree): pharmacological and clinical data. In: Lawson LD, Bauer R, editors. *Phytomedicines of Europe: Chemistry and Biological Activity*, ACS Symposium Series 691. Proceedings of the 212th National Meeting of the American Chemical Society; 1996 Aug; Orlando (FL). Washington (DC): American Chemical Society, 1998. p. 299–308.

Wuttke W, Gorkow C, Jarry H. Dopaminergic compounds in *Vitex agnus castus*. [in German]. In: Loew D, Rietbrock N (eds.). *Phytopharmaka in Forschung und klinischer Anwendung*. Darmstadt: Sterinkopff Verlag; 1995.

Clinical Studies on Chaste Tree (*Vitex agnus castus* L.)

Corpus Luteum Irregularities/Hyperprolactinemia

Author/Year	Subject	Design	Duration	Dosage	Preparation	Results/Conclusion
Merz *et al.*, 1996	Hyper-prolactinemia	O, PC, Cm (intra-individual comparison) n=20 healthy men	14-day treatment period for each phase with 7-day wash-out phase between phases	Phase 1: placebo Phase 2: One capsule 3x/day (120 mg/day) Phase 3: Two capsules 3x/day (240 mg/day) Phase 4: Four capsules 3x/day (480 mg/day)	Bionorica BNO1095 capsules containing 20 mg BP1095E1 extract [6–12:1 extract (spissum) (70% ethanol)] equivalent to 40 mg crude drug	Pharmacological data were obtained on the influence of 14-day vitex treatment on Thyroxin Releasing Hormone (TRH)-stimulated prolactin release compared to placebo. Significant increase (p=0.003) in prolactin levels in men receiving the lowest dose (120 mg per day), but slight reduction in prolactin level in those receiving higher dose. There were no significant dose-dependent changes in the 24-hour serum prolactin profile.
Milewicz *et al.*, 1993	Luteal phase defects due to hyper-prolactinemia	R, DB, PC n=37 women with luteal phase defects due to latent hyper-prolactinemia (ages 19–42 years old)	3 months	1 capsule vitex extract/day or 1 capsule placebo/evening	Strotan® soft-gel capsule containing 20 mg vitex fruit aqueous, alcoholic, dry native extract	After 3 months, vitex group experienced significant reduction in symptoms compared to placebo group. Significant reduction in prolactin release in response to TRH stimulation compared to placebo (p<0.0001). Mid-luteal progesterone levels, low at baseline, were normal after 3 months in vitex group. Luteal phase normalization and luteal progesterone synthesis normalization were seen in vitex group with no observable changes in these parameters in placebo group. No side effects were noted.
Propping *et al.*, 1991	Corpus luteum insufficiency, menstrual disorders, and PMS	O, MC, U n=1,592 women with corpus luteum insufficiency; including 418 with hypermenorrhea; 355 with polymenorrhea; 202 with secondary amenorrhea, 186 with dysmenorrhea; 175 with PMS, anovulation; 145 experiencing sterility; 66 with menorrhagia; 32 with disturbed menstruation (average age 32.9 years)	16 years (average treatment period, 6 months)	43 drops tincture/day	Agnolyt® vitex fruit tincture (Each 100 ml of aqueous-alcoholic solution contains 9 ml of 1:5 tincture)	In 90% of cases, physician's clinical observation assessment was good or satisfactory, with 33% of patients free of complaints and a positive response to treatment in 51% noted. Patients experienced relief at about 8–9 weeks after beginning treatment. Out of 145 patients who were trying to conceive during treatment period, 56 became pregnant. Adverse effects, including nausea, skin rashes, headaches, and dyspepsia, were reported by 2.4% of patients.
Propping and Katzorke, 1987	Corpus luteum insufficiency	O, U n=18 infertile normo-prolactinemic women (24–39 years old)	3 months	40 drops tincture/day	Agnolyt® vitex fruit tincture	Treatment was deemed successful in 13 of 18 patients (outcome was assessed by normalization of the mid-luteal progesterone level and by correction of pre-existing short menstrual cycle). 2 women became pregnant, and 11 patients had significantly improved serum progesterone values. There was a trend towards normalization of progesterone levels in 4 cases. These findings are indicative of corpus luteal function enhancement.

KEY: **C** – controlled, **CC** – case-control, **CH** – cohort, **CI** – confidence interval, **Cm** – comparison, **CO** – crossover, **CS** – cross-sectional, **DB** – double-blind, **E** – epidemiological, **LC** – longitudinal cohort, **MA** – meta-analysis, **MC** – multi-center, **n** – number of patients, **O** – open, **OB** – observational, **OL** – open label, **OR** – odds ratio, **P** – prospective, **PB** – patient-blind, **PC** – placebo-controlled, **PG** – parallel group, **PS** – pilot study, **R** – randomized, **RC** – reference-controlled, **RCS** – retrospective cross-sectional, **RS** - retrospective, **S** – surveillance, **SB** – single-blind, **SC** – single-center, **U** – uncontrolled, **UP** – unpublished, **VC** – vehicle-controlled.

Menstrual Cycle Irregularities

Author/Year	Subject	Design	Duration	Dosage	Preparation	Results/Conclusion
Bubenzer, 1993	Oligo-menorrhea, corpus luteum insufficiency, poly-menorrhea	O, U n=120 women with hormone imbalance syndromes	6 months		Strotan® soft-gel capsule containing 20 mg vitex fruit aqueous, alcoholic, dry native extract	Of the subjects, 63% had normalized cycle (most had extended follicular phase), and those with disturbed temperatures during their cycles normalized. Patients with very low progesterone benefited particularly. 29% became pregnant.
Loch et al., 1991	Menstrual irregularity	O, U n=2,447 women with a variety of menstrual disorders	9 years (average treatment period, 5 months)	42 drops tincture/day	Agnolyt® vitex fruit tincture	Both patients and physicians noted improvement of symptoms. Of the patients, 90% demonstrated very good, good, or satisfactory results; 2.3% experienced minor side effects.
Loch and Kaiser, 1990	Secondary amenorrhea	P, O, U n=15 female out-patients with secondary amenorrhea (17–29 years old)	6 1/2 months	40 drops tincture/day with some liquid in mornings apart from meals	Agnolyt® vitex fruit tincture	In 10 of 15 patients, the onset of menstruation was observed at about 6 months of treatment. Hormone values for progesterone and LH increased, while FSH decreased slightly or did not change. Authors concluded that Agnolyt® can be recommended for long-term treatment of secondary amenorrhea.
Bleier, 1959	Oligo-menorrhea, polymenor-rhea, menor-rhagia	O n=126 women (35 with oligomenor-rhea, 33 with poly-menor-rhea, 58 with menorrhagia)	2–3 months	15 drops, 3x/day with water 1/2 hour before meals	Agnolyt® vitex fruit tincture	In 58 patients with menorrhagia, a statistically significant shortening of bleeding period was achieved. In 33 patients with polymenorrhea, duration between periods lengthened (on average, from 20 days to 26 days). In 33 cases of oligomenorrhea, the average cycle was shortened from 39 to 31 days. Fourteen patients became pregnant.
Probst and Roth, 1954	Secondary amenorrhea, oligohy-pomenorrhea, cystic granular hyperplasia of endometrium, anovulatory cycle	O, Cm, U n=82 women (57 in vitex group; 25 in group combining vitex with estrogen)	5–24 months	15 drops vitex tincture, 3x/day vs. 1 tablet ethenyl estradiol, 3x/day with same vitex dosage	Alyt® vitex fruit tincture, same as Agnolyt® tincture of aqueous-alcoholic solution	Of women in vitex group 87.7% showed normalization of bleeding in menstrual cycle compared to 52% in the vitex/estradiol combination group. Of those women in vitex group, 100% were diagnosed with anovulatory cycle, 50% with secondary amenorrhea and 44% with oligo-hypomenorrhea experienced a distinct increase in the basal temperature curve. Only 16% of the women in the combination therapy group observed an increase in basal temperature. The authors concluded that vitex was particularly indicated in patients with deficient corpus luteum function.

Premenstrual Syndrome (PMS)

Author/Year	Subject	Design	Duration	Dosage	Preparation	Results/Conclusion
Schellenberg, 2001	PMS	R, DB, PC, PG n=170 women aver-age menstrual cycle = 28 days; average duration of menses = 4.5 days (average age 36 years)	3 menstrual cycles	One, 20 mg tablet/day	PreMens® (Ze440) extract tablets 40 mg (20 mg native dry extract, 20 mg lactose as excipient)	Improvement in vitex group in the main efficacy variables from baseline to end of third cycle in women's self assessment and physician's assessment of irritability, mood change, anger, headache, breast fullness, and other menstrual symptoms including bloating (p<0.001). Over half of women had 50% or greater improvement of symptoms. 4 women in vitex group and 3 in placebo group reported mild adverse events, none which caused discontinuation. Authors conclude that vitex fruit is a safe and effective treatment for relief of symptoms of PMS.
Loch et al., 2000	PMS	OL, MC n=1,634 women with PMS; data from 857 gynecologists (mean age 35.8 years)	3 menstrual cycles	One, 20 mg capsule, 2x/day	Femicur® capsules containing 1.6–3.0 mg dried extract [6.7–12.5:1] corresponding to 20 mg drug	93% reported PMS symptoms lessened or disappeared after vitex treatment over 3 menstrual cycles. Changes from baseline were recorded on questionnaires by physicians before treatment and after 3.0 cycles. Significant decrease of all symptoms. Of the patients, 42% reported that they no longer suffered from PMS; 51% showed a decrease in symptoms.

KEY: C – controlled, **CC** – case-control, **CH** – cohort, **CI** – confidence interval, **Cm** – comparison, **CO** – crossover, **CS** – cross-sectional, **DB** – double-blind, **E** – epidemiological, **LC** – longitudinal cohort, **MA** – meta-analysis, **MC** – multi-center, **n** – number of patients, **O** – open, **OB** – observational, **OL** – open label, **OR** – odds ratio, **P** – prospective, **PB** – patient-blind, **PC** – placebo-controlled, **PG** – parallel group, **PS** – pilot study, **R** – randomized, **RC** – reference-controlled, **RCS** – retrospective cross-sectional, **RS** - retrospective, **S** – surveillance, **SB** – single-blind, **SC** – single-center, **U** – uncontrolled, **UP** – unpublished, **VC** – vehicle-controlled.

Premenstrual Syndrome (PMS) (cont.)

Author/Year	Subject	Design	Duration	Dosage	Preparation	Results/Conclusion
Berger et al, 2000	PMS	P, MC n=43	8 menstrual cycles; including 2 baseline, 3 treatment, and 3 post-treatment	One, 20 mg tablet/day in the morning	PreMens® Ze440 tablet containing 20 mg vitex fruit, hydro-alcoholic, native dry extract, 6.0–12.0:1 (w/w)	Significant score reduction (42.5%) using the MMDQ (Moos Menstrual Distress Questionnaire) as the main effect parameter (p<0.001). Symptoms gradually returned after cessation of treatment. However, a difference from baseline remained (20%; p<0.001) up to 3 cycles thereafter.
Berger et al., 1999	Late luteal phase dysphoric disorder (PMS III –R)	C, E, MC n=132 women, 65 on oral contraceptives and 67 not on oral contraceptives (19–30 years old)	6 months (3 cycles followed by 3-month observation period)	One, 20 mg tablet/day in morning	PreMens® Ze440 tablet containing 20 mg vitex fruit, hydro-alcoholic, native dry extract, 6.0–12.0:1 (w/w)	Using Visual Analog Scale (VAS), the only marginal differences were observed between the contraceptive and non-contraceptive groups during the medication period and post-medication period. All clinically relevant reduction in VAS scores of approximately 60% of all patients was reached. Of all patients, 90% believed that vitex helped and 75% said they would use vitex in the future. A good use-risk ratio was determined for both groups. Clinically relevant score-values of PMS declined during the 3 cycle therapy and rose again thereafter.
Lauritzen et al., 1997	PMS	MC, C,R, Cm n=105 women with PMS; Agnolyt® group n=46, pyridoxine group n=59 after exclusion (18–45 years old)	3 months	Vitex group: 1 capsule Agnolyt®/day plus 1 capsule placebo/day. B6 group: 1 placebo capsule, 2x/day, on days 1–15; 1 B6 capsule, 2x/day, on days 16–35 of menstrual cycle.	Agnolyt® capsules containing 3.5–4.2 mg vitex native extract, 9.58–11.5:1 (w/w) vs. B6 capsules containing 100 mg pyridoxine HCL	Agnolyt® was superior to pyridoxine. On the premenstrual tension syndrome (PMTS) scale, vitex group had reduction in score points from 15.2 to 5.1 vs. 11.9 to 5.1 in B6 group. Of patients in vitex group, 77.1% vs. 60.6% of patients in B6 group showed improvement on Clinical Global Impression (CGI) scale. No serious adverse events were noted. Side effects included gastrointestinal complaints (equally distributed between both groups), skin reactions (two patients in vitex group), and transitory headache (one patient in vitex group).
Turner and Mills, 1993	PMS	R, DB, PC n=217 women (105 in vitex group, 112 in placebo group) with PMS (physiological symptoms)	3 months	600 mg, 3x/day vs. soya-based placebo	Vitex capsules (brand not stated)	Vitex was statistically more effective than placebo only in alleviating jitters and restlessness; there was no statistical significant difference for other PMS symptoms including impaired concentration, fluid retention, or pain.
Dittmar and Böhnert, 1992	PMS	O, MC, U n=1,542 women with PMS (13–62 years old)	166 days average treatment duration	40 drops/day in morning	Agnolyt® vitex fruit tincture	Of patients, 33% reported total relief of symptoms, 57% reported partial relief, 4% reported no improvement. On 5% no data were obtained, and 2% terminated treatment because of side effects. Physicians observed a positive response (good or very good) to treatment in 92% of patients.
Coeugniet et al., 1986	PMS	O, U n=36 women with PMS	3 months	40 drops/day	Agnolyt® vitex fruit tincture	After 3 months, physical and psychological alterations experienced during luteal phase of cycle were significantly reduced (p<0.5), including reduction in headaches, breast tenderness, bloating, fatigue, appetite, sweet cravings, nervousness, restlessness, anxiety, irritability, lack of concentration, depression, mood swings, and aggressiveness. Interval of luteal phase normalized from average of 5.4 days to 11.4 days and a diphasic cycle was established.

KEY: C – controlled, **CC** – case-control, **CH** – cohort, **CI** – confidence interval, **Cm** – comparison, **CO** – crossover, **CS** – cross-sectional, **DB** – double-blind, **E** – epidemiological, **LC** – longitudinal cohort, **MA** – meta-analysis, **MC** – multi-center, **n** – number of patients, **O** – open, **OB** – observational, **OL** – open label, **OR** – odds ratio, **P** – prospective, **PB** – patient-blind, **PC** – placebo-controlled, **PG** – parallel group, **PS** – pilot study, **R** – randomized, **RC** – reference-controlled, **RCS** – retrospective cross-sectional, **RS** - retrospective, **S** – surveillance, **SB** – single-blind, **SC** – single-center, **U** – uncontrolled, **UP** – unpublished, **VC** – vehicle-controlled.

Chaste Tree

Monograph

Other

Author/Year	Subject	Design	Duration	Dosage	Preparation	Results/Conclusion
Giss and Rothenburg, 1968	Acne vulgaris, acne indurate, acne conglobata, acne follicularis	C, Cm n=161 patients with acne (30% male; 70% female)	1–2 years (minimum 3-month treatment period)	20 drops tincture, 2x/day (morning and evening) for 4–6 weeks; then 15 drops daily for 1–2 years.	Agnolyt® vitex fruit tincture vs. standard acne therapy	118 patients received Agnolyt®, and 43 received standard acne therapy. Over 2 years, a statistically significant improvement of acne conditions was reported in the mostly female vitex group compared to placebo.

KEY: C – controlled, **CC** – case-control, **CH** – cohort, **CI** – confidence interval, **Cm** – comparison, **CO** – crossover, **CS** – cross-sectional, **DB** – double-blind, **E** – epidemiological, **LC** – longitudinal cohort, **MA** – meta-analysis, **MC** – multi-center, **n** – number of patients, **O** – open, **OB** – observational, **OL** – open label, **OR** – odds ratio, **P** – prospective, **PB** – patient-blind, **PC** – placebo-controlled, **PG** – parallel group, **PS** – pilot study, **R** – randomized, **RC** – reference-controlled, **RCS** – retrospective cross-sectional, **RS** - retrospective, **S** – surveillance, **SB** – single-blind, **SC** – single-center, **U** – uncontrolled, **UP** – unpublished, **VC** – vehicle-controlled.

Cranberry

Vaccinium macrocarpon Aiton

[Fam. *Ericaceae*]

OVERVIEW

Cranberry is a fruit native to North America, with almost 98% of the world's supply cultivated in natural and artificial bogs in the northern U.S. and Canada. Both indigenous Americans and colonists valued cranberry for its medicinal and nutritional properties. Cranberries are a high-value crop, ranking 40th in sales of all cash crops monitored by the U.S. Department of Agriculture's National Agricultural Statistical Service. Sales of cranberry dietary supplements ranked 10th in 1999 in total herb sales in U.S. food, drug, and mass-market retail outlets (increasing more than $12 million in 1999, a 15% jump from 1998). This figure reflects sales in supplement (usually capsule) form only, and does not include supplement sales in other retail channels (natural food, multilevel, mail-order, professional). It also does not reflect sales in the mainstream market for cranberry juice, which may be increasing due to consumers' growing recognition of cranberry's health benefits for the urinary tract system.

PRIMARY USES

• Reduction in UTI occurrence
• Kidney stones

OTHER POTENTIAL USES

• Treatment, UTI

NOTE: Cranberry juice may reduce the need for repeated antibiotic use in the treatment of recurrent UTIs and, therefore, reduce side effects, such as vulvovaginal candidiasis. However, recurrent UTIs require proper medical diagnosis and cranberry is not a substitute for antibiotics.

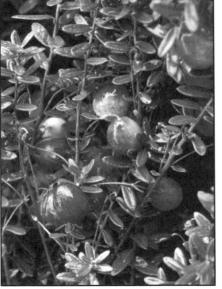

Photo © 2003 stevenfoster.com

PHARMACOLOGICAL ACTIONS

Inhibits adherence of bacteria to the lining of the bladder and urethra (at normal consumption levels); urinary antiseptic (at high levels of consumption).

DOSAGE AND ADMINISTRATION

Internal

Crude preparations

NOTE: The following juice doses are based on sweetened preparations unless otherwise noted. At least 10 clinical studies conducted on sweetened cranberry juice cocktail strongly suggest the safety and efficacy of this type of preparation. Some naturopathic authors suggest that sweeteners in the juice should be avoided or minimized, and recommend patients drink plenty of fluids (at least 2 liters daily) throughout the day. Authors recommending unsweetened juice generally suggest using capsules as unsweetened juice can be unpalatable.

Juice

TREATMENT OF UTI: 16–32 fl. oz. daily; at least 0.5 liters (approx 18 fl. oz.) of unsweetened juice daily.

PREVENTION OF UTI: 4–32 fl. oz. daily.

RENAL STONES: 8 fl. oz., 4 times daily for several days, then 8 fl. oz., twice daily for treatment and prophylaxis of renal stones that are more soluble in an acid milieu.

Concentrated Juice Extract

PREVENTION AND TREATMENT OF UTI: 300–400+ mg, 2–3 times daily.

CONTRAINDICATIONS

Potential contraindications of cranberry may be present with renal insufficiency and in persons with the potential for developing uric acid or calcium oxalate stones. However, cranberry juice containing very low amounts of oxalate was found to be safe for individuals with calcium stones. Ingesting large quantities of cranberry juice either reduced the incidence of stone formation or reduced urinary ionized calcium associated with calcium-containing renal stones.

PREGNANCY AND LACTATION: No known restrictions during pregnancy or lactation.

ADVERSE EFFECTS

None known at therapeutic dosage levels. At high dosages (more than 3–4 liters daily), diarrhea or mild gastrointestinal upset may occur.

DRUG INTERACTIONS

No known interactions with antibiotics or other drugs.

CLINICAL REVIEW

In 19 mostly uncontrolled clinical studies on cranberry including a total of 1,149 participants, all but two studies demonstrated some positive effect, primarily for urinary tract health. All of the studies investigated the effects of cranberry on the urinary tract system with the exception of one study on 13 patients with peri-stomal skin damage. Of three double-blind, placebo-controlled (DB, PC) studies performed on a total of 178 participants, two were conducted with statistically significant positive outcomes in favor of cranberry prophylaxis or treatment. One used a dry cranberry extract for reducing the occurrence of UTIs in women while the other addressed treatment of bacteriuria and pyuria in elderly women. A subsequent randomized, PC, crossover study using 17 elderly patients confirmed its successful use in reducing the frequency of bacteriuria. A DB, PC study did not find cranberry juice concentrate to be effective in preventing UTIs in 15 children (ages 2–18) with neurogenic bladders, nor did another single-blind, randomized, cross-over study performed on 21 children investigating ingestion of cranberry juice cocktail vs. water for antibacterial prophylaxis in pediatric neuropathic bladders. A Cochrane review evaluated randomized, controlled trials of cranberry juice in preventing urinary tract infections and found that the trials were generally of poor quality and included a large number of dropouts. The reviewers recommended that other cranberry products, such as capsules, may prevent dropouts and that further well-designed trials are necessary.

Cranberry

Vaccinium macrocarpon Aiton
[Fam. *Ericaceae*]

OVERVIEW

Cranberry is a fruit native to North America, with almost 98% of the world supply cultivated in the northern U.S. and Canada. Both indigenous Americans and colonists valued cranberry for its medicinal and nutritional properties. Cranberries are a high-value crop, ranking 40th in sales of all cash crops monitored by the U.S. Department of Agriculture's National Agricultural Statistical Service. Sales of cranberry dietary supplements ranked 10th in 1999 in total herb sales in U.S. food, drug, and mass-market retail outlets.

USES

Urinary tract infections (UTIs), including prevention, treatment, and decreasing occurrence; kidney stones.

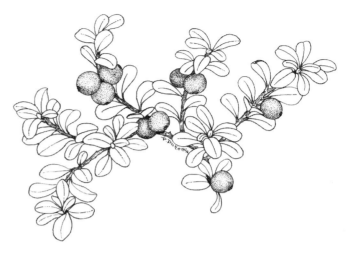

DOSAGE

Internal

NOTE: The following juice doses are based on sweetened preparations unless otherwise noted. Although some authors suggest that sweeteners in the juice should be avoided or minimized, clinical studies strongly suggest that these types of products are safe and effective. Additionally, patients should drink plenty of fluids (at least 2 liters daily) throughout the day. Authors recommending unsweetened juice generally suggest using capsules as unsweetened juice can be unpleasant tasting.

Juice

TREATMENT OF UTI: 16–32 fl. oz. daily or at least 17 fl. oz. of unsweetened juice daily.

PREVENTION OF UTI: 4–32 fl. oz. daily.

KIDNEY STONES: 8 fl. oz., 4 times daily for several days, then 8 fl. oz., twice daily for treatment and prevention of kidney stones that dissolve better in acid solutions.

Concentrated Juice Extract

PREVENTION AND TREATMENT OF UTI: 300–400 mg, 2–3 times daily.

CONTRAINDICATIONS

Consult a healthcare provider in cases of kidney insufficiency or tendency to develop uric acid or calcium oxalate stones.

PREGNANCY AND LACTATION: No known restrictions during pregnancy or lactation.

ADVERSE EFFECTS

No adverse effects occur at recommended dosages. High dosages (more than 3–4 liters or approximately 2.5-3.5 qt. daily) may cause diarrhea or mild gastrointestinal upset.

Caution: If no improvement in acute infection of the urinary tract occurs within the first 24 hours of herbal treatment, seek conventional medical treatment.

DRUG INTERACTIONS

No known interactions with antibiotics or other drugs.

Comments

When using a dietary supplement, purchase it from a reliable source. For best results, use the same brand of product throughout the period of use. As with all medications and dietary supplements, please inform your healthcare provider of all herbs and medications you are taking. Interactions may occur between medications and herbs or even among different herbs when taken at the same time. Treat your herbal supplement with care by taking it as directed, storing it as advised on the label, and keeping it out of the reach of children and pets. Consult your healthcare provider with any questions.

AMERICAN
BOTANICAL
COUNCIL

Cranberry

Vaccinium macrocarpon Aiton

[Fam. *Ericaceae*]

OVERVIEW

Cranberry, a fruit native to North America, is used by the Iroquois and the Cherokee Indians as a symbol of peace and friendship (Eck, 1990). Almost 98% of the world's supply is cultivated in natural and artificial bogs in the northern United States and Canada (Vandenberg and Parent, 1999). Both indigenous Americans and colonists valued cranberry, native to Massachusetts, for its medicinal and nutritional properties.

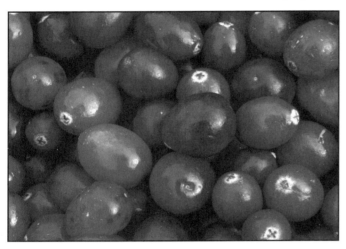

Photo © 2003 stevenfoster.com

Indigenous Americans used cranberries in poultices for treating wounds and blood poisoning. American sailors and colonists used cranberries to prevent scurvy, similar to the use of citrus by the British. They also used cranberries and their leaves for various conditions including blood disorders, stomach ailments, liver problems, fever, "cancers," swollen glands, and mumps. Cranberry has also been used traditionally to treat urinary tract infections (UTIs) (Avorn *et al.*, 1994). Cranberries are a high-value crop, ranking 40th in sales of all cash crops monitored by the U.S. Department of Agriculture's National Agricultural Statistical Service (USDA, 1999). Sales of cranberry dietary supplements ranked 10th in 1999 in total herb sales in food, drug, and mass-market retail outlets in the U.S., but dropped off the list of 20 leading herbs in 2001 (Blumenthal, 1999, 2001). This figure reflects sales in supplement (usually capsule) form only, and does not include supplement sales in other retail channels (natural food, multilevel, mail order, professional). It also does not reflect sales in the mainstream market for cranberry juice, which may be increasing due to consumers' growing recognition of cranberry's health benefits for the urinary tract system.

DESCRIPTION

Cranberry preparations consist of the ripe fruit of *Vaccinium macrocarpon* Aiton [Fam. *Ericaceae*]. U.S. Pharmacopeial-grade Cranberry Liquid Preparation is a bright red juice derived from the fruits of *V. macrocarpon* or *V. oxycoccos*, containing no added substances. Its pH is 2.5 ±0.1, with no more than 0.05% sorbitol, or 0.05% sucrose and, not less than 2.4% dextrose, 0.7% fructose, 0.9% quinic acid, 0.9% citric acid and 0.7% malic acid. The ratio of quinic acid to malic acid is not less than 1 (USP, 2002). The Brix level (measurement of sugar content of a solution) of single strength cranberry juice is a minimum 7.5% (US FDA, 1999).

PRIMARY USES

Urinary tract infection (UTI)
- Reduction in UTI occurrence (Walker *et al.*, 1997; Haverkorn and Mandigers, 1994; Gibson *et al.*, 1991)

Nephrolithiasis
- Management of kidney stones (Leaver, 1996; Light *et al.*, 1973; Sternlieb, 1963; Zinsser *et al.*, 1968)

OTHER POTENTIAL USES
- Treatment of UTI (Leaver, 1996; Avorn *et al.*, 1994; Papas *et al.*, 1966; Sternlieb, 1963)

NOTE: Cranberry juice may reduce the need for repeated antibiotic use in the treatment of recurrent UTIs and, therefore, reduce side effects, such as vulvovaginal candidiasis. However, recurrent UTIs require proper medical diagnosis and cranberry is not a substitute for antibiotics (Brown, 2000).

COMBINATION PREPARATIONS

Clinical and research experience has demonstrated positive results with cranberry in combination with herbs that have antibacterial activity (e.g., Chinese goldthread rhizome [*Coptis chinensis*] or goldenseal root [*Hydrastis canadensis*]) (Barney, 1996). Cranberry juice with bacteriostatic agents is recommended for long-term suppressive therapy of urinary infections in children suffering from recurrent bacterial infections. Cranberry is combined with buchu leaf (*Agathosma betulina*), three–leaved caper stem bark (*Crateva nurvala*), and/or uva ursi leaf (*Arctostaphylos uva-ursi*) for urinary antiseptic, anti-inflammatory, astringent, antilithic, bladder tonic, and diuretic actions (Bone and Morgan, 1999). There appears to be little need for concern about interactions with uva ursi leaf because therapeutic doses of cranberry are not high enough to acidify the urine (Yarnell, 1997). Taking cranberry juice along with beneficial intestinal bacteria, such as *Lactobacillus acidophilus,* may alleviate the discomfort caused by uropathogens while restoring normal microbial balance in the gut and in vaginal mucosal surfaces (Anon, 1991).

DOSAGE

Internal

Crude preparations

NOTE: The following juice doses are based on sweetened preparations unless otherwise noted. At least 10 clinical studies conducted on sweetened cranberry juice cocktail strongly suggest the safety and efficacy of this type of preparation (Jackson and

Hicks, 1997; Foda *et al.,* 1995; Avorn *et al.,* 1994; Haverkorn and Mandigers, 1994; Tsukada *et al.,* 1994; Gibson *et al.,* 1991; Kinney and Blount, 1979; Kahn *et al.,* 1967; Papas *et al.,* 1966; Bodel *et al.,* 1959). Some naturopathic authors suggest that sweeteners in the juice should be avoided or minimized, stating that consumers should not rely on sweetened cranberry juice cocktail, which contains only one-third juice mixed with water and sugar (Brown, 2000; Pizzorno and Murray, 1999; Yarnell, 1997). Capsules offer an alternative to unsweetened juice, which can be unpalatable (Brown, 2000; Yarnell, 1997). Additionally, some authors suggest patients drink plenty of fluids (at least 2 liters daily) throughout the day (Brown, 2000; Pizzorno and Murray, 1999).

Juice
TREATMENT OF UTI: 16–32 fl. oz. daily (Leaver, 1996; Papas *et al.,* 1966; Sternlieb, 1963); at least 0.5 liters (approx 18 fl. oz.) of unsweetened juice daily (Pizzorno and Murray, 1999).

PREVENTION OF UTI: 4–32 fl. oz. daily (Leaver, 1996; Avorn *et al.,* 1994; Gibson *et al.,* 1991; Simons *et al.,* 1992; Sternlieb, 1963).

RENAL STONES: 16–32 fl. oz. daily for treatment and prevention of renal stones that are more soluble in an acid environment (Leaver, 1996; Light, 1973; Sternlieb, 1963).

Concentrated Juice Extract
PREVENTION AND TREATMENT OF UTI: 300–400+ mg, 2–3 times daily (Brown 2000; Yarnell, 1997).

DURATION OF ADMINISTRATION
Internal
Crude Preparations
Since cranberry is a common food, there is no known limit on the duration of use. Clinical studies have lasted from 6–12 months, with one retrospective study lasting 28 months (Dignan *et al.,* 1998). The minimum time necessary to produce lowered pH for the treatment of UTI is 2–5 days (Kahn *et al.,* 1967; Fellers *et al.,* 1933), with studies showing optimal effect after 12–15 days (Rogers, 1991; Kinney and Blount, 1979; Nickey, 1975). Cranberry juice did not reduce the occurrence of bacteriuria with pyuria in elderly women until after 4–8 weeks of treatment (Avorn *et al.,* 1994).

CHEMISTRY
Cranberry fruit contains six known anthocyanins: cyanidin-3-galactoside, cyanidin-3-glucoside, cyanidin-3-arabinose, peonidin-3-galactoside, peonidin-3-glucoside, and peonidin-3-arabinose (Hong and Wrolstad, 1986; Sapers and Hargrave, 1987); tannins, catechins, flavonol glycosides, proanthocyanidins, organic acids such as quinic, malic, and citric acids, and sugars such as dextrose and fructose (Bone and Morgan, 1999; Coppola *et al.,* 1995; Leung and Foster, 1996). Cranberries also contain proanthocyanidins with A-type, double linkages (Foo *et al.,* 2000a, 2000b). The principle characteristics of an authentic single-strength cranberry juice are reported to be: total organic acids, 2.2–3.3 g/100 g; relative percentages of organic acids, 39% quinic, 32% citric, and 27% malic; total anthocyanins by pH differential, 19.0–53.3 mg/100 g; relative percentages of anthocyanidins, 57% cyanidin, 43% peonidin; total sugars, 3.6–5.0 g/100 g; relative percentages of sugars, 79% glucose, 21% fructose (Hong and Wrolstad, 1986).

PHARMACOLOGICAL ACTIONS
Human
At normal consumption levels (10 fluid ounces or 300 ml per day), cranberry inhibits bacterial adherence to the lining of the bladder and urethra (Avorn *et al.,* 1994; Yarnell, 1997). At high levels of consumption (50 to 133 fluid ounces or 1,500 to 4,000 ml per day) cranberry may act as a urinary antiseptic (Blatherwick, 1914; Blatherwick and Long, 1923; Fellers *et al.,* 1933; Nickey, 1975; Kinney and Blount, 1979; Bodel *et al.,* 1959; Bone and Morgan, 1999).

In vitro
Urinary tract effects
Inhibited adherence of *Escherichia coli* to uroepithelial cells (Sobota, 1984); inhibited adherence for gram-negative rods (Schmidt and Sobota, 1988); inhibited adherence of urinary *E. coli* isolates expressing type I fimbriae and type P fimbriae (Zafriri *et al.,* 1989); juice fraction selectively inhibited mannose-resistant adhesions produced by urinary isolates of *E. coli* (Ofek *et al.,* 1996); purified cranberry proanthocyanidins inhibited adherence of uropathogenic strains of P-fimbriated *E. coli* to isolated uroepithelial cells (Howell *et al.,* 1998); inhibits expression of P-fimbriae of *E. coli* (Ahuja *et al.,* 1998); inhibited adherence and colonization of some uropathogens including *E. coli* and *Enterococcus faecalis* (Habash *et al.,* 1999); oligomeric proanthocyanins and flavone-glycosides inhibited adherence of *E. coli* to human bladder cells (Walker *et al.,* 1999); cranberry proanthocyanidins with A-type linkages inhibited adhesion of uropathogenic strains of P-fimbriated *E. coli* to mannose-resistant adhesion (Foo *et al.,* 2000a and 2000b).

Cardiovascular effects
Cranberry inhibits oxidation of human low density lipoproteins (LDL) (Wilson *et al.,* 1999); cranberry juice vasodilates rat aortae *in vitro* (Maher *et al.,* 2000); consumption of cranberry juice increases *ex vivo* antioxidant capacity (Pedersen *et al.,* 2000); oligomeric and polymeric proanthocyanidins inhibit copper-induced oxidation of human LDL (Krueger *et al.,* 2000).

Cancer
Proanthocyanidin fractions have potential anticarcinogenic activity (Bomser *et al.,* 1996); cranberry products inhibited proliferation of MDA-MB-435 estrogen receptor-negative and MCF-7 estrogen receptor-positive human breast cancer cells in a dose-dependent manner (Guthrie, 2000).

Other antiadhesion effects
Anticoaggregates subgingival microbiota (Weiss *et al.,* 1998); inhibited adherence of *Helicobacter pylori* bacteria to human gastric mucus and underlying epithelial cells (Burger *et al.,* 2000).

Antimicrobial
Antimicrobial against *Saccharomyces bayanus* and *Pseudomonas fluorescens* (Marwan and Nagel, 1986); a 5x concentrate of cranberry juice adjusted to pH 7 inhibited growth of certain bacteria (*E. coli, Staphylococcus aureus, Pseudomonas aeruginosa*) (Lee *et al.,* 2000); inactivated polio virus type 1 (Konowalchuck and Speirs, 1978).

MECHANISM OF ACTION
Bacterial adherence to mucosal surfaces is generally considered to be the initial event in the pathogenesis of most infectious diseases due to bacteria in humans (Beachey, 1981; Sobota, 1984). UTIs occur most frequently because of adherence of *E. coli* via P-fimbriae. The usual initiating mechanism involves bacterial adhesion

to specific molecules on cell surfaces, followed by invasive disease. The tip proteins of *E. coli* lead to the initiation of UTI (Roberts, 1996).

Cranberry's actions occur through the following mechanisms:

- Inhibits adherence of *E. coli* to the lining of the bladder and urethra (Marwan and Nagel, 1986; Ofek, 1991; Schmidt and Sobota, 1988; Sobota, 1984; Zafriri, 1989) through preventing colonization of these sites (Ofek *et al.*, 1991).
- Interrupts the binding of type 1 and P fimbriae in the gut and the bladder (Zafriri, 1989).
- A bioassay, based upon inhibition of adherence of *E. coli* to human bladder cells, human erythrocytes, and guinea pig erythrocytes, determined that the main anti-adherence components in cranberry preparations are the oligomeric proanthocyanins (OPCs) and, to a lesser extent, a secondary group of lower-molecular-weight polyphenolic substances, including flavone-glycosides (Walker *et al.*, 1999; Howell *et al.*, 1998).

Proanthocyanidins may be metabolized before reaching the bladder, suggesting that other constituents could be responsible for reducing the risk of *E. coli* infection (Reid, 1999). No studies have yet been conducted on the absorption and metabolism of cranberry proanthocyanidins, yet there is evidence of absorption of grape procyanidins (Koga *et al.*, 1999, Harmand and Blanquet, 1978).

CONTRAINDICATIONS

Some authors have noted the potential contraindications of cranberry with renal insufficiency and in persons with the potential for developing uric acid or calcium oxalate stones (Rogers, 1991; Bone and Morgan, 1999). However, Brinkley *et al.* (1981) found that cranberry juice contained very low amounts of oxalate and was safe for individuals with calcium stones. Two small studies found that ingestion of large quantities of cranberry juice reduced incidence in stone formation or reduced urinary ionized calcium associated with calcium-containing renal stones (Zinsser *et al.*, 1968; Light *et al.*, 1973).

PREGNANCY AND LACTATION: No known restrictions during pregnancy or lactation (Brown, 2000; Yarnell, 1997).

ADVERSE EFFECTS

None known at therapeutic dosage levels. At high dosage (more than 3–4 liters daily), diarrhea or mild gastrointestinal upset (Olin *et al.*, 1994; Yarnell, 1997).

DRUG INTERACTIONS

No known interactions with antibiotics. Cranberry may enhance vitamin B12 absorption, which is useful for patients taking omeprazole, a drug used to treat ulcers (Brown, 2000).

AMERICAN HERBAL PRODUCTS ASSOCIATION (AHPA) SAFETY RATING

Not rated (McGuffin *et al.*, 1997).

REGULATORY STATUS

CANADA: Food (CFIA, 2000) or Natural Health Product (NHP) depending on label claim statement. In Canada, NHPs, also referred to as complementary medicines or traditional remedies, are subject to the Food and Drug Act and Regulations (Health Canada, 2000).

FRANCE: Food. No monograph in the *French Pharmacopoeia*.

GERMANY: Food. No German Commission E monograph (Blumenthal *et al.*, 1998). No monograph in the *German Pharmacopoeia* (DAB).

SWEDEN: Food. No products containing cranberry are listed in the Medical Products Agency (MPA) "Authorised Natural Remedies" (MPA, 2001).

SWITZERLAND: Food. No monograph in the *Swiss Pharmacopoeia*.

U.K.: Food. Not listed in the *General Sale List* (GSL). No monograph in the *British Pharmacopoeia*.

U.S.: Food (USDA, 1997) or dietary supplement depending on label claim statement (USC, 1994). Cranberry Liquid Preparation, for manufacturing purposes only, is official in the 20th edition of the *National Formulary* (NF) (USP, 2002).

CLINICAL REVIEW

Nineteen studies, mostly uncontrolled, are outlined in the table, "Clinical Studies on Cranberry," including a total of 1,149 participants. All but two studies (Schlager *et al.*, 1999; Foda *et al.*, 1995), demonstrate some positive effect primarily for urinary tract health. All studies investigated effects on the urinary tract system with the exception of one study on 13 patients with skin damage (Tsukada *et al.*, 1994). Of three double-blind placebo-controlled (DB, PC) studies performed on a total of 178 participants (Schlager *et al.*, 1999; Avorn *et al.*, 1994; Walker *et al.*, 1997), two were conducted with statistically significant positive outcomes in favor of cranberry prophylaxis or treatment. One used a dry cranberry extract for reducing the occurrence of UTIs in women (Walker *et al.*, 1997) while the other addressed treatment of bacteriuria and pyuria in elderly women (Avorn *et al.*, 1994). A subsequent randomized, PC, crossover study on 17 elderly patients, confirmed the findings of Avorn (Haverkorn and Mandigers, 1994). The third DB, PC study did not find cranberry juice concentrate to be effective in preventing UTI in 15 children (ages 2–18) with neurogenic bladder (Schlager *et al.*, 1999), nor did another single-blind, randomized, cross-over study performed on 21 participants, investigating ingestion of cranberry juice cocktail vs. water for antibacterial prophylaxis in pediatric neuropathic bladders (Foda *et al.*, 1995). This study also did not find cranberry juice concentrate to be effective in preventing UTIs. A Cochrane Collaboration review evaluated randomized, controlled trials of cranberry juice in preventing urinary tract infections and found that the trials were generally of poor quality and included a large number of dropouts. The reviewers recommended that other cranberry products, such as capsules, may prevent dropouts and that further well-designed trials are necessary (Jepson *et al.*, 2001).

BRANDED PRODUCTS

Azo-Cranberry® Capsules: PolyMedica Corporation / 11 State Street / Woburn, Massachusetts 01801/ U.S.A. / Tel: 781-933-2021 / www.polymedica.com. Capsules contain 450 mg dried cranberry extracted solids.

Ocean Spray® Cranberry Juice Cocktail: Ocean Spray Cranberries Inc./ One Ocean Spray Drive / Lakeville-Middleboro, MA 02349 / U.S.A. / Tel: (800) 662-3263 / www.oceanspray.com. Cocktail contains: filtered water, cranberry juice (cranberry juice and cranberry juice from concentrate), high fructose corn syrup, ascorbic acid (vitamin C).

Solaray®CranActin®: Nutraceutical Corporation / 1400 Kearns Blvd / Park City, Utah 84060 / U.S. / Tel.: (800) 669-8877 / www.neutraceutical.com. Capsules contain 400 mg dried cranberry extracted solids.

REFERENCES

Ahuja S, Kaack B, Roberts J. Loss of fimbrial adhesion with the addition of *Vaccinium macrocarpon* to the growth medium of P-fimbriated *Escherichia coli*. *J Urology* 1998;159:559–62.

Anon. Urinary tract infection and potential for natural treatment. *BioMed Newsletter* 1991;2(6):1–4.

Avorn J, Monane M, Gurwitz J, et al. Reduction of bacteriuria and pyuria after ingestion of cranberry juice. *JAMA* 1994;271(1): 751–4.

Barney P. The cranberry cure. *Herbs for Health* 1996 Nov/Dec;45–7.

Beachey E. Bacterial adherence: adhesion-receptor interactions mediating the attachment of bacteria to mucosal surface. *J Infect Dis* 1981;143(3):325–45.

Blatherwick N, Long M. Studies of urinary acidity II: The increased acidity produced by eating prunes and cranberries. *J Biol Chem* 1923;57:815–8.

Blatherwick N. The specific role of foods in relation to the composition of the urine. *Arch Int Med* 1914;14:409–450.

Blumenthal M. Herb market levels after five years of boom: 1999 sales in mainstream market up only 11% in first half of 1999 after 55% increase in 1998. *HerbalGram* 1999;47:64–5.

Blumenthal M. Herb sales down 15% in Mainstream Market. *HerbalGram* 2001;51:69.

Blumenthal M, Busse WR, Goldberg A, Gruenwald J, Hall T, Riggins CW, Rister RS (eds.). Klein S, Rister RS (trans.). *The Complete German Commission E Monographs—Therapeutic Guide to Herbal Medicines*. Austin, TX: American Botanical Council; Boston: Integrative Medicine Communication; 1998; 108.

Bodel P, Cotran R, Kass E. Cranberry juice and the antibacterial action of hippuric acid. *J Lab Clin Med* 1959;54:881–8.

Bomser J, Madhavi D, Singletary K, Smith M. *In vitro* anticancer activity of fruit extracts from *Vaccinium* species. *Planta Med* 1996;62:212–6.

Bone K, Morgan M. *Vaccinium macrocarpon* – Cranberry. *MediHerb Professional Review* 1999 Nov;Number 72:1–4.

Brinkley L, McGuire J, Gregory J, Pak C. Bioavailability of oxalate in foods. *Urology* 1981;17(6):534–8.

Brown D. Cranberry. In: *Herbal Prescriptions for Better Health*. Roseville, CA: Prima Publishing; 2000;71–76.

Burger O, Ofek I, Tabak M, Weiss E, Sharon N, Neeman I. A high molecular mass constituent of cranberry juice inhibits *Helicobacter pylori* adhesion to human gastric mucus. *FEMS Immunology and Medical Microbiology* 2000;29:295–301.

Canadian Food Inspection Agency (CFIA). Fresh Fruit and Vegetable Regulations, Canada Agricultural Products Act: Grades and Standards for Cranberries. Nepean, Ontario: Canadian Food Inspection Agency; 2000.

CFIA. See: Canadian Food Inspection Agency.

Coppola E, English N, Provost J, et al. Authenticity of cranberry products including non-domestic varieties. In: Nagy S, Wade R (eds.). *Methods to Detect Adulteration of Fruit-Juice Beverages*, Vol. 1. Auburndale, FL: Ag Science, Inc.; 1995;287–308.

Dignam R, Ahmed M, Kelly K, et al. The effect of cranberry juice on urinary tract infection rates in a long-term care facility. *Ann Long-Term Care* 1998;6(5):163–7.

Eck P. *The American Cranberry*. New Brunswick: Rutgers University Press. 1990.

Fellers C, Redmon B, Parrott E. Effect of cranberries on urinary acidity and blood alkali reserve. *J Nutrition* 1933;6(5):455-63.

Foda M, Middlebrook PF, Gatfield CT, et al. Efficacy of cranberry in prevention of urinary tract infection in a susceptible pediatric population. *Can J Urology* 1995;2(1):98–102.

Foo LY, Lu Y, Howell A, Vorsa N. The structure of cranberry proanthocyanidins which inhibit adherence of uropathogenic P-fimbriated *Escherichia coli in vitro*. *Phytochem* 2000a;54:173–81.

Foo LY, Lu Y, Howell A, Vorsa N. A-type proanthocyanidin trimers from cranberry that inhibit adherence of uropathogenic P-fimbriated *Escherichia coli*. *J Nat Prod Chem* 2000b; 63(9):1225–8.

Fourcroy J. Personal communication to K. Dinda; 2000.

Gibson L, Pike L, Kilbourn JP. Clinical Study: Effectiveness of cranberry juice in preventing urinary tract infections in Long-Term Care Facility patients. *J Naturopathic Med* 1991;2(1):45–7.

Guthrie N. Effect of cranberry juice and products on human breast cancer cell growth [abstract]. San Diego, CA: *Proc Exp Biol* 2000;April 14–18., San Diego, CA.

Habash MB, Van der Mei HC, Busscher HJ, Reid G. The effect of water, ascorbic acid, and cranberry derived supplementation on human urine and uropathogen adhesion to silicone rubber. *Can J Microbiol* 1999;45:691–4.

Harmand M, Blanquet P. The fate of total flavonolic oligomers (OFT) extracted from *Vitis vinifera* in the rat. *Eur J Drug Metab Pharmacokin* 1978;1:15–30.

Haverkorn M, Mandigers J. Reduction of bacteriuria and pyuria using cranberry juice [letter]. *JAMA* 1994;272(8):590.

Health Canada. Information: Natural Health Products in Canada – A History. Ottawa, Ontario: Health Canada; 2000 May.

Hong V, Wrolstad R. Cranberry juice composition. *J Assoc Off Anal Chem* 1986;69(2):199–207.

Howell AB, Vorsa N, Der Marderosian A, Foo LY. Inhibition of the adherence of P-fimbriated *Escherichia coli* to uroepithelial-cell surfaces by proanthocyanidin extracts from cranberries [letter]. *New Eng J Med* 1998;339(15):1085–6.

Jackson B, Hicks L. Effect of cranberry juice on urinary pH in older adults. *Home Healthcare Nurse* 1997;15(3):198–202.

Jepson RG, Mihaljevic L, Craig J. Cranberries for preventing urinary tract infections (Cochrane Review). In: *The Cochrane Library*. Oxford: Update Software 2001.

Kahn DH, Panariello VA, Saeli J, Sampson JR, Schwwartz E. Effect of cranberry juice on urine. *J Am Dietetic Assoc* 1967;51(3):251-4.

Kinney A, Blount M. Effect of cranberry juice on urinary pH. *Nursing Res* 1979;28(5):287–90.

Koga T, Moro K, Nakamori K, et al. Increase of antioxidative potential of rat plasma by oral administration of proanthocyanidin-rich extract from grape seeds. *J Agric Food Chem* 1999;47(5):1892–7.

Konowalchuk J, Speirs JI. Antiviral Effect of Commercial Juices and Beverages. *Appl Environ Microbiol* 1978 Jun; 35(6):1219-20

Kontiokari T, Sundquvist K, Nuutinen M et al. Cranberry-Lingonberry Juice and *Lactobacillus* GG Drink for the Prevention of urinary tract infections in women. *British Medical Journal* 2001;322:1–5.

Krueger C, Porter M, Wieba D, et al. Potential of cranberry flavonoids in the prevention of copper-induced LDL oxidation. Freising-Weihenstephan, Germany: *Polyphenols Communications*; 2000 Sept. 11–15, Freising-Weihenstephan, Germany.

Leaver R. Cranberry juice. *Prof Nurse* 1996;11(8):525–6.

Lee Y, Owens J, Thrupp L, Cesario T. Does cranberry juice have antibacterial activity? *JAMA* 2000;283(13):1691.

Leung AY, Foster S. Cranberry. In: *Encyclopedia of Common Natural Ingredients used in Food, Drugs, and Cosmetics*. New York: John Wiley & Sons, Inc. 1996;198–9.

Light I, et al. Urinary ionized calcium in urolithiasis. *Urology* 1973;1(1):67–70.

Maher M, Mataczynski H, Stefaniak H, Wilson T. Cranberry juice induces nitric-oxide-dependent vasodilatation *in vitro* and its infusion transiently reduces blood pressure in anesthetized rats. *J Medicinal Food* 2000;3(3):141–7.

Marwan A, Nagel C. Microbial inhibitors of cranberries. *J Food Sci* 1986;51(4):1009–13.

McGuffin M, Hobbs C, Upton R, Goldberg A. *American Herbal Product Association's Botanical Safety Handbook*. Boca Raton, FL: CRC Press; 1997.

Medical Products Agency (MPA). *Naturläkemedel: Authorised Natural Remedies* (as of January 24, 2001). Uppsala, Sweden: Medical Products Agency; 2001.

MPA. See: Medical Products Agency.

Nawar W. Cranberry seed oil: A new source of tocotrienols, omega-3 fatty acids, and other bioactive components [abstract]. Houston, TX: *International Conference and Exhibition on Nutraceuticals and Functional Foods*, 2000; Sept. 13–17, Houston, TX.

Nickey KE. Urinary pH: effect of prescribed regimes of cranberry juice and ascorbic acid [Academy/Congress Abstracts]. *Arch Phys Med Rehabil* 1975;56:556.

Ofek I, et al. Anti – *Escherichia* adhesion activity of cranberry and blueberry juices. *New Eng J Med* 1991;324(22):1599.

Ofek I, Goldhar J, Sharon N. Anti-*Escherichia coli* adhesion activity of cranberry and blueberry juices. In: Kahane and Ofek (eds.). *Toward Anti-adhesion Therapy for Microbial Diseases*. New York: Plenum Press; 1996;179–83.

Olin BR, Dombek C, Hulbert MK, Liberti L (eds.). Cranberry. In: *The Lawrence Review of Natural Products*. St. Louis, MO: Facts and Comparisons. 1994.

Papas P, Brusch C, Ceresia GC. Cranberry juice in the treatment of urinary tract infection. *Southwest Med J* 1966;47(1):17–20.

Pedersen C, Kyle J, Jenkinson A, et al. Effects of blueberry and cranberry juice consumption on the plasma antioxidant capacity of healthy female volunteers. *Eur J Clin Nutr* 2000;54:405–8.

Pizzorno JE, Murray MT, editors. Chronic interstitial cystitis. In: *Textbook of Natural Medicine*, Vol. 2, 2nd ed. New York: Churchill Livingstone; 1999;1186–9.

Reid G. Effect of cranberry consumption and probiotics on bacterial biofilm formation and infection. Houston, TX: *International Conference and Exhibition on Nutraceuticals and Functional Foods*; 2000 Sept;. 13–17.

Reid G. Potential preventive strategies and therapies in urinary tract infection [abstract]. *World J Urol* 1999;17:359–63.

Roberts, J. Tropism in bacterial infections: Urinary tract infections. *J Urol* 156: 1996;1552–9.

Rogers J. Clinical: Pass the cranberry juice. *Nursing Times* 1991;27(87):36–7.

Sapers G, Hargrave D. Proportions of individual anthocyanins in fruits of cranberry cultivars. *J Amer Soc Hortic Sci* 1987;112:100–4.

Schlager T, Anderson S, Trudell J, Hendley J. Effect of cranberry juice on bacteriuria in children with neurogenic bladder receiving intermittent catheterization. *J Pediatr* 1999;135(6):698–702.

Schmidt D, Sobota A. An examination of the anti-adherence activity of cranberry juice on urinary and non-urinary bacterial isolates. *Microbios* 1988;55:173–81.

Schultz A. Efficacy of cranberry juice and ascorbic acid in acidifying the urine in multiple sclerosis subjects. *J Community Health Nursing* 1984a;1(3):139–69.

Schultz A. Efficacy of cranberry on urinary pH. *J Community Health Nursing* 1984b;1:159–69.

Simons A, Hasselbring B, Castleman M. Urinary Tract Infection. In: *Before You Call the Doctor: Safe, Effective Self-Care for Over 300 Common Medical Problems.* New York, NY: Ballantine Books; 1992;431–4.

Sobota AE. Inhibition of bacterial adherence by cranberry juice: potential use for the treatment of urinary tract infections. *J Urol* 1984;131:1013–6.

Sternlieb P. Cranberry juice in renal disease [letter]. *New Eng J Med* 1963;268(1):57.

Tsukada K, Tokunaga K, Iwama T. Cranberry juice and its impact on peri-stomal skin conditions for urostomy patients. *Ostomy/Wound Manage* 1994;40(9):60–7.

United States Congress. Public Law 103–417: Dietary Supplement Health and Education Act of 1994. Washington, DC: 103rd Congress of the United States; 1994.

United States Department of Agriculture (USDA). Cranberries: 1998 Area Harvested, Yield and = Total [report]. Washington, DC: USDA National Agricultural Statistical Service (NASS); 1999.

United States Department of Agriculture (USDA). United States Standards for Grades of Fresh Cranberries for Processing: Effective August 24, 1957 (Reprinted January 1997). Washington, DC: United States Department of Agriculture–Fruit and Vegetable Division–Fresh Products Branch; 1997.

United States Food and Drug Administration (US FDA). Code of Federal Regulations, Title 21, Chapter I, Part 101, Sec. 101.30 percentage juice declaration for foods purporting to be beverages [Revised as of April 1, 1999]. Washington, DC: U.S. Government Printing Office via GPO Access; 1999;74–77.

United States Pharmacopeia (USP 25th Revision) - The National Formulary (NF 20th Edition). Rockville, MD: United States Pharmacopeial Convetion, Inc. 2002.

US FDA. See: United States Food and Drug Administration.

USC. See: United States Congress.

USDA. See: United States Department of Agriculture.

USP. See: *United States Pharmacopeia.*

Vandenberg J, Parent G. Profile of the Canadian Cranberry Industry. Ottawa, Ontario: Agriculture and Agri-Food Canada (AAFC) Market & Industry Services Branch; 1999 March 25, 1999.

Walker E, Barney D, Mickelsen JN, *et al.* Cranberry concentrate: UTI prophylaxis. *J Fam Pract* 1997;45(2):167–8.

Walker E, Mickelsen R, Mickelsen J. Identification and characterization of the active antiadherence factors from cranberry [Poster Session]. *American Society of Pharmacognosy Interim Meeting* April 29–May 1, 1999 *Program and Abstract Book* 1999;20.

Weiss E, Lev-Dor R, Kashamn Y, *et al.* Inhibiting interspecies coaggregation of plaque bacteria with a cranberry juice constituent. *J Am Dent Assoc* 1998;129(12):1719–923.

Wilson T, Porcari J, Maher M. Cranberry juice inhibits metal and non-metal initiated oxidation of human low-density lipoproteins *in vitro. Journal of Nutraceuticals, Functional & Medical Foods* 1999;2(2):5–14.

Yarnell E. Botanical medicine for cystitis. *Altern Complement Ther* 1997 Aug;269–75.

Zafriri D, Ofek I, Adar R, *et al.* Inhibitory activity of cranberry juice on adherence of type 1 and type P fimbriated *Escherichia coli* to eucaryotic cells. *Antimicrob Agents Chemother* 1989;33(1):92–8.

Zinsser H, *et al.* Management of infected stones with acidifying agents. *NY State J Med* 1968;68:301–10.

Clinical Studies on Cranberry (*Vaccinium macrocarpon* Aiton)

Urinary Tract Infection

Author/Year	Subject	Design	Duration	Dosage	Preparation	Results/Conclusion
Kontiokari et al., 2001	Urinary tract infection prevention	O, R, C n=150	12 months	50 ml of cranberry-lingonberry juice daily for 6 months or 100 ml of lactobacillus drink 5 days/wk for 1 year, or no intervention	Cranberry-lingonberry juice concentrate or lactobacillus drink	Cranberry juice, compared to lactobacillus or no intervention, significantly reduced the recurrence of urinary tract infections. The women had at least 1 recurrence at the following rates: 8 (16%) of the women in cranberry group, 19 (39%) in the lactobacillus group, and 18 (36%) in the control group. The cranberry group demonstrated a 20% reduction in absolute risk compared with the control group.
Schlager et al., 1999	Urinary tract system assessment of bacteriuria using preventive therapy	DB, PC, C n=15 children, 2–18 years, with neurogenic bladder	6 months (3-month crossover), receiving clean intermittent cathaterization	60 ml/day juice concentrate (equivalent to 300 ml cranberry juice cocktail)	Specially prepared unsweetened cranberry juice concentrate (Ocean Spray®) vs. cranberry Jell-O® placebo concentrate (Kraft Foods Inc.)	Cranberry concentrate had no effect on bacteriuria, and no significant difference was observed in the acidification of urine vs. placebo. Results suggest that cranberry juice may not be effective in preventing UTIs in children with neurogenic bladder receiving intermittent catheterization.
Dignam et al., 1998	Urinary tract system	RCS, LC n=538 nursing home patients with a history of UTIs	RCS: 28 months LC:16 months (8 months preintervention; 8 months intervention)	4 ounces juice/day or 450 mg/day	Commercial cranberry juice cocktail or Azo-Cranberry® capsules	In the cross-sectional study, symptomatic UTI rates were significantly reduced in long-term care residents. In the preintervention period of 19 months, there were 545 UTIs. For the full intervention period of 19 months, there were 164 UTIs. The Student T-test was used to compare average numbers of UTIs in preintervention with full intervention, yielding a T-value of 2.84, which is significant (p=0.0008). In the longitudinal cohort study of 113 residents for 16 months, the number of UTIs dropped from 103 in the preintervention period, to 84 during the intervention period. Although cranberry reduced the number of UTIs, the authors recommended additional well-controlled trials.
Walker et al., 1997	Urinary tract system prevention of UTIs	R, DB, PC, C n=10 women; 28–44 yrs with history of recurrent UTIs (at least 4 UTIs in the previous year or at least 1 during previous 3 months)	6 months (3 months cranberry; 3 months placebo). Treatment began after 10-day course of antibiotic therapy for symptomatic UTI. UTI treated with antibiotics was not counted in the study for enrollment criteria.	400 mg, 2x/day dry cranberry solids vs. placebo (dicalcium phosphate)	Solaray® CranActin®, each capsule contains 400 mg powdered cranberry solids	Using Student T-test and 99% confidence interval, daily consumption of cranberry extract was more effective than placebo in reducing the occurrence of UTIs (p<0.005).
Jackson and Hicks, 1997	Urinary tract system (effect on urinary pH)	PS, DCO, n=40 (21 completed study) Elderly men residing in nursing home with history of UTIs (mean age, 73 years)	3 months (4 weeks no juice, 4 weeks juice, 4 weeks no juice)	236.6 ml, 3x/day with meals	Cranberry juice (brand not stated)	Urinary pH during juice period was significantly lower than first and second non-juice periods. The findings support the claim that cranberry juice acidifies urine, even in moderate amounts. This study suggests that cranberry juice can be a home health nursing intervention to reduce risk of UTIs in the elderly.

KEY: C – controlled, **CC** – case-control, **CH** – cohort, **CI** – confidence interval, **Cm** – comparison, **CO** – crossover, **CS** – cross-sectional, **DB** – double-blind, **E** – epidemiological, **LC** – longitudinal cohort, **MA** – meta-analysis, **MC** – multi-center, **n** – number of patients, **O** – open, **OB** – observational, **OL** – open label, **OR** – odds ratio, **P** – prospective, **PB** – patient-blind, **PC** – placebo-controlled, **PG** – parallel group, **PS** – pilot study, **R** – randomized, **RC** – reference-controlled, **RCS** – retrospective cross-sectional, **RS** - retrospective, **S** – surveillance, **SB** – single-blind, **SC** – single-center, **U** – uncontrolled, **UP** – unpublished, **VC** – vehicle-controlled.

Urinary Tract Infection (cont.)

Author/Year	Subject	Design	Duration	Dosage	Preparation	Results/Conclusion
Foda et al., 1995	Urinary tract system	R, SB, C n=21 pediatric neuropathic bladder population prophylaxes receiving clean intermittent catheterization	12 months (6 months cranberry and 6 months water)	15 ml/kg/day cocktail for 6 months; 15 ml/kg/day with water for 6 months	Cranberry juice (brand not stated)	No difference between intervention periods (2-tailed, p=0.5566 [whole group]; p=0.2845 [antimicrobial subset]) with respect to infection. 12 patients dropped out for reasons related to cranberry (taste, caloric load, cost). Fewer infections were observed in 9 patients taking juice and in 9 taking water; no difference was noted in 3 Cranberry, on a daily basis, at 15 ml/kg, did not have any effect greater than water in preventing UTI. This study does not support use of cranberry for antibacterial prophylaxis in pediatric neuropathic bladders.
Avorn et al., 1994	Urinary tract system (effect on bacteriuria and pyuria)	R, DB, PC n=153 (elderly women, mean age 78.5 years)	6 months using clean-catch urine samples	300 ml/day vs. placebo	Ocean Spray® Cranberry Juice Cocktail, vs. cranberry-flavored, vitamin C-fortified placebo	After 4 to 8 weeks of regular intake, there was a significantly reduced (95% confidence interval, p=0.004) frequency of bacteriuria and pyuria in the cranberry group. Bacteriuria with pyuria occurred in 28.1% of urine specimens of placebo group compared to 15% in the cranberry group. Cranberry reduced pre-existing bacteria in the urinary tract. Average pH of urine in the cranberry group (6.0) was higher than in the placebo group (5.5). Patients in cranberry group with bacteriuria and pyuria were more likely to convert to non-bacteriuria pyuria than in control group.
Haverkorn and Mandigers, 1994	Urinary tract system	R, PC, C n=17 (elderly patients)	8 weeks (4 weeks cranberry; 4 weeks placebo)	15 ml, 2x/day in water	Cranberry juice diluted in water (brand not stated)	This study confirmed the findings of Avorn et al. (1994), suggesting that cranberry juice reduces the frequency of bacteriuria in elderly persons. 3 patients had bacteriuria all the time and 7 at no time during the study. The remaining 7 had fewer occurrences of bacteriuria during the cranberry treatment period (p=0.004). Increased diuresis is unlikely to be the cause of the decreased bacteriuria rate.
Gibson et al, 1991	Urinary tract system (prevention of UTI)	O n=28 (nursing home patients)	7 weeks	120–180 ml, ca./day	Cranberry Juice Cocktail, Ocean Spray®	Daily ingestion prevented UTIs in 19 of the 28 nursing home patients. The remaining 9 patients had trace or greater leukocytes and/or nitrates in all their urine and significant colony counts of Gram-negative bacilli. This study suggested that cranberry might be preventive rather than curative.
Rogers, 1991	Urinary tract system	U, MC n=16 girls with neuropathic bladders	2 weeks	180–240 ml, 2x/day for 1 week followed by 3x/day for one week	Cranberry juice (brand not stated)	All urine samples showed a reduction in both red and white cell counts, which suggests a significant reduction in infection. Urine samples from school group continued to culture *E. coli*, whereas cultures from hospital group showed a significant reduction of *E. coli*. Study suggests that cranberry juice is beneficial to children with neuropathic bladders, especially in the case of suspected infection or after bladder surgery. No statistics reported.
Schultz, 1984a	Urinary tract system (acidification of urine)	R, C n=8 (3 women, 5 men) with multiple sclerosis	41 days (20 days cranberry treatment, 24-hour washout, 20 days orange juice)	180 ml juice, 2x/day; plus 500 mg, 2x/day ascorbic acid	Cranberry juice vs. orange juice control (brand not stated)	Cranberry juice was significantly more effective than orange juice (p<0.001) in acidifying urine, and evening pH values were significantly lower (p<0.001) than morning pH values (N-580).
Kinney and Blount, 1979	Urinary tract system (effect on urinary pH)	R n=40 (21 women, 19 men, mostly students) (ages 20–35 years)	12 days	4 separate groups; 150, 180, 210 or 240 ml, 3x/day with meals	Specially prepared sweetened beverage containing 80% juice, Ocean Spray®	Significant reduction in mean urine pH (p<0.01) was observed from ingestion of cranberry juice in each of the experimental groups. Effect was not dose dependent, and there were no serious side effects.

KEY: **C** – controlled, **CC** – case-control, **CH** – cohort, **CI** – confidence interval, **Cm** – comparison, **CO** – crossover, **CS** – cross-sectional, **DB** – double-blind, **E** – epidemiological, **LC** – longitudinal cohort, **MA** – meta-analysis, **MC** – multi-center, **n** – number of patients, **O** – open, **OB** – observational, **OL** – open label, **OR** – odds ratio, **P** – prospective, **PB** – patient-blind, **PC** – placebo-controlled, **PG** – parallel group, **PS** – pilot study, **R** – randomized, **RC** – reference-controlled, **RCS** – retrospective cross-sectional, **RS** - retrospective, **S** – surveillance, **SB** – single-blind, **SC** – single-center, **U** – uncontrolled, **UP** – unpublished, **VC** – vehicle-controlled.

Cranberry

Monograph

Urinary Tract Infection   (cont.)

Author/Year	Subject	Design	Duration	Dosage	Preparation	Results/Conclusion
Nickey, 1975	Urinary tract system (effect on urinary pH)	n=10	15 days		Cranberry juice and ascorbic acid given alone and in combination (brand not stated)	Mean urinary pH reductions from baseline during administration of cranberry juice and ascorbic acid, alone and in combination. Greatest reduction occurring with combination, with occurrence of mean urinary pH of 5.5 and 5.0 or below. No statistic reported.
Light et al., 1973	Urinary tract system	U n=15 Patients with calcium-containing renal stones (n=10). Patients without calcium-containing renal stones (n=5).	Not stated	Stone-forming patients: 32 oz. daily Normal patients: 32–80 oz. daily	Cranberry juice (brand not stated)	In patients with calcium-containing renal stones, the urinary ionized calcium was reduced with cranberry juice by an average of 50% (p<0.001). No consistent change in total or ionized calcium excretion in normals by administration of up to 480 ml juice.
Kahn et al., 1967	Urinary tract system (effect on urinary pH and calcium excretion)	U n=4 healthy, infection-free men	7–11 days	1,500–4,000 ml/day, depending on subject's liquid tolerance, 1x/day	Cranberry Juice Cocktail Ocean Spray®	3 subjects demonstrated only transient decrease in pH and increase in titratable acidity, while fourth sustained these changes for 1 week. 2 subjects experienced progressive increase in urinary calcium, despite absence of sustained urinary acidification effect. Statistics are based on each subject, not on entire group.
Papas et al., 1966	Urinary tract system (treatment of acute UTI)	U n=60 44 women and 16 men with acute UTI (All patients were symptomatic, but only 38 fit colony count criterion of 100,000 organism/ml for UTI)	21 days	ca. 450ml/day	Commercial cranberry juice product (brand not stated)	After 3 weeks of cranberry therapy, a positive clinical response was reported in 53% (32/60) of UTI patients (no urogenital complaints and fewer than 100,000 bacteria per ml urine), while an additional 20% experienced moderate improvement. During the 6 weeks after treatment period, 61% experienced recurrence. Substantial decrease in bacterial count and alleviation of urogenital complaints was significant.
Bodel et al., 1959	Urinary tract system (effects on urine pH and hippuric acid excretion)	U n=5	24 hours	1,200–4,000 ml/day	Cranberry Juice Cocktail, Ocean Spray®	Hippuric acid content of urine increased by several grams a day. Only slight changes in urine pH were reported. Bacteriostatic activity decreases five-fold when urinary pH rises to 5.6. No statistics available.
Fellers et al., 1933	Urinary tract system (effect on urine pH)	U n=6 healthy men (22–27 years)	5 days	100–300 g/day	Fresh cranberries	Cranberry ingestion increased titratable acidity, organic acids, hippuric acid, hydrogen ion concentration, and ammonia in urine, while uric acid and urea nitrogen slightly decreased. Amount of hippuric acid in urine was directly proportional to weight of cranberries eaten.

Other

Author/Year	Subject	Design	Duration	Dosage	Preparation	Results/Conclusion
Tsukada et al., 1994	Dermatological improvement of skin complications from urostomies	U n=13 patients with peristomial skin conditions; (average, 61.5 years)	Average 6 months (3 weeks to 2 years)	160 ml, 1–2x/day	Cranberry juice, 50% concentration (brand not stated)	An improvement in skin condition in 6 patients with erythema, maceration, or pseudoepithelia hyperplasia (PEH) and in 2 patients with maceration or PEH. Study suggests that cranberry juice improves peristomial skin PEH and maceration. Improvement was not due to acidification of urine, as the pH of the fresh urine actually became unexpectedly more alkaline (p=0.0178).

KEY: C – controlled, **CC** – case-control, **CH** – cohort, **CI** – confidence interval, **Cm** – comparison, **CO** – crossover, **CS** – cross-sectional, **DB** – double-blind, **E** – epidemiological, **LC** – longitudinal cohort, **MA** – meta-analysis, **MC** – multi-center, **n** – number of patients, **O** – open, **OB** – observational, **OL** – open label, **OR** – odds ratio, **P** – prospective, **PB** – patient-blind, **PC** – placebo-controlled, **PG** – parallel group, **PS** – pilot study, **R** – randomized, **RC** – reference-controlled, **RCS** – retrospective cross-sectional, **RS** - retrospective, **S** – surveillance, **SB** – single-blind, **SC** – single-center, **U** – uncontrolled, **UP** – unpublished, **VC** – vehicle-controlled.

(This page intentionally left blank.)

Echinacea

Echinacea purpurea (L.) Moench, *E. pallida* (Nutt.) Nutt.,
E. angustifolia DC.

[Fam. *Asteraceae*]

OVERVIEW

The native American medicinal plant, echinacea, is one of the most popular herbs in the U.S. marketplace. Preparations made from several plant species and plant parts of the genus *Echinacea* constituted the top-selling herbal medicine in all channels of sales (mass market, multilevel, and natural food stores) in 1997, capturing 9% of the total market based on $3.6 billion of total sales. Echinacea preparations ranked fourth with retail sales of over $58 million in the mainstream market in 2000. While the main constituents in the different species and plant parts have pharmacological activity, the exact compounds responsible for the therapeutic value are unclear. For this reason it is important to note the taxonomic source and type of preparation for each clinical study.

PRIMARY USES

- Upper respiratory tract infections (URTIs) — Treatment

OTHER POTENTIAL USES

Internal
- Immune system stimulant
- Adjunct therapy in chronic candidiasis in women
- URTIs — Prevention

External
- Wound healing

PHARMACOLOGICAL ACTIONS

Internal
Promotes immunomodulatory activity. In animal studies: demonstrates antitumor activity in combination with *Thuja occidentalis* tips and *Baptisia tinctoria* rhizome; increases phagocytosis; increases serum leukocytes; stimulates granulocyte migration; stimulates cytokine production; protective effects on influenza A-virus infection in mice.

External
Protects against photodamage; promotes wound healing; increases total lymphocyte count with a decreased percentage of T-helper cells.

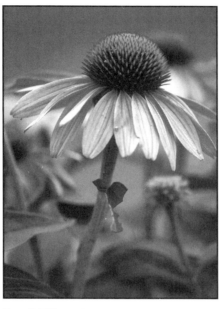

Photo © 2003 stevenfoster.com

DOSAGE AND ADMINISTRATION

The German Commission E recommends limiting the use of internal and external echinacea preparations to 8 weeks because the conditions for which echinacea preparations are used are usually relatively minor and transient. If symptoms still persist after 8 weeks of echinacea therapy, more aggressive treatment is presumably needed.

Internal

E. purpurea herb
EXPRESSED JUICE FROM FRESH AERIAL PARTS: (2.5:1), stabilized in 22% alcohol: 6–9 ml daily.

INFUSION: For upper respiratory and flu symptoms, 150–240 ml boiling water poured over about 1 g dried herb and steeped, covered, for 10–15 minutes, 5–6 times daily.

TINCTURE: 1:10 (*w/v*), in 65% (*v/v*) alcohol: 5 drops, 1–3 times daily. For acute conditions, 5 drops every 1/2–1 hr.

E. purpurea, *E. pallida*, *E. angustifolia* root
DRIED ROOT: 0.9–1 g, approximately 900 mg cut root 3 times daily.

INFUSION: 0.9 g root in 150 ml boiled water steeped for 10 min., several times daily between meals.

DECOCTION: 1 g in 150 ml water boiled for 10 min., 3 times daily.

FLUID EXTRACT: 1:1 in 45% alcohol: 0.5–1.0 ml 3 times daily.

TINCTURE: 1:5 (*g/ml*), ethanol 55% (*v/v*): 30–60 drops, approximately 1.5–5 ml, 3 times daily.

External
OINTMENT: Semisolid preparation containing at least 15% pressed juice in a base of petroleum jelly, or anhydrous lanolin, and vegetable oil applied locally.

POULTICE: Semisolid paste or plaster containing at least 15% pressed juice applied locally.

Echinacea

Clinical Overview

CONTRAINDICATIONS

Caution may be advised with internal echinacea preparations in cases of increased tendency for allergies, especially to members of the family *Asteraceae,* including arnica (*Arnica* spp.*),* chamomile (*Matricaria* spp.), marigold (*Calendula officinalis*), yarrow (*Achillea* spp.), ragweed (*Ambrosia* spp.), asters (*Aster tataricus*), and chrysanthemums (*Chrysanthemum* spp.). Based on theoretical considerations, the Commission E also advises using echinacea with caution in progressive systemic diseases such as tuberculosis, leukosis, collagenosis, multiple sclerosis, AIDS, HIV infection, and other autoimmune diseases. No contraindications are known for external echinacea preparations.

PREGNANCY AND LACTATION: No known restrictions. In a recent controlled trial, echinacea consumption by pregnant women showed no evidence of risk.

ADVERSE EFFECTS

Few adverse effects have been reported for internal and external echinacea preparations. Ingestion of an echinacea preparation made of *E. angustifolia* (whole plant) and *E. purpurea* root has been associated with anaphylaxis. It is possible that pollens might be present in echinacea preparations made with aerial parts and not in those preparations containing root material only.

DRUG INTERACTIONS

None known.

CLINICAL REVIEW

Of 21 studies on echinacea that included a total of 3,508 participants, all but three demonstrated positive effects for indications including cold, flu, upper respiratory tract infections (URTIs), candidiasis, and gestational safety. Five positive randomized, double-blind, placebo-controlled (R, DB, PC) studies, involving a total of 825 subjects, supported the use of specific and unique echinacea monopreparations for the treatment (incidence, severity, and/or duration) of acute upper respiratory or flu-like infections. The acute treatment was further supported by six additional R, DB, PC studies using combination preparations containing echinacea and other herbs. One R, DB, PC study on an echinacea monopreparation did not find measurable benefit for treatment of URTI symptoms, though this may be due to the low dose and lack of severity of the symptoms.

The prevention of URTIs was studied in five R, PC studies with a total of 1,209 subjects focused on the use of distinct mono-preparations and unique combination products. Two of these studies did not find a significant effect. Non-continuous administration of the treatment in one study may have been a factor, though the authors attributed the results to a sample size smaller than desired. In another study, the authors reported that the "treatment with fluid extract of *Echinacea purpurea* did not significantly decrease the incidence, duration or severity of colds and respiratory infections compared to placebo."

Other trials included a study on genital herpes that found no demonstrated effect. One R, PC study on immunology in athletes concluded that the echinacea group had no URTIs compared to placebo. Women using echinacea drops as an adjunct therapy in the treatment of chronic candidiasis showed a reduced recurrence rate. A study on the safety of echinacea during pregnancy found no statistical difference between echinacea and control groups.

A review of 13 R, DB, PC trials studying the treatment and prevention of URTIs evaluated the effectiveness of orally ingested echinacea preparations. The authors concluded that the published trials suggest echinacea may be beneficial for *treatment*, but the variation of preparations and compositions (including combination products containing other botanicals) makes recommending specific doses problematic. They claimed that there was very little evidence supporting the prolonged use of echinacea for *prevention* of URTIs. An assessment of the methodology of 26 controlled clinical trials concluded that the published clinical studies suggest that some preparations containing echinacea can be efficacious as immunomodulators. However, the evidence is insufficient to recommend an exact dosage or specific preparation for use. A review observed that despite contraindications in autoimmune diseases based on theoretical considerations (e.g., those suggested by Commission E), current clinical use and scientific evidence do not support limitations on long-term use of echinacea with particular auto-immune diseases. The author suggested echinacea should be considered an immunomodulator rather than an immunostimulant.

Echinacea

Echinacea purpurea (L.) Moench, *E. pallida* (Nutt.) Nutt., *E. angustifolia* DC.
[Fam. *Asteraceae*]

OVERVIEW

The native American medicinal plant echinacea is one of the most popular herbs in the U.S. marketplace. Preparations made from several plant species and parts of echinacea are used, including the above-ground parts, or the roots, stems or leaves from *Echinacea purpurea, E. pallida*, and/or *E. angustifolia*. While all of these species variations can be effective for treating different ailments, the exact chemical compounds responsible for the therapeutic effects are not yet known.

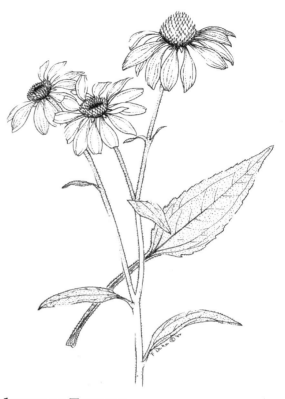

USES

Supportive care to treat colds and chronic infections of the upper respiratory tract.

DOSAGE

Consult your healthcare practitioner if symptoms have not improved within eight weeks.

E. purpurea herb
TINCTURE: 5 ml, 3 times daily.

E. purpurea, E. pallida, E. angustifolia root
DRIED ROOT: 900 mg, 3 times daily.

FLUID EXTRACT: 0.5–1.0 ml, 3 times daily.

TINCTURE: 30–60 drops, 3 times daily.

Echinacea preparations are also available as teas, capsules, and tablets.

CONTRAINDICATIONS

Consult your healthcare provider before ingesting echinacea preparations in cases of an increased tendency toward allergies to plants in the daisy family (*Asteraceae*), including arnica, chamomile, chrysanthemum, marigold, ragweed, and yarrow.

PREGNANCY AND LACTATION: There are no known restrictions for use during pregnancy or while breast-feeding.

ADVERSE EFFECTS

Rare cases of allergic reactions to plants in the family *Asteraceae* are the only known adverse effects of echinacea.

DRUG INTERACTIONS

There are no known drug interactions.

Comments

When using a dietary supplement, purchase it from a reliable source. For best results, use the same brand of product throughout the period of use. As with all medications and dietary supplements, please inform your healthcare provider of all herbs and medications you are taking. Interactions may occur between medications and herbs or even among different herbs when taken at the same time. Treat your herbal supplement with care by taking it as directed, storing it as advised on the label, and keeping it out of the reach of children and pets. Consult your healthcare provider with any questions.

AMERICAN BOTANICAL COUNCIL

The information contained on this sheet has been excerpted from *The ABC Clinical Guide to Herbs* © 2003 by the American Botanical Council (ABC). ABC is an independent member-based educational organization focusing on the medicinal use of herbs. For more detailed information about this herb please consult the healthcare provider who gave you this sheet. To order *The ABC Clinical Guide to Herbs* or become a member of ABC, visit their website at www.herbalgram.org.

Echinacea

Echinacea spp.

Echinacea purpurea (L.) Moench, *E. pallida* (Nutt.) Nutt., *E. angustifolia* DC.

[Fam. *Asteraceae*]

OVERVIEW

The medicinal plant echinacea, indigenous to the U.S., is one of the most popular herbs in the U.S. marketplace. The roots of several species were the most widely used medicines of Native Americans of the Great Plains. Ethnobotanist M.R. Gilmore noted, "Echinacea seems to have been used as a remedy for more ailments than any other plant" (Gilmore, 1911). Foster (1991) and Moerman (1998) have reviewed the ethnobotany of both the roots and leaves of various species of *Echinacea*. They were used by Native Americans for toothache, enlarged glands (mumps), sore throat, snakebite, coughs, burns, and as an analgesic. Eclectic medical physicians of the late 19th century employed *E. angustifolia* root for a variety of indications, both internally and externally, including sepsis (e.g., gangrene, boils, septicemia), foul mucous discharges, cancerous growths, typhoid, various types of fevers, and locally applied for chronic skin sores (Felter and Lloyd, 1898). They also used it for mitigation of the pain of gonorrhea and syphilis, as a local anesthetic, for snakebite and other venomous stings (Foster, 1991).

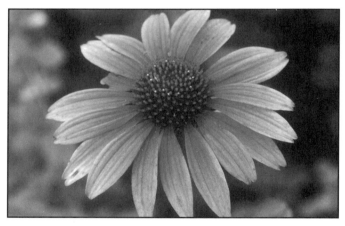

Photo © 2003 stevenfoster.com

Preparations made from several plant species and plant parts of the genus *Echinacea* constituted the top-selling herbal supplement sold in all U.S. channels of sales (mass market, multilevel, and natural food stores) in 1997, consisting of 9% of the total market based on $3.6 billion in total sales (Brevoort, 1998). In 2000, echinacea preparations ranked fourth in the mainstream market with retail sales of $58,422,932 (Blumenthal, 2001). While the main constituents of the different species and plant parts have pharmacological activity, the exact compounds responsible for echinacea's therapeutic value are unclear. For this reason, it is important to note the taxonomic source, plant part, and type of preparation for each clinical study (Parnham, 1999; Bauer 1999; Melchart and Linde, 1999).

DESCRIPTION

Nine species of the genus *Echinacea* have been classified taxonomically (Hobbs, 1994) although recent chemical and genetic research suggests possible reclassification of the genus to four species (Binns *et al.*, 2002). Echinacea preparations consist of any one or more of the plant parts from three *Echinacea* species [Fam. *Asteraceae*], including the fresh, above-ground parts (harvested at the time of flowering), the fresh or dried root of *E. purpurea* (L.) Moench, and the fresh or dried root of *E. pallida* (Nutt.) Nutt., and/or *E. angustifolia* D.C., and their preparations in effective dosage. Occasionally, the fresh or dried above-ground parts of *E. pallida*, collected at the time of flowering, are used but are often labeled incorrectly as "*E. angustifolia*" in the marketplace (Blumenthal *et al.*, 2000).

PRIMARY USES

Respiratory

- Treatment of symptoms and duration in upper respiratory tract infections (URTIs)

  E. purpurea herb and root (Brinkeborn, 1998; Hoheisel *et al.*, 1997; Bräunig *et al*, 1992)

  E. pallida root (Dorn *et al.,* 1997)

  E. angustifolia root (Galea *et al.*, 1996)

  E. purpurea and *E. angustifolia* stems and *E. purpurea* root (Lindenmuth and Lindenmuth, 2000)

  E. purpurea and *E. pallida* roots (Henneicke-von Zepelin *et al.*, 1999; Reitz *et al.*, 1990; Vorberg, 1984)

OTHER POTENTIAL USES

Internal

- Immune system stimulant

  E. purpurea (Berg *et al.*, 1998; Brinkeborn, 1999; Hoheisel *et al.*, 1997; Braunig *et al.*, 1992)

  E pallida (Dorn *et al.*, 1997)

- Adjunct therapy in chronic candidiasis in women

  E. pupurea (Coeugniet and Kuhnast *et al.,* 1986)

- Prevention of URTIs:

  E. purpurea (Grimm and Müller, 1999; Schöneberger *et al.*, 1992)

  E. angustifolia (Melchart *et al*, 1998)

  E. purpurea and *E. pallida* (Forth *et al.*, 1981)

  E. angustifolia herb and root combination (Schmidt *et al.*, 1990)

External

- Wound healing

  E. purpurea (Blumenthal *et al.*, 1998; WHO, 1999)

  E. pallida root (Speroni *et al.,* 1998)

  E. angustifolia root (Bradley, 1992)

DOSAGE
Internal
Crude Preparations
E. purpurea herb

JUICE: 6–9 ml daily expressed juice from fresh *E. purpurea* aerial parts 2.5:1, stabilized in 22% alcohol, (Bauer and Liersch, 1993; Blumenthal *et al.*, 1998).

INFUSION: For upper respiratory and flu symptoms, 150–240 ml boiling water poured over about 1 g dried herb and steeped covered, for 10–15 minutes, 5–6 times daily (Lindenmuth and Lindenmuth, 2000).

TINCTURE: 5 drops, 1–3 times daily 1:10 (*w/v*), in 65% (*v/v*) alcohol. For acute conditions, 5 drops every 1/2–1 hour (Bauer and Liersch, 1993).

E. purpurea, E. pallida, E. angustifolia root

DRIED ROOT: 0.9–1 g (approximately 900 mg) cut root, 3 times daily.

INFUSION: 0.9 g root in 150 ml boiled water steeped for 10 minutes, several times daily between meals (Bauer and Liersch, 1993; Wichtl and Bisset, 1994).

DECOCTION: 1 g in 150 ml water boiled for 10 minutes, 3 times daily (Bradley, 1992).

FLUID EXTRACT: 1:1 in 45% alcohol, 0.5–1.0 ml 3 times daily (Newall *et al.*, 1996; Bradley, 1992).

TINCTURE: 1:5 (*g/ml*), ethanol 55% (*v/v*) 30–60 drops, approximately 1.5–5 ml (Bradley, 1992), three times daily (Bauer and Liersch, 1993; ESCOP, 1999).

External
Crude Preparations
OINTMENT: Semisolid preparation containing at least 15% pressed juice in a base of petroleum jelly or anhydrous lanolin, and vegetable oil applied locally (Blumenthal *et al.*, 1998; Blumenthal *et al.*, 2000).

POULTICE: Semisolid paste or plaster containing at least 15% pressed juice, applied locally (Blumenthal *et al.*, 2000).

DURATION OF ADMINISTRATION
Internal and External
The German Commission E recommended use for no longer than eight weeks (Blumenthal *et al.*, 1998). NOTE: This duration limit has been misinterpreted as meaning that echinacea preparations may not be safe for use for longer than eight weeks, but this is not the case. This restriction was adopted by the Commission E due to its opinion that most conditions for which echinacea preparations are to be used are usually relatively minor and transient. Therefore, if therapy with echinacea has not succeeded within eight weeks, and symptoms still persist, more aggressive treatment is presumably needed.

CHEMISTRY
The constituents of echinacea preparations vary depending on the particular species and plant part used.

E. purpurea herb (i.e., aerial parts) and root both contain caffeic acid derivatives (0.6–2.1% in roots), including mainly cichoric acid (1.2–3.1% in the flowers), caffeic acid, caftaric acid, chlorogenic acid and 0.001–0.04% alkamides. *E. purpurea* herb also contains water-soluble polysaccharides (arabinoxylan and arabinogalactan types); fructans; 0.48% flavonoids of quercetin and kaempferol type; and 0.08–0.32% essential oil (Bauer, 1999;

Bauer and Liersch, 1993). *E. purpurea* root differs in containing polyacetylene derivatives; polysaccharides (fructosans, arabinogalactans); glycoproteins comprised of approximately 3% protein, of which the dominant sugars are 64–84% arabinose, 1.9–5.3% galactose, and 6% glucosamine, and up to 0.2% essential oil (Bauer 1999; Bauer and Liersch, 1993; ESCOP, 1999; Pietta *et al.*, 1998).

E. pallida herb contains caffeic acid derivatives including cichoric acid, caftaric acid, echinacoside, verbascoside, chlorogenic acid, and isochlorogenic acid; flavonoids (mainly rutoside); alkamides; and <0.1% essential oil (Bauer, 1998; Bauer and Liersch, 1993; Leung and Foster, 1996; Pietta *et al.*, 1998).

E. pallida root contains caffeic acid derivatives, mainly 0.7–1.0% echinacoside, followed by isochlorogenic acid, 6–*O*-caffeoylechinacoside, and chlorogenic acid; 0.2–2.0% essential oil comprised mainly of ketoalkynes and ketoalkenes, polyacetylenes, polysaccharides, and glycoproteins (Bauer, 1999; Bauer and Liersch, 1993; ESCOP, 1999; Pietta *et al.*, 1998). Methyl jasmonate, a naturally-occurring cellular signal molecule, increased content of alkamides and ketoalene/ynes (Binns, 2001).

E. angustifolia herb contains caffeic acid derivatives such as cichoric acid, echinacoside, verbascoside, chlorogenic acid, and isochlorogenic acid; flavonoids (mostly quercetin); alkamides; polysaccharides; and less than 0.1% essential oil (Bauer, 1998; Bauer and Liersch, 1993; Leung and Foster, 1996; Pietta *et al.*, 1998).

E. angustifolia root contains caffeic acid derivatives, mainly 0.3–1.7% echinacoside, followed by chlorogenic acid; an isochlorogenic acid and its characteristic constituent, cynarin; polysaccharides, including 5.9% inulin; glycoproteins comprised of approximately 3% protein, of which the dominant sugars are 64–84% arabinose, 1.9–5.3% galactose, and 6% glucosamines; 0.01–0.15% alkamides; and less than 0.1% essential oil (Bauer, 1998; Bauer, 1999; Bauer and Liersch, 1993; Pietta *et al.*, 1998).

PHARMACOLOGICAL ACTIONS
Echinacea's pharmacological activity is believed to result from the combined effect of several of its chemical constituents, found within the different species and parts of echinacea.

Internal
Human
E. angustifolia

Promotes immunomodulatory activity (Melchart *et al.*, 1994).

E. pallida

Exhibits immunomodulatory (Melchart *et al.*, 1994) and immunostimulant activity (Dorn *et al.*, 1997).

E. purpurea

Demonstrates immunomodulatory (Melchart *et al.*, 1994); immunostimulant (Berg *et al.*, 1998; Braunig *et al.*, 1992; Brinkeborn, 1999; Hoheisel *et al.*, 1997; Parnham, 1996); and antimycotic activity (Coeugniet and Kuhnast, 1986).

Animal
E. angustifolia and E. pallida

Demonstrate antitumor activity (Voaden *et al.*, 1972) in combination with *Thuja occidentalis* tips and *Baptisia tinctoria* rhizome (per oral application).

E. purpurea

Increases phagocytosis (Bauer, 1999; Roesler *et al.*, 1991; Wagner *et al.*, 1988; Mose, 1983); increases serum leukocytes (Bauer,

1999); stimulates granulocyte migration (Roesler *et al.*, 1991; Wildfeuer and Mayerhofer, 1994); stimulates cytokine production (Bauer, 1999; Burger *et al.*, 1997; Wagner *et al.*, 1985); protective effects on influenza A-virus infection in mice (Bodinet, 1999).

In vitro
E. purpurea

Enhances phagocytosis (Bauer, 1999); increases NO-production of macrophages (Bodinet, 1999); demonstrates natural killer cell action (See *et al.*, 1997); and enhances the cytotoxicity of macrophages against tumor cells (Stimpel *et al.*, 1984).

E. purpurea, E. angustifolia, E. pallida

Enhances antibody production (IgM, number of antibody-producing cells) (Beuscher *et al.*, 1995; Bodinet, 1999); induces cytokine production (IL-1, IL-6, TNFa, IFNab) (Beuscher *et al.*, 1995).

External
Human
E. angustifolia

Promotes wound-healing for skin inflammation and abrasions (Boon and Smith, 1999).

E. purpurea

Increases total lymphocyte count with a decreased percentage of T-helper cells in patients with eczema, neurodermatitis, candida, and herpes simplex (Boon and Smith, 1999).

E. purpurea, E. angustifolia, E. pallida

Protect against photodamage (Facino *et al.*, 1995).

Animal
E. pallida and *E. angustifolia*

Inhibit inflammation (Speroni *et al.*, 1998; Tubaro *et al.*, 1987; Tragni *et al.*, 1985).

E. pallida

Demonstrates cicatrizing and vulnerary activity (Speroni *et al.*, 1998).

MECHANISM OF ACTION

Although the mechanism of action for *Echinacea* spp. is not fully understood, the following are proposed:

- Binds polysaccharides to carbohydrate receptors on the cell surface of T-cell lymphocytes and macrophages (Wagner *et al.*, 1984; Mose *et al.*, 1983).
- Promotes tissue regeneration and reduces inflammation by inhibiting hyaluronidase production (Tragni *et al.*, 1985).
- Generates oxidative burst and selective cytokine production in macrophages, leading to specific toxicity to tumor cell lines (Luettig *et al.*, 1989; Stimpel *et al.*, 1984).
- A combination of three polysaccharides from *E. purpurea* cell cultures produced a substantial increase in the number of peripheral blood leukocytes, due to an increase in polymorphanuclear cells (PMNs) in mice (Roesler, 1991).
- Enhances phagocytosis by human neutrophils *in vitro* and in human studies (Mose, 1983; Parnham, 1996).

CONTRAINDICATIONS
Internal
Individuals with an increased tendency to have allergies, especially allergies to members of the family *Asteraceae* including arnica (*Arnica* spp.) flower, chamomile (*Matricaria* spp.) flower, marigold (*Calendula officinalis* L.) flower, yarrow (*Achillea* spp.) flower (Braun *et al.*, 1996); ragweed (*Ambrosia* spp.); asters (*Aster tataricus*); and chrysanthemum (*Chrysanthemum* spp.) (Blumenthal *et al.*, 2000). The Commission E noted that progressive systemic diseases such as tuberculosis, leukosis, collagenosis, multiple sclerosis, Acquired Immune Deficiency Syndrome (AIDS), Human Immunodeficiency Virus (HIV) infection, and other autoimmune diseases are contraindicated (Blumenthal *et al.*, 1998), though these cautions were made based on theoretical considerations and not on reports of adverse findings (Bone, 1997–98).

External
None known (Blumenthal *et al.* 1998).

PREGNANCY AND LACTATION: The Commission E found no known restrictions (Blumenthal *et al.*, 1998). Although consumption of most medications and herbs is contraindicated during the first trimester, one recent controlled trial showed no evidence of increased risk for pregnant women who consumed echinacea (*E. angustifolia* and *E. purpurea*) (Gallo *et al.*, 2000).

ADVERSE EFFECTS
There are few reported adverse effects for internal and external applications. Aanaphylaxis has been reported with ingestion of an echinacea preparation made of *E. angustifolia* (whole plant) and *E. purpurea* root (Mullins, 1998; Mullins and Heddle, 2002). It is possible that pollens might be present in echinacea preparations made with aerial parts and not in those preparations containing root material only. NOTE: One source suggests that hepatotoxic effects have been reported with the persistent use of echinacea, causing one source to caution against the simultaneous use of echinacea with known hepatotoxic agents (e.g., anabolic steroids, amiodarone, methotrexate, or ketoconazole) (Miller, 1998). However, the significance of this purported hepatotoxicity is questionable, since echinacea lacks the 1, 2 unsaturated necine ring system associated with hepatotoxic pyrrolizidine alkaloids (PAs) (Roeder *et al.*, 1984). PAs do not constitute a significant part of echinacea chemistry, and those PAs found in echinacea species are not of the saturated type. No known documentation of hepatotoxicity is associated with ingestion of echinacea.

DRUG INTERACTIONS
The Commission E stated that there are no known interactions (Blumenthal *et al.*, 1998). Several sources raise the issue of potential interactions with immunosuppressive drugs (e.g., cyclosporine and corticosteroids), but to date these concerns are speculative and lack clinical documentation (Brinker, 2001).

AMERICAN HERBAL PRODUCTS ASSOCIATION (AHPA) SAFETY RATING
CLASS 1: Herbs that can be consumed safely when used appropriately (McGuffin *et al.*, 1997).

REGULATORY STATUS
AUSTRIA: The combination *E. purpurea* and *E. pallida* root, *Thuja occidentalis* herb, and *Baptisia tinctoria* root is approved as a nonprescription drug.

CANADA: When labeled as a Traditional Herbal Medicine (THM) or as a homeopathic drug, echinacea root (*E. angustifolia, E. pallida, E. purpurea*) is regulated as a nonprescription drug, requiring premarket registration and assignment of a Drug Identification Number (DIN) (Health Canada, 1990, 1997, 2000; WHO, 1998).

FRANCE: The homeopathic mother tincture of the whole fresh plant, 1:10 (*w/v*) in 55% alcohol, is official in the *French Pharmacopoeia* (Ph.Fr.X) (Bauer and Liersch, 1993).

GERMANY: Approved by Commission E as a nonprescription drug (*E. purpurea* herb and *E. pallida* root) (Blumenthal *et al.*, 1998). The combination of *E. purpurea* and *E. pallida* root, *Thuja occidentalis* herb, and *Baptisia tinctoria* root has not yet been approved as a nonprescription drug. The homeopathic mother tincture of the whole fresh plant (*E. angustifolia* or *E. pallida*) or aerial parts (*E. purpurea*) and dilutions are official in the *German Homeopathic Pharmacopoeia* (HAB, 2000).

SWEDEN: Classified as a natural remedy, intended for self-medication, requiring advance application for marketing authorization (MPA, 2001; Tunón, 1999; WHO, 1998). A monograph for Echinagard® (Echinacin®), is published in the Medical Products Agency (MPA) "Authorised Natural Remedies" (MPA, 1997).

SWITZERLAND: Echinacea anthroposophical, homeopathic, and phytomedicines have positive classification (List D) by the *Interkantonale Konstrollstelle für Heilmittel* (IKS) and corresponding sales category D, with sale limited to pharmacies and drugstores, without prescription (Morant and Ruppanner, 2001; *Codex*, 2000/01; WHO, 1998).

U.K.: Herbal medicine in *General Sale List*, Schedule 1 (medicinal products requiring a full Product License), Table A (for internal or external use) (Bradley, 1992).

U.S.: Dietary supplement (USC, 1994). Homeopathic mother tincture, 1:10 (*w/v*) in 55% alcohol (*v/v*), is a Class C over-the-counter (OTC) drug official in the *Homeopathic Pharmacopoeia of the United States* (1991), Official Compendium (1992). Rhizome with roots, powdered root and powdered extract are subjects of botanical monographs in development for the USP-NF. Previews of the standards development were published in *Pharmacopeial Forum* (USP, 2002).

CLINICAL REVIEW

Twenty-one studies are outlined in the following table "Clinical Studies on Echinacea," including a total of 3,508 participants. All but three of these studies (Galea and Thacker, 1996; Melchart *et al.*, 1998; Vonau *et al.*, 2001), demonstrated positive effects for indications including cold, flu, upper respiratory tract infections (URTIs), candidiasis, and gestational safety. Five positive randomized, double-blind, placebo-controlled (R, DB, PC) studies, involving a total of 825 subjects, supported the use of echinacea monopreparations for the treatment (incidence, severity, and/or duration) of acute upper respiratory or flu-like infections (Brinkeborn *et al.*, 1998, 1999; Dorn *et al.*, 1997; Hoheisel *et al.*, 1997; Bräunig *et al.*, 1992). The acute treatment was further supported by six additional R, DB, PC studies using combination preparations of echinacea and other herbs (Lindenmuth and Lindenmuth, 2000; Henneicke-von Zepelin *et al.*, 1999; Reitz *et al.*, 1990; Dorn 1989; Vorberg and Schneider, 1989; Vorberg, 1984). One R, DB, PC study on an echinacea monopreparation did not find measurable benefit for treatment of URTI symptoms, though this may be due to the low dose and lack of severity of the symptoms (Galea and Thacker, 1996).

The prevention of URTIs was studied in a total of five R, PC studies with a total of 1,209 subjects, focused on the use of distinct monopreparations (Grimm and Müller, 1999; Melchart *et al.*, 1998; Schöneberger, 1992) and unique combination products (Schmidt *et al.*, 1990; Forth and Beuscher, 1981). Two of these studies concluded that echinacea did not significantly pre-

vent URTIs. In the Melchart (1998) study, the treatment was administered noncontinuously, which may have been a factor in the lack of positive results, although the authors attributed the results to a subject group that was smaller than desired. Grimm and Muller (1999) reported that the "treatment with fluid extract of *Echinacea purpurea* did not significantly decrease the incidence, duration or severity of colds and respiratory infections compared to placebo."

Other trials included a study on genital herpes that found no demonstrated effect (Vonau *et al.*, 2001). One R, PC study on immunology in athletes, concluded that the echinacea group had no URTIs compared to placebo (Berg *et al.*, 1998). Women using echinacea drops as an adjunct therapy in the treatment of chronic candidiasis showed a reduced recurrence rate (Coeugniet and Kuhnast *et al.*, 1986). A prospective, controlled study on the safety of echinacea during pregnancy found no statistical difference between the groups (Gallo *et al.*, 2000).

A review of 13 R, DB, PC trials studying the treatment and prevention of URTIs, evaluated the effectiveness of orally ingested echinacea preparations (Barrett *et al.*, 1999). The authors concluded that the published trials suggest echinacea may be beneficial for *treatment*, but the variation of preparations and compositions (including combination products containing other botanicals) makes recommending specific doses problematic. They claimed that there was little evidence supporting the prolonged use of echinacea for *prevention* of URTIs (Barrett *et al.*, 1999). An assessment of the methodology of 26 controlled clinical trials concluded that the published clinical studies suggest that some preparations containing echinacea can be efficacious as immunomodulators. However, the evidence is insufficient to recommend an exact dosage or specific preparation for use (Melchart *et al.*, 1994). A review by Bone (1997-1998) observed that despite contraindications in auto-immune diseases based on theoretical considerations (e.g., those suggested by Commission E), current clinical use and scientific evidence do not support limitations on long-term use of echinacea with particular auto-immune diseases. Bone suggested echinacea should be considered an immunomodulator rather than an immunostimulant.

BRANDED PRODUCTS*

Echinacea Plus®: Traditional Medicinals®, Inc. / 4515 Ross Road / Sebastopol, CA 95472 U.S.A. / / Tel: (707) 823-8911 / Fax: (800) 886-4349 / www.traditionalmedicinals.com. Each tea bag 1,095 mg of the flowering aerial parts of *E. purpurea* and *E. angustifolia*, 30 mg of Echinacea purpurea extract (6:1) and flavor components lemongrass leaf and spearmint leaf.

Echinacin®: Madaus AG / Ostermerheimer Strausse 198 / Köln, Germany / Tel: +49-22-18-9984-76 / Fax: +49-22-18-9987-21 / Email: b.londener@madaus.de. Expressed juice of the aerial parts of *Echinacea purpurea*, stabilized with 22% ethanol, by volume.

Echinaforce®: Bioforce AG / CH-9325 Roggwil TG/ Switzerland / Tel: +41 71 454 61 61 / Fax: +41 71 454 61 62 / E-mail: Info@bioforce.ch / www.bioforce.com. Each tablet contains 400 mg dried extract, concentrated from a hydroalcoholic mother tincture (1:10) of *E. purpurea* herb fresh-flowering tops (380 mg) and E. purpurea root (20 mg), plus inert excipients materials.

EchinaGuard®: Nature's Way Products, Inc. / 10 Mountain Spring Parkway / Springville, Utah 84663 / U.S.A. / Tel: (801) 489-1500 / www.naturesway.com. Expressed juice of the aerial parts of *Echinacea purpurea*, stabilized with 22% ethanol, by volume.

Esberitox® (prior to 1985): Schaper and Brümmer GmbH & Co. KG / Bahnhofstrasse 35 / 38259 Salzgitter / Ringelheim / Germany / Tel: +49-5341-30-70 / Fax: +49-5341-30-71-24 / Email: info@schaperbruemmer.de / www.schaper-bruemmer.com. Ethanolic extract of 7.5 mg of extracts of E. purpurea and E. pallida root (1:1), 2 mg of *Thuja occidentalis* herb, and 10 mg *Baptisia tinctoria* root and homeopathic dilutions of Apis mell. (D4), Crotalus (D6), Lachesis (D4), and Silicea (D4).

Esberitox® N1 Tablets (1985 formulation based on Esberitox®): Schaper and Brümmer GmbH & Co. KG. 7.5 mg of extracts of E. purpurea and *E. pallida* root (1:1), 2 mg of *Thuja occidentalis* herb, and 10 mg Baptisia tinctoria.

Esberitox® N2 Tablets (1990 formulation based on Esberitox® N1): Schaper and Brümmer GmbH & Co. KG. 7.5 mg of E. *purpurea* and *E. pallida* root (1:1), 2 mg of Thuja occidentalis herb, and 10 mg *Baptisia tinctoria* root. Subsequently changed sources of echinacea.

Resistan®: TRUW Arzneimittel Vertriebs GmbH / Ziethenstrasse 8 / 33330 Gutersloh / Germany / Tel: +49-52-41-3007-40 / www.truw.de. Each 100 mg of Resistan® contains: 12 g *Echinacea angustifolia*; 2.9 g *Eupatorium perfoliatum*; 2 g *Baptista tinctoria*; 2 g *Arnica montana* D2. Contains 13 vol. percent. (NOTE: this product is being reformulated and may change names.)

* American equivalents, if any, are found in the Product Table beginning on page 398.

REFERENCES

Barrett B, Vohmann V, Calabrese C. *Echinacea* for upper respiratory tract infection. *J Fam Pract* 1999;48(8):628–35.

Bauer R, Liersch R. *Echinacea*. In: Hänsel R, Keller H, Rimpler G. Schneider (eds.). *Hagers Handbuch der Pharmazeutischen Praxis,* 5th ed. Vol. 5. Drogen E–O. New York: Springer Verlag; 1993:1–34.

Bauer R. Chemistry, analysis and immunological investigations of *Echinacea* phytopharmaceuticals. In: Wagner, H. (ed.) *Immunomodulatory Agents from Plants*, Basel; Boston; Berlin: Birkhäuser Verlag; 1999:41–88.

Bauer R, Wagner H. *Echinacea* species as potential immunostimulatory drugs. In: Wagner H, Farnsworth N (eds.). *Economic and Medicinal Plants Research*, Vol. 5. New York: Academic Press; 1991;5:253–321.

Berg A, Northoff H, König D, *et al*. Influence of Echinacin (EC31) treatment on the exercise-induced immune response in athletes. *J Clin Res* 1998;1:367–80.

Beuscher N, Bodinet C, Willigmann I, Egert D. Immune-stimulating effect of several echinacea root extracts. [in German]. *Z Phytother* 1995;16:157–66.

Binns SE, Livesey JF, Arnason JT, Baum BR. Phytochemical variation in echinacea from roots and flowerheads of wild and cultivated populations. *J Agric Food Chem* 2002;50(13):3673–87.

Binns SE, Inparajah I, Baum BR, Arnason JT. Methyl jasmonate increases reported alkamides and ketoalkene/ynes in *Echinacea pallida* (Asteraceae). *Phytochemistry* 2001;57:417–20.

Blumenthal M, Busse WR, Goldberg A, Gruenwald J, Hall T, Riggins CW, Rister RS (eds.). Klein S, Rister RS (trans.). *The Complete German Commission E Monographs—Therapeutic Guide to Herbal Medicines*. Austin, TX: American Botanical Council; Boston: Integrative Medicine Communication; 1998;122–3.

Blumenthal M, Goldberg A, Brinckmann J. *Herbal Medicine: Expanded Commission E Monographs*. Newton, MA: Integrative Medicine Communications; 2000; 88–102.

Blumenthal M. Herb sales down 15 percent in mainstream market. *HerbalGram* 2001;51:69.

Bodinet K. Immune-pharmacological assessment of a plant derived immune-stimulator [dissertation]. [in German]. Ernst-Moritz-Arndt-Universitat Greifswald. 1999.

Bone K. Echinacea: When should it be used? *Eur J Herb Med* 1997–1998;3(3):13–7.

Boon H, Smith M. *The Botanical Pharmacy: The Pharmacology of 47 Common Herbs*. Kingston, Ontario: Quarry Health Books; 1999;103–13.

Bradley P (ed.). *Echinacea angustifolia radix*. In: *British Herbal Compendium*, Vol. 1. Dorset, England: British Herbal Medicine Association; 1992:81–91.

Bratman S, Kroll D. *The Natural Pharmacist: Clinical Evaluation of Medicinal Herbs and Other Therapeutic Natural Products*. Rocklin, CA: Prima Publishing; 1999:1–8.

Bräunig B, Knick E. Therapeutic experiences with *Echinacea pallida* for influenza-like infections. [in German]. *Naturheilpraxis* 1993;1:72–5.

Bräunig B, Dorn M, Limburg E, *et al*. *Echinacea purpurea radix* for strengthening the immune response in flu-like infections. [in German]. *Z Phytother* 1992;13:7–13.

Brevoort P. The booming US botanical market. *HerbalGram* 1998;44:33–40.

Brinkeborn R, Shah D, Degenring F. Echinaforce® and other *Echinacea* fresh plant preparations in the treatment of the common cold. A randomized, placebo controlled, double-blind clinical trial. *Phytomedicine* 1999;6(1):1–6.

Brinkeborn R, Shah D, Geissbuhler S, Degenring F. Echinaforce® in the treatment of acute colds: Results of a placebo-controlled, double-blind study carried out in Sweden. [in German] *Schweizensche Z Ganz Med* 1998;10(1):16-9.

Brinker F. *Herb Contraindications and Drug Interactions*, 3rd ed. Sandy, OR: Eclectic Medical Publications; 2001:84–5.

Bruneton J. *Pharmacognosy, Phytochemistry, Medicinal Plants*. Paris: Lavoisier Publishing; 1995:151.

Burger R, Torres A, Warren R, *et al*. *Echinacea*-induced cytokine production by human macrophages. *Int J Immunopharmacol* 1997;19(7):371–9.

Codex 2000/01. (Monographs): Floraceae *Echinacea* Kautabletten und Saft; Echinacin Salbe; Echinaforce Tabletten und Tropfen; Echinamed Tabletten; Similasan *Echinacea* Homöopathische Globuli; Wala *Echinacea* Anthroposophisches Mundspray; Esberitox N Tabletten. Schönbühl, Switzerland: Galenical Informations Systems; 2000.

Coeugniet E. Kühnast R. Recurrent candidiasis: adjutant immunotherapy with different formulations of Echinacin®. *Therapiewoche* 1986;36:3352–8.

Dorn M, Knick E, Lewith G. Placebo-controlled, double-blind study of *Echinacea pallida* radix in upper respiratory tract infections. *Complement Ther Med* 1997;5:40–2.

Dorn, M. Mitigation of flu-like effects by means of a plant immunostimulant. *Natur und Ganzheitsmedizin* 1989;2:314–9.

ESCOP. Echinacea—Proposal for the Summary of Product Characteristics. *Monographs on the Medicinal Uses of Plant Drugs*. Exeter, U.K.: European Scientific Cooperative on Phytotherapy; 1999.

Facino R, Carini M, Aldini G, *et al*. Echinacoside and caffeoyl conjugates protect collagen from free radical-induced degradation: a potential use of *Echinacea* extracts in the prevention of skin photo damage. *Planta Med* 1995;61(6):510–4.

Felter HW, Lloyd JU. *King's American Dispensatory*. Cincinnati, OH: The Ohio Valley Co.; 1898:673–77.

Forth H and Beuscher N. Influence of Esberitox on the frequency of the common cold. [in German]. *Z Allgemeinmed* 1981;57:2272–5.

Foster S. *Echinacea: Nature's Immune Enhancer*. Rochester, VT: Healing Arts Press; 1991:20–24.

Galea S, Thacker K. Double-blind prospective trial investigating the effectiveness of a commonly prescribed herbal remedy in altering the duration, severity and symptoms of the common cold. Unpublished. 1996.

Gallo M, Sarkar M, Au W, *et al*. Pregnancy outcome following gestational exposure to *Echinacea*: a prospective controlled study. *Arch Intern Med* 2000;160:3141–3.

General Sale List 1984–1994. Statutory Instrument (S.I.). The Medicines (Products other than Veterinary Drugs). London, UK: Her Majesty's Stationery Office; 1984; S.I. No. 769, as amended 1985; S.I. No. 1540, 1990; S.I. No. 1129, 1994; S.I. No. 2410.

Gilmore MR. Bureau of American Ethnological Association's Annual Report; 1911;33:368.

Grimm W, Muller H. A randomized controlled trial of the effect of fluid extract of *Echinacea purpurea* on the incidence and severity of colds and respiratory infections [see comments]. *Am J Med* 1999;106(2):138–43.

GSL. See: *General Sale List*.

HAB. See: *Homöopathisches Arzneibuch*.

Health Canada. *Drug Product Database (DPD)*. Ottawa, Ontario: Health Canada Therapeutic Products Programme; 2000.

Health Canada. *Drugs Directorate Guidelines: Traditional Herbal Medicines*. Ottawa, Ontario Canada: Minister of National Health and Welfare; Canada. 1990.

Health Canada. *Labeling Standard Echinacea Root*. Ottawa, Ontario: Health Canada Therapeutic Products Directorate; 1997 June 1;1–4.

Henneicke-von Zepelin H, Hentschel C, Schnitker J, Kohnen R, Kohler G, Wustenberg P. Efficacy and safety of a fixed combination phytomedicine in the treatment of the common cold (acute viral respiratory tract infection): results of a randomized, double blind, placebo controlled, multicenter study. *Curr Med Res Opin* 1999;15(3):214–27.

Hobbs C. Echinacea: A Literature Review. *HerbalGram* 1994;30:33–48.

Hoheisel O, Sandberg M, Bertram S, *et al*. Echinagard® treatment shortens the course of the common cold: a double-blind, placebo-controlled clinical trial. *Eur J Clin Res* 1997;9:261–8.

Homeopathic Pharmacopoeia of the United States — Revision Service Official Compendium from July 1, 1992. Falls Church, VA: American Institute of Homeopathy; 1991 June;3212-ECHN.

Homopathisches Arzneibuch. Echinacea. In: HAB 2000. Stuttgart, Germany: Deutscher Apotheker Verlag; 2000.

HPUS. See: *Homeopathic Pharmacopoeia of the United States.*

Leung A, Foster S. *Encyclopedia of Common Natural Ingredients Used in Food, Drugs, and Cosmetics,* 2nd ed. New York: John Wiley & Sons; 1996;216–9.

Lindenmuth G, Lindenmuth E. The efficacy of *Echinacea* compound herbal tea preparation on the severity and duration of upper respiratory and flu symptoms: a randomized, double-blind placebo-controlled study. *J Altern Comp Med* 2000;6(4):327–34.

Luettig B, Steinmuller C, Gifford G, *et al.* Macrophage activation by the polysaccharide arabinogalactan isolated from plant cell cultures of *Echinacea purpurea. J Natl Cancer Inst* 1989;81(9):669–75.

McGuffin M, Hobbs C, Upton R, Goldberg A (eds.). *American Herbal Products Association Botanical Safety Handbook.* Boca Raton, FL: CRC Press; 1997.

Medical Products Agency (MPA). *Naturläkemedel: Authorised Natural Remedies* (as of January 24, 2001). Uppsala, Sweden: Medical Products Agency; 2001.

Medical Products Agency (MPA). *Naturläkemedelsmonografi: Echinagard.* Uppsala, Sweden: Medical Products Agency; 1997.

Melchart D, Linde K, Worku F, *et al.* Immunomodulation with *Echinacea*—A systematic review of controlled clinical trials. *Phytomedicine* 1994;1:245–54.

Melchart D, Walther E, Linde K, *et al. Echinacea* root extracts for the prevention of upper respiratory tract infections: a double-blind, placebo-controlled randomized trial. *Arch Fam Med* 1998;7(6):541–5.

Melchart D, *et al.* Results of five randomized studies on the immunomodulatory activity of preparations of *Echinacea. J Altern Comp Med* 1995;1(2):145–60.

Melchart D, Linde K. Clinical investigations of *Echinacea* phytopharmaceuticals. In:. *Immunomodulatory Agents from Plants.* Wagner, H (ed.). Basel: Birkhauser Verlag; 1999:105–18.

Mengs U, Clare C, Poiley J. Toxicity of *Echinacea purpurea. Arzneimittelforschung* 1991;41(10):1076–81.

Miller L. Herbal medicinals: selected clinical considerations focusing on known or potential drug-herb interactions. *Arch Intern Med* 1998 Nov 9;158(20):2200–11.

Moerman D. *Native American Ethnobotany.* Portland, OR: Timber Press; 1998; 205-6.

Morant J, Ruppanner H (eds.). *Arzneimittel-Kompendium der Schweiz 2001.* Basel, Switzerland: Documed AG. 2001.

Mose JR. Effect of Echinacin on phagocytosis and natural killer cells. [in German]. *Med Welt* 1983;34(51–2):1463–7.

MPA. See: Medical Products Agency.

Mullins R. Echinacea–associated anaphylaxis. *Med J Aust* 1998;168(4):170–2.

Mullins RJ, Heddle R. Adverse reactions associated with echinacea: the Australian experience. *Ann Allergy Asthma Immunol* 2002 Jan;88(1):7–9.

Newall C, Anderson L, Phillipson J. *Herbal Medicines: A Guide for Health-Care Professionals.* London: The Pharmaceutical Press; 1996:101–3.

Parnham M. Benefit-risk assessment of the squeezed sap of the purple coneflower (*Echinacea purpurea*) for long-term oral immunostimulation. *Phytomedicine* 1996;3(1):95–102.

Parnham, M. Benefits and risks of the squeezed sap of the purple coneflower (*Echinacea purpurea*) for long-term oral immunistimulant therapy. In: Wagner H (ed.). *Immunomodulatory agents from plants.* Basel; Boston; Berlin: Birkhäuser Verlag; 1999:119-35.

Ph.Fr. See: *Pharmacopée Française.*

Pharmacopée Française (Ph.Fr.X). Moulins-lès-Metz, France: Maisonneuve SA; 1982–96.

Pietta P, Mauri P, Bauer R. MEKC analysis of different *Echinacea* species. *Planta Med* 1998; 64:649–52.

Pizzorno JE, Murray MT (eds.). *Textbook of Natural Medicine,* Vol. 1, 2nd ed. New York: Churchill Livingston; 1999: 703–11.

Reitz, HD. Immunomodulation with phytotherapeutic agents: a scientific study on the example of Esberitox®. [in German]. *Notebene Medici* 1990;20:362–6.

Richman A. Witkowski J. A wonderful year for herbs. *Whole Foods* 1996; Oct:52–60.

Richman A. Herb sales still strong. *Whole Foods* 1998; Oct:19–26.

Richman A. Herbs…by the numbers. *Whole Foods* 1997; Oct:20–28.

Roeder E, Wiedenfeld H, Hille Th, Britz-Kirstgen R. Pyrrolizidines in *Echinacea angustifolia* and *Echinacea purpurea. Deut Apoth Ztg.* 1984;124(45):2316–8.

Roesler J, Emmendorffer A, Steinmuller C, *et al.* Application of purified polysaccharides from cell cultures of the plant *Echinacea purpurea* to test subjects mediates activation of the phagocyte system. *Int J Immunopharmacol* 1991;13(7):931–41.

Scaglione F, Lund B. Efficacy in the treatment of the common cold of a preparation containing an echinacea extract. *Int J Immunother* 1995;21(4):163–6.

Schmidt U, Albrecht M, Schenk N. Botanical immunostimulant lowers frequency of influenzal infections [in German]. *Natur- und Ganzheitsmedizin* 1990;3:277–81.

Schöneberger D. The influences of immune-stimulating effects of pressed juice from *Echinacea purpurea* on the course and severity of colds: results of a double-blind study. [in German]. *Forum Immunol* 1992;8:2–12.

Schultz V, Hänsel R, Tyler V. *Rational Phytotherapy: A Physicians' Guide to Herbal Medicine.* New York: Springer-Verlag; 1997:259–60, 273–8.

See D, Berman S, Justis J, *et al.* A Phase I study on the safety of *Echinacea angustifolia* and its effect on viral load in HIV infected individuals. *JAMA* 1998;1(1):14–7.

See D, Broumand L, Sahl L, Tilles J. *In vitro* effects of echinacea and ginseng on natural killer and antibody-dependent cell cytotoxicity in healthy subjects and chronic fatigue syndrome or acquired immunodeficiency syndrome patients. *Immunopharmacol* 1997;35(3):229–35.

Speroni E, Crespi-Perellino, Guerra M, Mearelli F, Minghetti A. Skin effects of *Echinacea pallida* Nutt. root extract [oral presentation abstract]. *Fitoterapia* 1998;64(Suppl 5):36.

Stimpel M, Proksch A, Wagner H, Lohmann-Matthes M. Macrophage activation and induction of macrophage cytotoxicity by purified polysaccharide fractions from the plant *Echinacea purpurea. Infect Immun* 1984;46(3):845–9.

Stoll A, Renz J, Brack A. Antibacterial substances II. Isolation and constitution of echinacoside, a glycoside from the roots of *Echinacea angustifolia. Helv Chim Acta* 1950;33:1877–93.

Tragni E, Tubaro A, Melis S, Galli C. Evidence from two classic irritation tests for an anti–inflammatory action of a natural extract, Echinacea B. *Food Chem Toxicol* 1985;23(2):317–9.

Tubaro A, Tragni E, Del Negro P, *et al.* Anti-inflammatory activity of a polysaccharidic fraction of *Echinacea angustifolia. J Pharm Pharmacol* 1987;39(7):567–9.

Tunón H. Phytotherapie in Schweden. [in German]. *Z Phytother* 1999;20:269–77.

United States Congress. Public Law 103–417: *Dietary Supplement Health and Education Act of 1994* (S 7840). Washington, DC: 103rd Congress of the United States; October 25, 1994.

United States Pharmacopeia (USP 25th Revision) - The National Formulary (NF 20th Edition). Rockville, MD: United States Pharmacopeial Convention, Inc. 2002.

USC. See: United States Congress.

USP. See: United States Pharmacopeial.

Voaden D, Jacobson M. Tumor inhibitors. 3. Identification and synthesis of an oncolytic hydrocarbon form American coneflower roots. *J Med Chem* 1972;15:619–23.

Vonau B, Chard S, Mandalia S, *et al.* Does the extract of the plant *Echinacea purpurea* influence the clinical course of recurrent genital herpes? *International Journal of STD & AIDS* 2001;12:154–8.

Vorberg G. A double-blind study shows: The proven phytotherapeutic Esberitox® shortens the duration of symptoms. *Arztliche Praxis* 1984;36(6):97–8.

Vorberg G, Schneider B. Phythotherapeutic immunostimulator decreases the duration of influenza-like syndrome. Double-blind trial proves the enhancement of unspecific immune defense. [in German]. *Ärztliche Forschung* 1989;36:3–8.

Wacker A, Hilbig W. Virus-inhibition by *Echinacea purpurea.* [in German]. *Planta Med* 1978;33(1):89–102.

Wagner H, Jurcic K. Immunologic studies of plant combination preparations. *In vitro* and *in vivo* studies on the stimulation of phagocytosis. [in German]. *Arzneimittelforschung* 1991;41(10):1072–6.

Wagner H, Proksch A, Riess-Maurer I, *et al.* Immunostimulating action of polysaccharides (heteroglycans) from higher plants. [in German]. *Arzneimittelforschung* 1985;35(7):1069–75.

Wagner H, Proksch A, Riess-Maurer I, *et al.* Immunostimulant action of polysaccharides (heteroglycans) from higher plants. Preliminary communication. [in German]. *Arzneimittelforschung* 1984;34(6):659–61.

Wagner H, Breau W, Willer F, *et al. In vitro* inhibition of arachidonate metabolism by some alkamides and phenylated phenols. *Planta Med* 1989;55:566–7.

Wagner H. Search for potent immunostimulating agents from plants and other natural sources. In: Wagner H (ed.). *Immunomodulatory Agents from Plants.* Basel; Boston; Berlin: Birkhäuser Verlag; 1999:1–39.

Wagner H. Herbal immunostimulants for the prophylaxis and therapy of colds and influenza. *Eur J Herbal Med* 1997;3(1).

Wagner H, *et al.* Immunologically active polysaccharides of *Echinacea purpurea* cell cultures. *Phytochemistry* 1988;(27)1:119–26.

Weiss RF, Fintelmann V. *Herbal Medicine* 2nd ed. New York: Thieme; 2000:216–217.

WHO. See: World Health Organization.

Wichtl M, Bisset N (eds.). *Herbal Drugs and Phytopharmaceuticals.* Stuttgart: Medpharm Scientific Publishers; 1994:182–4.

Wildfeuer AT, Mayerhofer D. The effects of plant preparations on cellular functions in body defense. [in German]. *Arzneimittelforschung* 1994;44(3):361–6.

World Health Organization (WHO). 1999. *Herba Echinacea Purpureae Radix Echinacea* and *Radix Echinacea. WHO Monographs on Selected Medicinal Plants,* Vol. 1. Geneva: World Health Organization; 136–44; 125–35.

World Health Organization. *Regulatory Status of Herbal Medicines: A Worldwide Review.* Geneva, Switzerland: World Health Organization Traditional Medicine Programme; 1998:25–7.

Wüstenberg P, Henneicke von Zepelin H, Köhler G, Stammwitz U. Efficacy and mode of action of an immunomodulator herbal preparation containing echinacea, wild indigo, and white cedar. *Advs Ther* 1999;16(1):51–70.

Echinacea

Monograph

Cold/Flu/Upper Respiratory Tract Infection (URTI) Treatment

Author/Year	Subject	Design	Duration	Dosage	Preparation	Results/Conclusion
Brinkeborn et al., 1999	URTI symptoms	R, DB, PC (4 arm) n=246 subjects with colds	7 days from the start of acute URTI (1–2 days of symptoms)	2 tablets, 3x/day	Echinaforce® concentrate, special *E. purpurea* root preparation	Relative reduction in complaint index for 12 symptoms in the 4 groups differed significantly (p=0.015). Echinacea patients reductions in complaint index were significantly higher than in the placebo group (p=0.003 and p=0.020). Echinacea was concluded to be a low-risk, effective alternative for symptomatic acute treatment of the common cold.
Brinkeborn et al., 1998	URTI symptoms	R, DB, PC n=119	8 days from the start of acute URTI (1–2 days of symptoms)	Two, 400 mg tablets 3x/day	Echinaforce® tablet	Based on 12 symptoms, the "overall clinical picture" for the intention-to-treat was reduced in the treatment group from 9.0 to 4.1 (p=0.045), while the placebo group decreased from 8.8 to 5.3. Echinacea was concluded to be a low-risk, effective alternative for symptomatic acute treatment of the common cold.
Dorn et al., 1997	URTI symptoms	R, DB, PC n=160 (ages >18 years)	8–10 days from onset of flu-like respiratory symptoms	45 drops extract 2x/day (equivalent to 900 mg/day)	Brand not stated	The length of the illness decreased from 13 to 9.8 days (bacterial infections) and to 9.1 days (viral infections) compared to placebo (p=0.0001). The infection type was determined by lymphocyte and neutrophil counts in the blood. Echinacea appears to shorten the duration of URTIs.
Hoheisel et al., 1997	URTI symptoms	R, DB, PC n=120 with at least 3 infections in the past 6 months	10 days from the first sign of URTI, before full development	20 drops, every 2 hours on day 1, 20 drops, 3x/day thereafter	Echinaguard® extract	Of the echinacea group, 40% developed a "real cold" compared to 60% in the placebo group (p=0.044), while in 4 days symptoms improved for echinacea group compared to 8 days for the placebo group. Echinacea showed more rapid recovery in the intention-to-treat population (p<0.0001).
Galea and Thacker, 1996	URTI symptoms	R, DB, PC, P n=190	From the first sign of URTI through 10 days	250 mg capsule	*E. angustifolia* root dried (brand not stated)	8 symptoms were assessed and no measurable benefits were reported, attributed to the relatively low dose and lack of severity of the symptoms being measured.
Bräunig et al., 1992	Flu-like symptoms	R, DB, PC n=180 one group of 60 per preparation	From onset of flu-like respiratory symptoms until symptoms subsided	90 drops (450 mg)/day or 180 drops (900 mg)/day	*E. purpurea* root extract (1:5, 55% ethanol) (brand not stated)	Echinacea patients receiving 180 drops (900 mg) dose displayed statistically significant improvement (p<0.05) compared with placebo group in relieving symptoms and decreasing the duration of symptoms. The study suggests that dosage influences effectiveness.

Combination Preparations (Treatment)

Author/Year	Subject	Design	Duration	Dosage	Preparation	Results/Conclusion
Lindenmuth and Lindenmuth, 2000	Cold, flu-like, URTI symptoms	R, DB, PC n=95 with early symptoms of cold or flu, primarily females (mean age 39.7 years)	From first sign of flu-like symptoms through 6 days	5–6 cups tea first day of symptoms and titrating down 1 cup of tea/day for next 5 days (equivalent of 1,275 mg dried herb and root per tea bag serving)	Echinacea Plus® tea vs. Traditional Medicinals Eater's Digest® herbal tea (placebo)	Based on questionnaire on effectiveness of echinacea, duration of symptoms, and time taken for subjects to notice any changes in symptoms, echinacea group was shown to be statistically significant in effectiveness (p<0.001); duration (p<0.001); and in noticeable change in symptoms (p<0.001). Authors concluded that treatment with echinacea compound tea, given at early onset of symptoms was effective in relieving cold or flu symptoms in noticeably fewer days compared to placebo.
Henneicke-von Zepelin et al., 1999	Common cold (acute viral URTI)	R, DB, PC, MC (15 centers) n=238 patients (ages 18–70 years)	7–9 days once identified as having a common cold	3 tablets 3x/day	Esberitox® N2 tablet vs. placebo	The echinacea combination product was significantly better than placebo (p=0.0497), with highly statistically significant results in overall well-being (p=0.0048), rhinitis, and bronchitis scores. This study suggests this is a safe and effective treatment and notes the greatest benefits would be experienced if treatment is started as soon as possible after onset of the cold.

KEY: C – controlled, **CC** – case-control, **CH** – cohort, **CI** – confidence interval, **Cm** – comparison, **CO** – crossover, **CS** – cross-sectional, **DB** – double-blind, **E** – epidemiological, **LC** – longitudinal cohort, **MA** – meta-analysis, **MC** – multi-center, **n** – number of patients, **O** – open, **OB** – observational, **OL** – open label, **OR** – odds ratio, **P** – prospective, **PB** – patient-blind, **PC** – placebo-controlled, **PG** – parallel group, **PS** – pilot study, **R** – randomized, **RC** – reference-controlled, **RCS** – retrospective cross-sectional, **RS** - retrospective, **S** – surveillance, **SB** – single-blind, **SC** – single-center, **U** – uncontrolled, **UP** – unpublished, **VC** – vehicle-controlled.

Clinical Studies on Echinacea (*Echinacea* spp.) (cont.)

Combination Preparations (Treatment) (cont.)

Author/Year	Subject	Design	Duration	Dosage	Preparation	Results/Conclusion
Reitz, 1990	URTI symptoms and signs	R, DB, PC n=150	8 weeks initially, with monitoring for an additional year	One, 22.5 mg tablet 3x/day or placebo (vitamin C)	Esberitox® N1 tablet vs. placebo	Majority of symptoms and signs at 7 and 14 days were significantly better than placebo; nasal symptoms were most affected. No difference in result from blood work was reported.
Dorn, 1989	URTI symptoms and signs	R, DB, PC n=100	From 2 days of URTI onset	Day 1–2: 30 ml/day Day 3–6: 15 ml/day	Resistan® vs. placebo	Echinacea patients experienced a decrease in the length of illness and severity in 7 of 7 self-assessed symptoms compared to 4 of 7 in placebo group (p=0.001). The study suggests that taking the preparation as soon as symptoms first appear shortens duration of URTI.
Vorberg and Schneider, 1989	URTI symptoms and signs	R, DB, PC n=100	10 days beginning 2 days after onset of URTI	15–30 ml/day	Resistan® vs. placebo	Most symptoms were significantly better in the echinacea group compared to placebo at both 2 to 3 days and at 8 to 10 days. The results indicate echinacea has efficacy for the prevention and treatment of URTIs.
Vorberg, 1984	URTI symptoms and signs in patients suffering from common cold	R, DB, PC n=100	10 days	15 mg tablet 3x/day	Esberitox® tablet vs. placebo	Echinacea group reported significant superiority compared to placebo group in all examined parameters of common cold (p<0.001) including fatigue, reduced performance, runny nose, and sore throat.

Cold/Flu/URTI Prevention

Author/Year	Subject	Design	Duration	Dosage	Preparation	Results/Conclusion
Grimm and Müller, 1999	URTI occurrence	R, PC n=108 with history of 3 colds or respiratory infections in the preceding year (mean age echinacea group 42 years; mean age placebo group 38 years)	2 months	4 ml expressed juice 2x/day	E. purpurea fluid (expressed juice of aerial parts, brand not stated, though test material was provided by Madaus AG and it presumably is Echinacin®)	During 8-week treatment period, 35 (65%) of 54 patients in echinacea group and 40 (74%) of 54 patients in placebo group had at least one cold or respiratory infection (relative risk [RR]=0.88; 95% confidence interval [CI] [0.60, 1.22]). Average number of colds and respiratory infections per patient was 0.78 in echinacea group, and 0.93 in placebo group (difference=0.15; 95% CI [-0.12, 0.41], p=0.33). Median duration of colds and respiratory infections was 4.5 days in echinacea group and 6.5 days in placebo group (95% CI [-1, +3 days]; p=0.45). There were no significant differences between treatment groups in number of, duration, or severity of colds. Side effects were observed in 11 patients (20%) of echinacea group and in 7 patients (13%) of placebo group (p=0.44).
Melchart et al., 1998	URTI occurrence	R, DB, PC n=289 (ages 18–65 years)	12 weeks (M-F only)	50 drops E. angustifolia 2x/day or 50 drops E. purpurea 2x/day or placebo	E. angustifolia and E. purpurea roots extracts (1:11 in 30% ethanol) (brand not stated)	Participants in treatment group believed they had more benefit than placebo group (p=0.04). URTIs (at least one) were experienced by 32%, 29%, and 37% of E. angustifolia, E. purpurea, and placebo groups respectively, and onset was at 66, 69, and 65 days, respectively, with no significant differences in duration, incidence, or severity of URTIs. Noncontinuous administration of treatment was not addressed in the conclusion.
Schöneberger, 1992	URTI occurrence	R, DB, PC, MC n=108 patients with increased susceptibility to colds (suffered at least 3 colds in previous year) (ages 13–84 years)	2 months	4 ml 2x/day	Echinacin®	Echinacea group experienced decreased in URTI incidence in 35% (vs. 26%), decrease in duration of 5.34 days (vs. 7.54 days), increase in interval between infections of 40 days (vs. 25 days), and decreased severity of symptoms calculated as 78% (vs. 68%) compared with placebo. Patients with weakened defense (calculated as a T4/T8-ratio of less than 1.5) benefited most.

KEY: **C** – controlled, **CC** – case-control, **CH** – cohort, **CI** – confidence interval, **Cm** – comparison, **CO** – crossover, **CS** – cross-sectional, **DB** – double-blind, **E** – epidemiological, **LC** – longitudinal cohort, **MA** – meta-analysis, **MC** – multi-center, **n** – number of patients, **O** – open, **OB** – observational, **OL** – open label, **OR** – odds ratio, **P** – prospective, **PB** – patient-blind, **PC** – placebo-controlled, **PG** – parallel group, **PS** – pilot study, **R** – randomized, **RC** – reference-controlled, **RCS** – retrospective cross-sectional, **RS** - retrospective, **S** – surveillance, **SB** – single-blind, **SC** – single-center, **U** – uncontrolled, **UP** – unpublished, **VC** – vehicle-controlled.

Echinacea

Monograph

Combination Preparations (Prevention)

Author/Year	Subject	Design	Duration	Dosage	Preparation	Results/Conclusion
Schmidt et al., 1990	URTI occurrence	R, DB, PC n=609 college students	2 months	12 ml/day	Resistan® vs. placebo	Echinacea patients experienced 15% fewer primary infections, and relapses decreased by 27%, or relative risk reduction of 12%. Due to potential immuno-stimulant activity of other botanicals, the results could not be attributed to echinacea alone.
Forth and Beuscher, 1981	URTI occurrence	R, PC (not fully double-blind) n=95	16 weeks (November through February)	25 drops 3x/day or 1 mg tablet or placebo	Esberitox®	Patients had relative risk reduction of 49% overall, even though no apparent difference for other 7 symptoms was observed in all groups compared to placebo. However, improvement of nasal symptoms was significant.

Other

Author/Year	Subject	Design	Duration	Dosage	Preparation	Results/Conclusion
Vonau et al., 2001	Effect on clinical course of genital herpes	SC, P, DB, PC, CO n=50 (mean age 36.5 years)	1 year (6 months placebo, 6 months echinacea)	800 mg 2x/day	Echinaforce® tablet	No statistically significant benefit was shown for use of echinacea to treat frequently recurring genital herpes.
Gallo et al., 2000	Safety of gestational exposure to echinacea	P, C n=206 patients who used echinacea during pregnancy	Until birth or termination of the pregnancy n=112 (echinacea used during first trimester)	Range of 250–1,000 mg/day capsule or tablets taken by 114 females or range of 5–10 to 30 drops maximum/day taken by 76 females continuously for 5–7 days	Primarily *E. angustifolia* and *E. purpurea*; only one reported using *E. pallida* (brand not stated)	Of 206 subjects who used echinacea during pregnancy, there were 195 live births, 13 spontaneous abortions, and one therapeutic abortion, compared to the control group giving 198 live births, 7 spontaneous abortions, and 1 therapeutic abortion. These results indicated no statistical differences between the 2 groups in terms of pregnancy outcome, delivery method, maternal weight gain, gestational age, birth weight, or fetal distress. Rates of major malformation between study and control groups were not statistically different.
Berg et al., 1998	Exercise-induced immunological effects	R, PC, PG n=42 male athletes, 3 groups (mean age 27.5 years)	28 days (prior to triathlon)	40 drops 3x/day (8 ml/day) (n=14) or magnesium (n=13) or placebo (n=13)	Echinacin®	Echinacea facilitated IL-6 release and reduced SIL-2R release in serum and urine, significantly increased serum cortisol (one hour after the event), and may exert slight effects on natural killer cells and T-cells. Echinacea group did not report any URTIs compared to 7 total from 2 other groups, along with 6 reporting other infections.
Coeugniet and Kuhnast, 1986	Chronic candidiasis in females	OL, Cm (5-arm) n=203	10 weeks	30 drops 3x/day with cream for 6 days (n=60) or cream alone (6 days only) (n=43)	Echinacin® and econazole nitrate cream (antimycotic treatment)	Use of echinacea as adjunct therapy reduced recurrence rate 5–16% compared to women using only cream, who experienced a recurrence rate of 60.5%.

KEY: C – controlled, **CC** – case-control, **CH** – cohort, **CI** – confidence interval, **Cm** – comparison, **CO** – crossover, **CS** – cross-sectional, **DB** – double-blind, **E** – epidemiological, **LC** – longitudinal cohort, **MA** – meta-analysis, **MC** – multi-center, **n** – number of patients, **O** – open, **OB** – observational, **OL** – open label, **OR** – odds ratio, **P** – prospective, **PB** – patient-blind, **PC** – placebo-controlled, **PG** – parallel group, **PS** – pilot study, **R** – randomized, **RC** – reference-controlled, **RCS** – retrospective cross-sectional, **RS** - retrospective, **S** – surveillance, **SB** – single-blind, **SC** – single-center, **U** – uncontrolled, **UP** – unpublished, **VC** – vehicle-controlled.

Eleuthero

Eleuthrococcus senticosus (Rupr. & Maxim.) Maxim.
(syn. *Acanthopanax senticosus* [Rupr. & Maxim.] Harms)
[Fam. *Araliaceae*]

OVERVIEW

Eleuthero root has been widely known in the U.S. as "Siberian ginseng." It was first marketed in the U.S. in the late 1970s, and since become one of the top-selling herbal dietary supplements in the natural foods class of trade. It has been used in Traditional Chinese Medicine (TCM) for over two thousand years. From the 1940s through the 1960s, Soviet scientists conducted extensive clinical research on eleuthero in their search for a more abundant and economical alternative to Asian ginseng (*Panax ginseng*). Russian Olympic athletes, explorers, divers, sailors, and miners now use eleuthero as a preventive agent against stress-related illnesses.

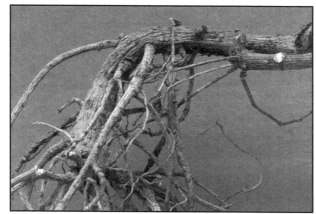

Photo © 2003 stevenfoster.com

PRIMARY USES

- Herpes simplex type II infections
- Influenza complications (possible prevention)
- Fatigue; debility; declining work capacity and concentration; convalescence; chronic fatigue syndrome; supportive therapy during radiation or chemotherapy
- Functional asthenia
- Selective memory improvement

OTHER POTENTIAL USES

- Cholesterol reduction; atherosclerosis
- Insomnia and other anxiety-like conditions
- Chronic inflammatory conditions
- Visual perception enhancement

PHARMACOLOGICAL ACTIONS

Increases lymphocyte count; tonifying; anti-stress activity; immunomodulatory effect on cellular immune system; tranquilizes central nervous system; reduces heart palpitations and headaches due to high-altitude hypoxia syndrome.

DOSAGE AND ADMINISTRATION

Use for one to three months followed by a two-month break. A repeat course is feasible.

POWDERED ROOT: 2–3 g daily.

DECOCTION: 9–27 g daily.

INFUSION: Pour 150 ml of boiling water over 2–3 g, steep for 5–10 minutes.

FLUID EXTRACT: 2–4 ml, 1–3 times daily [1:1 (*g/ml*), 33% ethanol]; or 2–8 ml per day [1:2 (*g/ml*)]; or 2–3 g daily powdered or cut root aqueous alcoholic extract.

TINCTURE: 10–20 ml, 1–3 times daily [1:5 (*g/ml*)].

NATIVE EXTRACT: 300–450 mg, 3 times daily [20:1 (*w/w*)]; or 2–3 tablets (150 mg native extract per tablet), twice daily.

STANDARDIZED DRY EXTRACT: (>1% eleutheroside E), 100–200 mg, 3 times daily.

CONTRAINDICATIONS

Some authorities recommend that patients with high blood pressure (especially greater than 180/90) should consult a healthcare provider before using eleuthero. This is based solely on a 35-year old report in the Russian literature of a study on patients with rheumatic heart lesions. Eleuthero should not be used during the acute phase of infections, although it may be used concurrently with antibiotics for the treatment of dysentery.

PREGNANCY AND LACTATION: No known restrictions.

ADVERSE EFFECTS

No side effects have been documented for eleuthero in healthy individuals. In rare cases, mild, transient diarrhea and sleep disturbances (if taken close to bedtime) may occur. In patients with rheumatic heart disease, side effects such as pericardial pain, headaches, and elevated blood pressure have been reported.

DRUG INTERACTIONS

Mutual potentiation when administered with the radioprotector drug adeturone. Potentiates effect of antibiotics monomycin and kanamycin in treatment of *Shigella* dysentery and *Proteus* enterocollitis. May interact with concurrently administered antipsychotic drugs, barbiturates, or sedatives (speculative). May produce enhanced effect on insulin and antidiabetic therapy; therefore, blood glucose levels should be monitored closely in diabetics because of possible hypoglycemic action.

CLINICAL REVIEW

In 9 studies on eleuthero that included over 1,984 participants, all but one demonstrated positive effects for therapeutic indications, including immune response, stress, fatigue, and cardiovascular health. Four double-blind, placebo-controlled (DB, PC) studies investigated the effects of eleuthero on concentration, selective memory, cognitive function and well-being, ergogenic parameters in athletes, immune protection against herpes simplex type II infection, and immunomodulatory measurements (e.g., T-cells) in healthy volunteers. A single-blind, PC study evaluated eleuthero's effects on work capacity, stamina, and fatigue in male athletes. In clinical studies on eleuthero extracts conducted in the former Soviet Union since the early 1960s, more than 2,100 normal and stressed human subjects were orally administered eleuthero root fluid extract, 33% ethanol. The studies examined the adaptogenic response of humans to adverse conditions such as heat, noise, motion, workload increase, and exercise. They also measured a significant improvement in auditory disturbances, increased mental alertness, work output, and quality of work under stress.

Eleuthero

Eleutherococcus senticosus (Rupr. & Maxim.) Maxim. (syn. *Acanthopanax senticosus* [Rupr. & Maxim.] Harms) [Fam. *Araliaceae*]

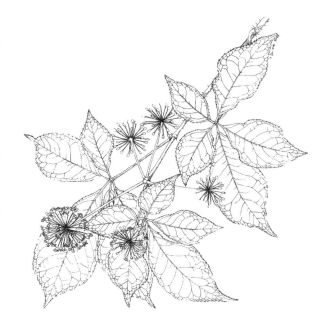

OVERVIEW

Eleuthero root has been used in Traditional Chinese Medicine for thousands of years, and has been known as "Siberian ginseng." Eleuthero is an "adaptogen," a mild substance that produces a normalizing effect on the body. It was first marketed in the U.S. in the late 1970s, and has since become one of the top-selling herbal dietary supplements.

USES

Herpes simplex type II infections; decrease in occurrence of influenza complications; fatigue; chronic inflammation; debility; decreased work and concentration; chronic fatigue syndrome; convalescence; functional asthenia; supportive therapy during radiation or chemotherapy; atherosclerosis; selective memory improvement.

DOSAGE

Use for one to three months, followed by a two-month break.

INFUSION (TEA): Pour 150 ml of boiling water over 2–3 g, steep for 5–10 minutes.

FLUID EXTRACT: 2–4 ml, 1 to 3 times daily [1:1].

FLUID EXTRACT: 2–8 ml daily [1:2].

TINCTURE: 10–20 ml, 1 to 3 times daily [1:5].

NATIVE EXTRACT: 300–450 mg, 3 times daily.

STANDARDIZED DRY EXTRACT: (21% eleutheroside E), 100–200 mg, 3 times daily.

CONTRAINDICATIONS

Although the use of eleuthero is generally considered quite safe, some authorities recommend that patients with high blood pressure (especially greater than 180/90) should consult a healthcare provider before using eleuthero. It should not be used during the acute phase of infections, although it may be used concurrently with antibiotics for the treatment of dysentery.

PREGNANCY AND LACTATION: There are no known restrictions for usage during pregnancy or while breast-feeding.

ADVERSE EFFECTS

No significant adverse effects have been reported in healthy individuals. However, on rare occasions eleuthero may cause mild, brief diarrhea or insomnia if taken too close to bedtime. In individuals with rheumatic heart disease, side effects such as headaches, elevated blood pressure, and pain in the pericardium (the sac that encloses the heart) have been reported.

DRUG INTERACTIONS

Eleuthero may increase the effects of certain antibiotics, including monomycin and kanamycin, and the radioprotective drug adeturone. Eleuthero may interact with antipsychotic drugs barbiturates, and sedatives (although these interactions are only speculative, not reported). Eleuthero may possibly increase the effect of insulin and diabetic drugs. Diabetics taking eleuthero and antidiabetic medication should be closely monitored.

Comments

When using a dietary supplement, purchase it from a reliable source. For best results, use the same brand of product throughout the period of use. As with all medications and dietary supplements, please inform your healthcare provider of all herbs and medications you are taking. Interactions may occur between medications and herbs or even among different herbs when taken at the same time. Treat your herbal supplement with care by taking it as directed, storing it as advised on the label, and keeping it out of the reach of children and pets. Consult your healthcare provider with any questions.

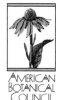

AMERICAN BOTANICAL COUNCIL

The information contained on this sheet has been excerpted from *The ABC Clinical Guide to Herbs* © 2003 by the American Botanical Council (ABC). ABC is an independent member-based educational organization focusing on the medicinal use of herbs. For more detailed information about this herb please consult the healthcare provider who gave you this sheet. To order *The ABC Clinical Guide to Herbs* or become a member of ABC, visit their website at www.herbalgram.org.

Eleuthero

Eleutherococcus senticosus (Rupr. & Maxim.) Maxim.
(syn. *Acanthopanax senticosus* [Rupr. & Maxim.] Harms)

[Fam. *Araliaceae*]

OVERVIEW

Eleuthero root has been widely known in the U.S. as "Siberian ginseng." It was first marketed in the U.S. in the late 1970s (Foster, 1991), and since become one of the top-selling herbal dietary supplements in the natural foods class of trade (Brevoort, 1998; Tyler, 1998). It has been used in Traditional Chinese Medicine (TCM) for over 2,000 years and is listed in the *Shen Nong Ben Cao Jing*, China's oldest pharmacopoeia, as well as in the pharmacopeia of Li Shih-Zhen of the Ming dynasty (Halstead and Hood, 1984). However, it was modern Russian researchers who popularized this herb in the West (Foster and Chongxi, 1992; Kenner and Requena, 1996). From the 1940s through the 1960s, Soviet scientists conducted extensive clinical research on eleuthero in their search for a more abundant and economical alternative to Asian ginseng (*Panax ginseng*). "Adaptogen" has traditionally been defined as a substance useful for both sick and healthy individuals, which

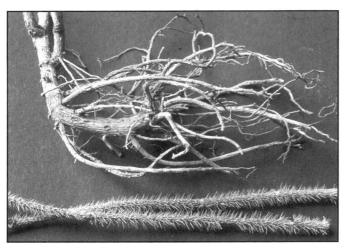

Photo © 2003 stevenfoster.com

improves dysfunction without side effects (Brekhman, 1980; Davydov and Krikorian, 2000; Farnsworth, *et al.*. 1985). In the case of eleuthero, "adaptogen" is defined as a substance that is innocuous and relatively free of side effects, has nonspecific actions, increases resistance to a wide range of environmental or other physical stressors, and may have a normalizing action in the body, irrespective of a diseased state (Brekhman, 1980). Russian Olympic athletes, explorers, divers, sailors, and miners have used eleuthero as a preventive agent against stress-related illnesses (Brekhman, 1980; Fulder, 1980). Eleuthero is official in Russia, China, France, and Germany (see "Regulatory Status" below). Scientific comparisons of eleuthero to the more familiar Asian ginseng ("true ginseng") underscored that they differ considerably chemically and pharmacologically, and cannot be considered interchangeable. Accordingly, the herb industry has

recommended that the common name "Siberian ginseng" be replaced with the more preferred common name "eleuthero" (Foster, 1992; McGuffin, 2001). Federal regulations now require that, "the common or usual name of ingredients of dietary supplements that are botanicals…shall be consistent with the names standardized in *Herbs of Commerce*, 1992 edition" (US FDA, 1999). This nomenclature has been accepted by the U.S. Food and Drug Administration.

DESCRIPTION

Eleuthero preparations consist of the dried roots and/or rhizomes of *Eleutherococcus senticosus* (Rupr. & Maxim.) Maxim. (syn. *Acanthopanax senticosus* [Rupr. & Maxim.] Harms [Fam. *Araliaceae*]), The dried root contains no less than 4% water-soluble extractive (BHP, 1996), and no less than 6% water- and ethanol-soluble extractive (DAB, 1999).

PRIMARY USES

Immunology

- Decrease in severity, duration, or frequency of attacks of herpes simplex type II infections (Williams, 1995)
- Decrease in the occurrence of influenza complications (Shadrin *et al.*, 1986)

Fatigue

- Tonic for invigoration and fortification in treatment of: fatigue, debility (Bradley, 1992; Blumenthal *et al.*, 1998), declining work capacity and concentration, convalescence (Blumenthal *et al.*, 1998); chronic fatigue syndrome and supportive therapy during radiation or chemotherapy (Brown, 2000)
- Functional asthenia (Bruneton, 1999)

Memory Disturbance

- Improvements in selective memory (Winther *et al.*, 1997)

OTHER POTENTIAL USES

- Decrease in total cholesterol, LDL cholesterol, and triglyceride levels (Szolomicki *et al.*, 2000); atherosclerosis (Golikov, 1963)
- Insomnia and other conditions characterized by anxiety-like behavior in modern Chinese medicinal use (as a single-herb remedy) (Chang, 1986). This is consistent with eleuthero's observed sedative activity, primarily in animal studies (Newall *et al.*, 1996)
- Chronic inflammatory conditions (Bradley, 1992)

Vision, perception

- Increased color perception level and functional stability level, enhanced spectral and contrast sensitivity and range of signal light visibility and increased speed of color discrimination (Sosuova, 1986)

DOSAGE

Internal

Crude Preparations

POWDERED ROOT: 2–3 g daily (Bradley, 1992), 1–4 g daily (MediHerb, 1994).

DECOCTION: 9–27 g (PPRC, 1997).

INFUSION: 150 ml of boiling water is poured over 2–3 g and steeped for 5–10 minutes (Blumenthal *et al.*, 1998).

FLUID EXTRACT: 1:1 (*g/ml*), 33% ethanol, 2–4 ml, 1–3 times daily (Pizzorno and Murray, 1999; Werbach and Murray, 2000), 1:2 (*g/ml*): 2–8 ml per day (MediHerb, 1994), 2–3 g daily powdered or cut root aqueous alcoholic extract (Blumenthal *et al.*, 1998).

TINCTURE: 1:5 (*g/ml*), 10–20 ml, 1–3 times daily (Pizzorno and Murray, 1999).

NATIVE EXTRACT: 20:1 (*w/w*), 300–450 mg, 3 times daily; tablets containing 150 mg native extract, 2–3 tablets, twice daily (PPRC, 1997).

Standardized Preparations

DRY EXTRACT: (>1% eleutheroside E), 100–200 mg, 3 times daily (Werbach and Murray, 2000).

NOTE: In healthy individuals, maintenance doses should be based on the lower end of the dosage range. For treatment of illness and high-stress situations, the upper end of the dosage range should be considered (MediHerb, 1994).

DURATION OF ADMINISTRATION

Some sources recommend a course of one month (Bradley, 1992) to three months (Blumenthal *et al.*, 1998) followed by a two month break (Bradley, 1992). A repeat course is feasible (Blumenthal *et al.*, 1998). While the issue has not been studied specifically, it is a general practice to temporarily halt herb consumption after a reasonable period when it is not considered essential for maintaining vital functions. This provides an opportunity to reassess the case and either stop its use completely, continue at a lower dose, or re-institute its use as before. Such a recommendation is not a limitation, but advice on its reasonable use, as opposed to assuming regular, ongoing consumption is necessary or appropriate.

CHEMISTRY

Eleuthero contains ca. 0.6–0.9% eleutherosides A-G in an approximate ratio of 8:30:10:12:4:2:1. Eleutheroside A is the sterol daucosterol; eleutheroside B is the phenylpropanoid syringin; eleutheroside C is the sugar methyl α-D-galactoside. Eleutheroside D is the lignan (-)-syringaresinol di-O-β-D-glucoside, and its diastereoisomer is eleutheroside E (Bradley, 1992; Farnsworth *et al.*, 1985). Eleuthero also contains immunostimulant polysaccharides (Fang *et al.*, 1985; Huang, 1999). An extensive review of the chemistry of eleuthero with 29 chemical structures has been published (Tang and Eisenbrand, 1992).

PHARMACOLOGICAL ACTIONS

Human

Increases lymphocyte count (Blumenthal *et al.*, 1998); adaptogen; tonic (BHP, 1996); anti-stress activity (Wagner *et al.*, 1994); immunomodulatory effect on the cellular immune system (Bohn *et al.*, 1987); tranquilizes central nervous system; reduces heart palpitations and headaches due to high-altitude hypoxia syndrome (Huang, 1999); increases phagocytic activity of neutro-cytes (Szolomicki *et al.*, 2000); increases the absolute numbers of immunocompetent cells, particularly T-cells, predominantly of the helper/inducer type, but also on cytotoxic and natural killer cells (Bohn *et al*, 1987); in TCM theory, reinforces and tonifies vital energy known as "*qi*," invigorates the function of the "spleen" and "kidney," and tranquilizes (Chang and But, 1986; PPRC, 1997).

Animal

Enhances endurance (Blumenthal *et al.* 1998); chemical-, biological-, and radioactive-protective (Collisson, 1991; Minkova and Pantev, 1987; Yonezawa *et al.*, 1989); antioxidant, antihypertensive, hypo/hyperglycemic activity (Farnsworth *et al.*, 1985; Hikino *et al.*, 1986; Medon *et al.*, 1981); sedative (Medon *et al.*, 1984); stress reduction (Takasugi *et al.*, 1985). Eleuthero's isolated glucosides protect against myocardial infarction and can lower blood sugar levels in normal and hyperglycemia-induced mice (Hikino *et al.*, 1986; Tang and Eisenbrand, 1992).

In vitro

Mutual potentiation of antiproliferative effects on leukemia cells when applied in combination with conventional antimetabolite drugs (Hacker and Medon, 1984); slight gamma radiation protection (Ben-Hur and Fulder, 1981); inhibition of hexobarbital metabolism in mice (Medon *et al.*, 1984).

MECHANISM OF ACTION

Most studies on eleuthero were conducted to investigate its adaptogenic effects. The chemical compounds and pharmacological actions of eleuthero support the theory that the primary benefit of an adaptogen is its protective and inhibitory action against free radicals (Davydov and Krikorian, 2000). The exact mechanisms of action of eleuthero and/or the significance of its constituents are not yet fully understood (MediHerb, 1993), despite numerous pharmacological investigations in human and animal models.

According to the literature, eleuthero acts via the following mechanisms:

- Increases immune system function by enhancement of T-cell activation (Wagner, 1985). Active principles responsible for its immunomodulation activities are not yet known (Wagner, *et al.*, 1994).

- Intensifies regeneration, *in vivo,* of subcellular structures and accelerates recovery during experimental myocardial infarction; may be related to the transformation of lipids into glycogen (Afanas'eva and Lebkova, 1987).

- May support and enhance adrenal function and the optimal functioning of the hypothalamic-pituitary-adrenal cortex axis (Baranov, 1982; Brekhman and Dardymov, 1969; Filaretov *et al.*, 1988; Kirilov, 1964). Greater energy and better reaction to stress are associated with optimal adrenal function.

- Maximizes the utilization of oxygen by working muscles, which prolongs the aerobic state (Asano *et al.,* 1986).

- Increases endurance and reduces activation of the adrenal cortex in response to stress (alarm phase reaction) and also has significant prophylactic effects on stress reactions (Brekhman and Kirillov, 1969; Czygan, 1984).

- *In vitro*, ethanolic fluid extract increases phagocytosis of *Candida albicans* by granulocytes and monocytes from healthy donors by 30–40% (Wildfeuer and Mayerhofer, 1994).

- *In vitro*, binds to progestin, mineralocorticoid, glucocorticoid receptors, and estrogen receptors, which could explain the observed glucocorticoid-like activity of the extract (Pearce *et al.*, 1982).
- Increases cAMP levels (Wagner *et al.*, 1994).

CONTRAINDICATIONS

The Commission E contraindicates eleuthero for patients with high blood pressure (Blumenthal *et al.*, 1998). This is based on a Russian study on patients with rheumatic lesions of the heart that recommended that eleuthero not be given to persons with blood pressure higher than 180/90 mm Hg (Mikunis *et al.*, 1966; Farnsworth *et al.*, 1985). However, there is no other literature available to support the contraindication of eleuthero in otherwise normal hypertensive patients. Based on Russian clinical experience, eleuthero should not be used during the acute phase of infections, though it is used to treat dysentery in combination with antibiotic use (MediHerb, 1994).

PREGNANCY AND LACTATION: No known restrictions (Brown, 2000; McGuffin *et al.*, 1997). An absence of teratogenicity with administration of eleuthero has been demonstrated in animals (Farnsworth *et al.*, 1985).

ADVERSE EFFECTS

No side effects have been documented for eleuthero in healthy individuals (Farnsworth *et al.*, 1985; Blumenthal *et al.*, 1998). In rare cases, mild, transient diarrhea has been reported. In rare cases, sleep disturbances have been reported (Hänsel, 1991; Brown, 2000). In patients with rheumatic heart disease, side effects such as pericardial pain, headaches, and elevated blood pressure have been reported (Werbach and Murray, 2000). Reports of neonatal/maternal androgenization ("hairy baby" syndrome) have been attributed to maternal ingestion of products labeled as "Siberian ginseng" (Koren *et al.*, 1990), though subsequent investigations determined the implicated product did not contain eleuthero but was adulterated with Chinese silk vine (*Periploca sepium*) (Awang, 1991; Awang, 1996b).

DRUG INTERACTIONS

There are few well-documented reports of interactions with eleuthero. Mutual potentiation of beneficial effects when eleuthero is administered with the radioprotector drug adeturone has been reported (Minkova and Pantev, 1987). Eleuthero potentiates effects of antibiotics monomycin and kanamycin in treatment of *Shigella* dysentery and *Proteus* enterocolitis (Brinker, 2001).

One case of unexplained elevated digoxin levels has been reported (McRae, 1996). It is unclear whether some unknown component of eleuthero was converted to digoxin *in vivo*, interfered with digoxin elimination, caused a false serum assay result, or was a result of a possible substituted herbal material, since the identity of the raw material was not confirmed and may have been another case of adulteration with Chinese silk vine (Awang, 1996a; 1996b). Possible interactions with prescription drugs warrants caution regarding the concomitant use of eleuthero and antipsychotic drugs, barbiturates, and sedatives (Medon, 1984); however, there are no actual reports to support this speculation. Eleuthero may produce an enhanced effect on insulin and antidiabetic therapy, at least theoretically (Brinker, 2001); diabetics should monitor blood glucose levels closely due to the potential hypoglycemic action.

AMERICAN HERBAL PRODUCTS ASSOCIATION (AHPA) SAFETY RATING

CLASS 1: Herbs that can be safely consumed when used appropriately (McGuffin *et al.*, 1997).

REGULATORY STATUS

CANADA: Drug Identification Number (DIN) assigned (Health Canada, 2001).

CHINA: One eleuthero-containing multi-ingredient product has schedule OTC status with a Drug Identification Number (DIN) assigned (Health Canada, 2001).

EUROPEAN UNION: Dried root official in the *European Pharmacopoeia*, 3rd ed. Supplement 2000 (Ph.Eur., 2000).

FRANCE: Traditional Herbal Medicine (THM) for specific indication (Bradley, 1992; Bruneton, 1999). Added to *French Pharmacopoeia* in 1996 (Bruneton, 1999; Ph.Fr., 1996).

GERMANY: Approved non-prescription drug of the German Commission E (Blumenthal *et al.*, 1998). Official in the *German Pharmacopoeia* (DAB, 1999).

RUSSIAN FEDERATION: Official in the *State Pharmacopoeia of the Union of Soviet Socialist Republics* since 1962 (Foster, 1991; Fulder, 1980; Schulz and Hänsel, 1996; USSR, 1990).

SWEDEN: As of January 2001, no eleuthero products are listed in the Medical Products Agency (MPA) "Authorised Natural Remedies" (MPA, 2001).

SWITZERLAND: No licensed herbal medicines containing eleuthero. No monograph in the *Swiss Pharmacopoeia*.

U.K.: Not included on the *General Sale List*, and no product licenses granted (Bradley, 1992; Newall *et al.*, 1996).

U.S.: Dietary supplement (USC, 1994).

CLINICAL REVIEW

Nine studies are outlined in the following table, "Clinical Studies on Eleuthero," conducted on 1,984 participants. All but one of these studies (Dowling *et al.*, 1996) demonstrate positive effects for immune response, stress, fatigue, and cardiovascular health. The table includes four double-blind, placebo-controlled (DB, PC) studies investigating the effects of eleuthero on concentration, selective memory, cognitive function, and well-being (Winther *et al.*, 1997); ergogenic parameters in athletes (Dowling *et al.*, 1996); immune protection against herpes simplex type II infection (Williams, 1995); and immunomodulatory measurements (e.g., T-cells) in healthy volunteers (Bohn *et al.*, 1987). A single-blind, placebo-controlled (SB, PC) study evaluated eleuthero's effects on work capacity, stamina, and fatigue in male athletes (Asano *et al.*, 1986). Clinical studies on eleuthero extracts have been extensively conducted in the former Soviet Union since the early 1960s. More than 2,100 normal and stressed human subjects were orally administered eleuthero root fluid extract, 33% ethanol. The studies examined the adaptogenic response of humans to adverse conditions such as heat, noise, motion, workload increase, and exercise. These studies also measured a significant improvement in auditory disturbances, increased mental alertness, work output, and quality of work under stress (Farnsworth *et al.*, 1985).

BRANDED PRODUCTS

Elagen: Eladon Ltd. / 63 High Street / Bangor, Gwynedd / LL57 1NR / U.K. / Tel: +44-01-24-83-7005-9 / www.elagen.com. Hydro-alcoholic dried extract (10:1) of *Eleutherococcus senticosus* root extract standardized root at 0.4% eleutheroside B and 0.4% eleutheroside E in 375 mg tablets. This product is now called Eleugetic®.

Eleukokk®: Pharma-Inter-Med / Am Born 19 / 22765 Hamburg / Germany. 10 g of test preparation consisted of 1.96 g eleuthero root ethanolic fluid extract 1:1 (0.20% (*w/v*) eleutheroside B, 1.30 g sorbitol water 70% (*w/v*), and 6.74 g dessert wine. This product is no longer available.

Maxim-L®: Omega Nutripharm. No manufacturer information available. Eleuthero root fluid extract with 30–34% ethanol (eleutherosides B and E present).

Medexport: Moscow, Russia. No manufacturer information available. Eleuthero root fluid extract Ph. USSR: 42-358-72, 335 ethanol. Each ml of fluid extract contains 75 mg of soluble extractive of *Eleutherococcus senticosus*, including 0.53 mg of syringin (eleutheroside B) and 0.12 mg of syringaresinol di-glucoside (eleutheroside D).

Taigutan® Eleuthero root fluid extract: Dr. Mewes Heilmittel GmbH / PF 1325 / 56194 Höhr-Grenzhausen / Germany / Tel: +49-02-62-49-4529-0 / Fax: +49-02-62-49-4529-1 / www.paesel.lorei.de. A 1:1 (*w/v*) extract in 35% (*v/v*) ethanol. Unable to confirm manufacturer.

REFERENCES

Afanas'eva T, Lebkova N. Effect of *Eleutherococcus* on the subcellular structures of the heart in experimental myocardial infarct. [in Russian]. *Biull Eksp Biol Med* 1987;103(2):212–5.

Asano K Takahashi T, Miyashita M, *et al.* Effect of *Eleutherococcus senticosus* extract on human physical working capacity. *Planta Med* 1986;3:175–7.

Awang D. Maternal use of ginseng and neonatal androgenization. *JAMA* 1991;266(3):363.

Awang D. Eleuthero. *CPJ* Oct 1996b;52–4.

Awang D. Siberian ginseng toxicity may be case of mistaken identity. *Canadian Med Assoc J* 1996a;155(9):1237.

Baranov A. Medicinal uses of ginseng and related plants in the Soviet Union: recent trends in the Soviet literature. *J Ethnopharm* 1982;6:339–53.

Ben-Hur E, Fulder S. Effect of *Panax ginseng* saponins and *Eleutherococcus senticosus* on survival of cultured mammalian cells after ionizing radiation. *Am J Chin Med* 1981;9(1):48–56.

Berdyshev V. Effect of the long-term intake of *Eleutherococcus* on the adaptation of sailors in the tropics. [in Russian]. *Voen Med Zh* 1981;(5):57–8.

BHP. See: *British Herbal Pharmacopoeia.*

Blumenthal M, Busse WR, Goldberg A, Gruenwald J, Hall T, Riggins CW, Rister RS (eds.). Klein S, Rister RS (trans.). *The Complete German Commission E Monographs—Therapeutic Guide to Herbal Medicines.* Austin, TX: American Botanical Council; Boston: Integrative Medicine Communication; 1998;124–5.

Bohn B, Nebe C, Birr C. Flow-cytometric studies with *Eleutherococcus senticosus* extract as an immunomodulatory agent. *Arzneiforschung* 1987;37(10):1193–6.

Bradley P (ed.). *British Herbal Compendium*, Vol. 1. Bournemouth, UK: British Herbal Medicine Association; 1992;89–91.

Brekhman II, Dardymov I. New substances of plant origin which increase nonspecific resistance. *Annu Rev Pharmacol* 1969;4:419–30.

Brekhman II, Kirillov O. Effect of *Eleutherococcus* on alarm-phase of stress. *Life Sci* 1969;8(3):113–21.

Brekhman II. *Man and Biologically Active Substances, The Effect of Drugs, Diet and Pollution on Health.* Oxford: Pergamon Press Ltd; 1980.

Brevoort P. The booming U.S. botanical market: a new overview. *HerbalGram* 1998;44:33–48.

Brinker F. *Herb Contraindications and Drug Interactions*, 3rd ed. Sandy, OR: Eclectic Medical Publications; 2001;86-87.

British Herbal Pharmacopoeia (BHP). Exeter, UK: British Herbal Medicine Association; 1996;74–5.

Brown D. *Herbal Prescriptions for Health & Healing.* Rocklin, CA: Prima Publishing; 2000;69–77.

Bruneton J. *Pharmacognosy, Phytochemistry, Medicinal Plants*, 2nd ed. Paris, France: Lavoisier Publishing; 1999;709–10.

Chang H, But P. *Pharmacology and Applications of Chinese Materia Medica.* Singapore: World Scientific; 1986;725–35.

Collisson R. Siberian ginseng (*Eleutherococcus senticosus*). *Br J Phytother* 1991;2(2):61–71.

Czygan F (ed.). *Biogene Arzneistoffe.* Wiesbaden, Germany; 1984;212–6, 220–2.

DAB. See: *Deutsches Arzneibuch.*

Davydor M, Krikorian AD. *Eleutherococcus senticosus* (Rupr. & Maxim.) Maxim. (Araliaceae) as an adaptogen: a closer look. *J Ethnopharmacol* 2000;72(3):345–393.

Deutsches Arzneibuch Ergänzungslieferung. Stuttgart, Germany: Deutscher Apotheker Verlag; 1999.

Dowling E, Redondo DR, Branch JD *et al.* Effect of *Eleutherococcus senticosus* on submaximal and maximal exercise performance. *Med Sci Sports Exerc* 1996;28(4):482–9.

European Pharmacopoeia (Ph.Eur. 3 Supplement 2000). Strasbourg, France: Council of Europe; 2000;762.

Fang J, Proksch A, Wagner H. Immunologically active polysaccharides of *Eleutherococcus senticosus.* *Phytochem* 1985;24(11):2619–22.

Farnsworth N, Kinghorn A, Soejarto D, Waller D. Siberian Ginseng (*Eleutherococcus senticosus*): Current status as an adaptogen. In: Wagner H, Hikino H, Farnsworth NR (eds.). *Economic and Medicinal Plant Research,* Vol. I. London, UK: Academic Press; 1985;155–215, 217–284.

Filaretov A, Bogdanova T, Podvigina T, Bogdanov A. Role of pituitary-adrenocortical system in body adaptation abilities. *Exp Clin Endocrinol* 1988;92(2):129-136.

Foster S (ed.). *Herbs of Commerce.* Austin, TX: American Herbal Products Assn.; 1992.

Foster S. *Siberian Ginseng—Eleutherococcus senticosus. Botanical Booklet Series* No. 302. Austin, TX: American Botanical Council; 1991.

Foster S, Chongxi Y. *Herbal Emissaries: Bringing Chinese Herbs to the West.* Rochester, VT: Healing Arts Press; 1992;73–9.

Fulder S. The drug that builds Russians. *New Scientist* 1980;576–9.

Golikov P. Influence of aqueous extracts of roots, stems and leaves of *Eleutherococcus senticosus* and *Panax ginseng* on the mental abilities of working humans. [in Russian]. *Mater K Izuch Zhen-shenya i Drug Lek Dal'nego Vostoka* 1963;5:233–5.

Hacker B, Medon P. Cytotoxic effects of *Eleutherococcus senticosus* aqueous extracts in combination with N6-(delta 2-isopentenyl)-adenosine and 1-beta-D-arabinofuranosylcytosine against L1210 leukemia cells. *J Pharm Sci* 1984;73(2):270–2.

Halstead BW, Hood LL. *Eleutherococcus senticosus (Siberian Ginseng): An Introduction to the Concept of Adaptogenic Medicine.* Taiwan, R.O.C.: Oriental Healing Arts Institute; 1984.

Hänsel R. *Phytopharmaka*, 2nd ed. Berlin, Germany: Springer Verlag; 1991;272-5.

Health Canada. Product Information: Enzymatic Therapy Vitamin B-12 Capsules with Non-Medicinal Liquid Liver Extract and Siberian Ginseng. In: *Drug Product Database* (*DPD*). Ottawa, Ontario: Health Canada Therapeutic Products Programme; 2001.

Hikino H, Takahashi M, Otake K, Konno C. Isolation and hypoglycemic activity of eleutherans A, B, C, D, E, F, and G: glycans of *Eleutherococcus senticosus* roots. *J Nat Prod* 1986;49(2):293–7.

Huang K. *The Pharmacology of Chinese Herbs*, 2nd ed. Boca Raton, FL: CRC Press; 1999;46–8.

Kaloeva Z. Effect of the glycosides of *Eleutherococcus senticosus* on the hemodynamic indices of children with hypotensive states. [in Russian]. *Farmakol Toksikol* 1986;49(5):73.

Kaptchuck T. The Organs of the Body: The Harmonious Landscape. In: *The Web That Has No Weaver: Understanding Chinese Medicine.* Chicago, Il: Congdon & Weed, Inc.; 1983;50–76.

Kenner D, Requena Y. *Botanical Medicine: A European Professional Perspective.* Brookline, MA: Paradigm Publications; 1996;132–3.

Kirilov O. The effect of fluid extract of *Eleutherococcus* root on the pituitary-adrenocortical system. [in Russian]. *Sib Otd Acad Nauk S.S.S.R.* 1964;23:3–5.

Kolomisvsky L. Control over adaptive reactions of cardiologic patients using small doses of *Eleutherococcus* extract. In: *New Data on Eleuthercoccus: Proceedings of the Second International Symposium on Eleutherococcus.* Moscow, Russia: Academy of Sciences of the USSR Far East Science Center; 1986;265–71.

Koren G, Randor S, Martin S, *et al.* Maternal ginseng use associated with neonatal androgenization. *JAMA.* 1990;264:86.

Leung A, Foster S. *Encyclopedia of Common Natural Ingredients Used in Food, Drugs, and Cosmetics*, 2nd ed. New York, NY: John Wiley & Sons, Inc; 1996;225–7.

McGuffin M, Hobbs C, Upton R, Goldberg A (eds.). *American Herbal Product Association's Botanical Safety Handbook.* Boca Raton: CRC Press; 1997;45.

McGuffin M, Kartesz J, Leung A, Tucker A (eds.). *Herbs of Commerce*, 2nd ed. Silver Spring, MD: American Herbal Products Assn; 2001.

McRae S. Elevated serum digoxin levels in a patient taking digoxin and Siberian ginseng. *Canadian Med Assoc J* 1996;155(3):293–5.

Medical Products Agency (MPA). Naturläkemedel: Authorised Natural Remedies (as of January 24, 2001). Uppsala, Sweden: Medical Products Agency; 2001.

MediHerb. *Eleutherococcus* — a herbal adaptogen, Part 1. *MediHerb Professional Newsletter*. 1993 Nov;Number 36.

MediHerb. *Eleutherococcus* — a herbal adaptogen, Part 2. *MediHerb Professional Newsletter*. 1994 Jan;Number 37.

Medon P, Thompson EB, Farnsworth NR. Hypoglycaemic effect and toxicity of *Eleutherococcus senticosus* following acute and chronic administration in mice. *Zhongguo Yao Li Xue Bao* 1981;2(4):281–5.

Medon P, Ferguson P, Watson C. Effects of *Eleutherococcus senticosus* extracts on hexobarbital metabolism *in vivo* and *in vitro*. *J Ethnopharmacol* 1984;10(2):235–41.

Minkova M, Pantev T. Effect of *Eleutherococcus* extract on the radioprotective action of adeturone. *Acta Physiol Pharmacol Bulg* 1987;13(4):66–70.

Mikunis R, Serkova V, Shirkova T. The effect of Eleutherococcus on some biomedical parameters of the blood in the combined treatment of patients with rheumatic lesions of the heart. *Lek Sredestva Dal'nego Vosto*ka 1966; 7:227–30.

MPA. See: Medical Products Agency.

Newall C, Anderson L, Phillipson J. *Herbal Medicines: A Guide for Health-care Professionals*. London, UK: The Pharmaceutical Press; 1996;141–4.

Novozhilov G, Sil'chenko K. Mechanism of adaptogenic effect of *Eleutherococcus* on the human body during thermal stress. [in Russian]. *Fiziol Cheloveka* 1985;11(2):303–6.

Pearce P, Zois I, Wynne K, Funder J. *Panax ginseng* and *Eleutherococcus senticosus* extracts — *in vitro* studies on binding to steroid receptors. *Endocrinol Jpn* 1982;29(5):567.

Ph.Eur. See: *European Pharmacopoeia*.

Ph.Fr. See: *Pharmacopée Française*.

Pharmacopée Française. (Ph.Fr.). Paris, France: Adrapharm; 1996.

Pharmacopoeia of the People's Republic of China (PPRC English Edition, 1997). Beijing, China: Chemical Industry Press; 1997;132–3, 272, 380–1.

Pizzorno JE, Murray MT, editors. *Textbook of Natural Medicine*, Volume 1, 2nd ed. New York: Churchill Livingstone; 1999;713–7.

PPRC. See: *Pharmacopoeia of the People's Republic of China*.

Schulz V, Hänsel R. *Rationelle Phytotherapie*, 3rd ed. Berlin, Germany: Springer Verlag. 1996;305-306.

Shadrin A *et al*. Estimation of prophylactic and immunostimulating effects of Eleutherococcus and Schisandra chinensis preparations. In: *New Data on Eleutherecoccus: Proceedings of the Second International Symposium on Eleutherococcus*. Moscow, Russia: Academy of Sciences of the USSR Far East Science Center;. 1986;289–93.

Sosnova T. The effect of *Eleutherococcus spinosus* on the color discrimination function of the optic analyzer in persons with normal trichromatic vision. [in Russian]. *Vestn Oftalmol* 1969;82(5):59–61.

Sosuova T. *Eleutherococcus* as a means to raise colour perception of locomotive engineers. In: *New Data on Eleuthercoccus: Proceedings of the Second International Symposium on Eleutherococcus*. Moscow, Russia: Academy of Sciences of the USSR Far East Science Center; 1986;258–64.

State Pharmacopoeia of the Union of Soviet Socialist Republics, 11th ed., Vols. 1 & 2 (USSR XI). Moscow, Russia: Medicina; 1990

Szolomicki S, Samochowiec L, Wójcicki J, Drozdzik M. The influence of active components of *Eleutherococcus senticosus* on cellular defense and physical fitness in man. *Phytother Res* 2000;14:30–5.

Takasugi N, Moriguchi T, Fuwa T, *et al*. Effect of *Eleutherococcus senticosus* and its components on rectal temperature, body and grip tones, motor coordination, and exploratory and spontaneous movements in mice under acute stress. *Shoyakugaku Zasshi* 1985;39(3):232–7.

Tang W, Eisenbrand G. *Chinese Drugs of Plant Origin: Chemistry, Pharmacology, and Use in Traditional and Modern Medicine*. New York, NY: Springer Verlag; 1992.

Tseitlin G, Saltanov A. Some parameters of antistress activity of *Eleutherococcus* extract in patients with Hodgkin's disease after splenectomy. [in Russian]. *Pediatriia* 1981;(5):25–7.

Tyler VE. Importance of European phytomedicinals in the American market: an overview. In.: Lawson LD, Bauer R (eds.). *Phytomedicines of Europe: Chemistry and Biological Activity*. Washington, DC: American Chemical Society; 1998;2–12.

United States Congress (USC). Public Law 103-417: *Dietary Supplement Health and Education Act of 1994*. Washington, DC: 103rd Congress of the United States; 1994.

United States Food and Drug Administration (US FDA). 21 CFR (Code of Federal Regulation, Title 21, Volume 2, Parts 100–169), Revised as of April 1, 1999. Washington, DC: Office of the Federal Register National Archives and Records Administration. 1999; 15–19.

US FDA. See: United States Food and Drug Administration.

USC. See: United States Congress.

USSR. See: *State Pharmacopoeia of the Union of Soviet Socialist Republics*.

Vereschchagin I. Treatment of dysentery in children with a combination of monomycin and *Eleutherococcus*. [in Russian]. *Antibiotiki* 1978;23(7):633–6.

Wagner H, Nörr H, Winterhoff H. Plant adaptogens. *Phytomedicine* 1994;1:63–76.

Wagner H. Immunostimulants from medicinal plants. In: Chang H, Yeung W, Tso W, Koo A (eds.). *Advances in Chinese Medicinal Material Research*. Singapore: World Scientific; 1985.

Werbach M, Murray M. *Botanical Influences on Illness: A Sourcebook of Clinical Research,* 2nd ed. Tarzana, CA: Third Line Press; 1994; 2000.

Wildfeuer A, Mayerhofer D. The effects of plant preparations on cellular functions in body defense. [in German]. *Arzneimittelforschung* 1994;44(1), Nr. 3:361–6.

Williams M. Immuno-protection against *Herpes simplex* type II infection by *Eleutherococcus* root extract. *Int J Altern Comp Med* 1995;13:9–12.

Winther K *et al*. Russian root (Siberian Ginseng) improves cognitive functions in middle-aged people, whereas *Gingko biloba* seems effective only in the elderly. (XVI World Congress of Neurology, Buenos Aires). *J Neurologic Sci* 1997;150:S90.

Yonezawa M Katch N, Takeda A. Radiation protection by Shigoka extract on split dose irradiation in mice. *J Radiation Res* 1989;30(3):247–54.

Zaikova M, Verba A, Snegireva M. *Eleutherococcus* in ophthalmology. [in Russian]. *Vestn Oftalmol* 1968;81(3):70–4.

Clinical Studies on Eleuthero (*Eleutherococcus senticosus* [Rupr & Maxim.] Maxim.)

Immunology

Author/Year	Subject	Design	Duration	Dosage	Preparation	Results/Conclusion
Szolomicki et al., 2000	Immunology	R, Cm n=50 healthy male volunteers	30 days	25 drops eleuthero 3x/day vs. 40 drops echinacea 3x/day	Taigutan® Eleuthero root fluidextract 1:1 (w/v) vs. Echinacin® echinacea herb fresh juice preparation	In cellular defense mechanism assays, the phagocytic activity of neutrocytes in the eleuthero group rose significantly, and the number of neutrocytes actively participating in phagocytosis increased. Authors conclude that eleuthero extractives affect cellular defense, physical fitness, and lipid metabolism.
Williams, 1995	Immune protection against herpes simplex type II infection	DB, R, PC (2 parallel groups) n=93 volunteers of the Herpes Association	6 months	375 mg 4x/day	Elagen® eleuthero standardized extract (eleutherosides B and E)	Effects on frequency, duration, and severity of recurrent episodes of herpes simplex type II infections were observed. Statistically significant results (p = 0.0002 to 0.0007) in the eleuthero group where 75% reported improvements in severity, duration, or frequency of attacks vs. 34% in the placebo group.
Shadrin et al., 1986	Immunology	PC n=1,376 students	Fall of 1981 during influenza epidemic	2 ml extract diluted into a sweetened tea/day	Eleuthero root fluid extract	Occurrence of typical influenza complications (pneumonia, bronchitis, maxillary sinusitis, otitis) in eleuthero group were lower (1.5 cases per 100 persons) vs. control group (3.2 cases per 100), a statistically significant difference (p<0.05).
Bohn et al., 1987	Immunology	DB, PC n=36 healthy volunteers	1 month (followed by a 6-month observation period)	10 ml fluidextract diluted in wine and sorbitol water 3x/day vs. dry wine with same ethanol content	Eleukokk® fluidextract (0.2% eleutheroside B w/v) vs. dry wine	Eleuthero improved non-specific immune reactivities as determined by quantitative flow-cytometry. Significant increase in the absolute numbers of immunocompetent cells, particularly T-cells, predominantly of the helper/inducer type, but also on cytotoxic and natural killer cells. A general enhancement of the activation state of T-lymphocytes was also observed.

Adaptogenic

Author/Year	Subject	Design	Duration	Dosage	Preparation	Results/Conclusion
Dowling et al., 1996	Adaptogen, stress, fatigue during submaximal and maximal aerobic exercise	DB, R, PC (2 parallel groups) n=20 male & female athletes (mean age 37 years)	2 months	3.4 ml/day, (6-week treatment, 2-week withdrawal)	Maxim–L® eleuthero fluidextract, 30–34% ethanol (eleutherosides B and E present)	No significant differences were observed between test and control groups in heart rate, oxygen consumption, expired-minute volume, respiratory exchange ratio, perceived exertion, and serum lactate. The authors concluded that ergogenic claims cannot be supported based on their results.
Kolomisvsky, 1986	Adaptive response to stress in cardiac patients, which activates protective forces to maintain homeostasis.	Cm n=147 cardiologic patients in 3 groups Group 1: n=42 (ages 23–72); Group 2: n=39 (ages 28–67); Group 3: n=66 (ages 23–56)	7–10 days	Group 1: Received conventional therapy (not defined). Group 2: 30 drops/day extract on empty stomach. Group 3: 15–35 drops/day	Eleuthero root fluid-extract (brand not stated) vs. usual treatment (not defined)	Group 1: Adaptive reaction background in non-eleuthero group did not improve. Group 2: Eleuthero extract showed an anti-stress effect and helped to normalize adaptive reactions. Group 3: When used to control adaptive reactions with activation therapy, eleuthero helped patients recover from stress state, resulting in significant increase in normal adaptive reactions.
Asano et al., 1986	Adaptogen, stress, fatigue	SB, PC, CO n=6 healthy male athletes (mean age 21.5 years)	8 days	2 ml extract or placebo 2x/day (morning and evening) 0.5 hours before meal	Medexport (eleuthero root fluid extract) or placebo	Significant increase in all parameters tested for eleuthero treatment period including maximal oxygen uptake (p<0.01), oxygen pulse (p<0.025), total work (p<0.005), and exhaustion time. Athletes in the eleuthero group showed a 23.3% (p<0.005) increase in total exercise duration and stamina compared to 7.5% in placebo group. Increase in total work appeared to be attributable to improvement of bodily oxygen metabolism reflected in the increase in maximal oxygen uptake and maximal oxygen pulse.

KEY: C – controlled, **CC** – case-control, **CH** – cohort, **CI** – confidence interval, **Cm** – comparison, **CO** – crossover, **CS** – cross-sectional, **DB** – double-blind, **E** – epidemiological, **LC** – longitudinal cohort, **MA** – meta-analysis, **MC** – multi-center, **n** – number of patients, **O** – open, **OB** – observational, **OL** – open label, **OR** – odds ratio, **P** – prospective, **PB** – patient-blind, **PC** – placebo-controlled, **PG** – parallel group, **PS** – pilot study, **R** – randomized, **RC** – reference-controlled, **RCS** – retrospective cross-sectional, **RS** - retrospective, **S** – surveillance, **SB** – single-blind, **SC** – single-center, **U** – uncontrolled, **UP** – unpublished, **VC** – vehicle-controlled.

Other

Author/Year	Subject	Design	Duration	Dosage	Preparation	Results/Conclusion
Winther et al., 1997	Neurology, psychiatry	DB, PC, R, C (4-armed) n=24 healthy volunteers	9 months (3 months eleuthero, 3 months ginkgo, 3 months placebo)	62.5 mg eleuthero root 2x/day or 28.2 mg *Ginkgo biloba* flavone glycosides 2x/day or placebo	Eleuthero root vs. ginkgo leaf extract (containing 28.2 mg ginkgo flavone glycosides and 7.2 mg terpene lactones) vs. placebo	At end of each 3-month dose period, concentration, selective memory, cognitive function, and well-being were measured. Significant improvements in selective memory of eleuthero group vs. placebo group (p<0.02) were demonstrated. No change in concentration was discovered in any group. Significant effects from eleuthero were also noted in feelings of well-being and levels of activity.
Sosuova, 1986	Opthalmology	PC n=232 healthy locomotive engineers (ages 24–45 years)	100 days	2 ml with 30 ml water, 1x/day (40 days treatment, 60 days no treatment)	Eleuthero root fluidextract (brand not stated)	Eleuthero increased color perception level, induced a one-and-a-half to two-fold increase in functional stability level, 30–50% rise in spectral and contrast sensitivity, 2.5–4.5% rise in range of signal light visibility and 10–15% increase in speed of color discrimination. The effects remained at this level throughout administration and 2–2.5 months after end of treatment period. The placebo group did not experience these changes in perception.

KEY: C – controlled, **CC** – case-control, **CH** – cohort, **CI** – confidence interval, **Cm** – comparison, **CO** – crossover, **CS** – cross-sectional, **DB** – double-blind, **E** – epidemiological, **LC** – longitudinal cohort, **MA** – meta-analysis, **MC** – multi-center, **n** – number of patients, **O** – open, **OB** – observational, **OL** – open label, **OR** – odds ratio, **P** – prospective, **PB** – patient-blind, **PC** – placebo-controlled, **PG** – parallel group, **PS** – pilot study, **R** – randomized, **RC** – reference-controlled, **RCS** – retrospective cross-sectional, **RS** - retrospective, **S** – surveillance, **SB** – single-blind, **SC** – single-center, **U** – uncontrolled, **UP** – unpublished, **VC** – vehicle-controlled.

Ephedra

Ephedra sinica Stapf

[Fam. *Ephedraceae*]

OVERVIEW

EDITOR'S NOTE: In an attempt to clarify the controversy surrounding the safety of ephedra, the following monograph devotes additional space to some of the safety, legal, and regulatory issues. These comments have been condensed for this clinical overview.

In Asian medicine, ephedra is the chief herbal drug for treatment of asthma and bronchitis. This herb is one of the oldest and most widely used Chinese herbs, having been employed for thousands of years in traditional Chinese medicine (TCM) as a primary component of multi-herb formulas prescribed to treat bronchial asthma, cold and flu, cough and wheezing, fever, chills, lack of perspiration, headache, and nasal congestion. Ephedra became controversial in the 1980s and 1990s due to its potential adverse effects and its increasing popularity as a major ingredient in herbal dietary supplements in the United States. As a result, in June 1997, the FDA issued proposed regulations on ephedra-containing dietary supplements that would limit the level of total ephedra alkaloids in herbal preparations to no more than 8 mg per dose, and no more than 24 mg total ingestion per day. However, the U.S. General Accounting Office (GAO) questioned the reliability of many of the adverse event reports (AER's) and criticized the apparent lack of science employed in formulating the proposed dosage limits of alkaloids. In February 2000, the FDA responded to GAO by announcing that it would withdraw portions of its proposed rules on duration of use and dosage levels. In August 2000, the Office of Women's Health (OWH) of the U.S. Department of Health and Human Services (HHS) held a two-day public hearing on the safety of ephedra in which testimony was presented by various scientific and medical experts who had conducted extensive reviews of the scientific and clinical literature on ephedra, as well as some who had conducted clinical investigations into the potential risks and benefits of ephedra for weight loss. That same panel also conducted the first comparison of incident rates of the adverse events at issue (e.g., stroke, heart attack, and seizure) in the general population and incident rates of the same events in ephedra consumers. The conclusion of the expert panel was that the analysis suggests that there was no evidence of increased risk, even using the most conservative of assumptions. In September 2000, the OWH issued a report recommending that additional research be conducted. Additionally, recent clinical research suggests that ephedra, in combination with other herbs, can be used safely in persons with normal blood pressure levels. Peer-reviewed scientific literature suggests that the risks of caffeine combined with ephedrine are outweighed by the benefits of achieving and maintaining a healthy weight. Further confirmation of that conclusion for herbal products containing caffeine and ephedrine awaits additional controlled clinical trials. Additional research into the use of ephedra as a weight loss aid appears to be warranted. In June 2002, the Secretary of HHS called for more research on ephedra to determine its safety and efficacy. Various athletic organizations have banned the use of ephedra supplements and ephedrine alkaloid-containing over-the-counter (OTC) drugs. Medical groups have stated that these items should be available by prescription only.

PRIMARY USES

- Mild bronchospasms in adults and children over the age of six (per approval in Germany)
- Bronchodilator in treatment of bronchial asthma
- Nasal congestion due to hay fever, allergic rhinitis, acute coryza (rhinitis), common cold, sinusitis
- Weight loss and thermogenesis

PHARMACOLOGICAL ACTIONS

Ephedrine and related alkaloids produce sympathomimetic effects, including vasoconstriction; increased heart rate; and stimulation of central nervous system. Ephedrine decreases gastric emptying, possibly contributing to reduction of food intake. Ephedra herb preparations are shown to produce dilated bronchi, and induce perspiration (diaphoretic), and diuresis (diuretic). Ephedra-caffeine herb combinations are shown to increase thermogenesis and weight loss in obese patients.

DOSAGE AND ADMINISTRATION

According to the German Commission E, ephedra preparations should only be used short-term because of tachyphylaxis and potential addiction. However, a recent analysis of available U.S. health and safety data showed no evidence of significant abuse or addiction to ephedra, despite decades of widespread use.

Crude Preparations

NOTE: According to U.S. herb industry labeling policy, the maximum adult daily dose for ephedra and ephedra-containing products is 100 mg total alkaloids.

DECOCTION: 1–6 g dried herb daily.

CHINESE PHARMACOPEIA DOSAGE: 1.5–9 g dried herb daily.

DRIED COMMINUTED HERB (for Commission E approved bronchial indications):

ADULT SINGLE DOSE: 15–30 mg total alkaloid, calculated as ephedrine.

DRIED COMMINUTED HERB (for Commission E approved bronchial indications) (cont.):

ADULT MAXIMUM DAILY DOSE: corresponding to 300 mg total alkaloid calculated as ephedrine.

CHILD SINGLE DOSE (over age 6): corresponding to 0.5 mg total alkaloid per kg of body weight.

CHILD MAXIMUM DAILY DOSE (over age 6): 2 mg total alkaloid per kg of body weight.

[NOTE: These children's dosages are based on the recommendations for licensed preparations for the approved bronchial indication in Germany only. Ephedra supplements in the U.S. are not recommended for children under the age of 18, according to industry labeling policy.]

FLUID EXTRACT: 1:1 (*g/ml*), 45% alcohol, 1–3 ml daily.

TINCTURE: 1:4 (*g/ml*), 45% alcohol, 6–8 ml daily. Maximum weekly dose: 48 ml.

NO OBSERVED ADVERSE EFFECT LEVEL BASED ON THE CANTOX TOXICOLOGICAL REVIEW: ephedra preparations equivalent to 30 mg total alkaloids per dose; 90 mg per day.

Purified alkaloids (i.e., OTC drugs)

For bronchodilation the maximum adult daily dose of ephedrine (or ephedrine hydrochloride) is 150 mg per day, and the maximum adult daily dose of pseudoephedrine (or pseudoephedrine hydrochloride) is 240 mg per day.

CONTRAINDICATIONS

Anxiety and restlessness, hypertension, glaucoma, impaired cerebral circulation, adenoma of prostate with residual urine accumulation, pheochromocytoma, thyrotoxicosis, pregnancy, anorexia, diabetes, heart disease, insomnia, stomach ulcers, children, renal failure. Patients with the following conditions or symptoms should consult a healthcare provider before using ephedra: difficulty urinating, prostate enlargement, thyroid disease, depression or other psychiatric condition, or if using a monoamine oxidase (MAO) inhibitor, any other prescription drug, or an OTC drug containing ephedrine, pseudoephedrine or phenylpropanolamine (PPA) (ingredients found in certain allergy, asthma, cough/cold, and weight control products). (PPA has been removed from the OTC market, but consumers might still possess older PPA-containing drug products.) Exceeding recommended dosage will not improve therapeutic benefits and may cause serious adverse health effects. Patients should discontinue use and call a health care professional immediately if they experience rapid heartbeat, dizziness, severe headache, shortness of breath, or other similar symptoms.

PREGNANCY AND LACTATION: Ephedra is not recommended for use during pregnancy or lactation.

ADVERSE EFFECTS

Insomnia, motor restlessness, irritability, headaches, nausea, vomiting, disturbances of urination, tachycardia; higher dosages (greater than the equivalent of 300 mg ephedra alkaloids per day) may produce a drastic increase in blood pressure, cardiac arrhythmia, and development of dependency. Isolated reports of adverse events, some serious, including stroke and death, have been received by the FDA. One highly publicized review of selected events reported to the FDA concluded that the adverse event reports (AERs) do not establish causality and cannot be used to quantify risk. Recent evidence submitted to the FDA shows no association between clinically significant adverse events and doses of under 100 mg of ephedra alkaloids per day.

An epidemiological analysis of the AERs showed no greater incidence of seizures, strokes, and myocardial infarctions (MIs) in persons consuming dietary supplements containing ephedrine alkaloids than that expected in the general U.S. population. In addition, the FDA advises that AERs alone do not provide a scientific basis for assessing the safety of dietary supplements containing ephedrine alkaloids.

DRUG INTERACTIONS

Actual or potential interactions may occur between orally ingested ephedrine alkaloids (mainly ephedrine and/or pseudoephedrine and not necessarily the herb ephedra itself) and:

ANTIHYPERTENSIVES (including ACE inhibitors and beta-blockers): May result in severe hypertension.

CARDIAC GLYCOSIDES OR HALOTHANE: Disturbs heart rhythm.

CORTICOSTEROIDS: Increase the clearance of dexamethasone, therefore decreasing its activity.

GUANETHIDINE: Antagonizes the hypotensive effect.

MAO-INHIBITORS (including tranylcypromine, pargyline, procarbazine, selegiline, phenelzine, and moclobemide): Significantly raise the sympathomimetic action of ephedrine.

METHYL XANTHINES (e.g., caffeine, theophylline): Increase thermogenesis and weight loss due to reduction in body fat when ephedrine is combined with xanthines, plus causes excessive nervous stimulation.

SECALE ALKALOID DERIVATIVES OR OXYTOCIN: May lead to hypertension.

URINARY ALKALIZERS (e.g., acetazolamide, sodium bicarbonate): Excrete more slowly (than with urinary acidifiers, e.g., ammonium chloride), due to effects of reabsorption from tubules in the kidneys.

CLINICAL REVIEW

There is one published clinical trial based on ephedra as a single ingredient. Most ephedra trials tested multi-ingredient formulations that include a caffeine-containing herb such as cola nut or guarana. At least 3 such trials on ephedra combination preparations suggest safe and effective use for weight loss. Several unpublished trials employed 4 different ephedra products (ephedra only, not combinations) on 300 subjects over a period of 6 weeks and 6 months to monitor weight loss and adverse effects, respectively. The studies concluded that ephedra appears to be safe, effective, and cost effective, and compares favorably with pharmaceutical weight loss agents, with a relatively low side effect profile. Ephedrine and caffeine combinations and a much-publicized Danish formula of ephedrine combined with caffeine and aspirin have demonstrated relative safety and efficacy in weight loss in clinical trials.

Ephedra

Ephedra sinica Stapf
[Fam. *Ephedraceae*]

DESCRIPTION

For thousands of years in Traditional Chinese Medicine, ephedra (*ma huang* in Chinese) has been a primary ingredient in formulas used to treat bronchial asthma, cold, flu, wheezing, fever, and chills. In the 1980s and 1990s ephedra became controversial because of its possible adverse effects and its growing popularity as a major ingredient in herbal dietary supplements in the U.S. The FDA has attempted to amend regulations since that time in an effort to reduce potential risk and misuse of this herb. Recent research and expert reviews have raised questions about how to evaluate the potential risks of ephedra use. Nevertheless, further research is warranted to assess the use of ephedra as a weight loss aid. In June 2002, the U.S. Department of Health and Human Services announced it would sponsor more research on ephedra's safety and efficacy.

USES

Mild bronchospasms in adults; asthma (bronchodilator); nasal congestion due to hay fever, allergic nasal inflammation, common cold, or sinusitis; weight loss; thermogenesis (burning of fatty tissue).

DOSAGE

NOTE: According to U.S. herb industry labeling policy, the maximum adult daily dose for ephedra and ephedra-containing products is 100 mg total alkaloids, while a safety review recommended a slightly lower dose of 90 mg total alkaloids per day.

Crude Preparations
DECOCTION (TEA): 1–9 g daily.

Purified alkaloids (i.e., OTC drugs)
For bronchodilation the maximum adult daily dose: 150 mg/day ephedrine; 240 mg/day pseudoephedrine

CONTRAINDICATIONS

Ephedra and products containing it should be avoided in cases of anxiety and restlessness, high blood pressure, glaucoma, reduced circulation to the brain, benign tumor of the prostate with residual urine accumulation, pheochromocytoma (a usually benign tumor that frequently produces high blood pressure), hyperthyroidism (over-active thyroid), pregnancy, anorexia, diabetes, heart disease, insomnia, stomach ulcers, kidney failure, and in children. Patients with the following should consult a healthcare provider before using ephedra: difficulty urinating, prostate enlargement, thyroid disease, depression or other psychiatric condition, or if using a monoamine oxidase (MAO) inhibitor drug, any other prescription or over-the-counter (OTC) drug containing ephedrine, pseudoephedrine, or phenylpropanolamine (PPA) (ingredients found in certain allergy, asthma, cough/cold, and weight control products). (PPA has been removed from the OTC market.) Exceeding recommended dosage will not improve therapeutic benefits and may cause serious adverse health effects. Patients should discontinue use and call a health professional immediately if they experience rapid heartbeat, dizziness, severe headache, shortness of breath, or other similar symptoms.

PREGNANCY AND LACTATION: Not recommended for use during pregnancy or lactation.

ADVERSE EFFECTS

Adverse effects include insomnia, motor restlessness, irritability, headaches, nausea, vomiting, disturbances of urination, rapid heart beat. Higher dosages (more than 300 mg of ephedra alkaloids per day) may produce drastic increase in blood pressure and cardiac arrhythmia. There are reports of serious adverse events, including stroke and death. However, FDA advises that adverse events reports cannot be used alone to scientifically determine the overall safety of ephedra.

DRUG INTERACTIONS

The herb ephedra and/or its alkaloids (e.g., ephedrine, pseudoephedrine) may cause a disturbance of heart rhythm when combined with cardiac glycoside drugs, or halothane; may increase stimulation of the nervous system when combined with MAO inhibitors; may reduce the blood pressure-lowering effect of guanethidine; may lead to hypertension when combined with secale alkaloid derivatives, or oxytocin; when combined with corticosteroids, may increase their effects. Patients should discuss the potential use of ephedra or ephedrine-containing alkaloid OTC drugs with their healthcare provider or pharmacist before using these products with any medicines.

Comments

When using a dietary supplement, purchase it from a reliable source. For best results, use the same brand of product throughout the period of use. As with all medications and dietary supplements, please inform your healthcare provider of all herbs and medications you are taking. Interactions may occur between medications and herbs or even among different herbs when taken at the same time. Treat your herbal supplement with care by taking it as directed, storing it as advised on the label, and keeping it out of the reach of children and pets. Consult your healthcare provider with any questions.

The information contained on this sheet has been excerpted from *The ABC Clinical Guide to Herbs* © 2003 by the American Botanical Council (ABC). ABC is an independent member-based educational organization focusing on the medicinal use of herbs. For more detailed information about this herb please consult the healthcare provider who gave you this sheet. To order *The ABC Clinical Guide to Herbs* or become a member of ABC, visit their website at www.herbalgram.org.

Ephedra

Ephedra sinica Stapf

[Fam. *Ephedraceae*]

OVERVIEW

EDITORS' NOTE: In an attempt to clarify the controversy surrounding the safety of ephedra, this monograph devotes additional space to some of the safety, legal, and regulatory issues. Thus, the "Overview" section is longer for ephedra than for other monographs in this publication.

In Asian medicine, ephedra (known in Chinese as *ma huang*) is the primary herbal drug for treatment of asthma and bronchitis. This herb is one of the oldest and most widely used Chinese herbs, having been employed for thousands of years in traditional Chinese medicine (TCM) as a primary component of multi-herb formulas prescribed to treat bronchial asthma, cold and flu, cough and wheezing, fever, chills, lack of perspiration, headache, and nasal congestion. Listed in the oldest comprehensive materia medica, *Shen Nong Ben Cao Jing* (ca. 100 C.E.), among the "middle class" herbs, ephedra is used to induce perspiration, and as an anti-allergy agent (Blumenthal and King, 1995; Bruneton, 1995; Der Marderosian, 1999; Huang, 1999; Leung and Foster, 1996; Weiss, 1988). Presently, ephedra is official in the national pharmacopeias of China, Germany, and Japan, while the isolated or synthesized alkaloids from the plant, primarily ephedrine and pseudoephedrine, are official in most countries.

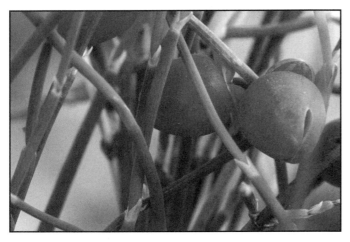

Photo © 2003 stevenfoster.com

Ephedra-containing dietary supplements have become increasingly popular in the past two decades as agents to help promote weight loss and athletic performance. A recent survey has suggested that 7% of the American adult population uses nonprescription drugs for weight loss, 2% using phenylpropanolamine (PPA) (no longer sold over-the-counter), and 1% using products containing ephedra (Blanck *et al.*, 2001). In a survey on herb use in the Minneapolis metro area, 230 people (61.2% of responders) said they had used herbs in the past 12 months; with 13.6% responding that they had used herbs for weight loss.

Forty-four (12.0%) said they used ephedra for a variety of reasons: 23 to boost energy; 20 for weight loss; 10 as a decongestant; 7 for asthma. Over half rated the ephedra effective or very effective (Harnack *et al.*, 2001).

Discussions of the safety and effectiveness of the herb ephedra are usually based on scientific research conducted on the isolated (sometimes synthesized) alkaloids in the herb (i.e., ephedrine and pseudoephedrine or their related isomers; see Chemistry section below). Both are approved by the U.S. Food and Drug Administration (FDA) as safe and effective over-the-counter (OTC) drug ingredients. Most of the scientific literature to date focuses on these alkaloids. Due to the popularity of the herb there is an increasing number of clinical studies being conducted on the herb itself, often in combination with other herbs. This review focuses on the herb itself, with reference to research on ephedrine and pseudoephedrine in the Pharmacology and Mechanisms sections, and others, as necessary.

The safety and the appropriate regulation of ephedra arose as controversial issues in the U. S. during the 1980–90's when the herb began to be used as a major ingredient in herbal dietary supplements intended to aid weight loss and exercise. Some products that were subsequently determined to be adulterated with synthetic ephedrine (e.g., Formula One®) or marketed as purportedly legal substitutes for the illicit drug Ecstasy (e.g., Herbal Ecstacy® and Ultimate Xphoria®) raised significant concerns among various state health authorities, health professionals, and responsible members of the herb and dietary supplement industry (Blumenthal and King, 1996). In 1994, increasing concerns about potential risks associated with the use of ephedra herbal products prompted the American Herbal Products Association (AHPA) and the National Nutritional Foods Association (NNFA) to issue a labeling policy for its member companies to set serving and daily intake limits as well as list contraindications for the herb on labels of ephedra-containing products (see Contraindications section below) (AHPA, 1994).

Health professionals also became increasingly concerned about the public health implications of ephedra and ephedra alkaloid-containing products, and several groups passed resolutions supporting the restriction of ephedra alkaloid-containing products. In May 1995 the Texas Medical Association (TMA) adopted a policy that ephedrine and ephedrine alkaloids should be prohibited from non-prescription foods, dietary supplements, or other OTC commercial products intended for public consumption, and that such products be made available by prescription only. In November 1998, TMA also proposed that such products be labeled to declare the amount of active ingredients of the substances with pharmacologic properties and that the products have accurate warning labels (TMA, n.d.). The American Medical Association (AMA) has adopted a similar policy (AMA, 2002, 2000).

In 1996, the Ohio legislature passed a law, supported by industry dietary supplement organizations, to appropriately regulate these products. Since that time, laws regulating ephedra that incorporate the AHPA and NNFA standards for formulation and labeling have been passed in Hawaii, Michigan, Washington, Oklahoma, and Nebraska.

In June 1997, the FDA issued proposed regulations on ephedra-containing dietary supplements that would limit the level of total ephedra alkaloids in herbal preparations to no more than 8 mg per dose, with no more than 24 mg per day (FDA, 1997). The proposal would have banned the combination of ephedra with other stimulants like caffeine or caffeine-containing herbs (including cola [*Cola nitida*], guarana [*Paullinia cupana* var. *sorbilis*], maté [*Ilex paraguariensis*]) in herbal products; would have prohibited the sale of ephedra products for use in weight loss or for athletic performance; would have restricted use of ephedra-containing herbal products to no more than seven days duration; and would have required warnings on all labels for products containing ephedra. The proposal also called for the ban of so called "street drug knockoffs" containing the herb ephedra or ephedrine alkaloids, to be used as replacements for illicit drugs; such copies of drugs are illegal under federal law. The proposed rule was based primarily on approximately 800 adverse event reports (AERs) submitted to FDA. Industry, scientific and medical experts, and many consumers criticized the proposed rule, often noting that the AERs were not a valid scientific basis for rulemaking, as was established by the FDA's own policies.

As a result of this criticism, Congress requested that the U.S. General Accounting Office (GAO), the government agency that monitors accountability of all federal agencies, conduct an audit of the scientific basis for FDA's proposed serving and daily intake limits, the proposed duration of use limit (seven days), including the ban on claims for weight loss and exercise, and FDA's cost/benefit analysis for the proposed rule. In August 1999, the GAO issued a 68-page report, *Dietary Supplements: Uncertainties in Analyses Underlying FDA's Proposed Rule on Ephedrine Alkaloids* (GAO, 1999). The report reveals deficiencies in the FDA's proposed rule on ephedra. GAO acknowledged that the AERs the FDA had received for ephedra raised concerns that warranted examination. At the same time, GAO questioned the reliability of many of the AERs and criticized the apparent lack of science employed in formulating the proposed dosage limits of alkaloids, the proposed duration limits, and ban on weight loss and exercise claims. As a result of this and other significant deficiencies, including a failure to establish that the proposed rule would have a public health benefit, the GAO recommended that the FDA not finalize the proposed rule unless it could develop a valid scientific basis and meet other requirements applicable to federal rulemaking.

In March 2000, the FDA responded to the GAO by withdrawing portions of its proposed rule on duration of use (including prohibitions against marketing ephedra for weight loss and exercise) and dosage levels. FDA simultaneously made public additional AERs on ephedra received since the publication of the June 1997 proposed rule, as well as reviews of those AERs by the FDA and outside consultants (FDA, 2000).

In August, the Office of Women's Health (OWH) of the U.S. Department of Health and Human Services (HHS) held a two-day public hearing on the safety of ephedra in which testimony was presented by various scientific and medical experts who had conducted extensive reviews of the scientific and clinical literature on ephedra, as well as some who had conducted clinical investigations into the safety and benefits of ephedra for weight loss. At the OWH hearing, the Ephedra Education Council (EEC, an industry group) presented the consensus views of a seven-member panel comprised of experts from various medical and scientific disciplines who concluded, based on reviews of both the published literature and the entire public record of more than 1,000 AERs submitted to the FDA, that there was no evidence of an association between ephedra and significant adverse events at the intake levels established by the AHPA's 1994 standards and subsequently adopted as law by several states. The panel's multi-disciplinary review of the AERs, which was subsequently submitted to the FDA as public comment, was critical of reviews performed by FDA consultants, one of which was subsequently published (Haller and Benowitz, 2000). One member of the EEC panel also conducted the first comparison of incident rates of the adverse events at issue (e.g., stroke, heart attack, and seizure) in the general population and incident rates of the same events in ephedra consumers. His conclusion was that the analysis suggests that there was no evidence of increased risk, even using the most conservative of assumptions (Kimmel, 2000). In September 2000 the OWH issued a report recommending that additional research be conducted (OWH, 2000).

The FDA's review of 140 AERs, reportedly associated with the ingestion of ephedra-containing dietary supplements, from the FDA's MedWatch program concluded that 43 (31%) of the AERs were "definitely" or "probably" associated with ephedra use (Haller and Benowitz, 2000). In response to a critical letter to the editor (Hutchins, 2001) the authors cautioned that their report "does not prove causation, nor does it provide quantitative information with regard to risk" (Hutchins, 2001). A subsequent evaluation concluded: "These reports, while possibly associating the use of herbal dietary supplements containing ephedra with side effects, do not in any way prove a causative relationship between herbal use and these problems. On the other hand, controlled studies of supplements containing ephedra provide considerable evidence of efficacy in weight loss and weight maintenance." (Heber and Greenway, 2002).

There have been several attempts to put the number of ephedra-related AERs and ephedra-using consumers into perspective, but there are no accurate or reliable data on how many consumers are using ephedra, how many doses have been consumed, or how many AERs are directly related to ephedra consumption. According to a survey by AHPA of 14 companies that manufactured and marketed ephedra-containing supplements there was a 700% increase in sales in ephedra-containing supplements in five years from 1995 to 1999, representing 425 million "servings" sold in 1995 rising to an estimated 3 billion servings in 1999, with total estimated sales of ephedra supplements equaling 6.8 billion servings (McGuffin, 2000). (Technically, dietary supplements are considered foods, not drugs, under federal law, and thus what would normally be considered a "unit dose" by a pharmacist or physician must be referred to in food language by members of the herb and supplement industries, hence the term "serving.") A total of 66 serious adverse events were reported to these 14 responding companies over the 5-year period from 1995 to 1999. Based on the estimate of more than 6.8 billion servings sold in the same 5-year period, these AERs represent a reporting rate of less than 10 such reports per billion servings sold. According to the survey, these sales statistics, based on a large but not total segment of ephedra manufacturers, show that although the reported sales of supplements containing ephedrine alkaloids has increased more than seven-fold in the past 5 years, there has been no commensurate increase of adverse events gathered by FDA (McGuffin, 2000).

Ephedra

Monograph

In October 2000, a group of industry trade associations petitioned the FDA to accept proposed limits of 100 mg ephedra alkaloids per day and a proposed warning label (AHPA *et al.,* 2000). In December 2000, Cantox Health Sciences International (CHSI), an independent Canadian research organization, concluded, on the basis of a quantitative method developed by the National Academy of Sciences, that 90 mg per day is a safe upper limit for the ingestion of ephedra alkaloids in normal, healthy individuals and that the lowest observed adverse effect level (LOAEL) is 150 mg per day (CHSI, 2000; Hathcock, 2001). The safety assessment was based on a review of all available clinical studies on the alkaloid ephedrine and the herb ephedra, plus pharmacological and other relevant studies. CHSI also reviewed the FDA's AER database but concluded that due to insufficient and inconsistent clinical data, these reports were not useful for assessing product safety. (The Council for Responsible Nutrition, a Washington, D.C.-based trade association of dietary supplement manufacturers and suppliers, commissioned the review.)

Some experts have suggested that the relative safety and potential benefits of ephedra-containing dietary supplements should be viewed within the broader public health context of the prevalence of obesity in America. In December 2001, the U.S. Surgeon General David Satcher, M.D. estimated that 300,000 Americans die each year from illnesses caused or exacerbated by obesity (Anon., 2001b). Satcher said that 62% of Americans are either overweight or obese, compared to 48% in 1980 (Anon., 2001a). A comprehensive review article of the scientific and medical literature of caffeine and ephedrine combinations in the treatment of obesity (Greenway, 2001) summed up the situation:

> Overweight and obesity are common problems affecting more than half the population, yet obesity is stigmatized by society. Therefore, it is not surprising that an effective weight loss product containing compounds with a long history of safe non-prescription use would be embraced enthusiastically by the public. When large numbers of the public are using any product, adverse events will inevitably occur, but the cause and effect relationship of these adverse events to the product use are usually unclear. Obesity is a disease that predisposes to diabetes, hypertension, and cardiovascular disease. These increased risks are reversed with weight loss. The peer-reviewed scientific literature suggests that the risks of caffeine and ephedrine are outweighed by the benefits of achieving and maintaining a healthy weight. Confirmation of that conclusion for herbal products containing caffeine and ephedrine awaits controlled clinical trials.

Recent clinical research, published after the Greenway (2001) review, suggests that ephedra, in combination with other herbs, produces significant weight loss with no clinically significant adverse effects in the study participants, and with small impact on blood pressure or heart rate (Boozer *et al.,* 2002; de Jonge *et al.,* 2001) and safety (Belfie *et al.,* 2001). Based on these findings, additional research into the use of ephedra as a weight loss aid appears to be warranted. In June 2002, the Secretary of HHS called for more research on ephedra to determine its safety and efficacy (HHS, 2002). Supporters and some prominent critics of ephedra agree that scientific reviews of the cases of the AERs on ephedra do not establish causality, thereby making additional clinical research the key to developing regulatory policy.

DESCRIPTION

Ephedra consists of the dried, young branchlets, harvested in the fall, of *Ephedra sinica* Stapf [Fam. *Ephedraceae*] or other equivalent *Ephedra* species (Blumenthal *et al.,* 1998; DAB, 1999), including *E. intermedia* Schrenk ex C.A. Mey. and *E. equisetina* Bunge (syn. *E. shennungiana* Tang) (PPRC, 1997). The Japanese Pharmacopeia requires that it contain not less than 0.6% total alkaloids, calculated as ephedrine (JSHM, 1993). The *Pharmacopoeia of the People's Republic of China* requires not less than 0.8% (PPRC, 1997), and the *German Pharmacopoeia* requires not less than 1% (DAB, 1999).

PRIMARY USES

Respiratory System
- Mild bronchospasms in adults and children over the age of six (Blumenthal *et al.,*1998)
- Bronchodilator in treatment of bronchial asthma (WHO, 1999)

Ear Nose and Throat
- Nasal congestion due to hay fever, allergic rhinitis, acute coryza (rhinitis), common cold, sinusitis (WHO, 1999)

Obesity/Weight Management
- Increased weight loss and thermogenesis (Boozer *et al.,* 2002, 2001; Belfie *et al.,* 2001; de Jonge *et al.,* 2001; Greenway, 2001; Liu *et al.,* 1995; Astrup *et al.,* 1986; Pasquali *et al.,* 1985)

OTHER POTENTIAL USES
- Uses in Traditional Chinese Medicine (TCM) include common cold marked by chilliness and mild fever, headache, stuffed and running nose, general aching, but no sweating; edema in acute nephritis; bronchial asthma (PPRC, 1997).
- Ephedra dietary supplements are frequently used by athletes as performance enhancing agents (This use is highly controversial and has been the subject of numerous athletic groups' attempts to ban or restrict dietary supplements containing ephedra for this application.) (IOC, 2001; Anon., 2001c; NCAA, 2001)

DOSAGE

Internal

Crude Preparations
NOTE: According to U.S. herb industry labeling policy, the maximum adult daily dose for ephedra and ephedra-containing products is 100 mg total alkaloids (AHPA, 2002).

DECOCTION: 1–6 g dried herb daily (WHO, 1999), 1.5–9 g dried herb daily (PPRC, 1997). NOTE: The yield of alkaloids is higher with hot water decoction than with extraction with ethanol and/or methanol (Noguchi *et al.,* 1978). In a decoction made with ephedra containing a range of a minimum of 0.8% alkaloids (according to the *Pharmacopoeia of the People's Republic of China*, PPRC) to 1.0% (according to the *German Pharmacopoeia*), the estimated range of alkaloids based on the WHO daily dosage range would be 8–60 mg and the range based on the PPRC dosage would be 12–90 mg.

DRIED COMMINUTED HERB (According to the German Commission E for approved bronchial indications): the adult single dose corresponds to 15–30 mg total alkaloid, calculated as ephedrine. The adult maximum daily dose corresponds to 300 mg total alkaloid calculated as ephedrine. For a child (over age 6) a single dose corresponds to 0.5 mg total alkaloid per kg of body weight. A child's maximum daily dose is 2 mg total alkaloid per kg of body weight (Blumenthal *et al.,* 1998). [NOTE: This children's dosage is based on the recommendation for licensed preparations for the approved bronchial indication in Germany only. Ephedra supplements in the U.S. are not recommended for children under the age of 18, according to industry labeling policy.]

FLUID EXTRACT: 1:1 (*g/ml*), 45% alcohol, 1–3 ml daily (WHO, 1999).

TINCTURE: 1:4 (*g/ml*), 45% alcohol, 6–8 ml daily (WHO, 1999). Maximum weekly dose: 48 ml (Denham, 1998).

NO OBSERVED ADVERSE EFFECT LEVEL BASED ON THE CANTOX TOXICOLOGICAL REVIEW: ephedra preparations equivalent to 30 mg total alkaloids per dose; 90 mg per day (CHSI, 2000).

Purified Ephedra Derivatives (i.e., OTC drugs):
For bronchodilation the maximum adult daily dose of ephedrine (or usually its salt form, ephedrine hydrochloride) is 150 mg per day (21 CFRa), and the maximum adult daily dose of pseudoephedrine (or its salt form pseudoephedrine hydrocholoride) is 240mg per day (21 CFRb). [NOTE: for comparison purposes, the maximum daily nonprescription oral dose of caffeine is 1,600 mg (Heber and Greenway, 2002).]

DURATION OF ADMINISTRATION
The Commission E monograph, published in 1991, recommended that ephedra preparations should be used only short-term because of tachyphylaxis and potential addiction. NOTE: A more recent analysis of the available U.S. health and safety data compiled by Edgar H. Adams, M.S., Sc.D., former director of the Division of Epidemiology and Statistical Analysis at the U.S. National Institute on Drug Abuse, indicates that there is no evidence of significant abuse of, or addiction to, ephedra despite decades of widespread use, concluding that any potential for addiction is low and does not rise to the level of regulatory concern that warrants scheduling (as is done with addictive narcotic drugs) (Adams, 2000). Nevertheless, as with other stimulant products that enhance athletic performance, products containing ephedra alkaloids are still banned by the International Olympic Committee for use by athletes competing in the Olympic games (IOC, 2001).

CHEMISTRY
The herb ephedra contains approximately 1.3% alkaloids composed mainly of ephedrine (up to 90%), pseudoephedrine, norephedrine, nor-pseudoephedrine, methylephedrine, and methylpseudoephedrine (Huang, 1999; Tang and Eisenbrand, 1992). These alkaloids are the primary active constituents. Other components include flavonoid glycosides; glycans (ephedrans); citric, malic, and oxalic acids; proanthocyanidins (condensed tannins); tannins and volatile oils (l-*a*-terpineol, limonene, and linalool) (Bruneton, 1995) but these compounds are not believed to exert much influence on the well established pharmacological effects of this herb.

PHARMACOLOGICAL ACTIONS
The pharmacological data cited below pertain to research conducted on the whole ephedra herb or its extracts, as well as to the isolated alkaloids ephedrine and pseudoephedrine, plus (as noted below) combinations of ephedrine and caffeine, or ephedrine and aspirin. Extensive clinical and pharmacological research has been conducted on ephedrine, usually its salt form, e.g. ephedrine hydrochloride (Astrup *et al.*, 1986; Tang and Eisenbrand, 1992), ephedrine and caffeine (Astrup *et al.*, 1991; Astrup *et al.*, 1992; Astrup and Toubro, 1993), and an ephedrine-caffeine-aspirin combination (Daly *et al.*, 1993). These results are probably directly relevant to the actions of the herb ephedra or its combinations with caffeine-containing herbs. One review on thermogenic agents states that the effects of ephedra and ephedrine are the same, except that ephedra is gentler and less likely to cause adverse effects, with the large body of scientific data on ephedrine being applicable to ephedra (Jones, 2001). A small clinical trial suggests similar pharmacokinetics between the ephedrine in ephedra and synthetic ephedrine (Gurley *et al.*, 1998). Research shows that ephedra alkaloids (e.g., ephedrine) from supplements containing ephedra *extracts* are absorbed more quickly than the alkaloids from preparations containing powdered ephedra herb, and thus products containing extracts probably exhibit absorption and disposition characteristics indistinguishable from those products containing isolated ephedra alkaloids (e.g., OTC drugs) (Gurley, 2000). For a detailed review of the clinical pharmacology of ephedrine, see Tang and Eisenbrand (1992), and for ephedrine combined with caffeine and/or aspirin, see Heber and Greenway (2002).

Human
- Ephedrine and related alkaloids produce sympathomimetic effects, including vasoconstriction, increased heart rate, and stimulation of central nervous system (Weiner, 1985).

- Ephedra herb preparations are shown to produce dilated bronchi (WHO, 1999), and induce perspiration (diaphoretic), and diuresis (diuretic) (PPRC, 1997).

- Increased thermogenesis and weight loss in obese patients (ephedra-caffeine herb combination) (Boozer *et al.*, 2002, 2001).

- Ephedrine stimulates brown adipose tissue (BAT) in rodents, but since humans possess relatively little BAT, ephedrine-induced thermogenesis happens mainly in skeletal muscle (Astrup, 1986).

- Ephedrine decreases gastric emptying, possibly contributing to reduction of food intake (Jonderko and Kucio, 1991).

An ephedrine-caffeine combination was found safe and effective in a pilot study on 32 obese adolescents, reducing weight more than 5% in 81% of the treatment group, compared to 31% in the placebo group (Molnar *et al.*, 2000).

An acute dose of a combination of ephedrine (30 mg) and aspirin (300 mg) produced greater post-prandial thermogenesis in 10 obese women for 160 minutes following a liquid meal than an acute dose of ephedrine (30 mg) alone. Aspirin alone did not produce this additional effect on thermogenesis in 10 lean women (Horton and Geissler, 1991) while ephedrine and aspirin normalized the post-prandial thermogenesis in obese women to levels equal to the lean (Geissler, 1993).

- Stimulation of central nervous system and cardiovascular parameters (i.e., increases in pulse rate, blood pressure, and serum glucose levels) have been documented when ephedrine and/or caffeine are given acutely either separately or together. According to a recent review of the peer reviewed literature, these side effects disappear with chronic use and are no longer present after 4 to 12 weeks, depending on the trial (Heber and Greenway, 2002).

There has been concern about the potential hypertensive effects of ephedra and its alkaloids. However, in one trial a proprietary ephedrine (20 mg) and caffeine (200 mg) preparation tested for its weight loss effects on 136 overweight normotensive or drug-controlled subjects with controlled hypertension, three doses of the product showed blood pressure-lowering effects over 6 weeks (Svendsen *et al.*, 1998). Systolic blood pressure was reduced 5.5 mm HG more in the controlled hypertensive subjects treated with the preparation than placebo in subjects treated with medication other than beta-blockers. The anti-hypertensive effect of the beta-blocker drug was not reduced by the caffeine-ephedrine combination. The normotensive patients treated with caffeine and ephedrine had a 4.4/3.9 mm HG greater drop in blood pressure than those treated with placebo. The mean loss of weight of 4 kg (8.8 lbs.) was significant for all groups.

- A recent review of ephedrine cites literature proposing it as an adjunct to cognitive restructuring and notes that ephedrine has been considered in reviews about non-prescription weight loss supplements, obesity management, energy balance, and obesity treatment (Heber and Greenway, 2002).

There has been recent concern about the use of dietary supplements containing the herb ephedra when used as performance enhancers in athletic activities. Although no studies are available on the herb ephedra in athletic performance, numerous clinical trials conducted at the Canadian Defence and Civil Institute of Environmental Medicine have measured the effects of ephedrine and caffeine combinations on exercise and related performance activities. These pilot studies have concluded that the combination of ephedrine (E) and caffeine (C), or ephedrine alone, produces the following effects in athletes or soldiers: (1) an improvement in anaerobic exercise performance is likely a result of both stimulation of the CNS by E and skeletal muscle by C (Bell *et al.* 2001); (2) although the metabolic rate in subjects was slightly increased with C+E treatment, it was sufficiently offset by increased heat loss mechanisms so that internal body temperature was not increased during moderate exercise in a hot, dry environment (Bell *et al.*, 1999a); (3) C+E improved performance of the Canadian Forces Warrior Test, a 3.2 km run wearing about 11 kg of battlefield uniform and equipment (Bell, Jacobs, 1999b); (4) C+E significantly prolonged exercise time to exhaustion compared to placebo, while neither C nor E treatments alone significantly changed time to exhaustion, the improved performance being attributed to increased CNS stimulation (Bell *et al.*, 1998); (5) the previously observed additive effects of C+E was not evident, with the primary ergogenic effect being attributed to E (Bell *et al.*, 2002); and (6) a lower dose (approx. 20% lower) of C+E than used previously resulted in an ergogenic effect similar in magnitude to that reported previously with a higher dose, and with a reduced incidence of negative side effects (vomiting and nausea) (Bell *et al.*, 2000).

Animal

- Ephedra herb prevents or relieves coughing and inhibits growth of bacteria in animal experiments, according to the Commission E (Blumenthal *et al.*, 1998);
- Ephedra stimulates the sympathetic nervous system in dogs (Huang, 1999), analogues of feruloyl-histamine, an alkaloid in ephedra *roots*, inhibit hypotension and histidine decarboxylase, is anti-ulcerous and anti-hepatoxic (Hikino *et al.*, 1984);
- Ephenadrines block ganglions (Hikino *et al.*, 1983);

- Pseudoephedrine relieves inflammation (Hikino *et al.*, 1980).

MECHANISM OF ACTION

All mechanistic data cited below pertain to isolated ephedra alkaloids.

- Ephedrine indirectly stimulates the sympathomimetic and central nervous systems (Blumenthal *et al.*, 1998). It has been shown to produce sympathomimetic effects (e.g., vasoconstriction and cardiac stimulation) by combining with α- and β-adrenergic receptors (WHO, 1999; Hardman *et al.*, 1996; Chang and But, 1986);
- The chemical structure of ephedrine resembles epinephrine (adrenaline) (Chang and But, 1986), though unlike epinephrine, it is completely absorbed from the intestine and has a much longer duration of action (Huang, 1999);
- Ephedrine triggers the release of endogenous catecholamines from post-ganglionic sympathetic fibers (Bruneton, 1995);
- Ephedrine relaxes bronchial muscles and acts as a bronchodilator by activating the β-adrenoceptors in the lungs (Weiner, 1985; Hardman *et al.*, 1996);
- Both ephedrine and pseudoephedrine inhibit norepinephrine uptake by nervous and nonnervous tissues (Chang and But, 1986);
- Ephedrine (i.v.) stimulates beta-1 receptors (stimulating heart rate), beta-2, and beta-3 receptors (stimulating glucose and oxygen consumption), insulin, and c-peptide (Jaedig and Henningsen, 1991).

CONTRAINDICATIONS

The Commission E noted the following contraindications: anxiety and restlessness, hypertension, glaucoma, impaired circulation of the cerebrum, adenoma of the prostate with residual urine accumulation, pheochromocytoma, and thyrotoxicosis (Blumenthal *et al.*, 1998). Additional contraindications include pregnancy, anorexia, diabetes, heart disease, insomnia, stomach ulcers, renal failure, and in children (Brinker, 2001).

The industry label warning for ephedra, currently being suggested as an official national standard by a group of dietary supplement industry trade organizations in a petition to the FDA, is as follows: "WARNING: Not intended for use by anyone under the age of 18. Do not use this product if you are pregnant or nursing. Consult a health care professional before using this product if you have heart disease, thyroid disease, diabetes, high blood pressure, depression or other psychiatric condition, glaucoma, difficulty in urinating, prostate enlargement, or seizure disorder, if you are using a monoamine oxidase inhibitor (MAO), or any other prescription drug, or you are using an over-the-counter drug containing ephedrine, pseudoephedrine or phenylpropanolamine (PPA) (ingredients found in certain allergy, asthma, cough/cold and weight control products). [PPA has been removed from the OTC market, but consumers might still possess older PPA-containing drug products.] Exceeding recommended serving will not improve results and may cause serious adverse health effects. Discontinue use and call a health care professional immediately if you experience rapid heartbeat, dizziness, severe headache, shortness of breath, or other similar symptoms." (AHPA *et al.*, 2000).

PREGNANCY AND LACTATION: Not recommended for use during pregnancy or lactation (Brinker, 2001; McGuffin *et al.*, 1997).

ADVERSE EFFECTS

According to the Commission E, the adverse effects of the herb ephedra include insomnia, motor restlessness, irritability, headaches, nausea, vomiting, disturbances of urination, and tachycardia. The commission also noted that higher dosages (presumably higher than the Commission E's recommended daily limit, equivalent to 300 mg ephedra alkaloids) may produce a drastic increase in blood pressure, cardiac arrhythmia, and development of dependency (Blumenthal et al., 1998). (See "Note" about dependency in "Duration of Administration" above.)

There have been isolated reports of adverse events, some serious, including stroke and death, in the published literature. Some are related to overdosing; others (e.g., possible myocarditis in a few case reports) are attributed to the consumption of relatively normal levels (Leikin and Klein, 2000; Zaacks et al., 1999).

In a recent review of FDA's AERs (926 cases reported to FDA between 1995 to 1997) focusing on 37 patients, ephedra use was temporarily related to stroke (16 patients, 3 deaths), myocardial infarction (10), or sudden death (11), noting that cardiovascular adverse effects were not limited to large doses (Samenuk et al., 2002). (This review relied on the same FDA database of AERs that had been previously analyzed and questioned for accuracy by the GAO.)

One highly publicized review of selected events reported to the FDA concluded that the AERs do not establish causality and cannot be used to quantify risk (Haller and Benowitz, 2000). This paper reviewed 140 reports of adverse events associated with the use of dietary supplements containing ephedra alkaloids submitted to the FDA between June 1, 1997, and March 31, 1999. The authors employed a standardized rating system for evaluating causation. They concluded that 43 (31%) cases were *definitely* or *probably* related to the use of ephedra-containing supplements, 44 cases (31%) deemed *possibly* related to the use of ephedra supplements, and 24 cases (17%) were considered unrelated. Of the adverse events that were assessed to be definitely, probably, or possibly related to the use of ephedra supplements, 47% involved cardiovascular symptoms and 18% involved the central nervous system. The most frequently reported adverse event was hypertension (17 reports), followed by palpitations, tachycardia, or both (13); stroke (10); and seizures (7). Ten events were associated with deaths, and 13 associated events resulted in permanent disability; these represent 26% of the definite, probable, and possible cases. In response to a critical letter to the editor (Hutchins, 2001) the authors cautioned that their report "does not prove causation, nor does it provide quantitative information with regard to risk" (Hutchins, 2001). A recent review concluded, "These reports, while possibly associating the use of herbal dietary supplements containing ephedra with side effects, do not in any way prove a causative relationship between herbal use and these problems." (Heber and Greenway, 2002).

More extensive evaluations of the entire FDA database of AERs have been submitted to the FDA, suggesting no association between clinically significant adverse events at doses of up to 100 mg per day (EEC, 2000; CHSI, 2000).

The AERs associated with ephedra have been analyzed from an epidemiological perspective suggesting no greater incidence of seizures, strokes, and myocardial infarctions (MIs) in persons consuming dietary supplements containing ephedrine alkaloids than that expected in the general U.S. population (Kimmel, 2000).

The Secretary of HHS, in a press release announcing plans to study ephedra, stated as follows:

> Adverse event reports regarding the use of dietary supplements containing ephedrine alkaloids have been received by the Food and Drug Administration (FDA) and have raised questions regarding the safety of these products. However, the FDA has advised that adverse event reports alone regarding dietary supplements containing ephedrine alkaloids do not provide a scientific basis for assessing the safety of these products and that there is need for further scientific research. (HHS, 2002).

Isolated ephedrine has been reported to cause urinary difficulty in men with benign prostatic hyperplasia and is believed to exacerbate angle-closure glaucoma (Dvorak et al., 1997), forming the basis for the contraindications for these conditions noted above. Other adverse effects documented for ephedrine in controlled conditions include agitation, insomnia, headache, weakness, palpitations, giddiness, tremors, and constipation; these effects were noted only with 50 mg dose given three times daily (total 150 mg per day), with amelioration during the duration of use, with no significant changes in pulse rate or blood pressure (Pasquali and Casimirri, 1993). The German phytomedicine authority R.F. Weiss, claims that the natural ephedrine found in ephedra is "better tolerated, causing fewer heart symptoms such as palpitation" than synthetic ephedrine (Weiss, 1988), although a revision of his book by another author suggests that patients use synthetic beta-sympathomimetics for bronchodilation due to the potential toxicity of ephedra (Weiss and Fintelmann, 2000).

DRUG INTERACTIONS

The following are actual or potential interactions of orally ingested ephedrine alkaloids (mainly ephedrine and/or pseudoephedrine, not necessarily the herb ephedra itself), with other substances. Documented interactions are derived mainly from human case studies or clinical trials, based on the alkaloid intake at various dosages.

ANTIHYPERTENSIVES, INCLUDING ACE INHIBITORS AND BETA-BLOCKERS: May be antagonized with resulting severe hypertension (speculative) (Brinker, 2001).

BROMOCRIPTINE: Dopaminergic activity may become increasingly toxic due to ephedra's sympathomimetic actions (speculative) (Brinker, 2001).

CARDIAC GLYCOSIDES OR HALOTHANE: Can cause arrhythmia (Brinker, 2001).

CORTICOSTEROIDS: Increases the clearance of dexamethasone, decreasing its activity (Brinker, 2001; Jubiz and Meikle, 1979).

GUANETHIDINE: Antagonizes the hypotensive effect (Brinker, 2001).

MAO-INHIBITORS (including tranylcypromine, pargyline, procarbazine, selegiline, phenelzine, and moclobemide) Significantly raise the sympathomimetic action of ephedrine (Brinker, 2001).

METHYL XANTHINES (e.g., caffeine, theophylline): Increase thermogenesis and weight loss with reduction in body fat when ephedrine is combined with xanthines, plus excessive nervous stimulation (noted in some case reports) (Brinker, 2001).

CAFFEINE: The alkaloids in ephedra combined with methylxanthines have been demonstrated to be synergistic on oxygen consumption in animals. A recent review noted both the caffeine and the catechins in various types of tea (*Camellia sinensis*), e.g., oolong tea, may interact with respect to respiration of brown adipose tissue, based on *in vitro* evidence. Catechins in green tea are synergistic with respect to oxygen consumption with caffeine, ephedrine, and the combination of caffeine and ephedrine; catechins inhibit catechol-*O*-methyl transferase, the enzyme that breaks down norepinephrine (Heber and Greenway, 2002).

SECALE ALKALOID DERIVATIVES OR OXYTOCIN: Develop hypertension (listed by German Commission E) (Blumenthal *et al.*, 1998).

SYMPATHOMIMETICS: May be potentiated when used with ephedra or ephedra alkaloids (speculative) (Brinker, 2001).

URINARY ALKALIZERS e.g., acetazolamide (Wilkinson and Beckett, 1968); sodium bicarbonate: Excrete more slowly than with urinary acidifiers (e.g., ammonium chloride), due to effects of reabsorption from tubules in the kidneys (Brinker, 2001).

AMERICAN HERBAL PRODUCTS ASSOCIATION (AHPA) SAFETY RATING

CLASS 2B: Not for use during pregnancy.

CLASS 2C: Not for use during nursing.

CLASS 2D: Contraindicated with anorexia, bulimia, and glaucoma; thyroid stimulant; not recommended for excessive or long-term use; may potentiate pharmaceutical MAO-inhibitors (McGuffin *et al.*,1997).

REGULATORY STATUS

AUSTRALIA: Ephedra, and products containing ephedra, are controlled substances listed in the Customs Prohibited Imports Regulations. Import permit required (TGA, 2001).

CANADA: Included in Drugs Directorate "List of Herbs Unacceptable as Non-medicinal Ingredients in Oral Use Products" (Health Canada, 1995). Ephedra Labeling Standard: Approved Schedule OTC drug with specific indications: (1) Traditional Herbal Medicine (THM) for relief of nasal congestion (cold, hayfever); (2) Traditional Herbal Nasal Decongestant. Dried young stem contains no less than 1.25% total alkaloids calculated as l-ephedrine (Health Canada, 1996). Also, permitted as a homeopathic drug. In either case requires premarket authorization and assignment of a Drug Identification Number (DIN) (Health Canada, 2001). In January, 2002 Health Canada issued a "voluntary recall" for ephedra- and ephedrine-containing products that are marketed for unapproved uses, e.g., appetite suppression, promoting weight loss, or increasing energy; or that contain over 8 mg ephedrine or a total dose of ephedrine alkaloids exceeding 32 mg per day (Lawlor, 2002).

CHINA: Dried herbaceous stem containing no less than 0.80% total alkaloids, calculated as ephedrine, official drug of the *Pharmacopoeia of the People's Republic of China* (PPRC, 1997).

FRANCE: Ephedra removed from *French Pharmacopoeia*. Isolated ephedrine is official (Bruneton, 1995).

GERMANY: Dried young whole or cut branchlet collected in autumn containing no less than 1.0% total alkaloids (as ephedrine) official in *German Pharmacopoeia* (DAB, 1999). Dried young branchlet is approved drug of the German Commission E (Blumenthal *et al.*, 1998).

JAPAN: Traditional Kampo medicine (Tsumura, 1996). Dried terrestrial stem containing no less than 0.15% total alkaloids (as ephedrine) official in *Japanese Pharmacopoeia* (JSHM, 1993).

SWEDEN: No products containing ephedra are presently registered in the Medical Products Agency's (MPA) "Authorized Natural Remedies," "Homeopathic Remedies" or "Drugs" listings (MPA, 2001a and 2001b).

SWITZERLAND: No monograph in the Swiss pharmacopeia. No ephedra-containing products are listed in the *Swiss Codex 2000/01* (Ruppanner and Schaefer, 2000). Since 1992, traditional Chinese medicine (TCM) has been made available as a primary health care option in the national HMO. Patients who choose TCM for their primary health care plan may receive traditional Chinese herbal medicines (which may contain ephedra) by prescription (Grüninger, 1992).

U.K.: Schedule III herb recommended to be limited for use by medical herbalists only (Denham, 1998).

U.S.: Dietary supplement (USC, 1994) and approved OTC drug ingredient, for bronchodilation (25 mg/dose orally up to 6 times per day, no limit on duration of use) and as a nasal decongestant (nasal spray) (21 CFR a-d).

CLINICAL REVIEW

Seven studies conducted on the herb ephedra (327 total participants) are summarized in the Table of Clinical Studies on Ephedra. One study on a preparation containing only powdered ephedra measured cardiovascular effects and pharmacokinetics (White *et al.*, 1997). However, few clinical trials are based on ephedra as a single ingredient. Most ephedra trials tested multi-ingredient formulations that include a caffeine-containing herb like cola nut (*Cola nitida*) (Boozer *et al.*, 2002; DeJong *et al.*, 2001; Greenway *et al.*, 2000) or guarana (*Paullinia cupana*) (Belfie *et al.*, 2001; Boozer *et al.* 2001). The Boozer *et al.*, 2002 and 2001 trials focused on weight loss and safety. One small randomized, crossover trial concluded that the pharmacokinetic properties of ephedrine in ephedra in dietary supplements were similar to those of synthetic ephedrine hydrochloride (Gurley *et al.*, 1998). At least three clinical studies have been conducted on the isolated alkaloid ephedrine for its use in weight loss (Liu *et al.*, 1995; Astrup *et al.*, 1986; Pasquali *et al.*, 1985), as summarized in the Table of Clinical Studies on Ephedra.

[EDITORS' NOTE: the following studies are not listed in the Table of Clinical Studies on Ephedra or the Table of Clinical Studies on Ephedrine.] Several unpublished trials employed four different ephedra products (ephedra only, not combinations) on 300 subjects over a period of six weeks and six months, to monitor weight loss and adverse effects respectively. The studies concluded that ephedra appears to be safe, effective, and cost-effective; and compares favorably with pharmaceutical weight loss agents, with a relatively low side effect profile (Huber, 2001). Clinical trials have been successfully conducted for weight loss using ephedrine and caffeine combinations (Astrup and Toubro, 1993; Astrup *et al.*, 1992, 1991) and a much-publicized Danish formula of ephedrine in combination with caffeine and aspirin demonstrated the relative safety and efficacy of this combination for weight loss (Daly *et al.*, 1993).

BRANDED PRODUCTS

DietMax®: NaturalMax Co./ Kal Inc., Div. Nutraceutical Corp., 1400 Kearns Blvd. / Park City, Utah 84060 / U.S.A. / Tel: (800) 669-8877 / www.nutraceutical.com. Each tablet contains 110 mg extract standardized to 8% ephedra alkaloids, equivalent to 5 mg ephedrine, 50 mg standardized kola nut extract (equivalent to 10 mg caffeine), 50 mg mustard seed powder, 50 mg spirulina, 50 mg ascorbic acid (vitamin C), potassium citrate 25 mg, magnesium aspartate 25 mg.

Escalation™: Enzymatic Therapy / 825 Challenger Drive / Green Bay, WI 54311 / U.S.A. / Tel: 920-469-1313 / www.enzy.com. Each capsule contains 250 mg cola (*Cola nitida*) nut extract containing 35 mg of caffeine alkaloids; 250 mg ephedra aerial part extract containing 15mg concentrated ephedrine group alkaloids in the form of herbal extracts; and 110 mg green tea (*Camellia sinensis*) leaf extract containing 15 mg of caffeine alkaloids.

Excel: Excel Corporation / Salt Lake City, UT: no information available.

Metabolife 356®: Metabolife International, 5070 Santa Fe Street / San Diego, CA 92109 / U.S.A. / Tel: (858) 490-5222 / www.metabolife.com. Each tablet contains 12 mg of ephedrine group alkaloids and 40 mg of caffeine alkaloids, combined with the following ingredients: Ma huang, Siberian ginseng (Eleuthero), lecithin, ginger root, damiana, sarsaparilla root, goldenseal, gotu kola, spirulina, algae, bee pollen, nettle leaf, royal jelly, bovine complex, 6 I.U. vitamin E, 75 mg magnesium chelate, 5 mg zinc chelate, and 75 mcg chromium picolinate.

Solaray® Ephedra: Nutraceutical Corp. Each capsule contains 375 mg powdered ephedra herb calculated at 4.8 mg ephedrine, 1.2 mg pseudoephedrine, 0.3 mg methyl-ephedrine per capsule.

Up Your Gas: National Health Products / 731 South Kirkman Road / Orlando, FL 32811 / U.S.A. / Tel: (407) 297-7671. Each capsule contains: 30 IU Vitamin E (as dl-alpha-tocopherol acetate); 255 mg calcium (as dicalcium phosphate and calcium carbonate); 4.5 mg magnesium (as magnesium carbonate); 5 mg potassium (as potassium bicarbonate); and 695 mg Up Your Gas Blend consisting of: guarana concentrate (seed), mahuang extract (*Ephedra sinica*) (stem) (285 mg of 6% alkaloid extract), ginseng extract (root), bee pollen, spirulina blue green algae, gotu kola (leaf), inosine monophosphate, pyridoxal-alpha-ketoglutarate, wheat grass, cayenne pepper (fruit), lipoic acid, co-enzyme Q-10, and octacosanol.

REFERENCES

21 CFRa [Code of Federal Regulations] Sect. 341.76 Food and Drug Administration, Department of Health and Human Services. Labeling of Bronchodilator Drug Products.

21 CFRb [Code of Federal Regulations] Sect. 341.80. Food and Drug Administration, Department of Health and Human Services. Labeling of Nasal Decongestant Drug Products.

21 CFRc [Code of Federal Regulations] Sect. 341.16 Food and Drug Administration, Department of Health and Human Services. Bronchodilator Active Ingredients.

21 CFRd [Code of Federal Regulations] Sect. 341.20. Food and Drug Administration, Department of Health and Human Services. Nasal Decongestant Active Ingredients.

Adams E. Statement of Edgar H. Adams, M.S., Sc.D. Submitted to FDA; Docket No. 98N–0148, cmt. 28, tab A: February 10, 1999.

AHPA. See: American Herbal Products Association.

American Herbal Products Association (AHPA). Policy Statement on *Ephedra sinica* (Ma huang). Austin, TX, 1994 Mar. 30.

American Herbal Products Association (AHPA), Consumer Healthcare Products Association, National Nutritional Foods Association, and Utah Natural Products Alliance. Citizens Petition to FDA on Ephedra Labeling. Oct. 25, 2000.

American Herbal Products Association (AHPA). Code of Ethics and Business Conduct. Silver Spring (MD): AHPA; 2002 Jul [cited 2002 Nov 13]. Available at: URL: http://www.ahpa.org/CodeJuly02.pdf.

Anonymous. NFL bans ephedrine, other stimulants. NFL News 2001c Sept 27. Available from:URL: http://www.nfl.com/news/2001/ephedrine092701.html.

Anonymous. Obesity becoming top threat to health. *Los Angeles Times* article published in *Austin American-Statesman*, Dec. 14, 2001a.

Anonymous. U.S. warning of death toll from obesity. Associated Press in *New York Times*. Dec. 14, 2001b.

Astrup A. Thermogenesis in human brown adipose tissue and skeletal muscle induced by sympathomimetic stimulation. *Acta Endocrinol* 1986(suppl.);278:1-32.

Astrup A, Breum L, Toubro S *et al.* The effect and safety of an ephedrine/caffeine compound compared to ephedrine, caffeine and placebo in obese subjects on an energy restricted diet. A double-blind trial. *Int J Obesity* 1992;16:269–77.

Astrup A, Madsen J, Holst JJ, Christensen NJ. The effect of chronic ephedrine treatment on substrate utilization, the sympathoadrenal activity, and energy expenditure during glucose-induced thermogenesis in man. *Metabolism* 1986;35(3):260–5.

Astrup A, Toubro S. Thermogenic, metabolic, and cardiovascular responses to ephedrine and caffeine in man. *Int J Obesity* 1993;17 (suppl):S41–3.

Astrup A, Toubro S, Cannon S *et al.* Thermogenic synergism between ephedrine and caffeine in healthy volunteers: A double-blind, placebo-controlled study. *Metabolism* 1991;40(3):323–9.

BAnz. See: *Bundesanzeiger*.

Belfie L, Petrie H, Chown S *et al.* Safety and effectiveness of an herbal dietary supplement containing ephedra (ma huang) and caffeine (guarana extract) when used in combination with a supervised diet and exercise intervention [presentation abstract]. *Obesity Research* 2001;9(S3):26.

Bell DG, McLellan TM, Sabiston CM. Effect of ingesting caffeine and ephedrine on 10-km run performance. *Med Sci Sports Exerc* 2002;34(2):344–9.

Bell DG, Jacobs I, Ellerington K. Effect of caffeine and ephedrine ingestion on anaerobic exercise performance. *Med Sci Sports Exerc* 2001;33(8):1399–403.

Bell DG, Jacobs I, McLellan TM, Zamecnik J. Reducing the dose of combined caffeine and ephedrine preserves the ergogenic effect. *Aviat Space Environ Med* 2000;71(4):415–9.

Bell DG, Jacobs I, McLellan TM, Miyazaki M, Sabiston CM. Thermal regulation in the heat during exercise after caffeine and ephedrine ingestion. *Aviat Space Environ Med* 1999a;70(6):583–8.

Bell DG, Jacobs I. Combined caffeine and ephedrine ingestion improves run times of Canadian forces warrior test. *Aviat Space Environ Med* 1999b Apr;70(4):325-9.

Bell DG, Jacobs I, Zamecnik J. Effects of caffeine, ephedrine and their combination on time exhaustion during high intensity exercise, *Eur J Appl Physiol* 1998:77:427-33.

Bensky D, Gamble A. *Chinese Herbal Medicine Materia Medica.* Revised (ed.). Seattle, WA: Eastland Press;1993.

Blanck HM, Khan LK, Serdula MK. Use of nonprescription weight loss products: results from a multistate survey. *JAMA* 2001;286(8):930-5.

Blumenthal M, Busse WR, Goldberg A, Gruenwald J, Hall T, Riggins CW, Rister RS (eds.). Klein S, Rister RS (trans.). *The Complete German Commission E Monographs—Therapeutic Guide to Herbal Medicines.* Austin, TX: American Botanical Council; Boston: Integrative Medicine Communication; 1998.

Blumenthal M, Goldberg A, Brinckmann J. *Herbal Medicine—Expanded Commission E Monographs.* Austin: American Botanical Council; Boston, MA: Integrative Medicine Communication; 2000.

Blumenthal M, King P. The agony of the ecstasy: Herbal high products get media attention. *HerbalGram* 1996; 37:20-24,32,49.

Blumenthal M, King P. Ma Huang: Ancient herb, modern medicine, regulatory dilemma. *HerbalGram* 1995;34:22–27,42–3,56–7.

Boozer CN, Daly PA, Homel P, Solomon JL, Blanchard D, Sanner JA, *et al.* Herbal ephedra/caffeine for weight loss: a 6-month randomized safety and efficacy trial. *Int J Obes* 2002;26:593-604.

Boozer C, Nasser J, Heymsfield S, Wang V, Chen G, Solomon J. An herbal supplement containing ma huang-guarana for weight loss: a randomized, double-blind trial. *Intl J Obesity* 2001 Mar;25(3):316–24.

Brinker F. *Herb Contraindications and Drug Interactions*, 3d ed. Sandy, OR: Eclectic Medical Publications; 2001:87–90.

Bruneton J. *Pharmacognosy, Phytochemistry, Medicinal Plants.* Paris, France: Lavoisier Publishing; 1995:711–4.

Bundesanzeiger (BAnz). *Monographien der Kommission E* (Zulassungs- und Aufbereitungskommission am BGA für den humanmed. Bereich, phytotherapeutische Therapierichtung und Stoffgruppe). Köln: Bundesgesundheitsamt (BGA); 1998.

Cantox Health Sciences International (CHSI). Safety assessment and determination of a tolerable upper limit for ephedra. December 2000. http://www.crnusa.org/CRNCantoxreportindex.html.

Chang H, But P (eds.). *Pharmacology and Applications of Chinese Materia Medica*, Vol. 1. Philadelphia, PA: World Scientific;1986:1119–24.

CHSI. See: Cantox Health Sciences International.

Code of Federal Regulations. See: 21 CFR.

DAB. See: *Deutsches Arzneibuch*.

Daly PA, Krieger DR, Dulloo AG *et al.* Ephedrine, caffeine, and aspirin: safety and efficacy for treatment of human obesity. *Int J Obesity* 1993;17 (suppl):S73–8.

De Jonge L, Frisard M, Blanchard D, Greenway F. Safety and efficacy of an herbal dietary supplement containing caffeine and ephedra for obesity treatment. *Obesity Research* 2001;9(S3):20.

Denham A. The 1968 Medicines Act – Schedule 3 herbs, and their use by practitioners. *Eur J Herbal Med* 1998;4(3):19–28.

Der Marderosian A (ed.). *The Review of Natural Products*. St. Louis: Facts and Comparisons; 1999.

Deutsches Arzneibuch (DAB 1999). Stuttgart, Germany: Deutscher Apotheker Verlag;1999.

Dvorak R, Starling RD, Calles-Escandon J *et al*. Drug therapy for obesity in the elderly. *Drugs Aging* 1997;11:338-51.

EEC. See: Ephedra Education Council.

Ephedra Education Council (EEC). Comments of the Expert Panel of the Ephedra Education Council on the Safety of Dietary Supplements Containing Ephedrine Alkaloids and on the Adverse Event Reports (AERs) and Health Assessments Released by the Food and Drug Administration (FDA) on April 3, 2000. Submitted to FDA; Docket No. 00N-1200: September 29, 2000.

FDA. See: Food and Drug Administration.

Fleming T. *PDR for Herbal Medicines*. Montvale, NJ: Medical Economics Co.; 1998.

Food and Drug Administration (FDA). Dietary Supplements Containing Ephedrine Alkaloids: Proposed Rule. *Federal Register* 1997;62(107):30678–717.

Food and Drug Administration (FDA). FDA announces the availability of new ephedrine and "street drug alternative" documents. *FDA Talk Paper*, 2000 Mar 31 [cited 2002 Jul 3]. Available from: URL: http://www.cfsan.fda.gov/~lrd/tpephedr.html.

GAO. See: General Accounting Office.

Geissler CA. Effects of weight loss, ephedrine and aspirin on energy expenditure in obese women. *Int J Obes Relat Metab Disord* 1993;17 (suppl. 1):S45-8.

General Accounting Office (GAO). Dietary Supplements: Uncertainties in Analyses Underlying FDA's Proposed Rule on Ephedrine Alkaloids. Washington, DC: United States General Accounting Office; 1999 July.

Greenway F. The safety and efficacy of pharmaceutical and herbal caffeine and ephedrine use as a weight loss agent. *Obesity Rev* 2001;2:199-211.

Greenway F, Raum W, DeLany J. The effect of an herbal dietary supplement containing ephedrine and caffeine on oxygen consumption in human. *J Alt Compl Med* 2000;6(6):553–5.

Grüninger T. Traditional Chinese Medicine in ENT. [in German]. *HMO Aktuell* 1992;3:3.

Gurley B. Extract versus herb: effect of formulation on the absorption rate of botanical ephedrine from dietary supplements containing Ephedra (ma huang). *Ther Drug Monitoring* 2000;22(4):497.

Gurley B, Gardner S, White L, Wang P. Ephedrine pharmacokinetics after the ingestion of nutritional supplements containing *Ephedra sinica* (ma huang). *Ther Drug Monit* 1998 Aug;20(4):439–45.

Haller C, Benowitz N. Adverse cardiovascular and central nervous system events associated with dietary supplements containing ephedra alkaloids. *N Engl J Med* 2000 Dec 21;343(25):1833–8.

Hardman J, Limbird L, Molinoff P, Ruddon R, Gilman A (eds.). *Goodman and Gilman's The Pharmacological Basis of Therapeutics*, 9th ed. New York: MacMillan Publishing;1996:221.

Harnack LJ, Rydell SA, Stang J. Prevalence of use of herbal products by adults in the Minneapolis/St. Paul, Minn, metropolitan area. *Mayo Clin Proc* 2001;76(7):688–94.

Hathcock JN. CRN's Cantox Report on the Quantitative Risk Assessment of Ephedra. *HerbalGram* 2001;53:31–3.

Health & Human Services (HHS). HHS announces plans to study ephedra: steps up enforcement of illegal ephedrine marketing [press release]. HHS; 2002 Jun 14 [cited 2002 Jul 3]. Available from: URL: http://www.hhs.gov/news/press/2002pres/20020614.html.

Health Canada. Ephedra. In: *Drug Product Database (DPD)*. Ottawa, Ontario: Health Canada Therapeutic Products Programme; 2001.

Health Canada. Ephedra. In: *Herbs Used as Non-medicinal Ingredients in Non-prescription Drugs for Human Use. Appendix II: List of Herbs Unacceptable as Non-medicinal Ingredients in Oral Use Products Subject to Part B.* Ottawa, Ontario: Health Canada Therapeutic Products Programme; 1995 Sept 22:6–15.

Health Canada. *Labelling Standard: Ephedra*. Ottawa, Canada: Health Canada Drugs Directorate; 1996:1–4.

Heber D, Greenway F. Herbal and Alternative Approaches to Obesity. In: Bray GA, Bouchard C (eds.). *Handbook of Obesity* 2d ed. New York: Marcel Dekker, 2002. (in press).

HHS. See: Health & Human Services.

Hikino H, Kiso Y, Ogata M, Konno C, *et al*. Pharmacological actions of analogues of feruloyl-histamine, an imidazole alkaloid of ephedra roots. *Planta Med* 1984;50(6):478–80.

Hikino H, Ogata K, Konno C, Sato S. Hypotensive actions of ephenadrines, macrocyclic spermine alkaloids of ephedra roots. *J Med Plant Res* 1983;48:290–3.

Hikino H, Konno C, Takata H, Tamada M. Anti-inflammatory principle of ephedra herbs. *Chem Pharm Bull* 1980;28:2900–4.

Horton TJ, Geissler CA. Aspirin potentiates the effect of ephedrine on the thermo-

genic response to a meal in obese but not lean women. *Int J Obes* 1991;15:359-66.

Hsu H. *Oriental Materia Medica*. Oriental Healing Arts Institute; 1986.

Huang K. *The Pharmacology of Chinese Herbs*, 2nd edition. Boca Raton, FL: CRC Press LLC; 1999:291–300.

Huber G. Preliminary results from clinical trials on ephedra dietary supplements (unpublished). Personal communication to M Blumenthal, Dec 18, 2001.

Hutchins GM. Dietary supplements containing ephedra alkaloids [letter]. *N Engl J Med* 2001 Apr 5;344(14):1095–6;discussion 1096–7.

Indian Pharmacopoeia (IP, 1996), Vol. I (A-O). Delhi, India: Controller of Publications Government of India Ministry of Health & Family Welfare; 1996:282–5.

International Olympic Committee (IOC). Prohibited classes of substances and prohibited methods 2001–2002. September, 2001. Available from: URL: http://www.wada-ama.org/asiakas/003/wada_english.nsf/Home?/OpenPage.

IOC. See: International Olympic Committee

IP. See: Indian Pharmacopoeia.

Jaedig S, Henningsen NC. Increased metabolic rate in obese women after ingestion of potassium, magnesium- and phosphate-enriched orange juice or injection of ephedrine. *Int J Obes* 1991;15:429-36.

Japanese Pharmacopoeia (JP XII). Tokyo, Japan: The Society of Japanese Pharmacopoeia; 1991.

Japanese Standards for Herbal Medicines (JSHM). Tokyo, Japan: Yakuji Nippo, Ltd.; 1993:107–8.

Jonderko K, Kucio C. Effect of anti-obesity drugs promoting energy expenditure, yohimbine and ephedrine, on gastric emptying in obese patients. *Aliment Pharmacol Ther* 1991;5:413-8.

Jones D. Thermogenesis: Theoretical and practical implications of thermogenic agents as aids to weight loss. Unpublished, 2001.

JP. See: Japanese Pharmacopoeia.

JSHM. See: Japanese Standards for Herbal Medicines.

Jubiz W, Meikle A. Alterations of glucocorticoid actions by other drugs and disease states. *Drugs* 1979;18:113–21.

Kimmel S. Summary of incidence of seizures, strokes, and myocardial infarctions in the population and estimations of risk in the population from ephedra products. Submitted to FDA; 2000 Aug [cited 2002 Jul 3]. Available from: URL: http://ephedrafacts.com/2.html.

Lawlor A. Health Canada recalls certain Ephedra products. *Globe and Mail*, Jan. 9, 2002.

Leikin J, Klein L . Ephedra causes myocarditis. *J Toxicol Clin Toxicol* 2000;38 (3):353–4

Leung A. Personal communication to M. Blumenthal. 1999, July 7th.

Leung A, Foster S. *Encyclopedia of Common Natural Ingredients Used in Food, Drugs and Cosmetics*, 2nd ed. New York, NY: John Wiley & Sons, Inc.; 1996.

Ling M, Piddlesden SJ, Morgan BP. A component of the medicinal herb ephedra blocks activation in the classical and alternative pathways of complement. *Clin Exp Immunol* 1995 Dec;102(3):582–8.

Liu Y, Toubro S, Astrup A, Stock M. Contribution of Beta-3-adrenoceptor activation to ephedrine-induced thermogenesis in humans. *Intl J Obesity* 1995;19:678–85.

McGuffin M. Statement before Department of Health & Human Services Office of Public Health & Sciences, Public Meeting on the Safety of Dietary Supplements Containing Ephedrine Alkaloids; 2000 Aug 8; Washington DC.

McGuffin M, Hobbs C, Upton R, Goldberg A. (eds.). *American Herbal Products Association's Botanical Safety Handbook* Boca Raton, FL: CRC Press; 1997.

Medical Products Agency (MPA). *Läkemedel: Läkemedelsnära Produkter* (registrerade homeopatiska produkter). Uppsala, Sweden: Medical Products Agency; 2001b.

Medical Products Agency (MPA). *Naturläkemedel: Authorised Natural Remedies* (as of January 24, 2001). Uppsala, Sweden: Medical Products Agency; 2001a.

Molnar D, Torok K, Erhardt E, Jeges S. Safety and efficacy of treatment with an ephedrine/caffeine mixture. The first double-blind placebo-controlled pilot study in adolescents. *In J Obes Relat Metab Disord* 2000;24(12):1573-8.

Morton J. *Major Medicinal Plants: Botany, Culture and Uses.* Springfield, IL: Charles C. Thomas; 1977.

MPA. See: Medical Products Agency.

Nasser J, *et al*. Efficacy trial for weight loss of an herbal supplement of ma huang and guarana. *FASEB J* 1999;13(5).

National Collegiate Athletic Association (NCAA) 2001–2002 NCAA banned-drug classes. Updated 2001 Aug 9. Available from: URL: http://www.ncaa.org/sports_sciences/drugtesting/banned_list.html.

NCAA. See: National Collegiate Athletic Association.

Noguchi M, Kubo M, Naka Y. Studies on the pharmaceutical quality evaluation of crude drug preparations used in the Oriental Medicine "Kampo". IV. Behavior of alkaloids in ephedra herb mixed with other crude drugs under decoction processes. [in Japanese]. *Yakugaku Zasshi* 1978;98(7):923–8.

Office on Women's Health. Safety of dietary supplements containing ephedrine alkaloids [report on public meeting of 8-9 Aug 2000]. The National Women's Health

Information Center; 2000 Sep [cited 14 Nov 2002]. Available at: http://www.4woman.gov/owh/public/report.htm.

OWH. See: Office on Women's Health.

Pasquali R, Casimirri F. Clinical aspects of ephedrine in the treatment of obesity. *Int J Obes Relat Metab Disord* 1993;17 (suppl 1):S65-8.

Pasquali R, Baraldi G, Cesari M *et al*. A controlled study using ephedrine in the treatment of obesity. *Intl J Obesity* 1985;9(2):93–8.

Pharmacopoeia of the People's Republic of China (PPRC 1997 English Edition). Beijing, China: Chemical Industry Press. 1997;92–93.

PPRC. See: *Pharmacopoeia of the People's Republic of China*.

Robbers J, Tyler V. *Tyler's Herbs of Choice: The Therapeutic Use of Phytomedicinals*. New York: Haworth Herbal Press; 1999;112–6.

Ruppanner H, Schaefer U (eds.). *Codex 2000/01 — Die Schweizer Arzneimittel in einem Griff*. Basel, Switzerland: Documed AG; 2000.

Samenuk D, Link MS, Homoud MK *et al*. Adverse cardiovascular events temporarily associated with ma huang, an herbal source of ephedrine. *Mayo Clin Proc* 2002;77:12-6.

Svendsen TL, Ingerslev J, Mork A. Is Letigen contraindicated in hypertension? A double-blind, placebo controlled multipractice study of Letigen administered to normotensive and adequately treated patients with hypersensitivity. *Ugeskr Laeger* 1998;160:4073-5, cited in Heber D, Greenway F. Herbal and Alternative Approaches to Obesity. In: Bray GA, Bouchard C (eds.) *Handbook of Obesity* 2d ed. NewYork: Marcel Dekker, 2002. (in press).

Tang W, Eisenbrand G. *Chinese Drugs of Plant Origin*. New York: Springer-Verlag; 1992;481–90.

Texas Medical Association. TMA Policy Compendium 260.057 Regulation of Ephedrine Products; 260.058 Labeling of Ephedrine Products. Austin, TX.

TGA. See: Therapeutic Goods Administration.

TMA. See: Texas Medical Association.

Therapeutic Goods Administration (TGA). *Commonly Asked Questions: Why are some substances available without a prescription overseas but are controlled substances in Australia?* Woden, Australia: TGA; 2001.

Tsumura Co., Ltd. Science and expert know how join forces to maintain the quality of raw herbs. *Kampo Today* 1996;1(3):1–2.

United States Congress (USC). Public Law 103–417: *Dietary Supplement Health and Education Act of 1994*. Washington, DC: 103rd Congress of the United States; 1994.

USC. See: United States Congress.

Weiner N. Norepinephrine, Epinephrine and the Sympathomimetic Amines. In: Goodman A *et al*. *Goodman and Gilman's The Pharmacological Basis of Therapeutics*, 8th edition. New York, NY: MacMillan; 1985;169–70.

Weiss R. *Herbal Medicine*. Beaconsfield, England: Beaconsfield Publishers; 1988.

Weiss R, Fintelmann V. *Herbal Medicine* 2nd ed. New York: Thieme; 2000:209.

White L,M, Gardner SF, Gurley BJ *et al*. Pharmacokinetics and cardiovascular effects of ma huang *(Ephedra sinica)* in normotensive adults. *J Clin Pharmacol* 1997;37:116–22.

WHO. See: World Health Organization.

Wilkinson GR, Beckett AH. Absorption, metabolism and excretion of the epinedrines in man. II. Pharmacokinetics. *J Pharm Sci* 1968 Nov;57(11):1933–8.

World Health Organization (WHO). Herba Ephedrae. In: *WHO Monographs on Selected Medicinal Plants*, Vol. 1. Geneva: World Health Organization; 1999:145–53.

Zaacks S, Klein L, Tan C, Rodriguez E, Leikin J. Hypersensitivity myocarditis associated with ephedra use. *J Toxicol Clin Toxicol* 1999;37(4):485–9.

Zhu Y. *Chinese Materia Medica*. Australia: Harwood Academic Publishers; 1998.

Clinical Studies on Ephedra (*Ephedra sinica* Stapf)

Metabolism and Weight Loss

Author/Year	Subject	Design	Duration	Dosage	Preparation	Results/Conclusion
Boozer et al., 2002	Weight loss and long-term safety: changes in blood pressure, heart function and body weight	R, DB, PC n=167 (BMI 31.8±4.1 kg/m²). Subjects were carefully selected by medical evaluation, excluding those consuming more than 500 mg caffeine/day and numerous other parameters.	6 months	2 tablets, 3x/day (equivalent to 90 mg/day ephedrine; 192 mg/day caffeine)	Tablets containing ephedra (15 mg ephedrine alkaloids) and kola nut (32 mg caffeine) (Custom made preparation)	The ephedra/caffeine combination versus placebo significantly increased weight loss (−5.3 vs −2.6 kg, p<0.001), and reduced body fat (−4.3 vs. −2.7 kg, p=0.02). LDL-cholesterol was lowered (−8 vs. 0 mg/dl, p=0.013) while HDL-cholesterol was raised (+2.7 vs. −0.3 mg/dl, p=0.004). These results occurred without significant adverse events and with minimal side effects in a carefully selected patient population.
Boozer et al., 2001	Weight loss and short-term safety	R, DB, PC n=48 overweight, weight-stable men and women (BMI>29 and <35 kg/m²)	8 weeks	2 tablets, 3x/day (equivalent to 72 mg/day ephedrine alkaloids; 240 mg/day caffeine)	Metabolife 356®	Herbal supplement versus placebo significantly increased loss of body weight (−4 vs −0.8 kg) and fat (−2.1% vs. 0.2%). Greater reductions in hip circumference and serum triglyceride levels were also seen with the herbal supplement versus placebo. Authors concluded this herbal supplement effectively promoted short-term weight and fat loss.
de Jonge et al., 2001	Weight loss	R, DB, PC n=40	3 months	70 mg of caffeine and 24 mg of ephedra, 3x /day	Brand not stated	After 3 months, the treatment group showed an 8% ± 0.4% (SD) rise in resting metabolic rate (RMR) compared to placebo (p<0.01). Weight loss with the treatment was 4 kg ± 4.2 kg compared to 0.7 kg ± 2.6 kg with placebo (p<0.05). An insignificant drop in pulse and blood pressure (4/1 mm Hg and 0.5 bpm) was observed with treatment. The study concluded that the caffeine and ephedra combination provided safe weight loss and increase in metabolic rate.
Greenway et al., 2000	Metabolism, oxygen consumption	DB, PC, CO n=10 obese females 41 ±4 years. Mean BMI 33kg/m²	45 minutes	2 capsules (10 mg caffeine; 5 mg ephedrine) or 2 placebo capsules	DietMax®	Herbal supplement increased peak oxygen consumption 0.178 ±0.03 (SEM) kcal/minutes (8.01 ±1.35 kcal minimum over 45 minutes) above baseline (p<0.0001); 2.0 ±0.56 kcal/min over 45 minutes compared to placebo (p<0.006). The significance of this result in weight loss requires more research.

Safety

Author/Year	Subject	Design	Duration	Dosage	Preparation	Results/Conclusion
Belfie et al., 2001	Weight loss and safety (changes in heart rate and blood pressure)	DB, PC n=21 obese men (BMI ≥ 30 kg/m²) (ages 19–34 years)	12 weeks	Ephedra alkaloids (20 mg) and guarana (200 mg caffeine) 3x/day vs. placebo	Herbal supplement containing ephedra alkaloids (20 mg) and guarana (200 mg caffeine); brand not stated	When taken in a controlled manner, the herbal supplement had only mild side effects, and did not influence the improvement in serum lipids. There was no impact on amount of adipose mass lost when diet and exercise were controlled. The authors suggest that any benefits of ephedra and caffeine supplements are likely the result of the anorectic effects.
Gurley et al., 1998	Pharmaco-kinetics	R, CO n=10 healthy volunteers (5 men, 5 women; 22–40 years; weight range 47–103 kg)	1 day for each of 4 phases with 1 week washout between phases	2 capsules of one of the commercial preparations or 25 mg ephedrine	Escalation™ or Excel or Up Your Gas or 25 mg ephedrine	Pharmacokinetic parameters were similar for botanical ephedrine and synthetic ephedrine hydrochloride. The authors suggest that the increased incidence of ephedra toxicity stems from accidental overdose often prompted by exaggerated off-label claims and a belief that "natural" medicinal agents are inherently safe, and not from differences in the absorption of botanical ephedrine compared with synthetic ephedrine.
White et al., 1997	Adverse effects, changes in blood pressure and heart rate and pharmaco-kinetics	Unstated n=12 normotensive non-smokers (ages 23–40 years)	20 hours	2 capsules (375 mg ea.) 4x/day	Solaray® capsules (375 mg E. sinica powdered herb each)	None of the 12 subjects experienced adverse effects. 6 patients showed an increased heart rate (78 bpm vs. 86 bpm). Results suggest that the use of ephedra herb powder is benign in a normotensive, young population in short-term use.

KEY: C – controlled, **CC** – case-control, **CH** – cohort, **CI** – confidence interval, **Cm** – comparison, **CO** – crossover, **CS** – cross-sectional, **DB** – double-blind, **E** – epidemiological, **LC** – longitudinal cohort, **MA** – meta-analysis, **MC** – multi-center, **n** – number of patients, **O** – open, **OB** – observational, **OL** – open label, **OR** – odds ratio, **P** – prospective, **PB** – patient-blind, **PC** – placebo-controlled, **PG** – parallel group, **PS** – pilot study, **R** – randomized, **RC** – reference-controlled, **RCS** – retrospective cross-sectional, **RS** - retrospective, **S** – surveillance, **SB** – single-blind, **SC** – single-center, **U** – uncontrolled, **UP** – unpublished, **VC** – vehicle-controlled.

Clinical Studies on Ephedrine

Thermogenesis and Weight loss

Author/Year	Subject	Design	Duration	Dosage	Preparation	Results/Conclusion
Liu *et al.*, 1995	Thermogenesis	SB, PC, CO n=9	5 days	30 mg ephedrine chloride with 0, 2.5, 5, or 10 mg nadolol/day, or placebo	Ephedrine chloride	Significant increase was found in thermogenesis, heart rate, systolic blood pressure, and plasma glucose. Ephedrine combined with nadolol maintained 43% thermogenesis without affecting heart rate and plasma glucose.
Astrup *et al.*, 1986	Glucose-induced thermo-genesis	C n=5	3 months	20 mg ephedrine hydrochloride, 3x/day	Ephedrine hydrochloride	Chronic treatment was found to enhance thermogenic response compared to acute treatment. Chronic ephedrine treatment sustained 10% elevation of meta-bolic rate. Plasma epinephrine levels were increased 87% during treatment.
Pasquali *et al.*, 1985	Weight loss	DB, PC n=46	3 months	25 mg or 50 mg ephedrine hydrochloride, 3x/day, or placebo	Ephedrine hydrochloride tablets	The study did not find significant weight loss benefit in unselected obese patients. The authors concluded ephedrine HCL might be useful in obese patients with defective thermogenesis.

KEY: C – controlled, **CC** – case-control, **CH** – cohort, **CI** – confidence interval, **Cm** – comparison, **CO** – crossover, **CS** – cross-sectional, **DB** – double-blind, **E** – epidemiological, **LC** – longitudinal cohort, **MA** – meta-analysis, **MC** – multi-center, **n** – number of patients, **O** – open, **OB** – observational, **OL** – open label, **OR** – odds ratio, **P** – prospective, **PB** – patient-blind, **PC** – placebo-controlled, **PG** – parallel group, **PS** – pilot study, **R** – randomized, **RC** – reference-controlled, **RCS** – retrospective cross-sectional, **RS** - retrospective, **S** – surveillance, **SB** – single-blind, **SC** – single-center, **U** – uncontrolled, **UP** – unpublished, **VC** – vehicle-controlled.

Ephedra

Monograph

(This page intentionally left blank.)

Evening Primrose Oil

Oenothera biennis L.

[Fam. *Onagraceae*]

OVERVIEW

Evening primrose is a plant native to North America, with its therapeutic use stemming from American indigenous medicine. Evening primrose oil (EPO) from the plant's seeds has been the subject of hundreds of scientific studies, which led to it becoming one of the most widely used botanical supplements today. EPO is sold in over 30 countries as a dietary supplement, drug, or food. In 2000, evening primrose oil ranked 10th of all herbal dietary supplements in U.S. food, drug, and mass-market retail outlets. Clinical studies have focused on its use in treating problems associated with essential fatty acid (EFA) deficiency: eczema, premenstrual syndrome (PMS), inflammation, and diabetic peripheral neuropathy. EPO is relatively high in EFAs, particularly gamma-linolenic acid (GLA) of which it contains 7–10%.

PRIMARY USES

- Atopic dermatitis
- Mastalgia, cyclical
- Lactation

OTHER POTENTIAL USES

- Atopic dermatitis in infants
- Diabetic neuropathy
- Dry eyes associated with Sjögren's syndrome
- Infant formula fortification
- Nutritional deficiencies (EFAs)
- Premenstrual syndrome symptoms
- Raynaud's disease
- Rheumatoid arthritis
- Seborrhoeic dermatitis (milk crust)
- Uremic skin symptoms

Photo © 2003 stevenfoster.com

PHARMACOLOGICAL ACTIONS

Improves EFA composition of plasma, erythrocyte, and platelet lipids and α-tocopherol levels in non-diabetic persons and Type 1 diabetic patients; increases total fat and EFA content of mother's milk; affects fatty acid composition of serum lipids and adipose tissue in men with low dihomo-gamma-linolenic acid (DGLA) levels; helps maintain normal cellular structures; serves as prostaglandin precursor.

DOSAGE AND ADMINISTRATION

EPO is a long-term therapy, so immediate results should not be expected. A patient may need to use EPO regularly for up to four months before a clinical response is observed. EPO appears to be safe for long-term use of at least one year.

Internal

ATOPIC DERMATITIS: 4–6 capsules (500 mg) twice daily (40 mg GLA per capsule).

CYCLICAL MASTALGIA: 6 capsules (500 mg) daily (40 mg GLA per capsule) for 4–6 months.

DIABETIC NEUROPATHY: 8–12 capsules (500 mg) daily.

LACTATION AID: 4 capsules (500 mg) twice daily, morning and evening.

RHEUMATOID ARTHRITIS: 10–20 capsules (500 mg) daily.

UREMIC SKIN SYMPTOMS: 2 capsules (500 mg) twice daily (45 mg GLA per capsule).

NOTE: EPO may be swallowed directly or may be taken with milk, another liquid, or with food. EPO taken with food may minimize any potential gastrointestinal side effects. Concurrent ingestion of the antioxidant vitamin E will protect EFAs from free radical damage and also prevent creation of counterproductive substances. Concurrent ingestion of a daily multiple vitamin may also provide nutritional cofactors (e.g., B6 and magnesium) required for EFA metabolism.

External

ATOPIC DERMATITIS: Water-in-oil emulsion containing 20% EPO, twice daily, applied topically to affected area for at least four weeks.

CONTRAINDICATIONS

Previous reports suggested that patients diagnosed with schizophrenia and/or those already receiving epileptogenic drugs such as phenothiazines should consult a healthcare provider before using EPO. However, a recently published analysis of clinical trials involving polyunsaturated fatty acids in the treatment of schizophrenia did not indicate a clear therapeutic or adverse effect of EPO supplements on schizophrenic patients.

PREGNANCY AND LACTATION: There are no known restrictions. Because LA, GLA, and DGLA are important components of human breast milk, EPO presumably may be taken while nursing. According to the World Health Organization (WHO), pregnant or lactating women should get 5% of their total daily caloric intake from EFAs.

ADVERSE EFFECTS

Adverse effects are rare at recommended dosages, and are reported by less than 2% of people using EPO for extended periods of time. Occasional adverse effects include headache, mild nausea, and abdominal bloating. Overdose symptoms include loose stools and abdominal pain.

DRUG INTERACTIONS

GLA may exacerbate temporal lobe epilepsy in schizophrenic patients being treated with epileptogenic drugs such as phenothiazines (however, this effect has not been confirmed). Steroids and nonsteroidal anti-inflammatory drugs may interfere with GLA metabolism, though this theoretical concern has not been proven. Steroids have been reported to inhibit the D6D enzyme, whereby the metabolism of LA to GLA is inhibited. For patients taking steroidal drugs, supplementation with a source of GLA such as EPO, borage oil, or black current oil may be beneficial.

CLINICAL REVIEW

In 22 clinical studies on evening primrose with a total of 1,154 participants, all but six demonstrated positive effects for indications including PMS, dermatological conditions, diabetic neuropathy, and arthritis. Seven double-blind, placebo-controlled (DB, PC) studies investigated the use of EPO in dermatological conditions, including uremic skin symptoms, chronic hand dermatitis, atopic dermatitis, chronic stable-plaque psoriasis, and psoriatic arthritis (PsA). Treatment of PMS symptoms was the subject of two DB, PC studies. Other DB, PC studies evaluated the effects of EPO in the treatment of cyclic mastalgia, diabetic neuropathy, rheumatoid arthritis, and menopausal hot flashes. EPO also was evaluated for its effect on fat composition and the content of human milk as well as on the survival time of patients with primary liver cancer. A recent study on pregnant, low-risk, nulliparous women measured pregnancy length and active-phase labor outcomes. A meta-analysis of nine PC studies on atopic eczema correlated clinical improvement with a rise in plasma EFAs. Improvement in reported itching symptoms was highly significant (p<0.01) compared to placebo. EPO showed a progressive effect, as well as a dose/response relationship in the 311 patients evaluated in the nine trials.

Evening Primrose Oil

Oenothera biennis L.
[Fam. *Onagraceae*]

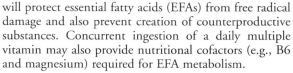

OVERVIEW

Evening primrose is a plant native to North America, with its therapeutic use stemming from American indigenous medicine. Evening primrose oil (EPO) from the plant's seeds has been the subject of hundreds of scientific studies, which has led to it becoming one of the most widely prescribed botanical medicines. Evening primrose oil (EPO) is relatively high in essential fatty acids, which play a major role in its effectiveness. In 2000, evening primrose oil ranked 10th of all herbal dietary supplements in U.S. food, drug, and mass-market retail outlets.

USES

Atopic dermatitis; painful breasts during menstruation; lactation; uremic skin symptoms; nutritional deficiencies (essential fatty acids); atopic dermatitis in infants; seborrhoeic dermatitis (milk crust); infant formula fortification; dry eyes associated with Sjögren's syndrome; Raynaud's disease; PMS symptoms; diabetic neuropathy; rheumatoid arthritis.

DOSAGE

ATOPIC DERMATITIS: 4–6 capsules (500 mg) twice daily [containing 40 mg GLA (gamma-linolenic acid) per capsule].

BREAST PAIN RELATED TO MENSTRUAL CYCLE: 6 capsules (500 mg) daily for four to six months [40 mg GLA per capsule].

DIABETIC NEUROPATHY: 8–12 capsules (500 mg) daily.

LACTATION AID: 4 capsules (500 mg) twice daily.

RHEUMATOID ARTHRITIS: 10–20 capsules (500 mg) daily.

UREMIC SKIN SYMPTOMS: 2 capsules (500 mg) twice daily [45 mg GLA per capsule].

NOTE: EPO may be swallowed directly or may be taken with milk, another liquid, or with food. EPO taken with food may minimize any potential gastrointestinal side effects. Concurrent ingestion of the antioxidant vitamin E will protect essential fatty acids (EFAs) from free radical damage and also prevent creation of counterproductive substances. Concurrent ingestion of a daily multiple vitamin may also provide nutritional cofactors (e.g., B6 and magnesium) required for EFA metabolism.

NOTE: EPO is a long-term therapy, so immediate results should not be expected. A patient may need to use EPO regularly for up to four months before a clinical response is observed. EPO appears to be safe for long-term use of at least one year.

CONTRAINDICATIONS

Some reports suggest that individuals diagnosed with schizophrenia and/or those already receiving epileptogenic drugs such as phenothiazines should consult a healthcare provider before using EPO. However, a recently published analysis of clinical trials involving polyunsaturated fatty acids in the treatment of schizophrenia indicates no clear positive effects of EPO supplementation on schizophrenic patients, but no adverse effects either.

PREGNANCY AND LACTATION: There are no known restrictions during pregnancy or lactation, and GLA, the essential fatty acid that EPO contains, is considered an important substance in human breast milk. According to the World Health Organization, 5% of pregnant women's total caloric intake should be from essential fatty acids.

ADVERSE EFFECTS

Adverse effects are rare at recommended dosages. Occasionally, headache, mild nausea, and abdominal bloating may occur. Overdose symptoms include loose stools and abdominal pain.

DRUG INTERACTIONS

There are no known drug interactions. Steroids and nonsteroidal anti-inflammatory drugs may potentially interfere with essential fatty acid metabolism.

Comments

When using a dietary supplement, purchase it from a reliable source. For best results, use the same brand of product throughout the period of use. As with all medications and dietary supplements, please inform your healthcare provider of all herbs and medications you are taking. Interactions may occur between medications and herbs or even among different herbs when taken at the same time. Treat your herbal supplement with care by taking it as directed, storing it as advised on the label, and keeping it out of the reach of children and pets. Consult your healthcare provider with any questions.

AMERICAN BOTANICAL COUNCIL

Evening Primrose Oil

Oenothera biennis L.

[Fam. *Onagraceae*]

OVERVIEW

Evening primrose is a plant native to North America. Traditionally, it was used externally to treat skin diseases and internally to treat breathing problems and arthritis (Manku *et al.,* 1982; Moerman, 1998; Willard, 1992). It was one of the first medicinal plants brought back to Europe by settlers in the 16th century (Willard, 1992). Evening primrose oil (EPO) has been the subject of hundreds of scientific studies, which led to it becoming one of the most widely used botanical medicines today (Brown, 1996). EPO is sold in over 30 countries as a dietary supplement, drug, or food (Chen, 1999). In 2000, evening primrose oil ranked 10th of all herbal dietary supplements in U.S. food, drug, and, mass-market retail outlets (Blumenthal, 2001). Clinical studies have focused on its use in treating problems associated with essential fatty acid (EFA) deficiency including atopic eczema, premenstrual syndrome, inflammation, and diabetic peripheral neuropathy. EPO is relatively high in essential fatty acids (EFAs), particularly gamma-linolenic acid (GLA, 7–10%) (Leung and Foster, 1996).

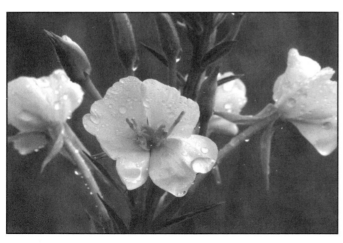

Photo © 2003 stevenfoster.com

DESCRIPTION

Evening primrose oil preparations consist of a clear, golden yellow, fixed oil extracted by cold expression, or solvent extraction, from the seeds of *Oenothera biennis* L. [Fam. *Onagraceae*] (Budavari *et al.,* 1996; Reynolds *et al.,* 1989), which first occur during the second year of plant growth. Evening primrose is a biennial herb, infertile for the first year (Schulz *et al.,* 1998).

PRIMARY USES

Dermatology

- Atopic dermatitis (Berth-Jones and Graham-Brown, 1993; Gehring *et al.,* 1999; Hederos and Berg, 1996; Schäfer and Kragballe, 1991)

Gynecology

- Mastalgia, cyclical (Wetzig, 1994; Gateley *et al.,* 1992; Cheung, 1999)
- Lactation (Cant *et al.,* 1991)

OTHER POTENTIAL USES

- Diabetic neuropathy (Keen *et al.,* 1993; Jamal and Carmichael, 1990)
- PMS symptoms (Khoo *et al.,* 1990; Ockerman *et al.,* 1986)
- Rheumathoid arthritis (Brzeski *et al.,* 1991)
- Nutritional deficiencies (essential fatty acids) (Brown, 1996)
- Dermatitis: seborrhoeic dermatitis (milk crust), and atopic dermatitis in infants (Schilcher, 1997)
- Infant formula fortification (Gibson and Rassias, 1990)
- Dry eyes associated with Sjögren's syndrome (Manthorpe *et al.,* 1990)
- Raynaud's disease (Brown, 1996; Chen, 1999)
- Uremic skin symptoms (Yoshimoto-Furuie *et al.,* 1999)

DOSAGE

Internal

ATOPIC DERMATITIS: 4–6 capsules (500 mg) twice daily (40 mg GLA per capsule) (Hederos and Berg, 1996; Schäfer and Kragballe, 1991; Schulz *et al.,* 1998).

CYCLICAL MASTALGIA: 6 capsules (500 mg) daily (40 mg GLA per capsule) for 4 –6 months (Cheung, 1999; Gateley *et al.,* 1992b; McFayden *et al.,* 1992).

DIABETIC NEUROPATHY: 8–12 capsules (500 mg) daily (Bratman and Kroll, 1999).

LACTATION AID: 500 mg capsules, twice daily, morning and evening (Cant *et al.,* 1991).

RHEUMATOID ARTHRITIS: 10–20 capsules (500 mg) daily (Bratman and Kroll, 1999).

UREMIC SKIN SYMPTOMS: 2 capsules (500 mg) twice daily (45 mg GLA per capsule) (Yoshimoto-Furuie *et al.,* 1999).

NOTE: Evening primrose oil may be swallowed directly or may be taken with milk, another liquid, or with food (Newall *et al.,* 1996). Evening primrose oil taken with food may minimize any potential gastrointestinal side effects. Concurrent ingestion of the antioxidant vitamin E will protect essential fatty acids (EFAs) from free radical damage and also prevent creation of counterproductive substances (Reddy *et al.,* 1994). Concurrent ingestion of a daily multiple vitamin may also provide nutritional cofactors (e.g., zinc, B6, and magnesium) required for EFA metabolism (Brown, 1996).

External

ATOPIC DERMATITIS: Water-in-oil emulsion containing 20% evening primrose oil, twice daily is applied topically to affected area for at least four weeks (Gehring *et al.*, 1999).

DURATION OF ADMINISTRATION

Internal

Evening primrose oil is a long-term therapy, and immediate results should not be expected. A patient may need evening primrose oil regularly for up to four months before a clinical response is observed (Gateley *et al.*, 1992b; Newall *et al.*, 1996). Evening primrose oil appears to be safe for long-term use, at least up to one year (Keen *et al.*, 1993).

CHEMISTRY

Evening primrose seed contains ca. 14% fixed oil (EPO), which is composed of ca. 65–75% linoleic acid (LA), 7–10% gamma-linolenic acid (GLA), plus oleic, palmitic, and stearic acids and steroids campesterol and β-sitosterol (Leung and Foster, 1996; Newall *et al.*, 1996).

PHARMACOLOGICAL ACTIONS

Human

Improves EFA composition of plasma, erythrocyte, and platelet lipids, and α-tocopherol levels in non-diabetic persons and Type 1 diabetic patients (van Doormaal *et al.*, 1988); increases total fat and EFA content of mother's milk (Cant *et al.*, 1991); affects fatty acid composition of serum lipids and adipose tissue in men with low dihomogammalinolenic acid (DGLA) levels (Abraham *et al.*, 1990); helps maintain normal cellular structures and is a precursor of prostaglandins (Chen, 1999). GLA functions as the precursor of DGLA, which is the parent of the 1-series prostanoids, and as a precursor of arachidonic acid, the parent of the 2-series prostanoids (Pizzorno and Murray, 1999).

Animal

Reduces chronic inflammation (Kunkel *et al.*, 1981); inhibits mammary tumor growth (Karmali and Marsh, 1985); has a beneficial effect on plasma lipids and protects against diabetic nephropathy (Barcelli *et al.*, 1990); anti-asthmatic at high doses (Dorsch and Schmidt, 1995); prevents reduced nerve conduction velocity in streptozotocin-induced diabetes mellitus in rats (Dines *et al.*, 1995); inhibits thromboxane A2 in diabetes (Dines *et al.*, 1996); antisecretory, anti-ulcerogenic, and cytoprotective in rats that exhibited gastric mucosal damage induced by varicose ulcerogenesis (al-Shabanah, 1997); inhibits binding of benzo(a)pyrene to cancerous skin cell DNA in mice exposed to a two-stage carcinogenesis model (Ramesh and Das, 1998); inhibits tumor growth in mice with transplanted mammary gland adenocarcinoma (Munoz *et al.*, 1999); alters fatty acid composition of immune system cells; immunomodulatory (Peterson *et al.*, 1999).

In vitro

Cytostatic activity on malignant cell lines (Botha and Robinson, 1986; Leary *et al.*, 1982); suppresses cancer cell proliferation of human osteogenic sarcoma cells (Booyens *et al.*, 1984).

MECHANISM OF ACTION

EFAs are required for the normal structure of all cell membranes in the human body. They are not synthesized endogenously and thus must be obtained from dietary sources (Brown, 1996; Chen, 1999). Major EFAs are linolenic acid (LA) and alpha-linolenic acid (ALA). Their metabolic products [long-chain polyunsaturated fatty acids including GLA, dihomogammalinolenic acid (DGLA), eicosapentaenoic acid (EPA), and docosahexaenoic acid (DHA)] are functionally essential and involved in prostaglandin biosynthetic pathways (Newall *et al*, 1996). LA is desaturated to GLA by the enzyme delta-6-desaturase (D6D). This conversion of LA to GLA by D6D is the rate-limiting step in the metabolic pathway for EFAs. Its activity is reduced/inhibited by increased demand caused by stress, aging, alcohol, smoking, diabetes, hypertension, and inflammatory diseases including arthritis, psoriasis, and others. In these circumstances, LA accumulates in the body, and an excess of LA may further limit the activity of the D6D enzyme (Giron *et al.*, 1989; Diboune, 1992). GLA is elongated to DGLA by the enzyme elongase and acts as a substrate for production of prostaglandins of series 1. It may also be desaturated to arachidoninc acid.

Actions of Evening Primrose Oil (EPO)

- Supplies GLA: The bioactivity of evening primrose oil is due primarily to its GLA content. By supplying GLA, it bypasses the rate-limiting step in the metabolism of LA. After ingestion of evening primrose oil, GLA is rapidly absorbed and then converts directly to DGLA and other prostaglandin precursors (Chen, 1999; Pizzorno and Murray, 1999).

- Acts on the prostanoid pathway (Croft *et al.*, 1984).

Actions of Essential Fatty Acids (EFA)

- Elevate levels of DGLA in plasma, neutrophils, and epidermal phospholipids. DGLA is the precursor of the anti-inflammatory substances 15-hydroxy-eicosatrienoic acid and prostaglandin E1 (Shafer and Kragballe, 1991).

- May reduce rheumatoid inflammation by metabolizing to the anti-inflammatory one-series prostaglandins and competitively inhibiting the synthesis of pro-inflammatory two-series prostaglandins and four-series leukotrienes (Joe and Hart, 1993).

- May inhibit papilloma formation *in vivo* by inhibiting the binding of benzo-(a)-pyrene to skin cell DNA and increasing the lipid peroxidation process (Ramesh and Das, 1998).

- Absorbed transdermally as well as internally (Houtsmuller and van der Berk, 1981).

CONTRAINDICATIONS

Previously not recommended for patients diagnosed with schizophrenia and/or those already receiving epileptogenic drugs such as phenothiazines, according to a data sheet produced by the leading marketer of evening primrose oil (Anon., 1994–95). However, a recently published analysis of clinical trials involving polyunsaturated fatty acids in the treatment of schizophrenia did not indicate a clear therapeutic or adverse effect of evening primrose oil supplements on schizophrenic patients (Joy, 2000).

PREGNANCY AND LACTATION: No known restrictions (Brown, 1996; McGuffin *et al.*, 1997). Non-teratogenic, based on animal studies (Anon., 1994–95; Horrobin, 1992). LA, GLA, and DGLA are important components of human breast milk, so it is reasonable to assume that evening primrose oil may be taken while nursing (Brown, 1996; Carter, 1988; Gibson and Rassias, 1990; Newall *et al.*, 1996). According to the World Health Organization, pregnant or lactating women should get 5% of their total daily caloric intake from EFAs (Chen, 1999).

ADVERSE EFFECTS

Adverse effects are rare at recommended dosages and are reported by less than 2% of people using evening primrose oil long-term (Brown, 1996; Chen, 1999). Occasional adverse effects include headache (Barber, 1988; Gateley *et al.*, 1992b; Hänsel *et al.*, 1993), mild nausea (Barber, 1988; Cheung, 1999; Gateley *et al.*, 1992b; Hänsel *et al.*, 1993), and abdominal bloating (Gateley *et al.*, 1992b). Overdose symptoms include loose stools and abdominal pain (Newall *et al.*, 1996).

DRUG INTERACTIONS

Early reports suggested that GLA might exacerbate temporal lobe epilepsy in schizophrenic patients being treated with epileptogenic drugs such as phenothiazines (Anon., 1994–95), though this possible effect has not been confirmed (Bratman and Kroll, 1999). Other reports have suggested that steroids and nonsteroidal anti-inflammatory drugs may interfere with GLA metabolism (Brenner, 1981), though this theoretical concern has not been proven (Brown, 1996). Steroids have been reported to inhibit the D6D enzyme, whereby the metabolism of LA to GLA is inhibited. For patients taking steroidal drugs, supplementation with a source of GLA such as evening primrose oil, borage oil (*Borago officinalis*), or black current oil (*Ribes nigrum*) may be beneficial (Marra and de Alaniz, 1990). In one clinical trial, 38 estrogen-dependent breast cancer patients showed a faster clinical response to tamoxifen after oral ingestion of GLA (as found in EPO) (Brinker, 2001).

AMERICAN HERBAL PRODUCTS ASSOCIATION (AHPA) SAFETY RATING

CLASS 1: Herbs that can be safely consumed when used appropriately (McGuffin *et al.*, 1997).

REGULATORY STATUS

CANADA: OTC schedule oral drug, requiring pre-market authorization and assignment of Drug Identification Number (DIN) (Health Canada, 2001).

FRANCE: Used in cosmetic products and toiletries (Bruneton, 1999).

GERMANY: Capsules containing 0.5 g evening primrose oil (corresponding to 40 mg GLA) are approved drugs for treatment and symptomatic relief of atopic eczema (Schulz *et al.*, 1998).

ITALY: No information available.

SWEDEN: Natural remedy for self-medication requiring marketing authorization by the Medical Products Agency (MPA) (Tunón, 1999; WHO, 1998). The only evening primrose-containing product listed in the "Authorised Natural Remedies" (Epogam®) was removed to the Deregistered Natural Remedies list in April of 2000 (MPA, 2001).

SWITZERLAND: Herbal medicine with positive classification (List D) by the *Interkantonale Kontrollstelle für Heilmittel* (IKS) and corresponding sales category D with sale limited to pharmacies and drugstores, without prescription (Morant and Ruppanner, 2001; *Codex*, 2000).

U.K.: Approved by the Department of Medicine for treatment of atopic eczema and mastalgia (Chen, 1999).

U.S.: Dietary supplement (USC, 1994).

CLINICAL REVIEW

Twenty-two studies are outlined in the following table "Clinical Studies on Evening Primrose," with a total of 1,154 participants. All but six of these studies (Whitaker *et al.*, 1996; Oliwiecki and Burton, 1994; Berth-Jones and Graham-Brown, 1993; Oliwiecki *et al.*, 1993; Dove *et al.*, 1999; Jenkins *et al.*, 1996) demonstrated positive effects for indications including PMS, dermatological conditions, diabetic neuropathy, and arthritis. The table includes seven double-blind, placebo-controlled (DB, PC) studies investigating the use of evening primrose oil in dermatological conditions including uremic skin symptoms (Yoshimoto-Furuie *et al.*, 1999), chronic hand dermatitis (Whitaker *et al.*, 1996), atopic dermatitis (Berth-Jones and Graham-Brown, 1993; Gehring *et al.*, 1999; Hederos and Berg, 1996), chronic stable-plaque psoriasis (Oliwiecki and Burton, 1994), and psoriatic arthritis (PsA) (Veale *et al.*, 1994). Treatment of PMS symptoms was the subject of two DB, PC studies (Khoo *et al.*, 1990; Ockerman *et al.*, 1986). Other subjects of DB, PC studies in the table included treatment of cyclic mastalgia (Cheung, 1999), diabetic neuropathy (Keen *et al.*, 1993; Jamal and Carmichael, 1990), rheumatoid arthritis (Brzeski *et al.*, 1991), menopausal hot flash (Chenoy *et al.*, 1994), effect on fat composition and content of human milk (Cant *et al.*, 1991), and the effect of survival time of patients with primary liver cancer (van der Merwe *et al.*, 1990). A recent study on pregnant, low-risk, nulliparous women measured pregnancy length and activephase labor outcomes (Dove *et al.*, 1999). A meta-analysis of nine PC studies on atopic eczema correlated clinical improvement with a rise in plasma essential fatty acids (Morse *et al.*, 1989). Improvement in reported itching symptoms was highly significant ($p<0.01$) compared to placebo. EPO showed a progressive effect as well as a dose/response relationship in the 311 atopic eczema patients evaluated in the nine trials. The protocol has been established for a systematic review of studies on EPO for the treatment of premenstrual syndrome (PMS), but it has not yet been concluded (Strid *et al.*, 2001).

BRANDED PRODUCTS

Efamast® 500 mg evening primrose oil: Scotia Pharmaceuticals Ltd. / Scotia House / Sterling / Scotland / FK9 4TZ / U.K. / http://fox.nstn.ca/~scotlib/index.html. 1 capsule contains 40 mg of GLA.

Efamol® 500 mg evening primrose oil: Scotia Pharmaceuticals Ltd. 75.0% linoleic acid (LA), 9.0% gamma-linolenic acid (GLA), 8.5% oleic acid (OE).

Efamol® Marine 500 mg: Scotia Pharmaceuticals Ltd. 430 mg evening primrose oil and 107 mg marine fish oil, providing 40 mg GLA, 20 mg EFA, 11 mg DHA, vitamin E.

Epogam® 500 mg EPO: Scotia Pharmaceuticals Ltd. 50 mg of GLA and 10 mg vitamin E per capsule.

Quest Vitamins: Quest Vitamins / 7080 River Road #129 / Richmond, BC / V6X 1X5 / Canada / Tel: (604) 273-0611 / Email: thartz@van.boehringer-ingelheim.com / www.questvitamins.com. Capsule containing 500 mg evening primrose oil.

Scotia Cream: Scotia Pharmaceuticals Ltd. Cream containing 0.1% beta-methasone valerate and 10% evening primrose oil.

REFERENCES

al-Shabanah O. Effect of evening primrose oil on gastric ulceration and secretion induced by various ulcerogenic and necrotizing agents in rats. *Food Chem Toxicol* 1997;35(1):769-75.

Anon. Data Sheet Compendium: Efamast®, Epogam®, Epogam® Pediatric (Searle). 1994–1995;1520-1.

Barber A. Evening primrose oil: a panacea? *Pharmaceut J* 1988;240:723-5.

Barcelli U, Weiss M, Beach D, Motz A, Thompson B. High linoleic acid diets ameliorate diabetic nephropathy in rats. *Am J Kidney Dis* 1990;16(3):244-51.

Behan P, Behan W, Horrobin D. The effect of high doses of essential fatty acids in the post-viral fatigue syndrome. *Acta Neurol Scand* 1990;82(3):209-16.

Berth-Jones J, Graham-Brown R. Placebo-controlled trial of essential fatty acid supplementation in atopic dermatitis [published erratum appears in *Lancet* 1993 Aug 28;342(8870):564] [see comments]. *Lancet* 1993;341(8860):1557-60.

Blumenthal M. Herb sales down 15% in mainstream market. *HerbalGram* 2001;51:69.

Booyens J, Engelbrecht P, le Roux S, *et al.* Some effects of the essential fatty acids linoleic acid and alpha-linolenic acid and of their metabolites gamma-linolenic acid, arachidonic acid, eicosapentaenoic acid, docosahexaenoic acid, and of prostaglandins A1 and E1 on the proliferation of human osteogenic sarcoma cells in culture. *Prostaglandins Leukot Med* 1984;14:15-33.

Botha J, Robinson K. Response of human mammary cell lines to gamma-linolenic acid, dihomo-gamma-linolenic acid and ethanol. *S Afr J Science* 1986;82:43.

Bratman S, Kroll D. Evening Primrose Oil. In: *Clinical Evaluation of Medicinal Herbs and Other Therapeutic Natural Products.* Rocklin, CA: Prima Publishing; 1999;1-6.

Brenner R. Nutritional and hormonal factors influencing desaturation of essential fatty acids. *Prog Lipid Res* 1981;20:41-8.

Brinker F. *Herb Contraindications and Drug Interactions*, 3rd ed. Sandy, OR: Eclectic Medical Publications; 2001:92-93.

Brown D. Evening Primrose In: *Herbal Prescriptions for Better Health.* Rocklin, CA: Prima Publishing; 1996;79-89.

Brzeski M, Madhok R, Capell H. Evening primrose oil in patients with rheumatoid arthritis and side-effects of non-steroidal anti-inflammatory drugs. *Br J Rheumatol* 1991;30(5):370-372.

Bruneton J. *Pharmacognosy, Phytochemistry, Medicinal Plants*, 2nd ed. Paris, France: Lavoisier Publishing 1999;157.

Budavari S, O'Neil M, Smith A, Heckelman P, Kinneary J (eds.). *The Merck Index – An Encyclopedia of Chemicals, Drugs, and Biologicals*, 12th ed. Whitehouse Station, NJ: Merck Research Laboratories; 1996;662-3.

Cant A, Shay J, Horrobin D. The effect of maternal supplementation with linoleic and gamma- linolenic acids on the fat composition and content of human milk: a placebo-controlled trial. *J Nutr Sci Vitaminol* 1991;37(6):573-9.

Carter J. Gamma-linolenic acid as a nutrient. *Food Tech* 1988;(6)7282.

Chen J. *Evening Primrose Oil Continuing Education Module.* Boulder, CO: New Hope Institute of Retailing in association with the University of Southern California School of Pharmacy; March 1999.

Chenoy R, Hussain S, Tayob Y, *et al.* 1994. Effect of oral gamma-linolenic acid from evening primrose oil on menopausal flushing. *BMJ* 1994;308:501-3.

Cheung K. Management of cyclical mastalgia in oriental women: pioneer experience of using gamma-linolenic acid (Efamast®) in Asia. *Aust N Z J Surg* 1999;69(7):492-4.

Codex 2000/01: Die Schweizer Arzneimittel in einem Griff. Basel, Switzerland: Documed AG; 2000;534-5.

Croft K, Beilin L, Mahoney D, *et al.* Dietary modification of platelet and renal prostaglandins. *Aust N Z J Med* 1984;14:448-52.

Diboune M, Ferard G, Igenbleek Y, *et al.* Composition of phospholipid fatty acids in red blood cell membranes of patients in intensive care units: effects of different intakes of soybean oil, medium-chain triglyceridess, and black-current seed oil. *J Parenter Enteral Nutr* 1992; 16(2):136-41.

Dines M, Cotter M, Cameron N. Nerve function in galactosemic rats: effects of evening primrose oil and doxazosin. *Eur J Pharm* 1995;281:301-9.

Dines K, Cotter M, Cameron N. Effectiveness of natural oils as sources of gamma-linolenic acid to correct peripheral nerve conduction velocity abnormalities in diabetic rats: modulation by thromboxane A2 inhibition. *Prostaglandins Leukot Essent Fatty Acids* 1996;55(3):159-65.

Dorsch W, Schmidt O. Antiasthmatic effects of gamma linolenic acid – high dose Evening Primrose Oil and Borage Oil stimulate allergen tachyphylaxis of sensitized guinea pigs and prevent allergen sensitization. *Phytomedicine* 1995;4:271-5.

Dove D, Johnson P. Oral evening primrose oil: Its effect on length of pregnancy and selected intrapartum outcomes in low-risk nulliparous women. *J Nurse-Midwifery* 1999;44(3):320-4.

Gateley C, Maddox P, Pritchard G, *et al.* Plasma fatty acid profiles in benign breast disorders. *Br J Surg* 1992a;79(5):407-9.

Gateley C, Miers M, Mansel R, Hughes L. Drug treatments for mastalgia: 17 years experience in the Cardiff Mastalgia Clinic. *J R Soc Med* 1992b;85(1):12-5.

Gehring W, Bopp R, Rippke F, Gloor M. Effect of topically applied evening primrose oil on epidermal barrier function in atopic dermatitis as a function of vehicle. *Arzneimittelforschung* 1999;49(II):635-42.

Gibson R, Rassias G. Infant nutrition and human milk. In: *Omega-6 Essential Fatty Acids: Pathophysiology and Roles in Clinical Medicine.* New York, NY: Alan R. Liss; 1990;283-93.

Giron M, Mataix F, Faus M, Suarez M. Effect of long-term feeding olive and sunflower oils on fatty acid composition and desaturation activities of liver microsomes. *Biochem Int* 1989; 19:645-56.

Hänsel R, Keller K. Rimpler H, Schneider G (eds.). *Hagers Handbuch der pharmazeutischen Praxis*, 5th ed., Vol. 5. Berlin, Germany: Springer Verlag; 1993;476-9.

Health Canada. *Drug Product Database* (DPD) *Product Information.* Ottawa, Ontario: Health Canada; 2001.

Hederos C, Berg A. Epogam® evening primrose oil treatment in atopic dermatitis and asthma. *Arch Dis Child* 1996;75(6):494-7.

Horrobin D. Evening primrose oil and premenstrual syndrome [letter; comment]. *Med J Aust* 1990;153(10):630-1.

Horrobin D, Ells K, Morse-Fisher N, Manku M. The effects of evening primrose oil, safflower oil and paraffin on plasma fatty acid levels in humans: choice of an appropriate placebo for clinical studies on primrose oil. *Prostaglandins Leukot Essent Fatty Acids* 1991;42:245-9.

Horrobin D. Nutritional and medical importance of gamma-linolenic acid. *Prog Lipid Res* 1992;31:163-94.

Houtsmuller U, van der Berk A. Effects of topical application of fatty acids. *Progress in Lipid Res* 1981;20:219-24.

Hughes L, Mansel R, Webster D. *Benign Disorders and Diseases of the Breast.* London, U.K.: Bailliere Tindall; 1989.

Jamal G *et al.* Gamma-linolenic acid in diabetic neuropathy [letter]. *Lancet* 1986;i:1098.

Jamal G, Carmichael H. The Effect of gamma-linolenic acid on human diabetic peripheral neuropathy: a double-blind placebo-controlled trial. *Diabetic Med* 1990;7(4):319-23.

Jenkins A, Green A, Thompson R. Essential fatty acid supplementation in chronic hepatitis B. *Aliment Pharmacol Ther* 1996;10(4):665-668.

Joe LA, Hart LL. Evening primrose oil in rheumatoid arthritis [see comments]. *Ann Pharmacother* 1993;27(12):1475-7.

Joy C, Mumby-Croft R, Joy L. Polyunsaturated fatty acid (fish or evening primrose oil) for schizophrenia. *Cochrane Database Syst Rev* 2000;(2):CD001257.

Karmali R, Marsh J. Antitumor activity in a rat mammary adenocarcinoma: the effect of cyclooxygenase inhibitors and immunization against prostaglandin E2. *Prostaglandins Leukot Med* 1985 Dec;20(3):283-6.

Keen H, Payan J, Allawi J, *et al.* Treatment of diabetic neuropathy with gamma-linolenic acid. The gamma-linolenic acid multicentre trial group. *Diabetes Care* 1993;16(1):8-15.

Khoo S, Munro C, Battistutta D. Evening primrose oil and treatment of premenstrual syndrome. *Med J Australia* 1990;153:189-92.

Kunkel S, Ogawa H, Ward P, Zurier RB. Suppression of chronic inflammation by evening primrose oil. *Prog Lipid Res* 1981;20:885-8.

Leary W, Robinson K, Booyens J, Dippenaar N. Some effects of gamma-linolenic acid on cultured human oesophageal carcinoma cells. *S Afr Med J* 1982;62:681-3.

Leung A, Foster S. *Encyclopedia of Common Natural Ingredients used in Food, Drugs and Cosmetic*s, 2nd edition. New York, NY: John Wiley & Sons, Inc; 1996;235-8.

Leventhal L, Boyce E, Zurier R. Treatment of rheumatoid arthritis with gamma linolenic acid. *Ann Intern Med* 1993;119(9):867-73.

Manku M, Horrobin D, Morse N. Reduced levels of prostaglandin precursors in blood of atopic patients: defective delta-6-desaturate function as a biochemical basis for atopy. *Prostaglandins Leukot Med* 1982;9:615-28.

Mansel R, Pye J, Hughes L. Effects of essential fatty acids on cyclical mastalgia and noncyclical breast disease. In: Horrobin D (ed.). *Omega-6 Essential Fatty Acids: Pathophysiology and Roles in Clinical Medicines.* New York, NY: Alan R. Liss; 1990;557-567.

Manthorpe R, Manthorpe T, Oxholm A, *et al.* Primary Sjörgren's Syndrome: New Concepts. In: Horrobin DF (ed.). *Omega-6 Essential Fatty Acids: Pathophysiology and Roles in Clinical Medicine.* New York: Alan R. Liss; 1990;239-53.

Marra CA, de Alaniz MJ. Mineralocorticoids modify rat liver delta 6 desaturase activity and other parameters of lipid metabolism. *Biochemistry-Iinternational* 1990 Nov; 22(3):483-93.

McFarlin B, Gibson M, O'Rear J, Harman P. A national survey of herbal preparation use by nurse-midwives for labor stimulation. *J Nurse-Midwifery* 1999;44(3):205-16.

McFayden I, Forrest AP, Chetty U, Raab G. Cyclical breast pain — some observations and the difficulties in treatment. *Brit J Clin Pract* 1992;46:161-4.

McGuffin M, Hobbs C, Upton R, Goldberg A (eds.). *American Herbal Products Association's Botanical Safety Handbook.* Boca Raton, FL: CRC Press; 1997;79.

Medical Products Agency (MPA). Naturläkemedel: Deregistered Natural Remedies (as of January 24, 2001). Uppsala, Sweden: Medical Products Agency; 2001.

MPA. See: Medical Products Agency.

Moerman D. *Native American Ethnobotany*. Portland, OR: Timber Press; 1998;361-2.

Morant J, Ruppanner H (eds.). Burgerstein EPO-Nachtkerzenöl-Kapseln; Dünner Biennol®; Sidroga Efamol® 500mg. In: *Arzneimittel-Kompendium der Schweiz®* 2001. Basel, Switzerland: Documed AG. 2001;154, 185, 428.

Morse P, Horrobin D, Manku M, *et al*. Meta-analysis of placebo-controlled studies of the efficacy of Epogam® in the treatment of atopic eczema. Relationship between plasma essential fatty acid changes and clinical response. *Br J Dermatol* 1989;121(1):75-90.

Munoz S, Piegari M, Guzman C, Eynard A. Differential effects of dietary Oenothera, *Zizyphus mistol*, and corn oils, and essential fatty acid deficiency on the progression of a murine mammary gland adenocarcinoma. *Nutrition* 1999;15(3):208-2.

Newall C, Anderson L, Phillipson J. *Herbal Medicines: A Guide for Health-care Professionals*. London, U.K.: The Pharmaceutical Press; 1996;110-3.

Ockerman P, Bachrack I, Glans S, Rassner S. Evening primrose oil as a treatment of premenstrual syndrome. *Recent Adv Clin Nutr* 1986;2:404-5.

Oliwiecki S, Armstrong J, Burton J, Bradfield J. The effect of essential fatty acids on epidermal atrophy due to topical steroids. *Clin Exp Dermatol* 1993;18(4):326-8.

Oliwiecki S, Burton J. Evening primrose oil and marine oil in the treatment of psoriasis. *Clin Exp Dermatol* 1994;19(2):127-9.

Peterson L, Thies F, Calder P. Dose-dependent effects of dietary gamma-linolenic acid on rat spleen lymphocyte functions. *Prostaglandins Leukot Essent Fatty Acids* 1999;61:19-24.

Pizzorno JE, Murray MT, editors. *Textbook of Natural Medicine, Vol 1. 2nd ed.* New York: Churchill Livingstone; 1999;138, 1129, 1210-1, 1527-8.

Puolakka J, Makarainen L, Viinikka L, Ylikorkala O. Biochemical and clinical effects of treating the premenstrual syndrome with prostaglandin synthesis inhibitors. *J Reprod Med* 1985;30(3):149-53.

Pye J, Mansel R, Hughes L. Clinical experience of drug treatments for mastalgia. *Lancet* 1985;2:373-7.

Ramesh G, Das U. Effect of evening primrose and fish oils on two-stage skin carcinogenesis in mice. *Prostaglandins Leukot Essent Fatty Acids* 1998;59:155-61.

Reddy A, *et al*. Dietary unsaturated fatty acids, vitamin E, curcumin and eugenol alter serum and liver lipid peroxidation in rats. *Nutr Res* 1994;14:1423-37.

Reichert R. Improvements in uremic pruritis with evening primrose oil. *Healthnotes Rev Complement Integr Med* 2000;7(1):23-34.

Reynolds J, *et al*. (eds.). *Martindale The Extra Pharmacopoeia, 29th ed.* London, UK: The Pharmaceutical Press; 1989;1570.

Rothman D, DeLuca P, Zurier R. Botanical lipids: Effects on inflammation, immune responses and rheumatoid arthritis. *Sem Arthritis Rheum* 1995;25(2):87-96.

Schäfer L, Kragballe K. Supplementation with evening primrose oil in atopic dermatitis: effect on fatty acids in neutrophils and epidermis. *Lipids* 1991;26(7):557-60.

Schalin-Karrila M, Mattila L, Jansen C, Uotila P. Evening primrose oil in the treatment of atopic eczema: effect on clinical status, plasma phospholipid fatty acids and circulating blood prostaglandins. *Br J Dermatol* 1987;117(1):11-9.

Schilcher H. *Phytotherapy in Paediatrics: Handbook for Physicians and Pharmacists.* Stuttgart, Germany: Medpharm Scientific Publishers; 1997;22-3.

Schulz V, Hänsel R, Tyler V. *Rational Phytotherapy: A Physicians' Guide to Herbal Medicine, 43rd ed.* Berlin, Germany: Springer Verlag; 1998.

Stevens E, Carrington A, Tomlinson D. Prostacyclin release in experimental diabetes: effects of evening primrose oil. *Prostaglandins Leukot Essent Fatty Acids* 1993;49(3):699-706.

Strid J, Jepson R, Moore V, Kleijnen J, Iasco SM. Evening Primrose Oil or other essential fatty acids for the treatment of pre-menstrual syndrome (PMS) (Cochrane Review). In: *The Cochrane Library*. Oxford: Update Software; 2001.

Tunón H. Phytotherapie in Schweden. *Z Phytother* 1999;20:269-77.

United States Congress (USC). Public Law 103-417: Dietary Supplement Health and Education Act of 1994. Washington, DC: 103rd Congress of the United States; 1994.

USC. See: United States Congress.

van der Merwe C, Booyens J, Joubert H, van der Merwe C. The effect of gamma-linolenic acid, an *in vitro* cytostatic substance contained in evening primrose oil, on primary liver cancer. A double- blind placebo controlled trial. *Prostaglandins Leukot Essent Fatty Acids* 1990;40(3):199-202.

van Doormaal J, Idema G, Muskiet A, *et al*. Effects of short-term high dose intake of evening primrose oil on plasma and cellular fatty acid compositions, alpha-toco-pherol levels, and erythropoiesis in normal and Type 1 (insulin-dependent) diabetic men. *Diabetologia* 1988;31(8):576-84.

Veale D, Torley H, Richards IM, *et al*. A double-blind placebo controlled trial of Efamol® Marine on skin and joint symptoms of psoriatic arthritis. *Br J Rheumatol* 1994;33(10):954-8.

Wetzig N. Mastalgia: a 3 year Australian study. *Aust N Z J Surg* 1994;64(5):329-31.

Whitaker D, Cilliers J, de Beer C. Evening primrose oil (Epogam®) in the treatment of chronic hand dermatitis: disappointing therapeutic results. *Dermatology* 1996;193(2):115-20.

Willard T. Evening primrose oil (EPO). In: *Textbook of Advanced Herbology.* Calgary, Canada: Wild Rose College of Natural Healing Ltd; 1992;191-4.

World Health Organization (WHO). *Traditional Medicine: Regulatory Situation of Herbal Medicines.* Geneva, Switzerland, World Health Organization Traditional Medicine Programme; 1998;25.

WHO. See: World Health Organization.

Wright S, Burton J. Oral evening primrose seed oil improves atopic eczema. *Lancet* 1982;2:1120-2.

Yoshimoto-Furuie K, Yoshimoto K, Tanaka T, *et al*. Effects of oral supplementation with evening primrose oil for six weeks on plasma essential fatty acid and uremic skin symptoms in hemodialysis patients. *Nephron* 1999;91:151-9.

Zurier R, Rossetti RG, Jacobson EW, *et al*. Gamma-linolenic acid treatment of rheumatoid arthritis. A randomized, placebo-controlled trial. *Arthritis Rheum* 1996;39(11):1808-17.

Clinical Studies on Evening Primrose (*Oenothera biennis* L.)

Breast Pain and PMS Symptoms

Author/Year	Subject	Design	Duration	Dosage	Preparation	Results/Conclusion
Cheung, 1999	Cyclical mastalgia	P n=32 women with disturbing cyclical mastalgia, median duration of pain 12 months, interfering with lifestyle (mean age 37 years)	3 months if symptoms improved; if symptoms did not completely resolve, additional 3 months (6 months total)	Six, 500 mg capsules/day (240 mg GLA/day)	Efamast® capsules (500 mg EPO providing 40 mg GLA per capsule)	An overall, clinically useful response rate of 97% was observed at 6 months. One-third and one-half of women were pain-free at end of 3 and 6 months, respectively. Side effects greater than expected (12%) though mild and did not interfere with treatment. Authors conclude that EPO should be recommended as first-line specific treatment for women with disturbing cyclical mastalgia.
Gateley et al., 1992b	Cyclical mastalgia	P n=85 women with cyclical mastalgia	17 years (4-month treatment periods)	Two, 500 mg capsules 6x/day (240 mg GLA/day)	Efamast® capsules (500 mg EPO providing 40 mg GLA per capsule)	A clinically useful response was obtained in 51 of 85 patients (54%) at 4 months. An additional 12 of 29 patients (41%) who failed to obtain a useful response from other therapies obtained a useful response from EPO as a second line treatment. EPO was less effective than danazol but showed equivalent efficacy to bromocriptine.
Wetzig, 1994	Cyclical and non-cyclical mastalgia with significant breast pain for more than 3 years	Cm n=170 (EPO group n=39) Australian women with cyclical or non-cyclical mastalgia (mean age 42 years)	3 years	Two, 500 mg capsules 2–3x/day	EPO 500 mg capsules, (brand not stated) or Vitamin B6 50–100mg 2x/day or Danazol 100 mg 2x/day tapering to 100 mg daily after pain control (tamoxifen dose not specified if resistant to danzol and progesterones)	10 out of 39 (26%) had complete pain relief. 70% of women who did not respond to treatment had cyclical pain. Response rates of vitamin B6 and EPO were no better than placebo effect. 67% of women taking danazol had complete response.
Khoo et al., 1990	PMS symptoms	DB, PC, R, CO n=38 women with PMS	6 months (crossover after 3 cycles)	Four, 500 mg capsules 2x/day (360 mg GLA/day)	Efamol® capsules (500 mg EPO providing 45 mg GLA) vs. placebo (500 mg liquid paraffin)	Substantial improvement in PMS symptoms for EPO and placebo suggesting a strong placebo effect. No significant differences in scoring of 10 PMS symptoms or menstrual symptoms between EPO and placebo. Authors conclude the improvement experienced by women with moderate PMS was solely placebo effect.
Ockerman et al., 1986	PMS symptoms	DB, PC n=36 women with severe PMS	3 months	One, 500 mg capsule	Efamol® capsules (500 mg EPO providing 45 mg GLA)	Statistically significant difference (p<0.01) between EPO group and placebo for moderate to complete relief of symptoms.

KEY: C – controlled, **CC** – case-control, **CH** – cohort, **CI** – confidence interval, **Cm** – comparison, **CO** – crossover, **CS** – cross-sectional, **DB** – double-blind, **E** – epidemiological, **LC** – longitudinal cohort, **MA** – meta-analysis, **MC** – multi-center, **n** – number of patients, **O** – open, **OB** – observational, **OL** – open label, **OR** – odds ratio, **P** – prospective, **PB** – patient-blind, **PC** – placebo-controlled, **PG** – parallel group, **PS** – pilot study, **R** – randomized, **RC** – reference-controlled, **RCS** – retrospective cross-sectional, **RS** - retrospective, **S** – surveillance, **SB** – single-blind, **SC** – single-center, **U** – uncontrolled, **UP** – unpublished, **VC** – vehicle-controlled.

Clinical Studies on Evening Primrose (*Oenothera biennis* L.)   (cont.)

Dermatological

Author/Year	Subject	Design	Duration	Dosage	Preparation	Results/Conclusion
Gehring et al., 1999	Atopic dermatitis	DB, VC, PC, R n=40	5 weeks (4-week treatment followed by 1 week no treatment)	Topical application to entire flexor side of forearm 2x/day	Amphiphilic oil-in-water emulsion containing 20% EPO vs. placebo (20% miglyol) and water-in-oil emulsion with 20% EPO vs. placebo (20% liquid paraffin)	Statistically significant stabilizing effect on barrier function was observed with EPO in water-in-oil emulsion (p<0.05) treatment vs. placebo, documented as a reduction in transepidermal water loss (TEWL). Peak effect not apparent until 5 weeks, including 1-week treatment-free period. Only water-in-oil emulsion proved to be an effective vehicle for EPO, demonstrating that choice in vehicle is an extremely important factor in the efficacy of topically applied EPO.
Yoshimoto-Furuie et al., 1999	Uremic skin symptoms (pruritus, erythema, dryness)	DB, PC, R n=16 male and female patients undergoing hemodialysis (ages 23–79 years)	6 weeks plus 6-week observation	Two, 500 mg capsules 2x/day (180 mg GLA/day)	Efamol® capsules (500 mg EPO providing 360 mg linoleic acid, 50 mg oleic acid, 45 mg GLA) vs. placebo (500 mg linoleic acid)	EPO group had statistically significant overall improvement vs. linoleic acid group (p<0.05). EPO group had significant increase in mean lipid plasma concentration of DGLA at weeks 6 and 12 compared to baseline (p<0.01). EPO group also had significant increases in plasma GLA levels in cholesterol ester (p<0.01) and triglyceride (p<0.05) fractions at 6 and 12 weeks.
Whitaker et al., 1996	Chronic hand dermatitis (>1 year duration)	DB, PC, R n=39	8 weeks each, with an 8-week follow-up period	Twelve, 500mg capsules/day for 16 weeks (600 mg GLA/day)	Epogam® capsules (500 mg EPO providing 50 mg GLA) vs. placebo (500 mg sunflower oil)	No statistical difference between orally ingested EPO and placebo groups for any parameters tested. Therapeutic value of EPO for chronic hand dermatitis was not superior to placebo.
Hederos and Berg, 1996	Children (ages 1–16 years) with atopic dermatitis who needed regular treatment with topical steroids (22 patients had asthma)	DB, PC, PG, R n=58	16 weeks	Four or six, 500 mg capsules 2x/day according to age (320–480 mg GLA/day)	Epogam® capsules (500 mg EPO providing 40 mg GLA w/10 mg vit. E) vs. placebo (500 mg sunflower oil with vitamin E)	EPO group had significantly increased plasma concentrations of EFAs (p<0.001). Both groups showed significant improvement from baseline symptoms (p<0.001–p<0.05) without a significant difference between placebo and EPO.
Oliwiecki and Burton, 1994	Chronic stable-plaque psoriasis	DB, PC, PG n=37 (ages 16–70 years)	28 weeks (4 week placebo then treatment, or placebo for 24 weeks)	Six, 500 mg capsules 2x/day (480 mg GLA/day)	Efamol® Marine capsules (430 mg EPO and 107 mg fish oil, providing 40 mg GLA, 20 mg EPA, 11 mg DHA, and 10 mg vitamin E) vs. placebo (paraffin)	No significant difference between EPO and placebo groups in plaque thickness or transepidermal water loss. In the clinical assessment, no significant difference in LAS (linear analogue measurement) was seen in erythema or scaling and overall severity scores. Mean LAS score for overall severity was significantly higher in EPO group at week 8 (p<0.05). Authors conclude that EPO combined with fish oil produces no significant improvement in chronic stable plaque psoriasis.
Veale et al., 1994	Dermatological; psoriatic arthritis (PsA)	DB, PC, R n=38	1 year (9-month treatment followed by 3 month placebo)	Twelve, 500mg capsules/day (480 mg GLA/day)	Efamol® Marine capsules (430 mg EPO and 107 mg fish oil, providing 40 mg GLA, 20 mg EPA, 11 mg DHA and 10 mg vitamin E) vs. placebo (paraffin and vitamin E)	EPO and fish oil combination appears to alter prostaglandin metabolism in patients with PsA though this study failed to prove that it could substitute for NSAID therapy. All measures of skin disease activity were unaffected by treatment and did not allow reduction in NSAID requirement. Authors conclude that the study did demonstrate metabolic effects on prostanoid and leukotriene metabolism, suggesting that larger doses might produce a clinical response.

KEY: C – controlled, **CC** – case-control, **CH** – cohort, **CI** – confidence interval, **Cm** – comparison, **CO** – crossover, **CS** – cross-sectional, **DB** – double-blind, **E** – epidemiological, **LC** – longitudinal cohort, **MA** – meta-analysis, **MC** – multi-center, **n** – number of patients, **O** – open, **OB** – observational, **OL** – open label, **OR** – odds ratio, **P** – prospective, **PB** – patient-blind, **PC** – placebo-controlled, **PG** – parallel group, **PS** – pilot study, **R** – randomized, **RC** – reference-controlled, **RCS** – retrospective cross-sectional, **RS** - retrospective, **S** – surveillance, **SB** – single-blind, **SC** – single-center, **U** – uncontrolled, **UP** – unpublished, **VC** – vehicle-controlled.

Dermatological   (cont.)

Author/Year	Subject	Design	Duration	Dosage	Preparation	Results/Conclusion
Berth-Jones and Graham-Brown, 1993	Atopic dermatitis	DB, PC, R, PG n=102 adults and children with 3 treatment limbs	16 weeks	Six, 500 mg capsules 2x/day (480 mg GLA/day) or six, 500 mg EPO & fish oil capsules 2x/day	Epogam® capsules (500 mg EPO, providing 321 mg LA, 40 mg GLA); Efamol® Marine capsules (430 mg EPO, 107 mg fish oil), vs. placebo (paraffin or olive oil)	No therapeutic effect was demonstrated for either EPO or EPO in combination with marine fish oil. No significant difference from placebo in mean improvement of any parameters used to monitor disease, severity including clinical severity scores (both Leicester score and Costa score systems used), percentage of skin affected, topical steroid requirement, and patient diaries.
Oliwiecki et al., 1993	Epidermal thinning	Cm, R n=24 healthy volunteers with 2 treatment limbs	3 weeks	Apply a thin layer of cream over an area of forearm 5 X 5 cm in diameter 2x/day	Scotia Cream A (0.1% beta-methasone valerate), Cream B (0.1% beta-methasone Valerate, 10% EPO), Cream C (10% arachis oil)	Concomitant administration of EPO and beta-methasone valerate did not prevent steroid-induced epidermal thinning, suggesting that steroid-induced epidermal thinning is not mediated by the inhibition of EFA release from cell membranes. EPO did not affect histological changes (e.g., absence of granular layer and flattening of rete ridges).
Schäfer and Kragballe, 1991	Atopic dermatitis	R (3 dose levels) n=15	10 weeks	4, 8, or 12 capsules/day (0.5g oil)	Quest Vitamins EPO capsules (500 mg EPO)	Supplementation at the highest dosage level, 6 g EPO/day, increased n-6 fatty acid level, especially DGLA by 15–60% in neutrophil and epidermal phospholipids (p<0.05). A beneficial shift in ratio between n-6 and monounsaturated fatty acids was also observed. Authors conclude that EPO at 6 g/day can effect moderate and favorable fatty acid changes in the epidermis of atopic dermatitis patients.

Other

Author/Year	Subject	Design	Duration	Dosage	Preparation	Results/Conclusion
Dove and Johnson, 1999	Pregnancy labor	R, PC, RS n=108	7 years, entering at different times (1991–98)	500 mg 3x/day for 1 week at week 37 of gestation, followed by 500 mg/day until labor	Brand not stated	No significant differences between EPO and placebo on age, Apgar score, days of gestation (p>.05). There was slight significant difference in birth weight (p = .043), with infants in EPO group averaging 156 g larger than those in control group. Women in EPO group had labor averaging 3 hours longer than for the placebo, and an increase in active-phase labor abnormalities including protracted active phase, prolonged rupture of membranes, increased oxytocin, and arrest of descent, some of which may be attributed to larger infant weight.
Jenkins et al., 1996	Liver damage due to chronic hepatitis B	PC, R n=20 patients with chronic hepatitis B	1 year	Four, 500 mg capsules 2x/day before meals	Efamol® capsules (500 mg EPO plus 10 mg vitamin E) vs. placebo (liquid paraffin)	EPO treatment showed no improvement over placebo in biochemical or histological indices of liver damage, or in rate of loss of circulating surface or e-antigen.
Chenoy et al., 1994	Menopausal hot flash (at least 3x daily)	DB, PC, R n=35 menopausal women (mean age EPO group 53.7 years; mean age placebo group 54.2 years)	6-month treatment periods	Four, 500 mg capsules 2x/day	Efamol® capsules (500 mg EPO with 10 mg natural vitamin E) vs. placebo (500 mg liquid paraffin)	The only significant improvement in EPO group was reduction in maximum number of nighttime flushes (p<0.05). Authors concluded that EPO provides no benefit over placebo in treatment of menopausal hot flashes.
Keen et al., 1993	Diabetic neuropathy	DB, PC, R, PG, MC n=111	1 year	500 mg capsule 12/day (480 mg GLA/day)	EF4- capsules (500 mg EPO providing 40 mg GLA)	EPO was significantly superior to placebo in relieving 13 of 16 parameters. Both neurological and conduction values improved significantly vs. placebo group. Researchers concluded that EPO may prevent deterioration and reverse the condition in patients with mild diabetic polyneuropathy.

KEY: C – controlled, **CC** – case-control, **CH** – cohort, **CI** – confidence interval, **Cm** – comparison, **CO** – crossover, **CS** – cross-sectional, **DB** – double-blind, **E** – epidemiological, **LC** – longitudinal cohort, **MA** – meta-analysis, **MC** – multi-center, **n** – number of patients, **O** – open, **OB** – observational, **OL** – open label, **OR** – odds ratio, **P** – prospective, **PB** – patient-blind, **PC** – placebo-controlled, **PG** – parallel group, **PS** – pilot study, **R** – randomized, **RC** – reference-controlled, **RCS** – retrospective cross-sectional, **RS** - retrospective, **S** – surveillance, **SB** – single-blind, **SC** – single-center, **U** – uncontrolled, **UP** – unpublished, **VC** – vehicle-controlled.

Evening Primrose Oil

Monograph

Other   (cont.)

Author/Year	Subject	Design	Duration	Dosage	Preparation	Results/Conclusion
Brzeski *et al.*, 1991	Rheumatoid arthritis and upper gastro-intestinal lesions due to non-steroidal anti-inflammatory drugs	DB, PC, P, R n=30 (mean age EPO group 60 years; mean age placebo group 61 years)	6 months	500 mg capsule 12/day (540 mg GLA/day)	Efamol® capsules (500 mg EPO plus 10 mg vitamin E) vs. placebo (olive oil)	EPO produced statistically significant reduction in morning stiffness but only small reduction in articular index. Only 23% (3/13) of EPO group could reduce NSAID dose and none could stop, similar to olive oil group. Of EPO group, 77% (10/13) showed a significant rise in plasma DGLA. Authors conclude that EPO cannot be substituted for non-steroidal anti-inflammatory drugs (NSAIDs) in patients with NSAID-induced upper gastrointestinal side effects.
Cant *et al.*, 1991	Effect on milk composition in nursing mothers	DB, PC, R n=36 breast-feeding women	8 months	Four, 500 mg capsules 2x/day (2,800 mg LA/day, 320 mg GLA/day)	Efamol® capsules (500 mg EPO) vs. placebo (liquid paraffin)	Total fat and EFA content in milk declined 17-23% in placebo group and increased an unspecified percentage in EPO group. This study demonstrates that supplementing the maternal diet with EPO changes milk fatty acid composition and may provide other beneficial effects by increasing fat content and energy content of breast milk while also increasing ratio of poly-unsaturated to saturated fats.
Jamal and Carmichael, 1990	Diabetic neuropathy	DB, PC, R n=22 patients with distal diabetic polyneuro-pathy	6 months	Two, 500 mg capsules 4x/day (360 mg GLA/day)	EPO (500-mg capsules providing 45 mg GLA) (brand not stated)	In comparison to placebo, patients in EPO group showed statistically significant increase in both median ($p<0.01$) and peroneal nerve conduction ($p<0.05$), as well as an improvement in neuropathy symptom scores ($p=0.001$) such as abnormal sensations of heat, cold, numbness, pain, weakness, and paresthesias.
van der Merwe *et al.*, 1990	Liver cancer	DB, PC, R n=62 patients with primary liver cancer	2 years, volunteers entering at different points during this period	500 mg capsule 36/day (1,440 mg GLA/day)	Efamol® capsules (500 mg EPO providing 40 mg GLA) vs. placebo (500 mg olive oil)	Mean survival time for EPO group was 58 vs. 42 days in placebo group. Effect of EPO on survival in primary liver cancer was not significantly better than placebo. In objective and subjective measurements, EPO scored better than placebo, but was not siginificant. EPO had a statistically significant beneficial effect on gamma-glutamyl transferase values, as a measure of liver function ($p=0.0192$).

KEY: C – controlled, **CC** – case-control, **CH** – cohort, **CI** – confidence interval, **Cm** – comparison, **CO** – crossover, **CS** – cross-sectional, **DB** – double-blind, **E** – epidemiological, **LC** – longitudinal cohort, **MA** – meta-analysis, **MC** – multi-center, **n** – number of patients, **O** – open, **OB** – observational, **OL** – open label, **OR** – odds ratio, **P** – prospective, **PB** – patient-blind, **PC** – placebo-controlled, **PG** – parallel group, **PS** – pilot study, **R** – randomized, **RC** – reference-controlled, **RCS** – retrospective cross-sectional, **RS** - retrospective, **S** – surveillance, **SB** – single-blind, **SC** – single-center, **U** – uncontrolled, **UP** – unpublished, **VC** – vehicle-controlled.

Feverfew

Tanacetum parthenium (L.) Sch. Bip. (syn. *Chrysanthemum parthenium* [L.] Bernh.)
[Fam. *Asteraceae*]

OVERVIEW

Feverfew is ranked 19th among herbal supplements sold in mainstream retail outlets in the U.S. It is used primarily for migraine prophylactic effects, and for concomitant nausea and vomiting. Many commercial feverfew preparations are standardized based on 0.1% to 0.2% parthenolide content. However, different commercial preparations can vary widely in parthenolide content depending upon the geographical location from which the seeds were derived, the vegetative cycle of the plant at the time of harvest, the parts of the plant used, and the duration and conditions of storage. Parthenolide, once believed to be the primary active constituent, is no longer considered principal; other, unknown compounds are believed to be responsible for feverfew's anti-migraine activity.

PRIMARY USES

- Migraine prophylaxis
- Nausea and vomiting associated with migraine

PHARMACOLOGICAL ACTIONS

Anti-nociceptive; anti-inflammatory; inhibits collagen-induced bronchoconstriction; anti-thrombotic potential; inhibits prostaglandin synthesis; inhibits serotonin release; inhibits mast cell release of histamine.

DOSAGE AND ADMINISTRATION

Optimal doses of feverfew for therapeutic benefits have not been established. However, an adult dose equivalent to 0.2–0.6 mg of parthenolide is recommended for migraine prophylaxis.

DRIED LEAVES: 50–150 mg per day, as indicated by the clinical studies.

FRESH LEAVES: 2.5 leaves per day, with or after food.

TINCTURE: (1:5, 25% ethanol) 5–20 drops per day.

NOTE: Clinical experience suggests that the beneficial effects of feverfew for migraine prophylaxis can usually be seen within 4–6 weeks of initiating treatment. However, the duration of treatment will vary for individual migraine sufferers. There are no long-term safety data because clinical studies showing positive results for the effects of feverfew on migraine prophylaxis have

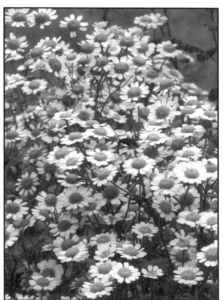

Photo © 2003 stevenfoster.com

been conducted for a brief duration of only 4–6 months. Therefore, it is recommended that patients on long-term therapy discontinue using feverfew for at least one month per year to evaluate efficacy and determine if continued treatment is necessary. The feverfew dose should be tapered gradually over the preceding month to prevent potential withdrawal symptoms.

CONTRAINDICATIONS

Feverfew is contraindicated for persons who are allergic to feverfew (*Tanacetum parthenium*) and other members of the family *Asteraceae*, including ragweed (*Ambrosia* spp.), chrysanthemums (*Chrysanthemum* spp.), marigolds (*Calendula officinalis*), chamomile (*Matricaria* spp.), yarrow (*Achillea* spp.), and daisies. Feverfew is not recommended for children under two years of age.

PREGNANCY AND LACTATION: Not for use in pregnancy and lactation. Feverfew is contraindicated during pregnancy because it may act as an emmenogogue in early pregnancy.

ADVERSE EFFECTS

Allergic contact dermatitis can result from handling fresh feverfew. Mouth ulceration and swelling of the tongue, lips, and oral mucosa have also been reported. Abdominal pains and indigestion have been reported for feverfew users who chewed the leaves over a period of years. Diarrhea, flatulence, nausea, and vomiting were rare, but important enough to discontinue treatment. Although long-term toxicity data are presently unavailable, no serious side effects have been noted in patients taking the plant for several years.

DRUG INTERACTIONS

No adverse side effects were noted in a large number of individuals taking feverfew in combination with other medications. Pharmacological studies suggest that, in theory, feverfew should not be ingested with anticoagulants or antiplatelet agents such as aspirin or warfarin. However, this recommendation is speculative and has yet to be substantiated by pharmacological or clinical data.

Feverfew

Clinical Overview

CLINICAL REVIEW

In six trials that included a total of 279 participants, 5 demonstrated positive effects in treating migraine. However, 1 trial examining feverfew's effects on arthritis found no apparent benefit. Three of the 5 migraine studies were randomized, double-blind, and placebo-controlled. In one of these studies, the participants used a feverfew extract, but did not experience a reduction in the number of migraine attacks; however, they were able to use fewer drugs during the period in which they took the feverfew. It has been theorized that the therapeutic effect of feverfew is due to an unidentified plant constituent that may have been lost or degraded in the extract made from feverfew material used in a study that did not produce positive results. In addition, the leaves of the plant used in the latter study were not cultivated from certified seeds. By comparison, the studies using dried feverfew leaf found a reduction in number and severity of migraine attacks. Feverfew consistently reduced vomiting and nausea associated with migraine. A recently published literature review concluded that the efficacy of feverfew for the prevention of migraine has not been established beyond reasonable doubt. In addition, one trial found that feverfew did not benefit women with rheumatoid arthritis.

Feverfew

Tanacetum parthenium (L.) Sch. Bip. (syn. *Chrysanthemum parthenium* [L.] Bernh.)
[Fam. *Asteraceae*]

OVERVIEW

Feverfew is usually collected when the plant is in bloom. However, different commercial preparations can vary widely in active ingredients depending on where the plant was growing, its condition at the time of harvest, and the parts of the plant used. Parthenolide is an active ingredient in feverfew that may be partly responsible for its effects in preventing and treating migraine headache, although scientists now believe that some other unidentified compound(s) may be responsible. Many feverfew products are standardized to contain between 0.1–0.2% parthenolide. Feverfew is ranked 19th among herbal supplements sold in mainstream retail outlets in the U.S.

USES

Migraine prevention; nausea and vomiting associated with migraine.

DOSAGE

To prevent migraine, take adult dose equal to 0.2–0.6 mg of parthenolide. Benefits usually begin within 4–6 weeks after starting treatment. The length of treatment will vary for individual migraine sufferers.

DRIED LEAVES: 50–150 mg per day, as indicated by clinical studies.

FRESH LEAVES: 2.5 leaves per day, with or after food.

TINCTURE: 5–20 drops per day [1:5, 25% ethanol].

CONTRAINDICATIONS

Consult a healthcare provider before using feverfew if you are allergic to this or other plants in the family *Asteraceae* such as ragweed, chrysanthemums, marigolds, chamomile, yarrow, and daisies. Feverfew is not recommended for children under 2 years of age.

PREGNANCY AND LACTATION: Feverfew should not be used during pregnancy or while breast-feeding.

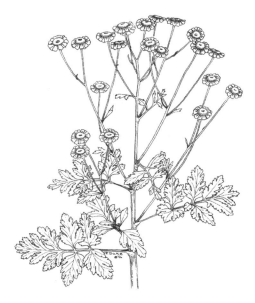

ADVERSE EFFECTS

No serious side effects have been noted in individuals taking feverfew for a period of years. Skin inflammation can result from handling fresh feverfew. Mouth ulcers and swelling of the tongue, lip, and the mucous membrane of the mouth may occur. Abdominal pains and indigestion have been reported for feverfew users who chewed the leaves over a period of years. Diarrhea, flatulence, nausea, and vomiting occur rarely.

DRUG INTERACTIONS

There are no known drug interactions. Theoretically, feverfew should not be ingested at the same time as blood-thinning (anticoagulant or antiplatelet) medications like aspirin or warfarin. However, this has not been scientifically proven in human studies.

Comments

When using a dietary supplement, purchase it from a reliable source. For best results, use the same brand of product throughout the period of use. As with all medications and dietary supplements, please inform your healthcare provider of all herbs and medications you are taking. Interactions may occur between medications and herbs or even among different herbs when taken at the same time. Treat your herbal supplement with care by taking it as directed, storing it as advised on the label, and keeping it out of the reach of children and pets. Consult your healthcare provider with any questions.

AMERICAN
BOTANICAL
COUNCIL

The information contained on this sheet has been excerpted from *The ABC Clinical Guide to Herbs* © 2003 by the American Botanical Council (ABC). ABC is an independent member-based educational organization focusing on the medicinal use of herbs. For more detailed information about this herb please consult the healthcare provider who gave you this sheet. To order *The ABC Clinical Guide to Herbs* or become a member of ABC, visit their website at www.herbalgram.org.

Feverfew
Tanacetum parthenium (L.) Sch. Bip.
[Fam. *Asteraceae*]

OVERVIEW

Traditionally, feverfew was used for a wide range of disorders including psoriasis, toothache, insect bites, rheumatism, vertigo, colic, cleansing the kidneys and bladder, stomach pain, menstrual problems, inflammation, and fever (Hobbs, 1989; Groenewegen *et al.*, 1992). The ancient Greeks called feverfew "parthenium" because, according to legend, it was used to save the life of someone who had fallen from the Parthenon, the Doric temple of the virgin goddess Athena on the Acropolis in Athens (Hobbs, 1989). However, its name may be more likely based on feverfew's traditional use for alleviating menstrual cramps in young girls (*parthenos* = virgin in Greek). Currently, feverfew is used primarily for migraine prophylactic effects, and for concomitant nausea and vomiting (Brown, 1995; ESCOP, 1996; Johnson *et al.*, 1985; Murphy *et al.*, 1988). Feverfew is ranked 19th among herbal supplements sold in mainstream retail outlets in the U.S. (Blumenthal, 2001).

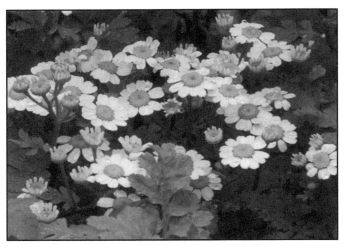

Photo © 2003 stevenfoster.com

DESCRIPTION

Feverfew preparations consist of the aerial parts or leaves of *Tanacetum parthenium* (L.) Sch. Bip. (syn. *Chrysanthemum parthenium* (L.) Bernh.) [Fam. *Asteraceae*], collected when the plant is in flower (Bradley, 1992; Reynolds, 1993; Newall *et al.*, 1996). The fresh leaves can also be chewed to obtain the purported therapeutic benefits (Newall *et al.*, 1996). Many commercial feverfew preparations are standardized based on parthenolide content (0.1% [French regulatory authorities] to 0.2% [Canadian authorities] are suggested as minimum contents for quality control purposes) (Bruneton, 1999; Evans, 1998). However, different commercial preparations can vary widely in parthenolide content depending upon the geographical location from which the seeds were derived, the vegetative cycle of the plant at the time of harvest, the parts of the plant used, and the

duration and conditions of storage (Bruneton, 1999; Evans, 1998; Heptinstall, 1992). No parthenolide was detected in feverfew grown in Mexico or Yugoslavia, and the feverfew in both countries contained eudesmolides and guaianolides as the primary constituents (Heptinstall *et al.*, 1992). Recent evidence indicates that the pharmacological activity of feverfew in the treatment and prophylaxis of migraines is not attributed to parthenolide content as was previously thought, but to other unidentified constituents (Awang, 1998a; de Weerdt *et al.*, 1996). In addition, parthenolide is not a unique constituent of feverfew (Heptinstall *et al.*, 1992); parthenolide is detected in 34 plant species (25 from *Asteraceae*, nine from *Magnoliaceae*) (Heptinstall *et al.*, 1992; Heptinstall and Awang, 1998). Therefore, parthenolide is used to ensure that the correct chemotype of *T. parthenium* is used, but it is not an assurance of the botanical identity or efficacy of feverfew products (Awang, 1998b). Since the active constituents are unknown, it is recommended that preparations containing the whole leaf (dried or fresh) should be used (Awang, 1998b; Heptinstall and Awang, 1998). Since parthenolide stability can vary with storage conditions, feverfew should be stored in a cool, dry, dark environment (Heptinstall *et al.*, 1992; Heptinstall and Awang, 1998).

PRIMARY USES

- Migraine prophylaxis (de Weerdt *et al.*, 1996; Palevitch *et al.*, 1997; Anderson *et al.*, 1988; Murphy *et al.*, 1988; Johnson *et al.*, 1985)
- Nausea and vomiting associated with migraine (Palevitch *et al.*, 1997; Murphy *et al.*, 1988; Johnson *et al.*, 1985)

DOSAGE

Optimal doses of feverfew for therapeutic benefits have not been established; however, an adult dose equivalent to 0.2–0.6 mg of parthenolide is recommended for migraine prophylaxis (ESCOP, 1996; Johnson *et al.*, 1985; Murphy *et al.*, 1988).

Internal
Crude Preparations
DRIED LEAF: 50–150 mg daily (Palevitch *et al.*, 1997; Murphy *et al.*, 1988; Johnson *et al.*, 1985).

FRESH LEAF: 2.5 leaves daily, with or after food (Newall *et al.*, 1996).

TINCTURE: 1:5, 25% ethanol, 5–20 drops daily (Bradley, 1992).

DURATION OF ADMINISTRATION
Internal
Crude Preparations
Prophylaxis benefit for migraine can usually be seen within four to six weeks of the initiation of treatment (Brown, 1995; Palevitch *et al.*, 1997). However, the duration of treatment will vary for individual migraine sufferers (Brown, 1995). Successful clinical studies involving feverfew for migraine prophylaxis have been conducted for durations of up to 46 months;

longer-term safety data are not presently available (Johnson *et al.,* 1985; Murphy *et al.,* 1988; Palevitch *et al.,* 1997). It is recommended that patients continuing long-term use should discontinue therapy for at least one month per year to evaluate efficacy and determine whether continuation is necessary (ESCOP, 1996; Baldwin *et al.,* 1987). The feverfew dose should be tapered gradually over the preceding month to prevent potential withdrawal symptoms (ESCOP, 1996; Baldwin *et al.,* 1987).

CHEMISTRY

The constituents of feverfew can vary depending upon the chemotype and the geographical location from which the seeds were derived (Heptinstall *et al.,* 1992). Constituents include sesquiterpene lactones including germacranolides—parthenolide (Bohlmann and Zdero, 1982; ESCOP, 1996; Hausen, 1992), eudesmolides—reynosin, and santamarin (Awang, 1989; Bohlmann and Zdero, 1982; Leung and Foster, 1996), guaianolides—canin and articanin (Bohlmann and Zdero, 1982; Bradley, 1992; Hausen, 1992; Leung and Foster, 1996). Parthenolide is usually the primary sesquiterpene lactone, but it is lacking in samples from Mexico and Yugoslavia (Heptinstall *et al.,* 1992). Additional sesquiterpenes and monoterpenes include camphor, β-farnesene, germacrene, chrysanthenyl acetate, α-pinene derivatives, bornyl acetate, bornyl angelate (Bohlmann and Zdero, 1982; Bradley, 1992; Newall *et al.,* 1996), pyrethrin (Newall *et al.,* 1996), flavonoids (Bruneton, 1999; Newall *et al.,* 1996; Williams *et al.,* 1995), tannins (Newall *et al.,* 1996), and melatonin (Murch *et al.,* 1997).

PHARMACOLOGICAL ACTIONS

Human

Antimigraine (Johnson *et al.,* 1985; Murphy *et al.,* 1988; Palevitch *et al.,* 1997); however, more information is needed. Although past studies have focused upon parthenolide as the active component responsible for antimigraine activity, a recent Dutch study determined an alcoholic feverfew leaf extract (containing an appropriate level of parthenolide) to be ineffective in migraine prophylaxis, challenging previous hypotheses (Awang, 1998b; de Weerdt *et al.,* 1996). The Dutch researchers suggest that another compound such as chrysanthenyl acetate, detected in significantly reduced amounts in the extract compared with the dried, whole plant material, may contribute to the anti-migraine activity due to its prostaglandin inhibition (de Weerdt *et al.,* 1996; Heptinstall and Awang, 1998).

Animal

Anti-nociceptive (Jain and Kulkarni, 1999); anti-inflammatory (Jain and Kulkarni, 1999); inhibits collagen-induced bronchoconstriction (Keery and Lumley, 1986).

In vitro

Anti-inflammatory (Williams *et al.,* 1995; Brown *et al.,* 1997); inhibits mast cell release of histamine (Hayes and Foreman, 1987); inhibits blood platelet secretion of serotonin (Heptinstall *et al.,* 1985; Groenewegen and Heptinstall, 1990); anti-thrombotic potential (Voyno-Yasenetskaya *et al.,* 1988; Groenewegen and Heptinstall, 1990; Löesche *et al.,* 1987); inhibits prostaglandin synthesis (Pugh and Sambo, 1988); inhibits serotonin release (Béjar, 1996; Marles *et al.,* 1992); inhibits eicosanoid synthesis (Sumner *et al.,* 1992); alters vascular responses (Barsby *et al.,* 1992, 1993a, 1993b); inhibits neutrophil phagocytosis (Williamson *et al.,* 1988); antibacterial (Hayes and Foreman, 1987); cytotoxic (O'Neill *et al.,* 1987).

MECHANISM OF ACTION

- May inhibit platelet behavior through the neutralization of sulphydryl groups on enzymes of proteins implicated in platelet aggregation and secretion (Heptinstall *et al.,* 1987).
- Sesquiterpene lactones and non-sesquiterpene lactones inhibit eicosanoid synthesis by inhibiting 5-lipoxygenase and cyclo-oxygenase in leukocytes (Sumner *et al.,* 1992). Tanetin may contribute to anti-inflammatory properties by inhibiting the generation of pro-inflammatory eicosanoids (Williams *et al.,* 1995; Hoult *et al.,* 1995).
- Parthenolide and other sesquiterpene lactones in extracts of fresh leaves appear to irreversibly and nonspecifically inhibit smooth muscle contractions (Barsby *et al.,* 1993a). In contrast, chloroform extracts of dried feverfew leaves, containing no parthenolide, produce reversible smooth muscle contractions via a selective open-channel block of voltage-dependent potassium channels (Barsby *et al.,* 1993b).
- Inhibits collagen-induced bronchoconstriction by inhibiting phospholipase A2 activity (Keery and Lumley, 1986).
- Parthenolide, and other sesquiterpene lactones inhibit serotonin release from bovine platelets. Serotonin has been implicated in the pathogenesis of migraines (Marles *et al.,* 1992).
- Parthenolide, michefuscalide, and chrysanthenyl acetate can inhibit prostaglandin synthetase, which catalyzes the conversion of arachadonic acid to prostaglandins (Pugh and Sambo, 1988).
- Extract inhibits histamine release from rat peritoneal mast cells (Hayes and Foreman, 1987).
- Blocks secretory activity in blood platelets and polymorphonuclear leukocytes (PMNs) (Heptinstall *et al.,* 1985).
- Inhibits the release of serotonin from platelets and platelet aggregation (Heptinstall *et al.,* 1985).
- Inhibits neutrophil phagocytosis and degranulation (Williamson *et al.,* 1988).
- Extract inhibits mitogen-induced, human peripheral-blood mononuclear cell proliferation and cytokine-mediated responses (O'Neill *et al.,* 1987).

CONTRAINDICATIONS

Feverfew is contraindicated when the patient is allergic to members of family *Asteraceae (Compositae)*, which includes feverfew (*Tanacetum parthenium*), ragweed (*Ambrosia* spp.), chrysanthemums (*Chrysanthemum* spp.), marigolds (*Calendula officinalis*), chamomile (*Matricaria* spp.), yarrow (*Achillea* spp.), and daisies (ESCOP, 1996, Hausen and Osmundsen, 1983; Newall *et al.,*1996). Not recommended for children under two years old (Awang, 1993). Contraindicated for presurgical patients due to possible anti-PAF activity (Brinker, 2001).

PREGNANCY AND LACTATION: Not for use in pregnancy or lactation (Awang, 1993). Contraindicated during pregnancy because it may act as an emmenagogue in early pregnancy (Brinker, 2001).

ADVERSE EFFECTS

Allergic contact dermatitis can occur when feverfew is handled (Brinker, 2001). Mouth ulceration and swelling of the tongue, lips, and oral mucosa have also been reported (Hausen, 1992;

Murphy *et al.*, 1988). Abdominal pains and indigestion have been reported for feverfew users who have chewed the leaves over a period of years (Hausen, 1992; Murphy *et al.*, 1988). Diarrhea, flatulence, nausea, and vomiting were rare, but resulted in the discontinuation of treatment (ESCOP, 1996; Hausen, 1992). Although long-term toxicity data are presently unavailable, no serious side effects have been noted in patients taking the plant for a period of years (Hausen *et al.*, 1992; Johnson *et al.*, 1985; Murphy *et al.*, 1988).

DRUG INTERACTIONS

No adverse side effects were noted in a large number of individuals taking feverfew together with other medications (ESCOP, 1996). Due to the pharmacology, speculative theories suggest that feverfew should not be consumed with anticoagulants or antiplatelet agents like aspirin or warfarin (Brinker, 2001; Bratman and Kroll, 1999). However, these theories have not been proven in a clinical or scientific setting (Boon and Smith, 1999).

AMERICAN HERBAL PRODUCTS ASSOCIATION (AHPA) SAFETY RATING

CLASS 2B: Not to be used during pregnancy (McGuffin *et al.*, 1997). NOTE: Mouth ulceration and gastric disturbances have been reported in 6–15% of users, usually in the first week of use (McGuffin *et al.*, 1997).

REGULATORY STATUS

CANADA: The Canadian Health Protection Branch has issued Drug Identification Numbers (DIN) to dried-leaf products containing a minimum of 0.2% parthenolide with certification of botanical identity. The Feverfew Leaf Labeling Standard permits the following indications: "Traditional Herbal Medicine (THM) to help prevent recurring migraine headaches and associated nausea and vomiting" (Awang, 1998b; Health Canada, 1997; Leung and Foster, 1996).

EUROPEAN UNION: Dried aerial part, containing not less than 0.2% of parthenolide, is official in the *European Pharmacopoeia* 3rd ed. Supplement 2001 (Ph.Eur., 2001).

FRANCE: THM approved for specific indications (Bradley, 1992). Fresh or dried aerial parts are official in the *French Pharmacopoeia* (ESCOP, 1996).

GERMANY: Not reviewed by the German Commission E. No monograph in the *German Pharmacopoeia* (DAB).

SWEDEN: Classified as a natural product (De Smet *et al.*, 1993). As of January 2001, no feverfew products are listed in the Medical Products Agency (MPA) "Authorised Natural Remedies" (MPA, 2001).

SWITZERLAND: No feverfew products are licensed herbal medicines. No monograph in the *Swiss Pharmacopoeia*.

U.K.: Not on the *General Sale List* and no product licenses granted (Bradley, 1992).

U.S.: Dietary supplement (USC, 1994). Dried leaf and dried powdered leaf are official in the *United States National Formulary* (USP, 2002).

CLINICAL REVIEW

Six trials are outlined in the following table "Clinical Studies on Feverfew", including a total of 279 participants. All five of the trials examining feverfew's effects on migraine demonstrate some positive effects, but one trial examining feverfew's effects on

arthritis found no apparent benefit. Three of the five migraine studies were randomized, double-blind, and placebo-controlled (R, DB, PC) (de Weerdt *et al.*, 1996; Murphy *et al.*, 1988; Johnson *et al.*, 1985). In one of these studies the participants used a feverfew extract but did not experience a reduction in the number of migraine attacks; however, they were able to use fewer drugs during the period they took the feverfew (de Weerdt *et al.*, 1996). Awang (1998b) has theorized that the therapeutic effect of feverfew is due to an unidentified plant constituent that may have been lost or degraded in the extract made from the feverfew material used in the de Weerdt (1996) study. Further, the leaves of the plant used in the study were not cultivated from certified seeds (Awang, 1998b). By comparison, the studies using dried feverfew leaf found a reduced number and severity of migraine attacks (Palevitch *et al.*, 1997; Murphy *et al.*, 1988; Johnson *et al.*, 1985). Feverfew consistently reduced vomiting and nausea associated with migraine (Palevitch *et al.*, 1997; Murphy *et al.*, 1988; Johnson *et al.*, 1985). A recently published literature review concludes that the efficacy of feverfew for the prevention of migraine has not been established beyond reasonable doubt (Pittler *et al.*, 2000). One trial found that feverfew did not benefit women with rheumatoid arthritis (Pattrick *et al.*, 1989).

BRANDED PRODUCTS

Studies conducted were based on generic, not specific products.

REFERENCES

Anderson D, Jenkinson P, Dewdney R, Blowers S, Johnson E, Kadam N. Chromosomal aberrations and sister chromatid exchanges in lymphocytes and urine mutagenicity of migraine patients: a comparison of chronic feverfew users and matched non-users. *Hum Toxicol* 1988;7(2):145–52.

Awang D. Feverfew fever: A headache for the consumer. *HerbalGram* 1993;29:34–36, 66.

Awang D. Feverfew (Herbal Medicine). *Can Pharm J* 1989;122(5):266–70.

Awang D. Parthenocide: The demise of a facile theory of feverfew activity. *J Herbs Spices Med Plants* 1998a;5(4):95–8.

Awang D. Prescribing therapeutic feverfew. *Integr Med* 1998b;1(1):11.

Baldwin C, Anderson L, Phillipson J. What pharmacists should know about feverfew. *Pharml J* 1987 Aug 29;237–9.

Barsby R, Knight D, McFadzean I. A chloroform extract of the herb feverfew blocks voltage-dependent potassium currents recorded from single smooth muscle cells. *J Pharm Pharmacol* 1993b;45(7):641–5.

Barsby R, Salan U, Knight D, Hoult J. Feverfew and vascular smooth muscle: extracts from fresh and dried plants show opposing pharmacological profiles, dependent upon sesquiterpene lactone content. *Planta Med* 1993a;59(1):20–5.

Barsby R, Salan U, Knight D, Hoult J. Feverfew extracts and parthenolide irreversibly inhibit vascular responses of the rabbit aorta. *J Pharm Pharmacol* 1992;44(9):737–40.

Béjar E. Parthenolide inhibits the contractile responses of rat stomach fundus to fenfluramine and dextroamphetamine but not serotonin. *J Ethnopharmacol* 1996;50(1):1–12.

Berry M. Feverfew. *Pharm J* 1994;(253):806–8.

Blumenthal M. Herb sales down 15% in mainstream market. *HerbalGram* 2001;51:69.

Blumenthal M, Busse WR, Goldberg A, Gruenwald J, Hall T, Riggins CW, Rister RS (eds.). Klein S, Rister RS (trans.). *The Complete German Commission E Monographs—Therapeutic Guide to Herbal Medicines*. Austin, TX: American Botanical Council; Boston: Integrative Medicine Communication; 1998;12.

Bohlmann F, Zdero C. Sesquiterpene lactones and other constituents from *Tanacetum parthenium*. *Phytochemistry* 1982;21:2543–9.

Boon H, Smith M. *The Botanical Pharmacy–The Pharmacology of 47 Common Herbs*. Quarry Health Books; 1999;133–9.

Bradley P (ed.). Feverfew monograph. In: *British Herbal Compendium*, Vol. 1. Dorset, England: British Herbal Medicine Association; 1992;81–91.

Bratman S, Kroll D. Feverfew (*Tanacetum parthenium*). *Clinical Evaluation of Medicinal Herbs and Other Therapeutic Natural Products*. Rocklin, CA: Prima Publishing; 1999;1–6.

Brinker F. *Herb Contraindications and Drug Interactions*, 3rd ed. Sandy, OR: Eclectic

Medical Publications; 2001;95.

Brown A, Edwards C, Davey M. Effects of extracts of *Tanacetum* species on human polymorphonuclear leucocyte activity *in vitro*. *Phytother Res* 1997;(11)479–84.

Brown D. Feverfew. In: *Herbal Prescriptions for Better Health–Your Up-to-date Guide to the Most Effective Herbal Treatments*. Rocklin, CA: Prima Health; 1995;91–5.

Bruneton, J. *Pharmacognosy, Phytochemistry, Medicinal Plants*. Paris: Lavoisier Publishing; 1999;361–3.

Collier H, Butt N, McDonald-Gibson W, Saeed S. Extract of feverfew inhibits prostaglandin biosynthesis. *Lancet* 1980;Oct 25;922–3.

De Smet P, Keller K, Hansel R, Chandler R. *Adverse Effects of Herbal Drugs* Vol. 2. Berlin: Springer-Verlag; 1993;81.

de Weerdt C, Bootsma H, Hendricks H. Herbal medicines in migraine prevention: Randomized double-blind placebo-controlled crossover trial of a feverfew preparation. *Phytomedicine* 1996;3(3):225–30.

ESCOP. See: European Scientific Cooperative on Phytotherapy.

European Pharmacopoeia. (Ph.Eur. 3rd Edition Supplement 2001). Strasbourg, France: Council of Europe; 2001;840–1.

European Scientific Cooperative on Phytotherapy. *ESCOP Monographs on the Medicinal Uses of Plant Drugs*. Exeter, U.K.: ESCOP; 1996 Mar;1–6.

Evans W. *Trease and Evans' Pharmacognosy Fourteenth Edition*. London: WB Saunders Company LTD; 1998;328.

Foster S. Feverfew. *Botanical Booklet Series No. 310*. Austin: American Botanical Council; 1996.

Groenewegen W, Hepstinall S. Amounts of feverfew in commercial preparations of the herb. *Lancet* 1986;1(8471):44–5.

Groenewegen W, Heptinstall S. A comparison of the effects of an extract of feverfew and parthenolide, a component of feverfew, on human platelet activity *in-vitro*. *J Pharm Pharmacol* 1990;42(8):553–7.

Groenewegen W, Knight D, Heptinstall S. Progress in the medicinal chemistry of the herb feverfew. *Prog Med Chem* 1992;29:217–38.

Hausen B, Osmundsen P. Contact allergy to parthenolide in *Tanacetum parthenium* (L.) Schultz- Bip. (feverfew, *Asteraceae*) and cross-reactions to related sesquiterpene lactone containing *Compositae* species. *Acta Derm Venereol* 1983;63(4):308–14.

Hausen B. Sesquiterpene Lactones–*Tanacetum parthenium*. *Adv Effects Herbal Drugs* 1992;255–60.

Hayes N, Foreman J. The activity of compounds extracted from feverfew on histamine release from rat mast cells. *J Pharm Pharmacol* 1987;39(6):466–70.

Health Canada. *Labeling Standard: Feverfew Leaf*. Ottawa, Ontario: Health Canada Therapeutic Products Directorate. August 6, 1997;1–3.

Heptinstall S, Awang D, Dawson B, Kindack D, Knight D, May J. Parthenolide content and bioactivity of feverfew (*Tanacetum parthenium* (L.) Schultz-Bip.). Estimation of commercial and authenticated feverfew products. *J Pharm Pharmacol* 1992;44:391–395.

Heptinstall S, Awang D. Feverfew: A review of its history, its biological and medicinal properties, and the status of commercial preparations of the herb. ACS Symposium Series 691. *Phytomedicines of Europe–Chemistry and Biological Activity* 1998; 158–75.

Heptinstall S, Groenewegen W, Spangenberg P, Loesche W. Extracts of feverfew may inhibit platelet behavior via neutralization of sulphydryl groups. *J Pharm Pharmacol* 1987;39(6):459–465.

Heptinstall S, White A, Williamson L, Mitchell J. Extracts of feverfew inhibit granule secretion in blood platelets and polymorphonuclear leucocytes. *Lancet* 1985;1(8437):1071–4.

Hobbs C. Feverfew. *Tanacetum parthenium*: A review. *HerbalGram* 1989;20:26–35.

Hoult J, Pang L, Bland-Ward P, et al. Inhibition of leucocyte 5-lipoxygenase and cyclo-oxygenase but not constitutive nitric oxide synthase by tanetin, a novel flavonol derived from feverfew, *Tanacetum parthenium*. *Pharm Sci* 1995;1:71–4.

Jain N, Kulkarni S. Antinociceptive and anti-inflammatory effects of *Tanacetum parthenium* L. extract in mice and rats. *J Ethnopharmacol* 1999;68(1–3):251–9.

Johnson E, Kadam N, Hylands D, Hylands J. Efficacy of feverfew as prophylactic treatment of migraine. *BMJ* 1985;291(6495):569–73.

Keery R, Lumley P. Does feverfew extract exhibit phospholipase A2 inhibitory activity *in vivo*? *Proc Brit Pharm Soc* 1986;Sept;10–18.

Leung A, Foster S. Feverfew. In: *Encyclopedia of Common Natural Ingredients*. New York: John Wiley and Sons, Inc.; 1996;246–7.

Löesche W, Mazurov A, Heptinstall S, et al. An extract of feverfew inhibits interactions of human platelets with collagen substrates. *Thromb Res* 1987;48(5):511–18.

Marles R, Kaminski J, Arnason J, et al. A bioassay for inhibition of serotonin release from bovine platelets. *J Nat Prod* 1992;55(8):1044–1056.

McGuffin M, Hobbs C, Upton R, Goldberg A (eds.). *American Herbal Products Association's Botanical Safety Handbook*. Boca Raton: CRC Press; 1997.

Medical Products Agency (MPA). Naturläkemedel: Authorised Natural Remedies (as of January 24, 2001). Uppsala, Sweden: Medical Products Agency; 2001.

MPA. See: Medical Products Agency.

Murch S, Simmons CB, Saxena PK. Melatonin in feverfew and other medicinal plants [letter]. *Lancet* 1997;350(9091):1598–9.

Murphy J, Heptinstall S, Mitchell J. Randomized double-blind placebo-controlled trial of feverfew in migraine prevention. *Lancet* 1988;2(8604):189–92.

Newall C, Anderson L, Phillipson J. Feverfew. *Herbal Medicines. A Guide for Healthcare Professionals*. London: The Pharmaceutical Press; 1996;119–21.

O'Neill L, Barrett M, Lewis G. Extracts of feverfew inhibit mitogen-induced human peripheral blood mononuclear cell proliferation and cytokine mediated responses: A cytotoxic effect. *Br J Clin Pharmacol* 1987;(23):81–3.

Palevitch D, Earon G, Carasso R. Feverfew (*Tanacetum parthenium*) as a prophylactic treatment for migraine: A double-blind placebo-controlled study. *Phytother Res* 1997;11:508–11.

Pattrick M, Heptinstall S, Doherty M. Feverfew in rheumatoid arthritis: a double blind, placebo controlled study. *Ann Rheum Dis* 1989;48(7):547–9.

Ph.Eur. See: *European Pharmacopoeia*.

Pittler M, Vogler B, Ernst E. Feverfew for preventing migraine (*Cochrane review*). *Cochrane Database Syst Rev* 2000;(3):CD002286

Pizzorno JE, Murray MT, editors. *Textbook of Natural Medicine*. Vol. 1, 2nd ed. New York: Churchill Livingston; 1999:975–7.

Pugh W, Sambo K. Prostaglandin synthetase inhibitors in feverfew. *J Pharm Pharmacol* 1988;40(10):743–5.

Reynolds J (ed.). *Martindale–The Extra Pharmacopoeia, Thirtieth Edition*. London: The Pharmaceutical Press; 1993;70.

Sumner H, Salan U, Knight D, Hoult J. Inhibition of 5-lipoxygenase and cyclo-oxygenase in leukocytes by feverfew. Involvement of sesquiterpene lactones and other components. *Biochem Pharmacol* 1992;43(11):2313–20.

United States Pharmacopeia (USP 25th Revision) *National Formulary* (NF 20th Edition). Rockville, MD: The United States Pharmacopeial Convention, Inc. 2002.

USP. See: *United States Pharmacopeia*.

Voyno-Yasenetskaya T, Loesche W, Groenewegen W, et al. Effects of an extract of feverfew on endothelial cell integrity and on cAMP in rabbit perfused aorta. *J Pharm Pharmacol* 1988;40(7):501–2.

Williams C, Hoult J, Harborne J, et al. A biologically active lipophilic flavonol from *Tanacetum parthenium*. *Phytochemistry* 1995;38(1):267–70.

Williamson L, Harvey D, Sheppard K, Fletcher J. Effect of feverfew on phagocytosis and killing of *Candida guilliermondii* by neutrophils. *Inflammation* 1988;12(1):11–6.

Clinical Studies on Feverfew (*Tanacetum parthenium* [L.] Schultz Bip.)

Migraine Prophylaxis

Author/Year	Subject	Design	Duration	Dosage	Preparation	Results/Conclusion
de Weerdt et al., 1996	Migraine	R, DB, PC, CO n=44 men and women with migraine at least 1x/month	9 months: 1 placebo capsule/day for 1 month; 4 months feverfew, and 4 months placebo	One, 143 mg capsule/day	Dried alcoholic extract of feverfew leaves providing 0.5 mg of parthenolide per capsule, prepared by investigators	Feverfew did not reduce the number of migraine attacks. However, patients taking feverfew had a tendency to use fewer symptomatic drugs during the period they took feverfew. Note: It is very likely that this extract and/or its method of preparation caused degradation of active constituents.
Palevitch et al., 1997	Migraine	R, DB, CO (there was also an O phase for the first 2 months) n=57 men and women with migraine	4 months (Group A: 3 months feverfew followed by 1 month placebo. Group B: 2 months feverfew followed by 1 month placebo, then an additional 1 month feverfew. No washout periods.)	One, 50 mg capsule 2x/day or placebo (chopped parsley)	50 mg of dried powdered leaves packed in gelatin capsules. 0.2% parthenolide content, prepared by investigators	Feverfew caused a significant (p<0.01) reduction in pain intensity (p<0.001). There was a significant (p<0.017–0.001) reduction in vomiting, nausea, sensitivity to noise, and sensitivity to light.
Anderson et al., 1988	Migraine	O, C, RS n=60 women with history of common or classical migraine for at least 2 years	30 of the patients had been using feverfew daily for at least 11 consecutive months; 30 of the patients were non-users	Varied, patients were self-dosing	This study examined blood and urine, and did not dispense feverfew. Patients self-administered raw feverfew leaves, or dried leaves in capsules or tablets	Prophylactic use of feverfew by migraine sufferers did not result in increases in chromosomal aberrations or sister chromatid exchanges in peripheral lymphocytes, nor did it produce mutagenic urine. The effect of feverfew on migraine was not examined.
Murphy et al., 1988	Migraine	R, DB, PC, CO n=60 men and women with migraine	9 months (1 month single-blind placebo-run-in, 4 months feverfew, 4 months placebo)	70–114 mg capsule/day (mean 82 mg) (amount of powder varied with the strength of the preparation, as judged by its anti-secretory activity) or placebo (dried cabbage)	Dried feverfew leaves in capsules (2.19 mmol parthenolide) prepared by investigators, or placebo	Feverfew was associated with reduced number and severity of attacks. However, the duration of the attacks was unaltered. Feverfew caused a significant reduction in nausea and vomiting (p<0.02). No serious side effects were reported.
Johnson et al., 1985	Migraine	R, DB, PC n=17 patients with migraine who had been self administering raw feverfew leaves daily for at least 3 months	6 months	One, 25 mg capsule 2x/day	Capsules contained 5 freeze-dried feverfew leaflets weighing 25.7 mg, prepared by investigators	Feverfew taken prophylactically reduced the frequency and severity of symptoms of migraine (p<0.02), but not the duration of attacks. Feverfew also reduced incidence of nausea/vomiting (p<0.05). During months 3–6 the patients taking dried feverfew had the same number of attacks as when they were taking fresh feverfew. In contrast, the patients taking the placebo had a relapse and experienced a significant increase in the frequency and severity of migraines and associated symptoms of nausea and vomiting.

Arthritis

Author/Year	Subject	Design	Duration	Dosage	Preparation	Results/Conclusion
Pattrick et al., 1989	Rheumatoid arthritis	R, DB, PC n=41 women with classical or definite rheumatoid arthritis (ages 28–65 years)	6 weeks	70–86 mg/day (mean 76 mg) or placebo (cabbage)	Dry, powdered leaf (equivalent to 2–3 μmol parthenolide), prepared by investigators	No differences observed between the groups. No apparent benefit from oral feverfew for rheumatoid arthritis.

KEY: C – controlled, **CC** – case-control, **CH** – cohort, **CI** – confidence interval, **Cm** – comparison, **CO** – crossover, **CS** – cross-sectional, **DB** – double-blind, **E** – epidemiological, **LC** – longitudinal cohort, **MA** – meta-analysis, **MC** – multi-center, **n** – number of patients, **O** – open, **OB** – observational, **OL** – open label, **OR** – odds ratio, **P** – prospective, **PB** – patient-blind, **PC** – placebo-controlled, **PG** – parallel group, **PS** – pilot study, **R** – randomized, **RC** – reference-controlled, **RCS** – retrospective cross-sectional, **RS** - retrospective, **S** – surveillance, **SB** – single-blind, **SC** – single-center, **U** – uncontrolled, **UP** – unpublished, **VC** – vehicle-controlled.

Flax

Linum usitatissimum L.

[Fam. *Linaceae*]

OVERVIEW

The crude form of flax is the dried, ripe seed of all varieties of *Linum usitatissimum* L. [Fam. *Linaceae*]. Commercial preparations include ground seed, gruel, and expressed oil. The oil is marketed in bottles or in soft-gel capsules. The seeds can be consumed raw or in baked foods. Flax has become popular in the mainstream market in many forms, including raw seeds, expressed oils, and as an ingredient in breads, muffins, cereals, and breakfast bars. It is estimated that 80% of Americans are deficient in the omega-3 essential fatty acids which flax provides. Flax oil contains 50–60% alpha-linolenic acid. Flax is also one of the most concentrated sources of lignans (phenolic resins found in many plants), containing 100 to 800 times the amount found in other foods.

PRIMARY USES

Internal

- Hyperlipidemia
- Atherosclerosis
- Breast cancer (may reduce risk of breast cancer and metastasis)
- Chronic constipation
- Colon damage by laxative abuse
- Irritable colon
- Diverticulitis
- Gastritis and enteritis

External

- Inflammation, local, as a poultice

OTHER POTENTIAL USES

- Lupus nephritis
- Osteoporosis (reduction of resorption rate)
- Prostate cancer (may reduce hormone and cell proliferation levels, may increase apoptosis)
- Rheumatoid arthritis

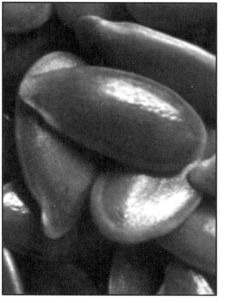

Photo © 2003 stevenfoster.com

PHARMACOLOGICAL ACTIONS

CRUDE PREPARATIONS: Laxative.

GROUND FLAX OR OIL PREPARATIONS: Develops brain function; lowers LDL serum cholesterol; antiplatelet aggregation; anti-inflammatory; antimetastatic; reduces proteinuria; increases creatinine clearance; reduces glomerulosclerosis.

DOSAGE AND ADMINISTRATION

Internal

CRUDE PREPARATIONS: Flax can be used continuously as a nutritional source, or as a bulk laxative.

BRUISED OR WHOLE SEED: 1 tablespoon (5 g) of whole, "bruised," or ground seed soaked in water and taken with a glassful of liquid 3 times daily. Grind the seeds to improve absorption of phytochemicals for therapeutic efficacy.

MUCILAGE (GRUEL): Soak 2–3 tablespoons of milled flaxseed in 200–300 ml water, strain after 30 minutes.

OIL: 1–2 tablespoons daily.

FLAX OIL CAPSULES: 3–6 capsules containing 1,000 mg each oil for general health maintenance.

GROUND SEED: 2.5 teaspoons, 2–3 times daily.

External

CATAPLASM (POULTICE): Semisolid paste containing 30–50 g flaxseed flour for a moist-heat direct application to the skin, used like a poultice as a counter-irritant. Draws blood to the surface to remove deep-seated inflammation. Flaxseed meal is traditionally mixed with mustard seed powder in this application.

COMPRESS OR FOMENTATION: A cloth is saturated with a hot, semisolid preparation containing 30–50 g flaxseed flour, folded, and applied firmly for a moist-heat direct application to the skin to relieve pain or inflammation.

NOTE: Flax oil and ground flaxseeds should be stored in air tight containers in a cool area away from direct sun light. Flax oil soft-gel capsules should be stored at room temperature in air tight bottles.

CONTRAINDICATIONS

Consult with a healthcare provider in cases of ileus of any origin.

PREGNANCY AND LACTATION: No known restrictions. Essential fatty acid (EFA) supplementation during pregnancy and nursing is beneficial for fetal and infant brain development and visual function.

ADVERSE EFFECTS

None known at therapeutic dosages when directions are followed (i.e., consumption of adequate amounts of liquid 1:10).

DRUG INTERACTIONS

As with any other mucilage, the whole or crushed seeds may inhibit the absorption of drugs or dietary nutrients. There are no known drug interactions for flax oil.

CLINICAL REVIEW

In 18 clinical studies on flax that included a total of 90,648 participants, all but two demonstrated positive effects for cardiovascular health, breast cancer, prostate cancer, lupus, and arthritis. One randomized, double-blind, placebo-controlled (R, DB, PC) study performed on 22 participants using flaxseed oil concluded that the duration of supplementation may have been too short to have an effect on rheumatoid arthritis or that missing co-factors may have interfered with the clinical outcomes of this study. Two R, DB crossover trials found that flaxseed baked in food products produced a significant decrease in LDL cholesterol and in retarding the rate of bone resorption. In another investigation, consumption of flaxseed oil had no effect on glycemic control or insulin secretion. A R, PC, single-blind, crossover trial found partially defatted flaxseed baked in food products reduced LDL serum cholesterol levels to concentrations associated with ingestion of full-fat flaxseed. One study found secondary prevention of heart attack. Two epidemiological reports found a reduction in the incidence of breast cancer or metastasis in women who used flaxseed oil. A recent pilot study with flaxseed and low-fat diet showed possible benefits in reducing testosterone and cancer cell proliferation rates and increased apoptosis.

Flax

Linum usitatissimum L.
[Fam. *Linaceae*]

OVERVIEW

Flax has become popular in the mainstream market in many forms: raw seeds; expressed oils; and as an ingredient in breads, muffins, cereals, and breakfast bars. Flaxseed oil provides the beneficial essential fatty acids in which 80% of Americans are deficient. Flax oil contains 50–60% alpha-linolenic acid and is also one of the most concentrated sources of lignans (phenolic resins found in many plants), containing 100 to 800 times the amounts found in other foods.

USES

Internal

Elevated lipid levels (e.g., high cholesterol); breast cancer (risk reduction); osteoporosis; lupus nephritis; rheumatoid arthritis, atherosclerosis; chronic constipation; irritable bowel and other colon disorders.

External

Local inflammation.

DOSAGE

Flax can be used long-term as a bulk laxative and as a nutritional supplement.

BRUISED OR WHOLE SEED: 1 tablespoon (5 g) of whole, "bruised," or ground seed soaked in water and taken with a glassful of liquid 3 times daily. Grinding the seeds improves absorption of plant nutrients.

MUCILAGE (GRUEL): Soak 2–3 tablespoons of milled flaxseed in 200–300 ml water, strain after 30 minutes.

OIL: 1–2 tablespoons daily.

FLAX OIL CAPSULES: 3–6 capsules containing 1,000 mg oil each for general health maintenance.

GROUND SEED: 2.5 teaspoons, 2–3 times daily.

COMPRESS OR FOMENTATION: Saturate cloth with a hot, semisolid preparation containing 30–50 g flaxseed flour. Fold and apply firmly for a moist-heat direct application to the skin to relieve pain or inflammation.

NOTE: Store flax oil and ground flaxseeds in air tight containers in a cool area away from direct sun light. Store flax oil soft-gel capsules at room temperature in air tight bottles.

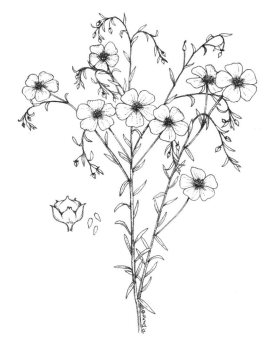

CONTRAINDICATIONS

Consult with a healthcare provider in cases of obstruction of bowels or painful, distended abdomen (ileus of any origin).

PREGNANCY AND LACTATION: There are no known restrictions for use during pregnancy or while breast-feeding.

ADVERSE EFFECTS

There are no known adverse effects for individuals using flaxseed at the suggested dosages when directions are followed [e.g., take with plenty of liquids (1 part flaxseed to 10 parts liquid)].

DRUG INTERACTIONS

Whole or crushed seeds produce a thick substance called mucilage which may affect the absorption of drugs or other nutrients taken simultaneously. There are no known drug interactions with flax oil.

Comments

When using a dietary supplement, purchase it from a reliable source. For best results, use the same brand of product throughout the period of use. As with all medications and dietary supplements, please inform your healthcare provider of all herbs and medications you are taking. Interactions may occur between medications and herbs or even among different herbs when taken at the same time. Treat your herbal supplement with care by taking it as directed, storing it as advised on the label, and keeping it out of the reach of children and pets. Consult your healthcare provider with any questions.

AMERICAN
BOTANICAL
COUNCIL

Flax

Linum usitatissimum L.
[Fam. *Linaceae*]

OVERVIEW

Flax has become popular in the mainstream market in many forms including raw seeds and expressed oils, and as an ingredient in breads, muffins, cereals, and breakfast bars (Blumenthal *et al.*, 2000). The oil from flaxseed, also called linseed, is one of the most concentrated plant sources of omega-3 fatty acids. It is also one of the most concentrated sources of lignans (phenolic resins found in many plants) containing 100–800 times the amount found in other foods (Mazur *et al.*, 1998; Mazur, 1998; Thompson *et al.*, 1991). Current research suggests that flax lignans are anti-atherogenic (Prasad, 1997), antioxidant, hypocholesterolemic, and anticarcinogenic (Nesbitt and Thompson, 1997). Flax, and some of its derivatives, is being studied for lowering LDL serum cholesterol, prevention of some cancers, and treatment of systemic lupus erythematosus (SLE). The largest flax producer is Canada (Haggerty, 1999). Flaxseed is an increasingly common ingredient in conventional foods, and is eaten either raw or in baked goods. Because phytochemicals (lignans and alpha-linolenic acid) from whole flaxseeds are poorly absorbed in the body, many people prefer to crush the seeds in order to obtain the optimal health benefit.

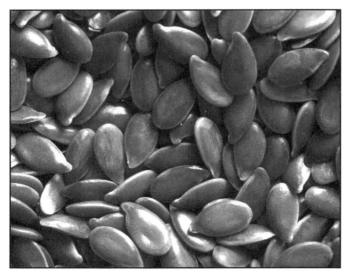

Photo © 2003 stevenfoster.com

DESCRIPTION

Flax preparations consist of the dried, ripe seed of all varieties of *Linum usitatissimum* L. [Fam. *Linaceae*] (Blumenthal *et al.*, 1998). The seeds can be consumed raw or in baked foods. Commercial preparations include ground seed, gruel, and expressed oil. The oil is marketed in bottles or in soft-gel capsules and contains 59% alpha-linolenic acid (ALA) (Bhatty, 1995).

PRIMARY USES

Internal
Cardiovascular
- Hyperlipidemia (Jenkins *et al.*, 1999; Arjmandi *et al.*, 1998a; Nestel *et al.*, 1997; Bierenbaum *et al.*, 1993; Cunnane *et al.*, 1995)
- Atherosclerosis (risk reduction) (Caughey *et al.*, 1996; Allman *et al.*, 1995; Bierenbaum *et al.*, 1993)

Breast Cancer
- May reduce risk of breast cancer and metastasis (Haggans *et al.*, 1999; Ingram *et al.*, 1997; Phipps *et al.*, 1993; Bougnoux *et al.*, 1994; Willett *et al.*, 1992)

Gastrointestinal
- Chronic constipation (Cunnane *et al.*, 1995; Blumenthal *et al.*, 1998)
- Colon damage by laxative abuse (Blumenthal *et al.*, 1998)
- Irritable colon (Blumenthal *et al.*, 1998)
- Diverticulitis (Blumenthal *et al.*, 1998)
- Gastritis and enteritis, as a mucilage (Blumenthal *et al.*, 1998)

OTHER POTENTIAL USES

Internal
- Osteoporosis (reduction of resorption rate) (Arjmandi *et al.*, 1998b)
- Lupus nephritis (Clark *et al.*, 1995)
- Prostate cancer (may reduce hormone and cell proliferation levels, may increase apoptosis) (Demark-Wahnefried *et al.*, 2001)
- Rheumatoid arthritis (Nordstrom *et al.*, 1995; Caughey *et al.*, 1996)

External
- Inflammation, local, as a poultice (Blumenthal *et al.*, 1998)

DOSAGE

Internal
Crude Preparations
BRUISED OR WHOLE SEED: 1 tablespoon (5 g) of whole, "bruised", or ground seed, is soaked in water, and taken with a glassful of liquid 3 times daily. It is usually preferable to grind the seeds to improve the absorption of phytochemicals and the resulting therapeutic efficacy. NOTE: The effect typically begins 18–24 hours later (ESCOP, 1997).

MUCILAGE (GRUEL): 2–3 tablespoons of milled flaxseed are soaked in 200–300 ml water and strained after 30 minutes.

OIL: 1–2 tablespoons daily (Blumenthal *et al.*, 1998)

FLAX OIL CAPSULES: 3–6 capsules containing 1,000 mg each oil for general health maintenance.

External

Crude Preparations

CATAPLASM (POULTICE): Semisolid paste containing 30–50 g flaxseed flour for a moist-heat direct application to the skin, used like a poultice as a counter-irritant. Draws blood to the surface to remove deep-seated inflammation. NOTE: Flaxseed meal is traditionally mixed with mustard seed powder in this application.

COMPRESS OR FOMENTATION: Cloth saturated with a hot semisolid preparation containing 30–50 g flaxseed flour. Folded and applied firmly for a moist-heat direct application to the skin to relieve pain or inflammation (Blumenthal et al., 1998).

NOTE ABOUT PROPER STORAGE: Flax oil and ground flaxseeds must be stored in air tight containers in a cool area away from direct sun. Flax oil soft-gel capsules can be stored at room temperature in air tight bottles.

DURATION OF ADMINISTRATION

Internal

Crude Preparations (from flaxseeds)

Flax can be used continuously as a nutritional source (Bhatty, 1995), or as a bulk laxative.

CHEMISTRY

Flaxseed contains 30–45% fixed oil, including triglycerides of alpha-linolenic, linoleic, oleic, stearic, palmitic, and myristic acids; 20–25% proteins; 3–10% mucilage, composed of neutral and acidic polysaccharides which, after hydrolysis, yield 8–10% galactose, 9–12% arabinose, 13–29% rhamnose, 25–27% xylose and galacturonic and about 30% mannuronic acids, sterols, and triterpenes (campesterol, stigmasterol, and sitosterol); 0.1–1.5% cyanogenic glycosides, mostly linustatin and neolinustatin and the monoglycosides linamarin and lotaustralin; and secoisolariciresinol diglucoside (SDG) (a precursor of lignans in mammals) (Bhatty, 1995; Budavari, 1996; ESCOP, 1997). A rapid RP-HPLC method was developed to quantify the lignan SDG in baked goods containing flaxseed or flax meal. Finely ground materials were found to have a significantly greater content of SDG than course materials (Muir and Westcott, 2000).

PHARMACOLOGICAL ACTIONS

Crude Preparations

Laxative (Cunnane et al., 1995; Blumenthal et al., 1998).

Ground Flax or Oil Preparations

Human

Develops brain function (Simopoulos, 1991); lowers LDL serum cholesterol (Jenkins et al., 1999; Arjmandi et al., 1998a; Bierenbaum et al., 1993); antiplatelet aggregation (Allman et al., 1995; Bierenbaum et al., 1993); anti-inflammatory (Caughey et al., 1996); antimetastatic (Bougnoux et al., 1994); reduces proteinuria; increases creatinine clearance; and reduces glomerulosclerosis (Clark et al., 1995).

Animal

Develops neurotransmission, neuromusculation, and cognition (Walker, 1967; Lamptey et al., 1976; Delion et al., 1994, 1996; Frances et al., 1995, 1996); may reduce breast and colon cancer risk (Serraino and Thompson, 1991, 1992a, 1992b; Jenab and Thompson, 1996); suppresses mammary tumor growth (Thompson et al., 1996); prevents atherosclerosis (Prasad, 1997); regulates fertility and sperm quality (Kelso et al. 1997; Arya and Caglj, 1993).

In vitro

Anti-cancer in human breast, lung, and prostate cells, and in mouse myeloma cells (Begin et al., 1986; Kumar and Das, 1995).

MECHANISM OF ACTION

- Stimulates bowels. Flax binds to water, mucilage swells, and stool volume increases (Weiss and Fintelmann, 2000; De Smet et al, 1997).
- Facilitates passage of feces through bowel through lubrication by the oil (Weiss and Fintelmann, 2000; De Smet et al., 1997).
- Supports and develops brain function by increasing levels of docosahexaenoic acid (DHA), the major component of cell membranes of cerebral cortex and myelin sheaths (Horrobin, 1982; Simopouls, 1991).
- Reduces cholesterol levels by increasing prostaglandins E1 and E3 (PGE1 and PGE3), which inhibit cholesterol synthesis and stimulate cholesterol movement across cell membranes (Horrobin, 1982).
- Reduces platelet aggregation by increasing levels of PGE1 and PGE3 (Horrobin, 1982).
- Reduces inflammation by lowering arachidonic acid levels and driving synthesis of series 1 and 3 prostaglandins (Horrobin, 1982).
- Increases concentrations of sex hormone binding globulin (SHBG) by lignans (Adlercreutz et al., 1987, 1992).
- Binds steroid hormones to its insoluble fiber, thereby reducing estrogen concentrations in circulation (Whitten and Shultz, 1988; Goldin et al., 1982).
- Protects against degenerative disease by supplying omega-3 essential fatty acids (EFAs) (Budwig, 1953).

CONTRAINDICATIONS

Ileus of any origin (flaxseeds) (Blumenthal et al., 1998).

PREGNANCY AND LACTATION: No known restrictions. EFA supplementation during pregnancy and nursing is beneficial for fetal and infant brain development and visual function (Simopoulos, 1991; Horrobin, 1982).

ADVERSE EFFECTS

None known at therapeutic dosages and following directions (i.e., consumption of adequate amounts of liquid, 1:10) (Blumenthal et al., 1998).

DRUG INTERACTIONS

As with any other mucilage, the whole or crushed seeds may negatively affect the absorption of other orally ingested drugs (Blumenthal et al., 1998), although this is mainly speculative (Brinker, 2001). May also inhibit absorption of dietary nutrients (McGuffin et al., 1997).

FLAX OIL: None known.

AMERICAN HERBAL PRODUCTS ASSOCIATION (AHPA) SAFETY RATING

CLASS 2D: Can be safely consumed with the following restriction: Take with at least 150 ml (6 ounces) liquid. Contraindicated in bowel obstruction (i.e., flaxseeds).

REGULATORY STATUS

AUSTRIA: Dried ripe seed official in the *Austrian Pharmacopoeia*, ÖAB (Meyer-Buchtela, 1999; Wichtl, 1997).

CANADA: Flaxseed is approved as a component of multiple-ingredient Schedule OTC (over-the-counter) Traditional Herbal Medicines (THMs), as a component of Schedule OTC nutritional agents, and as a single-ingredient homeopathic drug, all requiring premarket registration and assignment of a Drug Identification Number (DIN) (Health Canada, 2001).

CHINA: Dried ripe seed official in the *Pharmacopoeia of the People's Republic of China* (PPRC, 1997).

EUROPEAN UNION: Dried ripe seed official in the *European Pharmacopoeia* (Ph.Eur. 1997).

FRANCE: Dried ripe seed official in the *French Pharmacopoeia*, Ph.Fr.X (Bruneton, 1999).

GERMANY: Approved non-prescription drug of the German Commission E Monographs for both internal and external use (Blumenthal *et al.*, 1998). The gruel dosage form is an approved non-prescription drug of the *German Standard License* monographs (Braun *et al.*, 1996).

INDIA: Dried ripe seed official in the *Government of India Ayurvedic Pharmacopoeia of India* (API I, 1989) and is an approved single-drug dispensed in the Unani system of medicine (CCRUM, 1992).

SWEDEN: Component of multiple-herb products regulated as food without health claim (Tunón, 1999). As of January 2001, no flax products are listed in the Medical Products Agency (MPA) "Authorised Natural Remedies" (MPA, 2001).

SWITZERLAND: Dried, ripe seed official in the *Swiss Pharmacopoeia*, Ph.Helv. (Wichtl, 1997). Component of multiple-ingredient herbal medicines with positive classification (List D) by the *Interkantonale Kontrollstelle für Heilmittel* (IKS) and corresponding sales category D, with sale limited to pharmacies and drugstores, without prescription (Morant and Ruppanner, 2001; *Codex*, 2000/01).

U.K.: Linseed oil is on the *General Sale List*, Schedule 1 (medicinal product requiring a full product license), Table B (external use only) (GSL, 1994).

U.S.: Food or dietary supplement if structure-function label statement is made (USC, 1994).

CLINICAL REVIEW

Eighteen studies are outlined in the following table, "Clinical Studies on Flax" including a total of 90,648 participants. All but two of these studies (Nordstrom *et al.*, 1995; McManus *et al.*, 1996), demonstrated positive effects for cardiovascular health, breast cancer, prostate cancer, lupus, and arthritis. One randomized, double-blind, placebo-controlled (R, DB, PC) study performed on 22 participants using flaxseed oil concluded that the duration of supplementation may have been too short to have an effect on rheumatoid arthritis, or that missing co-factors may have interfered with the clinical outcomes of this study (Nordstrom *et al.*, 1995). Two R, DB crossover trials found that flaxseed baked in food products produced a significant decrease in LDL cholesterol and in retarding the rate of bone resorption (Arjmandi *et al.*, 1998a; Arjmandi *et al.*, 1998b). In another study, consumption of flaxseed oil had no effect on glycemic control or insulin secretion (McManus *et al.*, 1996). A R, PC, single-blind, crossover trial found partially defatted flaxseed baked in

food products reduced LDL serum cholesterol levels to concentrations associated with ingestion of full-fat flaxseed (Jenkins *et al.*, 1999). One study found secondary prevention of heart attack (De Lorgeril *et al.*, 1994). Two epidemiological reports found a reduction in the incidence of breast cancer or metastasis in women who used flaxseed oil (Bougnoux *et al.*, 1994; Willett *et al.*, 1992). One recent pilot study using flaxseed with and without a low-fat diet in older men with prostate cancer showed reduction in testosterone and prostate cancer cell proliferation rates and higher rates of apoptosis (Demark-Wahnefried *et al.*, 2001).

BRANDED PRODUCTS

Alena™: ENRECO / P.O. Box 186 / Newton, WI 53063-0186 / U.S.A. / Tel.: 800-962-9536 / Fax: 920-926-4224 / Email: info@enreco.com / www.enreco.com. Ground stabilized flaxseed, 1,450 mg omega-3 fatty acids per tablespoon.

REFERENCES

Aldercreutz H, Hockerstedt K, Bannwart C, *et al.* Effect of dietary components, including lignans and phytoestrogens, on enterohepatic circulation and liver metabolism of estrogens and on sex hormone binding globulin (SHBG). *J Steroid Biochem* 1987;27:1135–1144.

Aldercreutz H, Mousavi Y, Hockerstedt K. Diet and breast cancer. *Acta Oncol* 1992;31(2):175–81.

Allman, M, Pena M, Pang D. Supplementation with flax seed oil versus sunflower seed oil in healthy young men consuming a low fat diet: effects on platelet composition and function. *Eur J Clin Nutr* 1995;49(3):169–78.

API. See: *Ayurvedic Pharmacopoeia of India*.

Arjmandi B, Juma S, Lucas E, *et al.* Flaxseed supplementation positively influences bone metabolism in postmenopausal women. *J Am Nutraceutical Assn* 1998b;1(2):27–32.

Arjmandi B, Khan D, Juma S, *et al.* Whole flaxseed consumption lowers LDL-cholesterol and lipoprotein(a) concentrations in postmenopausal women. *Nutr Res* 1998a;18(7):1203–14.

Arya J, Caglj A. Exclusion of alpha-linolenic acid from diets for rats during several generations. I. Effect on reproduction and postnatal growth. *Arch-Latinoam-Nutr* 1993;43(2):123–31.

Ayurvedic Pharmacopoeia of India (API, Part I, Vol. I, 1st ed.). New Delhi, India: Government of India Ministry of Health and Family Welfare Department of Health; 1989;19.

Begin M, Ells G, Das U, *et al.* Differential killing of human carcinoma cells supplemented with n-3 and n-6 polyunsaturated fatty acids. *J Natl Cancer Inst* 1986;77(5):1053–62.

Bhatty RS. Nutrient Composition of Whole Flaxseed and Flaxseed Meal. In: Cunnane S and Thompson L. *Flaxseed in Human Nutrition*. Champaign, Ill: AOCS Press; 1995.

Bierenbaum, M, Reichstein R, Watkins T. Reducing atherogenic risk in hyperlipidemic humans with flaxseed supplementation: a preliminary report. *J Am Coll Nutr* 1993;12(5):501–4.

Blumenthal M, Busse WR, Goldberg A, Gruenwald J, Hall T, Riggins CW, Rister RS (eds.). Klein S, Rister RS (trans.). *The Complete German Commission E Monographs—Therapeutic Guide to Herbal Medicines*. Austin, TX: American Botanical Council; Boston: Integrative Medicine Communication; 1998.

Blumenthal M, Goldberg A, Brinckmann J (eds.). *Herbal Medicine – Expanded Commission E Monographs*. Newton, MA: Integrative Medicine Communications; 2000;201–4.

Bougnoux P, Koscielny S, Chajes V, *et al.* Alpha-linolenic acid content of adipose breast tissue: a host determinant of the risk of early metastasis in breast cancer. *Br J Cancer* 1994;70(2):330–4.

Braun R, Surmann P, Wendt R, Wichtl M, Ziegenmeyer J (eds.). *Standardzulassungen für Fertigarzneimittel – Text und Kommentar*, 11. Ergänzungslieferung. Stuttgart, Germany: Deutscher Apotheker Verlag; 1996 Feb;Zulassungsnummer 1099.99.99.

Brinker F. *Herb Contraindications and Drug Interactions* 3rd ed. Sandy, OR: Eclectic Medical Publications; 2001;96.

Bruneton J. *Pharmacognosy, Phytochemistry, Medicinal Plants*, 2nd ed. Paris, France: Lavoisier Publishing; 1999.

Budavari, S. (ed.). *The Merck Index: An Encyclopedia of Chemicals, Drugs, and Biologicals*, 12th ed. Whitehouse Station, NJ: Merck & Co, Inc; 1996.

Budwig J. *The principal function of respiration in relation to the autoxidation of nutrient* [in German]. Freiburg: Hyperion Verlag; 1953.

Caughey G, Mantzioris E, Gibson R, et al. The effect on human tumor necrosis factor alpha and interleukin 1 beta production of diets enriched in n-3 fatty acids from vegetable oils or fish oil. *Am J Clin Nutr* 1996;63(1):116–22.

CCRUM. See: Central Council for Research in Unani Medicine.

Central Council for Research in Unani Medicine (CCRUM). *Standardization of Single Drugs of Unani Medicine,* 1st Edition, Part II. New Delhi, India: Ministry of Health and Family Welfare, Government of India, CCRUM; 1992;276–81.

Clark W, Parbtani A, Huff M, et al. Flaxseed: A potential treatment of lupus nephritis. *Kidney Int* 1995;48(2):475–80.

Codex 2000/01: Die Schweizer Arzneimittel in einem Griff. Basel, Switzerland: Documed AG; 2000;111, 574, 578, 1039, 1402.

Cunnane S, Gangulis S, Menard C, et al. High alpha-linolenic acid flaxseed *(Linum usitatissimum):* some nutritional properties in humans. *Br J Nutr* 1993;69(2):443–453.

Cunnane SC, Hamadeh MJ, Liede AC, et al. Nutritional attributes of traditional flaxseed in healthy young adults. *Am J Clin Nutr* 1995;61(1):62–68.

de Lorgeril M, Renaud S, Mamelle N, et al. Mediterranean alpha-linolenic acid-rich diet in secondary prevention of coronary heart disease. *Lancet* 1994;343(8911):1454–9.

Delion S, Chalon S, Guilloteau D, et al. Alpha-linolenic acid dietary deficiency alters age-related changes of dopaminergic and serotoninergic neurotransmission in the rat frontal cortex. *J Neurochem* 1996;66:1582.

De Smet P, Keller K, Hansel R, et al. *Adverse effects of herbal drugs,* Vol. 2, Berlin, Germany: Springer-Verlag; 1997.

Delion S, Chalon S, Heralt J, et al. Chronic dietary alpha-linolenic acid deficiency alters dopaminergic and serotinergic neurotransmission in rats. *J Nutr* 1994;124(12):2466.

Demark-Wahnefried W, Price OT, Polzscik TJ et al. Pilot study of dietary fat restriction and flaxseed supplementation in men with prostate cancer before surgery: Exploring the effects of hormonal levels, prostate-specific antigen, and histopathological features. *Urology* 2001;58:47-52.

Erasmus U. Personal communication to T. Kunz. 2001.

ESCOP. 1997. "Lini semen." *Monographs on the Medicinal Uses of Plant Drugs.* Exeter, U.K.: European Scientific Cooperative on Phytotherapy; 1997.

Europäisches Arzneibuch, 3rd ed. (Ph.Eur.3). Stuttgart: Deutscher Apotheker Verlag; 1997.

Frances H, Monier C, Bourre J. Effects of dietary alpha-linolenic acid deficiency on neuromuscular and cognitive functions in mice. *Life Sci* 1995;57(21):1935.

Frances H, Monier C, Clement M, et al. Effect of dietary alpha-linolenic acid deficiency on habituation. *Life Sci* 1996;58(21):1805.

General Sale List (GSL). Statutory Instrument 1994 No. 2410 The Medicines (Products Other Than Veterinary Drugs) Amendment Order. London, U.K.: Her Majesty's Stationery Office (HMSO); 1994.

Goldin BR, Adlercreutz H, Gorbach SL, et al. Estrogen excretion patterns and plasma levels in vegetarian and omnivorous women. *N Eng J Med* 1982;307:1542–7.

GSL. See: *General Sale List.*

Haggans C, Hutchins A, Olson B, et al. Effect of flaxseed consumption on urinary estrogen metabolites in postmenopausal women. *Nutr Cancer* 1999;33(2):188–95.

Haggerty W. Flax: Ancient herb and modern medicine. *HerbalGram* 1999;45:51–7.

Health Canada. *Drug Product Database (DPD) Product Information.* Ottawa, Ontario: Health Canada; 2001.

Horrobin D. *Clinical Uses of Essential Fatty Acids.* London: Eden Press; 1982.

Ingram D, Sanders K, Kolybaba M, et al. Case-control study of phyto-estrogens and breast cancer. *Lancet* 1997;350(9083):990–4.

Jenab M, Thompson LU. The influence of flaxseed and lignans on colon carcinogenesis and β-glucuronidase activity. *Carcinogen* 1996;17(6):1343–8.

Jenkins D, Kendall C, Vidgen E, et al. Health aspects of partially defatted flaxseed, including effects on serum lipids, oxidative measures, and *ex vivo* androgen and progestin activity: a controlled crossover trial. *Am J Clin Nutr* 1999;69:395–402.

Kelley D, Branch L, Love J, et al. Dietary alpha-linolenic acid and immunocompetence in humans. *Am J Clin Nutr* 1991;53(1):40–6.

Kelso KA, Cerrolini S, Speake BK. Effects of dietary supplementation with alpha-linolenic acid on the phospholipid fatty acid composition and quality of spermatozoa in cockerel from 24 to 72 weeks of age. *J Reprod Fertil* 1997;110(1):53–9

Kumar G, Das U. Free radical-dependent suppression of growth of mouse myeloma cells by alpha-linolenic acid and eicosapentaenoic acid *in vitro. Cancer Lett* 1995;92:27.

Lamptey M, Walker B. A possible essential role for dietary linolenic acid in the development of the young rat. *J Nutr* 1976;106:86–93.

Mazur W. Phytoestrogen content in foods. In: Adlercreutz H. (ed.). *Phytoestrogens.* London: Bailliere Tindall; 1998;12(4):729-742.

Mazur WM, Rasku S, Salakka A, et al. Lignan and isoflavonoid concentrations in tea and coffee. *Br J Nutr* 1998;79:37-45.

McGuffin M, Hobbs C, Upton R, Goldberg A (eds.). *American Herbal Products Association's Botanical Safety Handbook.* Boca Raton, FL: CRC Press; 1997.

McManus R, Jumson J, Finegood D, et al. A comparison of the effects of n-3 fatty acids from linseed oil and fish oil in well-controlled type 1 diabetes. *Diabetes Care* 1996;19(5):463–7.

Medical Products Agency (MPA). Naturläkemedel: Authorised Natural Remedies (as of January 24, 2001). Uppsala, Sweden: Medical Products Agency; 2001.

Meyer-Buchtela E. *Tee-Rezepturen: Ein Handbuch für Apotheker und Ärzte.* Stuttgart, Germany: Deutscher Apotheker Verlag. 1999; Leinsamen.

Morant J, Ruppanner H (eds.). Bioforce Linoforce. In: *Arzneimittel-Kompendium der Schweiz®* 2001. Basel, Switzerland: Documed AG; 2001;728.

MPA. See: Medical Products Agency.

Muir AD, Westcott ND. Quantitation of the Lignan Secoisolariciresinol Diglucoside in Baked Goods Containing Flax Seed or Flax Meal. *J Agric Food Chem* 2000;48:4048-4052.

Nesbitt P, Thompson L. Lignans in homemade and commercial products containing flaxseed. *Nutr Cancer* 1997;29(3):222–7.

Nestel P, Pomeroy S, Sasahara T, et al. Arterial compliance in obese subjects is improved with dietary plant n-3 fatty acid from flaxseed oil despite increased LDL oxidizability. *Arterioscler Thromb Vasc Biol* 1997;17(6):1163–70.

Nordstrom D, Honkanen V, Nasu Y, et al. Alpha-linolenic acid in the treatment of rheumatoid arthritis. A double-blind, placebo-controlled and randomized study: flaxseed vs. safflower seed. *Rheumatol Int* 1995;14:231–4.

Ph.Eur. See: *Europäisches Arzneibuch.*

Pharmacopoeia of the People's Republic of China (PPRC English Edition Volume I 1997). Beijing, China: Chemical Industry Press; 1997;217.

Phipps W, Martini M, Lampe J, et al. Effect of flaxseed ingestion on the menstrual cycle. *J Clin Endocrin Metab* 1993;77(5):1215–9.

PPRC. See: *Pharmacopoeia of the People's Republic of China.*

Prasad K. Dietary flax seed in prevention of hypercholesterolemic atherosclerosis. *Atherosclerosis* 1997;132(1):69–76.

Serraino M, Thompson L. The effect of flaxseed supplementation on the initiation and promotional stages of mammary tumor genesis. *Nutr Cancer* 1992a;17(2):153–9.

Serraino M, Thompson L. Flaxseed supplementation and early markers of colon carcinogenesis. *Cancer Lett* 1992b;63(2):159–65.

Serraino M, Thompson L. The effect of flaxseed supplementation on early risk markers for mammary carcinogenesis. *Cancer Lett* 1991;60(2):135–42.

Simopoulos A. Omega-3 fatty acids in health and disease and in growth and development. *Am J Clin Nutr* 1991;54:438–63.

Thompson LU, Robb P, Serraino M, Cheung F. Mammalian lignan production from various foods. *Nutr Cancer* 1991;16:43-52.

Thompson LU, Rickard S, Orcheson L, Seidl MM. Flaxseed and its lignan and oil components reduce mammary tumor growth at a late stage of carcinogenesis. *Carcinogenesis* 1996;17(6):1373-1376.

Tunón H. Phytotherapie in Schweden. *Z Phytother* 1999;20:268–77.

United States Congress (USC). Public Law 103–417: Dietary Supplement Health and Education Act of 1994. Washington, DC: 103rd Congress of the United States; 1994.

USC. See: United States Congress.

Walker B. Maternal diet and brain fatty acids in young rats. *Lipids* 1967;2:497–500.

Weiss R, Fintelmann V. *Herbal Medicine.* Stuttgart: Thieme; 2000.

Whitten C, Shultz T. Binding of steroid hormones *in vitro* by water insoluble dietary fiber. *Nutr Res* 1988;8:1223–35.

Wichtl M (ed.). *Teedrogen und Phytopharmaka, 3. Auflage: Ein Handbuch für die Praxis auf wissenschaftlicher Grundlage.* Stuttgart, Germany: Wissenschaftliche Verlagsgesellschaft mbH. 1997;346-350.

Willet W, Hunter D, Stampfer M, et al. Dietary fat and fiber in relation to risk of breast cancer. An 8-year follow-up. *JAMA* 1992;268(15):2037–44.

Clinical Studies on Flax (*Linum usitatissimum* L.)

Cardiovascular

Author/Year	Subject	Design	Duration	Dosage	Preparation	Results/Conclusion
Jenkins et al., 1999	Effects on serum lipids, indicators of oxidation stress, and *ex vivo* sex hormone activities	R, SB, PC CO n=29 hyperlipidemic subjects (mean age 57 years)	3 periods: 1. 3 weeks treatment 2. 2 weeks wash-out 3. 3 weeks CO treatment	50 g/day	Partially defatted flaxseed meal baked in muffins	Significant reduction in total cholesterol (p=0.001), LDL serum cholesterol (p=0.001), and apolipoprotein (p=0.005) level with partially defatted flaxseed. No significant change in HDL cholesterol, serum protein carbonyl content, or *ex vivo* androgen or progestin activity with either treatment.
Arjmandi et al., 1998a	Effect on lipid profile	R, DB, CO n=38 severely hypercholesterolemic, post-menopausal women (mean age 56.3 years)	6 weeks treatment with flaxseed or sunflower seed; 2 weeks wash-out; 6 weeks CO to other seed	38 g/day	Flaxseed baked in bread and muffins or sunflower seed	Flaxseed significantly lowered LDL cholesterol (p<0.02) vs. sunflower seed. Serum Lp(a) decreased significantly with flaxseed (p<0.05). No effect on HDL cholesterol or triglycerides levels.
Nestel et al., 1997	Effect on arterial compliance	CC n=15 obese persons with markers of insulin resistance, mean BMI 30.4 kg/m² (mean age 54 years)	16 weeks (4 periods of 4 weeks each) 1. Saturated/high fat 2. Alpha-linolenic acid (ALA)/low fat 3. Oleic acid/low fat 4. High fat	2732 ± 533 kcal/3 days 20g ALA daily	Baked biscuits and muffins with purified deodorized flaxseed oil or Sunola oil (oleic acid-rich oil)	Significant increase in arterial compliance with flaxseed (p<0.0001) and with oleic acid (p<0.05). Significant decrease in mean arterial pressure with flaxseed (p<0.05) and with oleic acid (p<0.05). Significant decrease in HDL cholesterol with flaxseed (p<0.01) vs. oleic acid and control. Significant increase in insulin response with flaxseed vs. control (p=0.016).
Allman et al., 1995	Effect on platelet composition and function	R, P n=11 healthy non-smokers, mean BMI, < 30 kg/m² (mean age 22 years)	23 days	40 g/day flaxseed oil or sunflower oil	Flaxseed oil or sunflower oil	Improved platelet composition by 2x increase in platelet EPA (p<0.05) levels with ALA. Reduced platelet aggregation response (p<0.05) with alpha-linolenic acid.
De Lorgeril et al., 1994	Secondary prevention of myocardial infarction	R, MC, SB, P n=605 patients who had a myocardial infarction (MI) (n=302 treatment group; n=303 control group)	5 years	19 g/day	Flax-based spread substitution plus Mediterranean diet (rich in ALA)	Treatment group had 76% lower incidence of deaths due to MI and 70% lower mortality rate than control. 3x increase in omega-3 intake combined with decrease in saturated fat, cholesterol, and omega-6 intake reduces risk of second MI (adjusted risk rate=0.27; p=0.001).
Bierenbaum et al., 1993	Atherogenic risk	O n=15 subjects with hyperlipidemia on long-term vitamin E (800 IU/day) (mean age 52.2 years)	3 months	15 g/day plus 3 slices of 10% flaxseed bread	Ground flaxseed (flour) in diet	Significantly decreased both total cholesterol (p<0.01) and LDL cholesterol (p<0.01). Lack of effect on HDL cholesterol. ATP measurements suggest flax inhibits platelet aggregation.

KEY: C – controlled, **CC** – case-control, **CH** – cohort, **CI** – confidence interval, **Cm** – comparison, **CO** – crossover, **CS** – cross-sectional, **DB** – double-blind, **E** – epidemiological, **LC** – longitudinal cohort, **MA** – meta-analysis, **MC** – multi-center, **n** – number of patients, **O** – open, **OB** – observational, **OL** – open label, **OR** – odds ratio, **P** – prospective, **PB** – patient-blind, **PC** – placebo-controlled, **PG** – parallel group, **PS** – pilot study, **R** – randomized, **RC** – reference-controlled, **RCS** – retrospective cross-sectional, **RS** - retrospective, **S** – surveillance, **SB** – single-blind, **SC** – single-center, **U** – uncontrolled, **UP** – unpublished, **VC** – vehicle-controlled.

Clinical Studies on Flax (*Linum usitatissimum* L.) (cont.)

Breast Cancer

Author/Year	Subject	Design	Duration	Dosage	Preparation	Results/Conclusion
Haggans et al., 1999	Estrogen excretion	R, CO n=28 healthy post-menopausal women, non-smokers, mean BMI 23.9 kg/m² (mean age 68.3 years)	Three 7-week periods: 2 periods with flaxseed; 1 period as control	5–10 g/day (as single daily dose)	Raw, ground flaxseed vs. usual diet	Significant increase in urinary estrogen metabolites, 2-hydroxyestrogen (p<0.05) and 16-alpha-hydroxye-strone (p<0.0005). Suggests flaxseed may protect against breast cancer.
Ingram et al., 1997	Risk breast cancer	CC n=144 subjects with newly diag-nosed breast cancer vs. matched women with-out breast cancer living in the same ZIP code area (ages 30–84 years)	23 months	Not applicable	Dietary intake of phyto-estrogens	Substantial reduction in breast cancer risk among women with high intake of phytoestrogens, as assessed by significant increase in excretion of equol (p=0.009) and enterolactone (p=0.013).
Phipps et al., 1993	Effect on menstrual cycle and serum hormone concentration	R, CO n=18 healthy women with regular men-strual cycle length (25-30 days) (ages 20–34 years)	7 consecutive menstrual cycles	10 g/day 2x 5 g or 3x 3.33 g	Raw flaxseed powder	Flaxseed associated with longer luteal phase (p=0.002), increased longer luteal phase estradiol ratios, and few anovulatory cycles. Overall, decreased tendency for ovarian dysfunction, which possibly decreases risk for breast cancer.
Bougnoux et al., 1994	Assessment of ALA content in adipose breast tissue and metastasis	E, P n=121 patients with initially local-ized breast cancer	Followed for 31 months	Not applicable	Dietary intake of fatty acids	Predictive factors for occurrence of metastasis are related to large tumor size and low levels of ALA in adi-pose breast tissue of breast cancer patients. Suggests low levels of ALA have a role in the metastatic process *in vivo*.
Willett et al., 1992	Breast cancer risk	E, P n=89,494 registered nurses (ages 34–59 years)	8 years	Not applicable	Dietary intake of alpha-linolenic acid	No evidence of association between total fat intake and dietary fiber intake in middle-aged women.

KEY: C – controlled, **CC** – case-control, **CH** – cohort, **CI** – confidence interval, **Cm** – comparison, **CO** – crossover, **CS** – cross-sectional, **DB** – double-blind, **E** – epidemiological, **LC** – longitudinal cohort, **MA** – meta-analysis, **MC** – multi-center, **n** – number of patients, **O** – open, **OB** – observational, **OL** – open label, **OR** – odds ratio, **P** – prospective, **PB** – patient-blind, **PC** – placebo-controlled, **PG** – parallel group, **PS** – pilot study, **R** – randomized, **RC** – reference-controlled, **RCS** – retrospective cross-sectional, **RS** - retrospective, **S** – surveillance, **SB** – single-blind, **SC** – single-center, **U** – uncontrolled, **UP** – unpublished, **VC** – vehicle-controlled.

Flax

Monograph

Clinical Studies on Flax (*Linum usitatissimum* L.) (cont.)

Other

Author/Year	Subject	Design	Duration	Dosage	Preparation	Results/Conclusion
Demark-Wahnefried, 2001	Prostate cancer	PS n=25 men with prostate cancer (mean age 64 years)	Average 34 days (21–77 days)	30 g flaxseed meal (3 rounded Tblsp.)	Alena™	This study with and without a low-fat diet supplemented with flax showed significant decrease in total testosterone (p<0.001), lower cell proliferation rates, and higher apoptosis rates associated with short-term dietary intervention and flaxseed. PSA levels decreased among men who had biopsy Gleason sums of 6 or less and continued to rise among men with higher Gleason sums (despite evidence of lower rates of proliferation and higher rates of apoptosis).
Arjmandi et al., 1998b	Osteoporosis	R, DB, CO n=38 healthy, non-smoking, post-menopausal women not receiving hormone replacement therapy (mean age 56.3 years)	6 weeks treatment followed by 2-week wash-out followed by 6 weeks of treatment	38 g/day	Flaxseed or sunflower seed (control) baked in muffins and bread	Flaxseed treatment significantly lowered tartrate resistant acid phosphatase activity in serum (a marker of bone resorption) (p<0.05). No effect on insulin-like growth factor and insulin-like growth factor protein-3 concentration (serum bone-specific). No effect on total alkaline phosphatase activity (marker of bone formation), and 17b estradiol levels. Tendency to decrease urinary excretions of both hydrooxyproline and calcium. Flaxseed may not enhance bone formation, but may slow down the rate of bone resorption.
Caughey et al., 1996	Effect on cytokine production	Cm, PG n=15 healthy subjects (ages 24–44 years)	2 months	13.7 g/day ALA or 9 g/day fish oil (1.62 g EPA/day and 1.08 g DHA/day)	Flaxseed oil and flaxseed oil plus butter spread as dietary substitutions vs. sunflower oil	Vegetable oils rich in n-3 fatty acids inhibit TNF-alpha and IL-1-betasynthesis. This finding is significant, as these factors are implicated in inflammatory rheumatoid arthritis (p<0.05) and atherosclerosis (p<0.05).
McManus et al., 1996	Non-insulin dependent diabetes	R, DB, CO n=11 (mean age 61.8 years)	3 months	35 mg/kg/day	Flaxseed oil capsules or olive oil (control)	Neither oil significantly affected glycemic control or insulin secretion.
Clark et al., 1995	Lupus nephritis	O n=9 subjects with documented systemic lupus erythematosus, history of positive ANA, and with proteinuria >1 g/24 hours	17 weeks	Weeks 1–4: 15 g/day; Weeks 5–8: 15 g 2xday; Weeks 9–12: 15 g 3xday; Followed by 5-week wash-out period.	Crude flaxseed	Flaxseed was well-tolerated at 15 and 30 g/day, but not well-tolerated at 45 g/day. Total and LDL cholesterol levels and whole blood viscosity decreased significantly with 30 g/day. Reduction of serum creatine with 30 g and 45 g/day. Increase in creatinine clearance with 15 g and 30 g/day.
Nordstrom et al., 1995	Rheumatoid arthritis	R, DB, PC n=22 (mean age treatment group, 51 years; mean age control group, 53 years)	3 months	30 g/day	Flaxseed oil or safflower oil (control)	No statistical alterations or effects were found. Concluded supplementation may have been for too short of a term, or low intake of zinc impaired EFA conversion.
Cunnane et al., 1995	Nutritional status	R, CO n=10 healthy non-smokers (mean age 25 years)	1 month	50 g/day	Muffins with milled flaxseed or muffins without flaxseed	Significant reduction in total cholesterol (p<0.05) and LDL cholesterol (p<0.05) with flaxseed. No change in HDL cholesterol or triglycerides. Increased number of bowel movements (p<0.05) with flaxseed.

KEY: **C** – controlled, **CC** – case-control, **CH** – cohort, **CI** – confidence interval, **Cm** – comparison, **CO** – crossover, **CS** – cross-sectional, **DB** – double-blind, **E** – epidemiological, **LC** – longitudinal cohort, **MA** – meta-analysis, **MC** – multi-center, **n** – number of patients, **O** – open, **OB** – observational, **OL** – open label, **OR** – odds ratio, **P** – prospective, **PB** – patient-blind, **PC** – placebo-controlled, **PG** – parallel group, **PS** – pilot study, **R** – randomized, **RC** – reference-controlled, **RCS** – retrospective cross-sectional, **RS** - retrospective, **S** – surveillance, **SB** – single-blind, **SC** – single-center, **U** – uncontrolled, **UP** – unpublished, **VC** – vehicle-controlled.

Garlic

Allium sativum L.

[Fam. *Liliaceae*]

OVERVIEW

Garlic consists of various dosage forms of the fresh or carefully dried bulbs of *Allium sativum*. In the U.S. and Western Europe, most of garlic's popularity is based on the extensive traditional use of this herb, and on scientific research suggesting that cardiovascular benefits are associated with ingesting garlic as a conventional food and a dietary supplement. More than 3,000 scientific articles have been published on the chemistry, pharmacology, toxicology, and clinical uses of garlic.

PRIMARY USES

- Hyperlipidemia
- Atherosclerosis

OTHER POTENTIAL USES

- Hypertension, mild
- Peripheral arterial occlusive disease (PAOD)
- Decreased platelet function
- Colon cancer prevention
- Stomach cancer prevention
- Coughs, colds, catarrh, and rhinitis (These traditional uses are not supported by clinical trials.)

PHARMACOLOGICAL ACTIONS

Garlic reduces total cholesterol and serum triglycerides; elevates high density lipoproteins (HDL); prevents platelet aggregation and thrombus formation; stimulates fibrinolysis; prolongs clotting time; reduces low-density lipoprotein oxidation; reduces systolic and diastolic blood pressure; attenuates age- and blood pressure-related increases in aortic stiffness; has immunomodulating activity; reduces blood glucose levels; is antifungal and fungistatic against *Cryptococcus neoformans;* antioxidant; anticancer; antimicrobial; inhibits anion transport and sickle cell dehydration and restricts dense cell formation in sickle cell patients.

DOSAGE AND ADMINISTRATION

For the prevention of atherosclerosis and prophylaxis and treatment of peripheral arterial vascular diseases, long-term treatment is generally advised. Epidemiological findings support long-term, consistent use to aid in preventing stomach and intestinal cancers.

FRESH HERB: 4 g (1 clove) minced bulb daily.

INFUSION: 4 g in 150 ml of hot water.

FLUID EXTRACT: 4 ml [1:1 (*g/ml*)].

TINCTURE: 20 ml [1:5 (*g/ml*)].

GARLIC POWDER (standardized): 200–300 mg, 3 times daily.

AGE™ AGED GARLIC EXTRACT (standardized): 300–800 mg, 3 times daily, or 1–5 ml daily.

CONTRAINDICATIONS

None known according to the German Commission E and other European scientific bodies. According to the World Health Organization, patients with a known allergy to garlic and those taking warfarin (and presumably other anticoagulants) should use caution in ingesting garlic. However, a clinical trial on a proprietary aged garlic extract (AGE) showed no prolonged bleeding in patients taking warfarin. Reports of increased clotting time suggest that patients avoid garlic at least one week prior to surgery.

PREGNANCY AND LACTATION: There are no restrictions on using garlic during pregnancy and lactation. A controlled trial showed that garlic's major sulfur-containing volatile compounds are transmitted to human milk, leading to infants' improved drinking habits.

ADVERSE EFFECTS

Garlic odor may permeate the breath and skin. Gastrointestinal symptoms and intestinal flora changes or allergic reactions are rare. In separate single case reports, excessive ingestion of garlic was associated with postoperative bleeding, spontaneous spinal epidural hematoma, and platelet dysfunction. Occupational exposure to crushed garlic products and the topical application of garlic to treat wounds or infections may cause allergic contact dermatitis. For garlic and various generic garlic preparations, reported allergic reactions included burns, zosteriform dermatitis, induction of pemiphigus (blisters), allergic asthma and rhinitis, contact urticaria, and protein contact dermatitis; but no adverse effects were reported for AGE according to toxicological and clinical studies. Garlic preparations can increase clotting time, which is sometimes beneficial, but in some cases can contribute to an adverse event. Cross-sensitivity may occur with onions and tulips.

DRUG INTERACTIONS

Concurrent use of garlic and antiplatelet agents (e.g., aspirin) and anticoagulants (e.g., warfarin) might increase the potential for prolonged bleeding. One report showed that clotting time doubled for 2 patients taking warfarin and garlic simultaneously, although there was insufficient information to properly assess these cases. A controlled trial on AGE resulted in no interaction with warfarin. A small trial suggests possible serum reduction of saquinavir, an anti-HIV drug.

Garlic

Clinical Overview

CLINICAL REVIEW

Of 32 studies (45,694 total participants) on garlic's impact on cardiovascular and arterial health, cancer, immunity, and circulation, all but four demonstrated positive effects.

Two reviews concluded that garlic preparations might have small, positive, short-term effects (< 3 months) on lipids and promising antithrombic effects. Insignificant effects on blood pressure and no effect on glucose levels were observed. However, data was insufficient to draw conclusions about certain clinical cardiovascular outcomes (e.g. myocardial infarction), antithrombic activity, or cancer prevention. Due to the marginal quality and short duration of many trials and the unpredictable release and inadequate definition of active constituents of many garlic preparations used in the studies, conclusions regarding clinical significance are limited.

Lipid-lowering effect

Thirteen trials (795 participants) demonstrated a positive correlation between lipid-lowering effects and garlic oil, powder, or capsules. Six randomized, double-blind, placebo-controlled (R, DB, PC) studies and four DB studies supported garlic use in treating elevated lipid conditions including hyperlipidemia and hypercholesterolemia. One R, open, parallel group, comparison (O, PG, Cm) study (70 participants) found garlic powder to have a significant impact over garlic oil in lowering blood-lipid counts and blood pressure and in increasing a sense of overall well-being. An R, PC study involving 35 renal transplant patients found a garlic product to have positive effects on hyperlipidemia. One O study (82 participants) found a positive impact of garlic on coronary heart disease, in addition to its lipid-lowering effects.

A meta-analysis on garlic's effect on total serum cholesterol levels found a statistically significant reduction in total cholesterol levels. Another study assessed and subsequently reassessed clinical data from 952 patients and 16 trials and found that all data demonstrated a significant reduction of total cholesterol when comparing garlic to placebo. Three studies on the allicin-standardized garlic powder tablets failed to show a significant reduction in elevated serum cholesterol. It was later determined that allicin released from the tablets varied significantly, and that the lack of expected allicin release possibly led to negative results. A study of 24 brands of enteric-coated tablets found that 83% of the brands released less than 15% of their allicin potential. Subsequently, the researchers recommended that manufacturers standardize supplements to dissolution of allicin release, not to allicin potential. (For non-allicin products, e.g., AGE, the standardization is to bioavailable compounds, e.g., S-allycysteine [SAC].) In the most recent and comprehensive meta-analysis (13 R, DB, PC trials), researchers showed a significant difference (p<0.01; 5.8%) in the reduction of total cholesterol levels between baseline and placebo. The authors concluded that current evidence indicates that any specific lipid-lowering effect is small, and the clinical outcome may not be meaningful; however, there were several problems identified with the meta-analysis, indicating that conclusions can only be applied to the specific brands tested and not to the general effectiveness of garlic.

Antihypertensive effect

Two R, DB, PC studies and one R, O, PG, Cm study (159 total participants) showed garlic's antihypertensive effects. A systematic review and meta-analysis of 8 R, C trials (415 participants) was conducted to determine garlic's effect on blood pressure. Of the 7 trials that compared garlic with placebo, 3 demonstrated a significant reduction in systolic blood pressure (SBP), and 4 in diastolic blood pressure (DBP). The authors concluded that more rigorously designed trials might provide evidence to recommend hypertension treatment with garlic.

Antiplatelet effects

One R, DB, PC, crossover (CO) study and 2 DB, PC studies (214 total participants) indicate the potential use of garlic as a coronary disease preventative due to its positive impact on platelet functions.

Anti-atherosclerotic effect

Garlic's positive influence on arterial and fibrinolytic activities was shown in two studies (354 participants). The longest clinical trial on garlic to date, a R, DB, PC, 4-year study (152 participants), showed that garlic had an anti-atherosclerotic impact, decreasing age-related arterial plaque. In one epidemiological, cross-sectional, observational (E, CS, OB) study (202 participants), standardized garlic powder was found to have positive effects on arterial activities, including elastic vascular resistance, pulse wave velocity, and systolic blood pressure.

Anticancer/Chemoprevention

Anti-cancer and chemopreventative qualities of garlic were shown in 5 studies (44,044 subjects). One E study of 15 years demonstrated that stomach cancer incidents were reduced with use of raw and cooked garlic. Two E studies (42,325 subjects) found that garlic intake significantly decreased colon cancer risks. Two OB studies demonstrated garlic's chemopreventative potential through the improvement of arachidonic acid and acetaminophen metabolism. A meta-analysis of E studies on the association between garlic consumption and risk of stomach, colon, head and neck, lung, breast, and prostate cancers concluded that raw and cooked garlic use might have a protective effect against stomach and colorectal cancers.

Other

One pilot study involving 7 HIV+ patients demonstrated a positive impact on natural killer cell activity and improvement in conditions such as diarrhea, genital herpes, and candidiasis. One R, DB, PC study showed that garlic did not negatively impact bleeding potential in warfarin therapy patients. Garlic's impact on peripheral circulation was observed in two studies: one R, CO, Cm study showed immediate improvement in hand and foot circulation; and one DB, PC study showed a significant increase in walking distance in persons with peripheral arterial occlusive disease (PAOD). The latter was the only study to meet the Cochrane Library's inclusion criteria for its review on garlic use for PAOD. Because the one study reviewed was small, of short duration (12 weeks), and found no significant overall improvement in patients with PAOD, the Cochrane Review disagreed with the author's findings and concluded that further trials on garlic's effects on PAOD are warranted.

Garlic

Allium sativum L.
[Fam. *Liliaceae*]

OVERVIEW

In the U.S. and Western Europe, garlic is one of the most popular substances used to reduce various risks associated with heart disease. Most of garlic's popularity is based on the herb's well-known folk uses and scientific research on the benefits of garlic for heart health. These health-promoting benefits may be experienced by using garlic as both a food ingredient and a dietary supplement.

USES

For slightly reducing elevated levels of cholesterol in the blood; prevention of hardening of the arteries; improvement of blood flow; mild hypertension (high blood pressure); possible prevention of stomach and colon cancer; supportive therapy for peripheral arterial occlusive disease (PAOD, poor circulation to the legs causing tightness and pain in the calves when walking).

DOSAGE

Long-term treatment is generally advised in the prevention of atherosclerosis and in the prevention and treatment of peripheral arterial vascular diseases. Epidemiological findings (population studies) support long-term, consistent use for the possible prevention of stomach and intestinal cancers.

FRESH, MINCED GARLIC: 1 clove daily.

INFUSION: 1 clove in 150 ml of hot water.

GARLIC POWDER (standardized): 200–300 mg, 3 times daily (in pill or tablet form).

AGE™ AGED GARLIC EXTRACT (standardized): 300–800 mg, 3 times daily or 1–5 ml daily (in capsules).

CONTRAINDICATIONS

None known according to the German Commission E and other leading scientific bodies. According to the World Health Organization, patients with a known allergy to garlic and those taking anticoagulant drugs like warfarin (Coumadin®) should be cautious about ingesting garlic. Garlic should not be taken prior to surgery (at least one week) as it may interfere with blood clotting.

PREGNANCY AND LACTATION: There are no known restrictions during pregnancy or lactation. However, some of garlic's properties are transmitted to human milk, leading to improved drinking habits in infants.

ADVERSE EFFECTS

Being a commonly used food, garlic is relatively safe. Adverse effects are rare, but there may be gastrointestinal symptoms and changes to the intestinal flora (beneficial bacteria that aid in digestion). Allergic reactions have been reported for garlic and various generic preparations, but no adverse effects were reported for AGE according to toxicological and clinical studies. According to one report, garlic was associated with unusual bleeding after an operation. Garlic preparations can increase clotting time, which is sometimes beneficial, but in some cases can contribute to an adverse event. Also, garlic may produce a characteristic odor on the breath or skin.

DRUG INTERACTIONS

Taking garlic with antiplatelet agents, like aspirin, and anticoagulants, like warfarin, may increase the potential for prolonged bleeding.

Comments

When using a dietary supplement, purchase it from a reliable source. For best results, use the same brand of product throughout the period of use. As with all medications and dietary supplements, please inform your healthcare provider of all herbs and medications you are taking. Interactions may occur between medications and herbs or even among different herbs when taken at the same time. Treat your herbal supplement with care by taking it as directed, storing it as advised on the label, and keeping it out of the reach of children and pets. Consult your healthcare provider with any questions.

The information contained on this sheet has been excerpted from *The ABC Clinical Guide to Herbs* © 2003 by the American Botanical Council (ABC). ABC is an independent member-based educational organization focusing on the medicinal use of herbs. For more detailed information about this herb please consult the healthcare provider who gave you this sheet. To order *The ABC Clinical Guide to Herbs* or become a member of ABC, visit their website at www.herbalgram.org.

Garlic
Allium sativum L.
[Fam. *Lilaceae*]

OVERVIEW

In the United States and Western Europe, garlic is one of the most popular substances used to reduce various risks associated with cardiovascular disease. Most of garlic's popularity is based on the extensive traditional use of this herb and on scientific research suggesting that cardiovascular benefits are associated with ingesting garlic as both a conventional food and dietary supplement (Blumenthal *et al.*, 2000). Garlic preparations have been one of the top-selling herbal supplements on the U.S. market for many years (Brevoort, 1998), ranking third in retail sales in the mainstream market in 2000, and generating revenues over $61 million (Blumenthal, 2001). To date more than 3,000 scientific papers have been published investigating the activities of garlic and garlic compounds, including chemical, toxicological, pharmacological, clinical, and epidemiological studies (Amagase *et al.*, 2001). Garlic preparations with uniquely different chemical compositions, including powdered dried garlic products standardized to allicin yield and aged garlic extract (AGE™) products that are standardized to S-allylcysteine (SAC), have been the subject of numerous clinical studies. Determining which forms are the most effective remains controversial and is an ongoing subject of study and debate. Medical literature includes positive outcomes in clinical studies involving several types of garlic preparations.

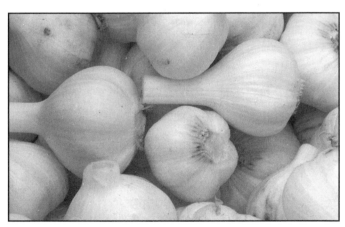

Photo © 2003 stevenfoster.com

DESCRIPTION

Garlic preparations consist of the fresh or dried bulbs (main bulb and secondary bulbs or cloves) of *Allium sativum* L. [Fam. *Lilaceae*], and various dosage forms (Blumenthal *et al.*, 1998). Garlic oil is not present in fresh or dried garlic bulbs; instead, the oil is produced by converting water-soluble thiosulfinates to oil-soluble sulfides via steam distillation. Aged garlic involves long-term extraction in dilute ethanol for up to 20 months, then drying; pickling garlic involves immersion in vinegar (5% acetic acid) (Amagase *et al.*, 2001; Lawson, 1998a).

PRIMARY USES
Cardiovascular
- Hyperlipidemia (Isaacsohn *et al.*, 1998; Lash *et al.*, 1998; McCrindle *et al.*, 1998; Steiner *et al.*,1996a, 1996b; Yeh *et al.*, 1995; De A Santos and Johns, 1995; Steiner and Lin, 1994; Jain *et al.*, 1993; Grünwald *et al.*, 1992; Holzgartner *et al.*, 1992; Mader, 1990; Vorberg *et al.*, 1990; Lau *et al.*, 1987; Bordia, 1981)
- Atherosclerosis (Koscielny *et al.*, 1999)

OTHER POTENTIAL USES
Cardiovascular
- Hypertension, mild (Steiner *et al.*, 1996; Auer *et al.*, 1990)
- Peripheral arterial occlusive disease (PAOD) (Koscielny *et al.*, 1999; ESCOP, 1997; Kiesewetter *et al.*, 1993b)

Hematology
- Decreased platelet function (Rahman and Billington, 2000; Steiner *et al.*, 2001; Steiner *et al.*, 1996; Kiesewetter *et al.*, 1991; Kiesewetter *et al.*, 1993a)

Chemopreventative
- Colon cancer preventative (Steinmetz *et al*, 1994; Witte *et al.,* 1996)
- Stomach cancer preventative (You *et al.*, 1989)

Miscellaneous
- Garlic has traditionally been used to relieve cough, colds, catarrh, and rhinitis, although clinical trials do not support such uses (ESCOP, 1997)

DOSAGE
Internal
Crude Preparations
FRESH HERB: 4 g daily (1 clove) minced bulb or equivalent preparations (Blumenthal *et al.*, 1998). [NOTE: Some authors have suggested that this dosage level should be revised downward to approximately 2,700 mg of fresh garlic, equivalent to the 900 mg of garlic powder used in some clinical trials that studied the ability of garlic to prevent and/or reverse atherosclerotic plaque build-up (Schulz *et al.*, 2001).]

INFUSION: 4 g in 150 ml of hot water (Blumenthal *et al.*, 2000).

FLUID EXTRACT: 1:1 (*g/ml*), 4 ml (Blumenthal *et al.*, 2000).

TINCTURE: 1:5 (*g/ml*), 20 ml (Blumenthal *et al.*, 2000).

Standardized Preparations
GARLIC POWDER (Kwai®): 200–300 mg, 3 times daily (Warshafsky *et al.*, 1993).

AGE ™ (Kyolic®) aged garlic extract: 300–800 mg, 3 times daily or 1–5 ml daily (Steiner 2001; Steiner *et al.*, 1996; Rahman and Billington, 2000; USP, 2002; Lau *et al.*, 1987).

DURATION OF ADMINISTRATION

Long-term treatment is generally advised in the prevention of atherosclerosis (Koscielny et al., 1999), and the prophylaxis and treatment of peripheral arterial vascular diseases (ESCOP, 1997). Epidemiological observations support the long-term consistent use for prevention of cancer in the stomach and intestines (You et al., 1989).

CHEMISTRY
Crude Preparations

Fresh garlic bulbs contain about 65% water, 28% carbohydrates (fructans), 2.3% organosulfur compounds (OSC), 2% protein, and 1.2% free amino acids. The main OSC in whole garlic are the cysteine sulfoxides (1% alliin and 0.1% cycloalliin) and the γ-glutamylcysteines (0.6% γ-glutamyl-S-trans-1-propenylcysteine and 0.4% γ-glutamyl-S-allylcysteine). When the bulb is bruised, crushed, chewed, or minced, the alliin, in the presence of the enzyme alliinase, is converted to allicin (ESCOP, 1997). One mg of alliin produces 0.458 mg of allicin, which is considered to be responsible for some of garlic's biological activity and is a precursor to some thiosulfinates, which also have been shown to be active (Lawson 1998a; Block, 1985; Bradley, 1992; Budavari, 1996; ESCOP, 1997). However, allicin is unstable and decomposes to other volatile sulfur compounds (the half-life of allicin is not more than 24 hours), so the extent of allicin's activity has been questioned. Intact garlic cloves (the sections that comprise the garlic bulb) also contain S-allylcysteine (SAC), but no allicin. SAC is formed from gamma-glutamyl cysteine catabolism and has been reported to contribute to the health benefits of some garlic preparations (Amagase et al., 2001). Fresh and aged garlic extract (AGE, see below) also contain steroidal saponins (Matsuura, 2001).

Standardized Preparations

Processed garlic preparations contain a variety of sulfur-containing compounds other than those found naturally in intact garlic cloves, depending on the conditions applied (Lawson, 1998a; Fenwick and Henley, 1985). Sulfur-containing compounds in commercial garlic preparations vary, depending on their manufacturing process. Powdered preparations of dried garlic contain alliin and compounds derived from its subsequent transformation, but no allicin. Enteric coatings protect these powdered preparations from conversion while in the stomach. Garlic oil yields neither alliin, nor allicin as the converting enzyme is destroyed by heat. It does contain diallyl disulfide, diallyl trisulfide, and allyl methyl trisulfide. Macerated garlic-derived oil contains vinyldithiins, ajoene, and diallyl trisulfides (Lawson, 1998a). Garlic extract and odorless AGE are listed in the *United States Pharmacopeia/National Formulary* (USP, 2002). The most abundant sulfur compound in AGE is SAC; it is standardized to not less than 0.05% SAC (USP, 2002).

PHARMACOLOGICAL ACTIONS
Human

Garlic reduces total cholesterol (TC) and serum triglycerides (TG) and elevates high density lipoproteins (HDL) (Auer et al., 1990; Barrie et al., 1987; Lau et al., 1987; Bordia, 1981; De A Santos and Johns, 1995; Silagy and Neil, 1994a); prevents platelet aggregation and thrombus formation (Rahman and Billington, 2000; Barrie et al., 1987; Kiesewetter et al., 1993a; Kiesewetter et al., 1993b; Legnani et al., 1993); stimulates fibrinolysis, prolongs clotting time (Chutani and Bordia, 1981;

Gadkari and Joshi, 1991; Harenberg et al., 1988; Legnani et al., 1993); reduces low-density lipoprotein (LDL) oxidation (Ide and Lau, 2001; Lau, 2001; Munday, 1999; Steiner and Lin, 1994; Harris et al., 1995; Phelps and Harris, 1993); reduces systolic blood pressure, diastolic blood pressure, and mean blood pressure from baseline (Steiner et al., 1996a, 1996b; De A Santos and Johns, 1995; Silagy and Neil, 1994b; Grünwald et al., 1992; Auer et al., 1990;); attenuates age- and blood pressure-related increases in aortic stiffness (Breithaupt-Grögler et al., 1997); stimulates peripheral microcirculation (Okuhara, 1994); is antifungal and fungistatic against *Cryptococcus neoformans*, the organism that causes cryptococcal meningitis (Anon., 1980; Davis et al., 1990); may decrease the risk of gastrointestinal cancers (Gail et al., 1998; You et al., 1991, 1989, 1988; Reuter et al., 1996; Buiatti et al., 1989; Lau, 1989); modulates immune system activity (Brosche and Platt, 1993; Kandil et al., 1988; Lawson, 1998a; Reuter et al., 1996); reduces blood glucose levels (Kiesewetter et al., 1991). Garlic does not inhibit *H. pylori* bacteria in the stomach (Graham et al., 1999). Although one study concluded that garlic extracts had no statistically significant impact on how far patients with peripheral vascular disease (PVD) can walk (Kiesewetter et al., 1993b), AGE has been reported to exhibit stimulation of peripheral circulation in human subjects (Okuhara, 1994; Kikuchi et al., 1994). One pilot clinical trial (Ohnishi et al., 2000) indicated an effect of AGE and other antioxidants in the potential treatment of sickle cell anemia patients.

Animal

Garlic lowers elevated levels of serum homocysteine (Yeh, 1999); lowers serum cholesterol and lipids (Bordia et al., 1975; Kamanna and Chandrasekhara, 1982; Chi et al., 1982); is antithrombotic (Bordia et al., 1975); increases fibrinolysis and clotting time (Bordia et al., 1975; Reuter et al., 1996); reduces blood pressure (Sial and Ahmad, 1982; Ruffin and Hunter, 1983); is antioxidant (Han et al., 1992; Lawson, 1998a); modulates immune system (Kyo et al., 1999, 1998; Lawson, 1998a; Reuter et al., 1996); reduces blood glucose levels and increases insulin levels (Augusti, 1975; Chang and Johnson, 1980); is antiallergenic (Kyo et al., 1997); exhibits antitumor activity against transitional cell carcinoma of the bladder with AGE (Lau et al., 1986; Riggs et al., 1997); reduces breast cancer incidence (Amagase and Milner, 1993; Liu et al., 1992; Kröning, 1964); decreases incidence of hepatic tumors in the *Bufo regularis* toad (El-Mofty et al., 1994).

In vitro
Antithrombotic

The rational clinical application of garlic necessitates demonstrating the association between garlic consumption and important clinical outcomes such as atherosclerosis. *In vivo* and *in vitro* studies suggest garlic extracts and several garlic constituents have a significant antithrombotic effect (Ariga et al., 1981; Boullin, 1981; Srivastava, 1986; Mohammed and Woodward, 1986). Garlic has been shown to increase fibrinolysis and prolong clotting time (Reuter et al., 1996). Adenosine in AGE and its constituents are the most potent antiplatelet constituents of garlic. Allicin was thought an active compound in garlic due to its highly reactive and oxidative characteristics, but it is rapidly metabolized in human blood (in *in vitro* culture) and therefore might not contribute to the *in vivo* antithrombotic effect of garlic (Freeman and Kodera, 1995; Koch and Lawson, 1996).

Ajoene is found in small amounts in garlic oil-macerates, but not in commercial garlic preparations and garlic powders.

Bioavailability of ajoene has not yet been established. Antithrombotic and vasodilatory actions of garlic might be due to adenosine deaminase and cyclic AMP phosphodiesterase, which can be found in garlic extracts. The decrease of thromboxane B2 (TXB2) levels is another possible explanation for garlic's antithrombotic effects. Most of the above explanations are based on *in vitro* and *in vivo* experiments (Berthold and Sudhop, 1998; Rahman and Billington, 2000; Bordia *et al.*, 1996; Agarwal 1996).

Koscielny *et al.* (1999) reported a slowing and reversal of atherosclerotic plaque formation. AGE has been shown to protect vascular endothelial cells against hydrogen peroxide-induced lipid peroxidation and biomembrane damage (Yamasaki *et al.*, 1994); prevent oxidized LDL-induced membrane damage, loss of cell viability, and lipid peroxidation (Ide and Lau, 1997b); and demonstrate antihypertensive activity (Lawson, 1998a; Steiner *et al.*, 1996; Koch *et al.*, 1992a; Sendl *et al.*, 1992).

Anticancer
Garlic inhibits the induction and growth of cancer (Milner, 1996; Lea, 1996). The effect on tumor initiation and promotion has been documented, and both the oil-soluble and water-soluble OSCs such as methyl propyl disulfide and propylene sulfide, SAC, S-allylmercaptocysteine (SAMC), and allicin reduce the proliferation of neoplasms and inhibit the development of liver glutathione S-transferase placental (GST-P) positive tumor foci and other indications of cancer in different organs. In contrast, OSCs such as diallyl sulfide, diallyl trisulfide, and allyl methyl trisulfide enhance the formation of liver tumor foci.

However, in rats, diallyl disulfide shows the following activities: inhibits the potential for colon and renal tumor development (Fukushima *et al.*, 1997); inhibits the growth of human prostate cancer cells (Pinto *et al.*, 1997a); demonstrates cytotoxic activity against MBT2 bladder tumor cells (Riggs *et al.*, 1997); is antiallergenic (Kyo *et al.*, 1997); stimulates macrophage activity, natural killer cells, and LAK cells. It may also increase production of interleukin (IL-2), tumor necrosis factor (TNF) and interferon gamma, which are cytokines associated with beneficial antitumor responses. AGE protects against the immunosuppression induced by chemo- and radiation therapy (Lamm and Riggs, 2000; Lau, 1989) and UV light (Reeve *et al.*, 1993a, 1993b).

Antimicrobial effects
Antibacterial activity against *Escherichia*, *Salmonella*, *Staphylococcus*, *Streptococcus*, *Klebsiella*, *Proteus*, *Bacillus*, *Mycobacterium*, *Clostridium*, and resistant strains (Adetumbi and Lau, 1983; Farbman *et al.*, 1993; Hughes and Lawson, 1991; Lawson 1998a; Reuter *et al.*, 1996); antifungal activity against *Candida* and *Cryptococcus* (Anon., 1980; Caporaso *et al.*, 1983; Hughes and Lawson, 1991; Lawson, 1998a); antiulcer/antibacterial against *Helicobacter pylori* (Sivam, 2001; Sivam *et al.*, 1997); antifungal, antiparasitic (Ankri and Mirelman, 1999). The main antimicrobial effect of allicin is limited when in direct exposure to the microorganisms due to its chemical reaction with enzymes (e.g., alcohol dehydrogenase, thioredoxin reductase) and RNA polymerase. This reaction can affect the essential metabolism of cysteine proteinase activity involved in the virulence of *Entamoeba histolytica*. An aqueous extract of garlic cloves, standardized for its thiosulfinate concentration tested positively for its antimicrobial activity against *H. pylori* (Sivam *et al.*, 1997). Minimum inhibitory concentration was 40 mcg thiosulfinate per ml. It is possible that the sensitivity of *H. pylori* to garlic extract at such low concentrations may be related to the reported low risk of stomach cancer in those populations with high allium vegetable intake. However, an uncontrolled trial involving 20 patients with positive urea breath tests, taking 300 mg tablets of dried garlic powder, three times daily for eight weeks, did not eradicate *H. pylori* (Fennerty *et al.*, 1999).

Hematology effects
In vitro studies (and a pilot clinical trial) have indicated an effect of AGE and other antioxidants in the potential treatment of sickle cell anemia patients (Ohnishi *et al.*, 2000, 2001; Ohnishi and Ohnishi, 2001).

MECHANISM OF ACTION
Lipid-lowering
- One possible mechanism is thought to be attributed to allicin/thiosulfinates (Lawson, 1998a; Reuter *et al.*, 1996) but a recent study revealed water-soluble OSC, e.g., SAC and SPC, may be the active compounds inhibiting cholesterol synthesis (Liu and Yeh, 2001). However, oil-soluble OSC, e.g., diallyl disulfide (DADS) and others, decomposed from thiosulfinates including allicin, actually killed the cells, thus indirectly inhibiting cholesterol synthesis (Liu and Yeh, 2001).
- Increases catabolism of fatty acid-containing lipids, especially triglycerides (Yeh *et al.*, 1995; Yeh and Yeh, 1994; Lawson, 1998a).
- Inhibits cholesterol biosynthesis at the level of β-hydroxy-β-methylglutaryl-CoA (HMG-CoA) reductase (Yeh *et al.*, 1995; Yeh and Yeh, 1994; Gebhardt *et al.*, 1994; Gebhardt, 1993).
- Inhibits cholesterol biosynthesis at later steps, as evidenced by accumulation of the cholesterol precursors, lanosterol and 7-dehydrocholesterol, although this latter effect may be of minor therapeutic significance (Gebhardt *et al.*, 1994; Gebhardt, 1993).
- Enhances palmitate-induced inhibition of cholesterol biosynthesis (Gebhardt, 1995).
- Inhibits cholesterol biosynthesis by targeting squalene monooxygenase, an enzyme that catalyzes the downstream pathway in cholesterol synthesis (*in vitro* study on fresh garlic extract) (Gupta and Porter, 2001).
- Lipid-lowering activity may be due to the presence of steroid saponins in fresh garlic and AGE, which may interfere with the absorption of total and LDL cholesterol from the intestine lumen, thereby reducing plasma levels (40–57% in test animals), without adversely affecting HDL levels. Saponins are known to inhibit intestinal absorption of cholesterol, suggesting possible hypocholesterolemic effect (Matsuura, 2001).

Antithrombotic
- Garlic inhibits platelet aggregation and stimulates fibrinolysis; this may be attributed to allicin/thiosulfinates at lower garlic doses and cycloalliin at higher garlic doses (*in vitro*) (Lawson, 1998a; Reuter *et al.*, 1996). However, since it is argued that allicin/thiosulfinates may not be bioavailable, other compounds may be responsible (Amagase *et al.*, 2001).
- Inhibits normal arachidonate metabolism (Ariga *et al.*, 1981; Makheja *et al.*, 1980; Makheja *et al.*, 1981; Reuter *et al.*, 1996).

- Inhibits the lipoxygenase and cyclo-oxygenase pathways of the arachidonic acid cascade, thereby inhibiting the synthesis of prostaglandins and thromboxanes (PGE2, PGD2, PGI2, TXB2) (Rahman and Billington, 2000; Reuter et al., 1996; Ariga et al., 1981; Makheja et al., 1981, 1980).
- Inhibits fatty acid lipoxygenase (Liu and Yeh, 2001; Reuter et al., 1996; Ariga et al., 1981; Makheja et al., 1981, 1980).
- Ajoene affects fibrinogen-induced human platelet aggregation and inhibits binding of fibrinogen to adenosine diphosphate (ADP) stimulated platelets in vitro (Reuter et al., 1996).

Antihypertensive
- Action is thought to be attributed to γ-glutamylcysteines and fructans; allicin is not involved (Lawson, 1998a; Reuter et al., 1996).
- γ-glutamylcysteines can inhibit angiotensin-converting enzyme (ACE), thus inhibiting angiotensin II (a hormone that increases vasoconstriction) (Lawson, 1998a; Sendl et al., 1992).
- Fructans can inhibit adenosine deaminase in isolated cells, thus increasing adenosine and its associated blood vessel dilatory activity (Lawson 1998a; Koch et al., 1992).
- Increases nitric oxide through activation of nitric oxide synthase activity (Das et al., 1995).

Antimicrobial
- Action is in vitro or externally thought to be attributed to allicin/thiosulfinates (Lawson, 1998a; Reuter et al., 1996).
- Allicin disrupts cellular metabolic processes in vitro through inactivation of proteins by oxidation of essential thiols to disulfide, competitive inhibition of enzymes containing cysteine in their active sites by reacting with the sulfhydryl (-SH) group, and noncompetitive inhibition of enzymes by reacting with -SH groups at allosteric sites (Adetumbi and Lau, 1983; Cavallito et al., 1944; Lawson, 1998a).
- Garlic extract inhibits H. pylori bacterial in vitro at moderate concentrations, thereby suggesting mechanism for antigastric ulcer effect (Sivam, 2001; Sivam et al., 1997).

Anticancer
- Action is thought to be attributed to any number of garlic compounds: SAC, SAMC, thiosulfinates, γ-glutamylcysteines, and other unknown compounds (Lawson, 1998a; Pinto et al., 1997b; Reuter et al., 1996, Amagase and Milner, 1993; Liu et al., 1992) although the thiosulfinates (e.g., allicin) are questioned due to their instability.
- Decreases the amount of nitrate-reducing bacteria in the stomach, thus reducing the formation of carcinogenic nitrosamines (Dion and Milner, 1996; Mei et al., 1985, 1982).
- Inhibits the induction and growth of cancer, which may be mediated by modulation of carcinogen metabolism (Lea, 1996).
- Stimulates macrophage activity, natural killer cells, and LAK cells, and might increase the production of IL-2, TNF, and interferon gamma, which are cytokines associated with beneficial antitumor response (Lamm and Riggs, 2000; Lau et al., 1991; Lau, 1989; Abdullah et al., 1989).

Antiallergenic
- Inhibits antigen-specific histamine release from mast cells in vitro (Kyo et al., 1997); decreases antigen-specific IgE mediated skin reactions in vivo (Kyo et al., 1997); and reduces antigen-specific, late-phase reaction by modulating the production and release of cytokines from activated T-lymphocytes in vivo (Kyo et al., 1997).

Antioxidant
- Action is thought to be attributed to primarily water-soluble OSC (e.g., SAC and SAMC) in addition to fructosyl-arginine, other Maillard reaction compounds in AGE, and other compounds (Ryu, 2001; Imai, 1994); some authors suggest action may be due to the allicin/thiosulfinates (Lawson, 1998a; Reuter et al., 1996).
- Decreases oxidation of LDL cholesterol in humans (Ide and Lau, 2001; Lau, 2001; Munday, 1999; Steiner and Lin, 1994; Harris et al., 1995; Phelps and Harris, 1993).
- Increases the activity of several enzymes (including glutathione peroxidase and catalase) involved in antioxidative processes and decreases the concentration of lipid peroxides in the blood (Ide and Lau, 1999; Steiner and Lin, 1994; Geng and Lau, 1997; Han et al., 1992).
- Increases intracellular glutathione (GSH) (a potent intracellular antioxidant and detoxifier), modulates the activity of the GSH redox cycle, and increases activity of superoxide dismutase (SOD, a potent intracellular antioxidant) activity (Ide and Lau, 2001; Wang et al., 1999; Hatono et al., 1996; Geng and Lau, 1997).

Immunomodulatory
- Action thought to be attributed to protein fraction of garlic (Moraika et al., 1993; Lau et al., 1991; Hirao et al., 1987).
- Inhibits activation of nuclear factor kappa B (NF-κB) in human T-cells that are involved in immune and inflammatory reactions (Geng et al., 1997).
- Increases phagocytosis, natural killer cell activity, antibody titer, and lymphocyte counts (Brosche and Platt, 1993; Kandil et al., 1988; Lawson, 1998a; Reuter et al., 1996).

Hematological (AGE)
- Inhibits anion transport and sickle cell dehydration (Ohnishi et al., 2001), restricts dense cell formation (Ohnishi and Ohnishi, 2001) and 4.0 mg/mL was shown to inhibit dense cell formation by 50% (Ohnishi et al., 2000). A U.S. patent has been granted to Wakunaga of America, Mission Viejo, CA for the "Therapeutic Uses of Specially Processed Garlic for Sickle Cell Disease" (Ohnishi and Tsuyoshi, 2001).
- Increased natural killer cell activity and improved helper suppressor T-cell ratios in AIDS patients (Abdullah et al., 1989).

CONTRAINDICATIONS
None known according to the German Commission E and other leading European scientific bodies (Blumenthal et al., 1998; ESCOP, 1997). The World Health Organization (WHO) cautions against the use of garlic by patients with a known allergy to garlic, and those taking warfarin (and presumably other anticoagulants) (WHO, 1999). However, AGE has been tested in a placebo-controlled, double-blind clinical trial in patients taking Coumadin® (warfarin); there was no demonstrated interaction

Garlic

Monograph

The ABC Clinical Guide to Herbs | 159

with Coumadin® and no prolonged bleeding (Rozenfeld *et al.*, 2000). Several case reports of increased clotting time suggest that patients should discontinue use prior to surgery (Brinker, 2001), usually by at least one week.

PREGNANCY AND LACTATION: None known (Blumenthal *et al.*, 1998; ESCOP, 1997). A controlled trial showed that major sulfur-containing volatiles from garlic are transmitted to breast milk, leading to improved drinking habits of infants (ESCOP, 1997; Mennella and Beauchamp, 1991). In Japan, AGE is an ingredient in pharmaceutical products that are used in nutritional nourishment for pregnant and lactating women.

ADVERSE EFFECTS

The most commonly reported adverse effect of garlic is that its odor may pervade the breath and skin (Blumenthal *et al.*, 1998). Raw garlic has a stronger odor and higher levels of high molecular weight sulfur compounds than cooked garlic, but malodorous breath tested in humans who ingested raw garlic showed higher levels of low molecular weight sulfur compounds and different constituents than those associated with common halitosis (Tamaki and Sonoki, 1999). Differences in the frequency of other adverse effects caused by various garlic preparations have not been completely determined (Mulrow *et al.*, 2000), such adverse effects being dependent upon the method of preparation. Gastrointestinal symptoms and changes to the intestinal flora or allergic reactions are rare but are occasionally reported (Lembo *et al.*, 1991). In separate, single-case reports, garlic was associated with postoperative bleeding (Burnham, 1995), spontaneous spinal epidural hematoma, and platelet dysfunction from excessive ingestion (Rose *et al.*, 1990). Occupational exposure to crushed garlic products and the topical application of garlic to treat wounds or skin infections may cause allergic contact dermatitis (Lee and Lam, 1991; Bojs and Svensson, 1998). Allergic reactions including burns (Roberge *et al.*, 1997), zosteriform dermatitis (Farrell and Staughton, 1996), induction of pemphigus (blisters) (Brenner and Wolf, 1994), allergic asthma and rhinitis, contact urticaria, and protein contact dermatitis have been reported for garlic and various generic garlic preparations (WHO, 1999; DeSmet, 1992), but no adverse effects were reported for AGE according to toxicological and clinical studies (Miyoshi *et al.*, 1984; Nakagawa *et al.*, 1984, 1980; Sumiyoshi *et al.*, 1984). Cross-sensitivity may occur with onions and tulips (Siegers, 1992; WHO, 1999). Garlic preparations can increase clotting time (Chutani and Bordia, 1981; Gadkari and Joshi, 1991; Harenberg *et al.*, 1988; Legnani *et al.*, 1993), which is sometimes beneficial, but in some cases, can contribute to an adverse event.

DRUG INTERACTIONS

Concurrent use of garlic and antiplatelet agents (e.g., aspirin) and anticoagulants (e.g., warfarin) might increase the potential for prolonged bleeding. One report showed that clotting time (International Normalization Ratio) doubled for two patients taking warfarin and garlic simultaneously (Sunter, 1991); however, this report lacks adequate data to assess causality (Rotblatt and Ziment, 2001). Further, a controlled clinical trial on AGE showed no interactions with warfarin (Rozenfeld, 2000). Another trial on nine HIV-negative individuals produced significant decreases in serum levels of the anti-HIV drug saquinavir (Piscitelli *et al.*, 2002); however, this study has design problems rendering the results uninterpretable.

AMERICAN HERBAL PRODUCTS ASSOCIATION (AHPA) SAFETY RATING

CLASS 2C: Not to be used while nursing (McGuffin *et al.*, 1997). However, a controlled trial indicated a positive therapeutic use during lactation (ESCOP, 1997; Mennella and Beauchamp, 1991).

REGULATORY STATUS

CANADA: Drug or possibly "New Drug" if claims made. Food in absence of claims (HPB, 1993). Schedule OTC "Herbal and Natural Products" and "Homoeopathic Products" have marketing authorization with Drug Identification Numbers (DIN) assigned (Health Canada, 2001).

EUROPEAN UNION: Powder, freeze-dried, or low temperature dried (<65°C), containing not less than 0.45% allicin, official in *European Pharmacopoeia* 3rd ed. Suppl. 2001 (Ph.Eur., 2001).

FRANCE: Traditional Herbal Medicine (THM) permitted for treatment of minor circulatory disorders (Bradley, 1992). Essential oil is dispensed as an aromatherapy drug (Goetz, 1999).

GERMANY: Fresh or carefully dried bulb is approved by Commission E as non-prescription drug (Blumenthal *et al.*, 1998). Fresh bulb for preparation of mother tincture official in the *German Homoeopathic Pharmacopoeia* (GHP, 1993).

GHANA: Monograph for fresh whole bulb occurs in *Ghana Herbal Pharmacopoeia* (GHP, 1992).

INDIA: Bulb and oil are approved single drugs dispensed in Unani system of medicine (CCRUM, 1997).

JAPAN: OTC drug for fatigue (Okada and Miyagaki, 1983). AGE approved for nourishment of pregnant and lactating women.

SWEDEN: Classified as 'Natural Remedy' for self-medication requiring pre-marketing authorization from Medical Products Agency (MPA). One product (e.g. Bio-Garlic Pharma Nord) is listed in the "Authorised Natural Remedies" with the approved indication "Traditionally used for the relief of cold symptoms" (MPA, 2001a; Tunón, 1999). Homoeopathic dilutions (e.g., Radiotron AB) are also registered drugs (MPA, 2001b).

SWITZERLAND: Powdered garlic in tablets, standardized powdered extract in tablets, oily macerate in capsules, and multiple-herb preparations containing standardized garlic extract have positive classification (List D) by the *Interkantonale Kontrollstelle für Heilmittel* (IKS) and corresponding sales category D, with sales limited to pharmacies and drugstores, without prescription (Morant and Ruppanner, 2001). Twenty-eight garlic phytomedicines and two homoeopathic medicines are listed in the *Swiss Codex* 2000/01 (Ruppanner and Schaefer, 2000).

U.K: Herbal medicine on the *General Sale List* (GSL), Table A (internal or external use), Schedule 1 (requires full product license) (GSL, 1989).

U.S.: Dietary Supplement (USC, 1994). Fresh or dried compound bulbs, powdered garlic, fluidextract and extract are official in the U.S. *National Formulary* 19th edition (USP, 2002). Tincture of mature bulb, 1:10 (*w/v*) in 55% alcohol (*v/v*), is a Class C OTC drug of the *Homoeopathic Pharmacopoeia of the United States* (HPUS, 1989).

CLINICAL REVIEW

Thirty-two studies, including 45,694 participants, are outlined in the following table, "Clinical Studies on Garlic." All but four of the studies (Berthold *et al.*, 1998; Isaacsohn *et al.*, 1998; McCrindle *et al.*, 1998; Simons *et al.*, 1995) demonstrated positive effects on conditions including cardiovascular and arterial health, cancer, immunity, and circulation. Studies from the table are categorized and discussed in the following six sections. In addition to the studies in the table, this Clinical Review discusses numerous reviews and meta-analyses that are not listed in the table.

Based on the Agency for Healthcare Research and Quality's (AHRQ) review and summary of clinical studies on garlic (Mulrow *et al.*, 2000), researchers concluded that garlic preparations may have small, positive, short-term effects (less than three months) on lipids, and promising antithrombic effects. However, the data was insufficient to draw conclusions about certain clinical cardiovascular outcomes (e.g., myocardial infarction), antithrombic activity, or cancer prevention. No effects on glucose or insulin sensitivity, or consistent decreases in blood pressure were found. Case-control studies suggest that consuming large amounts of garlic in the diet may reduce the risks of laryngeal, gastric, colorectal, and endometrial cancers, and adenomatous colorectal polyps (Mulrow, *et al.*, 2000). A subsequent review of 45 randomized trials by some of the same researchers concluded that the trials suggest possible small short-term benefits of garlic preparations on some lipid and antiplatelet factors, insignificant effects on blood pressure, and no effect on glucose levels (Ackermann *et al.*, 2001). Conclusions regarding clinical significance are limited due to the marginal quality and short duration of many trials, as well as the unpredictable release and inadequate definition of active constituents in many of the garlic preparations used in the studies.

Lipid-lowering effect

Thirteen trials involving a total of 795 participants demonstrated a positive correlation between garlic oil, powder, or capsule intake and lipid-lowering effects. Six randomized, double-blind, placebo-controlled (R, DB, PC) studies (Yeh *et al.*, 1995; Jain *et al.*, 1993; Rotzsch *et al.*, 1992; Auer *et al.*, 1990; Mader *et al.*, 1990; Vorberg *et al.*, 1990), as well as two DB, multi-center studies (Grünwald *et al.*, 1992; Holzgartner *et al.*, 1992) supported the use of garlic in treating elevated lipid conditions including hyperlipidemia and hypercholesterolemia. Three studies showed the positive impact of taking Kyolic® capsules specifically for improving hypercholesterolemia conditions (Steiner *et al.*, 1996; Steiner and Lin, 1994; Lau *et al.*, 1987). One R, open, parallel group, comparison (O, PG, Cm) found garlic powder to have a significant impact over garlic oil on lowering blood lipid counts and blood pressure, as well as increasing the overall sense of well-being in 70 subjects (De A Santos and Johns, 1995). An R, PC study involving 35 renal transplant patients found the garlic product, Pure-Gar®, to have positive effects on hyperlipidemia (Lash *et al.*, 1998). One O study involving 82 subjects (Bordia, 1981) found garlic to have, in conjunction with the lipid-lowering effects, a positive impact on patients with coronary heart disease.

A meta-analysis on the effect of garlic on total serum cholesterol levels found a statistically significant reduction in total cholesterol levels (Warshafsky *et al.*, 1993). Another analysis assessed clinical data from 952 patients and 16 trials, indicating a decrease in total cholesterol levels (Silagy and Neil, 1994b). A subsequent reanalysis of all data still demonstrated a significant reduction of total

cholesterol compared to placebo (Warshafsky *et al.*, 1993). Three studies on the allicin-standardized garlic powder tablets (Kwai®) failed to show a significant reduction in elevated serum cholesterol (Isaacsohn *et al.*, 1998; McCrindle *et al.*, 1998; Simons *et al.*, 1995). It was later determined that the allicin release from the tablets varied significantly, and that negative studies were possibly due to the lack of expected allicin release (Lawson *et al.*, 2001). A study of 24 brands of enteric-coated tablets found that 83% of the brands released less than 15% of their allicin potential (Lawson and Wang, 2001). Therefore, the researchers recommend that manufacturers standardize supplements to dissolution of allicin release, not to allicin potential. (For non-allicin releasing products, e.g., AGE, the standardization is to other compounds, e.g., SAC.) In a recent, comprehensive meta-analysis of 13 R, DB, PC trials researchers demonstrated a significant difference (p<0.01) in the reduction of total cholesterol levels between baseline and placebo, equivalent to a 5.8% reduction in total cholesterol levels. The authors concluded that current evidence indicates that any specific lipid-lowering effect is small, and the clinical outcome may not be meaningful (Stevinson *et al.*, 2000). However, there were several problems identified with the meta-analysis, indicating that the conclusions can only be attributed to the specific brands tested and not the effectiveness of garlic in general. In particular, the brand used in 10 of the trials did not protect allinase from exposure to gastric acid. Another tested supplement was spray-dried, resulting in the loss of alliin. The study on the garlic oil that showed no effect utilized a form that has demonstrated low bioavailability; therefore the conclusions of the meta-analysis need to be considered within this context (Lawson, 2001). Several of these products are not standardized to a bioavailable marker compound. Clinical studies with positive outcomes using AGE standardized with bioavailable SAC have shown significant levels of SAC in human blood during the study period (Steiner and Li, 2001).

Antihypertensive effect

Two R, DB, PC studies and one R, O, PG, Cm study (159 total participants) demonstrated the antihypertensive effects of garlic (De A Santos and Johns, 1995; Jain *et al.*, 1993; Auer *et al.*, 1990). A systematic review and meta-analysis of randomized controlled trials was conducted to determine the effect of garlic on blood pressure. Eight trials, including 415 participants, were identified. Of the seven trials that compared the effect of garlic with a placebo, three demonstrated a significant reduction in systolic blood pressure (SBP), and 4 in diastolic blood pressure (DBP). The authors concluded that more rigorously designed trials can provide evidence to recommend the clinical application of garlic in the treatment of hypertension (Silagy and Neil, 1994b).

Antiplatelet effects

One R, DB, PC, crossover (CO) study and 2 DB, PC studies involving a total of 214 subjects indicate the potential use of garlic as a coronary disease preventative due to its positive impact on platelet functions (Steiner and Li, 2001; Kiesewetter *et al.*, 1991; 1993a).

Anti-atherosclerotic effect

In the longest clinical trial on garlic to date, garlic's ability to prevent and possibly reverse atherosclerosis was tested in a R, DB, PC, four-year study in which 152 men and women were given 900 mg garlic powder as tablets (Kwai®) per day (Koscielny *et al.*, 1999). The subjects possessed significant plaque buildup and at least one additional cardiovascular risk factor (e.g., high LDL levels, hypertension, diabetes, and/or history of smoking). After the four years, garlic subjects had an average 2.6% reduction in plaque volume while the placebo group's plaque increased 15.6%. Researchers concluded that garlic has a preventive and possibly curative role in arteriosclerosis therapy. In one epidemiological, cross-sectional, observational (E, CS, OB) study with 202 participants, standardized garlic powered was found to have positive effects on arterial activities including elastic vascular resistance, pulse wave velocity, and systolic blood pressure (Breithaupt-Grogler, 1997).

Anticancer/Chemoprevention

Anti-cancer and chemopreventative qualities of garlic were demonstrated in five studies involving a total of 44,044 subjects. One E study spanning over a period of 15 years, demonstrated that raw and cooked garlic use had a significant impact on decreasing stomach cancer incidents (You *et al.*, 1989). Two other E studies found that garlic intake significantly decreased the risk of colon cancer in 42,325 participants (Witte *et al.*, 1996; Steinmetz *et al.*, 1994). Garlic's chemopreventative potential was demonstrated in two OB studies through the improvement of arachidonic acid and acetaminophen metabolism (Dimitrov and Bennink, 1997; Gwilt *et al.*, 1994). Case-control studies suggest that consuming large amounts of garlic in the diet may reduce the risks of laryngeal, gastric, colorectal, and endometrial cancers and adenomatous colorectal polyps (Mulrow, *et al.*, 2000).

Several reviews of E studies have examined the cancer-preventive effect of garlic, including garlic ingested as a food (Dorant *et al.*, 1993; Fleischauer *et al.*, 2000). A meta-analysis of the epidemiological evidence on the association between garlic consumption and risk of stomach, colon, head and neck, lung, breast, and prostate cancers concluded that raw and cooked garlic consumption might have a protective effect against stomach and colorectal cancers (Fleischauer *et al.*, 2000). An earlier review of *in vitro*, *in vivo*, epidemiologic, and case-control studies suggested that the evidence is not conclusive to support chemoprevention in humans, but further research is warranted (Dorant *et al.*, 1993); however, this review preceded much of the salient research in this area.

Other

One pilot study involving 7 HIV+ patients demonstrated a positive impact on natural killer cell activity as well as improvement in conditions such as diarrhea, genital herpes, and candidiasis (Abdullah *et al.,* 1989). One R, DB, PC study showed that garlic did not negatively impact bleeding potential in patients undergoing warfarin therapy (Rozenfeld, *et al.*, 2000). Two studies involving 92 subjects demonstrated garlic's positive impact on peripheral circulation: one R, CO, Cm study showed an immediate improvement in hand and foot circulation (Okuhara, 1994); and one DB, PC study involving 80 subjects with peripheral arterial occlusive disease (PAOD) showed a significant increase in walking distance (Kiesewetter *et al.,* 1993b). This last study was the only study to meet the inclusion criteria established by the Cochrane Library for its review on the use of garlic for PAOD. The Cochrane Review concluded that further trials on garlic's effectiveness on PAOD are warranted because the one study reviewed was small, of short duration (12 weeks), and found no significant overall improvement in patients with PAOD. The discrepancy between the conclusions of the study and those of the review is a result of the study's analysis of the mean difference between the garlic and placebo groups instead of analyzing the mean change within the groups' pre- and post-treatment.

BRANDED PRODUCTS*

AGE™ (Aged Garlic Extract): Wakunaga of America Co., Ltd. / 23501 Madero / Mission Viego, CA 92691 / U.S.A. / Tel: (800) 421-2998 / www.kyolic.com. This refers to a proprietary garlic extract with stable sulfure compounds standardized to bioavailable components (e.g., SAC) in various types of formulations. See Kyolic® below.

Höfel's® Garlic Pearles One-A-Day: Seven Seas Ltd., a division of the Merck Group / Hedon Road / Marfleet / Hull / England / HU9 5NJ / U.K. / Tel.: +44-1482-37-5234 / Fax: +44-1482-37-4345 / Email: info@hofels.com or Info@Seven-Seas.ltd.uk / www.hofels.com. A gelatin or glycerin capsule containing 2 mg garlic oil, and soybean oil.

Kwai® forte 300 mg LI 111: 1. Lichtwer Pharma AG / Wallenroder Strasse 8-14 / 13435 Berlin / Germany / Tel: +49-30-40-3700 / Fax: +49-30-40-3704-49 / www.lichtwer.de. One sugar-coated tablet (dragée) contains: garlic bulb powder 300 mg. Other components: lactose monohydrate, cellulose, highly dispersive silicon dioxide, magnesium stearate, castor oil, Macrogol 6000, Hypromellose, saccharose, talcum, gelatin, Povidon K25, carnauba wax, bleached wax, yellow quinoline E104, indigo carmine E132.

Kwai®N LI 111: Lichtwer Pharma AG. One tablet contains 100 mg dried powder from *Allium sativum* (garlic bulb) standardized to contain 1.3% allicin (yielding 0.6% allicin). Inactive ingredients: lactose, magnesium stearate, powdered cellulose, colloidal anhydrous silica, methylhydroxypropylcellulose, polyethylene glycol 6000, castor oil, talc, polyvinylpyrrolidone 25, sucrose, gelatin, quinoline yellow E 104, indigotine E 132, carnauba wax, cera alba.

Kyolic® Liquid: Wakunaga of America Co., Ltd. Aged Garlic Extract™ in water and residual alcohol from extraction.

Kyolic® Reserve: Wakunaga of America Co., Ltd. 600 mg Aged Garlic Extract™ per capsule.

Kyolic® Super Formula 100: Wakunaga of America Co., Ltd. 300 mg Aged Garlic Extract™ per capsule plus whey.

Kyolic® Super Formula 101: Wakunaga of America Co., Ltd. 270 mg Aged Garlic Extract™ per capsule, plus brewer's yeast, kelp, and whey.

Kyolic® Super Formula 102: Wakunaga of America Co., Ltd. 350 mg Aged Garlic Extract™ per capsule, plus food enzymes: amylase, protease, lipase, and cellulase (30 mg).

Kyolic® Super Formula 103: Wakunaga of America Co., Ltd. 220 mg Aged Garlic Extract™ per capsule, plus Ester C® (105 mg), *Astragalus membranaceous* (100 mg), and calcium (23 mg).

Kyolic® Super Formula 104: Wakunaga of America Co., Ltd. 300 mg Aged Garlic Extract™ per capsule, plus 190 mg lecithin.

Kyolic® Super Formula 105: Wakunaga of America Co., Ltd. 200 mg Aged Garlic Extract™ per capsule, plus beta-carotene (6 mg), vitamin C (120 mg), vitamin E (60 IU), selenium (25 mg), and green tea (45 mg).

Kyolic® Super Formula 106: Wakunaga of America Co., Ltd. 300 mg Aged Garlic Extract™ per capsule, plus hawthorn berry (50 mg), cayenne pepper (10 mg), and vitamin E (100 IU).

Pure-Gar® Garlic Powder A-2000: Essentially Pure Ingredients™, c/o Pure Gar L.P. / 21411 Prairie Street / Chatsworth, CA 91311 / U.S.A. / Tel: (800) 537-7695 /

www.essentiallypure.com. Dried powder from *Allium sativum* (garlic bulb): allicin yield 2,000 ppm min.; total thiosulfinates yield 2,100 ppm minimum; allian 7,500 ppm minimum; gamma-glutamylcysteines 10,000 ppm minimum.

Pure-Gar® Garlic Powder A-5000: Essentially Pure Ingredients™ / 21411 Prairie Street / Chatsworth, CA 91311 / U.S.A. / Tel: 818-739-6046 / www.essentiallypure.com. Dried powder from *Allium sativum* (garlic bulb): allicin yield 5,000 ppm minimum; total thiosulfinates yield 5,000 ppm minimum; allian 11,000 ppm minimum; gamma-glutamylcysteines 10,000 ppm minimum; total sulfur 6,500 ppm minimum.

Pure-Gar® Garlic Powder A-8000: Essentially Pure Ingredients™. Dried powder from *Allium sativum* (garlic bulb): allicin yield 8,000 ppm minimum; total thiosulfinates yield 8,000 ppm minimum; allian 18,000 ppm minimum; gamma-glutamylcysteines 8,000 ppm minimum.

Pure-Gar® Garlic Powder A-10000: Essentially Pure Ingredients™. Dried powder from *Allium sativum* (garlic bulb): allicin yield 10,000 ppm minimum; total thiosulfinates yield 10,000 ppm minimum; allian 23,000 ppm minimum; gamma-glutamylcysteines 8,000 ppm minimum.

Sapec®: Lichtwer Pharma AG. 300 mg tablet of dried garlic powder standardized to contain 1.3% allicin (yielding 0.6% allicin).

Tegra®: Hermes Fabrick Pharma / Georg-Kalb-Str. 5-8 / 82049 Grosshesselohe / Germany. Steam-distilled garlic oil (does not contain allicin, fructans, agrinine, or gamma-glutamylcysteines).

*American equivalents, if any, are found in the Product Table beginning on page 398.

REFERENCES

Abdullah TH, Kirkpatrick DV, Carter J. Enhancement of natural killer cell activity in AIDS with garlic. *Deutsche Z Onkol* 1989;21:52–3.

Ackermann RT, Mulrow CD, Ramirez G, Gardner CD, Morbidoni L, Lawrence VA. Garlic shows promise for improving some cardiovascular risk factors. *Arch Int Med* 2001;161(6):813–24.

Adetumbi MA, Lau BHS. *Allium sativum* (garlic)—a natural antibiotic. *Med Hypoth* 1983;12(3):227–37.

Agarwal K. Therapeutic actions of garlic constituents. *Med Res Rev* 1996;16(1):111–24.

Amagase H, Milner JA. Impact of various sources of garlic and their constituents on 7,12-dimethylbenz[a]anthracene binding to mammary cell DNA. *Carcinogenesis* 1993;14(8):1627–31.

Amagase H, Petesch BL, Matsuura H, Kasuga S, Itakura Y. Intake of garlic and its bioactive components. *J Nutr* 2001;131 Suppl 3:955S–62S.

Ankri S, Mirelman D. Antimicrobial properties of allicin from garlic. *Microbes Infect* 1999;1(2):125–9.

Anonymous. Garlic in cryptococcal meningitis: a preliminary report of 21 cases. *Chin Med J* 1980;93(2):123–6.

Ariga T, Oshiba S, Tamada T. Platelet aggregation inhibitor in garlic [letter]. *Lancet* 1981 Jan 17;1(8212):150–1.

Auer W, Eiber A, Hertkorn E, Hoehfeld E, Koehrle U, Lorenz A, et al. Hypertension and hyperlipidemia: garlic helps in mild cases. *Br J Clin Pract* 1990; 69 Suppl:3–6.

Augusti K. Studies on the effect of allicin (diallyl disulfide-oxide) on alloxan diabetes. *Experientia* 1975;31(11):1263–5.

Barrie SA, Wright JV, Pizzorno JE. Effects of garlic oil on platelet aggregation, serum lipids, and blood pressure in humans. *J Orthomolec Med* 1987;2(1):15–21.

Belman S. Onion and garlic oils inhibit tumor promotion. *Carcinogenesis*. 1983;4(8):1063–5.

Berthold HK, Sudhop T. Garlic preparations for prevention of atherosclerosis. *Curr Opin Lipidol* 1998;9(6):565–9.

Berthold HK, Sudhop T, von Bergmann K. Effect of a garlic oil preparation on serum lipoproteins and cholesterol metabolism: a randomized controlled trial. *JAMA* 1998;279(23):1900–2.

BHP. See: *British Herbal Pharmacopoeia*.

Block E. The chemistry of garlic and onions. *Sci Am 1985;*252(3):114–9.

Blumenthal M. Herb sales down 15% in mainstream market. *HerbalGram* 2001;51:69.

Blumenthal M, Goldberg A, Brinckmann J, editors. *Herbal Medicine – Expanded Commission E Monographs*. Austin (TX); American Botanical Council: Newton (MA): Integrative Medicine Communications; 2000. p. 139–48.

Blumenthal M, Busse WR, Goldberg A, Gruenwald J, Hall T, Riggins CW, Rister R, editors. Klein S, Rister R (trans.). *The Complete German Commission E Monographs: Therapeutic Guide to Herbal Medicines*. Austin (TX): American Botanical Council; Boston (MA): Integrative Medicine Communication: 1998. p. 134.

Bojs G, Svensson A. Contact allergy to garlic used for wound healing. *Contact Dermatitis* 1998;18(3):179–81.

Bordia A, Arora SK, Kathari LK, Jain KC, Rathore BS, Rathore AS, et al. The protective action of essential oils of onion and garlic in cholesterol-fed rabbits. *Atherosclerosis* 1975;22(1):103–9.

Bordia A. Effect of garlic on blood lipids in patients with coronary heart disease. *Am J Clin Nutr* 1981; 34:2100–3.

Bordia T, Mohammed N, Thomson M, Ali M. An evaluation of garlic and onion as antithrombotic agents. *Prostaglandins Leukot Essent Fatty Acids* 1996;54(3):183–6.

Boullin DJ. Garlic as a platelet inhibitor [letter]. *Lancet* 1981 Apr 4;1(8223):776–7.

Bradley PR, editor. *British Herbal Compendium Volume I — A Handbook of Scientific Information on Widely Used Plant Drugs*. Exeter, U.K.: British Herbal Medicine Association (BHMA); 1992. p. 105–8.

Breithaupt-Grögler K, Ling M, Boudoulas H, Belz GG. Protective effect of chronic garlic intake on elastic properties of aorta in the elderly. *Circulation* 1997;96(8):2649–55.

Brenner S, Wolf R. Possible nutritional factors in induced pemphigus [review]. *Dermatology* 1994;189(4):337–9.

Brevoort P. The booming US botanical market. *HerbalGram* 1998;44:33–40.

Brinker R. *Herb Contraindications and Drug Interactions* 3d ed. Sandy (OR): Eclectic Medical Publications; 2001. p. 99–101.

British Herbal Pharmacopoeia (BHP). Exeter, U.K.: British Herbal Medicine Association; 1996. p. 85–6.

Brosche T, Platt D. About the immunomodulatory effect of garlic (*Allium sativum*) [in German]. *Med Welt* 1993;44:309–13.

Brown D. *Herbal Prescriptions for Better Health*. Rocklin (CA): Prima Publishing; 1996. p. 97–109.

Budavari S, editor. *The Merck Index: An Encyclopedia of Chemicals, Drugs, and Biologicals,* 12th ed. Whitehouse Station (N.J.): Merck & Co, Inc; 1996. p. 741.

Buiatti E, Palli D, Decarli A, Amadori D, Avellini C, Bianchi S, et al. A case-control study of gastric cancer and diet in Italy. *Int J Cancer* 1989;44(4):611–6.

Burnham BE. Garlic as a possible risk for postoperative bleeding [letter]. *Plast Recontr Surgery* 1995;95(1):213.

Caporaso N, Smith S, Eng R. Antifungal activity in human urine and serum after ingestion of garlic (*Allium sativum*). *Antimicrob Agents Chemother* 1983;23(5):700–2.

Cavallito C, Buck J, Suter C. Allicin, the antibacterial principle of *Allium sativum*. II. Determination of the chemical structure. *J Am Chem Soc* 1944;66:1952–4.

CCRUM. See: Central Council for Research in Unani Medicine.

Central Council for Research in Unani Medicine (CCRUM). *Allium sativum*. In: *Standardisation of Single Drugs of Unani Medicine*, 1st edition, Part III. New Delhi, India: Central Council for Research in Unani Medicine, Ministry of Health & Family Welfare, Government of India; 1997 August. p. 199–204.

Chadha Y et al., editors. *The Wealth of India—A Dictionary of Indian Raw Materials & Industrial Products—Volume-I:A*. New Delhi, India: Publications & Information Directorate, Council of Scientific and Industrial Research (CSIR); 1952–88. p. 181–7.

Chang M, Johnson M. Effect of garlic on carbohydrate metabolism and lipid synthesis in rats. *J Nutr* 1980;110(5):931–6.

Chi MS, Koh ET, Stewart TJ. Effects of garlic on lipid metabolism in rats fed cholesterol or lard. *J Nutr* 1982;112(2):241–8.

Chutani SK, Bordia A. The effect of fried versus raw garlic on fibrinolytic activity in man. *Atherosclerosis* 1981;38:417–21.

Das I, Khan NS, Sooranna SR. Potent activation of nitric oxide synthetase by garlic: a basis for its therapeutic applications. *Curr Med Res Opinion* 1995;13(5):257–63.

Davis LE, Shen J-K, Cai Y. Antifungal activity in human cerebrospinal fluid and plasma after intravenous administration of *Allium sativum*. *Antimicrob Agents Chemother* 1990;34(4):651–3.

De A Santos OS, Johns RA. Effects of garlic powder and garlic oil preparations on blood lipids, blood pressure and well-being. *Br J Clin Res* 1995;6:91–100.

Dimitrov NV, Bennink MR. Modulation of arachidonic acid metabolism by garlic extracts. In: Lanchance PP, editor. *Nutraceuticals: Designer Foods III Garlic, Soy and Licorice*. Trubell (CT): Food & Nutrition Press; 1997. p. 199–202.

Dion ME, Milner JA. Formation and bioactivation of nitrosomorpholine is inhibited by S-allylcysteine. *FASEB J* 1996;10(3):A498.

Dorant E, van de Brandt PA, Goldbohm RA, Hermus RJJ, Sturmans F. Garlic and its significance for the prevention of cancers in humans: a critical view. *Br J Cancer* 1993;67(3):424–9.

Elbl G. Biochemical investigations of plant-derived inhibitors of the Angiotensin I-converting enzymes (ACE), especially the phytomedicinals *Lespedeza capitata* (Michx.) und *Allium ursinum* [dissertation] [in German]. University of Munich; 1991.

El-Mofty MM, Sakr SA, Essawy A, Gawad HSA. Preventative action of garlic. *Nutr Cancer* 1994;21(1):95–100.

ESCOP. See: European Scientific Cooperative on Phytotherapy.

European Scientific Cooperative on Phytotherapy. "*Allii sativi bulbus*." *Monographs on the Medicinal Uses of Plant Drugs*. Exeter, U.K.: European Scientific Cooperative on Phytotherapy; 1997 Jul.

Europäisches Arzneibuch (Ph.Eur.). Stuttgart: Deutscher Apotheker Verlag; 1999;754–5.

European Pharmacopoeia (Ph.Eur. 3rd ed. 1997 - Supplement 2001). Strasbourg, France: Council of Europe. 2001. p. 883–4.

Farbman KS, Barnett ED, Bolduc GR, Klein JO. Antibacterial activity of garlic and onions: a historical perspective. *Pediatric Infect Disease J* 1993;12(7):613–4.

Farrell AM, Staughton RCD. Garlic burns mimicking *Herpes zoster*. *Lancet* 1996 April 27;347:1195.

Fennerty MB, Lieberman DA, Vaikil N, Margaret N, Faigel DO, Helfand M. Effectiveness of *Helicobacter pylori* therapy in a clinical practice setting. *Arch Intern Med* 1999;159(14):1562–6.

Fenwick GR, Hanley AB. The genus *Allium*—Part 2. *CRC Crit Rev Food Sci Nutr* 1985;22(4):273–377.

Fleischauer AT, Poole C, Arab L. Garlic consumption and cancer prevention: meta-analysis of colorectal and stomach cancers. *Am J Clin Nutr* 2000;72(4):1047–52.

Freeman F, Kodera Y. Garlic Chemistry: Stability of S-(2-Propenyl) 2-Propene-1-sulfinothioate (Allicin) in blood, solvents, and simulated physiological fluids. *J Agric Food Chem* 1995;43:2332–8.

Fukushima S, Takada N, Hori T, Wanibuchi H. Cancer prevention by organosulfur compounds from garlic and onion. *J Cell Biochem Suppl* 1997;27:100–5.

Gadkari JD, Joshi VD. Effect of ingestion of raw garlic on serum cholesterol level, clotting time, and fibrinolytic activity in normal subjects. *J Postgrad Med* 1991;37(3):128–31.

Gail MH, You WC, Chang YS, Zhang L, Blot WJ, Brown LM, et al. Factorial trial of three interventions to reduce the progression of precancerous gastric lesions in Shandong, China: design issues and initial data. *Control Clin Trials* 1998;19(4):352–69.

Gebhardt R. Multiple inhibitory effects of garlic extracts on cholesterol biosynthesis in hepatocytes. *Lipids* 1993;28(7):613–9.

Gebhardt R, Beck H, Wagner K. Inhibition of cholesterol biosynthesis by allicin and ajoene in rat hepatocytes and HepG2 cells. *Biochim Biophys Acta* 1994;1213(1):57–62.

Gebhardt R. Amplification of palmitate-induced inhibition of cholesterol biosynthesis in cultured rat hepatocytes by garlic-derived organosulfur compounds. *Phytomedicine* 1995;2(1):29–34.

General Sale List (GSL). Statutory Instrument 1989 No. 969 — The Medicines (Products Other Than Veterinary Drugs) Amendment Order 1989. London, U.K.: Her Majesty's Stationery Office (HMSO). 1989.

Geng Z, Lau BHS. Aged garlic extract modulates glutathione redox cycle and superoxide dismutase activity in vascular endothelial cells. *Phytother Res* 1997;2:54–6.

Geng Z, Rong Y, Lau BHS. S-allyl cysteine inhibits activation of nuclear factor kappa B in human T cells. *Free Radical Biol Med* 1997;23(2):345–50.

German Homoeopathic Pharmacopoeia (GHP), 1st ed. 1978 with supplements through 1991. Translation of the German "*Homöopathisches Arzneibuch* (HAB 1), Amtliche Ausgabe." Stuttgart, Germany: Deutscher Apotheker Verlag; 1993. p. 39–40.

Ghana Herbal Pharmacopoeia (GHP). Accra, Ghana: Policy Research and Strategic Planning Institute (PORSPI); 1992. p. 59–61.

GHP. See: *German Homoeopathic Pharmacopoeia* or *Ghana Herbal Pharmacopoeia*.

Goetz P. Phytotherapie in Frankreich. *Zeitschrift für Phytotherapie* 1999;20:320–8.

Graham DY, Anderson S-Y, Lang T. Garlic or jalapeño peppers for treatment of *Helicobacter pylori* infection. *Am J Gastroent* 1999;94(5):1200–2.

Grünwald J, Heede J, Koch H, Albrecht R, Knudsen O, Ramussen N, et al. Effects of garlic powder tablets on blood lipids and blood pressure—the Danish Multicenter Kwai® Study. *Eur J Clin Res* 1992;3:179–86.

GSL. See: *General Sale List*.

Gupta N, Porter TD. Garlic and garlic-derived compounds inhibit human squalene monooxygenase. *J Nutr* 2001.131(6):1662–7.

Gwilt PR, Lear CL, Tempero MA, Birt DD, Grandjean AC, Ruddon RW, et al. The effect of garlic extract on human metabolism of acetaminophen. *Cancer Epidemiol Biomarkers Prev* 1994;3(2):155–60.

Han N, Liu B, Wang M. Effect of allicin on antioxidases in mice. *Acta Nutr Sinica*

1992;14:107–8.

Harenberg J, Giese C, Zimmermann R. Effect of dried garlic on blood coagualtion, fibrinolysis, platelet aggregation, and serum cholesterol levels in patients with hyperlipoproteinemia. *Atherosclerosis* 1988;74(3):247–9.

Harris WS, Windsor SL, Lickteig J. Garlic and lipoprotein resistance to oxidation. *Z Phytother Abstr* 1995;16:15.

Hatono S, Jimenez A, Wargovich, MJ. Chemopreventative effect of S-allylcysteine and its relationship to the detoxification enzyme glutathione S-transferase. *Carcinogenesis* 1996;17(5)1041–4.

Health Canada. Garlic. In: *Drug Product Database (DPD)*. Ottawa, Ontario: Health Canada Therapeutic Products Programme; 2001.

Health Protection Branch. *HPB Status Manual*. Ottawa, Ontario: Health Protection Branch; 1993 February 19. p. 82.

Hirao Y, Sumioka I, Nakagami S, Yamamoto M, Hatono S, Yoshida S, et al. Activation of immunoresponder cells by the protein fraction from aged garlic extract. *Phytother Res* 1987;1(4):161–4.

Holzgartner H, Schmidt U, Kuhn U. Comparison of the efficacy and tolerance of a garlic preparation vs. bezafibrate. *Arzneimittelforschung* 1992;42(12):1473–7.

Homoeopathic Pharmacopoeia of the United States (HPUS) — Revision Service Official Compendium from July 1, 1992. Falls Church (VA): American Institute of Homeopathy; 1989. p. 0081:ALLS.

HPB. See: Health Protection Branch.

HPUS. See: *Homoeopathic Pharmacopoeia of the United States*.

Hughes BG, Lawson LD. Antimicrobial effects of *Allium sativum* L. (garlic), *Allium ampeloprasu*m (elephant garlic), and *Allium cepa* L. (onion), garlic compounds and commercial garlic supplement products. *Phytother Res* 1991;5:154–8.

Ide N, Lau BHS. Garlic compounds inhibit low density lipoprotein (LDL) oxidation and protect endothelial cells from oxidized LDL-induced injury. *FASEB J* 1997a;11(3):A122.

Ide N, Lau BH. Garlic compounds minimize intracellular oxidative stress and inhibit nuclear factor-kappa b activation. *J Nutr* 2001;131 Suppl 3:1020S–6S.

Ide N, Lau BH. Garlic compounds protect vascular endothelial cells from oxidized low density lipoprotein-induced injury. *J Pharm Pharmacol* 1997b;49:908–11.

Ide N, Lau BH. S-allylcysteine attenuates oxidative stress in endothelial cells. *Drug Dev Industr Pharm* 1999;25(5):619–24.

Imai J, Ide N, Nagae S, Moriguchi T, Matsuura H, Itakura Y. Antioxidant and radical scavenging effects of aged garlic extract and its constituents. *Planta Medica* 1994;60(5):417–20.

Isaacsohn JL, Moser M, Stein EA, Dudley K, Davey JA, Liskov E, et al. Garlic powder and plasma lipids and lipoproteins: a multicenter, randomized, placebo-controlled trial. *Arch Intern Med* 1998;158(11):1189–94.

Jain AK, Vargas R, Gotzkowsky S, McMahon FG. Can garlic reduce levels of serum lipids? A controlled clinical study. *Am J Med* 1993;94(6):632–5.

Jepson RG, Kleijnen J, Leng GC. Garlic for peripheral arterial occlusive disease [review]. *Cochrane Database Syst Rev* 2000;2:CD000095.

Kamanna VS, Chandrasekhara N. Effect of garlic (*Allium sativum* linn) on serum lipoproteins and lipoprotein cholesterol levels in albino rats rendered hypercholesterolemic by feeding cholesterol. *Lipids* 1982;17(7):483–8.

Kandil O, Abdullah T, Tabuni AM, Elkadi A. Potential role of *Allium sativum* in natural cytotoxicity. *Arch AIDS Res* 1988;1:230–1.

Kiesewetter H, Jung F, Mrowietz C, Pindur G, Heiden M, Wenzel E, et al. Effects of garlic on blood fluidity and fibrinolytic activity: a randomised, placebo-controlled, double-blind study. *Br J Clin Pract Suppl* 1990;69 Suppl:24–9.

Kiesewetter H, Jung F, Pindur G, Jung EM, Mrowietz C, Wenzel E. Effect of garlic on thrombocyte aggregation, microcirculation, and other risk factors. *Int. J Clin Pharmacol Ther Toxicol* 1991;29(4):151–5.

Kiesewetter H, Jung F, Jung EM, Mrowietz C, Koscielny J, Wenzel E. Effect of garlic on platelet aggregation in patients with increased risk of juvenile ischaemic attack. *Eur J Clin Pharmacol* 1993a;45(4):333–6.

Kiesewetter H, Jung F, Jung EM, Blume J, Mrowietz C, Birk A, et al. Effects of garlic coated tablets in peripheral arterial occlusive disease. *Clin Investig* 1993b;71(5):383–6.

Kikuchi N, Nishimura Y, Tsukamoto C, Kawashima Y, Ochiai H, Hayashi Y, et al. Clinical effects of Leopin-5 (LE-5) and Garlic Extract (GE) on peripheral microcirculation. *Jpn J New Remedies Clin* 1994;43(1):146–58.

Koch H. "Hormonwirkungen" bei Allium-arten: historische berichte und moderne wissenschaftliche erkenntnisse. *Z Phytother* 1992a;13:177–188.

Koch HP, Jäger W, Hysek J, Körpert B. Garlic and onion extracts: in vitro inhibition of adenosine deaminase. *Phytother Res* 1992b;6:50–2.

Koch HP, Lawson LD, editors. *Garlic: The Science and Therapeutic Application of Allium sativum L. and Related Species*, 2nd ed. Baltimore (MD): Williams & Wilkins Publishing Co; 1996. p. 135-212.

Koscielny J, Klüssendorf D, Latza R, Schmitt R, Radtke H, Siegel G, Kiesewetter H. The antiatherosclerotic effect of *Allium sativum*. *Atherosclerosis* 1999;144(1):237–49.

Kröning F. Garlic as an inhibitor for spontaneous tumors in mice. *Acta Unio Int Cancrum* 1964;20:855–6.

Kyo E, Uda N, Kasuga S, Itakura Y, Sumiyoshi H. Garlic as an immunostimulant. In: Wagner H, editor. *Immunomodulatory Agents from Plants*. Basel, Switzerland: Birkhäuser Verlag; 1999. p. 273–88.

Kyo E, Uda N, Suzuki A, Kakimoto M, Ushijima M, Kasuga S, et al. Immunomodulation and antitumor activities of aged garlic extract. *Phytomed* 1998;5(4):259–67.

Kyo E, Uda N, Kakimato M, Yokoyama K, Ushijima M, Sumioka I, et al. Anti-allergic effects of aged garlic extract. *Phytomedicine* 1997;4(4):335–40.

Lamm DL, Riggs DR. The potential applications of *Allium sativum* (garlic) for the treatment of bladder cancer. *Urol Clin North Am* 2000;27(1):157–62.

Lash JP, Cardoso LR, Mesler PM, Walczak DA, Pollak R. The effect of garlic on hypercholesterolemia in renal transplant patients. *Transplant Proc* 1998;30(1):189–91.

Lau BHS. Suppression of LDL oxidation by garlic. *J Nutr* 2001;131 Suppl 3:985S–8S.

Lau BHS. Detoxifying, radioprotective and phagocyte-enhancing effects of garlic. *Internat Clin Nutr Rev* 1989;9(1):27–31.

Lau BHS, Lam F, Wang-Cheng R. Effect of an odor-modified garlic preparation on blood lipids. *Nutr Res* 1987;7:139–49.

Lau BHS, Woolley JL, Marsh CL, Barker GR, Koobs DH, Torrey RR. Superiority of intralesional immunotherapy with *Corynebacterium parvum* and *Allium sativum* in the control of murine transitional cell carcinoma. *J Uro* 1986;136(3):701–5.

Lau BHS, Yamasaki T, Grindley DS. Garlic compounds modulate macrophage and T-lymphocyte functions. *Mol Biother* 1991;3(2):103–7.

Lawson LD. Effect of garlic on serum lipids [letter]. *JAMA* 1998b;280(18):1568.

Lawson LD. Garlic: A Review of its Medicinal Effects and Indicated Active Compounds. In: Lawson L, Bauer R, editors. *Phytomedicines of Europe: Chemistry and Biological Activity.* Washington, DC: American Chemical Society; 1998a. p. 176–209.

Lawson LD. Garlic for total cholesterol reduction [letter]. *Ann Intern Med* 2001;135(1):65–6.

Lawson L. Garlic powder for hyperlipidemia—analysis of recent negative results. *Quart Rev Nat Med* 1998c;187–9.

Lawson LD, Ransom DK, Hughes BG. Inhibition of whole blood platelet-aggregation by compounds in garlic clove extracts and commercial garlic products. *Thromb Res* 1992;65(2):141–56.

Lawson LD, Wang ZJ. Low allicin release from garlic supplements: a major problem due to the sensitivities of alliinase activity. *J Agric Food Chem* 2001;49(5):2592–9.

Lawson LD, Wang ZJ, Papadimitriou D. Allicin release under simulated gastrointestinal conditions from garlic powder tablets employed in clinical trials on serum cholesterol. *Planta Med* 2001;67(1):13–8.

Lea MA. Organosulfur compounds and cancer [review]. *Adv Exp Med Biol* 1996;401:147–54.

Lee TY, Lam TH. Contact dermatitis due to topical treatment with garlic in Hong Kong. *Contact Dermatitis* 1991;24(3):193–6.

Legnani C, Frascaro M, Guazzaloca G, Ludovici S, Cesarano G, Coccheri S. Effects of a dried garlic preparation on fibrinolysis and platelet aggregation in healthy subjects. *Arzneimittelforschung* 1993;43(2):119–22.

Lembo G, Balato N, Patruno C, Auriccho L, Ayala F. Allergic contact dermatitis due to garlic (*Allium sativum*). *Contact Dermatitis* 1991;25(5):330–1.

Liu J, Lin RI, Milner JA. Inhibition of 7,12-dimethylbenz[a]anthracene-induced mammary tumors and DNA adducts by garlic powder. *Carcinogenesis* 1992;13(10):1847–51.

Liu L, Yeh YY. Water-soluble organosulfur compounds of garlic inhibit fatty acid and triglyceride synthesis in cultured rat hepatocytes. *Lipids* 2001;36(4):395–400.

Mader FH. Treatment of hyperlipidemia with garlic-powder tablets. Evidence from the German Association of General Practitioners' multicenter placebo-controlled double-blind study. *Arzneimittelforschung* 1990;40(10):1111–6.

Makheja AN, Vanderhoek JY, Bryant RW, Bailey JM. Altered arichidonic acid metabolism in platelets inhibited by onion or garlic extracts. *Adv Prostaglandin Thromboxane Res* 1980;6:309–12.

Makheja AN, Low CE, Bailey JM. Biological nature of platelet inhibitors from *Allium cepa*, *Allium sativum*, and *Auricularia polytricha*. *Thromb Haemostasis* 1981;46:148.

Matsuura H. Saponins in garlic as modifiers of the risk of cardiovascular disease. *J Nutr* 2001;131 Suppl:1000S–5S.

McCrindle BW, Helden E, Conner WT. Garlic extract therapy in children with hypercholesterolemia. *Arch Pediatr Adolesc Med* 1998;152(11):1089–94.

McGuffin M, Hobbs C, Upton R, Goldberg A, editors. *American Herbal Product Association's Botanical Safety Handbook*. Boca Raton (FL): CRC Press; 1997. p. 6.

Medical Products Agency (MPA). *Naturläkemedel: Authorised Natural Remedies* (as of January 24, 2001). Uppsala, Sweden: Medical Products Agency; 2001a.

Medical Products Agency (MPA). Läkemedelsnära Produkter; Homeopatika: Företag med registrerade homeopatika. Uppsala, Sweden: Medical Products Agency;

2001b.

Mei X, Wang M, Xu H, Pan X, Gao C, et al. Garlic and gastric cancer: the influence of garlic on the level of nitrate and nitrite in gastric juice. *Acta Nutri Sin* 1982;4:53–6.

Mei X, Wang M, Li T, Gao C, Han N, et al. Garlic and gastric cancer. II. The inhibitory effect of garlic on nitrate-reducing bacteria and their production of nitrite in gastric juice. *Acta Nutr Sin* 1985;7:173–7.

Mennella JA, Beauchamp GK. Maternal diet alters the sensory qualities of human milk and the nursling's behavior. *Pediatrics* 1991;88(4):737–44.

Milner JA. Garlic: its anticarcinogenic and antitumorigenic properties. *Nutr Rev* 1996 Nov;54(11 Pt 2):S82–6.

Miyoshi A, Hasegawa Y, Yamamoto T, Omata S, Harada H, Nakazawa S, et al. Effect of KYOLEPIN on various unexplained complaints which often accompany internal disease. *Treatment and New Medicine* 1984;21:1806–20.

Mohammed SF, Woodward SC. Characterization of a potent inhibitor of platelet aggregation and release reaction isolated from *Allium sativum* (garlic). *Thromb Res* 1986;44(6):793–806.

Morant J, Ruppanner H, editors. *Arzneimittel-Kompendium der Schweiz®* 2001. Basel, Switzerland: Documed AG; 2001. pp. 89, 169, 217, 1341, 1348.

Morioka N, Sze LL, Morton DL, Irie RF. A protein fraction from aged garlic extract enhances cytotoxicity and proliferation of human lymphocytes mediated by interleukin-2 and concanavalin A. *Cancer Immunol Immunother* 1993;37(5):316–22.

MPA. See: Medical Products Agency.

Mulrow C, Lawrence V, Ackermann R, Ramirez G, Morbidoni L, Aguilar C, et al. *Evidence Report/Technology Assessment Number 20—Garlic: Effects on Cardiovascular Risks and Disease, Protective Effects Against Cancer, and Clinical Adverse Effects.* Rockville (MD): Agency for Healthcare Research and Quality (AHQR); 2000 Oct; Pub No. 01-E023.

Munday JS, James KA, Fray LM, Kirkwood SW, Thompson KG. Daily supplementation with aged garlic extract, but not raw garlic, protects low density lipoprotein against *in vitro* oxidation. *Atherosclerosis* 1999;143:399–404.

Nakagawa S, Masamoto K, Sumiyoshi H, Harada H. Acute toxicity test of garlic extract [in Japanese]. *J Toxicol Sci* 1984;9(1):57–60.

Nakagawa S, Masamoto K, Sumiyoshi H, Kunihoro K, Fuwa T. Effect of raw and extracted-aged garlic juice on growth of young rats and their organs after peroral administration (author's translation) [in Japanese]. *J Toxicol Sci* 1980;5(1):91–112.

Neil HAW, Silagy CA, Lancaster T, Hodgeman J, Vos K, Moore JW, et al. Garlic powder in the treatment of moderate hyperlipidaemia: a controlled trial and meta-analysis. *J R Coll Physicians Lond* 1996;30(4):329–34.

Ohnishi ST, Ohnishi T. In vitro effects of aged garlic extract and other nutritional supplements on sickle erythrocytes. *J Nutr* 2001;131 Suppl 3:1085S–925.

Ohnishi ST, Ohnishi T, Ogunmola GB. Green tea extract and aged garlic extract inhibit anion transport and sickle cell dehydration in vitro. *Blood Cells, Molecules, and Diseases* 2001;27(1):148–57.

Ohnishi ST, Ohnishi T, Ogunmola GB. Sickle cell anemia: a potential nutritional approach for a molecular disease. *Nutrition* 2000;16:330–8.

Ohnishi T, Tsuyoshi N, inventors. Wakunaga of America Co., Ltd., assignee. Therapeutic uses of specially processed garlic for sickle cell disease. U.S. Patent 6,254,871. 2001 Jul 3. Available at: http://patft.uspto.gov/netahtml/searchbool.html.

Okada K, Miyagaki H. Effect of Kyoleopin (KLE) on fatigue and non-specific complaints: clinical study. *The Clinical Report* 1983;17:2173–83.

Okuhara T. A clinical study of garlic extract on peripheral circulation [in Japanese]. *Jap Pharmacol Therapeu* 1994;22(8):3695–701.

Phelps S, Harris WS. Garlic supplementation and lipoprotein oxidation susceptibility. *Lipids* 1993;28(5):475–7.

Ph.Eur. See: *Europäisches Arzneibuch* or *European Pharmacopoeia*.

Pinto J, Qiao C, Xing J, Suffaletto B, Rivlin RS, Heston W. Garlic constituents modify expression of biomarkers for human prostatic carcinoma cells. *FASEB Journal* 1997a;11(3): A439.

Pinto JT, Qiao C, Xing J, Rivlin RS, Protomastro ML, Weissler ML, et al. Effects of garlic thioallyl derivatives on growth, glutathione concentration, and polyamine formation of human prostate carcinoma cells in culture. *Am J Clin Nutr* 1997b;66(2):398–405.

Piscitelli SC, Burstein AH, Welden N et al. The effect of garlic supplements on the pharmacokinetics of saquinavir. *Clin Infect Dis* 2002;34(2):234–8.

Rahman K, Billington D. Dietary supplementation with aged garlic extract inhibits ADP-induced platelet aggregation in humans. *J Nutr* 2000;130(11):2662–5.

Reeve VE, Bosnic M, Rozinova E, Boehm-Wilcox C. A garlic extract protects from ultraviolet B (280–320 nm) radiation-induced suppression of contact hypersensitivity. *Photochem Photobiol* 1993a;58(6):813–7.

Reeve VE, Bosnic M, Rozinova E, Boehm-Wilcox C. Protection from UVB (280–320NM) radiation induced suppresion of contact hypersensitivity by a garlic extract. *Photochem Photobiol* 1993b;57 Suppl:29–30.

Reuter H, Koch H, Lawson L. In: *Garlic: The Science and Therapeutic Application of*

Allium sativum L. and Related Species. Baltimore (MD): Williams and Wilkins: 1996. p. 135–212.

Riggs DR, DeHaven JI, Lamm DL. *Allium sativum* (garlic) treatment for murine transitional cell carcinoma. *Cancer* 1997;79(10):1987–94.

Roberge RJ, Leckey R, Spence R, Krenzelok EJ. Garlic burns of the breast. *Am J Emerg Med* 1997;15(5):548.

Rose KD, Croissant PD, Parliament CF, Levin MB. Spontaneous spinal epidural hematoma with associated platelet dysfunction from excessive garlic ingestion: a case report. *Neurosurgery* 1990;26(5):880–2.

Rotblatt M, Ziment I. *Evidence-Based Herbal Medicine*. Philadelphia (PA): Hanley & Belfus; 2001. p. 193–200.

Rotzsch W, Richter V, Rassoul F, Walper A. Postprandial lipemia under treatment with *Allium sativum*. Controlled double-blind study of subjects with reduced HDL2-cholesterol [in German]. *Arzneimittelforschung* 1992;42(10):1223–7.

Rozenfeld V, Sisca TS, Callahan AK, Crain JL. Double-blind, randomized, placebo-controlled trial of aged garlic extract in patients stabilized on warfarin therapy [poster]. Las Vegas, NV: American Society of Health-System Pharmacists Midyear Clinical Meeting; 2000 December 3–7.

Ruffin J, Hunter SA. An evaluation of the side effects of garlic as an antihypertensive agent. *Cytobios* 1983;37:85–9.

Ruppanner H, Schaefer U, editors. *Codex 2000/01 — Die Schweizer Arzneimittel in einem Griff*. Basel, Switzerland: Documed AG; 2000.

Ryu K, Ide N, Matsuura H, Itakura Y. N alpha-(1-Deoxy-D-fructos-1-yl)-L-Arginine, and antioxidant compound indentified in aged-garlic extract. *J Nutr* 2001;131 Suppl 3:972S–6S.

Sendl A, Elbl G, Steinke B, Redl K, Breu W, Wagner H. Comparative pharmacological investigations of *Allium ursinum* and *Allium sativum*. *Planta Med* 1992;58:1–7.

Schulz V, Hänsel R, Tyler V. *Rational Phytotherapy*. 4th ed. Berlin: Springer-Verlag; 2001. p. 147.

Sial AY, Ahmad SI. Study of the hypotensive action of garlic extract in experimental animals. *J Pak Med Assoc* 1982;32(10):237–9.

Siegers CA. *Allium sativum*. In: De Smet PA et al., editors. *Adverse Effects of Herbal Drugs, Vol. 1*. Berlin, Germany: Springer-Verlag; 1992. p. 73–6.

Silagy C, Neil A. Garlic as a lipid lowering agent—a meta-analysis. *J R Coll Physicians Lond* 1994a;28(1):39–45.

Silagy CA, Neil HA. A meta-analysis of the effect of garlic on blood pressure. *J Hypertens* 1994b;12(4):463–8

Simons LA, Balasubramaniam S, von Konigsmark M, Parfitt A, Simons J, Peters W. On the effect of garlic on plasma lipids and lipoprotein in mild hypercholesterolaemia. *Atherosclerosis* 1995;113(2):219–25.

Sivam GP. Protection against *Helicobacter pylori* and other bacterial infections by garlic. *J Nutr* 2001;131 Suppl 3:1106S–8S.

Sivam GP, Lampe JW, Ulness B, Swanzy SR, Potter JD. *Helicobacter pylori* in vitro susceptibility to garlic (*Allium sativum*) extract. *Nutr Cancer* 1997;27(2):118–21.

Srivastava KC. Evidence for the mechanism by which garlic inhibits platelet aggregation. *Prostaglandins Leukotrienes Med* 1986;22(3):313–21.

Steiner M, Khan AH, Holbert D, Lin RI-S. A double-blind crossover study in moderately hypercholesterolemic men that compared the effect of aged garlic extract and placebo administration on blood lipids. *Am J Clin Nutr* 1996;64(6):866–70.

Steiner M, Li W. Aged garlic extract, a modulator of cardiovascular risk factors: a dose-finding study on the effects of AGE on platelet functions. *J Nutr* 2001;131 Suppl 3:980S–4S.

Steiner M, Lin RI. Cardiovascular and lipid changes in response to aged garlic extract ingestion [abstract]. *J Am Col Nutr* 1994;13(5):524.

Steiner M, Lin RS. Changes in platelet function and susceptibility of lipoproteins to oxidation associated with administration of aged garlic extract. *J Cardiovascular Pharmacol* 1998;31(6):904–8.

Steinmetz KA, Kushi LH, Bostick RM, Folsom AR, Potter JD. Vegetables, fruit, and colon cancer in the Iowa Women's Health Study. *Am J Epidemiol* 1994;139(1):1–15.

Stevinson C, Pittler MH, Ernst E. Garlic for treating hypercholesterolemia. *Ann Intern Med* 2000;133:420–9.

Sumiyoshi H, Kanezawa A, Masamoto K, Haroda H, Nakagami S, Yokota A, et al. Chronic toxicity test of garlic extract in rats [in Japanese]. *J Toxicol Sci* 1984;9(1):61–75.

Sunter WH. Warfarin and garlic [letter]. *Pharm J* 1991;246:722.

Tamaki T, Sonoki S. Volatile sulfur compounds in human expiration after eating raw or heat-treated garlic. *J Nutr Sci Vitaminol* 1999;45:213–22.

Tunón H. Phtyotherapie in Schweden. *Zeitschrift für Phytotherapie* 1999;20:268–77.

United States Congress (USC). Public Law 103–417: Dietary Supplement Health and Education Act of 1994. Washington, DC: 103rd Congress of the United States; 1994.

United States Pharmacopeia (USP 25th Revision) — *The National Formulary* (NF 20th Edition). Rockville, MD: United States Pharmacopeial Convention, Inc. 2002.

USC. See: *United States Congress*.

USP. See: *United States Pharmacopeia*.

Vorberg G, Schneider B. Therapy with garlic: results of a placebo-controlled, double-blind study. *Br J Clin Pract Suppl* 1990;44(69):7–11.

Wang BH, Zuzel KA, Rahman K, Billington D. Treatment with aged garlic extract protects against bromobenzene toxicity to precision cut rat liver slices. *Toxicology* 1999;132(2–3):215–25.

Warshafsky S, Kamer RS, Sivak SL. Effect of garlic on total serum cholesterol—a meta-analysis. *Ann Intern Med* 1993;119 (7 Pt 1):599–605.

Weisberger A, Pensky J. Tumor inhibition by a sulfhydryl-blocking agent related to an active principle of garlic (*Allium satiuum*). *Cancer Res* 1958;18:1301–8.

WHO. See: World Health Organization.

Witte JS, Longnecker MP, Bird CL, Lee ER, Frankl HD, Haile RW. Relation of vegetable, fruit, and grain consumption to colorectal adenomatous polyps. *Am J Epidemiol* 1996;144(11):1015–25.

World Health Organization (WHO). "*Bulbus Allii Sativi*." *WHO Monographs on Selected Medicinal Plants*, Vol. 1. Geneva: World Health Organization; 1999. p. 16–27.

Yamasaki T, Li L, Lau BHS. Garlic compounds protect vascular endothelial cells from hydrogen peroxide-induced oxidant injury. *Phytother Res* 1994;8:408–12.

Yeh, YY, Lin RIS, Yeh SM, Evans S. Cholesterol lowering effects of aged garlic extract supplementation on free-living hypercholesterolemic men consuming habitual diets. *J Am Col Nutr* 1995;13:545.

Yeh YY, Liu L. Cholesterol-lowering effect of garlic extracts and organosulfur compounds: human and animal studies [review]. *J Nutr* 2001;131 Suppl 3:989S–93S.

Yeh YY, Yeh SM. Garlic reduces plasma lipids by inhibiting hepatic cholesterol and triacylglycerol synthesis. *Lipids* 1994;29(3):189–93.

Yeh YY, Yeh SM, Lim HS, Picciano MF. Garlic extract reduces plasma concentration of homocysteine in rats rendered folic acid deficiency. *FASEB J* 1999;13(4):A232;209.12.

You WC, Chang YS, Yang ZT, Zhang L, Xu GW, Blot WJ, et al. Etiological research on gastric cancer and its precursor lesions in Shandong, China. *IARC Sci Publ* 1991;105:33–8.

You WC, Blot WJ, Chang YS, Ershow A, Yang ZT, An Q, et al. Allium vegetables and reduced risk of stomach cancer. *J Natl Cancer Inst* 1989;81(2):162–4.

You WC, Blot WJ, Chang YS, Ershow AG, Yang ZT, An Q, et al. Diet and high risk of stomach cancer in Shandong, China. *Cancer Res* 1988;48(12):3518–23.

Clinical Studies on Garlic (*Allium sativum* L.)

Cardiovascular
Hyperlipidemia/Hypercholesterolemia/Hypertension/Related Risk Factors

Author/Year	Subject	Design	Duration	Dosage	Preparation	Results/Conclusion
Berthold et al., 1998	Hypercholesterolemia (mean TC 291 mg/dl and mean LDL 207 mg/dl)	R, DB, PG n=25 (diet not controlled)	12 weeks following a 4-week washout period	5 mg, 2x/day or placebo (with meals)	Tegra® garlic oil (oil bound to b-cyclodextrin for slow release)	The garlic preparation did not influence serum lipoproteins, cholesterol, absorption, or cholesterol synthesis. Garlic oil could not be recommended for hypercholesterolemia. The study was criticized for slow-release aspect that has been found to greatly reduce total absorption and because the oil preparation contained a different chemical profile than preparations used in other studies.
Isaacsohn, 1998	Hyperlipidemia (LDL<160 mg/dL; TG <350 mg/dL)	R, PC, PG, MC n=50 (n=28 taking garlic; n=22 taking placebo) subjects on the NCEP Step I diet 8 weeks before and during treatment	12 weeks	300 mg, 3x/day	Sapec®, Kwai® garlic powder	No significant lipid or lipoprotein changes between the two groups. Compliance to diet was same for both groups; however, effect of diet on lipid/lipoprotein levels prior to treatment may have influenced treatment. Another factor possibly influencing the results is the alleged change made to the tablets' enteric coating in 1992–1993 (Lawson, 1998).
Lash et al., 1998	Hyperlipidemia in renal transplant patients (TC>185 mg/dl; LDL> 160 mg/dl)	R, PC n=35 (garlic n=19; placebo n=16) (NCEP Step I diet during treatment)	12 weeks	680 mg, 2x/day	Pure-Gar®	At 6 weeks, there was a significant decrease from baseline of 14 mg/dL in TC (p<0.05) and 12 mg/dL in LDL (p<0.05). Authors noted that although garlic showed benefit, patients still required drug therapy to treat hyperlipidemia. They suggested that garlic may be used to decrease the required dosage of HMG-CoA reductase inhibitors.
McCrindle et al., 1998	Hypercholesterolemia in children (TC >185 mg/dL)	R, DB, PC n=30 (garlic n=15; placebo n=15) NCEP Step 2 diet for 6 months prior to treatment	8 weeks	300 mg, 3x/day	Kwai® garlic powder	There was no significant reduction attributed to garlic for cardiovascular risk factors, with the exception of a small increase in apolipoprotein A-I levels. Authors note that adult studies have yielded positive results.
Steiner et al., 1996	Hypercholesterolemia (men) (TC=220–280 mg/dL)	DB, PC, C n=41	6 months, crossed over for 4 months (placed on NCEP Step I diet 4 weeks prior to start/ throughout)	3 capsules (800 mg each) 3x/day	Kyolic® AGE capsules vs. placebo capsules	Total cholesterol (TC) levels were reduced 6.1–7% compared to placebo period or baseline (p=0.0001), respectively. No difference noted for total glycerides (TG) or HDL (p=0.004). LDL decreased 4% and systolic blood pressure (SBP) decreased 5.5% (p=0.0001) with the garlic and modes decreased in diastolic blood pressure (DBP). Authors concluded AGE garlic supplementation has beneficial effects on lipid profile and BP in moderately hypercholesterolemic patients.
Yeh et al., 1995	Hypercholesterolemia (TC=220–285 mg/dL)	DB, PC, R n=34 (garlic n=17; placebo n=17) men (35–55 years old)	5 months	3 capsules, (800 mg each) 3x/day	Kyolic® AGE capsules vs. placebo capsules containing common food ingredient	At 4th and 5th month, TC levels in AGE group 6% and 7% lower, respectively, than baseline value and no change in placebo group. Plasma HDL-cholesterol and triglyceride levels not altered by AGE or placebo. Compared with placebo, LDL-cholesterol level significantly lower in AGE group (145 ± 25 vs. 165 ± 24 mg/dl). AGE supplementation has significant mild cholesterol lowering effect in hypercholesterolemic men.
De A Santos and Johns, 1995	Garlic powder vs. garlic oil on blood lipids, blood pressure, and well-being	R, O, PG, Cm n=70 (garlic powder n=36; or garlic oil n=34)	16 weeks	200 mg, 3x/day	Garlic powder: Kwai® (tablet), Garlic oil: Höfel's® Original Garlic Oil Capsules	Lipid-lowering effect for garlic powder=11% vs. 3% for oil. LDL lowered by 16% vs. 1% respectively. HDL did not change significantly and TG did not change. Also noted was a decrease in blood pressure with garlic powder but not for oil. Well-being assessment improved for powder but not for oil. Garlic powder appears to be superior to oil in reducing cholesterol, BP, and improved well-being.

KEY: **C** – controlled, **CC** – case-control, **CH** – cohort, **CI** – confidence interval, **Cm** – comparison, **CO** – crossover, **CS** – cross-sectional, **DB** – double-blind, **E** – epidemiological, **LC** – longitudinal cohort, **MA** – meta-analysis, **MC** – multi-center, **n** – number of patients, **O** – open, **OB** – observational, **OL** – open label, **OR** – odds ratio, **P** – prospective, **PB** – patient-blind, **PC** – placebo-controlled, **PG** – parallel group, **PS** – pilot study, **R** – randomized, **RC** – reference-controlled, **RCS** – retrospective cross-sectional, **RS** - retrospective, **S** – surveillance, **SB** – single-blind, **SC** – single-center, **U** – uncontrolled, **UP** – unpublished, **VC** – vehicle-controlled.

Garlic

Monograph

Cardiovascular (cont.)
Hyperlipidemia/Hypercholesterolemia/Hypertension/Related Risk Factors (cont.)

Author/Year	Subject	Design	Duration	Dosage	Preparation	Results/Conclusion
Simons et al., 1995	Hypercholesterolemia (mild to moderate) (5.5–8.05 mmol/L)	R, DB, PC, CO n=28	12 weeks after 28 day baseline dietary period; 28 day washout at end	300 mg, 3x/day	Kwai® garlic powder	No demonstrable effect of garlic on oxidizabilty of LDL, on ratio of plasma lathosterol/cholesterol (a measure of cholesterol synthesis), nor on LDL receptor expression in lymphocytes. No effect on ingestion of lipids and lipoproteins.
Steiner and Lin, 1994	Hypercholesterolemia (TC=230–290 mg/dL)	DB, CO, R n=45 men (30–70 years old)	10 months	700 mg, 3 capsules, 3x/day	Kyolic® AGE capsules vs. placebo capsules	66% of subjects in garlic group showed modest reduction (about 8%) of total and LDL cholesterol but no change in HDL. Significant reductions in measured platelet adhesion (34–58%) and aggregation (10–25%). Study suggests that AGE supplementation has beneficial effects on lipids, especially platelets, that may lead to cardiovascular risk reduction.
Jain et al., 1993	Serum lipids, lipoproteins, glucose, and blood pressure	R, DB, PC n=42	12 weeks	300 mg, 3xday, or placebo	Garlic powder in tablet form	Experimental group experienced a 6% reduction in TC (p<0.01) vs. placebo group (1%) reduction. LDL decreased 11% and 3% respectively (p<0.05). No changes in HDL, TG, serum glucose, or blood pressure noted (subjects were normotensive).
Grünwald et al., 1992	Hypercholesterolemia (TC>6.5 mmol/L)	DB, MC n=48	18 weeks	200 mg, 3x/day Subjects maintained a normal diet and medications	Kwai® garlic powder	After garlic treatment and compared to baseline, mean serum TC decreased by 8% (p<0.001); LDL decreased by a non-significant 5%; HDL increased by 5%; LDL:HDL improved by 12% (p<0.05); TG levels decreased by a non-significant 11%. 23 patients with mild hypertension experienced a significant decrease of 7% in SBP (p<0.05) and a non-significant 4% in DBP.
Holzgartner et al., 1992	Hyperlipoproteinemia (TC or TG >250 mg/ml) garlic vs. Bezafibrate	R, DB, MC, Cm n=98 (6-week pre-phase treatment w/placebo and NCEP Step 1 diet)	12 weeks (NCEP Step 1 diet maintained throughout study)	900 mg/day or 600 mg Bezalfibrate/day.	Garlic powder preparations equivalent to Sapec®, Kwai® garlic powder	Compared to baseline, both medications caused a significant decrease in TC (26%) (p<0.001), LDL (32%) (p<0.001), and TG (30%) (p<0.01), as well as a significant increase in HDL (51%) (p<0.001) with no difference between their efficacies. No differences were observed between the two regimens.
Rotzsch et al., 1992	Alimentary hypertriglyceridemia (after intake of fatty meals)	R, DB, PC n=24	6 weeks	300 mg/day or placebo and fatty meal	Sapec®, Kwai® garlic powder; fatty meal contained 100g butter	The postprandial increase of TG was reduced significantly in garlic group, and was up to 35% less compared to placebo. HDL-2 cholesterol tended to increase with garlic more than placebo.
Auer et al., 1990	Mild hypertension (DBP 95–104 mmHg; TC >250; TG>200)	R, DB, PC, C n=47 (garlic n=24; placebo n=23) (n=21 taking blood pressure medication)	12 weeks (after 7 week acclimation period)	200 mg/day or placebo	Kwai® garlic powder	Results indicated 13% decrease in DBP in garlic group vs. 4% for placebo (p<0.01). SBP decreased by 11% in garlic compared with 5% in the placebo group (p<0.05). Serum cholesterol and TG were significantly decreased after 8 and 12 weeks in garlic group vs. placebo (p<0.05).
Mader et al., 1990	Hyperlipidemia (TC >200mg/dL)	R, DB, PC, PG, MC n=221 (garlic n=111; placebo n=110)	16 weeks	200 mg/day or placebo	Kwai® garlic powder	Experimental group experienced a 12% reduction in TC vs. a 3% reduction in placebo group (p<0.001). TG decreased by 17% vs. 2% respectively (p<0.0001). The best effect was noted in patients with TC levels 251–300 mg/dL.
Vorberg et al., 1990	Hypercholesteriolemia	R, DB, PC, PG n=40 (garlic n=20; placebo n=20)	16 weeks	300 mg, 3x/day	Sapec®, Kwai® garlic powder	Garlic group resulted in a significantly lower TC (p<0.001), TG (p<0.05), BP (p<0.001), than placebo. A self-evaluation revealed a greater feeling of "well being" (p<0.05).

KEY: C – controlled, **CC** – case-control, **CH** – cohort, **CI** – confidence interval, **Cm** – comparison, **CO** – crossover, **CS** – cross-sectional, **DB** – double-blind, **E** – epidemiological, **LC** – longitudinal cohort, **MA** – meta-analysis, **MC** – multi-center, **n** – number of patients, **O** – open, **OB** – observational, **OL** – open label, **OR** – odds ratio, **P** – prospective, **PB** – patient-blind, **PC** – placebo-controlled, **PG** – parallel group, **PS** – pilot study, **R** – randomized, **RC** – reference-controlled, **RCS** – retrospective cross-sectional, **RS** - retrospective, **S** – surveillance, **SB** – single-blind, **SC** – single-center, **U** – uncontrolled, **UP** – unpublished, **VC** – vehicle-controlled.

Clinical Studies on Garlic (*Allium sativum* L.) (cont.)

Cardiovascular (cont.)
Hyperlipidemia/Hypercholesterolemia/Hypertension/Related Risk Factors (cont.)

Author/Year	Subject	Design	Duration	Dosage	Preparation	Results/Conclusion
Lau, et al., 1987	Hypercholes-terolemia and hypertriglyc-erides	DB, C, CC n=15	6 months	1 g/day	Kyolic® AGE capsules	Serum cholesterol level (220–440 mg/dl) significantly dropped (12–31%) with AGE compared to baseline. Serum LDL and triglycerides were also significantly reduced (p<0.05) with AGE.
Bordia, 1981	Blood lipids in subjects with coronary heart disease	O (n=20) healthy volunteers or (n=62) patients with coronary heart disease	10 months	0.25 mg/kg of body weight/day or placebo	Garlic essential oil in gelatin capsules	Patients taking garlic experienced a decrease in serum cholesterol (p<0.05) and LDL (p<0.05), while an increase was observed in the HDL fraction (p<0.05).

Arterial and Fibrinolytic Activity

Author/Year	Subject	Design	Duration	Dosage	Preparation	Results/Conclusion
Steiner and Li, 2001	Effects on platelet function	DB, CO, PC, R n=34 normal healthy men and women	44 weeks (6-week base-line period; 18-week sup-plementation, 18-week crossover; 2-week washout)	3 capsules (800 mg each) 3x/day 1st 6 weeks; 800 mg, 6x/day 2nd 6 weeks; 800 mg, 9x/day 3rd 6 weeks	Kyolic® AGE capsules vs. placebo capsules	Compared with baseline and placebo, threshold level of platelet aggregation was significantly increased, i.e., AGE significantly (p<0.05) inhibited platelet aggregation, espe-cially induced by collagen and epinephrine. Adherence of platelets inhibited by AGE in dose-dependent manner. AGE exerted selective inhibition on platelet aggregation and adhesion, suggesting potential use as cardiovascular disease prevention.
Koscielny et al., 1999	Arterial plaque (in patients with advanced athero-sclerotic plaque)	R, DB, PC n=152	4 years	300 mg, 3x/day	Kwai® garlic powder	In placebo the atherosclerotic plaque (in carotid and femoral artery) increased by 15.6% over 4 years while decreasing 2.6% in experimental group (p<0.0001). Garlic diminished the age-related decrease in plaque volume by 6–13% over 4 years (p<0.001). Assessed by high-resolution ultrasound. Results substantiate a pre-ventive and curative role for garlic powder for athero-sclerosis.
Breithaupt-Grogler, 1997	Age-related stiffening of the aorta (healthy adults)	E, CS, OB n=202 (matching pairs technique)	≥2 years	≥300 mg/day	Standardized garlic powder	Pressure-standardized elastic vascular resistance was lower in garlic groups than age-matched controls (p<0.0001). Pulse wave velocity (PWV) correlated with age (r=0.44 garlic, r=0.52 control) and systolic blood pressure (SBP) (r=0.48 garlic group, r=0.54 control group) for both groups, but in garlic group an increase in age or SBP was associated with a smaller rise in PWV vs. controls. No difference noted in blood pres-sure, heart rate, and plasma lipid levels in both groups. Chronic garlic powder consumption attenuated age-related increase in aortic stiffness.
Kiesewetter et al., 1993a	Platelet aggregation (juvenile ischemic attack)	DB, PC, PG n=60	4 weeks (following a 4-week washout period)	200 mg, 4x/day or placebo	Kwai® garlic powder	A significant decrease (p<0.01) in circulatory platelet aggregates (down 10.3%) and spontaneous platelet aggregates (down 56.3%) was observed in garlic group. Garlic group also decreased in DBP, plasma viscosity, and serum cholesterol.
Kiesewetter et al., 1991	Platelet aggregation	DB, PC n=120	4 weeks	400 mg, 2x/day or placebo	Garlic powder	Observations in garlic group include spontaneous platelet aggregation disappearance, increase of 47.6% microcirculation of the skin, 3.2% decrease in plasma viscosity, mean DBP decrease from 74 to 67 (p<0.05), and a drop in the mean fasting blood glucose concen-tration from 89.4 to 79.

KEY: **C** – controlled, **CC** – case-control, **CH** – cohort, **CI** – confidence interval, **Cm** – comparison, **CO** – crossover, **CS** – cross-sectional, **DB** – double-blind, **E** – epidemiological, **LC** – longitudinal cohort, **MA** – meta-analysis, **MC** – multi-center, **n** – number of patients, **O** – open, **OB** – observational, **OL** – open label, **OR** – odds ratio, **P** – prospective, **PB** – patient-blind, **PC** – placebo-controlled, **PG** – parallel group, **PS** – pilot study, **R** – randomized, **RC** – reference-controlled, **RCS** – retrospective cross-sectional, **RS** – retrospective, **S** – surveillance, **SB** – single-blind, **SC** – single-center, **U** – uncontrolled, **UP** – unpublished, **VC** – vehicle-controlled.

Garlic

Monograph

Anticancer/Chemoprevention

Author/Year	Subject	Design	Duration	Dosage	Preparation	Results/Conclusion
Dimitrov and Bennink, 1997	Effect on arachidonic acid metabolism	PS, O n=8 healthy female volunteers	3 months	10 mL extract/day mixed with orange or V8 juice in morning	Kyolic® aged garlic hydroalcoholic liquid extract	Compared to baseline, after 3 months of taking Kyolic® substantial decrease in serum PGE2 levels in majority of subjects. Results indicate that ethanol-water soluble extract is capable of modulating PGE2 and PGF2a.
Witte et al., 1996	Colon cancer	E, CC n=488	4 years	≥3 servings/week	Serving size unspecified	A reduction of 37% occurrence in pre-cancerous cells and colorectal polyps was observed. (Odds ratio = 0.63.)
Gwilt et al., 1994	Effect on metabolism of acetaminophen	O n=16 males (healthy, non-smoking)	3 months	10 ml extract/day mixed with 120 ml orange juice	Kyolic® aged garlic hydroalcoholic liquid extract plus acetaminophen (500 mg Tylenol®)	Garlic treatment had no discernible effect on oxidative metabolism, but was associated with slight increase in sulfate conjugation of acetaminophen. Study suggests that AGE has limited potential as a chemopreventive agent.
Steinmetz et al., 1994	Colon cancer	E, CH n=41,837	5 years	≥ 1 servings/week	Unspecified as to the quantity of a serving size	The study showed that risk of colon cancer in women ages 55–69 decreased with garlic consumption (rr=0.68).
You et al., 1989	Stomach cancer	E n=564 patients with stomach cancer, n=1,131 controls	15 years	0 kg/year; 0.1–1.5 kg/y; >1.5 kg/y	Raw and cooked garlic	Significant trends were shown for the decrease of stomach cancer with garlic use. Odds ratio (95% CI) for highest compared with lowest garlic consumption was 0.7 (0.4–1.0, p=0.03).

Other

Author/Year	Subject	Design	Duration	Dosage	Preparation	Results/Conclusion
Rozenfeld et al., 2000	Bleeding potential of combined garlic and warfarin therapy	DB, PC, R n=8 patients (INR therapeutic for at least 2 months)	4 weeks	1,200 mg/day or placebo	Kyolic® AGE capsules	All patients took Coumadin®. No INR differences between groups noted (p>0.05). Compared to baseline, no significant changes in INR values within each group (p>0.05). No patients developed urine or stool bleeding. Kyolic® did not worsen side effects of Coumadin®.
Okuhara, 1994	Peripheral circulation	Cm, CO, R n=12 healthy male volunteers	5 months (Jan~May 1994)	Single-administration test: 1.6 ml GE or GEC/day or continuous administration test: 0.8 ml GE or GEC 2 x/day	Kyolic® aged garlic hydroalcoholic liquid extract (GE) vs. heat-treated liquid preparation of garlic (GEC)	After single administration, skin temperatures in GE (garlic) group peaked at 60 minutes on backs of hands (p<0.01) and 90 minutes on backs of feet (p<0.01). In GEC (control) group, peaked at 30 minutes on backs of hands and feet. After 14 days continuous use, higher skin temperatures in GE group on backs of hands and feet and on only backs of feet in GEC group. Study suggests improved blood flow with GE.
Kiesewetter et al., 1993b	Intermittent claudication (Peripheral Arterial Occlusive Disease Stage II)	DB, PC n=80	12 weeks	200 mg, 4x/day or placebo	Kwai® garlic powder	A significant increase (p<0.05) was observed in walking distance by the 5th week and correlated to a simultaneous decrease in spontaneous platelet aggregation in garlic group vs. placebo. Garlic group also had decrease in diastolic blood pressure (DBP), plasma viscosity, and serum cholesterol.
Abdullah et al., 1989	Effects on natural killer (NK) cell activity in HIV+ patients	PS n=7	12 weeks	5 g/day 1st 6 weeks; 10 g/day 2nd 6 weeks	Aged processed garlic preparation: Special Garlic Preparation (SGP)	After 6 weeks, 6 of 7 qualified patients had normal NK activity, and all had normal NK activity at 12 weeks. Helper/suppressor ratio improved in 4 of 7 patients. Conditions of diarrhea, genital herpes, candidiasis and pansinusitis with recurrent fever also improved during the study.

KEY: **C** – controlled, **CC** – case-control, **CH** – cohort, **CI** – confidence interval, **Cm** – comparison, **CO** – crossover, **CS** – cross-sectional, **DB** – double-blind, **E** – epidemiological, **LC** – longitudinal cohort, **MA** – meta-analysis, **MC** – multi-center, **n** – number of patients, **O** – open, **OB** – observational, **OL** – open label, **OR** – odds ratio, **P** – prospective, **PB** – patient-blind, **PC** – placebo-controlled, **PG** – parallel group, **PS** – pilot study, **R** – randomized, **RC** – reference-controlled, **RCS** – retrospective cross-sectional, **RS** - retrospective, **S** – surveillance, **SB** – single-blind, **SC** – single-center, **U** – uncontrolled, **UP** – unpublished, **VC** – vehicle-controlled.

Ginger

Zingiber officinale Roscoe

[Fam. *Zingiberaceae*]

OVERVIEW

Ginger has been used for millennia as a common spice, food, and medicine, and has been mentioned in ancient Indian, Chinese, and Greco-Roman medical texts. Ginger dietary supplements have become increasingly popular in the past decade to help allay nausea associated with motion sickness. Ginger is used frequently as an alternative to antihistamines and anticholinergics, and as a prophylactic for motion sickness when side effects from pharmaceuticals warrant them unsuitable or intolerable for use. Ginger has also been investigated as an antiemetic for postoperative nausea and nausea induced by chemotherapy.

PRIMARY USES

- Motion sickness

OTHER POTENTIAL USES

- Hyperemesis gravidarum
- Chemotherapy-induced nausea
- Morning sickness
- Nausea, postoperative
- Osteoarthritis

PHARMACOLOGICAL ACTIONS

Antiemetic; antiplatelet aggregation; anti-inflammatory.

DOSAGE AND ADMINISTRATION

For motion sickness, take every 4 hours as needed.

FRESH OR DRIED RHIZOME: 2–4 g daily.

POWDERED DRY EXTRACT: 500 mg, 30 minutes before travel, and then 500 mg every 4 hours until end of travel.

INFUSION OR DECOCTION: 0.25–1.0 g in 150 ml boiled water, up to 3 times daily.

FLUID EXTRACT: 0.25–1.0 ml, 3 times daily [1:1 (*g/ml*)].

TINCTURE: 1.25–5.0 ml, 3 times daily [1:5 (*g/ml*)].

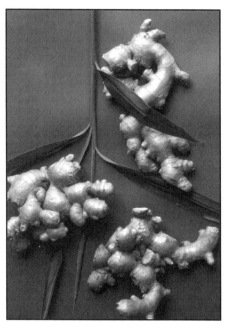

Photo © 2003 stevenfoster.com

CONTRAINDICATIONS

Patients with gallstones should consult a healthcare provider before using ginger.

PREGNANCY AND LACTATION: Fresh ginger is safe when used appropriately. It has traditionally been used to prevent morning sickness during the first trimester. Caution is advised against using excessive dosages of dried ginger during pregnancy.

ADVERSE EFFECTS

None known.

DRUG INTERACTIONS

None known. Reports of interaction with warfarin are anecdotal and not substantiated by documented case reports. Nevertheless, the narrow therapeutic index of warfarin warrants the cautious use of ginger in conjunction with it. Ginger does not appear to affect absorption of concurrent medications.

CLINICAL REVIEW

Of 21 studies that included a total of 2,669 participants, all but four of the trials showed positive effects for indications including motion sickness, postoperative nausea, cardiovascular conditions, and osteoarthritis. Nine of the studies are randomized, double-blind, and placebo-controlled (R, DB, PC); two of these studies concluded that ginger significantly reduces the incidence of motion sickness. One study found that two grams of ginger does not significantly change bleeding time, platelet count, or platelet aggregation. Two studies demonstrated that ginger is as effective as metoclopramide in reducing post-operative nausea. Two trials resulted in no significant reduction in post-operative nausea. Two demonstrated some effect from ginger in the treatment of osteoarthritis. Three R, DB, comparison trials were conducted on a total of 1,577 participants: all found that a standardized ginger preparation is equally or more effective than dimenhydrinate (Dramamine®), with better tolerability and fewer side effects, as a prophylaxis for motion sickness. One R, DB, cross-over trial found that ginger diminishes or eliminates symptoms of hyperemesis gravidarum, a severe form of morning sickness during pregnancy, while another R, DB, PC study suggested the safety and efficacy of ginger in reducing nausea during the first trimester of pregnancy. An early R, PC, single-blind, comparison study showed ginger to be superior to both placebo and dimenhydrinate (Dramamine®) in preventing motion sickness in patients with nausea induced in a tilted, rotating chair. A recent meta-analysis of six R, DB, PC studies concluded that ginger is a "promising antiemetic herbal remedy, but the clinical data to date are insufficient to draw firm conclusions."

Ginger

Zingiber officinale Roscoe
[Fam. *Zingiberaceae*]

OVERVIEW

Ginger has been used for millennia as a common spice, food, and medicine and is mentioned in the medical texts of Indian, Chinese, and Greco-Roman traditions. Ginger dietary supplements have become increasingly popular in the past decade and are used to help calm the nausea associated with motion sickness. China and India have cultivated ginger since ancient times and remain the world's leading producers.

USES

Motion sickness; morning sickness associated with pregnancy; hyperemesis gravidarum (excessive vomiting associated with pregnancy); chemotherapy-induced nausea; nausea after surgery; osteoarthritis.

DOSAGE

For motion sickness, take every 4 hours as needed.

FRESH OR DRIED GINGER: 2–4 g daily.

POWDERED DRY EXTRACT: 500 mg, 30 minutes before travel, and then 500 mg every 4 hours until end of travel.

INFUSION OR DECOCTION: 0.25–1.0 g in 150 ml boiled water, up to 3 times daily.

FLUID EXTRACT: 0.25–1.0 ml, 3 times daily [1:1 (*g/ml*)].

TINCTURE: 1.25–5.0 ml, 3 times daily [1:5 (*g/ml*)].

CONTRAINDICATIONS

Consult a healthcare provider before using ginger in cases of gallstones or gall bladder diseases.

PREGNANCY AND LACTATION: Fresh ginger is safe when used in moderation. Women have used ginger to prevent or treat morning sickness during the first trimester. However, pregnant women should use caution in taking excessive daily dosages of more than two grams of dried ginger and should consult their healthcare provider regarding the use of ginger or any dietary supplements during pregnancy or while nursing.

ADVERSE EFFECTS

Fresh and raw ginger in its natural form are not known to cause adverse side effects.

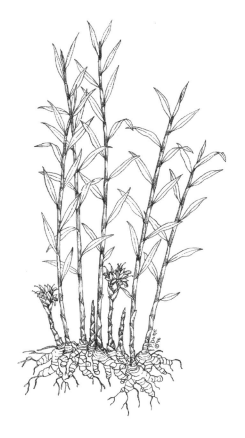

DRUG INTERACTIONS

There are no known drug interactions. According to anecdotal reports, ginger may interact with the blood-thinning drug warfarin (Coumadin®, Sofarin), but this has not been scientifically proven. Nevertheless, caution should be used when taking warfarin and ginger simultaneously. Ginger does not seem to affect the absorption of other drugs when taken at the same time.

Comments

When using a dietary supplement, purchase it from a reliable source. For best results, use the same brand of product throughout the period of use. As with all medications and dietary supplements, please inform your healthcare provider of all herbs and medications you are taking. Interactions may occur between medications and herbs or even among different herbs when taken at the same time. Treat your herbal supplement with care by taking it as directed, storing it as advised on the label, and keeping it out of the reach of children and pets. Consult your healthcare provider with any questions.

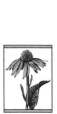

AMERICAN BOTANICAL COUNCIL

The information contained on this sheet has been excerpted from *The ABC Clinical Guide to Herbs* © 2003 by the American Botanical Council (ABC). ABC is an independent member-based educational organization focusing on the medicinal use of herbs. For more detailed information about this herb please consult the healthcare provider who gave you this sheet. To order *The ABC Clinical Guide to Herbs* or become a member of ABC, visit their website at www.herbalgram.org.

Ginger

Zingiber officinale Roscoe

[Fam. *Zingiberaceae*]

OVERVIEW

Ginger has been used for millennia as a common spice, food, and medicine; and was described in ancient Indian, Chinese, and Greco-Roman medical texts (Langner *et al.*, 1998). Ginger dietary supplements have become increasingly popular in the past decade to help allay nausea associated with motion sickness. In 2000, ginger sales ranked 17th of all herbal supplements sold in U.S. mainstream retail stores (Blumenthal, 2001). Ginger is frequently used as an alternative to antihistamines and anticholinergics, and as a prophylactic for motion sickness when side effects from pharmaceuticals warrant them unsuitable or intolerable for use (Robbers and Tyler, 2000). Ginger has also been investigated as an antiemetic for postoperative nausea and nausea induced by chemotherapy (Arfeen *et al.*, 1995; Meyer *et al.*, 1995). China and India have cultivated ginger since antiquity and remain the world's leading producers of ginger (Blumenthal *et al.*, 2000; USP, 1998).

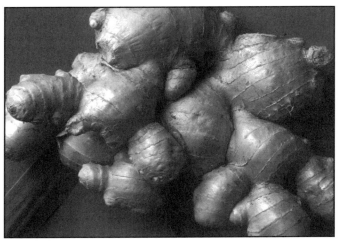

Photo © 2003 stevenfoster.com

DESCRIPTION

Ginger preparations consist of the peeled, finger-long, fresh or dried rhizome of *Zingiber officinale* Roscoe [Fam. *Zingiberaceae*] (Blumenthal *et al.*, 2000). Preparations include decoctions and infusions (teas), powdered ginger capsules, liquid extracts, tinctures, and candies made from ginger syrup or crystallized ginger (Blumenthal *et al.*, 2000). Some ginger products are standardized to 0.8% essential oils (McCaleb *et al.*, 2000).

PRIMARY USES

Gastrointestinal
- Motion sickness (Careddu *et al.*, 1999; Riebenfeld and Borzone, 1999; Schmid *et al.*, 1994; Grøntved *et al.*, 1988; Grøntved and Hentzer, 1986; Mowrey and Clayson, 1982)

OTHER POTENTIAL USES
- Hyperemesis gravidarum (Fischer-Rasmussen *et al.*, 1990)
- Chemotherapy-induced nausea (Meyer *et al.*, 1995)
- Morning sickness (Vutyavanich *et al.*, 2001)
- Nausea, postoperative (Bone *et al.*, 1990; Phillips *et al.*, 1993)
- Osteoarthritis (Altman and Marcussen, 2001; Bliddal *et al.*, 2000)

DOSAGE

Internal

Crude Preparations

FRESH OR DRIED RHIZOME: 2–4 g daily (Blumenthal *et al.*, 1998).

POWDERED DRY EXTRACT: 500 mg, 30 minutes before travel, and then 500 mg every 4 hours until end of travel (Riebenfeld and Borzone, 1999; Tenne, 1999).

INFUSION OR DECOCTION: 0.25–1.0 g in 150 ml boiled water, up to 3 times daily.

FLUID EXTRACT: 1:1 (*g/ml*), 0.25–1.0 ml 3 times daily (Blumenthal *et al.*, 1998).

TINCTURE: 1:5 (*g/ml*), 1.25–5.0 ml 3 times daily.

DURATION OF ADMINISTRATION

Internal

For motion sickness, at least 30 minutes before travel and every 4 hours as needed (Tenne, 1999).

CHEMISTRY

Ginger rhizome contains 4.0–10.0% oleoresin composed of nonvolatile, pungent principles (phenols such as gingerols and their related dehydration products, shogaols); nonpungent fats and waxes; 1.0–3.3% volatile oils, of which 30–70% are sesquiterpenes, mainly β-bisaolene, (-)zingiberene, β-sesquiphellandrene, and (+)arcurcumene; monoterpenes, mainly geranial and neral; 40–60% carbohydrates, mainly starch; 9–10% proteins and free amino acids; 6–10% lipids composed of triglycerides, phosphatidic acid, lecithins, and free fatty acids; vitamin A; niacin; and minerals (BHP, 1996).

PHARMACOLOGICAL ACTIONS

Crude Preparations

Human

Antiemetic (Grøntved and Hentzer, 1986; Grøntved *et al.*, 1988; Mowrey and Clayson, 1982; Fischer-Rasmussen *et al.*, 1990; Bone *et al.*, 1990; Phillips *et al.*, 1993; Meyer *et al.*, 1995); antiplatelet aggregation (Bordia *et al.*, 1997; Verma *et al.*, 1993; Srivastava, 1989).

Animal

Antiemetic (Chang and But, 1987); reduces chemotherapy-induced vomiting in dogs (Sharma *et al.*, 1997); enhances bile secretion; works as an antiulcer agent; enhances gastrointestinal motility; suppresses gastric contraction (Yamahara *et al.*, 1990); strengthens cardiac muscle (Shoji *et al.*, 1982); inhibits cholesterol synthesis (Tanabe *et al.*, 1993).

In vitro

Antiplatelet aggregation (Bordia *et al.*, 1997; Surh *et al.*, 1998); stimulates calcium uptake in skeletal and cardiac muscles (Kobayashi *et al.*, 1987); antibacterial (Mascolo *et al.*, 1989); antifungal (Endo *et al.*, 1990); antirhinoviral (Denyer *et al.*, 1994); anti-schistosomal (Adewunmi *et al.*, 1990); antioxidant (Cao *et al.*, 1993; Zhou and Xu, 1992); anti-atherosclerotic (Fuhrman *et al.*, 2000); anti-inflammatory (Surh *et al.*, 1998); chemopreventative (Surh *et al.*, 1998).

STANDARDIZED PREPARATIONS

Human

Antiemetic (Careddu *et al.*, 1999; Riebenfeld *et al.*, 1999; Schmid *et al.*, 1994); anti-inflammatory (Srivastava, 1989; Bliddel *et al.*, 2000).

MECHANISM OF ACTION

- Acts directly at the gastric level and not on the central nervous system for anti-nausea effect (Holtman *et al.*, 1989).

- Increases gastrointestinal motility, but does not seem to influence gastric emptying rate (Philips *et al.*, 1993; Meyer *et al.*, 1995).

- Reduces stimuli in gastrointestinal tract by absorbent property, blocking nausea feedback loop between brain stem and tract (Mowrey and Clayson, 1982).

- Inhibits cyclo-oxygenase and lipo-oxygenase pathways, inhibiting both prostaglandin and leukotriene synthesis (Verma *et al.*, 1993; Srivastava and Mustafa, 1992; Srivastava, 1989).

- Inhibits thromboxane synthetase; inhibits conversion of arachidonic acid (AA) to thromboxane (TXA2); decreases platelet aggregation (Bordia *et al.*, 1997; Verma *et al.*, 1993; Backon, 1991). Ginger's effect on thromboxane synthetase activity is dose dependent, or occurs with fresh ginger only. Up to 2 g of dried ginger is unlikely to cause platelet dysfunction when used therapeutically (Lumb, 1994).

- Inhibits prostaglandin PGE2 and leukotriene LTB4 synthesis, producing an anti-inflammatory effect (Kiuchi *et al.*, 1992; Srivastava and Mustafa, 1992; Srivastava, 1989).

CONTRAINDICATIONS

According to the German Commission E, patients with gallstones should consult a healthcare provider before use (Blumenthal *et al.*, 1998).

PREGNANCY AND LACTATION: A recent clinical trial reported no adverse effects of ginger use in pregnancy (Vutyavanich *et al.*, 2001). However, the Commission E previously contraindicated ginger during pregnancy based on *in vitro* research on single compounds from ginger (Blumenthal *et al.*, 1998); and the American Herbal Products Association advised against its therapeutic use during pregnancy (McGuffin *et al.*, 1997), based in part on the Commission E contraindication, but there is little clinical evidence to support these precautions when used in normal doses.

ADVERSE EFFECTS

None known (Blumenthal *et al.*, 1998).

DRUG INTERACTIONS

None known (Blumenthal *et al.*, 1998). Reports of interaction with warfarin are anecdotal and speculative and not substantiated by documented case reports (Heck *et al.*, 2000). Nevertheless, the narrow therapeutic index of warfarin warrants the cautious use of ginger in conjunction with warfarin. Ginger does not appear to affect absorption of concomittant medications (Philips *et al.*, 1993; Meyer *et al.*, 1995).

AMERICAN HERBAL PRODUCTS ASSOCIATION (AHPA) SAFETY RATING

Fresh root

CLASS 1: Can be safely consumed when used appropriately.

Dried root

CLASS 2B: Not to be used during pregnancy based on *in vitro* research and cautions from Chinese texts related to excessive use of dried ginger. See Contraindications/Pregnancy and Lactation Section.

CLASS 2D: Persons with gallstones should consult a practitioner prior to use.

NOTE: The classifications and concerns for this herb are based upon therapeutic use and may not be relevant to its consumption as a spice (McGuffin *et al.*, 1997).

REGULATORY STATUS

AUSTRIA: Dried rhizome official in the *Austrian Pharmacopoeia*, ÖAB (Meyer-Buchtela, 1999; Wichtl, 1997).

AUSTRALIA: Ginger is permitted as an active ingredient in listable Therapeutic Goods. High single dose of crude ginger (2 g and above) and/or highly concentrated extracts (25:1 or higher) are subject to required label warnings (TGA, 2000).

BELGIUM: Traditional Herbal Medicine (THM) accepted for specific indication as digestive aid (Bradley, 1992).

CANADA: Food, Drug, or New Drug depending on label claim statements (HPB, 1993). When labeled as a Traditional Herbal Medicine (THM) or as a homeopathic drug, ginger is regulated as a non-prescription drug requiring pre-market registration and assignment of a Drug Identification Number (DIN) (Health Canada, 1995, 2001).

CHINA: Dried ginger, fresh ginger, ginger tincture, and ginger fluid extract are all official preparations of the *Pharmacopoeia of the People's Republic of China* (PPRC, 1997).

EUROPEAN UNION: Dried rhizome official in the *European Pharmacopoeia*, Third edition, Supplement 2001 (Ph.Eur., 2001).

FRANCE: Food. No monograph in the *French Pharmacopoeia*.

GERMANY: Dried rhizome, for preparation as tea or other equivalent galenical dosage forms, is an approved nonprescription drug of the German Commission E monographs (Blumenthal *et al.*, 1998). Dried rhizome is official in the *German Drug Codex* (DAC, 1993) and in the *German Pharmacopoeia* (DAB, 1999). The dried rhizome, for preparation of alcoholic mother tincture and liquid dilutions, is official in the *German Homoeopathic Pharmacopoeia* (GHP, 1993).

INDIA: Dried rhizome official in the Government of India *Ayurvedic Pharmacopoeia* of India, First edition, volume I (API I,

1989) and fresh rhizome official in API, First edition, volume II (API II, 1999). Dried rhizome also occurs in the *Indian Herbal Pharmacopoeia* (IHP II, 1999).

JAPAN: Dried rhizome and powdered dried rhizome official in *Pharmacopoeia of Japan* (JSHM, 1993).

SWEDEN: Classified as foodstuff. As of January 2001, no ginger products are listed in the Medical Products Agency (MPA) "Authorised Natural Remedies" (MPA, 2001).

SWITZERLAND: Dried rhizome official in the *Swiss Pharmacopoeia*, Ph.Helv. (Meyer-Buchtela, 1999; Wichtl, 1997). Dried powdered rhizome in capsule has positive classification (List D) by the *Interkantonale Kontrollstelle für Heilmittel* (IKS) and corresponding sales category D with sale limited to pharmacies and drugstores, without prescription (Morant and Ruppanner, 2001).

U.K.: Herbal medicine on *General Sale List*, Schedule 1, Table A (Bradley, 1992). Dried rhizome official in the *British Pharmacopoeia*, BP 1993 (ESCOP, 1996; Newall *et al.*, 1996). Strong Ginger Tincture and Weak Ginger Tincture official preparations of the *British Pharmacopoeia* (BP, 1980).

U.S.: Generally recognized as safe (GRAS) (US FDA, 1998). Dietary supplement (USC, 1994). Dried rhizome and powdered dried rhizome official in the *United States National Formulary*, 19th edition (USP, 2002).

CLINICAL REVIEW

Twenty-one studies (2,669 total participants) are outlined in the following table, "Clinical Studies on Ginger." All but four (Bliddal *et al.*, 2000; Janssen *et al.*, 1996; Arfeen *et al.*, 1995; Vislyaputra *et al.*, 1998) demonstrated positive effects for indications including motion sickness, postoperative nausea, cardiovascular conditions, and osteoarthritis. Nine of the studies were randomized, double-blind, and placebo-controlled (R, DB,PC); two of these (Grøntved *et al.*, 1986 and 1988) concluded that ginger significantly reduced the incidence of motion sickness. One study (Lumb, 1994) found that 2 g of ginger did not significantly change bleeding time, platelet count, or platelet aggregation. Two studies demonstrated that ginger was as effective as metoclopramide in reducing postoperative nausea (Bone *et al.*, 1990; Phillips *et al.*, 1993). Two trials resulted in no significant reduction in postoperative nausea (Vislyaputra *et al.*, 1998; Arfeen *et al.*, 1995). Two studies demonstrated some effect from ginger in the treatment of osteoarthritis (Altman and Mercussen, 2001; Bliddel *et al.*, 2000). Three R, DB, comparison (Cm) trials (1,577 participants), found that Zintona® (standardized ginger preparation) was equally or more effective than dimenhydrinate (Dramamine®), with better tolerability and fewer side effects as a prophylaxis for motion sickness (Careddu *et al.*, 1999; Riebenfeld and Borzone, 1999; Schmid *et al.*, 1994). One R, DB, crossover trial (Fischer-Rasmussen *et al.*, 1990) found ginger diminished or eliminated symptoms of hyperemesis gravidarum, a severe form of morning sickness during pregnancy; and a recent R, DB, PC trial showed that ginger reduced nausea in pregnant women during the first trimester with no adverse effects on birth rates or newborns (Vutyavanich *et al.*, 2001). An early R, PC, single-blind, Cm study (Mowrey and Clayson, 1982) showed ginger to be superior to both placebo and dimenhydrinate in preventing motion sickness in patients with nausea induced in a tilted, rotating chair. A recent meta-analysis of six R, DB, PC studies concluded that ginger is a "promising antiemetic herbal remedy, but the clinical data to date are insufficient to draw firm conclusions" (Ernst and Pittler, 2000).

BRANDED PRODUCTS*

Blackmores custom powdered ginger capsules: Blackmores Ltd. / 23 Roseberry Street / Balgowlah / NSW 2093 / Australia / Tel: +61-29-95-1011-1 / Fax: +61-29-94-9195-4 / www.blackmores.com. Capsules contain 500 mg of ginger powder BP 1988 custom made according to standards of the *British Pharmacopoeia* of 1988.

EV. EXT 33: Ferrosan A/S / Sydmarken 5 / 2860 Soeborg / Denmark / Tel: +45-3969-2111 / Fax: +45-3969-6518 / www.ferrosan.com. Chinese ginger standardized to hydroxy-methoxy phenyl compounds (HMP) formulated in soft gelatin capsules.

EV. EXT 77: Ferrosan A/S. Each capsule contains 255 mg extract from 2,500–4,000 mg dried ginger rhizomes and 500–1,500 mg dried galanga [*Alpinia galanga*] rhizomes.

Martindale powdered ginger capsules: Martindale Pharmaceuticals Pty. Ltd. / Hubert Road / Brentwood / Essex / CM14 4LZ / U.K. / Tel: +44-01-27-72-6660-0 / Fax: +44-01-27-78-4897-6 / Email: mail@martindalepharma.co.uk / www.martindalepharma.co.uk. Capsules contain 500 mg powdered ginger rhizome.

Zintona®: Dalidar Pharma c/o BioDar Ltd. / Yavne Technology Park / P.O. Box 344 / Yavne 81103 / Israel / Tel: +972-08-942-0930 / Fax: +972-08-942-0928 / Email: dalidar@dalidar.com / www.dalidar.com. Ginger powder standardized to min. 1.4% volatile oils and min. 2.0 mg gingerols and shogaols in a capsule containing 250 ginger material. (As per 7th Supplement, USP-NF 18).

*American equivalents, if any, are found in the Product Table beginning on page 398.

REFERENCES

Adewunmi, C, Oguntimein B, Furu P. Molluscicidal and antischistosomal activities of *Zingiber officinale*. *Planta Med* 1990; 56(4):374–6.

Altman RD, Marcussen KC. Effects of a ginger extract on knee pain in patients with osteoarthritis. *Arthritis Rheum*. 2001 Nov;44(11):2531-8.

API. See: Ayurvedic Pharmacopoeia of India.

Arfeen Z *et al.* A double-blind randomized controlled trial of ginger for the prevention of postoperative nausea and vomiting. *Anaesth Intensive Care* 1995;23(4):449–52.

Ayurvedic Pharmacopoeia of India (API, Part I, Volume I, 1st Edition). New Delhi, India: Government of India Ministry of Health and Family Welfare Department of Health; 1989;103–4.

Ayurvedic Pharmacopoeia of India (API, Part I, Volume II, 1st Edition). New Delhi, India: Government of India Ministry of Health and Family Welfare Department of Indian System of Medicine & Homeopathy; 1999;12–4.

Backon J. Ginger as an antiemetic: possible side effects due to its thromboxane synthetase activity. *Anaesthesia* 1991;46:705–6.

Bliddal H, Rosetzsky A, Schlichting P, *et al.* A randomized, placebo-controlled crossover study of ginger extracts and ibuprofen in osteoarthritis. *Osteoarthr Cartil* 2000;8:9–12.

Blumenthal M. Herb sales down 15% in mainstream market. *HerbalGram* 2001;51:69.

Blumenthal M, Busse WR, Goldberg A, Gruenwald J, Hall T, Riggins CW, Rister RS (eds.). Klein S, Rister RS (trans.). *The Complete German Commission E Monographs—Therapeutic Guide to Herbal Medicines*. Austin, TX: American Botanical Council; Boston: Integrative Medicine Communication; 1998;135-136.

Blumenthal M, Goldberg A, Brinckmann J (eds.). *Herbal Medicine: Expanded Commission E Monographs*. Austin TX: American Botanical Council; Newton MA: Integrative Medicine Communications; 2000;153-9.

Bone, K. Ginger. *Brit J Phytother* 1997;4(3):110–20.

Bone M, Wilkinson D, Young J, McNeil J, Charlton S. Ginger root—a new antiemetic. The effect of ginger root on postoperative nausea and vomiting after major gynecological surgery. *Anaesthesia* 1990;45:669–71.

Bordia A, Verma S, Srivastava K. Effect of ginger (*Zingiber officinale* Rosc.) and fenugreek (*Trigonella foenumgraecum* L.) on blood lipids, blood sugar, and platelet aggregation in patients with coronary artery disease. *Prostaglan Leukotrien Ess Fatty Acids* 1997;56(5):379–84.

BP. See: *British Pharmacopoeia.*

Bradley P (ed.). *British Herbal Compendium*, Vol. I. A Handbook of Scientific Information on Widely Used Plant Drugs. Dorset, U.K.: British Herbal Medicine Association (BHMA); 1992;113–4.

British Herbal Pharmacopoeia (BHP). Exeter, U.K.: British Herbal Medicine Association; 1996.

British Pharmacopoeia (BP 1980 Vol. II). London, U.K.: Her Majesty's Stationery Office (HMSO); 1980;835.

Bruneton, J. *Pharmacognosy, Phytochemistry, Medicinal Plants.* Paris: Lavoisier Publishing; 1995.

Budavari S. (ed.). *The Merck Index: An Encyclopedia of Chemicals, Drugs, and Biologicals,* 12th ed. Whitehouse Station, N.J.: Merck & Co, Inc; 1996.

But, P *et al.* (eds.). 1997. *International Collation of Traditional and Folk Medicine.* Singapore: World Scientific.; 1997;210–1.

Cao Z, Chen Z, Guo P *et al.* Scavenging effects of ginger on superoxide anion and hydroxyl radical. *Chung-kuo chung yao tsa chih* (China Journal of Chinese Materia Medica) 1993;18(12):750–1.

Careddu P *et al.* Motion Sickness in Children: Results of a double-blind study with ginger (Zintona®) and Dimenhydrinate. *Euro Phytother* 1999;6(2):102–7.

Chang H, But P. *Pharmacology and Applications of Chinese Materia Medica.* World Scientific, Singapore: World Scientific; 1987.

DAB. See: *Deutsches Arzneibuch.*

DAC. See: *Deutscher Arzneimittel-Codex.*

Denyer C, Jackson P, Loakes D. Isolation of antirhinoviral sesquiterpenes from ginger (*Zingiber officinale*) *J Nat Prod* 1994;57(5):658–62.

Deutscher Arzneimittel-Codex (DAC 1986, 5. Ergänzung 1993). Stuttgart, Germany: Deutscher Apotheker Verlag; 1993;I-030:1–4.

Deutsches Arzneibuch (DAB Ergänzungslieferung 1999). Stuttgart, Germany: Deutscher Apotheker Verlag; 1999;Ingwerwurzelstock.

Endo K, Kanno E, Oshima Y. Structures of antifungal diarylheptenones, gingerenones A,B,C and isogingerenone B, isolated from the rhizomes of *Zingiber officinale.* *Phytochemistry* 1990;29(3):797–9.

Ernst E, Pittler M. Efficacy of ginger for nausea and vomiting: a systematic review of randomized clinical trials. *Br J Anaesth* 2000;84(3):367–71.

ESCOP. See: European Scientific Cooperative on Phytotherapy.

European Pharmacopoeia (Ph.Eur., 3rd edition Supplement 2001). Strasbourg, France: Council of Europe. 2001;886-887.

European Scientific Cooperative on Phytotherapy. *ESCOP Monographs on the Medicinal Uses of Plant Drugs.* Exeter, U.K.: ESCOP; March 1996;1–7.

Fischer-Rasmussen, W, Kjaer S, Dahl C, Asping U. Ginger treatment of hyperemesis gravidarum. *Eur J Obstet Gynecol Reprod Biol* 1990; 38(1):19–24.

Fuhrman BB, Rosenblat M, Hayek T, *et al.* Ginger extract consumption reduces plasma cholesterol, inhibits LDL oxidation and attenuates development of atherosclerosis in atherosclerotic, apolipoprotein e-deficient mice. *J Nutr* 2000;130:1124–31.

Fulder S, Tenne M. Ginger as an anti-nausea remedy in pregnancy: The issue of safety. *HerbalGram* 1996;38:47–50.

German Homeopathic Pharmacopoeia (GHP) 5th Supplement 1991 to the 1st edition 1978. Translation of the German "Homöopathisches Arzneibuch (HAB 1), 5. Nachtrag 1991, Amtliche Ausgabe." Stuttgart, Germany: Deutscher Apotheker Verlag. 1993;399-401.

Ghana Herbal Pharmacopoeia (GHP). 1992. Accra, Ghana: Policy Research and Strategic Planning Institute (PORSPI); 1992.

GHP. See: *German Homoeopathic Pharmacopoeia.*

Grøntved A, and Hentzer E. Vertigo-reducing effect of ginger root. A controlled clinical study. *ORL J Otorhinolaryngol Relat Spec* 1986;48(5):282–6.

Grøntved A, Brask T, Kambskard J, Hentzer E. Ginger root against seasickness. A controlled trial on the open sea. *Acta Otolaryngol (Stockh)* 1988; 105(1–2):45–9.

Health Canada. *Drug Product Database (DPD).* Ottawa, Ontario: Health Canada Therapeutic Products Programme; 2001.

Health Canada. *Drugs Directorate Guidelines: Traditional Herbal Medicines.* Ottawa, Ontario: Minister of National Health and Welfare. October 1995.

Health Protection Branch (HPB*). HPB Status Manual.* Ottawa, Ontario: Health Protection Branch; Feb19, 1993;86.

Heck A, DeWitt B, Lukes A. Potential interactions between alternative therapies and warfarin. *Am J Health Syst Pharm* 2000 Jul 1;57(13):1221–7.

Holtmann, S, Clarke A, Scherer H, Hohn M. The anti-motion sickness mechanism of ginger. A comparative study with placebo and dimenhydrate. *Acta Otolaryngol (Stockh)* 1989;108(3–4):168–74.

HPB. See: Health Protection Branch.

IHP: See: *Indian Herbal Pharmacopoeia.*

Indian Herbal Pharmacopoeia (IHP, Volume II). Jammu Tawi, India: Regional Research Laboratory – Council of Scientific & Industrial Research (CSIR); 1999;162–73.

Iwu M. *Handbook of African Medicinal Plants.* Boca Raton: CRC Press; 1990;263–5.

Janssen P, Meyboom S, van Staveren W, *et al.* Consumption of ginger (*Zingiber officinale* Roscoe) does not affect *ex vivo* platelet thromboxane production in humans. *Euro J Clin Nutr* 1996;50:772–4.

Japanese Pharmacopoeia, 12th ed. (JP XII). 1993. Tokyo: Government of Japan Ministry of Health and Welfare—Yakuji Nippo, Ltd; 1993;125–6.

Japanese Standards for Herbal Medicines (JSHM). Tokyo, Japan: Yakuji Nippo, Ltd; 1993;125–6.

JSHM. See: *Japanese Standards for Herbal Medicines.*

Kada T, Morita K, Inoue T. Anti-mutagenic action of vegetable factors on the mutagenic principle of tryptophan pyrolysate. *Mutat Res* 1978;53(3):351–3.

Kapoor L. 1990. *Handbook of Ayurvedic Medicinal Plants.* Boca Raton: CRC Press; 1990;341–42.

Karnick C. 1994. *Pharmacopoeial Standards of Herbal Plants,* Vol. 1. Delhi: Sri Satguru Publications; 1994;347–8.

Kiuchi F, Iwakami S, Shibuya M *et al.* Inhibition of prostaglandin and leukotriene biosynthesis by gingerols and diarylheptanoids. *Chem Pharm Bull* 1992;40:387–91.

Kobayashi M, Shoji N, Ohizumi Y. Gingerol, a novel cardiotonic agent, activates the Ca++ pumping ATPase in skeletal and cardiac sarcoplasmic reticulum. *Biochim Biophys Acta* 1987;903:96–102.

Lange D, Schippmann U. *Trade Survey of Medicinal Plants in Germany—A Contribution to International Plant Species Conservation.* Bonn: Bundesamt für Naturschutz; 1997;83–4.

Langner E, Greifenberg S, Gruenwald J. Ginger: History and Use. *Advances in Ther* 1998 Jan/Feb;15(1):25–44.

Leung A, Foster S. *Encyclopedia of Common Natural Ingredients Used in Food, Drugs, and Cosmetics,* 2nd ed. New York: John Wiley & Sons, Inc; 1996.

Lumb, A. Effect of dried ginger on human platelet function. *Thromb Haemost* 1994; 71(1):110–1.

Mascolo N, Jain R, Jain S, *et al.* Ethnopharmacological investigation of ginger (*Zingiber officinale*). *J Ethnopharmacol* 1989;27:129–40.

McCaleb RS, Leigh E, Morien K. *The Encyclopedia of Popular Herbs.* Boulder CO: Herb Research Foundation; Roseville CA: Prima Publishing; 2000.

McGuffin M, Hobbs C, Upton R, Goldberg A. *American Herbal Product Association's Botanical Safety Handbook.* Boca Raton: CRC Press; 1997.

Medical Products Agency (MPA). *Naturläkemedel: Authorised Natural Remedies* (as of January 24, 2001). Uppsala, Sweden: Medical Products Agency; 2001.

Meyer K, Schwartz J, Crater D, Keyes B. *Zingiber officinale* (ginger) used to prevent 8-MOP associated nausea. *Dermatol Nurs* 1995;7(4):242–4.

Meyer-Buchtela E. *Tee-Rezepturen — Ein Handbuch für Apotheker und Ärzte.* Stuttgart, Germany: Deutscher Apotheker Verlag; 1999; Inggwerwurzelstock.

Mowrey D, Clayson D. Motion sickness, ginger, and psychophysics. *Lancet* 1982;1(8273):655–7.

Morant J, Ruppanner H (eds.). Chrisana Zintona®. In: *Arzneimittel-Kompendium der Schweiz®* 2001. Basel, Switzerland: Documed AG. 2001;1455.

MPA. See: Medical Products Agency.

Nagabhushan M, Amonkar A, Bhide S. Mutagenicity of gingerol and shogaol and antimutagenicity of zingerone in Salmonella/microsome assay. *Cancer Lett* 1987;36(2):221–3.

Namakura H and Yamamoto T. Mutagen and anti-mutagen in ginger, *Zingiber officinale.* *Mutat Res* 1982;103(2):119–26.

Newall C, Anderson L, Phillipson J. *Herbal Medicines: A Guide for Health-care Professionals.* London, U.K.: The Pharmaceutical Press; 1996;135–7.

Pace, J. Oral ingestion of encapsulated ginger and reported self-care actions for the relief of chemotherapy-associated nausea and vomiting. *Diss Abstr Int (Sci)* 1987;7; 47(8):3297.

Ph.Eur. See: *European Pharmacopoeia.*

Pharmacopoeia Helvetica, 7th ed. Vol. 1–4. (Ph.Helv.VII). 1987. Bern: Office Central Fédéral des Imprimés et du Matériel; 1987.

Pharmacopoeia of the People's Republic of China (PPRC English Edition, 1997). Beijing, China: Chemical Industry Press; 1997.

Phillips S, Ruggier R, Hutchinson S. *Zingiber officinale* (ginger)—an anti-emetic for day case surgery. *Anaesthesia* 1993;48(8):715–7.

Pinco RG, Israelsen L. 1995. European-American Phytomedicines Coalition Citizen Petition to Amend FDA's OTC Drug Review Policy Regarding Foreign Ingredients. 1995; Jul. 24.

PPRC. See: *Pharmacopoeia of the People's Republic of China.*

Reineccius G. (ed.). 1994. *Source Book of Flavors,* 2nd ed. New York; London: Chapman & Hall; 1994;295–9.

Riebenfeld D, Borzone L. Randomized Double-Blind Study Comparing Ginger (Zintona®) and Dimenhydrinate in Motion Sickness. *European Phytotherapy* 1999;6(2):98–101.

Riebenfeld D, Borzone L. Randomized double-blind study to compare the activities and tolerability of Zintona® and dimenhydrinate in 60 subjects with motion sickness. (Unpublished report, *Pharmaton*, Lugano, Switz.); 1986.

Robbers J, Tyler V. *Tyler's Herbs of Choice: The Therapeutic Use of Phytomedicinals*. New York: Haworth Herbal Press; 2000.

Schilcher, H. 1998. The Present State of Phytotherapy in Germany. *Deutsche Apotheker Zeitung* 138 Jahrgang, No. 3, 1998 Jan;15:144–9.

Schmid R, Schick T, Steffen S, Tschopp A, Wilk T. Comparison of Seven Commonly Used Agents for Prophylaxis of Seasickness. *J Travel Med* 1994;1(4):203–6.

Sharma S, Kochupillai V, Gupta S, et al. Antiemetic efficacy of ginger (*Zingiber officinale*) against cisplatin-induced emesis in dogs. *J Ethnopharmacol* 1997;57:93–6.

Shoji N, Iwasa A, Takemoto T. Cardiotonic Principles of Ginger (*Zingiber officinale* Roscoe). *J Pharmaceut Sci* 1982;71(10):1174–5.

Srivastava K, Mustafa T. Ginger (*Zingiber officinale*) in Rheumatism and Musculoskeletal Disorders. *Med Hypoth* 1992;39:342–8.

Srivastava K. Effect of onion and ginger consumption on platelet thromboxane production in humans. *Prostaglandins Leukot Essent Fatty Acids* 1989; 35(3):183–5.

Stewart J, Wood M, Wood C, Mims M. Effects of ginger on motion sickness susceptibility and gastric function. *Pharmacol* 1991;41(2):111–20.

Stott J, Hubble M, Spencer M. A double-blind comparative trial of powdered ginger root, Hyosine (sic) Hydrobromide and Cinnarizinein the prophylaxis of motion sickness induced by cross-coupled stimulation. Advisory Group for Aerospace Research and Development, Conference Proceedings; 1985;372, 39:1–6.

Surh YS, Lee E, Lee JM. Chemoprotective properties of some pungent ingredients present in red pepper and ginger. *Mutat Res* 1998;402:259–67.

Taber C. *Taber's Cyclopedic Medical Dictionary*, 9th ed. Philadelphia, PA: F.A. Davis Company; 1962;G–18.

Tanabe M, Chen Y, Saito K, Kano Y. Cholesterol biosythesis inhibitory component from *Zingiber officinale* Roscoe. *Chem Pharm Bull(Tokyo)* 1993 April;41(4):710–3.

Tenne M (Dalidar Pharma). Personal communication to A. Goldberg. May 25, 1999.

TGA. See: Therapeutic Goods Administration.

Therapeutic Goods Administration. New Listable Substances and Existing Substances with Changed Conditions. Woden, Australia:Therapeutic Goods Administration; May 2000;1–8.

United States Congress (USC). Public Law 103-417: Dietary Supplement Health and Education Act of 1994. Washington, DC: 103rd Congress of the United States; 1994.

United States Food and Drug Administration (U.S. FDA). *Code of Federal Regulations*, Title 21, Part 182 – Substances Generally Recognized as Safe. Washington, DC: Office of the Federal Register National Archives and Records Administration; 1998;427–33.

United States Pharmacopeia (USP 25th Revision) – *The National Formulary* (NF 20th Edition). Rockville, MD: United States Pharmacopeial Convention, Inc. 2002.

United States Pharmacopeia (USP) *Consumer Information*. 1998. U.S. Rockville, MD: U.S. Pharmacopeial Convention; 1998.

US FDA. See: United States Food and Drug Administration.

USC. See: United States Congress.

USP. See: *United States Pharmacopoeia*.

Verma, S, J Singh J, Khamesra R, Bordia A. Effect of ginger on platelet aggregation in man. *Indian J Med Res* 1993;98:240–2.

Visalyaputra S, Petchpaisit N, Somcharoen K. The efficacy of ginger root in the prevention of postoperative nausea and vomiting after outpatient gynecological laparoscopy. *Anaesthesia* 1998; 53:486–510.

Vutyavanich T, Kraisarin T, Ruangsri RA. Ginger for nausea and vomiting in pregnancy: randomized, double-masked, placebo-controlled trial. *Obstet Gynecol* 2001; 97(4):577–82.

Wichtl M (ed.). *Teedrogen und Phytopharmaka, 3. Auflage: Ein Handbuch für die Praxis auf wissenschaftlicher Grundlage*. Stuttgart, Germany: Wissenschaftliche Verlagsgesellschaft mbH. 1997;631–633.

Wichtl M, Bisset N (eds.). 1994. *Herbal Drugs and Phytopharmaceuticals*. Stuttgart: Medpharm Scientific Publishers; 1994.

Wood C, Manno J, Wood M, et al. Comparison of efficacy of ginger with various antimotion sickness drugs. *Clin Res Pract Drug Reg Aff* 1988;6:129–36.

Yamahara J, Huang Q, Li Y, et al. Gastrointestinal motility enhancing effect of ginger and its active constituents. *Chem Pharmaceut Bull* 1990;38(2):430–1.

Zhou Y, Xu R. Antioxidative effect of Chinese drugs. *Chung-kuo chung yao tsa chih (China Journal of Chinese Materia Medica)* 1992;17(6):368–9, 373.

Clinical Studies on Ginger (*Zingiber officinale* Roscoe)

Kinetosis (Motion Sickness)

Author/Year	Subject	Design	Duration	Dosage	Preparation	Results/Conclusion
Careddu et al., 1999	Children with history of motion sickness	R, DB, Cm n=28 (ages 4–8 years)	2 days	Ages 3–6 years: 250 mg 1/2 hour before trip, followed by 250 mg every 4 hours as necessary; 6 years and older: 500 mg using above formula; or 1/2–1 capsule (12.5–25mg) dimenhydrinate 1/2 hour before the trip and if necessary 1 capsule every 4 hours	Zintona® vs. dimen-hydrinate	Significantly better therapeutic effectiveness in ginger-treated group than dimenhydrinate-treated group. Physician ratings reported good results in 100% of subjects taking ginger, and 31% of subjects taking dimenhydrinate. Ginger reduced symptoms within 30 minutes, and this difference was highly significant ($p < 0.0001$). None of the children taking ginger had any adverse side effects, while 69% of cases in the dimenhydrinate group had adverse effects from the drug, and this difference was also highly significant ($p < 0.0001$).
Riebenfeld and Borzone, 1999	Sea sickness in passengers on a cruise ship	R, DB, Cm n=60 (ages 10–77 years; mean age 31 years)	7 months	500 mg, 1/2 hour before embarkation, followed by 500 mg every 4 hours over a 48-hour period, or 100 mg of dimenhydrinate, 1/2 hour before embarkation followed by 100 mg every 4 hours over a 48-hour period	Zintona® vs dimen-hydrinate	Significantly improved total motion sickness score ($p<0.005$). Ginger is as effective as dimenhydrinate for treatment of motion sickness, with greater tolerability and lower incidence (13.3% vs. 40%) of side effects ($p<0.001$).
Schmid et al., 1994	Sea sickness in tourists on a whale-watching safari	R, DB, Cm n=1,489 (ages 16–65 years)	3 months	Group 1: 500 mg, 2 hours prior to departure, 500 mg, during trip, if needed. Group 2: 500 mg, after dinner on evening before trip, 500 mg, 2 hours prior to departure	Zintona®	Ginger showed equal potency to 7 common pharmaceutical drugs for sea sickness, and better effectiveness than scopolamine transdermal patch ($p=0.14$). As neither clinically relevant nor significant differences were found between products used, personal preference should be followed as to the medication taken as prophylaxis for seasickness.

KEY: C – controlled, **CC** – case-control, **CH** – cohort, **CI** – confidence interval, **Cm** – comparison, **CO** – crossover, **CS** – cross-sectional, **DB** – double-blind, **E** – epidemiological, **LC** – longitudinal cohort, **MA** – meta-analysis, **MC** – multi-center, **n** – number of patients, **O** – open, **OB** – observational, **OL** – open label, **OR** – odds ratio, **P** – prospective, **PB** – patient-blind, **PC** – placebo-controlled, **PG** – parallel group, **PS** – pilot study, **R** – randomized, **RC** – reference-controlled, **RCS** – retrospective cross-sectional, **RS** - retrospective, **S** – surveillance, **SB** – single-blind, **SC** – single-center, **U** – uncontrolled, **UP** – unpublished, **VC** – vehicle-controlled.

Kinetosis (Motion Sickness) (cont.)

Author/Year	Subject	Design	Duration	Dosage	Preparation	Results/Conclusion
Stewart et al., 1991	Motion sickness and gastric function	PC, Cm Phase 1 motion sickness, n=8; Phase 2 motion sickness, n=8; Phase 3 motion sickness, n=4; Phase 4 gastric function, n=8	14 hours	Phase 1: 500 mg or 1,000 mg ground ginger root or 0.6 mg scopolamine HBr or placebo on separate test days; Phase 2 One 1,000 mg fresh ginger root capsule or placebo Phase 3: 940 mg ground ginger or placbo Phase 4: Two, 250 mg capsules ginger or placebo	Phase 1: ground ginger root Phase 2: fresh ginger (capsules prepared by researchers) Phase 3: ground ginger Phase 4: 250 mg of ginger capsules	Powdered ginger partially inhibited tachygastria but did not enhance the EGG amplitude. Did not significantly alter gastric function during motion sickness or possess antimotion sickness activity.
Grøntved et al., 1988	Seasickness in naval cadets unaccustomed to sailing	R, DB, PC n=80 (median age 17 years)	4 hours	1 g	Powdered ginger capsules (brand not stated) vs. placebo	Ginger significantly reduced tendency to vomit and experience cold sweats (p<0.05). No side effects reported in both groups.
Grøntved and Hentzer, 1986	Vertigo and nystagmus (healthy volunteers who received caloric stimulation of the vestibular system)	R, DB, CO, PC n=48	6 days	1 g/day	Powdered ginger capsules (brand not stated)	Ginger significantly reduced the induced vertigo better than placebo (p<0.05). No statistically significant action upon the duration or maximum slow phase velocity of nystagmus.
Mowrey and Clayson, 1982	Motion sickness produced by a motor driven, tilted, revolving chair	R, Cm, PC, SB n=36 volunteer subjects with self-rated extreme or very high susceptibility to motion sickness (ages 18–20 years)	31 minutes	Single dose of 2 capsules (940 mg total)	Powdered ginger capsules (brand not stated)	Ginger is superior to both placebo and dimenhydrinate (p<0.05) in preventing the gastrointestinal symptoms of experimentally-induced motion sickness in highly susceptible individuals.

KEY: C – controlled, **CC** – case-control, **CH** – cohort, **CI** – confidence interval, **Cm** – comparison, **CO** – crossover, **CS** – cross-sectional, **DB** – double-blind, **E** – epidemiological, **LC** – longitudinal cohort, **MA** – meta-analysis, **MC** – multi-center, **n** – number of patients, **O** – open, **OB** – observational, **OL** – open label, **OR** – odds ratio, **P** – prospective, **PB** – patient-blind, **PC** – placebo-controlled, **PG** – parallel group, **PS** – pilot study, **R** – randomized, **RC** – reference-controlled, **RCS** – retrospective cross-sectional, **RS** - retrospective, **S** – surveillance, **SB** – single-blind, **SC** – single-center, **U** – uncontrolled, **UP** – unpublished, **VC** – vehicle-controlled.

Clinical Studies on Ginger (*Zingiber officinale* Roscoe) (cont.)

Nausea During Pregnancy

Author/Year	Subject	Design	Duration	Dosage	Preparation	Results/Conclusion
Vutyavanich et al., 2001	Hypermesis gravidarum (women with nausea and vomiting in early pregnancy)	R, DB, PC n=70	7 days	One, 250 mg capsule 4x/day	Fresh, baked ginger root ground into powder (prepared by researchers)	Significant median change in nausea scores with ginger post-therapy (p=0.014). Significant reduction in nausea scores with ginger on day 4 of only treatment (p=0.0348). Significant improvement in patients' subjective response with ginger (p<0.001). No adverse effect with ginger on pregnancy outcomes.
Fischer-Rasmussen et al., 1990	Hyperemesis gravidarum	R, DB, CO n=30 pregnant women admitted to hospital before 20 weeks of gestation with symptoms 2x/day (ages 18–39 years)	4 days	One, 250 mg capsule 4x/day	Powdered ginger capsules (brand not stated)	Ginger diminished or eliminated symptoms of hyperemesis gravidarum. Statistically significant preference for ginger. Reduced degree of nausea and number of attacks of vomiting. No side effects observed.

Postoperative Nausea

Author/Year	Subject	Design	Duration	Dosage	Preparation	Results/Conclusion
Vislyaputra et al., 1998	Gynecological diagnostic laparoscopy	R, DB, PC, Cm n=120 (ages 20–40 years)	24 hours	Four, 500 mg capsules ginger, or 1.25 mg droperidol, or placebo	Powdered ginger capsules (prepared by researchers) vs. placebo vs. droperidol IV	No significant reduction in incidence of postoperative nausea and vomiting. Severity of nausea and frequency of vomiting within 24 hours were not statistically different with ginger root capsules or the combination of ginger root and droperidol.
Arfeen et al., 1995	Day case gynecological laparoscopy	R, DB, PC n=108 (ages 18–75 years)	3 hours	One-time dose before surgery of 10 mg diazepam (orally) plus either 1–2 capsules (500 mg ea.) powdered ginger or placebo	Blackmores Ltd. BP 1988 custom powdered ginger capsules vs. placebo	Ginger in doses of 0.5 or 1.0 g given with oral diazepam premedication one hour prior to surgery was found ineffective in reducing the incidence of postoperative nausea and vomiting. Incidence of nausea and vomiting increased slightly, but insignificantly (nausea, p=0.2; vomiting, p=0.15), with increasing dose of ginger.
Phillips et al., 1993	Day case gynecological laparoscopy	R, P, DB, PC, Cm n=120 (ages >16 years)	24 hours	Two, 500 mg capsules ginger, or 10 mg metoclopramide	Martindale Pharmaceuticals powdered ginger capsules vs. placebo vs. metoclopramide	Ginger similarly reduced incidence of nausea and vomiting as metoclopramide. Oral administration of 1 g of ginger reduced incidence of nausea and vomiting by 50% and appears to be as effective as metoclopramide, 10 mg when given by mouth one hour before anesthesia. Ginger is an effective and promising prophylactic antiemetic without toxic effects, which may be especially useful in day case surgery.
Bone et al., 1990	Major gynecological surgery	R, DB, PC, Cm n=60 (ages 16–65 years)	24 hours	0.5 g ginger or 10 mg metoclopramide injection or placebo	Powdered ginger capsules (brand not stated) vs. placebo vs. metoclopramide	Statistically fewer recorded incidences of nausea for ginger compared with placebo (p<0.05). Numbers of incidences of nausea in ginger vs. metoclopramide groups were similar.

KEY: **C** – controlled, **CC** – case-control, **CH** – cohort, **CI** – confidence interval, **Cm** – comparison, **CO** – crossover, **CS** – cross-sectional, **DB** – double-blind, **E** – epidemiological, **LC** – longitudinal cohort, **MA** – meta-analysis, **MC** – multi-center, **n** – number of patients, **O** – open, **OB** – observational, **OL** – open label, **OR** – odds ratio, **P** – prospective, **PB** – patient-blind, **PC** – placebo-controlled, **PG** – parallel group, **PS** – pilot study, **R** – randomized, **RC** – reference-controlled, **RCS** – retrospective cross-sectional, **RS** - retrospective, **S** – surveillance, **SB** – single-blind, **SC** – single-center, **U** – uncontrolled, **UP** – unpublished, **VC** – vehicle-controlled.

Clinical Studies on Ginger (*Zingiber officinale* Roscoe) (cont.)

Cardiovascular

Author/Year	Subject	Design	Duration	Dosage	Preparation	Results/Conclusion
Bordia et al., 1997	Platelet aggregation in patients with coronary artery disease with history of myocardial infarction (76 months)	PC n=60	3 months	4 g ginger daily for 3 months or single dose of 10 g ginger vs. 5 g (2 x 2.5 g) fenugreek daily for 3 months vs. placebo	Powdered ginger capsules (prepared by researchers) vs. fenugreek vs. placebo	Powdered ginger in dose of 4 g/day did not affect ADP and epinephrine-induced platelet aggregation. However, single dose of 10 g powdered ginger after 4 hours produced a significant reduction in platelet aggregation (p<0.05).
Janssen et al., 1996	Platelet thromboxane production	R, PC, multiple CO n=18 healthy volunteers (mean age 22 years)	3 x 2 weeks	15 g daily raw ginger root vs. 40 g daily stem ginger	Vanilla custard with either 15 g raw ginger root or 40 g stem ginger	Daily treatment with either 15 g ginger root or 40 g stem ginger mixed in custard for 14 days did not affect maximum *ex vivo* platelet thromboxane B2 production (p=0.616).
Lumb, 1994	Platelet function	R, DB, PC, CO n=8 healthy male volunteers	24 hours	Single dose of 4 capsules (2 g total) dried ginger powder	Dried ginger power (capsules prepared by researchers)	No significant differences in bleeding time, platelet count, or platelet aggregation. 2 g dried ginger unlikely to cause platelet dysfunction when used therapeutically.
Verma et al., 1993	Platelet aggregation induced by fatty diet (fed 100 g butter x 7 days)	R, PC n=20 healthy males (ages 30–50 years)	1 week	Four, 625 mg capsules 2x/day with meals	Powdered ginger capsules, 625 mg (prepared by researchers)	Ginger significantly decreased platelet aggregation (p<0.001) when taken with fatty meals. Serum cholesterol and triglyceride levels remained unchanged from ginger.
Srivastava, 1989	Thromboxane synthesis	CC, Cm n=12	1 week	5 g/day	Raw fresh ginger	Ginger inhibited eicosanoid biosynthesis. Ginger consumption produced 37% inhibition (p<0.1) on TxB2 production in serum.

Other

Author/Year	Subject	Design	Duration	Dosage	Preparation	Results/Conclusion
Altman and Marcussen, 2001	Osteoarthritis (OA) of the knee	R, DB, PC, MC, PG n=247 men and women with OA of the knee (ages ≥ 18 years)	6 weeks preceeded by 1 week washout period	One, 255 mg capsule 2x/day or placebo	EV. EXT 77, (each capsule contains 255 mg extract from 2,500– 4,000 mg dried ginger and 500–1,500 mg dried galanga [Alpinia galanga] rhizomes) or placebo	Ginger extract produced greater reduction in the primary efficacy variable, knee pain on standing, compared with placebo (63% vs. 50%; p= 0.048). Ginger extract also produced a greater response in the secondary efficacy variables compared with placebo, when analyzing mean values: reduction in knee pain after walking 50 ft (15.1 mm vs. 8.7 mm on a visual analog scale; p=0.016), reduction in the Western Ontario and McMaster Universities OA composite index (12.9 mm vs. 9.0 mm on a visual analog scale; p=0.087). The researchers concluded that this highly purified and standardized ginger extract statistically significantly reduced symptoms of OA of the knee. The ginger extract had a moderate effect and a good safety profile with usually mild g.i. adverse events in 59 patients (45%) in the ginger group compared to 21 (16%) in placebo group. An accompanying editorial noted possible lack of effective blinding (ginger patients were told of ginger's pungent taste), although the trial was otherwise well designed; nevertheless, the editorial notes ginger's beneficial effects were "small and inconsistent."
Bliddal et al., 2000	Osteoarthritis	R, PC, DB, CO, Cm n=56 (mean age 66 years)	10 weeks	170 mg ginger extract 2x/day or 400 mg ibuprofen 2x/day	EV. EXT 33 (ginger extract) vs. ibuprofen vs. placebo	Statistically significant effect demonstrated by explorative statistical methods in the first period of treatment before cross-over, but not following crossover periods. Caution should be observed in the interpretation of a cross-over study of ginger extract. The study concluded that 400 mg/day ibuprofen found to be more efficacious on pain level and function than 170 mg ginger (p<0.0001). The 3-week period of therapy and the single dosage level of ginger used may have been insufficient to discover all of ginger's effects.

KEY: **C** – controlled, **CC** – case-control, **CH** – cohort, **CI** – confidence interval, **Cm** – comparison, **CO** – crossover, **CS** – cross-sectional, **DB** – double-blind, **E** – epidemiological, **LC** – longitudinal cohort, **MA** – meta-analysis, **MC** – multi-center, **n** – number of patients, **O** – open, **OB** – observational, **OL** – open label, **OR** – odds ratio, **P** – prospective, **PB** – patient-blind, **PC** – placebo-controlled, **PG** – parallel group, **PS** – pilot study, **R** – randomized, **RC** – reference-controlled, **RCS** – retrospective cross-sectional, **RS** - retrospective, **S** – surveillance, **SB** – single-blind, **SC** – single-center, **U** – uncontrolled, **UP** – unpublished, **VC** – vehicle-controlled.

Other (cont.)

Author/Year	Subject	Design	Duration	Dosage	Preparation	Results/Conclusion
Meyer et al., 1995	Extra-corporeal chemotherapy (photo-pheresis) nausea associated with oral psoralen (8-MOP) therapy	O, Cm n=11	Not reported	Single dose of three, 530 mg capsules, 30 minutes prior to 8-MOP ingestion	Powdered ginger capsules (brand not stated)	Significantly reduced nausea induced by psoralen (8-MOP) therapy when taken 30 minutes prior to 8-MOP ingestion. Did not affect 8-MOP absorption or therapeutic effectiveness.

KEY: C – controlled, **CC** – case-control, **CH** – cohort, **CI** – confidence interval, **Cm** – comparison, **CO** – crossover, **CS** – cross-sectional, **DB** – double-blind, **E** – epidemiological, **LC** – longitudinal cohort, **MA** – meta-analysis, **MC** – multi-center, **n** – number of patients, **O** – open, **OB** – observational, **OL** – open label, **OR** – odds ratio, **P** – prospective, **PB** – patient-blind, **PC** – placebo-controlled, **PG** – parallel group, **PS** – pilot study, **R** – randomized, **RC** – reference-controlled, **RCS** – retrospective cross-sectional, **RS** - retrospective, **S** – surveillance, **SB** – single-blind, **SC** – single-center, **U** – uncontrolled, **UP** – unpublished, **VC** – vehicle-controlled.

(This page intentionally left blank.)

Ginkgo

Ginkgo biloba L.
[Fam. *Ginkgoaceae*]

OVERVIEW

Ginkgo is the oldest living species of tree on earth, dating back to the Paleozoic period (more than 225 million years ago). A standardized extract of ginkgo leaf is one of the most frequently used phytomedicines in Europe and has been one of the 10 best-selling herbs in the U.S. for about 6 years. *Ginkgo biloba* extract (GBE) is approved in Germany for treatment of cerebral insufficiency (memory loss that occurs with conditions such as Alzheimer's and vascular or multi-infarct dementia, as well as other conditions), tinnitus (ringing in the ears), vertigo, and intermittent claudication (poor circulation to the lower legs). In the U.S., ginkgo is widely used as a complementary therapy for Alzheimer's disease and vascular dementia. Ginkgo preparations consist of the dried green leaf of *Ginkgo biloba* L. [Fam.

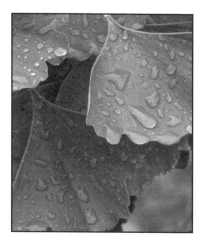

Photo © 2003 stevenfoster.com

Ginkgoaceae]. The dry extract is pharmaceutically prepared using a 35–67:1 ratio of dried leaves to final extract (50:1 is the average level at which the leading German product is based). Standardization is carried out to 22–27% ginkgo flavonol glycosides (e.g., flavones quercetin, kaempferol, and isorhamnetin) and 5–7% terpene lactones (ginkgolides and bilobalide). In Germany, the content of ginkgolic acid is limited to a concentration of 5 ppm. The scientific literature shows little or no support for clinical benefits of other dosage forms of crude ginkgo leaf or low concentration extracts made from the leaf.

PRIMARY USES

- Cerebral insufficiency: memory deficit, poor concentration, depression, and headache resulting from demential syndromes; attention and memory loss that occur with Alzheimer's disease and multi-infarct dementia
- Vertigo and tinnitus (ringing in the ear) of vascular and involutional origin
- Peripheral vascular disease: improvement of pain-free walking distance in Peripheral Arterial Occlusive Disease in Stage II according to Fontaine (intermittent claudication)

in a regimen of physical therapeutic measures, in particular walking exercise

OTHER POTENTIAL USES

- Sexual dysfunction associated with SSRI use
- Control of acute altitude sickness symptoms and vascular reactivity to cold exposure
- Protective action in hypoxia
- Acute cochlear deafness

PHARMACOLOGICAL ACTIONS

Improvements in: cognition, working memory, short-term visual memory in dementia, short-term memory in cerebral insufficiency, social functioning in people with dementia, concentration in people with dementia, attention in people with dementia, tinnitus in people with dementia, intermittent claudication, activities of daily living (ADL) scores in people under 60 years old, mood and sleep in older individuals; increases in alpha wave brain activity; decreases in theta wave activity; inhibits binding of platelet activating factor (PAF) to platelets resulting in inhibited platelet aggregation and increased blood fluidity; reduces thrombosis, inflammation, allergy, and bronchoconstriction.

DOSAGE AND ADMINISTRATION

The German Commission E makes the following recommendations: for chronic cognitive disorders, a minimum of 8 weeks with administration for more than 3 months subject to medical review; for intermittent claudication, not less than 6 weeks; for vertigo and tinnitus (vascular origin), use for more than 6–8 weeks has no therapeutic benefit.

Clinical studies suggest the following duration: for cerebral insufficiency, 4 weeks to one year as observed in clinical trials—improvements are usually seen after 8–12 weeks of treatment; 24 weeks for peripheral vascular disease.

DRY EXTRACT (STANDARDIZED): 40–60 mg in solid pharmaceutical form 2–3 times daily to treat dementia syndromes (120–240 mg/day); or 40–60 mg dry extract 2–3 times daily to treat intermittent claudication, vertigo, and tinnitus (120–160 mg/day).

CONTRAINDICATIONS

Ginkgo should not be used in persons who have a history of allergy to ginkgo. It is also contraindicated in bleeding disorders due to increased bleeding potential associated with chronic use (6–12 months) or before elective surgery. The 120 mg dosage should not be used in children under 12 years. Clinicians are advised to use all necessary precautionary measures in administering ginkgo extracts for treatment of depressive mood and headache not associated with demential syndromes since these conditions have not been sufficiently investigated.

PREGNANCY AND LACTATION: No known restrictions.

ADVERSE EFFECTS

Rare cases of stomach or intestinal upsets, headaches, or allergic skin reactions have been documented. Ginkgo has also been reported to cause dizziness and palpitations. In higher than recommended doses, diarrhea, nausea, vomiting, restlessness, and weakness may occur. Several case reports of bleeding associated with ginkgo use have been reported, including two reports of subdural hematoma, one report of subarachnoid hemorrhage, one report of intracerebral hemorrhage, and one report of anterior chamber bleeding in the eye (hyphema).

DRUG INTERACTIONS

Ginkgo extract may potentiate MAO-inhibiting drugs but the evidence is conflicting.

Ginkgo preparations may enhance the effect of antiplatelet agents (e.g., aspirin); in one case, a spontaneous hyphema occurred after combined intake of ginkgo and aspirin. Ginkgo may enhance the effect of warfarin, although no interaction was shown in a controlled trial. However, the true risks of these interactions are somewhat speculative and difficult to characterize due to the nature and limited number of existing reports. Ginkgo may also potentiate the effect of thiazide diuretics by increasing capillary permeability; however, no clinical relevance has been established as yet for this finding.

CLINICAL REVIEW

More than 120 clinical studies have been published on standardized ginkgo extract. Of 35 studies (3,541 participants) outlined in the table, "Clinical Studies on Ginkgo," only 2 trials found negative results: 1 study on dementia and 1 study on tinnitus. The remaining 33 studies demonstrated positive effects for indications including Alzheimer's disease and dementia, peripheral vascular disease (intermittent claudication), asthma, acute mountain (altitude) sickness, deafness, adjunct therapy in colorectal cancer, sexual dysfunction, and depression.

Eighteen studies (1,672 participants) supported the use of ginkgo in treating dementia due to cardiovascular insufficiency, Alzheimer's disease, or multi-infarct dementia; to slow the clinical deterioration of patients with dementia; or to improve cognitive symptoms. Of these 18 studies, 5 were randomized, double-blind, placebo-controlled, multi-center (R, DB, PC, MC) studies (663 participants); 11 were R, DB, PC (898 participants); and 2 were R, DB, PC, crossover (CO) studies (111 participants).

Three R, DB, PC studies (264 participants) showed positive results for treatment of peripheral arterial insufficiency/intermittent claudication with ginkgo.

Of the remaining studies investigating the use of ginkgo for various disorders, one R, DB, PC study (20 participants) found inconclusive results in the use of ginkgo for moderately severe depression; one R, DB, PC, CO study (8 participants) showed

positive effects for hypoxia; three DB, PC studies (110 participants) found positive effects on altitude sickness; one R, DB, PC, MC study (103 patients) found ginkgo improved the evolution of tinnitus; one R, DB, C study (20 participants) found ginkgo superior to nicergoline for acute cochlear deafness; one PC study (61 patients) reported positive effects in asthma; one open-labeled study (63 participants) found positive effects for sexual dysfunction secondary to antidepressant use; one Phase II study (32 participants) suggests a good benefit-risk ratio of ginkgo combined with 5-FU therapy as second-line treatment for advance colorectal cancer; and one DB study (12 participants) investigating the effect of ginkgo extract on brain electrophysiology found significant pharmacological effects on the central nervous system; and one R, DB, PC, CO study (21 participants) concluded that warfarin and ginkgo do not interact.

NOTE: the reviews and meta-analyses discussed below are not listed in the table of Clinical Studies on Ginkgo.

In a review of 40 clinical studies conducted through 1991 on the use of ginkgo for symptoms associated with cerebral insufficiency, eight R, DB, PC trials met the inclusion criteria. All but one concluded that ginkgo extract was as effective as co-dergocrine and superior to placebo. Ginkgo was well-tolerated, and side-effects compared favorably to five studies assessing Hydergine®, another widely-used product for cerebral insufficiency. Ginkgo and Hydergine® were deemed equally effective for treatment of cerebral insufficiency.

In a review and meta-analysis of the scientific literature, researchers evaluated the effects of treatment with ginkgo extract on objective measures of cognitive function in elderly patients with vascular dementia, cognitive impairment, or both. Only 4 out of 50 articles met inclusion criteria. Standardized ginkgo extract produced a significant effect size of 0.40 on cognitive function in Alzheimer's ($p<0.0001$) comparable with the findings of a trial on donepezil. A comparison review of placebo-controlled efficacy studies evaluated the clinical relevance of acetylcholinesterase inhibitors and ginkgo special extract EGb 761 with respect to Alzheimer's dementia. The study concluded that EGb 761 and second generation cholinesterase inhibitors are equally effective in treating mild to moderate Alzheimer's dementia. A meta-analysis of nine DB, PC trials found that ginkgo extract was more effective for dementia than placebo, with few adverse side effects. A review of trials on the use of ginkgo for clinical improvement of memory and other cognitive functions concluded that ginkgo produces a significant therapeutic benefit; however, long-term studies have not evaluated ginkgo's sustained benefits in cognitive function, especially if drug therapy is subsequently interrupted. A Cochrane Review of 33 trials concluded that they showed "promising evidence" for treating dementia. The Cochrane Review concluded that in one identified trial on ginkgo and age-related macular degeneration, a beneficial effect was observed. However, the author encourages additional research due to the small number of patients included in the trial.

One meta-analysis of eight R, DB, PC studies concluded that ginkgo is effective for intermittent claudication but questioned the clinical relevance based on the modest size of the overall treatment effect.

Ginkgo

Ginkgo biloba L.
[Fam. *Ginkgoaceae*]

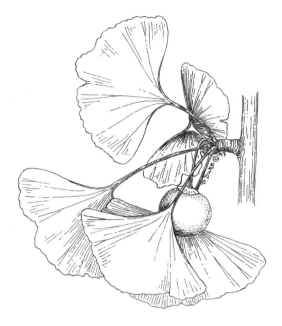

OVERVIEW

Ginkgo, the oldest living species of tree on earth, is more than 225 million years old. A standardized extract of ginkgo leaf is presently one of the most frequently used plant-based medicines in Europe. In the U.S., it has been one of the 10 best-selling herbs for more than five years. In Germany, ginkgo is also an approved therapy for the treatment of memory loss in conditions such as Alzheimer's, ringing in the ears, dizziness, and poor circulation in the lower legs resulting in pain during walking (intermittent claudication).

USES

Poor memory, poor concentration, depression, and headache occurring with dementia diagnosed by a health-care practitioner; attention and memory loss in Alzheimer's; ringing in ears (tinnitus); dizziness or whirling sensation (vertigo); peripheral vascular disease including poor circulation to the lower legs (intermittent claudication).

OTHER POTENTIAL USES

Sexual dysfunction associated with use of SSRI drugs (selective serotonin reuptake inhibitors); control of acute symptoms of altitude sickness and vascular reactivity to cold exposure; protective action in hypoxia (insufficient oxygen in the body); acute deafness related to the cochlea (part of the inner ear).

DOSAGE

DRY EXTRACT (STANDARDIZED): a total of 120–240 mg per day, taken in dosage forms (e.g., tablets or capsules) of 40–60 mg each, 2 or 3 times daily to treat dementia; or a daily total of 120–160 mg, taken in 40–60 mg doses, 2 or 3 times daily to treat intermittent claudication, vertigo, and ringing in the ears (tinnitus).

CONTRAINDICATIONS

Ginkgo should not be used before elective surgery or in persons who are allergic to ginkgo or have a bleeding disorder. The 120 mg dosage should not be used in children under 12 years.

PREGNANCY AND LACTATION: No known restrictions.

ADVERSE EFFECTS

Stomach or intestinal upsets, headaches, or allergic skin reactions occur rarely. Dizziness and pounding heartbeat may also occur. Isolated cases of bleeding (subdural hematoma, subarachnoid hemorrhage, intracerebral hemorrhage, anterior chamber bleeding in the eye [hyphema]) have been reported, but these reactions are extremely rare.

DRUG INTERACTIONS

Ginkgo extract may possibly increase the effects of monoamine oxidase inhibiting (MAOI) drugs. Ginkgo preparations may increase the effect of blood-thinning drugs such as aspirin and warfarin. Gingko may also enhance the effect of thiazide diuretics.

Comments

When using a dietary supplement, purchase it from a reliable source. For best results, use the same brand of product throughout the period of use. As with all medications and dietary supplements, please inform your healthcare provider of all herbs and medications you are taking. Interactions may occur between medications and herbs or even among different herbs when taken at the same time. Treat your herbal supplement with care by taking it as directed, storing it as advised on the label, and keeping it out of the reach of children and pets. Consult your healthcare provider with any questions.

AMERICAN
BOTANICAL
COUNCIL

The information contained on this sheet has been excerpted from *The ABC Clinical Guide to Herbs* © 2003 by the American Botanical Council (ABC). ABC is an independent member-based educational organization focusing on the medicinal use of herbs. For more detailed information about this herb please consult the healthcare provider who gave you this sheet. To order *The ABC Clinical Guide to Herbs* or become a member of ABC, visit their website at www.herbalgram.org.

Ginkgo

Patient Information Sheet

Ginkgo
Ginkgo biloba L.
[Fam. *Ginkgoaceae*]

OVERVIEW

Ginkgo is the oldest living species of tree on earth, dating back to the Paleozoic period, over 225 million years ago. The medicinal use of ginkgo leaf is first mentioned in Chinese medicine in the Ming dynasty in 1436 (Foster, 1996). A standardized extract of ginkgo leaf is one of the most clinically tested and frequently prescribed phytomedicines in Europe, and has been one of the 10 best-selling herbal dietary supplements in the U.S. for about six years (Blumenthal *et al.,* 1998, 2001). *Ginkgo biloba* extract (GBE) is approved in Germany for the treatment of cerebral insufficiency (memory loss that occurs with conditions such as Alzheimer's disease, vascular or multi-infarct dementia, and other conditions), tinnitus (ringing in the ears), vertigo, and intermittent claudication (poor circulation to the lower legs). In the U.S, ginkgo is used widely as a complementary therapy for Alzheimer's disease and vascular dementia (Oken *et al.,* 1998). For comprehensive detailed reviews, see DeFeudis (1998) and McKenna *et al.* (2001).

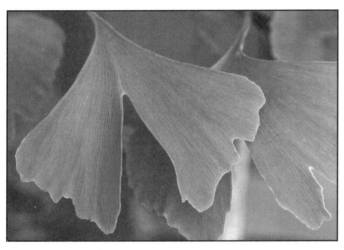

Photo © 2003 stevenfoster.com

DESCRIPTION

Ginkgo preparations are derived from the dried, green leaf of *Ginkgo biloba* L. [Fam. *Ginkgoaceae*]. Ginkgo extracts are usually manufactured using acetone and water, and subsequent purification steps, without addition of concentrates or isolated ingredients. The dry extract is prepared pharmaceutically using a 35–67:1 ratio of dried leaves to final extract (50:1 is the average level at which the leading German product is based). Standardization is carried out to 22–27% ginkgo flavonol glycosides (e.g., the flavones quercetin, kaempferol, and isorhamnetin) and 5–7% terpene lactones (ginkgolides and bilobalide). In Germany, the content of ginkgolic acid is limited to a concentration of 5 parts per million (ppm). Scientific literature gives little or no support of the clinical benefits of other dosage forms

of crude ginkgo leaf or low concentration extracts made from the leaf (Blumenthal *et al.*, 2000).

PRIMARY USES

Neurology

- Cerebral insufficiency:
  The German Commission E approved ginkgo for the following symptoms resulting from demential syndromes: memory deficit, poor concentration, depression, dizziness, tinnitus, and headache (Blumenthal *et al.,*1998)

  Treatment of attention and memory loss that occur with Alzheimer's disease and multi-infarct dementia (Arrigo, 1986; Brautigam *et al.*, 1998; Grässel, 1992; Halama *et al.*, 1988; Hofferberth, 1994; Hofferberth, 1989; Kanowski *et al.*, 1997; Kleijnen and Knipschild, 1992; Le Bars *et al.*, 1997; Oken *et al.*, 1998; Rigney *et al.*, 1999; Taillandier *et al.*, 1986; Vesper and Hansgen, 1994; Wesnes *et al.*, 1987)

- Vertigo and tinnitus (ringing in the ear) of vascular and involutional origin (Morgenstern and Biermann, 2002; Meyer, 1986; Dubreuil, 1986)

Vascular Disease

- Peripheral vascular disease: improvement of pain-free walking distance in Peripheral Arterial Occlusive Disease in Stage II according to Fontaine (intermittent claudication) in a regimen of physical therapeutic measures, in particular walking exercise (Bauer, 1984; Peters *et al.*, 1998; Schweizer and Hautmann, 1999; Pittler and Ernst, 2000) approved by Commission E (Blumenthal *et al.*, 1998)

OTHER POTENTIAL USES

- Sexual dysfunction secondary to selective serotonin reuptake inhibitor (SSRI) use (Cohen and Bartlik,1998)
- Control of acute altitude sickness and vascular reactivity to cold exposure (Leadbetter *et al.*, 2001; Roncin *et al.*, 1996)
- Protective action in hypoxia (Schaffler and Reeh, 1985)
- Acute cochlear deafness (Dubreuil, 1986)

DOSAGE

Internal

Standardized Preparations

DRY EXTRACT: total of 120–240 mg solid pharmaceutical form per day, administered in small doses (e.g., 40–60 mg) 2–3 times daily to treat dementia syndromes (Blumenthal *et al.*, 1998), or total of 120–160 mg dry extract per day, administered in doses of 40–60 mg 2–3 times daily to treat intermittent claudication, vertigo, and tinnitus (Blumenthal *et al.*, 1998; WHO, 1999).

DURATION OF ADMINISTRATION

German Commission E made the following recommendations: for chronic cognitive disorders, a minimum of eight weeks with administration for more than three months subject to medical review; for intermittent claudication, not less than six weeks; for vertigo and tinnitus (vascular origin), use for more than six to eight weeks has no therapeutic benefit (Blumenthal et al., 1998).

Clinical studies suggest the following duration: for cerebral insufficiency, four weeks to one year as observed in clinical trials (Kanowski et al., 1997; Grässel, 1992; Le Bars et al., 1997; Taillandier et al., 1986; Hofferberth, 1994; Vesper and Hansgen, 1994; Brautigam et al., 1998; Halama et al., 1988; Hofferberth, 1989; Wesnes et al., 1987; Arrigo, 1986; Rigney et al., 1999). Improvements are typically seen after eight to twelve weeks of treatment; 24 weeks for peripheral vascular disease (Bauer, 1984; Peters et al., 1998; Schweizer and Hautmann, 1999; Pittler and Ernst, 2000).

CHEMISTRY
Standardized Preparations
The active constituents in ginkgo extract are unique diterpene lactones, ginkgolides A, B, C, and J, and the sesquiterpene lactone bilobalide (WHO, 1999). Standardized dry ginkgo extract contains 22–27% ginkgo flavonol glycosides (based on flavones like quercetin, kaempferol, and isorhamnetin) and 5–7% terpene lactones of which 2.9% is bilobalide and 3.1% the ginkgolides A, B, and C (Kleijnen and Knipshild, 1992). The relative amounts of the various flavonoids or the ginkgolide and bilobalide components of the terpenoids may vary across different commercial preparations (Sticher, 1993). Ginkgo extract contains trace amounts of ginkgolic acid, a potential allergen, which is limited to a maximum of 5 ppm by German authorities (Blumenthal et al., 1998). Extensive reviews of ginkgo chemistry have been written (Van Beek, 1998; Tang and Eisenbrandt, 1992; Braquet, 1988,1989).

PHARMACOLOGICAL ACTIONS
Humans
Improves cognition (Rigney et al., 1999; Le Bars et al., 1997); improves working memory (Rigney et al., 1999); improves short-term visual memory in people with dementia (Brautigam et al., 1998); improves short-term memory in people with cerebral insufficiency (Grässel, 1992); improves social functioning in people with dementia (Le Bars et al., 1997); improves concentration in people with dementia (Vesper and Hansgen, 1994); improves attention in people with dementia (Hofferberth, 1989); improves tinnitus in people with dementia (Halama et al., 1988; Arrigo, 1986); improves intermittent claudication (Pittler and Ernst 2000; Schweizer and Hautmann, 1999; Peters et al., 1998; Bauer, 1984); increases alpha wave brain activity and decreases theta wave activity (Brown, 1997); improves activities of daily living (ADL) scores in people under 60 years old, and improves mood and sleep in older individuals (Cockle et al., 2000). Inhibits binding of platelet activating factor (PAF) to platelets, which inhibits platelet aggregation and increases blood fluidity (Jung et al., 1990; Guinot et al., 1989); reduces thrombosis, inflammation, allergy, and bronchoconstriction (Smith et al., 1996), increases pancreatic β-cell function with increased insulin and C-peptide levels (Kudolo, 2000).

Animal
Protects against cerebral ischemia (WHO, 1999; Larssen et al., 1978; Rapin et al., 1986; Le Poncin-Lafitte et al., 1980); decreases cerebral edema induced by trauma or toxins (Chatterjee and Gabard, 1984; Otani et al., 1986; Borzeix, 1985; Blumenthal et al., 1998); improves memory and learning (WHO, 1999; Winter, 1991); increases arteriolar diameter in the pia mater and increases cerebral blood flow by intravenous infusion (WHO, 1999; Krieglstein et al., 1986).

In vitro
Inhibits lipid peroxidation (Cott, 1995); flavonoids and terpenoid constituents are antioxidant and free radical scavenging (Pincemail et al., 1989; WHO, 1999); attacks oxygen free radicals (Sastre et al., 1998); inhibits monoamine oxidase A and B (White et al., 1996) but more recent research has shown that ginkgo does not inhibit MAO in vivo (Fowler et al., 2000; Porsolt, 2000); inhibits platelet aggregation (Van Beek et al., 1998); protects against apoptosis (Ahlemeyer and Krieglstein, 1998); protects against cerebral hypoxia (Oberpichler et al., 1988; Krieglstein, 1995; Blumenthal et al., 1998).

MECHANISM OF ACTION
Ginkgolides (primarily ginkgolide B)
• Inhibit platelet activating factor (PAF) (WHO, 1999; Bracquet, 1988, 1989; Oberpichler, 1990).
• Inhibit 3'5'-cyclic GMP phosphodiesterase, leading to endothelium relaxation (WHO, 1999; DeFeudis, 1991).

Flavonoid fraction (especially quercetin)
• Increases serotonin release and uptake (Ahlemeyer and Krieglstein, 1998).
• Inhibits age-related reduction of muscarinergic cholinoceptors and alpha-adrenoceptors, and stimulates choline uptake in the hippocampus (DeFeudis, 1998; Blumenthal et al., 1998).
• Acts as a free-radical scavenger (Smith et al, 1996).
• Inhibits nitric oxide formation, which may cause its neuroprotective effects. Pre-treatment (15 days) with ginkgo reduced significantly, in a dose-dependent manner, post-ischemic brain MDA levels and post-ischemic brain edema (Calapai et al., 2000).
• Antagonism of PAF, antioxidant and metabolic actions, and effects on neurotransmitters may be due to the flavonoids and terpenoids, acting together or separately (Logani et al., 2000).

CONTRAINDICATIONS
Ginkgo should not be used by persons who have a history of allergy to the herb (this is considered rare) (Blumenthal et al., 1998; Brinker, 2001). It is also contraindicated in bleeding disorders due to increased bleeding potential associated with chronic use (6–12 months) or before elective surgery (Brinker, 2001). The product sheet of the leading ginkgo preparation (EGb 761) notes that the 120 mg dosage should not be used in children under 12. In addition, it recommends to use all necessary precautionary measures in administering ginkgo extracts for treatment of depressive mood and headache not associated with demential syndromes since these conditions have not been sufficiently investigated (Schwabe, 2001).

PREGNANCY AND LACTATION: According to Commission E, no known restrictions (Blumenthal et al., 1998) although no long-term studies have been conducted on pregnant or lactating woman.

ADVERSE EFFECTS
In general, ginkgo extract has produced few adverse effects in clinical trials, with effects for ginkgo being the same as for

placebo. Rare cases of stomach or intestinal upsets, headaches, or allergic skin reaction have been documented (Blumenthal *et al.*, 1998). Ginkgo has also been reported to cause dizziness and palpitations. Several case reports of bleeding associated with ginkgo use have been reported, including two reports of subdural hematoma (Rowin and Lewis, 1996; Gilbert, 1997), one report of subarachnoid hemorrhage (Vale, 1998), one report of intracerebral hemorrhage (Matthews, 1998), and one report of anterior chamber bleeding in the eye (hyphema) (Rosenblatt and Mindel, 1997). However, animal experiments have suggested a protective effect of ginkgo extract on subarachnoid hemorrhage-induced vasospasm and vasculopathy (Kurtsoy *et al.*, 2000).

DRUG INTERACTIONS
MAO-Inhibition
A safety review suggested that ginkgo extract may potentiate MAO-inhibiting drugs (McGuffin *et al.*, 1997), but the evidence is questionable. Recent studies have concluded that ginkgo does not inhibit MAO *in vivo*, and that a different mechanism may be responsible for some of ginkgo's effects on the central nervous system (Fowler *et al.*, 2000; Porsolt *et al.*, 2000).

Anticoagulants and antiplatelet drugs
Interaction with drugs inhibiting blood coagulation cannot be excluded. A single case of a spontaneous hyphema after combined intake of a ginkgo-containing pharmaceutical preparation and aspirin has been documented (Rosenblatt and Mindel, 1997). However, in a placebo-controlled double-blind study carried out in 50 subjects over a period of 7 days, interactions of ginkgo special extract EGb 761 (daily dose 240 mg) with acetyl salicylic acid (aspirin, daily dose 500 mg) could not be demonstrated (Schwabe, 2001). There is a single case of an intracerebral hemorrhage after concomitant intake of warfarin and ginkgo described in the literature (Matthews, 1998). However, further investigation revealed that the patient received two other drugs (amiodarone and lovastatin) with known interactions with warfarin (Schwabe, 1998). A recent randomized, double-blind, placebo-controlled crossover study has concluded that ginkgo does not interact with warfarin (Engelsen *et al.*, 2002).

Diuretics
One old case report of intravenous use of ginkgo (300 mg/day) speculated the possibility that ginkgo may potentiate the effect of thiazide diuretics by increasing capillary permeability, but the clinical relevance, if any, is not clear (Lagrue *et al.*, 1986). A review of this case suggests that ginkgo did not increase capillary permeability but decreased the shock-induced hyperpermeability (Busse, 2001).

Anticonvulsants
One paper reported the presence of a potential neurotoxin (4'-*O*-methylpyroxidine) in both the ginkgo leaf and seed; the author suggests that ginkgo should thus be used with caution by epileptic patients being treated with anticonvulsants (Arenz *et al.*, 1996). However, an analysis of this case report shows that the toxic concentration of this compound after oral administration of ginkgo is 11 mg/kg of body weight (BW). Thus, the toxic dose is an estimated 11,000 times higher than the maximum daily dose of commercial ginkgo extract (60 mcg) corresponding to 1 mcg/kg BW (Leistner, 1997). Further, the bilobalide in ginkgo has anticonvulsant effects (Sasaki *et al.*, 1995). Thus, there is no clinical evidence to support cautions regarding use of ginkgo extract with anticonvulsants.

Antidepressant
Ginkgo can offset sexual dysfunction symptoms in patients taking antidepressants (SSRIs, MAOIs, and tricyclics) (Brinker, 2001).

Other
Use of ginkgo for 12–18 months potentiated papaverine intracavernosal injections in men where papaverine alone was previously ineffective (Sikora *et al.*, 1989). Use of ginkgo before and after kidney transplant helped prevent PAF-induced organ rejection when used with cyclosporine (Brinker, 2001). In one case report, ginkgo used with trazodone resulted in coma that was immediately resolved by injection of 1 mg flumazenil (Brinker, 2001).

AMERICAN HERBAL PRODUCTS ASSOCIATION (AHPA) SAFETY RATING
CLASS 1: Herbs that can be safely consumed when used appropriately.

REGULATORY STATUS
ARGENTINA: Standardized extracts (Ginkgo NF) are approved for peripheral and cerebrovascular disorders.

AUSTRIA: A standardized extract (EGb 761) is approved for cerebral and nutritional insufficiencies, dementia, intermittent claudication, and supportive treatment of hearing deficits.

BRAZIL: Standardized extracts (Ginkgo NF) are approved for cerebrovascular deficits; peripheral vascular disorders; neurosensorial disorders of vascular origin in the ears, eyes, and nose, and migraine headaches.

CANADA: New Drug if claims made. Extract form is unacceptable as food ingredient (HPB, 1993). Permitted as a homeopathic drug requiring premarket authorization and assignment of a Drug Identification Number (DIN). Thirty-two ginkgo homeopathic preparations are listed in the Drug Product Database (DPD) (Health Canada, 2001).

DENMARK: Standardized ginkgo extracts (most of which comply with Ginkgo NF) are approved for memory and concentration deficits, tiredness, continuing dizziness, and tinnitus in the elderly, tendency to cold extremities, and intermittent claudication.

FRANCE: Marketed under the brand name Tanakan® (EGb 761) is a prescription medication (Itil *et al.*, 1996). The standardized extract (EGb 761) is approved for treating symptoms of cerebral insufficiencies, intermittent claudication, Raynaud's disease, certain dizziness and/or tinnitus syndromes, and retinal conditions due to probable ischemia.

GERMANY: Only semi-purified normalized (standardized) dry extracts (35–67:1) with less than 5 ppm ginkolic acids are approved drugs of the German Commission E; Active Ingredient Classification ASK No. 05939 (Blumenthal *et al.*, 1998). Dry extract, (35–67:1) is official in the *German Pharmacopoeia*, standardized to contain no less than 22.0% and no more than 27.0% flavone glycosides, as well as no less than 5.0% and no more than 7.0% terpene lactones, of which 2.8–3.4% are ginkgolides A, B, and C and 2.5–3.2% are bilobalide (DAB, 2000). Licensed for the treatment of cerebral dysfunction with attendant memory loss, dementia, poor concentration, etc., plus vertigo and tinnitus of vascular origin, and for intermittent claudication (Blumenthal *et al.*, 1998). Marketed both as a prescription and a nonprescription drug.

MEXICO: Standardized extracts (Ginkgo NF) are approved for treating diminished mental capacities, demential syndromes, dizziness, and tinnitus.

SPAIN: A standardized extract (Ginkgo NF) is approved for cerebral insufficiencies (such as dizziness, headache, and memory deficits), and peripheral vascular disorders.

SWEDEN: Classified as Natural Remedy, requiring premarket authorization. As of January, 2001, six ginkgo products are listed in the Medical Products Agency (MPA) "Authorised Natural Remedies," and a monograph is published with the approved indication: "Herbal remedy for the treatment of long-standing symptoms in elderly people such as difficulties of memory and concentration, vertigo, tinnitus and feeling of tiredness. Prior to treatment other serious conditions should have been ruled out by doctor" (MPA, 1998, 2001; Tunón, 1999).

SWITZERLAND: Herbal medicine with positive classification (List D) by the *Interkantonale Konstrollstellefar Heilmittel* (IKS) and corresponding sales Category D with sale limited to pharmacies and drugstores, without prescription (Morant and Ruppanner, 2001; Ruppanner and Schaefer, 2000). There are nine ginkgo monopreparation phytomedicines, nine polypreparations and three ginkgo homeopathic preparations listed in the *Swiss Codex 2000/01* (Ruppanner and Schaefer, 2000). Standardized ginkgo extracts, most of which comply with Ginkgo NF, are approved for concentration difficulties, forgetfulness, and dizziness (due to arteriosclerotic complaints).

U.K.: Not entered in the *General Sale List* (GSL). Standardized extracts, are available.

U.S.: Dietary supplement (USC, 1994). Dried leaf containing no less than 0.8% flavonol glycosides is official in the *National Formulary* 19th edition (USP 25-NF 20, 2002). Standardized extracts are commonly sold.

CLINICAL REVIEW

More than 120 clinical studies have been published on standardized ginkgo extract. The table "Clinical Studies on Ginkgo" outlines 35 studies including 3,541 participants. Two trials found negative results: one on dementia (Van Dongen *et al.*, 2000) and one on tinnitus (Drew and Davies, 2001). The remaining 33 studies found positive effects for indications including Alzheimer's disease and dementia, peripheral vascular disease (intermittent claudication), asthma, acute mountain (altitude) sickness, deafness, adjunct therapy in colorectal cancer, sexual dysfunction, and depression.

Eighteen studies involving a total of 1,672 participants supported the use of ginkgo in treating dementia due to cardiovascular insufficiency, Alzheimer's disease, or multi-infarct dementia, or to slow the clinical deterioration of patients with dementia or to improve cognitive symptoms. Of these 18 studies, five were randomized, double-blind, placebo controlled, multi-center (R, DB, PC, MC) studies involving a total of 663 participants (Le Bars *et al.*, 1997; Kanowski *et al.*, 1997; Grässel, 1992; Vesper and Hansgen, 1994; Taillandier *et al.*, 1986); 11 were R, DB, PC with a total of 898 participants (Brautigam *et al.*, 1998; Hofferberth, 1994, 1989; Halama, 1991; Rai *et al.*, 1991; Schmidt *et al.*, 1991; Brüchert *et al.*, 1991; Eckmann, 1990; Vorberg *et al.*, 1989; Halama *et al.*, 1988; Wesnes *et al.*, 1987); and two were R, DB, PC, crossover (CO) studies involving a total of 111 participants (Rigney *et al.*, 1999; Arrigo, 1986).

Three R, DB, PC studies (Bauer, 1984; Peters *et al.*, 1998; Schweizer and Hautmann, 1999), with a total of 264 participants, focused on ginkgo for treatment of peripheral arterial insufficiency/intermittent claudication, with positive results.

Of the remaining studies investigating the use of ginkgo for various disorders, one R, DB, PC study (20 participants) found inconclusive results for the use of ginkgo for moderately severe depression (Halama, 1990); one R, DB, PC, CO study (8 participants) found positive effects for hypoxia (Schaffler and Reeh 1985); two R, DB, PC studies and one DB, PC study on altitude sickness (total 110 participants) had positive results (Gertsch *et al.*, 2002; Roncin *et al.*, 1996; Leadbetter *et al.*, 2001); one R, DB, PC, MC study (Meyer, 1986) on 103 patients found ginkgo improved the evolution of tinnitus; one R, DB, C study (20 participants) (Dubreuil, 1986) found ginkgo superior to nicergoline for acute cochlear deafness; one PC study of 61 patients with asthma reported positive effects (Li *et al.*, 1997); one open-labeled study (63 participants) investigating sexual dysfunction secondary to antidepressant use found positive effects (Cohen and Bartlik, 1998); one Phase II study (32 participants) suggests a good benefit-risk ratio of ginkgo combined with 5-FU therapy as second line treatment for advance colorectal cancer (Hauns et al., 2001); and one DB study (12 participants) investigating the effect of ginkgo extract on brain electrophysiology found that pharmacological effects on the central nervous system are statistically significant when compared to placebo (Itil *et al.*, 1996). One R, DB, PC, CO study (21 participants) concluded that warfarin and ginkgo do not interact (Engelsen *et al.*, 2002).

NOTE: the reviews and meta-analyses discussed below are not listed in the table "Clinical Studies on Ginkgo." In a review of 40 clinical studies conducted through 1991 on the use of ginkgo for symptoms associated with cerebral insufficiency, eight R, DB, PC trials of the 40 studies met inclusion criteria for a well-designed study (Kleijnen and Knipschild, 1992). All but one (Hartmann and Frick, 1991) of these eight studies concluded that ginkgo extract was as effective as co-dergocrine and superior to placebo. Symptoms most often reported improved were concentration and memory, anxiety, dizziness, tinnitus, and headache. Ginkgo was well-tolerated and side effects compared favorably to five studies assessing Hydergine®, another widely-used product for cerebral insufficiency. Ginkgo and Hydergine® were deemed equally effective for treatment of cerebral insufficiency.

A recent Cochrane review of 33 trials on ginkgo extract found that the trials showed "promising evidence of improvement in cognition and function" (Birks *et al.*, 2002).

In a review and meta-analysis of the scientific literature, researchers evaluated the effects of treatment with ginkgo extract on objective measures of cognitive function in elderly patients with vascular dementia, cognitive impairment, or both (Oken *et al.*, 1998). Of more than 50 articles, only four met reasonable inclusion criteria for adequate clinical trial design, with a total of 212 subjects in each of the placebo and ginkgo treatment groups (Le Bars *et al.*, 1997; Hofferberth, 1994; Kanowski *et al.*, 1997; Wesnes *et al.*, 1987). Standardized ginkgo extract produced a significant effect size of 0.40 on cognitive function in Alzheimer's (p<0.0001) comparable with the findings of a trial on donepezil (Rogers *et al.*, 1998). The clinical trials reviewed did not determine whether there is improvement in noncognitive behavior or daily function. A comparison review of PC efficacy studies evaluated the clinical relevance of acetylcholinesterase inhibitors and ginkgo special extract EGb 761 for Alzheimer's dementia. The study concluded that EGb 761 and second generation cholinesterase inhibitors are equally effective in treating mild to moderate Alzheimer's dementia (Wettstein, 2000). A meta-analysis of nine DB, PC trials found ginkgo extract more effective for dementia than placebo, with few adverse side effects (Ernst and Pittler, 1999). A review of trials on ginkgo use for clinical improvement of memory and other cognitive functions found that ginkgo produces a significant therapeutic benefit; however, long-term studies have not evaluated its sustained benefits in cognitive function, especially if drug therapy is subsequently interrupted. The author cites the need for further studies to test the relative efficacy of different doses of ginkgo (Soholm, 1998).

The Cochrane Review selected R, controlled trials (C) that studied ginkgo and age-related macular degeneration. The review concluded that in the one identified trial on that condition, a beneficial effect was observed on 20 patients. However, the author encourages additional research due to the small number of patients included in the trial (Evans, 2000).

One meta-analysis of eight R, DB, PC studies (Pittler and Ernst, 2000) concluded that ginkgo is effective for intermittent claudication but questioned the clinical relevance based on the modest size of the overall treatment effect; patients in the ginkgo groups had a longer distance of pain-free walking than those in the placebo groups (average increase of 34 meters).

Shortly after completion of this monograph, a new study on ginkgo extract for cognitive abilities in healthy older adults (over 60) was published finding no significant improvement in various measured parameters at a dose of 120 mg/day for four weeks (Solomon et al., 2002). Previously, at least four trials of various sizes and designs had suggested that ginkgo extract did contribute to increased mental performance in asymptomatic subjects (Mix and Crews, 2002; Stough et al., 2001; Mix and Crews, 2000).

The most comprehensive review of research and clinical information on ginkgo is compiled by DeFeudis (1998).

BRANDED PRODUCTS*

Bio-Biloba®: Pharma Nord ApS / Sadelmagervej 30-32, DK-7100 / Vejle / Denmark / Tel: +43-75-85-7400 / Fax: +43-75-85-7474 / www.pharmanord.com.

Concentrated Ginkgo leaf liquid: Quindao Fengyi Biotechnology Limited. Contact information not available. Each milliliter contains 14.5 mg flavone glycosides and 2.8 mg terpene lactones.

EGb-761: Dr. Willmar Schwabe Pharmaceuticals / International Division / Willmar Schwabe Str. 4, D-76227 / Karlsruhe / Germany / Tel: +49-721-4005 ext. 294 / www.schwabepharma.com / Email: melville-eaves@schwabe.de. The standardized mono-extract of dried leaves from ginkgo (50:1) consists of 24% ginkgo flavonol glycosides and 6% terpene lactones, of which 2.9% is bilobalide and 3.1% is the ginkgolides A, B, and C. Contains less than 5 ppm ginkgolic acids and conforms to the German Commission E requirements for GBE.

Geriaforce®: CH-9325 Roggwil TG / Switzerland / Tel: +41 71 454 61 61 / Fax: +41 71 454 61 62 / www.bioforce.com / Email: info@bioforce.ch. Each tablet contains an ethanolic extract of fresh leaves 1:4, with a content of flavonol glycosides of 0.20 mg/ml and ginkgolides 0.34 mg/ml.

Ginkgold®: Nature's Way Products, Inc. / 10 Mountain Spring Parkway / Springville, Utah 84663 / U.S.A. / Tel: (801) 489-

1500 / www.naturesway.com. The standardized mono-extract (EGb-761) of dried leaves from ginkgo (50:1) consists of 24% ginkgo flavonol glycosides and 6% terpene lactones, of which 2.9% is bilobalide and 3.1% is the ginkgolides A, B, and C. Contains less than 5 ppm ginkgolic acids and conforms to the German Commission E requirements for GBE.

Kaveri®: Lichtwer Pharma AG / Wallenroder Strasse 8-14 / 13435 / Berlin / Germany / Tel: +49-30-40-3700 / Fax: +49-30-40-3704-49 / www.lichtwer.de. Prepared from the standardized mono-extract (LI-1370) of dried leaves from ginkgo (50:1) containing at least 25% flavonol glycosides and 6% terpene lactones. Contains less than 5 ppm ginkgolic acids and conforms to the German Commission E requirements for GBE.

LI-1370: Lichtwer Pharma AG, Berlin, Germany. The standardized mono-extract of dried leaves from ginkgo (50:1) contains at least 25% flavonol glycosides and 6% terpene lactones (Vesper and Hansgen, 1994) and conforms to the German Commission E specifications. Contains less than 5 ppm ginkgolic acids and conforms to the German Commission E requirements for GBE.

Rökan®: Spitzner GmbH / Postfach 763, 76261 Ettlingen, Germany / Tel. +49 72 43 – 106 01 / Fax +49 72 43 – 106 333 / www.spitzner.de / Email: info@spitzner.de. The standardized mono-extract (EGb-761) of dried leaves from ginkgo (50:1) consists of 24% ginkgo flavonol glycosides and 6% terpene lactones, of which 2.9% is bilobalide and 3.1% is the ginkgolides A, B, and C. Contains less than 5 ppm ginkgolic acids and conforms to the German Commission E requirements for GBE.

Tanakan®: 4. Beaufor-Ipsen / Paris, France / Tel.: +33 (0) 1 44 30 42 15 / Fax: +33 (0) 1 44 30 42 04 / www.beaufour-ipsen.com/ / Email: contact.web@beaufour-ipsen.com. The standardized mono-extract (EGb-761) of dried leaves from ginkgo (50:1) consists of 24% ginkgo flavonol glycosides and 6% terpene lactones, of which 2.9% is bilobalide and 3.1% is the ginkgolides A, B, and C. Contains less than 5 ppm ginkgolic acids and conforms to the German Commission E requirements for GBE.

Tebonin® forte: Dr. Willmar Schwabe Pharmaceuticals. The standardized mono-extract (EGb-761) of dried leaves from ginkgo (50:1) consists of 24% ginkgo flavonol glycosides and 6% terpene lactones, of which 2.9% is bilobalide and 3.1% is the ginkgolides A, B, and C. Contains less than 5 ppm ginkgolic acids and conforms to the German Commission E requirements for GBE.

*American equivalents, if any, are found in the Product Table beginning on page 398.

REFERENCES

Ahlemeyer B, Kriegelstein J. Neuroprotective effects of *Ginkgo biloba* extract. In: Lawson L, Bauer R, editors. *Phytomedicines of Europe chemistry and biological activity*. Washington D.C.: American Chemical Society; 1998. p. 210–220.

Arenz A, Klein M, Fiehe K, Groß J, Drewke C, Hemscheidt T, Leistner E. Occurrence of neurotoxic 4'-o-methylpyridoxine in *Ginkgo biloba* leaves, ginkgo medications and Japanese ginkgo food. *Planta Med* 1996;62:548–51.

Arrigo A. Treatment of chronic cerebrovascular insufficiency with *Ginkgo biloba* extract. *Therapiewoche* 1986;36:5208–18.

Bauer U. 6-Month double-blind randomised clinical trial of *Ginkgo biloba* extract versus placebo in two parallel groups in patients suffering from peripheral arterial insufficiency. *Arzneimittelforschung* 1984;34(6):716–20.

Birks J, Grimley EJ, Van Dongen M. *Ginkgo biloba* for cognitive impairment and dementia [Cochrane Review]. In: *The Cochrane Library*, Issue 4, 2002. Oxford. Update Software.

Blume J, Kieser M, Hölscher U. Placebo-controlled double blind study on the efficacy of *Ginkgo biloba* special extract EGb 761 in maximum-level trained patients with intermittent claudication. *VASA* 1996;25(3):265–74.

Blume J, Kieser M, Hölscher U. Efficacy of *Ginkgo biloba* special extract EGb 761 in peripheral arterial occlusive disease. *Fortschr Med(Originalien)* 1998;116:137–43.

Blumenthal M. Herb Sales Down 15% in Mainstream Market. *HerbalGram* 2001;51:69.

Blumenthal M, Busse WR, Goldberg A, Gruenwald J, Hall T, Riggins CW, Rister RS, editors. Klein S, Rister RS (trans.). *The Complete German Commission E Monographs— Therapeutic Guide to Herbal Medicines.* Austin (TX): American Botanical Council; Boston (MA): Integrative Medicine Communication; 1998. p. 136–8.

Blumenthal M, Goldberg A, Brinckmann J. *Herbal Medicine—Expanded Commission E Monographs.* Newton (MA): Integrative Medicine Communications; 2000. p. 160–9.

Borzeix M. Effects of *Ginkgo biloba* extract on two types of cerebral oedema. In: Agnoli A *et al.*, editors. *Effects of Ginkgo biloba extract on organic cerebral impairment.* London: John Libbey; 1985. p. 51–6.

Braquet P. *Ginkgolides- Chemistry, Biology, Pharmacology and Clinical Perspectives* (Vol. 1). Barcelona, Spain: J.R. Prous Science Publishers; 1988.

Braquet P. *Ginkgolides- Chemistry, Biology, Pharmacology and Clinical Perspectives* (Vol. 2). Barcelona, Spain: J.R. Prous Science Publishers; 1989.

Brautigam MRH, Blommaert FA, Verleye G, Castermans J, Jansen Steur ENH, Kleijnen J. Treatment of age-related memory complaints with *Ginkgo biloba* extract: a randomized double blind placebo-controlled study. *Phytomedicine* 1998;5(6):425–34.

Brinker F. *Herb Contraindications and Drug Interactions.* 3d ed. Sandy (OR): Eclectic Medical Publications; 2001. p. 103–7.

Brown D. *Ginkgo biloba* extract for age-related cognitive decline and early-stage dementia—a clinical overview. *Q Rev Nat Med* Summer 1997:91–6.

Brüchert E, Heinrich SE, Ruf-Kohler P. Efficacy of LI 1370 in older patients with cerebral insufficiency [in German]. *Munch Med Wschr* 1991;133(l):9–14.

Bruneton J. *Pharmacognosy, Phytochemistry, Medicinal Plants.* 2nd ed. Paris: Lavoisier Publishing;1995. p. 329–44.

Busse WR. (Wilmar Schwabe). Personal communication to M. Blumenthal. Oct. 11, 2001.

Calapai G, Crupi A, Firenzuoli F, Marciano MC, Squadrito F, Inferrera G, et al. Neuroprotective effects of *Ginkgo biloba* extract in brain ischemia are mediated by inhibition of nitric oxide synthesis. *Life Sciences* 2000;67:2673–83.

Chatterjee S, Gabard B. Effect of an extract of *Ginkgo biloba* on experimental neurotoxicity. *Arch Pharmacol* 1984;325 Suppl:327.

Cockle S, Kimber S, Hindmarch L. The effects of *Ginkgo biloba* extract (LI 1370) Supplementation on activities of daily living in free-living older volunteers: A questionnaire survey. *Human Psychopharmacology: Clinical and Experimental* 2000;15:227–235.

Cohen AJ, Bartlik B. *Ginkgo biloba* for antidepressant-induced sexual dysfunction. *J Sex Marital Ther* 1998;24(2):139–43.

Cott J. NCDEU update. Natural product formulations available in Europe for psychotropic indications. *Psychopharmacol Bull* 1995;31(4):745–51.

DAB. See: *Deutsches Arzneibuch.*

DeFeudis F. *Ginkgo biloba Extract (EGb 761): From Chemist to the Clinic.* Weisbaden, Germany: Ullstein Medical Verlagsgesellschaft; 1998.

DeFeudis F. *Ginkgo biloba Extract (EGb 761): Pharmacological Activities and Clinical Applications.* Paris: Elsevier, Editions Scientifiques; 1991. p. 1187.

Deutsches Arzneibuch (DAB ErgAanzungslieferung 2000). Stuttgart, Germany: Deutscher Apotheker Verlag. 2000.

Dr. Willmar Schwabe GmbH & Co. Expert information: Tebonin® forte 40 mg. Karlsruhe (Germany):Schwabe; 2001.

Dr. Willmar Schwabe GmbH & Co. Personal communication. Sep 17, 1998.

Drew S, Davies E. Effectiveness of *Ginkgo biloba* in treating tinnitus: double blind, placebo controlled trial. *BMJ* 2001 Jan 13;322(7278):73.

Dubreuil C. Therapeutic trial in acute cochlear deafness. Comparative study with *Ginkgo biloba* extract and nicergoline [in French]. *Presse Med* 1986 Sep 25;15(31):1559–61.

Eckmann VF. Cerebral insufficiency—treatment with *Ginkgo biloba* extract. Time of onset of the effect in a double-blind study involving 60 inpatients [in German]. *Fortschr Med* 1990;108(29):557–60.

Engelsen J, Nielsen JD, Winther K. Effect of coenzyme Q10 and Ginkgo biloba on warfarin dosage in stable, long-term warfarin treated outpatients [letter]. *Thromb Haemost* 2002;87(6):1075–6.

Ernst E, Pittler MH. *Ginkgo biloba* for dementia—a systematic review of double-blind, placebo-controlled trials. *Clin Drug Invest* 1999;17(4):301–8.

Evans JR. *Ginkgo biloba* extract for age-related macular degeneration [review]. *Cochrane Database Syst Rev* [serial online]. 2001 [cited 2001 Apr 17];(1):[10 screens]. Available from: URL: http://www.update-software.com/cochrane/.

Foster S. *Ginkgo-Ginkgo biloba.* Botanical booklet No. 304. Austin (TX): American Botanical Council; 1996.

Fowler JS, Wang G-J, Volkow ND, Logan J, Franceshi D, Franceshi M, et al. Evidence that *Ginkgo biloba* extract does not inhibit MAO A and B in living human brain. *Life Sci* 2000;66(9):141–6.

Gertsch JH, Seto TB, Mor J, Onopa J. Ginkgo biloba for the prevention of severe acute mountain sickness (AMS) starting one day before rapid ascent. *High Alt Med Biol* 2002;3(1):29-37.

Gilbert GJ. *Ginkgo biloba* [letter]. *Neurol* 1997 Apr;48:1137.

Grässel E. Effect of *Ginkgo biloba* extract on mental performance. Double-blind study using computerized measurement conditions in patients with cerebral insufficiency [in German]. *Fortschr Med* 1992 Feb 20;110(5):73–6.

Guinot P, Caffrey E, Lambe R, Darragh A. Tanakan® inhibits platelet-activating-factor induced platelet aggregation in healthy male volunteers. *Haemostasis* 1989;19(4):219–23.

Halama P. Judgement of well-being and psychometric test in patients from a neurological practice treated with ginkgo [in German]. *Munch Med Wschr* 1991;133 Suppl 1:S19–S22.

Halama P. What does the special extract do (EGb 761)? Treatment with *Ginkgo biloba* in patients with cerebral insufficiency and refractory depressive symptoms. Results of a placebo-controlled, randomized double-blind pilot study [in German]. *Therapiewoche* 1990;40(51/52):3760–5.

Halama P, Bartsch G, Meng G. Disturbances of cerebral performance of vascular origin. Randomized double-blind study of the effectiveness of *Gingko biloba* extract [in German]. *Fortschr Med* 1988; 106(19):408–12.

Hartmann A, Frick M. Wirkung eines Ginkgo-Spezial-extraktes auf psychometrische Parameter bei Patienten mit vasculär bedingter Demenz [in German]. *Münchener Medizinische Wochenschrift* 1991;133 Suppl 1:S23–S25. Cited in Kleijnen J, Knipschild P. *Ginkgo biloba* for cerebral insufficiency. *Br J Clin Pharmac* 1992a;34:352–8.

Hauns B, Häring B, Köhler S, Mross K, Unger C. Phase II study of combined 5-flourouracil/ *Ginkgo biloba* extract (GBE 761 ONC) therapy in 5-flourouracil pretreated patients with advanced colorectal cancer. *Phytother Res* 2001 Feb;15:34–8.

Health Canada. *Ginkgo biloba.* In: *Drug Product Database (DPD).* Ottawa, Ontario: Health Canada Therapeutic Products Programme. 2001.

Health Protection Branch. *Ginkgo biloba.* In: *HPB Status Manual.* Ottawa, Ontario: Health Protection Branch. 19. February 1993;87–88.

Hofferberth B. The effect of *Ginkgo biloba* extract on neurophysiological and psychometric measurement results in patients with cerebro-organic syndrome. A double-blind study versus placebo [in German]. *Arzneimittelforschung* 1989;39(8):918–22.

Hofferberth B. The efficacy of EGb 761 in patients with senile dementia of the Alzheimer type, a double-blind, placebo-controlled study on different levels of investigation. *Hum Psychopharmacol* 1994;9:215–22.

HPB. See: Health Protection Branch.

Itil TM, Eralp E, Tsambis E, Itil KZ, Stein U. Central nervous system effects of *Ginkgo biloba,* a plant extract. *Am J Ther* 1996;3:63–73.

Jung F, Mrowietz C, Kiesewetter H, Wenzel E. Effect of *Gingko biloba* on fluidity of blood and peripheral microcirculation in volunteers. *Arzneimittelforschung* 1990 May;40(5):589–93.

Kanowski S, Herrmann WM, Stephan K, Wierich W, Hörr R. Proof of efficacy of the *Ginkgo biloba* special extract EGb 761 in outpatients suffering from mild to moderate primary degenerative dementia of the Alzheimer type or multi-infarct dementia. *Phytomedicine* 1997;4(1):3–13.

Kim YS, Pyo MK, Park KM, Park PH, Hahn BS, Wu SJ,et al. Antiplatelet and antithrombic effects of a combination of ticlopidine and *Ginkgo biloba* ext (Egb 761). *Thromb Res* 1998;91(1):33–8.

Kleijnen J, Knipschild P. *Ginkgo biloba* for cerebral insufficiency. *Br J Clin Pharmac* 1992;34:352–8.

Krieglstein J. Neuroprotective effects of *Ginkgo biloba* constituents. *Euro J Pharm Sci* 1995;3:39–48.

Krieglstein J, Beck T, Seibert A. Influence of an extract of *Ginkgo biloba* on cerebral blood flow and metabolism. *Life Sci* 1986;39:2327–34.

Kudolo GB. The effect of 3-month ingestion of *Ginkgo biloba* extract on pancreatic β-cell function in response to glucose loading in normal glucose tolerant individuals. *J Clin Pharmacol* 2000;40:647–54.

Kurtsoy A, Canbay S, Oktem IS, Akdemir H, Koc RK, Menku A, Tucer B. Effect of EGb 761 on vasospasm in experimental subarachnoid hemorrhage. *Res Exp Med (Berl)* 2000 Feb;199(4):207–15.

Larssen R, Dupeyron J, Boulu R. Modéles d'ischémie cérébrale expérimentale par microsphéres chez le rat. Étude de l'effet de deux extraits de *Ginkgo biloba* et du naftidrofuryl. *Therapie* 1978;33:651–60.

Le Bars PL, Katz MM, Berman N, Itil TM, Freedman AM, Schatzberg AF. A placebo-controlled, double-blind, randomized trial of an extract of *Ginkgo biloba* for dementia. North American EGb Study Group. *JAMA* 1997;278(16):1327–32.

Le Poncin-Lafitte M, Rapin J, Rapin JR. Effects of *Ginkgo biloba* on changes induced by quantitative cerebral microembolization in rats. *Archives Intl Pharmacodynam* 1980;243(2):236–44.

Leadbetter G, Maakestad K, Olson, S, Hackett, P. *Ginkgo biloba* reduces the incidence and severity of acute mountain sickness [abstract]. *High Altitude Medicine and Biology.* 2001;2(1):110.

Ginkgo

Monograph

Leistner E, Arnez A. Expert advice: Safety and toxicology of *Ginkgo biloba* [in German]. *Phytotherapie* 1997;18(4):230–1.

Li MH, Zhang HL, Yang BY. Effects of ginkgo leave concentrated oral liquor in treating asthma [in Chinese]. *Zhonggou Zhong Xi Yi Jie He Za Zhi* 1997 Apr;17(4):216–8.

Logani S, Chen MC, Tran T, Le T, Raffa RB. Actions of *Ginkgo biloba* related to potential utility for the treatment of conditions involving cerebral hypoxia. *Life Sciences* 2000;67:1389–96.

Matthews MK. Association of *Ginkgo biloba* with intracerebral hemorrhage [letter]. *Neurol* 1998;50:1933–4.

McGuffin M, Hobbs C, Upton R, Goldberg A, editors. *American Herbal Products Association's Botanical Safety Handbook*. Boca Raton (FL): CRC Press; 1997.

McKenna DJ, Jones K, Hughes K. Efficacy, safety, and use of *Ginkgo biloba* in clinical and preclinical applications. *Alt Ther* 2001;7(5):70–90.

Medical Products Agency (MPA). *Naturlakemedel: Authorised Natural Remedies* (as of January 24, 2001). Uppsala, Sweden: Medical Products Agency. 2001.

Medical Products Agency (MPA). *Naturitikemedelsmonografin: Semper AB Anjo GB 8 Ginkgo Tabletter och mixtur, Lichtwer Pharma Gink-Yo Tabletter*. Uppsala, Sweden: Medical Products Agency. 1998.

Meyer B. Multicenter randomized double-blind drug vs. placebo study of the treatment of tinnitus with *Ginkgo biloba* extract [in French]. *Presse Med* 1986;15(31):1562–4.

Mix J, Crews D. A double-blind, placebo-controlled, randomized trial of *Ginkgo biloba* extract EGb 761® in a sample of cognitively intact older adults: neuropsychological findings. *Hum Psychopharmacol Clin Exp* 2002;17:267–77.

Mix J, Crews D. An examination of the efficacy of *Ginkgo biloba* extract EGb 761 on theneuropsychological functioning of cognitively intact older adults. *J Alternative and Complementary Med* 2000;6:219–29.

Morant J, Ruppanner H, editors. *Arzneimittel-Kompendium der Schweiz & 2001/02* Publikumsausgabe. Basel, Switzerland: Documed AG. 2001. pp. 338, 555–6.

Morgenstern C, Biermann E. The efficacy of Ginkgo special extract EGb 761 in patients with tinnitus. *Int J Clin Pharmacol Ther* 2002;40(5):188–97.

MPA. See: Medical Products Agency.

Oberpichler H. PAF-antagonist ginkgolide B reduces postischemic neuronal damage in rat brain hippocampus. *J Cereb Blood Flow Metab* 1990;10(1):133–5.

Oberpichler H, Beck T, Abdel-Rahman MM, Bielenberg GW, Krieglstein J. Effects of *Ginkgo biloba* constituents related to protection against brain damage caused by hypoxia. *Pharmacol Res Commun* 1988;20(5):349–68.

Oken BS, Storzbach DM, Kaye JA. The efficacy of *Ginkgo biloba* on cognitive function in Alzheimer disease. *Arch Neurol* 1998;55(11):1409–15.

Otani M, Chatterjee SS, Gabard B, Kreutzberg GW. Effect of an extract of *Ginkgo biloba* on triethyltin-induced cerebral edema. *Acta Neuropathol* (Berl) 1986;69(1–2):54–65.

Peters H, Kieser M, Hölscher U. Demonstration of the efficacy of *Ginkgo biloba* special extract EGb 761® on intermittent claudication—a placebo-controlled, double-blind multicenter trial. *VASA* 1998;27(2):106–10.

Pincemail J, Dupuis M, Nasr C, Hans P, Haag-Berrurier M, Anton R, et al. Superoxide anion scavenging effect and superoxide dismutase activity of *Ginkgo biloba* extract. *Experientia* 1989;15;45(8):708–12.

Pittler MH, Ernst E. *Ginkgo biloba* extract for the treatment of intermittent claudication: A meta-analysis of randomized trials. *Am J Med* 2000 Mar;108:276–81.

Porsolt RD, Roux S, Drieu K. Evaluation of a *Ginkgo biloba* extract (EGb 761) in functional tests for monoamine oxidase inhibition. *Arzneimittelforschung* 2000;50(3):232–5.

Rai GS, Shovfin C, Wesnes KA. A double-blind, placebo controlled study of *Ginkgo biloba* extract (Tanakan®) in elderly outpatients with mild to moderate memory impairment. *Curr Med Res Opin* 1991;12(6):350–5.

Rapin JR, LePoncin-Lafitte M. Cerebral glucose consumption. The effect of *Ginkgo biloba* extract [in French]. *Pressemed* 1986 Sept 21;15(31):1494–7.

Rigney U, Kimber S, Hindmarch I. The effects of acute doses of standardized *Ginkgo biloba* extract on memory and psychomotor performance in volunteers. *Phytother Res* 1999;13(5):408–15.

Rogers SL, Doody RS, Mohs RC, Friedhoff LT. A 24-week, double-blind, placebo-controlled trial of donepezil in patients with Alzheimer's disease. Donepezil Study Group. *Neurology* 1998 Jan;50(1):136–45.

Roncin JP, Schwartz F, D'Arbigny P. EGb 761 in control of acute mountain sickness and vascular reactivity to cold exposure. *Aviat Space Environ Med* 1996;67(5):445–52.

Rong Y, Geng Z, Lau BHS. *Ginkgo biloba* attenuates oxidative stress in macrophages and endothelial cells. *Free Radical Bio Med* 1996;20(1):121–7.

Rosenblatt M, Mindel J. Spontaneous hyphema associated with ingestion of *Ginkgo biloba* extract [letter]. *N Engl J Med* 1997 Apr;336(15):1108.

Rowin J, Lewis SL. Spontaneous bilateral subdural hematomas associated with chronic *Ginkgo biloba* ingestion. *Neurol* 1996;46(6):1775–6

Ruppanner H, Schaefer U (eds.). *Codex 2000/01 - Die Schweizer Arzneimittel in einem Griff*. Basel, Switzerland: Documed AG. 2000. pp. 179, 433, 1247–50.

Sasaki K, Hatta S, Wada K, Ohshika H, Haga M. Anticonvulsant activity of bilobalide, a sequiterpene in *Ginkgo biloba* L. leaves against chemical-induced and electroshock-induced convulsions in mice. *Res Comm Biolog Psychol Psych* 1995;20(3&4):145–56.

Sastre J, Milan A, Garcia de la Asuncion J, et al. A *Ginkgo biloba* extract (EGb 761) prevents mitochondrial aging by protecting against oxidative stress. *Free Radic Biol Med* 1998;24(2):298–304.

Schaffler K, Reeh PW. Double-blind study of the hypoxia-protective effect of a standardized *Ginkgo biloba* preparation after repeated administration in healthy volunteers [in German]. *Arzneimittelforschung* 1985;35(8):1283–6.

Schmidt U, Rabinovici K, Lande S. Effect of a *Ginkgo biloba* special extract on well-being in cerebral insufficiency [in German]. *Manch Med Wschr* 1991;133(l):15–8.

Schwabe. See: Dr. Willmar Schwabe GmbH & Co.

Schweizer J, Hautmann C. Comparison of two dosages of *Ginkgo biloba* extract EGb 761 in patients with peripheral arterial occlusive disease Fontaine's stage IIb. A randomised, double-blind, multicentric clinical trial. *Arzneimittelforschung* 1999;49(II):900–4.

Sikora R, Sohn M, Deutz F-J, et al. *Ginkgo biloba* extract in the therapy of erectile dysfunction. *J Urol* 1989;141:188A.

Smith PF, Maclennan K, Darlington CL. The neuroprotective properties of *Ginkgo biloba*: a review of the possible relationship to platelet-activating factor (PAF) [review]. *J Ethnopharmacol* 1996;50(3):131–139.

Soholm B. Clinical improvement of memory and other cognitive functions by *Ginkgo biloba*: review of relevant literature. *Adv Ther* 1998;15(1):54–65.

Sticher O. Quality of ginkgo preparations. *Planta Med* 1993;59:2–11.

Stough C, Clarke J, Lloyd J, Nathan PJ. Neuropsychological changes after 30-day *Ginkgo biloba* administration in healthy participants. *Int J Neuropsychopharmacol* 2001;2:131–4.

Taillandier J, Ammar A, Rabourdin JP, Ribeyre JP, Pichon J, Niddam S, et al. *Ginkgo biloba* extract in the treatment of cerebral disorders due to aging. A longitudinal multicenter double-blind placebo controlled drug trial [in French]. *Presse Med* 1986;15(31):1583–7.

Tang W, Eissenbrandt G. *Chinese Drugs of Plant Origin: Chemistry, Pharmacology, and Use in Traditional and Modern Medicine*. New York (NY): Springer Verlag; 1992.

Tunón H. Phtyotherapie in Schweden [in German]. *Z Phytotherapie* 1999;20:268–77.

United States Congress (USC). Public Law 103-417: Dietary Supplement Health and Education Act of 1994. Washington, DC: 103rd Congress of the United States. 1994.

United States Pharmacopeia (USP 25th Revision)—The National Formulary (NF# 20th Edition). Rockville, MD: United States Pharmacopeial Convention, Inc. 2002.

USC. See: United States Congress.

USP. See: *United States Pharmacopeia*.

Vaes LP, Chyka PA. Interactions of warfarin with garlic, ginger, ginkgo, or ginseng: Nature of the evidence. *Ann Pharmacother* 2000 Dec;34(12):1478–82.

Vale S. Subarachnoid hemorrhage associated with *Ginkgo biloba* [letter]. *Lancet* 1998 Jul 4;352(9121):36.

Van Beek TA, Bombardelli E, Morazzoni P, Peterlongo F. *Ginkgo biloba* L. *Fitoterapia* 1998;69(3):195–244.

Van Dongen MCJM, van Rossurn E, Kessels AGH, Sielhorst HJG, Knipschild PG. The efficacy of ginkgo for elderly people with dementia and age-associated memory impairment: new results of a randomized clinical trial. *J Am Geriatr Soc* 2000;48(10):1183–94.

Vesper J, Hansgen K-D. Efficacy of *Ginkgo biloba* in 90 outpatients with cerebral insufficiency caused by old age. *Phytomedicine* 1994;1:9–16.

Vorberg G, Schenk N, Schmidt U. The efficacy of a new *Ginkgo biloba* extract in 100 patients with cerebral insufficiency. *Herz Gefäße* 1989;9:396–401.

Wearies K, Simmons D, Rook M, Simpson P. A double-blind placebo-controlled trial of Tanakan® in the treatment of idiopathic cognitive impairment in the elderly. *Hum Psychopharmacol* 1987;2:159–69.

Wesnes K, Simmons D, Rook M, Simpson P. A Double-blind Placebo-controlled Trial of Tanakan in the Treatment of Idiopathic Cognitive Impairment in the Elderly. *Hum Psychopharmacol* 1987;2:159–69.

Wettstein A. Cholinesterase inhibitors and ginkgo extracts—are they comparable in the treatment of dementia? Comparison of published placebo-controlled efficacy studies of at least six months' duration. *Phytomedicine* 2000;6(6):393–401.

White HL, Scates PW, Cooper BR. Extracts of *Ginkgo biloba* leaves inhibit monoamine oxidase. *Life Sci* 1996;58(16):1315–21.

WHO. See: World Health Organization.

Winter E. Effects of an extract of *Ginkgo biloba* on learning and memory in mice. *Pharmacol Biochem Behav* 1991;38:109–14.

World Health Organization (WHO). Folium Ginkgo. In: WHO *Monographs on Selected Medicinal Plants*, Vol. 1. Geneva: World Health Organization; 1999. p. 154–67.

Clinical Studies on Ginkgo (*Ginkgo biloba* L.)

Cerebral Insufficiency (Alzheimer's Disease, Multi-infarct Dementia, Cerebro-Organic Syndrome)

Author/Year	Subject	Design	Duration	Dosage	Preparation	Results/Conclusion
Van Dongen et al., 2000	Dementia and age-associated memory impairment (AAMI)	R, DB, PC, MC, PG n=196 older patients with mild to moderate dementia or AAMI; intention to treat analysis	Total 24 weeks. Patients randomized to usual dose, high dose, or placebo for 3 months, then randomized again for next 3 months	80 mg, 2x/day or 120 mg, 2x/day or placebo	EGb-761	In 24 weeks, ginkgo group showed no improvement compared to placebo in outcome measures (neuro-psychological testing, digit memory span, verbal learning, depressive mood, self-evaluated health and memory, and behavioral evaluation). No benefit was seen for higher dose or extended duration of ginkgo. Ginkgo did not benefit any subgroups. Authors concluded that ginkgo is not effective to treat mild to moderate dementia or AAMI.
Rigney et al., 1999	Memory and psychomotor performance	R, DB, PC, CO (5-way) n=31 asymptomatic individuals (30-59 years old)	Each treatment was taken for 2 days and separated by a washout period of 5 days or more	50 mg, 3x/day; or 100 mg 3x/day; or 120 mg, 1x/day in a.m.; or 240 mg/day in a.m.; or placebo	Kaveri® LI 1370 (50 mg film-coated tablets)	Ginkgo produced a non-significant cognitive improvement in overall word recall (short-term working-memory task) (p=0.318) and significantly increased integrative capacity of the central nervous system (based on the critical flicker fusion threshold test) (p=0.043). There was no improvement in choice reaction time. Authors concluded that improvements in asymptomatic controls are most pronounced for working memory, and in individuals over 50 years of age.
Brautigam et al., 1998	Cerebral insufficiency	R, DB, PC n=197 elderly patients with cognitive impairment	6 months	1.9 ml, 3x/day undiluted; or 1.9 ml, 3x/day (1:1 dilution) or placebo	Geriaforce® (liquid extract)	Low-dose ginkgo treatment significantly improved short-term visual memory more than high dose or placebo treatment (based on contrast statistical analysis of the Benton Test of Visual Retention-Revised task) (p=0.0076). There was no improvement in the following parameters: attention or concentration (based on Expended Mental Control Test); short-term memory or learning curve (based on Rey Test part 2). Overall, ginkgo had limited efficacy in this battery of subjective and objective tests. [Note: The ginkgo extract used in this trial is not phyto-equivalent with the 2 preparations upon which most of the studies on ginkgo have been conducted.]
Kanowski et al., 1997	Dementia	R, DB, PC, MC, P n=156 elderly patients with Alzheimer's disease or multi-infarct dementia	6 months	120 mg 2x/day or placebo	EGb-761 (120 mg capsule)	Per protocol and intent-to-treat analyses significantly favored EGb-761 over placebo (p=0.012). Clinical Global Impressions scores, a measure of psycho-pathological assessment, increased 15% (p<0.05). Syndrom-Kurztest, for the assessment of attention and memory, improved 20% (p<0.05). Overall, EGb-761 was well-tolerated and effective in treatment of Alzheimer's disease and multi-infarct dementia.
Le Bars et al., 1997	Dementia	R, DB, PC, MC, P n=202 elderly patients with mild to severe Alzheimer's disease or mulit-infarct dementia	13 months	40 mg, 3x/day or placebo	Ginkgold® (EGb-761 40 mg tablet)	Patients receiving ginkgo had no significant change in ADAS-Cog score (evaluates memory, language skill, and orientation), but by comparison there was significant worsening in placebo group (p=0.04). Patients taking ginkgo had mild improvement on GERRI test, (assesses daily living and social behavior) while placebo group had significant worsening (p=0.04). Both groups had slight worsening in CGIC, (assesses overall psychopathology). It was concluded that ginkgo is safe and capable of stabilizing or improving cognitive performance and social functioning of demented patients for 6 months to 1 year.
Hofferberth, 1994	Dementia	R, DB, PC n=40 elderly patients with Alzheimer's disease	3 months	80 mg per day (2x 40 mg) or placebo	EGb-761 film-coated tablets (Tebonin® forte)	Of individuals treated with ginkgo, 90.5% had significant improvement in memory and attention as assessed by Syndrom-Kurztest total value at end of study (p=0.00017). Improvements were seen in all 5 subsets of the SCAG (cognitive disturbances, emotional disturbances, lack of drive, social behavior, and somatic disturbances) (p<0.01). Authors concluded treatment improved memory, attention, psychopathology, psychomotor performance, functional dynamics, and neurophysiology after one month. Ginkgo was well-tolerated.

KEY: ADAS-Cog – Alzheimer's Disease Assessment Scale-cognitive subscale, **C** – controlled, **CC** – case-control, **CGIC** – Clinical Global Assessment of Change, **CH** – cohort, **CI** – confidence interval, **Cm** – comparison, **CO** – crossover, **CS** – cross-sectional, **DB** – double-blind, **E** – epidemiological, **GERRI** – Geriatric Evaluation by Relative's Rating Instrument, **GLC** – concentrated ginkgo leaf product, **LC** – longitudinal cohort, **MA** – meta-analysis, **MC** – multi-center, **MMSE** – Mini Mental Status Exam, **n** – number of patients, **O** – open, **OB** – observational, **OL** – open label, **OR** – odds ratio, **P** – prospective, **PB** – patient-blind, **PC** – placebo-controlled, **PG** – parallel group, **PS** – pilot study, **QPEG** –quantitative pharmaco-electroencephalogram, **R** – randomized, **RC** – reference-controlled, **RCS** – retrospective cross-sectional, **RS** - retrospective, **S** – surveillance, **SB** – single-blind, **SC** - single-center, **SCAG** – Sandoz Clinical Assessment Scale, **SKT** – Syndrom-Kurztest, **U** – uncontrolled, **UP** – unpublished, **VC** – vehicle-controlled, **WAIS** – Wechsler Adult Intelligence Scale.

Ginkgo

Monograph

Clinical Studies on Ginkgo (*Ginkgo biloba* L.) (cont.)

Cerebral Insufficiency (Alzheimer's Disease, Multi-infarct Dementia, Cerebro-Organic Syndrome) (cont.)

Author/Year	Subject	Design	Duration	Dosage	Preparation	Results/Conclusion
Vesper and Hansgen, 1994	Cerebral insufficiency	R, DB, PC, MC n=86 elderly patients with cerebral insufficiency	3 months	50 mg, 3x/day or placebo	Kaveri® LI 1370 (50 mg film-coated tablets)	Target parameters and results were established with help of computer diagnostics and demonstrated improved reaction time, concentration (p<0.05), and mental flexibility (p<0.05), and improved memory (p<0.05), improved concentration power (p<0.05) after several weeks of ginkgo treatment.
Grässel, 1992	Cerebral insufficiency	R, DB, PC, MC n=53 elderly patients with cerebral insufficiency	24 weeks	80 mg, 2x/day or placebo	Rökan® EGb-761 (80 mg film-coated tablets)	Computer aided measurements revealed improved short-term memory and learning rate after treatment for 6 weeks or 24 weeks, respectively.
Brüchert et al., 1991	Cerebral insufficiency	R, DB, PC n=209 patients with typical symptoms of cerebral insufficiency	3 months	50 mg, 3x/day or placebo	Kaveri® LI 1370 (50 mg film-coated tablets)	After 12 weeks, statistically significant improvements were demonstrated on 8 out of 11 typical symptoms. In ginkgo group, period for figure connection test was improved by 25% vs. only 14% in placebo group (p<0.01) Both physicians and patients judged highly significant differences between ginkgo and placebo.
Halama, 1991	Dementia of degenerative or vascular origin	R, DB, PC n=42 patients with presenile, senile, and arteriosclerotic dementia	3 months	50 mg, 3x/day or placebo	Kaveri® LI 1370 (50 mg film-coated tablets)	After 12 weeks, significant differences between ginkgo and placebo group for 7 out of 11 typical symptoms. Ginkgo group was significantly faster in carrying out figure configuration test after 6 and 12 weeks. Authors concluded that ginkgo treatment resulted in improvement in cerebral functional capacity in patients with degenerative and vascular dementia.
Rai et al., 1991	Memory impairment	R, DB, PC, P n=27 elderly patients with mild to moderate memory impairment	6 months	40 mg, 3x/day or placebo	Tanakan® EGb-761 (40 mg tablets)	Ginkgo improved performance on digit-copying subtest of Kendrick battery at both 12 (p=0.022) and 24 (p=0.017) weeks, and improved speed of response on computerized classification task (p=0.02591), and mean reaction time (p=0.0502). Although the digit recall task at 24 weeks showed much lower scores (p=0.032), further analysis indicated that ginkgo has beneficial effects on mental efficiency.
Schmidt et al., 1991	Cerebral insufficiency	R, DB, PC n=99 patients with cerebral insufficiency	3 months	150 mg/day or placebo	Kaveri® LI 1370 (50 mg film-coated tablets)	After only 4 weeks, 8 of 12 typical symptoms of cerebral insufficiency improved significantly (p<0.05 to p<0.01) compared to placebo. Ginkgo was very well-tolerated.
Eckmann, 1990	Cerebral insufficiency	R, DB, PC n=58 patients with cerebral insufficiency with leading symptom of depressive mood.	6 weeks	160 mg/day or placebo	LI 1370 liquid form	Marked differences in improvement of 11 of 12 symptoms in ginkgo group compared to placebo group. Largest number of improvements observed between 2nd and 4th week of treatment.
Hofferberth, 1989	Cerebro-organic syndrome	R, DB, PC n=36 elderly patients with cerebro-organic syndrome	2 months	40 mg, 3x/day or placebo	Rökan® EGb-761 (40 mg film-coated tablets)	Psychometric tests showed improved visual response speed with reduced saccade (eye movement) duration and latency (Saccade test) (p<0.0001), and improved reaction time (Vienna determination test and trail making test) (p<0.0001). Researchers concluded ginkgo is well-tolerated and of clinical efficacy.
Vorberg et al., 1989	Cerebral insufficiency	R, DB, PC n=96 patients with typical symptoms of cerebral insufficiency	3 months	15 ml, 3x/day (112 mg/day) or placebo	LI 1370 liquid form (Kaveri®)	Severity of symptoms improved in ginkgo group by 50% compared to only 25% with placebo. Statistically significant differences between ginkgo and placebo could be demonstrated for these symptoms: loss of memory, lack of concentration, anxiety, dizziness, and headache (p<0.05 to p<0.001).

KEY: **ADAS-Cog** – Alzheimer's Disease Assessment Scale-cognitive subscale, **C** – controlled, **CC** – case-control, **CGIC** – Clinical Global Assessment of Change, **CH** – cohort, **CI** – confidence interval, **Cm** – comparison, **CO** – crossover, **CS** – cross-sectional, **DB** – double-blind, **E** – epidemiological, **GERRI** – Geriatric Evaluation by Relative's Rating Instrument, **GLC** – concentrated ginkgo leaf product, **LC** – longitudinal cohort, **MA** – meta-analysis, **MC** – multi-center, **MMSE** – Mini Mental Status Exam, **n** – number of patients, **O** – open, **OB** – observational, **OL** – open label, **OR** – odds ratio, **P** – prospective, **PB** – patient-blind, **PC** – placebo-controlled, **PG** – parallel group, **PS** – pilot study, **QPEG** –quantitative pharmaco-electroencephalogram, **R** – randomized, **RC** – reference-controlled, **RCS** – retrospective cross-sectional, **RS** - retrospective, **S** – surveillance, **SB** – single-blind, **SC** - single-center, **SCAG** – Sandoz Clinical Assessment Scale, **SKT** – Syndrom-Kurztest, **U** – uncontrolled, **UP** – unpublished, **VC** – vehicle-controlled, **WAIS** – Wechsler Adult Intelligence Scale.

Clinical Studies on Ginkgo (*Ginkgo biloba* L.) (cont.)

Cerebral Insufficiency (Alzheimer's Disease, Multi-infarct Dementia, Cerebro-Organic Syndrome) (cont.)

Author/Year	Subject	Design	Duration	Dosage	Preparation	Results/Conclusion
Halama et al., 1988	Cerebro-vascular insufficiency	R, DB, PC n=40 elderly patients with mild to medium cere-brovascular insufficiency	3 months	40 mg, 3x/day or placebo	Tebonin® forte EGb-761 (40 mg film-coated tablets)	After 12 weeks of ginkgo treatment, there was significant improvement in SCAG scale (p=0.00005), dizziness, (p<0.001), tinnitus (p=0.035), and lessened indifference to surroundings.
Wesnes et al., 1987	Idiopathic cognitive impairment	R, DB, PC n=54 elderly patients with idiopathic cognitive impairment	3 months	40 mg, 3x/day or placebo	Tanakan® EGb-761 (40 mg film-coated tablets)	Treatment improved cognitive function and mental efficiency based on a battery of computerized and pen-cil-and-paper tasks (number matching, p=0.0183; word recognition, p=0.026), and increased interest in everyday life. Researchers concluded that ginkgo may be potentially helpful in treating early stages of primary degenerative dementia.
Taillandier et al., 1986	Cerebral insufficiency	R, DB, PC, MC n=166 elderly patients with cerebral insufficiency	12 months	2 ml, 3x/day (160 mg /day), or placebo	Tanakan® EGb-761 liquid form (40 mg/ml)	Scores on geriatric clinical evaluation scale test (measuring intellectual functions, mood, social insertion, and neurosensory disorders) were improved after 3 months of ginkgo treatment (p<0.05) and reached 17% improvement for placebo (p=0.01). Authors concluded that ginkgo is effective in ameliorating cerebral disorders due to aging.
Arrigo, 1986	Cerebro-vascular insufficiency	R, DB, PC, CO n=80 elderly patients with chronic cere-brovascular insufficiency	45 days drug; 15 days wash-out; vs. 45 days control; 15 days wash-out	40 mg, 3x/day or placebo	Tebonin® forte EGb-761	Ginkgo improved memory (p<0.0001), logical thinking, and vigilance, based on WAIS (p<0.01), a Word Recognition task and a Memory Table (p<0.0001). In addition, ginkgo lessened headache, dizziness, tinnitus, visual impairment, and asthenia, based on self-assessment by patients.

Peripheral Vascular Disease (Intermittent Claudication)

Author/Year	Subject	Design	Duration	Dosage	Preparation	Results/Conclusion
Schweizer and Hautmann, 1999	Peripheral Arterial Occlusive Disease; Fontaine's Stage IIb	R, DB, MC, P n=74	6 months	120 mg/day (n=38); 240 mg/day (n=36)	Rökan®	Pain-free walking distance improved with both 120 mg and 240 mg treatments, with a mean increase of 60.6 meters, and 107 meters, respectively (p=0.0253). The superiority of the higher dose was statistically significant and demonstrated a substantial therapeutic benefit.
Peters et al., 1998	Intermittent claudication	R, DB, PC, MC n=111	6 months	40 mg, 3x/day or placebo	Tebonin® forte EGb-761 40 mg film-coated tablets	Ginkgo group experienced a significant decrease of pain associated with walking and increased walking distance, at 8 (p=0.017), 16 (p=0.007), and 24 (p=0.016) weeks.
Bauer, 1984	Peripheral arterial insufficiency, Fontaine's Stage IIb	R, DB, PC, PG n=79	6 months	40 mg, 3x/day or placebo	Rökan® EGb-761 40 mg film-coated tablets	Ginkgo group experienced decreased pain associated with walking, improved walking distance, and increased limb perfusion. Ginkgo was concluded to be a beneficial clinical treatment.

KEY: ADAS-Cog – Alzheimer's Disease Assessment Scale-cognitive subscale, **C** – controlled, **CC** – case-control, **CGIC** – Clinical Global Assessment of Change, **CH** – cohort, **CI** – confidence interval, **Cm** – comparison, **CO** – crossover, **CS** – cross-sectional, **DB** – double-blind, **E** – epidemiological, **GERRI** – Geriatric Evaluation by Relative's Rating Instrument, **GLC** – concentrated ginkgo leaf product, **LC** – longitudinal cohort, **MA** – meta-analysis, **MC** – multi-center, **MMSE** – Mini Mental Status Exam, **n** – number of patients, **O** – open, **OB** – observational, **OL** – open label, **OR** – odds ratio, **P** – prospective, **PB** – patient-blind, **PC** – placebo-controlled, **PG** – parallel group, **PS** – pilot study, **QPEG** –quantitative pharmaco-electroencephalogram, **R** – randomized, **RC** – reference-controlled, **RCS** – retrospective cross-sectional, **RS** - retrospective, **S** – surveillance, **SB** – single-blind, **SC** - single-center, **SCAG** – Sandoz Clinical Assessment Scale, **SKT** – Syndrom-Kurztest, **U** – uncontrolled, **UP** – unpublished, **VC** – vehicle-controlled, **WAIS** – Wechsler Adult Intelligence Scale.

Ginkgo

Monograph

Clinical Studies on Ginkgo (*Ginkgo biloba* L.) (cont.)

Respiratory Conditions (Asthma and Acute Mountain [Altitude] Sickness)

Author/Year	Subject	Design	Duration	Dosage	Preparation	Results/Conclusion
Gertsch et al., 2002	Acute mountain sickness (AMS)	R, DB, PC n=26 sea level residents	1 day prior to ascent	60 mg or placebo, 3x/day	*Ginkgo biloba* extract (brand not stated)	Participants traveled by air from sea level to 4,205 meters over 3 hrs with 1 hr at 2,835 m. Ginkgo group showed significantly lower median Lake Louise Self-report scores (LLSR) than placebo (4, range 1–8 vs. 5, range 2–9, p=0.03). Ginkgo lowered the incidence of AMS but this effect was not deemed statistically significant compared with placebo (58.3% vs. 92.9%, p=0.07). Authors conclude pretreatment with ginkgo one day prior to rapid ascent may reduce severity of AMS.
Leadbetter et al., 2001	Acute mountain sickness (AMS)	DB, PC n=40	5 days prior to ascent	120 mg or placebo, 2x/day	*Ginkgo biloba* extract (brand not stated)	Ginkgo reduced the incidence and severity of AMS when taken 5 days prior to an ascent of 4,300 meters. The ginkgo group demonstrated a decrease in incidence of AMS of 33% compared with 68% in the placebo group (p<0.02).
Li et al., 1997	Asthma	PC n=61	2 months	45 g crude herb, 10 ml, 3x/day (15 g/10 ml) (equates to 1,400 mg of standard - extract) or placebo	Concentrated ginkgo leaf liquid product (produced by Quindao Fengyi Biotechnology Limited). Contains 14.5 mg/ml flavone glycosides and 2.8 mg/ml terpene lactones	Improved airway reactivity test at 4 and 8 weeks (p<0.05). Improved pulmonary function test at 8 weeks (p<0.05) including forced expiratory volume and peak expiratory flow rate.
Roncin et al., 1996	Control of acute mountain (altitude) sickness (AMS) and vascular reactivity to cold exposure	R, DB, PC n=44	30 days	80 mg, 2x/day or placebo	Tanakan® EGb-761 80 mg tablets	Ginkgo was effective in preventing AMS. No individuals receiving prophylactic experienced AMS, compared to 41% taking placebo (p=0.0014). Respiratory symptoms of altitude sickness occurred in 13.6% of the ginkgo group (p=0.000012), compared to 81.8% of the placebo group. Of ginkgo subjects, 18% reported moderate or severe impairment of diuresis at high altitude compared with 77% of placebo subjects. Ginkgo also reduced vasomotor disorders of the extremities, as demonstrated by plethysmography (p<10–8) and questionnaire (p<10–9). Authors concluded ginkgo treatment was effective.

Tinnitus and Acute Cochlear Deafness

Author/Year	Subject	Design	Duration	Dosage	Preparation	Results/Conclusion
Drew and Davies, 2001	Tinnitus	DB, PC n=956	12 weeks	50 mg, 3x/day or placebo	LI 1370 or placebo	The researchers concluded that 50 mg ginkgo extract LI 1370 given 3 times daily for 12 weeks is no more effective than placebo. This conclusion was based upon participant's assessment of tinnitus before, during, and after treatment.
Meyer, 1986	Tinnitus	R, DB, PC, MC n=103 patients with recent tinnitus (appearing within the previous 12 months)	13 months	2 ml, 2x/day or placebo	Rökan® EGb-761 liquid form	Ginkgo treatment significantly improved symptoms of tinnitus compared to placebo (p=0.05). The time before disappearance or distinct improvement in 50% of tinnitus cases was 70 days in ginkgo group, compared to 119 days for placebo. Authors concluded that treatment with ginkgo improves the evolution of tinnitus.

KEY: ADAS-Cog – Alzheimer's Disease Assessment Scale-cognitive subscale, **C** – controlled, **CC** – case-control, **CGIC** – Clinical Global Assessment of Change, **CH** – cohort, **CI** – confidence interval, **Cm** – comparison, **CO** – crossover, **CS** – cross-sectional, **DB** – double-blind, **E** – epidemiological, **GERRI** – Geriatric Evaluation by Relative's Rating Instrument, **GLC** – concentrated ginkgo leaf product, **LC** – longitudinal cohort, **MA** – meta-analysis, **MC** – multi-center, **MMSE** – Mini Mental Status Exam, **n** – number of patients, **O** – open, **OB** – observational, **OL** – open label, **OR** – odds ratio, **P** – prospective, **PB** – patient-blind, **PC** – placebo-controlled, **PG** – parallel group, **PS** – pilot study, **QPEG** –quantitative pharmaco-electroencephalogram, **R** – randomized, **RC** – reference-controlled, **RCS** – retrospective cross-sectional, **RS** - retrospective, **S** – surveillance, **SB** – single-blind, **SC** - single-center, **SCAG** – Sandoz Clinical Assessment Scale, **SKT** – Syndrom-Kurztest, **U** – uncontrolled, **UP** – unpublished, **VC** – vehicle-controlled, **WAIS** – Wechsler Adult Intelligence Scale.

Clinical Studies on Ginkgo (*Ginkgo biloba* L.) (cont.)

Tinnitus and Acute Cochlear Deafness (cont.)

Author/Year	Subject	Design	Duration	Dosage	Preparation	Results/Conclusion
Dubreuil, 1986	Acute cochlear deafness	R, DB, C n=20 individuals with acute cochlear deafness (partial or complete) within the preceding week	30 days	4 ml liquid ginkgo extract 2x/day or 2 tablets nicergoline 3x/day	Rökan® EGb-761 or nicergoline	Ginkgo was superior over nicergoline, an alpha-blocker commonly prescribed for the same indication. By day 10, ginkgo group had an average gain of 30 decibels/frequency, compared to a 21-decibel gain with nicergoline treatment. By day 30, ginkgo patients had gained on average 34 decibels/frequency, compared to 23 decibels for nicergoline patients. After one month of treatment, ginkgo group registered a total gain exceeding the nicergoline group by 67 decibels, (6-15 decibels, depending on frequency). The small sample size demands cautious conclusions; however, ginkgo demonstrated much greater efficacy than nicergoline. Therapeutic results were obtained as early as day 10; however, several weeks of treatment are suggested to consolidate the result.

Other

Author/Year	Subject	Design	Duration	Dosage	Preparation	Results/Conclusion
Engelsen et al., 2002	Drug interaction (long-term warfarin use in patients with recurrent venous thromboembolism, mechanical heart valves) or chronic atrial fibrillation)	R, DB, PC, CO n=21	4 weeks each phase with 2 week washout between each phase	100 mg ginkgo daily, 100 mg coenzyme Q10 daily or placebo	Bio-Biloba® (Ginkgo); Bio-Quinone® (CoQ10); placebo	The stability was confirmed by linear regression of INR values and geometric mean doses of warfarin did not change during treatment. The study concluded that CoQ10 and ginkgo do not interact with warfarin.
Hauns et al., 2001	Advanced colorectal cancer	Phase II n=32	Every 3 weeks, for 4 treatments (12 weeks)	350 mg ginkgo as a 30-minute i.v. infusion (days 1–6) followed by 500 mg/m2/d 5-FU as a 30-minute i.v. infusion (days 2–6)	EGb-761 and 5-Fluorouracil (5-FU)	The results suggested a good benefit-risk ratio of combining 5-FU and EGb 761 therapy as the second line treatment. Patients showed an overall response rate of 6.3%, with the disease progressing in 22 patients. Of these, the disease progressed in 17 patients after one course of treatment, 2 patients after 3 treatments, and 3 patients after 4 treatments. The study saw no change in 8 patients and a partial response in 2 patients.
Cohen and Bartlik, 1998	Sexual dysfunction secondary to SSRI use	O n=63	1 month	Average dose: 207 mg/day 40-60-120 mg, 2x/day (dosage range: 40–60 mg, 4x/day to 120 mg 2x/day)	Ginkgo extract (brand not stated) 40 or 60 mg capsules	Ginkgo was 84% effective in treating antidepressant-induced sexual dysfunction predominantly caused by selective serotonin reuptake inhibitors. Women were more responsive than men, with relative success rates of 91% versus 76%. Ginkgo had positive effects on desire, excitement, orgasm, and resolution phases of the sexual response cycle.
Itil et al., 1996	Effect on electro-physiological characteristics of the central nervous system	R, DB, PC, CO n=12	Acute treatment followed by a minimum 3-day washout	40 mg/day or 120 mg/day or 240 mg/day or placebo	Ginkgold® EGb-761	The higher doses had more pharmacological effects than the 40 mg dose, and the 120 or 240 mg dose may be clinically more beneficial (changes in alpha activity, p=0.002; change in coefficient of CEEG response, p=0.008). Ginkgo extract has electrophysiological effects in the central nervous system similar to other well-known cognitive activators.

KEY: **ADAS-Cog** – Alzheimer's Disease Assessment Scale-cognitive subscale, **C** – controlled, **CC** – case-control, **CGIC** – Clinical Global Assessment of Change, **CH** – cohort, **CI** – confidence interval, **Cm** – comparison, **CO** – crossover, **CS** – cross-sectional, **DB** – double-blind, **E** – epidemiological, **GERRI** – Geriatric Evaluation by Relative's Rating Instrument, **GLC** – concentrated ginkgo leaf product, **LC** – longitudinal cohort, **MA** – meta-analysis, **MC** – multi-center, **MMSE** – Mini Mental Status Exam, **n** – number of patients, **O** – open, **OB** – observational, **OL** – open label, **OR** – odds ratio, **P** – prospective, **PB** – patient-blind, **PC** – placebo-controlled, **PG** – parallel group, **PS** – pilot study, **QPEG** –quantitative pharmaco-electroencephalogram, **R** – randomized, **RC** – reference-controlled, **RCS** – retrospective cross-sectional, **RS** - retrospective, **S** – surveillance, **SB** – single-blind, **SC** - single-center, **SCAG** – Sandoz Clinical Assessment Scale, **SKT** – Syndrom-Kurztest, **U** – uncontrolled, **UP** – unpublished, **VC** – vehicle-controlled, **WAIS** –Wechsler Adult Intelligence Scale.

Other (cont.)

Author/Year	Subject	Design	Duration	Dosage	Preparation	Results/Conclusion
Halama, 1990	Depression	R, DB, PC n=20 elderly patients with moderately severe depression	2 months	80 mg, 3x/day or placebo. Patients continued taking existing anti-depressive medication (75–100 mg/day Stangyl®, n=12; 75–100 mg/day Ludiomil®, n=5; 50–75 mg/day Pertrofan®, n=3).	Tebonin® forte EGb-761 (40 mg tablets)	Severity of depression lessened in 3 patients, was unchanged in 4, and became worse in 3 patients. Placebo-treated groups showed no lessened depression, while depression remained unchanged in 5 and worsened in 5 patients. Authors conclude that results are inconclusive.
Schaffler and Reeh, 1985	Hypoxia	R, DB, PC, CO n=8	5 weeks drug; 2-week washout, 1 week placebo	4 ml (80 drops), 2 ml 2x/day or placebo	Tebonin® forte EGb 761 liquid form	The oculomotor system was used to test effectiveness of ginkgo. Hypoxia-induced increase of corneoretinal resting potential and the augmented respiratory drive were reduced. Compared with placebo, saccadic eye movements and choice reaction times were significantly reduced under cumulative hypoxic stress. These findings were interpreted as indicative of a protective action against hypoxia, relevant to the treatment of cardiovascular insufficiency.

KEY: ADAS-Cog – Alzheimer's Disease Assessment Scale-cognitive subscale, **C** – controlled, **CC** – case-control, **CGIC** – Clinical Global Assessment of Change, **CH** – cohort, **CI** – confidence interval, **Cm** – comparison, **CO** – crossover, **CS** – cross-sectional, **DB** – double-blind, **E** – epidemiological, **GERRI** – Geriatric Evaluation by Relative's Rating Instrument, **GLC** – concentrated ginkgo leaf product, **LC** – longitudinal cohort, **MA** – meta-analysis, **MC** – multi-center, **MMSE** – Mini Mental Status Exam, **n** – number of patients, **O** – open, **OB** – observational, **OL** – open label, **OR** – odds ratio, **P** – prospective, **PB** – patient-blind, **PC** – placebo-controlled, **PG** – parallel group, **PS** – pilot study, **QPEG** –quantitative pharmaco-electroencephalogram, **R** – randomized, **RC** – reference-controlled, **RCS** – retrospective cross-sectional, **RS** - retrospective, **S** – surveillance, **SB** – single-blind, **SC** - single-center, **SCAG** – Sandoz Clinical Assessment Scale, **SKT** – Syndrom-Kurztest, **U** – uncontrolled, **UP** – unpublished, **VC** – vehicle-controlled, **WAIS** – Wechsler Adult Intelligence Scale.

Ginseng, American
Panax quinquefolius L.
[Fam. *Araliaceae*]

OVERVIEW

Ginseng is one of the most widely used medicinal herbs with at least six species used in traditional systems of medicine. Most world production and trade of ginseng involves two species: Asian ginseng (*Panax ginseng*) and American ginseng (*P. quinquefolius*). The U.S. exports up to two million pounds of cultivated ginseng roots annually and approximately 132,000 pounds of wild ginseng, primarily to China. Wisconsin produces 97% of all U.S.-grown ginseng. American ginseng consumption in the U.S. trails far behind that of Asian ginseng and eleuthero (also called Siberian ginseng, *Eleutherococcus senticosus*). Besides being sold as a dietary supplement, American ginseng's primary use is as an ingredient in beverages. Compared to the scores of clinical trials on Asian ginseng, few clinical studies have been conducted on American ginseng. Each species of ginseng has similar but distinct chemical profiles, and therefore exhibits different pharmacological and clinical activity.

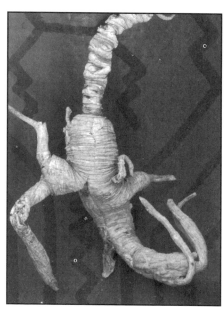

Photo © 2003 stevenfoster.com

PRIMARY USES

- Reduces postprandial glycemia in non diabetics and in patients with type 2 diabetes

OTHER POTENTIAL USES

- Possible reduction of ventilation and increased oxygen consumption ability during submaximal exercise (based on small trial)
- Possible benefit in mental performance (proofreading) based on small trial
- In Traditional Chinese Medicine (TCM), American ginseng is used for various tonic purposes

PHARMACOLOGICAL ACTIONS

ROOT POWDER: Reduced postprandial glycemia in type 2 diabetes mellitus and in nondiabetic subjects.

ROOT EXTRACT: Acted on the Fourier components of the radial artery pulse, increased respiratory endurance in exercise.

DOSAGE AND ADMINISTRATION

For therapeutic effectiveness, American ginseng is probably optimally used continuously over an extended period of time, although published clinical trials over 90 days are lacking.

DECOCTION: 3–6 g dried root simmered in 720–960 ml water for approximately 45 minutes; alternatively, 2–9 g simmered.

INFUSION: 150–240 ml boiling water poured over 1–2 g dried root and steeped for 20 minutes.

DRY ROOT POWDER: 3 g daily for postprandial glycemia in type 2 diabetes mellitus.

DRY EXTRACT: 330 mg, 3 times daily for improving physical endurance during work.

CONTRAINDICATIONS

None known.

PREGNANCY AND LACTATION: None known.

ADVERSE EFFECTS

None known.

DRUG INTERACTIONS

None known. Diabetics may need to monitor insulin levels due to hypoglycemic action.

CLINICAL REVIEW

In 6 clinical studies on American ginseng that included a total of 126 participants, all but one (ergonomic response to intense excercise) demonstrated positive effects on athletic performance, diabetes, and circulation. One double-blind, placebo-controlled (DB, PC) study and one PC, crossover (CO) study reported beneficial effects of an American ginseng root powder on postprandial glycemia in type 2 diabetes mellitus subjects. A subsequent randomized, PC, crossover study revealed that powdered American ginseng reduced postprandial glycemia in healthy individuals. Improved athletic performance was the focus of two small PC studies; one study showed no positive effect, and the other resulted in reduced ventilation requirements and increased ability to consume oxygen in submaximal exercise. One small comparative, PC study examined the effects of ginseng on psychomotor skills and found Asian and American ginseng to have equal effects on improving proofreading, error-detection, and mood-fatigue.

Ginseng, American

Panax quinquefolius L.
[Fam. *Araliaceae*]

OVERVIEW

Medicinal use of Asian ginseng (*Panax ginseng*) dates back at least 5,000 years in Asia. American ginseng is produced in North America from a plant that has similar but different chemistry and slightly different biological activity. In the U.S., it is used in a wide range of tonic, energy, and immune-stimulating dietary supplements.

USES

Promotes blood sugar metabolism in healthy people and persons with type 2 (non-insulin dependent) diabetes.

DOSAGE

In general, short-term use may not be beneficial, so continued use over an extended period of time is usually recommended. However, American ginseng was shown in clinical trials to be effective in lowering blood sugar levels directly after meals in both healthy and diabetic (type 2) persons when taken during or just after the meal.

DECOCTION (TEA): Simmer 3–6 g dried root in 720–960 ml water for approximately 45 minutes; alternatively, simmer 2 to 9 g.

INFUSION (TEA): Pour 150–240 ml boiling water over 1–2 g dried root and steep for 20 minutes.

DRY ROOT POWDER: 3 g daily for regulation of postprandial (after meal) glycemia (blood sugar level) in type 2 diabetes mellitus (non-insulin dependent diabetes).

DRY EXTRACT: 330 mg, 3 times daily, for improvement of oxygen uptake during moderate exercise.

CONTRAINDICATIONS

None known.

PREGNANCY AND LACTATION: None known.

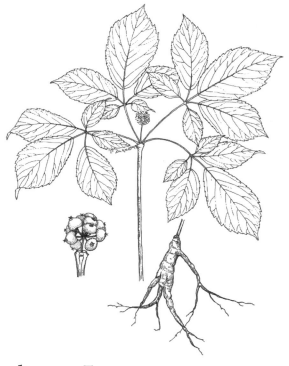

ADVERSE EFFECTS

None known.

DRUG INTERACTIONS

None known. Diabetics may need to monitor insulin levels because of the blood sugar-lowering effect.

Comments

When using a dietary supplement, purchase it from a reliable source. For best results, use the same brand of product throughout the period of use. As with all medications and dietary supplements, please inform your healthcare provider of all herbs and medications you are taking. Interactions may occur between medications and herbs or even among different herbs when taken at the same time. Treat your herbal supplement with care by taking it as directed, storing it as advised on the label, and keeping it out of the reach of children and pets. Consult your healthcare provider with any questions.

AMERICAN BOTANICAL COUNCIL

Ginseng, American

Panax quinquefolius L.

[Fam. *Araliaceae*]

OVERVIEW

Ginseng is one of the most widely used medicinal herbs with at least six species used in traditional systems of medicine. Most world production and trade of ginseng involves two species: Asian ginseng (*Panax ginseng*) and American ginseng (*P. quinquefolius*) (AAFC, 2000). According to TRAFFIC USA (the division of the World Wildlife Fund that monitors the status of threatened and endangered species), no other plant better represents the cultural and economic value of medicine harvested from the wild in North America than American ginseng (Robbins, 1997). The U.S. Department of Commerce (USDOC) measures ginseng production separately from other herbs due to its significant economic value. The U.S. exports up to two million pounds of cultivated ginseng roots annually (USDOC, 1995; USFWS, 1999a) and approximately 132,000 pounds of wild ginseng, primarily to China (Robbins, 1997; USDOC, 2000). Wisconsin produces 97% of all U.S.-grown ginseng. In 1998, Canada produced over 60% of the world supply of American ginseng (approximately four million pounds annually), the U.S. produced approximately 30%, and China produced the balance (approximately 7%). China remains the largest consumer of American ginseng (Xiao, 2000).

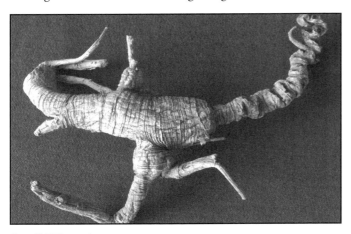

Photo © 2003 stevenfoster.com

Native to North America, American ginseng is used in traditional indigenous medicine, particularly by the Cherokee, Creek, Iroquois, Menominee, Ojibwa, Pawnee, and Seneca tribes (Foster, 1999; Heffern, 1976; Moerman, 1998). In 1718, Canadian Jesuits began organizing the collection of American ginseng from the wild for export to China (Rafinesque, 1830), where in 1765, during the Qing dynasty, it was added to the *Supplement to the Grand Materia Medica* (a.k.a., *Omissions from Ben Cao Gang Mu*), by Zhao Xuemin (Bensky *et al.,* 1986; Foster and Chongxi, 1992). American ginseng (*xi yang shen*) has since become integrated into Traditional Chinese Medicine (TCM) with indications for use distinctly different from those of Asian

ginseng (*ren shen*) (Awang, 1998; Xiao, 2000). American ginseng became official in the *United States Pharmacopeia* (USP) in 1842. It was removed from the USP in 1882, but its popular use by American Eclectic medical doctors and homeopaths continued (Felter and Lloyd, 1898; Foster, 1999; HPUS, 1992; Millspaugh, 1892; Scudder, 1891). Its primary use was as a stomach tonic, though it was also used for nervous exhaustion from overwork (Felter and Lloyd, 1898; Scudder, 1891). By the late 19th century, American ginseng was already a threatened species due to overcollecting, and extensive cultivation efforts began (Millspaugh, 1892; USFWS, 1977; Wood *et al.,* 1926). In 1947, the cultivation of American ginseng also began in China, but did not become large-scale until 1980 (AAFC, 1998; Xiao, 2000). American ginseng consumption in the U.S. trails far behind that of Asian ginseng and eleuthero (previously called Siberian ginseng, *Eleutherococcus senticosus*). Besides being sold as a dietary supplement, American ginseng's primary use is as an ingredient in beverages. Compared to the scores of clinical trials on Asian ginseng, few clinical studies have been conducted on American ginseng (see table below). Each species of ginseng has similar but distinct chemical profiles, and therefore exhibits different pharmacological and clinical activity.

DESCRIPTION

American ginseng root consists of the mature, dried, (usually) cultivated root of *Panax quinquefolius* L. [Fam. *Araliaceae*], harvested in the fall, separated from rhizomes, dried at low temperature, and containing no less than 1.0% of ginsenoside Rb1 as determined by HPLC (PPRC, 2000). American ginseng is harvested usually after a minimum of five years growth, although many roots cultivated in North America are harvested after four years. The highest-quality dried roots break with a somewhat soft and waxy fracture, while immature or undersized roots dry hard and glassy (USDA, 1978). Plant maturity can be determined before harvesting using two methods: counting the number of leaves (a.k.a., prongs) and/or removing soil where the stem joins the root to count the number of bud scale scars on the root. A single scar is produced every autumn after the plant's stem falls (USFWS, 1999b). In December 1998, China issued quality control standards for American ginseng and its products entitled *Grade and Quality Standards of Products of Processed American Ginseng* (State Standard of People's Republic of China, 1998).

PRIMARY USES

Endocrinology

- Reduces postprandial glycemia in non-diabetics and type 2 diabetes patients (Vuksan *et al.,* 2001, 2000a, 2000b)

OTHER POTENTIAL USES

Sports Medicine

- May improve cardio-respiratory endurance during submaximal work (reduced ventilation and increased oxygen consumption ability) (Goode *et al.,* 1993)

Cognition

- May improve mood-fatigue, may improve proofreading error detection (Johnson *et al.,* 1980)

Traditional Chinese Medicine (TCM)

- Deficiency of *qi* (diminished function of the internal organs and lowered body resistance); deficiency of *yin* (lack of body fluid, vital essence and blood, often resulting in endogenous heat); *internal-heat* (heat syndrome typically manifested by fever, night sweating, thirst, and constipation); cough and asthma; phlegm mixed with the blood; dysphoria and tiredness; diabetes; dry mouth and throat (PPRC, 2000). (These are terms and concepts used in TCM and may not always be correlated easily to Western biomedical terminology.)

DOSAGE
Internal
Crude Preparations

DECOCTION: 3–6 g dried root simmered in 720–960 ml water for approximately 45 minutes (PPRC, 2000; Yen, 1992). Other sources recommend simmering 2–9 g (Bensky *et al.*, 1986; Foster and Chongxi, 1992).

INFUSION: 150–240 ml boiling water poured over 1–2 g cut, dried root and steeped for 20 minutes (Xiao-fan and Liscum, 1996).

ROOT POWDER (DRY): 1–3 g in capsules 40 minutes prior to meal for normalization of blood sugar in postprandial glycemia with or after meal (Vuksan *et al.*, 2001).

WHOLE ROOT POWDER: 3 g daily for postprandial glycemia in type 2 diabetes mellitus (Vuksan *et al.*, 2000a).

DRY EXTRACT: 330 mg, 3 times daily for improving physical endurance during work (Goode *et al.*, 1993).

DURATION OF ADMINISTRATION

According to previous Eclectic medical use, American ginseng does not have an immediate effect and short-term use provides little benefit. Thus, continued use over an extended period of time is usually recommended (Felter and Lloyd, 1898). However, recent clinical trials have demonstrated an almost immediate effect in blood sugar metabolism when taken before meals (Vuksan *et al.,* 2001, 2000a).

CHEMISTRY

American ginseng has a chemical profile distinct from that of Asian ginseng. Its concentration of ginsenosides varies considerably depending on root age, month of harvest, method of drying, and method of analysis (Court *et al.*, 1996; Reynolds, 1998). Studies identified 3.0–7.3% dammarane-type triterpene glycosides (saponins) including 1.22–1.6% ginsenoside Rb1, 0.02–0.27% ginsenoside Rb2, 0.18–0.29% ginsenoside Rc, 0.09–0.8% ginsenoside Rd, 0.9–1.1% ginsenoside Re, 0.12–0.2% ginsenoside Rg1; oleanolic acid derived ginsenoside: 0.1–0.25% ginsenoside Ro (Chuang *et al.*, 1995; Li *et al.*, 1996; Yen, 1992); 0.78% malonyl (m) ginsenosdes: 0.78% m-Rb1, 0.20% m-Rb2, 0.24% m-Rc, 0.14% m-Rd (Ren and Chen, 1999); dammarane-type triterpene oligoglycosides: quinquenosides I, II, III, IV, V (Yoshikawa *et al.*, 1998); acetylenic alcohols: panaxynol, falcarindiol, panaxydol, and panaxytriol (Wang *et al.*, 2000); a homodimeric protein quinqueginsin (Wang and Ng, 2000); and 0.04–0.97% volatile oil (Zheng *et al.*, 1989).

Due to the potential adulteration of American ginseng with Asian ginseng in the marketplace, methods have been developed to differentiate the two species. For example, 24(R)-pseudo-ginsenoside-F11 is a characteristic constituent of American ginseng but occurs only in minute quantities in Asian ginseng, whereas ginsenoside-Rf is the characteristic constituent of Asian ginseng that is lacking in American ginseng (Chan *et al.*, 2000; Dou *et al.*, 1998; Shaw and But, 1995; Wenkui *et al.*, 2000). Malonyl ginsenosides are found at much lower levels in Asian ginseng, at 10% total ginsenoside content compared to 40% total ginsenoside content in American ginseng (Awang, 2000). Thorough reviews of ginseng chemistry have been or will soon be published (Court, 2000; Chen *et al.*, 2003).

PHARMACOLOGICAL ACTIONS
Human

American ginseng whole root powder reduced postprandial glycemia in type 2 diabetes mellitus and in nondiabetic subjects (Vuksan *et al.*, 2000a; 2000b). American ginseng root powder reduced glycemia in healthy individuals (Vuksan *et al.*, 2001). American ginseng total extract demonstrated specific effect on the Fourier components of the radial artery pulse, confirming TCM descriptions (Wang *et al.*, 1994), and increased respiratory endurance in exercise (Goode *et al.*, 1993).

Traditional Chinese Medicine (TCM) Actions

Dispel *wind* (exogenous pathogenic factor with symptoms such as upper respiratory catarrh with headache and urticaria) and remove *heat* (symptoms such as fever, flushed face, thirst); relieve cough and resolve *phlegm* (secretions of the respiratory system) (PPRC, 2000).

Animal

American ginseng root stimulated copulatory behavior in male rats (Murphy *et al.*, 1998); aqueous extract possessed significant gastricmodulating effect on brain neuronal activity in rats (Yuan *et al.*, 1998a, 1998b); methanolic American ginseng extract exhibited liver-protective effect against D-galactosamine- and lipopolysaccharide-induced injury in mice (Yoshikawa *et al.*, 1998); aqueous American ginseng extract significantly exhibited hypoglycemic activity in mice (Oshima *et al.*, 1987); inhibitory effect on the cerebral cortex and moderately stimulates subcortical centers (Bensky *et al.*, 1986); saponin extract decreased plasma glucose levels in resting rats (Martinez and Staba, 1984). Research on fractions and isolated constituents have been conducted, yielding results which may or may not be consistent with studies on whole American ginseng extracts: isolated saponins significantly elevated total and maximum heat production and improved cold tolerance in rats (Wang and Lee, 2000); pseudo-ginsenoside-F11 antagonized scopolamine-induced memory impairment in mice and rats (Li *et al.*, 1999); ginsenoside Rb1 prevented scopolamine-induced amnesia in rats (Benishin *et al.*, 1991).

In vitro

American ginseng root extract showed effective antioxidant activity in both lipid and aqueous mediums by chelation of metal ions and free radical scavenging (Kitts *et al.*, 2000); ethanolic extract showed nicotinic activity by displacement of 3H-(-)nicotine from human brain cerebral cortex membranes (Lewis *et al.*, 1999); inhibited thrombin-induced endothelin release in cultured human umbilical vein endothelial cells (Yuan *et al.*, 1999); ethyl acetate American ginseng extract inhibited nitrite production by inducible nitric oxide synthase (iNOS) (Wang *et al.*, 2000);

isolated quinqueginsin inhibited human immunodeficiency virus-1 reverse transcriptase (Wang and Ng, 2000); standardized extract and breast chemotherapeutic drugs synergistically inhibited MCF-7 breast cancer cell growth (Duda *et al.*, 1999); extract exhibited estrogenic activity in MCF-7 breast cancer cells (Duda *et al.*, 1997).

MECHANISM OF ACTION

The mechanisms of action of American ginseng are not fully understood. Some suggested mechanisms include:

Animal

- Reduced plasma prolactin levels and significantly stimulated copulatory behavior due to ginseng-induced alterations in dopaminergic neurotransmission (Murphy *et al.*, 1998). Research also suggests that American ginseng's apparent increase of the male sexual arousal response is the result of relaxing and vasodilating the corpus cavernosum, allowing greater erectile performance, which appears to occur by means of an interaction with nitric oxide synthase (Nocerino *et al.*, 2000).
- Regulated GABAergic neurotransmission (Yuan *et al.*, 1998a; Yuan *et al.*, 1998b).

In vitro

- Facilitated the release of acetylcholine (ACh) from hippocampal slices (ginsenoside Rb1, isolated from American ginseng roots and fibers), which is associated with an increased uptake of choline into nerve endings. The ability of Rb1 to prevent memory deficit in animal experiments may be related to ACh metabolism in the central nervous system (Benishin *et al.*, 1991).

CONTRAINDICATIONS

None known.

Traditional Chinese Medicine (TCM) Contraindications
Cold-Damp Stomach (condition marked by intolerance of cold and abdominal distention) (Bensky *et al.*, 1986).

PREGNANCY AND LACTATION: No known restrictions (McGuffin *et al.*, 1997).

ADVERSE EFFECTS

None known.

DRUG INTERACTIONS

None known. Insulin levels in diabetic patients may need monitoring due to American ginseng's blood sugar modulating effect.

AMERICAN HERBAL PRODUCTS ASSOCIATION (AHPA) SAFETY RATING

CLASS 1: Herbs that can be safely consumed when used appropriately (McGuffin *et al.*, 1997).

REGULATORY STATUS

CANADA: Food, if no therapeutic claims are made, and New Drug if drug claims are made (HPB, 1993) except as per the Traditional Herbal Medicine (THM) Policy. Permitted as a THM, if the claim(s) are supported by traditional references, requiring premarket authorization and assignment of a Drug Identification Number (DIN) (Health Canada, 1999). Also, permitted as a homeopathic over-the-counter (OTC) drug with premarket authorization and assignment of a DIN (Health Canada, 2001).

CHINA: Regulated as a drug, which must meet the State Standard of People's Republic of China 1998: Grade and Quality Standards of American Ginseng. American ginseng dried roots and teas are Class 3 materials (herbal pharmaceuticals). American ginseng capsules are also Class 3 drugs, but require additional premarket licenses and inspection from the Ministry of Health (AAFC, 1998; Xiao, 2000).

FRANCE: No official monograph for this species of *Panax*.

GERMANY: No official monograph for this species of *Panax*.

ITALY: No official monograph for this species of *Panax*.

JAPAN: Used in traditional Kampo medicine (Rister, 1999). Before May 23, 2000, American ginseng was considered a drug; now deregulated by Japan's Ministry of Health and Welfare, and may be sold as a food product without medical efficacy claims (USDS, 2000).

SWEDEN: Possible Natural Remedy for self-medication requiring advance application for marketing authorization. As of January 2001, no American ginseng products have been listed in the Medical Products Agency (MPA) "Authorised Natural Remedies" (MPA, 2001). Food, if no therapeutic claims are made.

SWITZERLAND: No official monograph for this species of *Panax*.

U.K.: Entered in *General Sales List*, Table A (internal or external use) of Schedule 1 (subject to a full product license) (GSL, 1994).

U.S.: Dietary supplement (USC, 1994). The homeopathic tincture (1X) of the fresh or dried root is an OTC Class C drug of the *Homeopathic Pharmacopoeia of the United States* (HPUS, 1992).

CLINICAL REVIEW

Six studies are outlined in the following table, "Clinical Studies on American Ginseng," including a total of 126 participants. All but one of the studies (Morris *et al.*, 1996), demonstrated positive effects on diabetes, circulation, or oxygen utilization during athletic performance. One double-blind placebo-controlled (DB, PC) study and one PC crossover (CO) study reported beneficial effects of American ginseng root powder on postprandial glycemia in type 2 diabetes mellitus subjects (Vuksan *et al.*, 2000a; 2000b). A subsequent randomized, PC, CO study evaluated the effects of powdered American ginseng on postprandial glycemia in healthy individuals (Vuksan *et al.*, 2001). These subjects experienced a reduction in postprandial glycemia. Improved athletic performance was the focus of two PC studies (Goode *et al.*, 1993; Morris, 1996). One small comparison, PC study examined the effects of ginseng on psychomotor skills and found Asian and American ginseng to have equal effects on improving proofreading error-detection and mood-fatigue (Johnson *et al.*, 1980). All these studies are small and need confirmation in larger trials. The evidence on American ginseng's ability to lower postprandial blood sugar levels in both healthy individuals and type 2 diabetics in one dose is mounting but needs validation in larger, longer-term studies.

BRANDED PRODUCTS

Chai-Na-Ta® CNT2000™ capsules: Chai-Na-Ta Corp., 5965 205A Street / Langley, BC / V3A 8C4 / Canada / Tel.: (800) 406-7668 / Fax (604) 533-8891 / www.chainata.com. One capsule, standardized to 6% genenosides, contains 500 mg of 3-year-old Ontario-grown, dried and ground American ginseng root, standardized to 6% ginsenosides.

REFERENCES

AAFC. See: Agriculture and Agri-Food Canada.

Agriculture and Agri-Food Canada (AAFC). Ginseng and Nutraceuticals in China. Ottawa, ON: Agriculture and Agri-Food Canada; 1998, Sept.

Agriculture and Agri-Food Canada (AAFC). Special Crops: Canadian Ginseng Profile. Ottawa, ON: Agriculture and Agri-Food Canada; 2000; Available at: http://www.agr.ca/misb/spcrops/gin_e.html.

Awang D. The neglected ginsenosides of North American ginseng (*Panax quinquefolius* L.). *J Herbs Spices & Med Plants* 2000;7(2):103–9.

Awang D. The anti-stress potential of North American ginseng (*Panax quinquefolius* L.). *J Herbs, Spices & Med Plants* 1998;6(2):87–91.

Benishin C, Lee R, Wang L, Liu H. Effects of ginsenoside Rb1 on central cholinergic metabolism. *Pharmacology* 1991;42(4):223–9.

Bensky D, Gamble A, Kaptchuck T. *Chinese Herbal Medicine Materia Medica*. Seattle, WA: Eastland Press; 1986;518.

Chan T, But P, Cheng S, *et al.* Differentiation and authentication of *Panax ginseng, Panax quinquefolius*, and ginseng products by using HPLC/MS. *Annl Chem* 2000;72(6):1281–7.

Chen YJ, Wu CF, Awang DVC, *et al. Ginsenosides: The Chemistry, Pharmacology, and Clinical Perspectives.* 2003 [in press].

Chuang W, Wu H, Sheu S, *et al.* A comparative study on commercial samples of Ginseng Radix. *Planta Med* 1995;61:459–65.

Court W. *Ginseng: The Genus Panax.* Amsterdam: Harwood Academic Publishers; 2000.

Court W, Reynolds L, Hendel J. Influence of root age on the concentration of ginsenosides of American ginseng (*Panax quinquefolium*). *Can J Plant Sci* 1996;76:853–5.

Dou D, Hou W, Chen Y. Studies on the characteristic constituents of Chinese ginseng and American ginseng. *Planta Med* 1998;64:585–6.

Duda R, Zhong Y, Navas V, *et al.* American ginseng and breast cancer therapeutic agents synergistically inhibit MCF-7 breast cancer cell growth. *J Surg Oncol* 1999;72(4):230–9.

Duda R, Taback B, Navas V, Zhong Y, Slomovic B, Alvarez J. Comparison of estrogenicity of *Panax quinquefolium* and *Panax ginseng* in MCF-7 breast cancer cells (meeting abstract). *Proc Annu Meet Am Assoc Cancer Res* 1997;38:A756.

Felter H, Lloyd J. *King's American Dispensatory*, 18th edition, 3rd revision. Cincinnati, OH: The Ohio Valley Co.; 1898;1429–30.

Foster S. *American Ginseng Panax quinquefolius.* Austin, TX: American Botanical Council; Botanical Series No. 308;1999.

Foster S, Chongxi Y. *Herbal Emissaries: Bringing Chinese Herbs to the West.* Rochester, VT: Healing Arts Press; 1992;102–12.

General Sale List (GSL). Statutory Instrument 1994 No. 2410 – The Medicines (Products Other Than Veterinary Drugs). Amendment Order 1994. London, U.K.: Her Majesty's Stationery Office (HMSO). 1994.

Goode R, Chatha D, Baker J, *et al.* The Effects of Ginseng on Physical Performance in Human Subjects. Toronto, ON: University of Toronto Dept. of Physiology, Faculty of Medicine and School of Physical and Health Education; 1993.

GSL. See: General Sale List.

Health Canada. *Listing of Drugs Currently Regulated as New Drugs*—Revised April 1999. Ottawa, ON: Health Canada; 1999, April;11, 21–2.

Health Canada. Product Information: *Aralia quinquefolia.* In: *Drug Product Database (DPD).* Ottawa, ON: Health Canada Therapeutic Products Programme; 2001.

Health Protection Branch (HPB). Ginseng. In: *HPB Status Manual.* Ottawa, ON: Health Protection Branch; 1993, Feb. 19;89.

Heffern R. The Use of North American Ginseng. In: *The Complete Book of Ginseng.* Millbrae, CA: Celestial Arts; 1976;81–9.

Homeopathic Pharmacopoeia of the United States (HPUS) Revision Service Official Compendium from July 1, 1992. Washington, DC: Homeopathic Pharmacopoeia Convention of the United States; 1992;0201—ARQU.

Hou J. The chemical constituents of ginseng plants. *Comparative Med East and West* 1977;5(2):123–45.

HPB. See: Health Protection Branch.

HPUS. See: *Homeopathic Pharmacopoeia of the United States.*

Johnson A, Jiang N, Stuba E. Whole ginseng effects on human response to demands for performance. *Proceedings of the 3rd International Ginseng Symposium*, Sept. 8–10;1980. Seoul Korea: Korea Ginseng Research Institute.

Kitts D, Wijewickreme A, Hu C. Antioxidant properties of a North American ginseng extract. *Mol Cell Biochem* 2000;203(1–2):1–10.

Lewis R, Wake G, Court G, *et al.* Non-ginsenoside nicotinic activity in ginseng species. *Phytother Res* 1999;13(1):59–64.

Li T, Mazza G, Cottrell A, Gao L. Ginsenosides in roots and leaves of American ginseng. *J Agric Food Chem* 1996;44:717–20.

Li Z, Guo Y, Wu C, Li X, Wang J. Protective effects of pseudoginsenoside-F11 on scopolamine-induced memory impairment in mice and rats. *J Pharm Pharmacol* 1999;51(4):435–40.

Martinez B, Staba E. The physiological effects of *Aralia, Panax* and *Eleutherococcus* on exercised rats. *Jpn J Pharmacol* 1984;35(2):79–85.

McGuffin M, Hobbs C, Upton R, Goldberg A (eds.). *American Herbal Products Association's Botanical Safety Handbook.* Boca Raton, FL: CRC Press; 1997;82.

Medical Products Agency (MPA). *Naturläkemedel: Authorised Natural Remedies* (as of January 24, 2001). Uppsala, Sweden: Medical Products Agency. 2001.

Millspaugh C. *Medicinal Plants.* Philadelphia, PA: John C. Yorston & Co.; 1892;276–9.

Moerman D. *Native American Ethnobotany.* Portland, OR: Timber Press; 1998;376–7.

Morris A, Jacobs I, McLellan T, *et al.* No ergogenic effect of ginseng ingestion. *Int J Sport Nutr* 1996;(6):263–71.

MPA. See: Medical Products Agency.

Murphy L, Cadena R, Chavez D, Ferraro J. Effect of American ginseng (*Panax quinquefolium*) on male copulatory behavior in the rat. *Physiol Behav* 1998;64(4):445–50.

Nocerino E, Amato M, Izzo A. The aphrodisiac and adaptogenic properties of ginseng. *Fitoterapia* 2000, Aug;71(0):S1–S5.

Oshima Y, Sato K, Hikino H. Isolation and hypoglycemic activity of quinquefolans A, B, and C, glycans of *Panax quinquefolium* roots. *J Nat Prod* 1987;50(2):188–90.

Pharmacopoeia of the People's Republic of China (PPRC 2000 English Edition). Beijing, China: Chemical Industry Press. 2000;183–84.

PPRC. See: *Pharmacopoeia of the People's Republic of China.*

Rafinesque C. *Medical Flora: Manual of the Medical Botany of the United States of America,* Volume II. Philadelphia, PA: Samuel C. Atkinson; 1830;53.

Ren G, Chen F. Simultaneous quantification of ginsenosides in American ginseng (*Panax quinquefolium*) root powder by visible/near-infrared reflectance spectroscopy. *J Agric Food Chem* 1999;47(7):2771–5.

Reynolds L. Effects of drying on chemical and physical characteristics of American ginseng (*Panax quinquefolius* L.). *J Herbs, Spices & Med Plants* 1998;6(2):9–21.

Rister RS. American Ginseng. In: *Japanese Herbal Medicine: The Healing Art of Kampo.* Garden City Park, NY: Avery Publishing Group; 1999;23–4.

Robbins C. *Panax quinquefolius* popularity prompts probe. *Medicinal Plant Conservation* 1997, Nov.1;4:13–5.

Scudder J. *The American Eclectic Materia Medica and Therapeutics.* Cincinnati, OH: John M. Scudder; 1891;454.

Shaw P, But P. Authentication of *Panax* species and their adulterants by random-primed polymerase chain reaction. *Planta Med* 1995;61:466–9.

Sontaniemi E, Haapakoski E, Rautio A. Ginseng therapy in non-insulin-dependent diabetic patients. *Diabetes Care* 1995;18:1373–5.

State Standard of People's Republic of China. *Grade and Quality Standards of Products of Processed American Ginseng.* Beijing, China: Standards Press of China; 1998;GB/T 17356.1–17356.5.

United States Congress (USC). Public Law 103–417: Dietary Supplement Health and Education Act of 1994. Washington, DC: 103rd Congress of the United States; 1994.

United States Department of Agriculture (USDA). Farmers Bulletin Number 2201: Growing Ginseng. Washington, DC: United States Department of Agriculture; 1978, June.

United States Department of Commerce (USDOC). Ginseng: United States Exports by Type and Unit Value. Washington, DC: U.S. Department of Commerce. 1995, April;83–85.

United States Department of Commerce (USDOC). Ginseng Roots, Fresh or Dried, Whether or not Cut, Crushed or Powdered. U.S. Domestic Exports: November 2000 and 2000 YTD, not Seasonally Adjusted; December 1999 and 1999 YTD, not Seasonally Adjusted. Washington, DC: U.S. Department of Commerce; 2000.

United States Department of State (USDS). Deregulation of Herbs Used as Dietary Supplements. Country: Japan. Washington, DC: U.S. & Foreign Commercial Service and U.S. Department of State; June 12, 2000; Available at: http://www.csjapan.doc.gov/imi0006/herb.html.

United States Fish and Wildlife Service (USFWS). News Release: Status Review of American Ginseng Plant. Washington, DC: Department of the Interior: U.S. Fish and Wildlife Service; 1977, Aug. 11;INT:4735–77.

United States Fish and Wildlife Service (USFWS). U.S. Fish and Wildlife Service Announces First-Ever Export Restrictions for Ginseng Roots. Washington DC: U.S. Fish and Wildlife Service International Affairs; 1999a. Available at: http://international.fws.gov/global/ginsenpr.html.

United States Fish and Wildlife Service (USFWS). How to Determine the Age of Ginseng Plants. Washington DC: U.S. Fish and Wildlife Service International Affairs; 1999b. Available at: http://international.fws.gov/global/ginseng.html.

United States Fish and Wildlife Service (USFWS). Convention Permit Applications for Ginseng. Washington DC: U.S. Fish and Wildlife Service International Affairs; 1999c. Available at: http://international.fws.gov/animals/gingfind.html.

USC. See: United States Congress.

USDA. See: United States Department of Agriculture.

USDOC. See: United States Department of Commerce.

USDS. See: United States Department of State.

USFWS. See: United States Fish and Wildlife Service.

Vuksan V, Sievenpiper J, Wong J, *et al.* American ginseng (*Panax quinquefolius* L.) attenuates postprandial glycemia in a time-dependent but not dose-dependent manner in healthy individuals. *Am J Clin Nutr* 2001;73:753–8.

Vuksan V, Sievenpiper, J, Koo, V, *et al.* American ginseng (*Panax quinquefolius* L.) reduces postprandial glycemia in nondiabetic subjects and subjects with type 2 diabetes mellitus. *Arch Intern Med* 2000a;160:1009–13.

Vuksan V, Stavro MP, Sievenpiper JL, *et al.* Similar postprandial glycemic reductions with escalation of dose and administration time of American ginseng in type 2 diabetes. *Diabetes Care* 2000b;23(9):1221–6.

Wang C, Lee T. Effect of ginseng saponins on cold tolerance in young and elderly rats. *Planta Med* 2000;66:144–7.

Wang C, Shiao Y, Kuo Y, *et al.* Inducible nitric oxide synthase inhibitors from *Saposhnikovia divaricata* and *Panax quinquefolium*. *Planta Med* 2000;66:644–7.

Wang H, Ng T. Quinqueginsin, a novel protein with anti-human immunodeficiency virus, antifungal, ribonuclease and cell-free translation-inhibitory activities from American ginseng roots. *Biochem Biophys Res Commun* 2000;269(1):203–8.

Wang W, Chen H, Hsu T, Wang Y. Alteration of pulse in human subjects by three Chinese herbs. *Am J Chin Med* 1994;22(2):197–203.

Wenkui L., Chungang G., Hongjie Z. *et al.* Use of High-Performance Liquid Chromatography—Tandem Mass Spectrometry to Distinguish *Panax ginseng* C.A. Meyer (Asian Ginseng) and *Panax quinquefolius* L. (North American Ginseng). *Anal Chem* 2000;72:5417—5422.

Wood G, Bache F. *Panax*, U.S. In: *The Dispensatory of the United States of America*, 11th edition. Philadelphia, PA: J.B. Lippincott and Co; 1858;575–6.

Wood H, LaWall C, Youngken H, *et al. The Dispensatory of the United States of America*, 21st edition. Philadelphia, PA: J.B. Lippincott Co.; 1926;1316.

Xiao M. *The Canadian Ginseng Industry: Preparing for the 21st Century.* Ottawa, ON: Agriculture and Agri-Food Canada; 2000–02–07.

Xiao-fan Z, Liscum G. *Chinese Medicinal Teas.* Boulder, CO: Blue Poppy Press, Inc.; 1996;269–70.

Yen K. *The Illustrated Chinese Materia Medica—Crude and Prepared.* Taipei, Taiwan: SMC Publishing Inc.; 1992;53.

Yoshikawa M, Murakami T, Yashiro K, *et al.* Bioactive saponins and glycoside. XI. Structures of new dammarane-type triterpene oligoglycosides, quinquenosides I, II, III, IV, and V, from American ginseng, the roots of *Panax quinquefolium* L. *Chem Pharm Bull* (Tokyo); 1998;46(4):647–54.

Yuan C, Attele A, Wu J, Liu D. Modulation of American ginseng on brainstem GABAergic effects in rats. *J Ethnopharm* 1998a;62(3):215–22.

Yuan C, Attele A, Wu J, *et al. Panax quinquefolium* L. inhibits thrombin-induced endothelin release *in vitro*. *Am J Chin Med* 1999;27(2–3):331–8.

Yuan C, Wu J, Lowell T, Gu M. Gut and brain effects of American ginseng root on brainstem neuronal activities in rats. *Am J Chin Med* 1998b;26(1):47–55.

Zheng Y, Zhang C, Li X, Guo S. A comparison between Chinese *Panax quinquefolius* and imported *Panax quinquefolius*—analysis of composition of essential oil in *Panax quinquefolius*. [in Chinese]. *Yao Hsueh Hsueh Pao* 1989;24(2):118–21.

Clinical Studies on American Ginseng (*Panax quinquefolius* L.)

Athletic Performance

Author/Year	Subject	Design	Duration	Dosage	Preparation	Results/Conclusion
Morris et al., 1996	Ergogenic response of ginseng to intense exercise	PC, CO n=8	1 week	8 or 16 mg/kg body weight	American ginseng root purified extract vs. placebo (brand not stated)	No significant intergroup differences in any measured parameters (oxygen uptake, heart rate, time to exhaustion, mean lactate concentration, rating of perceived exertion during submaximal ergometer exercise).
Goode et al., 1993	Sub-maximal and maximal performance as measured by oxygen consumption and ventilation	R, PC n=39 (mean age 22.5 years)	90 days	3 capsules per day of 330 mg; 2 with breakfast and 1 at supper	American ginseng root extract, encapsulated (brand not stated) vs. placebo (wheat flour)	Significant reduction (p<0.01) in ventilation during submaximal exercise in post-test results compared to pretest values for entire ginseng group and compared to no significant change in placebo group. Increased ability to consume oxygen, especially in those who were less fit (not significant).

Diabetes

Author/Year	Subject	Design	Duration	Dosage	Preparation	Results/Conclusion
Vuksan et al., 2001	Postprandial glycemia in healthy individuals	R, PC, CO, Cm n=12	1 day	16 treatments: 2 capsules (1 g), 4 capsules (2 g), 6 capsules (3 g) or placebo at 40, 20, 10, or 0 minutes before 25 g oral glucose challenge	Chai-Na-Ta® capsules containing 500 mg 3-year old, dried and ground American ginseng root vs. placebo capsules (corn flour)	Ginseng reduced postprandial glycemia in nondiabetic subjects. Ginseng significantly lowered glycemia over last 45 minutes of test after doses of 1, 2, or 3 g compared to placebo (p<0.05). No significant differences among three doses. Glycemia in last hour of test and area under the curve significantly lower when ginseng was administered 40 minutes before challenge than when administered 20, 10, or 0 minutes before challenge (p<0.05). Reductions were time-dependent and not dose-dependent, even though one of the doses (3 g) is relatively higher than normal.
Vuksan et al., 2000a	Postprandial glycemia in nondiabetic individuals and individuals with type 2 diabetes mellitus	R, DB, PC n=19 (mean age nondiabetics 34 years; mean age diabetics 62 years)	4 weeks	3 g/day, 40 minutes before or w/25 g oral glucose	Chai-Na-Ta® Ontario-grown American ginseng root capsules vs. placebo (corn flour)	Type 2 diabetes mellitus subjects: ginseng significantly (p<0.05) lowered incremental glycemia; 22% ± 17% with glucose challenge and 19% ± 22%, 40 minutes before glucose challenge. Nondiabetic subjects: ginseng significantly (p<0.05) lowered incremental glycemia 18% ± 31% when taken 40 minutes before glucose challenge, but no difference when taken with glucose challenge.
Vuksan et al., 2000b	Postprandial glycemia in individuals with type 2 diabetes mellitus	R, PC, CO n=10 type 2 diabetic individuals (6 males, 4 females) (age 63± 2 years)	16 doses (at least 3 day washout between each dose)	3, 6, 9 g ginseng or placebo, 120, 80, 40, or 0 minutes before receiving glucose challenge	Chai-Na-Ta® Ontario-grown American ginseng root encapsulated or placebo (corn flour)	Treatment with 3, 6, 9 g American ginseng significantly lowered incremental glycemia (p<0.05). Reductions, however, occurred independent of the dose used. This effect was seen irrespective of the time of administration.

Psychomotor Response

Author/Year	Subject	Design	Duration	Dosage	Preparation	Results/Conclusion
Johnson et al., 1980	Effect of whole ginseng on mental performance	DB, PC, Cm n=38 dental students 4 arms: Arm 1: n=8 males, 1 female Arm 2: n=5 males Arm 3: n=13 males, 1 female Arm 4: n=10 males (approximately 25 years old)	Over 32 days	All arms: Approximately 2 g/dose, 8–14 doses over 30 days	4 arms: Arm 1: Asian red ginseng root (*Panax ginseng*) Arm 2: North American white ginseng root (*P. quinquefolius*) Arm 3: Eleuthero (a.k.a., Siberian ginseng) root (*Eleutherococcus senticosus*) Arm 4: Placebo	Both species of ginseng and eleuthero improved proofreading error detection, while only Korean and American ginseng improved mood-fatigue. None significantly affected mathematical performance and final grade performance, or the urinary concentrations of catecholamines.

KEY: **C** – controlled, **CC** – case-control, **CH** – cohort, **CI** – confidence interval, **Cm** – comparison, **CO** – crossover, **CS** – cross-sectional, **DB** – double-blind, **E** – epidemiological, **LC** – longitudinal cohort, **MA** – meta-analysis, **MC** – multi-center, **n** – number of patients, **O** – open, **OB** – observational, **OL** – open label, **OR** – odds ratio, **P** – prospective, **PB** – patient-blind, **PC** – placebo-controlled, **PG** – parallel group, **PS** – pilot study, **R** – randomized, **RC** – reference-controlled, **RCS** – retrospective cross-sectional, **RS** – retrospective, **S** – surveillance, **SB** – single-blind, **SC** – single-center, **U** – uncontrolled, **UP** – unpublished, **VC** – vehicle-controlled.

(This page intentionally left blank.)

Ginseng, Asian

Panax ginseng C.A. Meyer (syn. *P. schinseng* T. Nees)

[Fam. *Araliaceae*]

OVERVIEW

Asian ginseng is one of the most economically important medicinal herbs in world trade. In the U.S., ginseng ranks second in total sales in food, drug, and mass market retail stores with sales in 2000 totaling $62.5 million. The medical use of ginseng dates back thousands of years, though the first written account of its use appears in *Shen-nung pen-ts'ao-ching*, the first *Chinese Materia Medica*, believed to have been compiled during the Late Han Dynasty in the first century C.E. Ginseng has remained an important medicine in the health care systems of China, Japan, and Korea and has also become a leading product in European and U.S. herbal supplements.

PRIMARY USES

- Adaptogen and general tonic
- Increased athletic performance and endurance (although several more recent studies have not resulted in positive outcomes for performance enhancement)
- Immunomodulatory effects

OTHER POTENTIAL USES

- Non-insulin dependent diabetes mellitus
- Menopausal symptoms
- Aphrodisiac; erectile dysfunction and fertility
- Improved cognitive function and mental performance (although the effects on psychological wellbeing in normal healthy young adults were not confirmed in a later study)
- Possible reduction of risk of gastric cancer, as well as cancer of the, lungs, ovaries, larynx, esophagus, and pancreas
- Maintained CD4+ T-cell counts and delayed resistance to zidovudine in HIV positive patients taking Korean red ginseng combined with zidovudine
- Improved pulmonary function in treatment of severe, chronic respiratory disease; additive effect of antibiotic treatment for respiratory tract infection

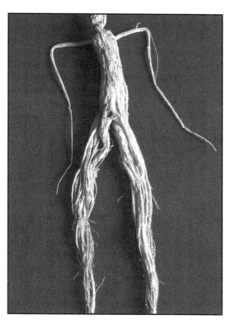

Photo © 2003 stevenfoster.com

TRADITIONAL CHINESE MEDICINE (TCM)

INDICATIONS

White Ginseng (Renshen)

Prostration with impending collapse marked by cold limbs and faint pulse; diminished function of the spleen with loss of appetite; cough and dyspnea due to diminished function of the lung; thirst due to impairment of body fluid; diabetes caused by internal heat; general weakness with irritability and insomnia in chronic diseases; impotence or frigidity; heart failure and cardiogenic shock.

Red Ginseng (Hongshen)

Collapse tendency due to asthenia; cool limbs and weak pulse; *qi* (vital force) cannot control blood; uterine bleeding; cardiac failure and cardiogenic shock.

NOTE: In TCM, the terms "spleen" and "lung" do not correlate to the western system of anatomy, but are part of a system of classification defined by their functions and relationships. Also, in TCM, herbs are rarely used as monopreparations and almost always used in combinations; it is therefore difficult to attribute the traditional uses of ginseng to the pharmacology of this herb alone as the actions of other herbs used in classic formulas may have an additive or synergistic effect.

PHARMACOLOGICAL ACTIONS

RED GINSENG ROOT: long-term, immunomodulating effect in human immunodeficiency virus (HIV) patients; improves parameters of rigidity and tumescence in erection, early detumescence, libido, and satisfaction.

STANDARDIZED EXTRACT: increases natural killer cell activity; immunomodulatory effects; reduces plasma total cholesterol and triglycerides and elevated HDL levels.

POWDERED ROOT: significantly increases mean platelet count.

DOSAGE AND ADMINISTRATION

Ginseng can generally be used up to three months, with a repeated course of treatment possible.

DRIED ROOT, POWDERED: 1–2 g daily for up to three months.

DECOCTION: 3–9 g dried root simmered in 720–960 ml water for approximately 45 minutes.

INFUSION: 150–250 ml boiling water poured over 1–2 g fine cut or powdered root, steeped covered for 10 minutes, then strained.

FLUID EXTRACT: 1–6 ml daily [1:2 (*g/ml*)].

DRY EXTRACT: 2, 100 mg capsules daily taken with liquid at breakfast or 1 capsule with breakfast and 1 capsule with lunch [standardized to 4% ginsenosides].

CONTRAINDICATIONS

No known contraindications according to the Commission E and the World Health Organization (WHO). The *British Herbal Compendium* (BHC) contraindicates ginseng for patients with acute illnesses, hypertension, or who use excessive amounts of stimulants, particularly caffeine-containing beverages.

PREGNANCY AND LACTATION: No known restrictions according to the American Herbal Products Association and the Commission E, but controlled, long-term safety studies are lacking. The BHC contraindicates ginseng in pregnancy, even though ginseng is not teratogenic *in vivo*. NOTE: In Traditional Chinese Medicine (TCM), ginseng root is included in prescriptions given during pregnancy, labor, and postpartum.

ADVERSE EFFECTS

None known. Although a few adverse effects have been reported in the literature, given the long and safe history of use, widespread modern use, and clinical trials, most authoritative experts conclude that Asian ginseng is not associated with serious adverse effects if taken at the recommended dosages.

DRUG INTERACTIONS

Two cases of interaction between ginseng and phenelzine, a monoamine oxidase inhibitor, have been reported, although the clinical significance of this interaction is not yet known. Diabetic patients may need to adjust their insulin dosages because ginseng may reduce blood glucose levels slightly. Positive synergistic effects of ginseng combined with zidovudine in HIV patients have been reported. In one case report, an interaction with warfarin resulted in a subtherapeutic decrease in clotting time (International Normalization Ratio). The BHC cautions against using ginseng with stimulants, including excessive amounts of caffeine.

CLINICAL REVIEW

More than 60 clinical studies on ginseng have been published with most using a dry extract (G115®) standardized to 4% total ginsenosides at a daily dosage of 200 mg. The drug-to-extract ratio is approximately 5:1 (*w/w*) so that 200 mg of extract corresponds to about 1 g of dried root. Of 29 clinical studies on Asian ginseng root that included a total of 12,037 participants, all but five demonstrated positive effects for indications including cancer prevention, diabetes, immune support, fatigue, menopause, and circulation. Five double-blind, placebo-controlled (DB, PC) trials investigated the ergogenic and anti-fatigue effects of ginseng extract on physical performance. Six DB, PC studies examined the effect of ginseng on psychological functions. Ginseng's immunomodulatory activity is the subject of three DB, PC studies. One DB, PC study investigated the effect of ginseng on newly diagnosed non-insulin-dependent diabetes. Ginseng's effect on erectile dysfunction and fertility in men was the focus of two studies. A review in a popular newsletter has raised issues regarding the design and results of some of these studies.

In a meta-analysis of studies on the general effectiveness of Asian ginseng on physical performance in young healthy volunteers, nine of the 16 clinical trials reviewed concluded that the "ginseng" preparation used in the trials had a positive effect. However, the analysis has been criticized because it did not differentiate between five different types of "ginseng." Another review of 16 clinical trials involving ginseng's effect on exercise performance in athletes and other healthy subjects was criticized for statistical and design problems and for methodological problems such as inadequate sample size and lack of DB, PC paradigms. These studies were conducted on ginseng combined with other ingredients (e.g., herbs, vitamins) and, in some cases, did not specify dose, duration, or specific parameters of the ginseng preparation. The authors of this review concluded that future trials should rectify design flaws so that a reasonable conclusion can be made about the effect of ginseng on physical performance. Another paper suggests that increasing dosage levels to be consistent with those used historically in TCM and in recent pharmacological experiments in animals would produce more positive outcomes in clinical trials measuring the ergonomics and other activities of ginseng.

Ginseng, Asian

Panax ginseng C.A. Meyer (syn. *P. schinseng* T. Nees)
[Fam. *Araliaceae*]

OVERVIEW

Asian ginseng is one of the most economically important medicinal herbs in world trade; in the U.S., ginseng ranks second in total sales in food, drug, and mass market retail stores with sales in 2000 totaling $62.5 million. Ginseng root is indigenous to northern mountainous regions of China, Korea, and parts of the Russian Federation. In Asia, the medical use of ginseng dates back thousands of years, and it has remained an important drug in the health care systems of China, Japan, and Korea.

PRIMARY USES

May increase athletic performance and endurance; immunomodulating effects; fatigue.

OTHER POTENTIAL USES

Non-insulin dependent diabetes mellitus; menopausal symptoms; erectile or fertility problems; improves cognitive function and mental performance; possibly reduces risk of gastric, lung, ovarian, larynx, esophagus, and pancreas cancers; improves lung function; increases antibiotic effect for respiratory tract infection.

DOSAGE

Ginseng can generally be used for up to three months followed by a repeated course of treatment.

DRIED ROOT, POWDERED: 1–2 g daily for up to three months.

DECOCTION: Simmer 3–9 g dried root in 720–960 ml water for approximately 45 minutes.

INFUSION: Pour 150–250 ml boiling water over 1–2 g finely cut or powdered root, steep covered for 10 minutes, then strain.

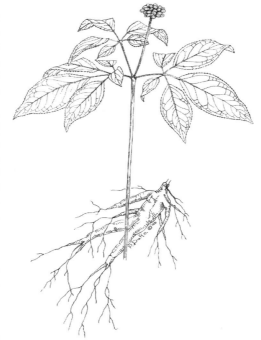

FLUID EXTRACT: 1–6 ml daily [1:2 (*g/ml*)].

DRY EXTRACT: Take 2, 100 mg capsules daily with liquid at breakfast; or 1 capsule with breakfast and 1 capsule with lunch [standardized to 4% ginsenosides].

CONTRAINDICATIONS

Consult with a healthcare provider before using Asian ginseng in cases of acute illnesses, high blood pressure (hypertension), and when using large amounts of stimulants like caffeine-containing beverages.

PREGNANCY AND LACTATION: No known restrictions although some authorities say that ginseng root should not be used during pregnancy. In Traditional Chinese Medicine, ginseng root is used during pregnancy, labor, and postpartum, in combinations containing other herbs.

ADVERSE EFFECTS

None known.

DRUG INTERACTIONS

Patients taking phenelzine (an MAO inhibitor), warfarin (an anticoagulating drug), or zidovidin (an HIV drug) should consult with a healthcare provider before using ginseng. Diabetic patients may need to adjust their insulin dosages because ginseng may lower blood glucose levels. Use with caution when taking with significant amounts of stimulants such as coffee, sugar, and caffeine-containing teas.

Comments

When using a dietary supplement, purchase it from a reliable source. For best results, use the same brand of product throughout the period of use. As with all medications and dietary supplements, please inform your healthcare provider of all herbs and medications you are taking. Interactions may occur between medications and herbs or even among different herbs when taken at the same time. Treat your herbal supplement with care by taking it as directed, storing it as advised on the label, and keeping it out of the reach of children and pets. Consult your healthcare provider with any questions.

AMERICAN
BOTANICAL
COUNCIL

The information contained on this sheet has been excerpted from *The ABC Clinical Guide to Herbs* © 2003 by the American Botanical Council (ABC). ABC is an independent member-based educational organization focusing on the medicinal use of herbs. For more detailed information about this herb please consult the healthcare provider who gave you this sheet. To order *The ABC Clinical Guide to Herbs* or become a member of ABC, visit their website at www.herbalgram.org.

Ginseng, Asian

Panax ginseng C.A. Meyer (syn. *P. schinseng* T. Nees)
[Fam. *Araliaceae*]

OVERVIEW

Asian ginseng is one of the most economically important medicinal herbs in world trade (Iqbal, 1993; Ma, 1999). In the U.S., ginseng ranks second in total sales in food, drug, and mass market retail stores with sales in 2000 totaling $62.5 million (Blumenthal, 2001). The U.S. Department of Commerce (USDOC) tracks ginseng imports due to the herb's significant economic value. The U.S. imports over 1 million pounds of cultivated Asian ginseng roots annually mainly from China, Hong Kong, and Korea (USDOC, 2000). The quantity and value of finished ginseng consumer products imported into the U.S. from Europe and Asia are significant. In Germany, ginseng is one of the few economically important herbal drugs listed separately in the *Foreign Trade Statistics*. A considerable amount of ginseng is value-added (i.e., processed into finished products) in Germany, and then exported mostly to France, Italy, and Argentina (Lange and Schippmann, 1997). A recent study by the American Botanical Council's Ginseng Evaluation Program, found that the quality control regarding standardized ginseng products was reasonably consistent over five separate lots of 13 different products (Hall *et al.*, 2001).

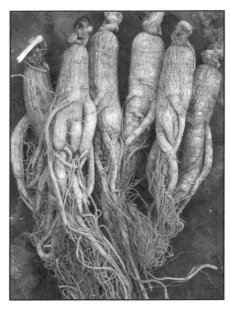

Photo © 2003 stevenfoster.com

Asian ginseng (*Panax ginseng*) is indigenous to northern mountainous regions of China and Korea and far eastern regions of the Russian Federation (Blumenthal *et al.*, 2000). Though Asian ginseng is cultivated in China, Japan, Korea and Russia (Siberia), the Republic of Korea, and China are the main producers and exporters of the herb (Iqbal, 1993).

In Asia, the medical use of ginseng dates back thousands of years, though the first written account of its use appears in *Shen-nung pen-ts'ao-ching*, the first *Chinese Materia Medica*, believed to have been compiled during the Late Han Dynasty in the first century C.E. (Hu, 1977). Ginseng has remained an important medicine in the health care systems of China, Japan, and Korea (JSHM, 1993; PPRC, 1997). Asian ginseng has also become integrated into European medicine (Morant and Ruppanner, 2001; Blumenthal *et al.*, 2000; DAB, 1999; ÖAB, 1990; Ph.Eur., 2001). In Sweden, ginseng represents the top-selling category of all registered natural remedies (Tunón, 1999). An extensive review of the detailed chemistry, mechanisms of action, pharmacology, therapeutics, and related information on *P. ginseng* was recently published, stating that since 1960 more than 4,000 research articles have been published in the scientific literature covering Asian ginseng (Court, 2000). Another review has focused on the ginsenosides, the primary active constituents, and includes biological effects noted in pharmacological and clinical studies on ginsenosides from ginseng root and aerial parts (leaves, flowers, fruits) (Chen *et al.*, 2002).

DESCRIPTION

White ginseng root (also referred to in the literature by its pharmaceutical name, *Radix Ginseng*) consists of the mature dried root of *Panax ginseng* C.A. Meyer [Fam. *Araliaceae*], collected in autumn and dried in the sun (PPRC, 1997). Before drying, the root is washed, and the rhizomes are removed (JSHM, 1993). White ginseng root contains no less than 0.4% of combined ginsenosides Rg1 and Rb1, calculated with reference to the dried root (Ph.Eur., 2001), or no less than 1.5% of total ginsenosides calculated as ginsenoside Rg1 (Blumenthal *et al.*, 1998; DAB, 1999). Red ginseng root (*Radix Ginseng Rubra*) is produced by steaming the raw root at 98–100°C for two to three hours (Kim *et al.*, 2000), then drying. The concentration of the major ginsenosides (Rb1, Rb2, Rc, Rd, Re, Rf, Rgl) are slightly higher in white ginseng than red ginseng (Yun, 1996).

PRIMARY USES

* Adaptogen and general tonic (Amato *et al.*, 2000; Court, 2000)

Fatigue and physical performance

* Increased athletic performance and endurance (Le Gal, 1996; Van Schepdael, 1993; Cherdrungsi and Rungroeng, 1995), (although several more recent studies have not resulted in positive outcomes for performance enhancement [Bahrke and Morgan, 1994, 2000])

Immunology

* Immunomodulatory effects (Scaglione *et al.*, 1990, 1996; Srisurapanon *et al.*, 1997)

OTHER POTENTIAL USES

Diabetes

* Non-insulin dependent diabetes mellitus (Sotaniemi *et al.*, 1995)

Gynecology

* Menopausal symptoms (Wickland *et al.*, 1994; Reinold 1990)

Male Reproductive Health
- Aphrodisiac (Amato *et al.*, 2000); erectile dysfunction and fertility (Salvati *et al.*, 1996; Choi *et al.*, 1995)

Mental Health
- Improved cognitive function and mental performance (Sørenson *et al.*, 1996; Smith *et al.*, 1995; Rosenfeld, 1989; Von Ardenne *et al.*, 1987; D'Angelo *et al.*, 1986; Fulder *et al.*, 1984; Dorling, 1980; Johnson *et al.*, 1980), although the effects on psychological well-being in normal healthy young adults were not confirmed in a later study (Cardinal and Engels, 2001).

Oncology
- Possible reduction of risk of gastric cancer, as well as cancer of the, lungs, ovaries, larynx, esophagus, and pancreas (Kakizoe, 2000; Yun and Choi,1998; Yun and Choi, 1995; Yun and Choi, 1990)
- Maintained CD4+ T-cell counts and delayed resistance to zidovudine in HIV + patients taking Korean red ginseng combined with zidovudine (Cho *et al.*, 2001).

Respiratory System
- Improved pulmonary function in treatment of severe, chronic respiratory disease (Gross *et al.*, 1995); additive effect of antibiotic treatment for respiratory tract infection (Scaglione *et al.*, 2001, 1994)

Ginseng root extracts and/or isolated ginsenosides have been studied clinically for the following indications with some positive results: general quality of life, adaptogenic activity and physical stress, anti-aging effects, aphrodisiac effects, memory and intellectual skills, diabetes, various types of cancers, angiocardiopathy and other cardiovascular parameters, hepatitis, peptic ulcer, aplastic anemia, atherosclerosis, and others (Court, 2000; Chen *et al.*, 2003).

TRADITIONAL CHINESE MEDICINE (TCM) INDICATIONS

White Ginseng (Renshen)
Prostration with impending collapse marked by cold limbs and faint pulse; diminished function of the spleen with loss of appetite; cough and dyspnea due to diminished function of the lung; thirst due to impairment of body fluid; diabetes caused by internal heat; general weakness with irritability and insomnia in chronic diseases; impotence or frigidity; heart failure and cardiogenic shock (PPRC, 1997).

Red Ginseng (Hongshen)
Collapse tendency due to asthenia; cool limbs and weak pulse; *qi* (vital force) cannot control blood; uterine bleeding; cardiac failure and cardiogenic shock (PPRC, 1997).

NOTE: In TCM, the terms "spleen" and "lung" do not correlate to the Western system of anatomy, but are part of a system of classification defined by their functions and relationships. Also, in TCM, herbs are rarely used as monopreparations and almost always used in combinations (Kaptchuk, 1983); it is therefore difficult to attribute the traditional uses of ginseng to the pharmacology of this herb alone as the actions of other herbs used in classic formulas may have an additive or synergistic effect.

DOSAGE

Internal

Crude Preparations
DRIED ROOT, POWDERED: 1–2 g daily for up to three months (Blumenthal *et al.*, 1998).

DECOCTION: 3–9 g dried root simmered in 720–960 ml water for approximately 45 minutes (PPRC, 1997).

INFUSION: 150–250 ml boiling water poured over 1–2 g fine cut or powdered root, steeped covered for 10 minutes, then strained (Blumenthal *et al.*, 1998, 2000).

FLUID EXTRACT: 1:2 (*g/ml*): 1–6 ml daily (Bone, 1998).

NOTE: The German Commission E specifies cut root for teas, powder, or equivalent preparations (Blumenthal *et al.*, 1998). In an infusion of coarsely powdered root, the yield of total ginsenosides at 10 minutes steeping time is 64%, and the yield is 73% at 15 minutes. If decocted, the yield of ginsenosides is 69% at 5 minutes and 77% at 15 minutes. A cold maceration will yield 71% at 60 minutes (Meyer-Buchtela, 1999).

Standardized Preparations
DRY EXTRACT: Standardized to 4% ginsenosides, 2x100 mg capsules daily taken with liquid at breakfast, or 1 capsule with breakfast and 1 capsule with lunch (Morant and Ruppanner, 2001).

NOTE: Much of the pharmacological and clinical research conducted on the leading 4% standardized ginseng extract (G115®) suggests that 200 mg of this extract, yielding 8 mg ginsenosides per day, is an optimal dose (Soldati, 2000). However, a review of historical literature and recent pharmacological investigations conducted in Asia suggests that significantly higher doses (3–9 g of dried root, equivalent to as much as 80–240 mg ginsenosides per day) are possibly warranted (Dharmananda, 2002).

DURATION OF ADMINISTRATION
According to the German Commission E, ginseng can generally be used up to three months, with a repeated course of treatment possible (Blumenthal *et al.*, 1998).

CHEMISTRY
Ginseng root contains up to 40 dammarane- and oleanane-type saponins, polyacetylene derivatives, and polysaccharides (Chen *et al.*, 2003; Court, 2000; Fukuda *et al.*, 2000; Tang and Eisenbrand, 1992). Saponins are believed to be the primary active components of ginseng, with characteristic dammarane-type saponins divided into two major groups based on their aglycones; (1) 20(S)-protopanaxadial: ginsenosides Rb1, Rb2, Rc, and Rd; and (2) 20(S)-protopanaxatriol: ginsenosides Re, Rf, Rg1, and Rg2 (Kwon *et al.*, 2000). Ginsenoside Ro is an oleanane-type saponin (WHO, 1999). Ginseng also contains alkaloids, phenols, amino acids, polypeptides, proteins, and other constituents (Court, 2000).

Raw (white) ginseng root contains 0.56–0.95% ginsenoside Rb1, 0.52–0.74% ginsenoside Rb2, 0.48–0.72% ginsenoside Rc, 0.26–0.46% ginsenoside Rd, 0.38–0.64% ginsenoside Re, 0.11% ginsenoside Rf, 0.39–0.61% ginsenoside Rg1 and 0.13% ginsenoside Rg2 (Chuang *et al.*, 1995; Kim *et al.*, 2000; Kwon *et al.*, 2000) 0.005% volatile oil (Yen, 1992).

Steamed (red) ginseng root, depending on the temperature used during steaming, contains 0.12–0.5% ginsenoside Rb1, 0.1–0.44% ginsenoside Rb2, 0.17–0.57% ginsenoside Rc, 0.14–0.27% ginsenoside Rd, 0.02–0.3% ginsenoside Re, 0.1–0.12% ginsenoside Rf, 0.22–0.35% ginsenoside Rg1,

0.2–0.3% ginsenoside Rg2, 0.24–1.32% ginsenoside Rg3, 0.15–0.64% ginsenoside Rg5, 0.14–0.23% ginsenoside F4 (Kim *et al.*, 2000). Ginsenosides Rg3, Rg5, and F4, do not occur in white ginseng and are formed as a product of the steaming process.

A high-performance liquid chromotography-tandem mass spectrometry method was developed to distinguish between *P. ginseng* (Asian ginseng) and *P. quinquefolius* (American ginseng). This method differentiates between American ginseng containing 24(R)-pseudoginsenoside F11 in excess of 0.1% (*w/w*) in the dried root and Asian ginseng containing trace levels of less than 0.00001% (Wenkui *et al.*, 2000).

Ginsenosides are quite stable: They were identified in 1,200 year-old root samples from Japan (Court, 2000).

PHARMACOLOGICAL ACTIONS

Pharmacological studies on Asian ginseng are numerous and are summarized in recent publications (Chen *et al.*, 2003; Court, 2000; Tang and Eisenbrand, 1992).

Human
Red ginseng root
Demonstrated a long-term, immunomodulating effect in human immunodeficiency virus (HIV) patients (Cho *et al.*, 1997); improved parameters of rigidity and tumescence in erection, early detumescence, libido, and satisfaction (Choi *et al*, 1995).

Standardized extract
Increased natural killer cell activity (Scaglione *et al.*, 1996); showed significant immunomodulatory effects (Scaglione *et al.*, 1990); reduced plasma total cholesterol and triglycerides, and elevated HDL levels (Yamamoto *et al.*, 1983).

Powdered root
Significantly increased mean platelet count (Chang *et al.*, 1980).

Animal
Increased resistance in coldness test and immobilization test in rodents (Blumenthal *et al.*, 1998); increased oxidative capacity of the skeletal muscle in rats (standardized extract) (Ferrando *et al.*, 1999); demonstrated hormone-like and cholesterol-lowering effects, promoted vasodilation, acted as anxiolytic, and antidepressant (Choi *et al.*, 1995; Chong *et al.*, 1988); prevented cancer-causing effects of DMBA, uerethane, and aflatoxin in newborn mice (Yun *et al.*, 1993); inhibited alcohol-induced amnesia in rats (Lee *et al.*, 2000); enhanced thermogenic capacity (Wang and Lee, 2000); enhanced energy metabolism (Avakian *et al.*, 1984); protected against irradiation damage (Takeda *et al.*, 1981, 1982); reduced injuries and inflammation caused by eccentric muscle contractions in rats (de Oliveira *et al.*, 2001); Ginseng Total Saponin (GTS) fraction inhibited striatal dopamine release stimulated by local infusion of nicotine in male rats (Shim *et al.*, 2000).

In vitro
ANTI-TUMOR: Isolated ginsenoside Rg3 demonstrated antiproliferative activity in human prostate cancer cell line (Liu *et al.*, 2000); isolated ginsenosides have shown antitumor effects in human and mouse tumor cells (Molnar *et al.*, 2000).

BRONCHO-RELAXING: Ginsenosides induced relaxation of human bronchial smooth muscle via stimuation of nitric oxide generation, mainly from airway epithelium and cyclic GMP synthesis, possibly explaining the anti-asthmatic effect of ginseng (Kawatani *et al.*, 2000).

TRADITIONAL CHINESE MEDICINE (TCM)
ACTIONS
According to the concepts inherent in TCM, the actions of ginseng are explained in terms of TCM's energetics model as follows:

White Ginseng (Renshen)
Reinforces vital energy (*qi*), remedies collapse and restores normal pulse, benefits the spleen and lung, promotes production of body fluid, calms the nerves (PPRC, 1997). NOTE: "spleen" in TCM is not the specific anatomical organ known in Western medicine; in TCM, "organs" are discussed with reference to their functions and relationships to other organs, substances and other body parts. In most cases, the term "spleen" in TCM refers to the entire digestive system.

Red Ginseng (Hongshen)
Replenishes vital essence (*jing*), promotes blood circulation and relieves collapse, reinforces *qi* and stanches bleeding (PPRC, 1997).

MECHANISM OF ACTION
- Some research suggests that ginseng acts through both the hypothalamus-pituitary-adrenal axis and partly through its immunomodulatory activity (WHO, 1999).
- *In vitro*, isolated ginsenosides have shown a chemical structure-dependent immunomodulating effect by enhancing the activity of natural killer cells and ADCC (antibody-dependent cell-mediated cytotoxicity) activities, the effect being structure-dependent (Molnar *et al.*, 2000).
- For male impotence, ginseng saponins appear to depress blood prolactin levels, causing increased libido (WHO, 1999), suggesting that ginseng may have an effect at different levels of the hypothalamus-pituitary-testes axis (Salvati *et al.*, 1996).
- Based on animal experiments, pretreatment with either ginseng extract or its isolated saponins block methamphetamine- or cocaine-induced behavioral activity. Ginseng Total Saponins (GTS) inhibits striatal dopamine release stimulated by local infusion of nicotine, suggesting that ginseng may act on presynaptic nicotinic acetylcholine receptors (nAChRs), or receptor-operated Na+ channels in dopaminergic nerve terminals, though not on voltage-sensitive ion channels (Shim *et al.*, 2000).
- Red ginseng total saponin's (RGTS) inhibition of alcohol-induced amnesia in rats is dependent on catecholaminergic but not serotonergic neuronal activity (Lee *et al.*, 2000).
- Depressant and stimulant effects on the central nervous system by the two main ginsenosides, Rb1 and Rg1, (Chong and Oberholzer, 1988) indicate that the pharmacological actions of individual ginsenosides may work in opposition. In rats with selective hippocampal lesions, red ginseng ameliorates learning and memory deficits through its effect on the CNS which may be partly due to its effects on hippocampal formation (Zhong *et al.*, 2000).

CONTRAINDICATIONS
The Commission E and World Health Organization (WHO) report that there are no known contraindications for Asian ginseng (Blumenthal *et al.*, 1998; WHO, 1999). The *British Herbal Compendium* (BHC) contraindicates ginseng in acute illnesses, hypertension, and with use of stimulants, particularly caffeine-containing beverages (Bradley, 1992).

PREGNANCY AND LACTATION: No known restrictions are noted by the American Herbal Products Association (McGuffin *et al.*, 1997) and the Commission E (Blumenthal *et al.*, 1998), but controlled, long-term safety studies have not been conducted. The BHC contraindicates ginseng in pregnancy. The WHO monograph states that the safety of ginseng use during pregnancy has not been established, but it has been shown that ginseng is not teratogenic *in vivo* (WHO, 1999). NOTE: In TCM, ginseng root is included in prescriptions given during pregnancy, labor, and postpartum (Hu, 1977).

ADVERSE EFFECTS

There is some confusion about the relative safety of Asian ginseng in the scientific literature. After evaluating various reports published prior to 1991, the Commission E determined that there was not sufficient basis for supporting definitive adverse reactions, concluding that there were none known (Blumenthal *et al.*, 1998). One paper suggests that the relative safety of ginseng is supported by the contention that the dose required to produce adverse effects is about 1,000 times the normal effective dose (Chandler, 1988).

The WHO states, "Various researchers who studied Radix Ginseng extracts using conventional toxicological methods in five different animal models reported no acute or chronic toxicity of the extract. On the basis of Radix ginseng's long use, and the relative infrequency of significant demonstrable side-effects, it has been concluded that the use of Radix Ginseng is not associated with serious adverse effects if taken at the recommended dose" (WHO, 1999). The BHC states that "Numerous studies have confirmed the safety of Ginseng; no significant toxicity or drug interactions have been reported." (Bradley, 1992). Another leading manual for professionals (Newall *et al.*, 1996) cites a report from Japan in which Asian ginseng was administered to more than 500 people in the course of two studies with no adverse side effects reported. There is considerable difficulty in evaluating individual case reports on ginseng due to a lack of information on dose, duration, species of ginseng (reports sometimes inadequately refer to "ginseng" without citing the specific type or species) and other simultaneous medication (Newall *et al.*, 1996).

Despite the relative safety of Asian ginseng, reports surface in the literature regarding potential adverse reactions. Many writers continue to uncritically cite an uncontrolled study (Siegel, 1979) in which 133 people reportedly using some form of "ginseng" (type or identity not determined) were studied for potential adverse reactions. About 10% (14) reported hypertension, nervousness, irritability, insomnia, morning diarrhea, and related symptoms, which the author labeled as the "Ginseng Abuse Syndrome" (GAS). All subjects reporting these symptoms were determined to have taken abnormally large amounts of "ginseng" (up to 15 g per day), many with concomitantly large levels of caffeine, prompting the author to suggest a potential ginseng-caffeine synergy. The study has been discredited for being uncontrolled, for not having confirmed the identity of the purported ginseng products ingested, and because most of the symptoms of GAS are also associated with consumption of large amounts of caffeine (Blumenthal, 1991).

Other adverse effects are reported. WHO cites two cases of mydriasis, disturbance in accommodation, and dizziness that were reported from ingestion of relatively large doses (3–9g) of an unspecified ginseng product (Lou *et al.*, 1989). There is one report of vaginal bleeding resulting from the vaginal application

of a "ginseng face cream" (Hopkins *et al.*, 1988). The composition of the cream was not analyzed to determine the identity of the purported ginseng contents and what level of ginseng may have been present; it is probable that other cosmetic ingredients in the preparation, intended and approved for safety in facial dermal application, but not for mucous epithelia, were responsible. The WHO discusses reports suggesting potential estrogen-like effects in premenopausal and postmenopausal women after use of ginseng. Seven cases of mastalgia as well as increased libido in premenopausal women have been reported; however, subsequent pharmacological studies on a standardized ginseng extract suggest that there is no interaction of ginseng constituents with either cytosolic estrogen receptors isolated from mature rat uterus or progesterone receptors from human myometrium. Additionally, clinical studies on a standardized ginseng extract show that ginseng does not alter male and female hormone levels (WHO, 1999).

DRUG INTERACTIONS

The Commission E reported none known (Blumenthal *et al.*, 1998). The WHO monograph cites two cases of ginseng interaction with phenelzine, a monoamine oxidase inhibitor, although the clinical significance of this interaction has yet to be determined. Diabetic patients may need to adjust insulin dosage because ginseng may reduce blood glucose levels slightly (WHO, 1999). Positive synergistic effects of ginseng combined with zidovudine in HIV patients have been reported (Cho *et al.*, 1994). There is one case report of an interaction with warfarin resulting in a subtherapeutic decrease in clotting time (International Normalization Ratio) (Morreale and Janetsky, 1997). However, in a recent study on rats, the pharmacokinetics and pharmacodynamics of warfarin were not significantly altered with the addition of a decoction of ginseng (2 g/kg), twice daily over five days (Zhou *et al.*, 1999). The BHC cautions against using ginseng with stimulants, including excessive caffeine (Bradley, 1992). A freeze-dried hot water extract of ginseng reduced blood alcohol levels 35.2% 40 minutes after the last drink of alcohol (Brinker, 2001). Case reports and pharmacological studies suggest that ginseng saponins can alleviate some of the adverse effects of glucocorticoid drugs (e.g., prednisolone) without significantly compromising the anti-inflammatory effect of the drug (Chen *et al.*, 2003). In a clinical study ginseng extract (100 mg 2x daily) increased bacterial clearance from lungs in acute attacks of chronic bronchitis when combined with amoxicillin and clavulanic acid more than when the antimicrobial drugs were used (Brinker, 2001).

TRADITIONAL CHINESE MEDICINE (TCM) DRUG INTERACTIONS

According to the *Chinese Pharmacopoeia*, ginseng is incompatible with the root and rhizome of hellebore (*Veratrum nigrum* and presumably other species of *Veratrum*); however, the nature of this incompatibility is not explained (PPRC, 1997). NOTE: *Veratrum* species are not found in herbal products in the North American market.

AMERICAN HERBAL PRODUCTS ASSOCIATION (AHPA) SAFETY RATING

CLASS 2D: Contraindicated in hypertension (McGuffin *et al.*, 1997).

AUSTRIA: Official in the *Austrian Pharmacopoeia* (ÖAB, 1990) (Meyer-Buchtela, 1999; Wichtl and Bisset, 1994).

CANADA: Food, if no therapeutic claims are made, and New Drug if drug claims are made (HPB, 1993) except as per the Traditional Herbal Medicine (THM) Policy. Permitted as an over–the–counter (OTC) THM, if the claim(s) are supported by traditional references, requiring premarket authorization and assignment of a Drug Identification Number (DIN) (Health Canada, 1999). Also, permitted as an OTC homeopathic drug with premarket authorization and assignment of a DIN (Health Canada, 2001).

CHINA: Both white and red (steamed) dried root are official drugs in the *Pharmacopoeia of the People's Republic of China* (PPRC, 1997).

EUROPEAN UNION: Dried root containing not less than (NLT) 0.4% of combined ginsenosides Rg1 and Rb1 is official in the *European Pharmacopoeia* (Ph.Eur., 2001). The homeopathic mother tincture and dilutions thereof are also allowed in veterinary medicinal products for all food-producing animal species (EMEA, 1999).

FRANCE: Official in the *French Pharmacopoeia* (Ph.Fr.X) (WHO, 1999). Traditional Herbal Medicine for self-medication with specific indications (Bradley, 1992; Goetz, 1999).

GERMANY: Dried root containing a minimum of 1.5% ginsenosides, official in the *German Pharmacopoeia* (DAB, 1999). Dried main and lateral root, and root hairs containing a minimum of 1.5% ginsenosides, used for preparation as tea, powder, or equivalent galenical preparations, is an approved nonprescription drug of the Commission E monographs (Blumenthal *et al.*, 1998).

JAPAN: Dried root with rootlets removed is official in the *Japanese Pharmacopoeia,* and powdered root is official in the *Japanese Herbal Medicine Codex* (JSHM, 1993).

REPUBLIC OF KOREA: Quality standards for ginseng extracts are published in the Korean Food Standard Code (KMHW, 1999; Kwon *et al.*, 2000; Lee *et al.*, 1999), which maintains specific guidelines for manufacturing and for ginseng product approvals (KMHW, 2000). All herbal drugs must meet the requirements of the *Korean Pharmacopoeia*, the National Institute of Health, and the Ministry of Public Health and Social Affairs (WHO, 1998).

RUSSIAN FEDERATION: Official in the *State Pharmacopoeia of the Union of Soviet Socialist Republics* (Ph USSR X) (Bradley, 1992; Reynolds *et al.*, 1989).

SWEDEN: Classified as Natural Remedy for self-medication requiring advance application for marketing authorization. A *Panax ginseng* monograph is published in the Medical Products Agency (MPA) "Authorized Natural Remedies," which lists five registered monopreparations (e.g., Gericomplex® and Ginsana®) with the approved indication: "Traditionally used as a tonic in case of decreased performance such as fatigue and sensation of weakness" (MPA, 1999 & 2001; Tunón, 1999). Food, if no therapeutic claims are made.

SWITZERLAND: Official in the *Swiss Pharmacopoeia* (Ph.Helv.) (Meyer-Buchtela, 1999; WHO, 1999). Positive classification (List D) by the *Interkantonale Kontrollstelle für Heilmittel*, and corresponding sales Category D with sale limited to pharmacies and drugstores, without prescription (Morant and Ruppanner, 2001; Ruppanner and Schaefer, 2000; WHO, 1998).

U.K.: Entered in *General Sale List*, Table A (internal or external use) of Schedule 1 (subject to a full Product License) (GSL, 1994).

U.S.: Dietary supplement (USC, 1994). Asian ginseng root and powdered Asian ginseng root, powdered Asian Ginseng extract, and ginseng tablets are official in the *U.S. National Formulary* (USP, 2002). A monograph for Asian ginseng root, dry extract, in capsules is in development (USPC, 2000).

CLINICAL REVIEW

More than 60 clinical studies on ginseng have been published with most using a dry extract (G115®) standardized to 4% total ginsenosides at a daily dosage of 200 mg. Its drug-to-extract ratio is approximately 5:1 (*w/w*) so that 200 mg of extract corresponds to about 1 g of dried root (Bone, 1998).

Twenty-nine studies are outlined in the table, "Clinical Studies on Asian Ginseng," including a total of 12,037 participants. All but five of these studies (Engels and Wirth, 1997; Engels *et al.*, 1996; Srisurapanon *et al.*, 1997; Sørenson *et al.*, 1996; Smith *et al.*, 1995) demonstrated positive effects for indications including cancer prevention, diabetes, immune support, fatigue, menopause, and circulation. The table includes 15 double-blind, placebo-controlled (DB, PC) studies. Five of these investigated the ergogenic and anti-fatigue effects of ginseng extract on physical performance (Cherdrungsi and Rungroeng, 1995; Engels *et al.*, 1996; Engels and Wirth, 1997; Le Gal *et al.*, 1996; Van Schepdael, 1993). Six DB, PC studies examined the effect of ginseng on psychological functions (D'Angelo *et al.*, 1986; Dorling, 1980; Forgo *et al.*, 1981; Fulder *et al.*, 1984; Johnson *et al.*, 1980; Sørenson *et al.*, 1996). Ginseng's immunomodulatory activity is the subject of three DB, PC studies (Scaglione *et al.*, 1990, 1997; Srisurapanon *et al.*, 1997). One DB, PC study investigated the effect of ginseng on newly diagnosed non-insulin-dependent diabetes (Sotaniemi *et al.*, 1995). Ginseng's effect on erectile dysfunction and fertility in men was the focus of two studies (Choi *et al.*, 1995; Salavati *et al.*, 1996).

A review in a popular newsletter has raised issues regarding the design and results of some of these studies (Schardt, 1999). A recent meta-analysis questioned the general effectiveness of Asian ginseng on physical performance in young, healthy volunteers (Vogler *et al.*, 1999). The meta-analysis acknowledged that nine of the 16 clinical trials reviewed concluded the "ginseng" preparation used in the trials had a positive effect. However, this review has been criticized because the authors included five different types of "ginseng": Asian, American, Japanese (*P. japonicus*), Vietnamese (*P. vietnamensis*) and eleuthero (also known as Siberian ginseng) (*Eleutherococcus senticosus*). Such reviews should focus on a homogeneous substance or in this case, one species of an herb, especially since the reviewers themselves acknowledged the chemical differences among the species (Hoegler, 2001a).

In another review (Bahrke and Morgan, 2000), researchers examined 16 clinical trials involving athletes and other healthy subjects who tested ginseng's effect on exercise performance. Criticizing the current level of ginseng research, the review's authors discussed statistical and design problems, and methodological problems such as inadequate sample size and lack of DB, PC paradigms. Studies were conducted on ginseng combined with other ingredients (e.g., herbs, vitamins), and in some cases did not specify dose, duration, or specific parameters of the ginseng preparation. The authors of this review concluded that future trials should rectify design flaws so that a reasonable conclusion can be made about the effect of ginseng on physical performance. Another paper suggests that increasing dosage levels to be consistent with those used historically in TCM and in recent pharmacological experiments in animals would produce more positive outcomes in clinical trials measuring the ergonomic and other activities of ginseng (Dharmananda, 2002).

BRANDED PRODUCTS*

Dansk Droge Ginseng tablets: Dansk Droge A/S / Industrigrenen 10 / 2635 / Ishoj / Copenhagen / Denmark / Tel: +43-56-5656 / Fax: +43-56-5600. 100 mg or 200 mg ginseng root (ginseng composition not stated).

G115®: Pharmaton Natural Health Products / P.O. Box 368 / Ridgefield, CT 06877 / U.S.A. / Tel: 800-451-6688 / Fax: 203-798-5771 / www.pharmaton.com / Email: askpharmaton@rdg.boehringer-ingelheim.com.

Gerimax® Ginseng extract: Dansk Droge A/S / Industrigrenen 10 / 2635, Ishoj, Copenhagen / Denmark / Tel: +43-56-5656 / Fax: +43-56-5600. Internal composition of tablet not disclosed in study.

Ginsana® G115 capsules: Pharmaton Natural Health Products. One capsule contains 100 mg of standardized (4% total ginsenosides) ginseng root extract G115®. Dry extract is approximately 5:1 (*w/w*) so that 200 mg extract corresponds to about 1 g of dried root.

Pharmaton® capsules: Pharmaton Natural Health Products. One capsule contains 40 mg of standardized (4% total ginsenosides) ginseng root extract G115®, 26 mg dimethyl aminoethanol bitartrate, 4,000 I.U. vitamin A, 2 mg vitamin B1, 2 mg vitamin B2, 1 mg vitamin B6, 1 mcg vitamin B12, 60 mg vitamin C, 400 I.U. vitamin D, 10 mg vitamin E, 15 mg niacinamide, 2.8 mg copper sulphate monohydrate, 3.1 mg manganese sulphate monohydrate.

PKC 167/79: Pharmaton S.A. / CH-6903 / Lugano / Switzerland / Tel: +41-91-610-3111. Each capsule contains 100 mg of ginseng extract derived from an aqueous solution. Investigational product only, not available.

*American equivalents, if any, are found in the Product Table beginning on page 398.

REFERENCES

Amato M, Izzo A, Nocerino E. The aphrodisiac and adaptogenic properties of ginseng. *Fitoterapia* 2000;71:S1-S5.

Ando T, Muraoka T, Yamasaki N, Okuda H. Preparation of antilipolytic substance from *Panax ginseng*. *Planta Med* 1980;38:18–23.

Avakian E, *et al.* Effect of *Panax ginseng* extract on energy metabolism during exercise in rats. *Planta Med* 1984;50:151–4.

Bahrke M, Morgan W. Evaluation of the ergogenic properties of ginseng. *Sports Med* 1994;18(4):229–48.

Bahrke M, Morgan W. Evaluation of the ergogenic properties of ginseng. *Sports Med* 2000;29(2):113–33.

Blumenthal M. Debunking the "ginseng abuse syndrome". *Whole Foods* 1991 March:89–91.

Blumenthal M. Herb sales down 15% in mainstream market. *HerbalGram* 2001;51:69.

Blumenthal M, Busse WR, Goldberg A, Gruenwald J, Hall T, Riggins CW, Rister RS (eds.). Klein S, Rister RS (trans.). *The Complete German Commission E Monographs—Therapeutic Guide to Herbal Medicines.* Austin, TX: American Botanical Council; Boston: Integrative Medicine Communication; 1998; 138–9.

Blumenthal M, Goldberg A, Brinckmann J (eds.). *Herbal Medicine—Expanded Commission E Monographs.* Newton, MA: Integrative Medicine Communications; 2000;170–7.

Bone K. Ginseng—The Regal Herb, Part 1. *MediHerb Pro Rev* 1998 May;62:1–4.

Ginseng The Regal Herb, Part 2. *MediHerb Pro Rev* 1998 June;63:1–4. Ginseng— The Regal Herb, Part 3. *MediHerb Pro Rev* 1998 July;64:1–4.

Bradley P (ed.). *British Herbal Compendium: A handbook of scientific information on widely used plant drugs.* Dorset, England: British Herbal Medicine Association; 1992.

Brinker F. *Herb Contraindications and Drug Interactions* 3d ed. Sandy, OR: Eclectic Medical Publications, 2001;107–9.

Cardinal BJ, Engels HJ. Ginseng does not enhance psychological well-being in healthy, young adults: results of a double-blind, placebo-controlled, randomized clinical trial. *J Am Diet Assoc* 2001 Jun;101(6):655–60.

Chang Y, Park C., Noh, H. The effect of *Panax ginseng* on the postoperative radiation complication in cervical cancer patients. *Seoul J Med* 1980;(21):187–93.

Chen YJ, Wu CF, Awang DVC, *et al. Ginsenosides: The Chemistry, Pharmacology, and Clinical Perspectives.* 2003 [in press].

Cherdrungsi P, Rungroeng K. Effects of standardized ginseng extract and exercise training on aerobic and anaerobic exercise capacities in humans. *Korean J Ginseng Sci* 1995;(19):93–100.

Cho YK, Lee HJ, Sung H *et al.* Long-term intake of Korean red ginseng in HIV-1-infected patients: development of resistance mutation to zidovudine is delayed. *Intl Immunopharmacol* 2001;1:1295–1305.

Cho Y, Lee H, Oh W, Kim Y. Long term immunological effect of ginseng on HIV-infected patients. *Abstr Gen Meet Am Soc Microbiol* 1997;97:247. (Abstract No. E44).

Cho Y, Kim Y, Choi M, *et al.* The effect of red ginseng and Zidovudine on HIV patients. Int Conf AIDS; 1994;10(1):215. (Abstract No. PB0289).

Choi H, Seong D, Rha K. Clinical efficacy of Korean red ginseng for erectile dysfunction. *Int J Impot Res* 1995;7(3):181–6.

Choi K, Seong D. Effectiveness for erectile dysfunction after the administration of Korean red ginseng. *Korean J Ginseng Sci* 1995;19:17–21.

Chong S, Oberholzer V. Ginseng—is there a use in clinical medicine? *Postgrad Med J* 1988;64:841–6.

Chuang W, Wu H, Sheu S, *et al.* A comparative study on commercial samples of Ginseng Radix. *Planta Med* 1995;61:459–65.

Chung C, *et al.* Isolation and hypoglycaemic activity of panaxans A, B, C, D, and E, glycans of *Panax ginseng* roots. *Planta Med* 1984;38:18–23.

Coon JT, Ernst E. *Panax ginseng*: a systematic review of adverse effects and drug interactions. *Drug Saf* 2002;25(5):323–44.

Court W. *Ginseng: The Genus* Panax. Amsterdam: Harwood Scientific Publishers; 2000.

D'Angelo L, Grimaldi R, Caravaggi M *et al.* Double-blind, placebo-controlled clinical study on the effect of a standardized Ginseng extract on psychomotor performance in healthy volunteers. *J Ethnopharmacol* 1986;16(1):15–22.

DAB. See: *Deutsches Arzneibuch*.

De Oliveira ACC, Perez AC, Merino G *et al.* Protective effects of *Panax ginseng* on muscle injury and inflammation after eccentric exercise. *Compar Biochem Physiol* 2001;C(130):369–77.

De Smet PAGM, Keller K, Hansel R, Chandler RF. *Adverse Effects of Herbal Drugs 2.* New York: Springer-Verlag, 1993.

Deutsches Arzneibuch (DAB). Ginsengwurzel. In: *Deutsches Arzneibuch* Ergänzungslieferung 1999. Stuttgart, Germany: Deutscher Apotheker Verlag; 1999.

Dharmananda S. The nature of ginseng: Traditional use, modern research, and the question of dosage. *HerbalGram* 2002;54:34–51.

Dörling E. Do ginsenosides influence the performance? Results of a double-blind study. *Notabene Medici* 1980;10(5):241–6.

EMEA. See: European Agency for the Evaluation of Medicinal Products.

Engels H, Said J, Wirth J. Failure of chronic ginseng supplementation to affect work performance and energy metabolism in healthy adult females. *Nutr Res* 1996;16(8):1295–1305.

Engels H, Wirth J. No ergogenic effects of ginseng (*Panax ginseng* C.A. Meyer) during graded maximal aerobic exercise. *J Am Diet Assoc* 1997;97(10):1110–5.

European Agency for the Evaluation of Medicinal Products (EMEA). Ginseng Summary Report. London, UK: European Agency for the Evaluation of Medicinal Products: Committee for Veterinary Medicinal Products; 1999 Aug;EMEA/MRL/669/99-FINAL.

European Pharmacopoeia (Ph.Eur. 2001). Ginseng radix. In: *European Pharmacopoeia* 3rd edition Supplement 2001. Strasbourg, France: Council of Europe; 2001;887–9.

Ferrando A, Vila L, Voces J, *et al.* Effects of a standardized *Panax ginseng* extract on the skeletal muscle of the rat: a comparative study in animals at rest and under exercise. *Planta Med* 1999;65:239–44.

Forgo L, Kayasseh L, Staub J. Effect of a standardized Ginseng extract on general well-being, reaction-time, pulmonary function and the sex hormones. [in German]. *Medizinische Welt* 1981;32:751–6.

Fukuda N, Tanaka H, Shoyama Y. Isolation of the pharmacologically active saponin ginsenoside Rb1 from ginseng by immunoaffinity column chromatography. *J Nat Prod* 2000;63:283–5.

Fulder S, Kataria M, Gethyn-Smith B. A double-blind clinical trial of *Panax ginseng* in aged subjects. *Proceedings of the 4th International Ginseng Symposium.* Daejeon, Korea: Korea Ginseng & Tobacco Research Institute; 1984 Sept 18–20.

General Sale List (GSL). Ginseng. In: *Statutory Instrument 1994 No. 2410: The Medicines (Products Other than Veterinary Drugs). General Sale List.* London, UK: Her Majesty's Stationery Office (HMSO); 1994;No.2410.

Goetz P. Phytotherapie in Frankreich. *Z Phytother* 1999;20:320–8.

Gross D, Krieger D, Efrat R, Dayan M. Ginseng extrakt G115® for the treatment of chronic respiratory diseases. *Schweiz Z Ganzheits Med* 1995;29–33.

GSL. See: *General Sale List.*

Hall T, Lu Z-Z, Yat PN *et al.* Evaluation of Consistency of Standardized Asian Ginseng Products in the Ginseng Evaluation Program. *Herbalgram* 2001;52:31–47

Han K, Choe S, Kim H, *et al.* Effect of red ginseng on blood pressure in patients with essential hypertension and white coat hypertension. *Am J Chin Med* 1998;26(2):199–209.

Han K, *et al.* Studies on the antioxidant components of Korean ginseng. III. Identification of phenolic acids. *Arch Pharmacol Res* 1983;4:54–8.

Health Canada. *Listing of Drugs Currently Regulated as New Drugs*—Revised April 1999. Ottawa, ON: Health Canada; 1999 April 11;21–2.

Health Canada. Product Information: *Panax ginseng.* In: *Drug Product Database (DPD).* Ottawa, ON: Health Canada Therapeutic Products Programme; 2001.

Health Protection Branch (HPB). Ginseng. In: *HPB Status Manual.* Ottawa, ON: Health Protection Branch; 1993 Feb 19;89.

Hoegler N. Researchers Claim Ginseng Lacks "Compelling Evidence". *HerbalGram.* 2001a; 52:20.

Hoegler N. Review Questions Ginseng's Role in Exercise. *HerbalGram.* 2001b; 52:21.

Hopkins MP, Androff L, Benninghoff AS. A case of post menopausal bleeding attributed to the use of topical ginseng is reported. Ginseng appears to have an estrogen-like effect on genital tissues. *Am J Obstet Gynecol* 1988 Nov;159(5)1121-2.

Hou, J. The Chemical Constituents of Ginseng Plants. *Comp Med East and West* 1977;123–45.

HPB. See: Health Protection Branch.

Hu S. A contribution to our knowledge of ginseng. *Am J Chinese Med* 1977;5(1):1–23.

Iqbal M. Medicinal Plants: Ginseng. In: *International Trade in Non-wood Forest Products: An Overview.* Rome, Italy: Food and Agriculture Organization (FAO) of the United Nations. 1993 Nov; Chapter XI Medicinal Plants; Section 5.13.

Japanese Standards for Herbal Medicines (JSHM). Monographs: Ginseng Radix JP XII; Ginseng Radix Pulverata Japanese Herbal Medicine Codex. In: *Japanese Standards for Herbal Medicines.* Tokyo, Japan: Yakuji Nippo LTD.; 1993;127–8.

Johnson A, Jiang N, Staba EJ. Whole ginseng effects on human response to demands for performance. *Proceedings of the 3rd International Ginseng Symposium.* Seoul Korea: Korea Ginseng Research Institute; 1980 Sept. 8–10.

JSHM. See: Japanese Standards for Herbal Medicines.

Kakizoe T. Asian studies of cancer chemoprevention: latest clinical trials. *Eu J Cancer* 2000;36:1303–9.

Kawatani K, Nakata J, Tamaoki J *et al.* Ginsenoside-induced relaxation of human bronchial smooth muscle via release of nitric oxide. *Br J Pharmacol* 2000;130(8):1859–64.

Kim W, Kim J, Han S, *et al.* Steaming of ginseng at high temperature enhances biological activity. *J Nat Prod* 2000;63:1702–4.

KMHW. See: Korean Ministry of Health and Welfare.

Korean Ministry of Health and Welfare (KMHW). *Korean Food Standards Code.* Seoul, Korea: The Korean Ministry of Health; 1999;423.

Korean Ministry of Health and Welfare (KMHW). Major Programs for Health and Welfare: Pharmaceuticals Approval System. Seoul, Korea: The Korean Ministry of Health; 2000. Available at: http://www.mohw.go.kr/html/e0003050102.html

Kwon J, Kim K, Belanger J, Parel J. A novel application of microwave-assisted process to the fast extraction of soluble ginseng components. Taegu, Korea: Kyungpook National University Department of Food Science and Technology; 2000.

Lange D, Schippmann U. Trade Survey of Medicinal Plants in Germany—A Contribution to International Plant Species Conservation. Bonn, Bundesamt für Naturschutz; 1997;69–72.

Le Gal M, Cathebras P, Strüby K. Pharmaton® capsules in the treatment of functional fatigue: A double-blind study versus placebo evaluated by a new methodology. *Phytother Res* 1996;10:49–53.

Lee S, Lee G, Kwon J. Optimization of extraction conditions for soluble ginseng components using microwave extraction system under pressure. *J Korean Soc Food Sci Nutr* 1999;28(2):409–16.

Lee S, Moon Y, You K. Effects of red ginseng saponins and nootropic drugs on impaired acquisition of ethanol-treated rats in passive avoidance performance. *J Ethnopharmacol* 2000;69(1):1–8.

Liu C, Xiao P. Recent advances on ginseng research in China. *J Ethnopharmacol*

1992;(36):27–38.

Liu W, Xu S, Che C. Anti-proliferative effect of ginseng saponins on human prostate cancer cell line. *Life Sci* 2000;67(11):1297–306.

Ma Q. Ginseng roots. In: Asia-Pacific Forestry Sector Outlook Study: Volume I – Socio-Economic, Resources and Non-Wood Products Statistics. Rome, Italy: Food and Agriculture Organization (FAO) of the United Nations; 1999.

McGuffin M, Hobbs C, Upton R, Goldberg A (eds.). *American Herbal Products Association's Botanical Safety Handbook.* Boca Raton, FL: CRC Press; 1997;81.

Medical Products Agency (MPA). Naturläkemedel: Authorised Natural Remedies (as of January 24, 2001). Uppsala, Sweden: Medical Products Agency; 2001.

Medical Products Agency (MPA). Naturläkemedelsmonografi: *Panax ginseng.* Uppsala, Sweden: Medical Products Agency; 1999.

Meyer-Buchtela E. Ginsengwurzel. In: *Tee-Rezepturen—Ein Handbuch für Apotheker und Ärzte.* Stuttgart, Germany: Deutscher Apotheker Verlag; 1999.

Molnar J, Szabo D, Pusztai R, *et al.* Membrane associated antitumor effects of crocine-, ginsenoside- and cannabinoid deriviates. *Anticancer Res* 2000;20(2A):861–867.

Morant J, Ruppanner H (eds.). *Arzneimittel-Kompendium der Schweiz® 2001/02 Publikumsausgabe.* Basel, Switzerland: Documed AG; 2001.

Morreale A, Janetsky K. Probable interaction between warfarin and ginseng. *Am J Health Sys Pharm* 1997;54(6):692–3.

MPA. See: Medical Products Agency.

ÖAB. See: *Österreichisches Arzneibuch.*

Österreichisches Arzneibuch (ÖAB). Wien, Österreich: Verlag der Österreichischen Staatsdruckerei. 1990.

Petkov V, Mosharrof A. Effects of standardized ginseng extract on learning, memory, and physical capabilities. *Am J Chin Med* 1987;(15):19–29.

Ph.Eur. See: *European Pharmacopoeia.*

Ph.Fr. See: *Pharmacopée Française.*

Ph.Helv. See: *Pharmacopoeia Helvetica.*

Pharmacopée Française Xe Édition (Ph.Fr.X). Moulins-les-Metz: Maisonneuve S.A: 1983–1990.

Pharmacopoeia Helvetica (Ph.Helv.VII). Office Central Fédéral des Imprimés et du Matériel: Bern; 1987;7(1–4).

Pharmacopoeia of the People's Republic of China (PPRC English Edition 1997 Volume I). Beijing, China; Chemical Industry Press; 1997;151–3.

Pieralisi G, Ripari P, Vecchiet L. Effects of a standardized ginseng extract combined with dimethylaminoethanol ditartrate, vitamins, minerals, and trace elements on physical performance during exercise. *Clin Ther* 1991;13(3):373–82.

PPRC. See: *Pharmacopoeia of the People's Republic of China.*

Quiroga H, Imbriano A. The effect of *Panax ginseng* extract on cerebrovascular deficits. *Orientacion Med* 1979;1208:86–87.

Quiroga H. Comparative double-blind study of the effect of Ginsana® G115 and Hydergine on cerebrovascular deficits. *Orientacion Medica* 1981;1281:201–2.

Reinold E. The use of ginseng in gynecology. [in German]. *Natur-und Ganzheits Med* 1990;4:131–4.

Reynolds J, Parfitt K, Parsons A, Sweetman S (eds.). Ginseng. In: *Martindale: The Extra Pharmacopoeia* 29th ed. London, UK: The Pharmaceutical Press; 1989;1574.

Rosenfeld M, Nachtajler S, Schwartz G, *et al.* Evaluation of the efficacy of a standardized ginseng extract in patients with psychophysical asthenia and neurological disorders. *La Semana Medica* 1989;173(9):148–54.

Ruppanner H, Schaefer U (eds.). *Codex 2000/01 — Die Schweizer Arzneimittel in einem Griff.* Basel, Switzerland: Documed AG; 2000.

Saito H, Yoshida Y, Takagi K. Effect of *Panax ginseng* root on exhaustive exercise in mice. *Jap J Pharm* 1974;24:119–27.

Salvati G, *et al.* Effects of *Panax ginseng* C.A. Meyer saponins on male fertility. *Panminerva Med* 1996;38(4):249–54.

Sandberg, Finn. Clinical effects of ginseng preparation. *Department of Pharmacognosy, Biomedicum,* 23. Sweden; 1974.

Sankary T. Controlled clinical trials of Anginlyc, Chinese herbal immune enhancer, in HIV seropositives. *Int Conf AIDS* 1989;5:496. (Abstract No. B.596).

Scaglione F, Cattaneo G, Alessandria M, Cogo R. Efficacy and safety of the standardized ginseng extract G115® for potentiating vaccination against common cold and/or fluenza syndrome. *Drugs Exp Clin Res* 1996;22(2):65–72. [Corrected; published erratum appears in 22(6):338.]

Scaglione F, Cogo R, Cocuzza C, Arcidiacono M, Beretta A. Immunomodulatory effects of *Panax ginseng* C.A. Meyer (G115®) on alveolar macrophages from patients suffering with chronic bronchitis. *Internat J Immunother* 1994;10(1):21–4.

Scaglione F, *et al.* Immunomodulatory effects of two extracts of *Panax ginseng* C.A. Meyer. *Drugs Exp Clin Res* 1990;16(10):537–42.

Scaglione F, Weiser K, Alessandria M. Effects of the standardized ginseng extract G115® in patients with chronic bronchitis: a non-blinded, randomized, comparative pilot study. *Clin Drug Invest* 2001;21(1):41–5.

Schardt D. Ginseng. *Nutrition Action Healthletter,* May 1999:10-11.

Siegel RK. Ginseng abuse syndrome: problems with the panacea. *JAMA* Apr 13;241(15):1614–5.

Shim I, Javaid J, Kim S. Effect of ginseng total saponin on extracellular dopamine release elicited by local infusion of nicotine into the striatum of freely moving rats. *Planta Med* 2000;66(8):705–8.

Shin H, Kim J, Yun T, *et al*. The cancer-preventive potential of *Panax ginseng*: a review of human and experimental evidence. *Cancer Causes Control* 2000;11(6):565–76.

Singh V, Agarwal S, Gupta B. Immunomodulatory activity of *Panax ginseng* extract. *Planta Med* 1984;50: 462–5.

Smith K, Engels H, Martin J, Wirth J. Efficacy of a standardized ginseng extract to alter psychological function characteristics at rest and during exercise stress. *Med Sci Sport Exerc* 1995;(27):147.

Soldati F. Panax ginseng: Standardization and biological activity. In: Cutler SJ, Cutler HG. *Biologically Active Natural Products: Pharmaceuticals*. Boca Raton, FL: CRC Press, 2000;209–32.

Sotaniemi E, Haapakoski E, Rautio A. Ginseng therapy in non-insulin-dependent diabetic patients. *Diabetes Care* 1995;18(10):1373–5.

Sørenson H, Sonne J. A double-masked study of the effects of ginseng on cognitive functions. *Curr Ther Res* 1996 Dec;57(12):959–68.

Srisurapanon S, Apibal S, Siripol R *et al*. The effect of standardized ginseng extract on peripheral blood leucocytes and lymphocyte subjects: a preliminary study in young healthy adults. *J Med Assoc Thai* 1997;(80):S81–5.

State Pharmacopoeia of the Union of Soviet Socialist Republics, 10th ed. (USSR X). Moscow: Ministry of Health of the U.S.S.R; 1973.

Takeda A, Katoh N, Yonezawa M. 1982. Restoration of radiation injury by ginseng. III. Radioprotective effect of thermostable fraction of ginseng extract on mice, rats and guinea pigs. *J Radiat Res* (Tokyo). 1982;23(2):150–67.

Takeda A, Yonezawa M, Katoh N. Restoration of radiation injury by ginseng. I. Responses of X- irradiated mice to ginseng extract. *J Radiat Res* (Tokyo). 1981;22(3):323–35.

Tang W, Eisenbrand G. *Chinese Drugs of Plant Origin: Chemistry, Pharmacology, and Use in Traditional and Modern Medicine*. Berlin: Springer-Verlag, 1992;711–51.

Tunón H. Phytotherapie in Schweden. *Z Phytother* 1999;20:268–77.

United States Congress (USC). Public Law 103–417: Dietary Supplement Health and Education Act of 1994. Washington, DC: 103rd Congress of the United States; 1994.

United States Department of Commerce (USDOC). Ginseng Roots, Fresh or Dried, Whether or Not Cut, Crushed or Powdered. U.S. Imports for Consumption: November 2000 and 2000 YTD, not Seasonally Adjusted; December 1999 and 1999 YTD, not Seasonally Adjusted. Washington, DC: U.S. Department of Commerce; 2000.

United States Pharmacopeia (USP 25th Revision) – National Formulary (NF 20th Edition). Rockville, MD: United States Pharmacopeial Convention, Inc. 2002.

United States Pharmacopeial Convention (USPC). Monographs In-Process Revision: Powdered Asian Ginseng Extract; Asian Ginseng Capsules; Asian Ginseng Tablets. *Pharmacopeial Forum*; 2000 May–June;26(3):453–6, 775–8.

USC. See: United States Congress.

USDOC. See: United States Department of Commerce.

USP. See: *United States Pharmacopeia*.

USPC. See: United States Pharmacopeial Convention.

Van Schepdael P. The effects on capacity of ginseng G115® in sports of endurance. [in French]. *Acta therapeutica*. 1993;19:337–47.

Vogler B, Pittler M, Ernst E. The efficacy of ginseng: a systematic review of randomised clinical trials. *Eur J Clin Pharmacol* 1999;55:567–75.

Von Ardenne M, Klemm, W. Measurements of the increase in the difference between the arterial and venous Hb-O saturation obtained with daily administration of 200 mg standardized ginseng extract G115® for four weeks. *Panminerva Med* 1987;(29)2:143–50.

Wang L, Lee T. Effect of ginseng saponins on cold tolerance in young and elderly rats. *Planta Med* 2000;66(2):144–7.

Wenkui L., Chungang G., Hongjie Z. *et al*. Use of High-Performance Liquid Chromatography—Tandem Mass Spectrometry to Distinguish *Panax ginseng* C.A. Meyer (Asian Ginseng) and *Panax quinquefolius* L. (North American Ginseng). *Anal Chem* 2000;72:5417—5422.

WHO. See: World Health Organization.

Wichtl M, Bisset N (eds.). *Herbal Drugs and Phytopharmaceuticals: A Handbook for Practice on a Scientific Basis*. Stuttgart, Germany: Medpharm Scientific Publishers; 1994;236–8.

Wiklund I, Lindgren R, Mattson L, Limoni C. Ginsana® G115 has a beneficial effect on quality of life in postmenopausal women: results from a randomized, placebo-controlled study. University of Gothenburg and Linkoping, Sweden; 1994.

Williams M. Immuno-protection against herpes simplex type II infection by *Eleutherococcus* root extract. *Int J Altern Comp Med* 1995;(13):9–12.

World Health Organization (WHO). Radix Ginseng. In: *WHO Monographs on Selected Medicinal Plants* Vol. 1. Geneva, Switzerland: World Health Organization; 1999;168–82.

World Health Organization (WHO). *Regulatory Situation of Herbal Medicines: A Worldwide Review*. Geneva, Switzerland: World Health Organization; 1998;44–5.

Yamamoto M, Uemura T, Nakama S *et al*. Serum HDL-cholesterol-increasing and fatty liver-improving actions of *Panax ginseng* in high cholesterol diet-fed rats with clinical affect on hyperlipidemia in man. *Am J Chin Med* 1983;11(1–4):96–101.

Yen K. *The Illustrated Chinese Materia Medica Crude and Prepared*. Taipei: SMC Publishing Inc.; 1992;40.

Yun T. Saponin contents and anticarcinogen effect of ginseng depending on types and ages in mice. *Chung Kuo Yao Li Hsueh Pao* 1996;17(4):293–8.

Yun T, Choi S. Non-organ specific cancer prevention of ginseng: a prospective study in Korea. *Int J Epidemiol* 1998;27(3):359–64.

Yun T, Choi S. Preventative effect of ginseng intake against various human cancers: A case-control study on 1987 pairs. *Cancer Epidemiol Biomarkers Prev* 1995 June;(4):401–8.

Yun T, Choi S. A case-control study of ginseng intake and cancer. *Int J Epidemiol* 1990 Dec;19(4):871–6.

Yun T, Choi S, Lee Y. Cohort study on ginseng intake and cancer for population over 40-year-old in ginseng production areas (a preliminary report). (Meeting Abstract (201993):132.) Berlin: *Second International Cancer Chemo Prevention Conference*; 1993.

Zhong YM, Nishijo H, Uwano T, *et al*. Red ginseng ameliorated place navigation deficits in young rats with hippocampal lesions and aged rats. *Physiol Behav* 2000;69(4–5):511–25.

Zhou M, Chan KW, Ng LS, *et al*. Possible influences of ginseng on the pharmacokinetics and pharmacodynamics of warfarin in rats. *J Pharm Pharmacol* 1999; 51-175-180. Cited in Brinker F. *Herb Contraindications and Drug Interactions*, 3rd ed. Sandy, OR: Eclectic Medical Publications; 2001:109.

Zuin M, Battezzati P, Camisasca M, *et al*. Effects of a preparation containing a standardized ginseng extract combined with trace elements and multivitamins against hepatotoxin-induced chronic liver disease in the elderly. *J Int Med Res* 1987;15(5):276–81.

Clinical Studies on Asian Ginseng (*Panax ginseng* C.A. Meyer)

Cancer Prevention

Author/Year	Subject	Design	Duration	Dosage	Preparation	Results/Conclusion
Yun and Choi, 1998	Cancer prevention	P, CC n=4,587 (mean age 55.5 years)	5 years (1987–92)	Varied	Ginseng root soup (boiled 3 hours), fresh ginseng root extract, and other dosage forms	Intake of ginseng correlated with an overall 60% reduction in risk of dying of any type of cancer compared to non-users. Fresh ginseng extract showed the strongest protective effect, with 69% risk reduction compared to non-users. The risk of gastric and lung cancers was also reduced significantly (67% and 70% protection, respectively).
Yun and Choi, 1995	Cancer prevention	E, CC n=3,974 case control study on 1,987 pairs (average ages men= 53.2 years, women=49.8 years)	67 weeks	Varied	Red ginseng root, white ginseng root powder, dried white ginseng extract, fresh white ginseng extract (brands not stated)	Relative risk of cancer in ginseng group was 50% lower than for non-users. Red ginseng users had the lowest risk. Subjects taking ginseng for one year decreased the rate of cancer incidence by 36% compared to 69% in those who used ginseng for 5 years or more. In those who had used ginseng less than 50 times in their lifetime the reduction was 45%, while those who had used ginseng over 500 times had a 72% reduction. Most protective against cancer of the ovaries, larynx, esophagus, pancreas, and stomach. No significant effect on breast, cervical, bladder, or thyroid cancer.
Yun and Choi, 1990	Cancer prevention	E, CC n=1,810 905 pairs, (average ages, men= 51 years, women=48 years)	5 years	Varied	Red ginseng root, white ginseng root powder, dried white ginseng extract, fresh white ginseng extract (brands not stated)	Of the cases, 62% had history of ginseng intake compared to 75% of controls; 0.56 odds ratio (OR) (p<0.01) of cancer in relation to ginseng intake. A dose-response relationship was observed. The higher the ginseng intake, the lower the risk of cancer. The extract and powder were found to be the most effective forms in reducing the OR.

Diabetes

Author/Year	Subject	Design	Duration	Dosage	Preparation	Results/Conclusion
Sotaniemi et al., 1995	Non-insulin-dependent diabetes mellitus (type 2)	DB, PC, R, MC n=36 type II diabetic patients; 3 parallel groups. Average age of 100 mg group=59 years, and 200 mg group=57 years	2 months	1 tablet/day containing 100 mg ginseng/day or 200 mg ginseng/day or placebo	Dansk Droge tablets containing 100 mg ginseng root or 200 mg ginseng root (ginseng composition not stated)	Compared with baseline, both ginseng groups experienced significant improvement (p<0.05) in physical performance, mood, reduced fasting blood glucose levels, serum aminoterminal propeptide (PIIINP) of type 2 procollagen concentration; also experienced lowered glycated hemoglobin. But no improvement in memory or sleep. Hemoglobin A1c (HbA1c) significantly improved (p<0.05) in patients receiving 200 mg ginseng daily.

Fatigue/Ergogenic Effects

Author/Year	Subject	Design	Duration	Dosage	Preparation	Results/Conclusion
Engels and Wirth, 1997	Maximal aerobic exercise	DB, PC n=36 healthy men, mean age 37 years, 3 parallel groups	8 weeks	2 or 4 capsules/day containing 100 mg extract each or placebo	Ginsana® G 115, 100 mg ginseng extract standardized to 4% ginsenosides	No significant effect on oxygen consumption, respiratory exchange ratio, blood lactic acid concentration, or heart rate (p>0.05). Study does not support claims that ginseng extract is an ergogenic aid to support submaximal and maximal aerobic exercise.
Engels et al., 1996	Athletic performance parameters	DB, PC, R n=19 healthy women, 21–35 years, 2 parallel groups	8 weeks	2 capsules/day containing 100 mg extract each or placebo	Ginsana® G 115	Athletic performance parameters measured included maximal work performance, oxygen uptake, respiratory exchange rate, blood lactate, and heart rate during graded cycle ergometry test to exhaustion. No significant intergroup differences in any of the measured parameters (p>0.05).
Le Gal et al., 1996	Functional fatigue	DB, PC, R n=232 age 25–60 years	42 days	1 capsule containing 40 mg ginseng extract G115, 2x/day or placebo	Pharmaton® capsules	Compared to placebo, ginseng group noticed improvements in tested parameters including fatigue score at 21 days, but no significant differences noted until day 42 (p=0.023).

KEY: C – controlled, **CC** – case-control, **CH** – cohort, **CI** – confidence interval, **Cm** – comparison, **CO** – crossover, **CS** – cross-sectional, **DB** – double-blind, **E** – epidemiological, **LC** – longitudinal cohort, **MA** – meta-analysis, **MC** – multi-center, **n** – number of patients, **O** – open, **OB** – observational, **OL** – open label, **OR** – odds ratio, **P** – prospective, **PB** – patient-blind, **PC** – placebo-controlled, **PG** – parallel group, **PS** – pilot study, **R** – randomized, **RC** – reference-controlled, **RCS** – retrospective cross-sectional, **RS** - retrospective, **S** – surveillance, **SB** – single-blind, **SC** – single-center, **U** – uncontrolled, **UP** – unpublished, **VC** – vehicle-controlled.

Clinical Studies on Asian Ginseng (*Panax ginseng* C.A. Meyer) (cont.)

Fatigue/Ergogenic Effects (cont.)

Author/Year	Subject	Design	Duration	Dosage	Preparation	Results/Conclusion
Cherdrungsi and Rungroeng, 1995	Maximal oxygen uptake, leg muscle strength, body fat, resting heart rate	DB, PC n=41 healthy students, 4 parallel groups	2 months	150 mg extract, 2x/day with exercise or placebo with exercise	Asian ginseng extract (extract composition not stated)	Body fat significantly decreased in both ginseng groups compared with baseline (p<0.05): subjects in the ginseng group without exercise improved maximal oxygen uptake, resting heart rate, and leg strength compared with the placebo group without exercise (p<0.05).
Van Schepdael, 1993	Effect on physical capacity and endurance	DB, PC, CO n=43 male triathletes	20 weeks during training	1 capsule containing 100 mg extract, 2x/day	Ginsana® G 115	During first 10-week period, no significant changes were observed. In the second 10-week period, ginseng treatment appeared to prevent loss of physical fitness determined by measurement of oxygen uptake and oxygen pulse.

Immunology

Author/Year	Subject	Design	Duration	Dosage	Preparation	Results/Conclusion
Cho et al., 1997	HIV	O, C n=26 HIV-infected patients	40–57 months with follow-up period of 41–69 months	5,400 mg/day	Korean red ginseng root powder (brand not stated)	Markers including CD4+ T-cells, serum beta2-microglobulin, soluble CD8 antigen (sCD8), and ICD p24 antigen were measured every 6 months and compared to control group. The sCD8 significantly decreased (p<0.01) in ginseng group. Study suggests that Korean red ginseng has definite long-term, immunomodulating effect without side effects on HIV-infected patients.
Srisurapanon et al., 1997	Immunomodulation parameters	DB, PC n=20 healthy men, age range 21–22, 2 parallel groups	2 months	3 capsules containing 100 mg extract/day	Ginsana® G 115	No significant intergroup differences in any tested parameters including total and differential leukocyte count, lymphocyte subpopulations CD3, CD4, CD8, CD4/8 ratio, CD19, CD25.
Scaglione et al., 1996	Immune response to flu vaccine	DB, PC, R, MC n=227 volunteers, mean age 48 years	3 months with an influenza vaccine at week 4	1 capsule containing 100 mg extract, 2x/day or placebo	Ginsana® G 115	Ginseng group experienced a significant immune response to flu vaccine with a significant rise in antibody levels and number of natural killer (NK) cells. Compared to placebo, ginseng group had significantly fewer (p<0.0001) cases of common cold or influenza. Antibody titres (p<0.0001) and NK cell activity (p<0.0001) significantly higher in ginseng group.
Scaglione et al., 1990	Immunomodulatory effects	DB, PC, Cm n=60 healthy volunteers, 3 parallel groups	8 weeks	One, 100 mg capsule G115, 2x/day or one, 100 mg capsule PKC 167/79, 2x/day or placebo	Ginsana® G115 vs. PKC 167/79 (an aqueous ginseng extract) vs. placebo	After 8 weeks, blood samples from both ginseng groups showed significant increase in intracellular killing of polymorphonuclear leukocytes, phagocytosis, and total number of T3 and T4 lymphocytes compared with baseline and placebo, though a more significant and earlier response was seen in the G115 group. Authors concluded that ginseng extract stimulates the human immune system and that the standardized extract was more effective than the aqueous extract.

Menopausal Symptoms

Author/Year	Subject	Design	Duration	Dosage	Preparation	Results/Conclusion
Wickland et al., 1994	Quality of life of post-menopausal women	R, PC n=NA	4 months	1 capsule containing 100 mg extract, 2x/day or placebo	Ginsana® G 115	No major impact on vasomotor symptoms. Significantly superior to placebo in enhancing aspects of well-being: vitality, alertness, mood, and relieving somatic symptoms.
Reinold, 1990	Menopausal symptoms	O, PC n=49	3 months	1 capsule containing 100 mg extract, 2x/day or placebo	Ginsana® G115	Good to very good effects on headache, dizziness, adynamia, asthenia, depression, and sleep disturbances. Unwanted side effects did not arise from taking the preparation. No changes observed in speculum exams and cytological smears from the cervix and vaginal wall.

KEY: C – controlled, **CC** – case-control, **CH** – cohort, **CI** – confidence interval, **Cm** – comparison, **CO** – crossover, **CS** – cross-sectional, **DB** – double-blind, **E** – epidemiological, **LC** – longitudinal cohort, **MA** – meta-analysis, **MC** – multi-center, **n** – number of patients, **O** – open, **OB** – observational, **OL** – open label, **OR** – odds ratio, **P** – prospective, **PB** – patient-blind, **PC** – placebo-controlled, **PG** – parallel group, **PS** – pilot study, **R** – randomized, **RC** – reference-controlled, **RCS** – retrospective cross-sectional, **RS** - retrospective, **S** – surveillance, **SB** – single-blind, **SC** – single-center, **U** – uncontrolled, **UP** – unpublished, **VC** – vehicle-controlled.

Ginseng, Asian

Monograph

Psychomotor Response/Circulatory System

Author/Year	Subject	Design	Duration	Dosage	Preparation	Results/Conclusion
Sørenson and Sonne, 1996	Effect on cognitive functions	DB, PC, R n=112 healthy volunteers (> 40 years), 2 parallel groups	8–9 weeks	400 mg extract/day or placebo	Gerimax®	Ginseng group had non-significant tendency to faster speed of simple reactions and significantly improved abstract thinking skills compared with placebo (p<0.02). No significant differentiation in concentration, memory, or subjective experience.
Smith et al., 1995	Effect on mood and perception	PC n=19 women, 2 parallel groups	2 months	1 capsule containing 100 mg extract, 2x/day or placebo	Ginsana® G115	No significant intergroup differences in tested parameters including mood profile and rating of perceived exertion after submaximal and maximal ergometer exercise.
Rosenfeld, 1989	Psycho-physical asthenia, depressive syndrome and neurological disorder	PC n=50 24 men, 26 women (mean age 39.7 years)	56 days, 2 week wash-out or placebo	1 capsule containing 100 mg extract, 2x/day or placebo	Ginsana® G115	G115® led to clinical improvement evidenced by the positive results of the psychometric tests used: Toulouetes (changes in total scores) (p<0.01); Wechsler-Bellevue test (intelligence and cognition function) (p<0.01); SCAG questionnaire (p<0.01).
Von Ardenne and Klemm, 1987	Oxygen status of human body in the elderly	C n=6 (venous), n=10 (arterial)	1 month	1 capsule containing 100 mg extract, 2x/day or placebo	Ginsana® G115	Increase in the resting pO_2 uptake and O_2 transport to the organs and tissues of the body from 100% before treatment to 129% after.
D'Angelo et al., 1986	Psychomotor performance	DB, PC n=32 healthy male volunteers (20–24 years old)	3 months	1 capsule containing 100 mg extract, 2x/day or placebo	Ginsana® G 115	Compared to baseline, ginseng and placebo group experienced favorable effects on attention, processing, integrated sensory-motor function, and auditory reaction time. Significant intergroup differences (p<0.05) in favor of ginseng compared to placebo in mental arithmetic test.
Fulder et al., 1984	Mental performance	DB, PC, CO n=49 with depression and reduced abilities associated with elderly senescence	20 days (10 days ginseng, 10 days placebo, with 3-week wash-out period between)	1,500 mg dried root/day or placebo	Korean red ginseng root (brand not stated)	Small improvements were noted in mood and well-being. Based on analog scales, subjects reported increased energy and alertness, but slightly worse sleep and reduced happiness. However, highly significant improvements were seen in the most objective and accurate tests of the trial: reactivity, speed, and coordination at the tapping test, and the visual, auditory, and disjunctive reaction timer. The authors concluded that ginseng can increase function in senile individuals.
Forgo et al., 1981	Effect on mental and physical functions	DB, PC n=120 60 men, 60 women, Divided by sex (male vs. female) and age, 30–39 years vs. 40–60 years)	3 months	1 capsule containing 100 mg extract, 2x/day or placebo	Ginsana® G 115	Significant difference between groups in favor of ginseng in self-assessment for women, ages 30–39 years (p=0.01). Significant changes in reaction capacity, pulmonary function, and self-assessment in patients ages 40–60 years. No significant difference in tests for mood, well-being, or general health.
Dörling, 1980	Effects on physical and mental performance	DB, PC n=60 22–80 years	90 days	1 capsule containing 100 mg extract, 2x/day or placebo	Ginsana® G 115	Improvements in reaction time to visual and auditory stimuli, coordination, respiratory quotients, and length of recovery phase.
Johnson et al., 1980	Effect on mental performance	DB, PC, Cm n=38	30 days	Approximately 2 g/day	Asian red ginseng root, or American ginseng root or eleuthero root (Siberian ginseng)	All 3 types of ginseng improved proofreading performance, while only Asian and American improved mood-fatigue. None significantly affected mathematical performance or final grade performance, nor did they affect urinary concentrations of catecholamines.

KEY: C – controlled, **CC** – case-control, **CH** – cohort, **CI** – confidence interval, **Cm** – comparison, **CO** – crossover, **CS** – cross-sectional, **DB** – double-blind, **E** – epidemiological, **LC** – longitudinal cohort, **MA** – meta-analysis, **MC** – multi-center, **n** – number of patients, **O** – open, **OB** – observational, **OL** – open label, **OR** – odds ratio, **P** – prospective, **PB** – patient-blind, **PC** – placebo-controlled, **PG** – parallel group, **PS** – pilot study, **R** – randomized, **RC** – reference-controlled, **RCS** – retrospective cross-sectional, **RS** - retrospective, **S** – surveillance, **SB** – single-blind, **SC** – single-center, **U** – uncontrolled, **UP** – unpublished, **VC** – vehicle-controlled.

Reproductive System, Male

Author/Year	Subject	Design	Duration	Dosage	Preparation	Results/Conclusion
Salvati et al., 1996	Fertility in men	O, C n=66 20 normal controls; 30 with idiopathic low sperm count, 16 with low sperm count due to varicocele	3 months	4,000 mg extract/day	Brand not stated	After 3 months, all 3 groups showed a rise in sperm count, total testosterone, sperm motility, free testosterone, and dihydrotestosterone (DHT) levels. Normal control subjects showed lowest increases. Prolactin levels fell in all 3 groups.
Choi et al., 1995	Erectile dysfunction	PC, Cm n=90 patients with erectile dysfunction	3 months	3 groups: 1,800 mg/day extract or 25 mg/day trazodone or placebo	Red ginseng extract (brand not stated), vs. trazodone or placebo	Compared to trazodone and placebo, ginseng caused significant improvements (p<0.05) in parameters of rigidity and tumescence in erection, early detumescence, libido, and patient satisfaction. No significant changes found in frequency of coitus, premature ejaculation, or morning erection.

Respiratory System

Author/Year	Subject	Design	Duration	Dosage	Preparation	Results/Conclusion
Scaglione et al., 2001	Acute bacterial attacks of chronic bronchitis (ACB)	R, Cm, PS n=75 (44 completed study) patients with acute attacks of chronic bronchitis (ages >18 years)	9 days	Initially 875 mg amoxicillin and 125 mg clavulanic acid 2x daily for 9 days then one group received antibiotic with 100 mg standardized ginseng extract G115 2x daily, the other group received antibacterial treatment only.	Ginsana® G 115	Both groups responded positively to treatment. In ginseng group, bacterial clearance was significantly faster than in the subjects receiving antibacterials alone. Statistically significant differences between treatment groups were observed on days 4, 5, 6, and 7 (p=0.0049, p=0.0104, p=0.0175, p=0.0182, respectively). Borderline trend seen on day 8 (p=0.0554). Log rank test showed significant difference after analysis of time to clearance of infection (chi^2=6.2127, p=0.0127). The authors concluded that due to the sample size, definitive conclusions could not be drawn, but the study suggests that patients with ACB may heal faster if ginseng is given with antibacterial treatment.
Gross et al., 1995	Severe chronic respiratory diseases	C, PS n=120 patients with severe chronic respiratory disease (mean age 67 years)	3 months	1 capsule containing 100 mg extract, 2x/day or placebo	Ginsana® G115	Improvement demonstrated in pulmonary functions, oxygenation capacity and walking capacity. Forced vital capacity increased from 32.1% to 72.8% (p<0.05), forced expiratory volume from 34.75% to 47.3% (p<0.05), and peak expiratory flow from 37.5% to 47.2% (p<0.01). Distance walked in 6 minutes increased from 600 m to 1,123 m.
Scaglione et al., 1994	Chronic bronchitis	SB, PC n=40 patients with smoker's chronic bronchitis	2 months	1 capsule containing 100 mg extract/12 hours or placebo	Ginsana® G 115	Intracellular killing of alveolar macrophages increased significantly by the eighth week in the treatment group but not in the control group. The study concluded G115 restored and increased the activity of alveolar macrophages in patients with chronic bronchitis (p<0.001).

KEY: **C** – controlled, **CC** – case-control, **CH** – cohort, **CI** – confidence interval, **Cm** – comparison, **CO** – crossover, **CS** – cross-sectional, **DB** – double-blind, **E** – epidemiological, **LC** – longitudinal cohort, **MA** – meta-analysis, **MC** – multi-center, **n** – number of patients, **O** – open, **OB** – observational, **OL** – open label, **OR** – odds ratio, **P** – prospective, **PB** – patient-blind, **PC** – placebo-controlled, **PG** – parallel group, **PS** – pilot study, **R** – randomized, **RC** – reference-controlled, **RCS** – retrospective cross-sectional, **RS** - retrospective, **S** – surveillance, **SB** – single-blind, **SC** – single-center, **U** – uncontrolled, **UP** – unpublished, **VC** – vehicle-controlled.

Ginseng, Asian

Monograph

(This page intentionally left blank.)

Goldenseal

Hydrastis canadensis L.
[Fam. *Ranunculaceae*]

OVERVIEW

Goldenseal is ranked among the top herbal supplements sold in natural food stores in the U.S. and is often combined with echinacea. In 2000, sales of goldenseal ranked 12th in the natural food trade. In 1998, sales of products that contain both goldenseal and echinacea ranked fifth in mainstream stores at $69.7 million. Despite goldenseal's popularity, clinical studies have been conducted only on its alkaloid, berberine. The fact that goldenseal is not widely used in Europe may account for the lack of clinical research. Goldenseal's medicinal value is believed to be due primarily to the alkadoidal constituents berberine and hydrastine.

PRIMARY USES

[EDITORS' NOTE: Since there are no published clinical trials scientifically documenting the safe and effective use of goldenseal preparations in humans, despite significant *empirical* data, the editors have refrained from suggesting any primary uses.]

Berberine

- Diarrhea
- Ocular trachoma infections (external)

OTHER POTENTIAL USES

Goldenseal

- Dyspepsia
- Gastritis
- Menorrhagia
- Eyewashes (external, diluted non-alcoholic extracts)

PHARMACOLOGICAL ACTIONS

Anti-diarrheal; anti-microbial; antiparasitic; decreases systemic and pulmonary vascular resistence and left ventricular end-diastolic pressure; increases stroke index, cardiac index and left ventricular ejection fraction; suppresses ventricular premature contractions (VPC) without severe side effects.

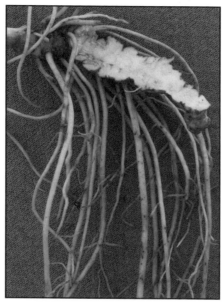

Photo © 2003 stevenfoster.com

DOSAGE AND ADMINISTRATION

It may take up to a few days to a week for the herb to produce benefits.

Internal

DRIED RHIZOME AND ROOT: 0.5–1.0 g, 3 times daily.

TINCTURE: 2–4 ml [1:10, 60% ethanol].

FLUID EXTRACT: 0.3–1 ml [1:1, 60% ethanol].

External

EYEWASH: 2 drops in each eye, 3 times daily [0.2% sterile aqueous berberine solution, or aqueous non-alcoholic goldenseal preparation].

CONTRAINDICATIONS

Goldenseal should not be used in cases of kidney disease, including kidney failure, due to inadequate urinary excretion of its alkaloids. It should be avoided in acute inflammation of the stomach, based on a case report in which a bitters formula enhanced gastric acid secretions. Contraindicated in cases of jaundice in newborns.

PREGNANCY AND LACTATION: Not for use during pregnancy. Berberine can increase bilirubin in neonates, possibly leading to neonatal jaundice. It may also have uterine stimulant activity. Although there are no known contraindications during lactation, use of goldenseal or berberine during nursing should be avoided until further research has been conducted.

ADVERSE EFFECTS

At recommended doses, goldenseal is considered nontoxic; berberine has also been well-tolerated in therapeutic doses.

DRUG INTERACTIONS

Goldenseal can potentially antagonize the anticoagulant activity of heparin. Studies in mice and rats have indicated hemodynamic properties of berberine, including an increase in the number of thrombocytes, decrease in the activity of factor XIII, and the promotion of blood coagulation.

CLINICAL REVIEW

Although modern controlled clinical studies on goldenseal are lacking, there have been studies published on one of its principal alkaloids, berberine. Five clinical studies on berberine that included a total of 465 participants all demonstrated positive effects for indications including diarrhea, ocular infections, and cardiovascular conditions, although the safety of cardiac conditions (e.g., ventricular arrhythmias) is not adequately established. Human studies on berberine have shown that it is poorly absorbed from the small intestines, and therefore its antimicrobial action is only locally effective (i.e. in the gut). Since berberine is excreted in the urine, it may have an antimicrobial effect in the kidneys or urinary tract. In clinical evaluations, berberine has been shown to be efficacious at stimulating bile and bilirubin secretion, improving symptoms of chronic cholecystitis, and normalizing elevated tyramine levels in persons with cirrhosis of the liver. Berberine is reportedly effective as an adjunct to cancer therapy. Clinical studies on berberine have confirmed that it is effective for acute diarrhea. Externally, it has been shown to be useful as an eyewash in treating trachoma, an infectious eye disease.

Goldenseal

Hydrastis canadensis L.
[Fam. *Ranunculaceae*]

OVERVIEW

Goldenseal is ranked among the top herbal supplements sold in natural food stores in the U.S. and is often combined with the herb echinacea (*Echinacea* spp.). In 1998, sales of products that contain both goldenseal and echinacea ranked 5th in mainstream stores at $69.7 million. In 2000, sales of goldenseal ranked 12th in the natural food trade. Goldenseal's medicinal actions are thought to be due to its primary active constituents, berberine and hydrastine. Goldenseal is often used by consumers for self-medication of upper respiratory tract infections associated with cold and flus although there is no scientific data to support this use.

PRIMARY USES OF BERBERINE

Internal
Diarrhea

External
Ocular (eye) trachoma infections (in special preparations usually in developing countries).

POTENTIAL USES OF GOLDENSEAL

[EDITORS' NOTE: Since there are no published clinical trials scientifically documenting the safe and effective use of goldenseal preparations in humans, despite significant *empirical* data, the editors have refrained from suggesting any primary uses.]

Internal
Stomach upset (dyspepsia, gastritis).

External
Eyewashes (using water or glycerine-based, diluted non-alcoholic preparations).

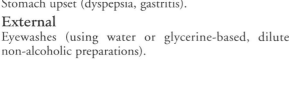

DOSAGE

NOTE: It may take up to a few days to a week for the herb to produce benefits.

DRIED RHIZOME AND ROOT: 0.5–1.0 g, 3 times daily.

TINCTURE: 2–4 ml [1:10, 60% ethanol].

FLUID EXTRACT: 0.3–1 ml [1:1, 60% ethanol].

EYEWASH: 2 drops in each eye, 3 times daily [0.2% sterile aqueous (non-alcoholic) berberine solution, or non-alcoholic, water-based goldenseal liquid preparations].

CONTRAINDICATIONS

Goldenseal should not be used in cases of kidney disease, including kidney failure due to inadequate urinary excretion of its alkaloids. It should be avoided in acute inflammation of the stomach. It is contraindicated in cases of jaundice in newborns.

PREGNANCY AND LACTATION: Not for use during pregnancy. Berberine can increase bilirubin in newborn babies, possibly leading to neonatal jaundice. It may have a stimulant effect on the uterus. Although there are no known contraindications during breast-feeding, use of goldenseal and berberine should be avoided during breast feeding until further research has been conducted.

ADVERSE EFFECTS

At recommended doses, goldenseal is considered nontoxic; berberine has also been well-tolerated in therapeutic doses.

DRUG INTERACTIONS

Goldenseal may antagonize the anticoagulant (blood-thinning) activity of heparin.

Comments

When using a dietary supplement, purchase it from a reliable source. For best results, use the same brand of product throughout the period of use. As with all medications and dietary supplements, please inform your healthcare provider of all herbs and medications you are taking. Interactions may occur between medications and herbs or even among different herbs when taken at the same time. Treat your herbal supplement with care by taking it as directed, storing it as advised on the label, and keeping it out of the reach of children and pets. Consult your healthcare provider with any questions.

AMERICAN
BOTANICAL
COUNCIL

The information contained on this sheet has been excerpted from *The ABC Clinical Guide to Herbs* © 2003 by the American Botanical Council (ABC). ABC is an independent member-based educational organization focusing on the medicinal use of herbs. For more detailed information about this herb please consult the healthcare provider who gave you this sheet. To order *The ABC Clinical Guide to Herbs* or become a member of ABC, visit their website at www.herbalgram.org.

Goldenseal

Hydrastis canadensis L.

[Fam. *Ranunculaceae*]

OVERVIEW

Goldenseal is ranked among the top herbal supplements sold in natural food stores in the U.S. (Blumenthal *et al.*, 1998) and it is often combined with echinacea (*Echinacea* spp.). In 2000, sales of goldenseal products ranked 12th in the natural food trade (NBJ, 2001). In 1998, sales of products that contain both goldenseal and echinacea, ranked fifth in mainstream stores, at $69.7 million (Blumenthal, 2001). Despite goldenseal's popularity, clinical studies have been conducted on only one of its principal alkaloids, berberine. Berberine, hydrastine, and related isoquinoline alkaloids are the primary constituents thought responsible for goldenseal's medicinal activity. Goldenseal is not used widely in Europe, and this may be the reason for the lack of clinical research (Tyler, 1998). Ethnomedical use dates to the Cherokee Indians, who used goldenseal root to treat skin diseases and sore or inflamed eyes. The Iroquois used the root for diarrhea, digestion, whooping cough, and pulmonary problems (Foster, 1996; Moerman, 1998). In the latter part of the 19th century, Eclectic physicians used goldenseal preparations primarily for acute or subacute inflammation of the mucous membranes (Felter and Lloyd, 1898), chronic inflammation of the stomach, and atonic dyspepsia associated with alcoholism (Blumenthal, 2001). Goldenseal root was official in the *United States Pharmacopeia* starting from 1860 (Lloyd, 1929), and up to five different preparations were listed in the USP until the 10th revision in 1926 (Boyle, 1991).

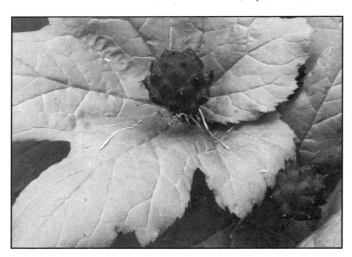

Photo © 2003 stevenfoster.com

Due to its relatively high price, some "goldenseal" products sold in the U.S. may contain "goldenseal herb", made with the leaves of the plant containing approximately 10% of the alkaloid levels usually found in the root. Some products have been known to be adulterated with the low cost goldthread root (*Coptis chinensis*) from China, a plant containing significant levels of berberine. Wild goldenseal was named a "threatened" species by CITES (Convention in Trade in Endangered Species) in 1997, thereby limiting its trade in international commerce (Bannerman, 1997). About 15–30% of domestic supplies of goldenseal are derived from cultivated sources within the U.S. (McGuffin, 1999).

DESCRIPTION

Goldenseal consists of the root and rhizome of *Hydrastis canadensis* L. [Fam. *Ranunculaceae*]. Its name derives from the seal-like scars on the rhizomes that are yellow or golden in color (Lloyd and Lloyd, 1884–85). The *United States Pharmacopeia* stipulates that the root and rhizome material must contain no less than 2.0% hydrastine and no less than 2.5% berberine (USPF, 2000).

PRIMARY USES

[EDITORS' NOTE: Since there are no published clinical trials documenting scientifically the safe and effective use of goldenseal preparations in humans, despite significant *empirical* data, the editors have refrained from suggesting any primary uses.]

Berberine (Pharmaceutical Preparations)
Internal
Gastrointestinal
- Diarrhea (Gupte, 1975; Khin *et al.*, 1985; Rabbani *et al.*, 1987)

External
Ophthalmic
- Ocular trachoma infections (Babbar *et al.*, 1982; Kholsa *et al.*, 1992 Mohan *et al.*, 1982)

OTHER POTENTIAL USES

Goldenseal
Internal
Gastrointestinal
- Dyspepsia (Bradley, 1992; Upton, 2001)
- Gastritis (Bradley, 1992)

Gynecology
- Menorrhagia (Bradley, 1992)

External
- Eyewashes (Bradley, 1992)

DOSAGE

Internal
DRIED RHIZOME AND ROOT: 0.5–1.0 g, 3 times daily (Bradley, 1992).

TINCTURE: (1:10, 60% ethanol), 2–4 ml (Bradley, 1992).

FLUID EXTRACT: (1:1, 60% ethanol), 0.3–1 ml (Bradley, 1992).

External
EYEWASH: (0.2% sterile aqueous [non-alcoholic] berberine solution) 2 drops are placed in each eye, 3 times daily (Kholsa *et al.*, 1992).

DURATION OF ADMINISTRATION

It may take up to a few days to a week for the herb to produce benefits. No known limitations on use (Tierra, 1998).

CHEMISTRY

The active ingredients of goldenseal are isoquinoline alkaloids, mainly hydrastine and berberine (Bruneton, 1999). Other constituents include canadaline, canadine, hydrastidine, isohydrastidine, (S)-corypalmine, (S)-isocorypalmine, berberastine, 1-α-hydrastine, and chlorogenic acid (Bradley, 1992; Upton, 2001).

PHARMACOLOGICAL ACTIONS

The following actions are primarily related to berberine, a constituent of goldenseal, and therefore, depending on berberine content, the pharmacological actions of goldenseal products may vary from those actions listed below.

Humans (berberine)

ANTI-DIARRHEAL: In cholera patients, berberine reduced cyclic adenosine by 77% (Khin et al., 1985). In diarrhea due to *Vibrio cholerae* and *Escherichia coli*, berberine reduced stool volume 30–50% without side effects (Rabbani, 1996).

ANTIPARASITIC: In children with giardiasis, berberine demonstrated effectiveness compared with metronidazole without side effects (Gupte et al., 1975).

CARDIOVASCULAR: Decrease in systemic and pulmonary vascular resistance and left ventricular end-diastolic pressure; increase in stroke index, cardiac index, and left ventricular ejection fraction (Marin-Neto et al., 1988); suppression of ventricular premature contractions without severe side effects (Huang, 1990b).

Animal (berberine)

Stimulates immune function (Rehman et al., 1999); antiparasitic in hamsters with *L. donovani* amastigotes (Ghosh et al., 1985); anti-chlamydial effects in ocular trachoma (Babbar et al., 1982); positively inotropic and mild vasodilating effects in anesthesized dogs with ischemic left ventricular failure (Huang et al., 1992); anti-inflammatory, inhibits vascular permeability and swelling induced by drugs (Zhang and Shen, 1989).

In vitro (goldenseal)

The total extract of goldenseal demonstrated bactericidal activity against six strains of microorganism, including *Staphylococcus aureus*, *Streptococcus sanguis*, *Escherichia coli*, *Pseudomonas aeruginosa*, with a killing time of 4–30 minutes against all of the examined strains (Scazzochio et al., 2001).

In vitro (berberine)

Berberine is antimicrobial (Scazzocchio et al., 1998); inhibits smooth muscle contraction (Baldazzi et al., 1998); anti-inflammatory, inhibits platelet aggregation, platelet adhesion induced by ADP, and arachidonic acid; inhibits thrombus formation, inhibits collagen-induced thromboxane A2 release from platelets, and lowers plasma level of PGI2 in rabbits (Ckless et al., 1995; Wu and Liu, 1995; Huang et al., 1991; Muller and Ziereis, 1994; Misik et al., 1995).

Antiparasitic, amoebicidal at 0.5–1.0 mg/ml; preliminary results indicate cysticidal activity (Subbaiah and Amin, 1967); cardiovascular antiarrhythmic and proarrhythmic action in the cardiac muscle of dogs (Riccioppo, 1993); increases coronary artery flow (Huang, 1990a); bacteriostatic at low doses and a bacteriocide at higher doses (Bruneton, 1999).

MECHANISM OF ACTION

The following mechanisms primarily describe the action of berberine:

- Increases antigen-specific immunoglobulin (IgM) production *in vivo*, demonstrated in goldenseal (Rehman et al., 1999).
- Blocks α_1 and α_2. These receptors mediate smooth muscle contraction (Baldazzi et al., 1998).
- Anti-diarrheal activity may result from the inhibition of intestinal ion secretion, inhibition of toxin formation, and inhibition of smooth muscle contraction in addition to antimicrobial effects (Birdsall and Kelly, 1997).
- Inhibits ventricular tachyarrhythmias through potassium channel blocking effects (Hua and Wang, 1994).
- Anti-trachomal through stimulating protective mechanism in the host (Babbar et al., 1982).
- Stimulates bile secretion and bilirubin discharge (Birdsall and Kelly, 1997).

CONTRAINDICATIONS

Goldenseal should not be used in cases of kidney disease, including kidney failure due to inadequate urinary excretion of its alkaloids. It should probably be avoided in acute inflammation of the stomach, based on a case report in which a bitters formula enhanced gastric acid secretions. It is contraindicated in cases of jaundice in newborns. One study in rats found berberine displaced bilirubin from serum albumin which may lead to kernicterus (nuclear jaundice) (Brinker, 2001).

PREGNANCY AND LACTATION: Not for use during pregnancy (Brinker, 2001; McGuffin et al., 1997). Berberine can increase bilirubin in neonates, possibly leading to neonatal jaundice (Hobbs, 2000; Upton, 2001). It may also demonstrate uterine-stimulant activity, since this has been demonstrated in its constituents berberine, canadine, hydrastine, and hydrastinine (Farnsworth, 1975). There are no known contraindications during lactation, but goldenseal's use should be avoided during lactation until further research has been conducted.

ADVERSE EFFECTS

At recommended doses, goldenseal is considered nontoxic; berberine has also been well-tolerated in therapeutic doses (De Smet et al., 1992; Newall et al., 1996).

DRUG INTERACTIONS

Goldenseal can potentially antagonize the anticoagulant activity of heparin. Studies in mice and rats have indicated hemodynamic properties of berberine, including an increase in the number of thrombocytes, decrease in the activity of factor XIII, and the promotion of blood coagulation (Ziablitskii et al., 1996).

AMERICAN HERBAL PRODUCTS ASSOCIATION (AHPA) SAFETY RATING

CLASS 2B: Not to be used during pregnancy (McGuffin et al., 1997).

REGULATORY STATUS

The following apply to goldenseal preparations, not berberine:

CANADA: Acceptable as a drug but unacceptable as a non-medicinal ingredient in oral use products (Health Canada, 1995a; HPB, 1993). Not permitted as single-ingredient Traditional Herbal Medicine (THM) and may not be used at over 300 mg/day as component of multi-ingredient THMs (Health Canada, 1995b). Acceptable indications: Bitter digestive in multiple ingredient products (up to 75 mg/day), and as mild antiseptic in topical THM multiple-ingredient products (up to 15%) (HPB, 1993). As a single active ingredient, not acceptable for internal use except in homeopathic dilution (HPB, 1993; Health Canada 2001)

FRANCE: Official in *French Pharmacopoeia* (Bradley, 1992; Newall *et al.*, 1996; Reynolds *et al.*, 1989).

GERMANY: Dried underground parts official in German *Homöopathisches Arzneibuch* (HAB 1) containing no less than 3.0% alkaloids, calculated as berberine (GHP, 1993). Homeopathic indications: D1–D4 for chronic nasal catarrh; uterine hemorrhages, leucorrhea, and tonic (Roth *et al.*, 1984).

SWEDEN: Natural product for external use (De Smet *et al.*, 1993). No products containing goldenseal are presently registered in the Medical Products Agency's (MPA) "Authorized Natural Remedies," "Homeopathic Remedies," or "Drugs" listings (MPA, 2001a, 2001b).

SWITZERLAND: In homeopathic dilutions, approved as a component of multi-ingredient homeopathic drugs classified by the *Interkantonale Kontrollstelle für Heilmittel* (IKS) as List D medicinal products with sales limited to pharmacies and drugstores, without prescription (Morant and Ruppanner, 2001; Ruppanner and Schaefer, 2000).

U.K.: *General Sale List*, Schedule 1 (requires full Product License), Table A (internal or external use) (Bradley, 1992; Newall *et al.*, 1996).

U.S.: Dietary supplement (USC, 1994). Subject of botanical monograph in development for the *U.S. National Formulary* containing no less than 2.0% hydrastine and no less than 2.5% berberine (USP, 2002). The 1X mother tincture of rhizome and roots, 65% alcohol *v/v*, is a Class C over-the-counter drug official in the *Homeopathic Pharmacopoeia of the United States* (HPUS, 1996).

CLINICAL REVIEW

Although modern, controlled clinical trials on goldenseal are lacking, some studies have been published on the alkaloid berberine. It is not generally possible or prudent to attempt to explain the activity of an herb based on the research on one of its primary active constituents. However, in the case of goldenseal, where no modern human trials are available in the literature, the research on the isolated alkaloid is indicative of the proposed activity of goldenseal and is consistent with the herb's empirically-determined uses. Five studies are outlined in the following table, "Clinical Studies on Berberine," including a total of 465 participants. All of these studies demonstrated positive effects for indications including diarrhea, ocular infections, and cardiovascular conditions. However, there may be questions regarding the safety of *intravenous* administration of berberine for cardiac conditions (e.g., ventricular arrhythmias) due to occurrence of *torsades de pointes* in 4 of 12 patients receiving 0.2mg/kg berberine i.v. (Marin-Neto *et al.*, 1988). A comprehensive review of the car-diovascular effects of berberine suggest possible clinical usefulness in the treatment of arrhythmias and/or heart failure (Lau *et al.*, 2001). There is no evidence that this issue is related to the oral use of lower goldenseal. Human studies on berberine have shown that it is absorbed poorly from the small intestines. Therefore, its antimicrobial action is only effective locally, i.e., in the gut. Berberine is excreted in the urine, so it may have some antimicrobial effect in the kidneys or urinary tract (Bergner, 1996). Berberine has also been tested clinically and shown to be efficacious at stimulating bile and bilirubin secretion, improving symptoms of chronic cholecystitis, and normalizing elevated tyramine levels in persons with cirrhosis of the liver (Watanabe *et al.*, 1982). Berberine is reportedly effective as an adjunct to cancer therapy (Liu *et al.*, 1991). Clinical studies on berberine have confirmed that it is effective for acute diarrhea (Sack and Froehlich, 1982; Kamat, 1967). Externally, it has been shown useful as an eyewash in treating trachoma, an infectious eye disease (Mohan *et al.*, 1982).

BRANDED PRODUCTS

Studies on berberine were conducted with generic, not specific, products.

REFERENCES

Babbar O, Chhatwal V, Ray I, *et al.* Effect of berberine chloride eye drops on clinically positive trachoma patients. *Indian J Med Res* 1982;76(suppl.):83–8.

Baird AW, Taylor CT, Brayden DJ. Non-antibiotic anti-diarrheal drugs: factors affecting oral bioavailability of berberine and loperamide in intestinal tissue. *Adv Drug Del Rev* 1997; 23:111–20.

Baldazzi C, Leone M, Casini M, Tita B. Effects of the major alkaloid of *Hydrastis canadensis* L., berberine, on rabbit prostate strips. *Phytotherp Res* 1998;12:589–91.

Bannerman JE. Goldenseal in World Trade: Pressures and Potentials. *HerbalGram* 1997;41:51–52.

Bergner P. Goldenseal and the common cold: The antibiotic myth. *Med Herbalism* 1996, 7a;8(4):1, 4–6.

Birdsall T, Kelly G. Berberine: Therapeutic potential of an alkaloid found in several medicinal plants. *Alt Med Rev* 1997;2:94–103.

Blumenthal M. Goldenseal. In: Gladstar R, Hirsch P (eds.). *Planting the Future: Saving Our Medicinal Herbs*. Rochester, VT: Healing Arts Press; 2001;111–22.

Blumenthal M, Busse WR, Goldberg A, Gruenwald J, Hall T, Riggins CW, Rister RS (eds.). Klein S, Rister RS (trans.). *The Complete German Commission E Monographs—Therapeutic Guide to Herbal Medicines*. Austin, TX: American Botanical Council; Boston: Integrative Medicine Communication; 1998;12.

Boyle W. *Official Herbs: Botanical Substances in the United States Pharmacopeias: 1820–1990*. East Palestine, OH: Buckeye Naturopathic Press; 1991.

Bradley PR (ed.). *British Herbal Compendium*, Vol. 1: *A Handbook of Scientific Information on Widely Used Plant Drugs*. Dorset, U.K.: British Herbal Medicine Association; 1992.

Brinker F. *Herb Contraindications and Drug Interactions*, 3rd ed. Sandy, OR: Eclectic Medical Publications; 2001;110–111.

Bruneton J. *Pharmacognosy, Phytochemistry, Medicinal Plants*. Paris: Lavoisier Publishing; 1999;361–3.

Ckless K, Schlottfeldt JL, Pasqual M, *et al.* Inhibition of *in-vitro* lymphocyte transformation by the isoquinoline alkaloid berberine. *J Pharm Pharmacol* 1995;47:1029–31.

De Smet P, Keller K, Hänsel R, Chandler RF (eds.). *Adverse Effects of Herbal Drugs 1*. Berlin, Germany: Springer Verlag; 1992.

Duke J. *CRC Handbook of Medicinal Herbs*. Boca Raton, FL: CRC Press, inc.; 1985; 238–9.

De Smet P, Keller K, Hänsel R, Chandler RF (eds.). *Adverse Effects of Herbal Drugs 2*. Berlin, Germany: Springer Verlag; 1993.

Farnsworth NR. Potential value of plants as sources of new antifertility agents I. *J Pharm Sci* 1975;64:535–98.

Felter HW and Lloyd JU. *King's American Dispensatory*. Cincinnati: The Ohio Valley Co.; 1898.

Foster S. *Goldenseal–Hydrastis canadensis*. Botanical Booklet No. 309. Austin, TX: American Botanical Council; 1996.

German Homeopathic Pharmacopoeia (GHP). Translation of the German

Homöopathisches. Arzneibuch (HAB 1), 1st edition 1978 *with five supplements through 1991.* Stuttgart, Germany: Deutscher Apotheker Verlag; 1993.

GHP. See: *German Homeopathic Pharmacopoeia.*

Ghosh AK., Bhattacharyya FK, Ghosh DK. Leishmania donovani: Amastigote inhibition and mode of action of berberine. *Exp Parasitol* 1985;60:404–13.

Gupte S. Use of berberine in treatment of giardiasis. *Am J Dis Child* 1975;129:866.

Hardin J, Arena J. *Human Poisoning from Native and Cultivated Plants.* 2nd ed. Durham, North Carolina: Duke University Press; 1974.

Health Canada. Hydrastis. In: *Drug Product Database (DPD) Product Information.* Ottawa, Ontario: Health Canada Therapeutic Products Programme. 2001.

Health Canada. Herbs used as non-medicinal ingredients in nonprescription drugs for human use — Appendix II: List of herbs unacceptable as non-medicinal ingredients in oral use products subject to part B. Ottawa, Ontario: Health Canada Drugs Directorate Bureau of Nonprescription Drugs. 1995a.

Health Canada. Bureau of Nonprescription Drugs: Medicinal Herbs in Traditional Herbal Medicines — Appendix I: Herbs That Are Restricted or Not Accepted as Medicinals in THMs. Ottawa, Ontario: Minister of National Health and Welfare, Canada. 1995b.

Health Protection Branch. *HPB Status Manual.* Ottawa, Ontario: Health Protection Branch. February 19, 1993.

Homeopathic Pharmacopoeia of the United States. HPUS Revision Service Official Compendium from July 1, 1992. Falls Church, VA: American Institute of Homeopathy. December 1996.

HPB. See: Health Protection Branch.

HPUS. See: *Homeopathic Pharmacopoeia of the United States.*

Hobbs C. Drug lore: Golden seal in early American medical botany. *Pharm Hist* 1990;32(2):79–82.

Hobbs C. Personal communication to M. Blumenthal; October 30, 2000.

Hua Z., Wang XL. Inhibitory effect of berberine on potassium channels in guinea pig ventricular myocytes. [in Chinese]. *Yao Hsueh Hsueh Pao* 1994;29:576–80.

Huang CG, Chu ZL, Yang ZM. Effects of berberine on synthesis of platelet TXA2 and plasma PGI2 in rabbits. [in Chinese]. *Chung Kuo Yao Li Hsueh Pao* 1991;12:526–8.

Huang W. The role and mechanism of berberine on coronary arteries. [in Chinese]. *Chung Hua Hsin Hsueh Kuan Ping Tsa Chih* 1990a;18:231–4.

Huang W. Ventricular tachyarrhythmias treated with berberine. [in Chinese]. *Chng Hua Hsin Hsueh Kuan Ping Tsa Chih* 1990b;18:155–6,190.

Huang WM, Yan H, Jin JM, *et al.* Beneficial effects of berberine on hemodynamics during acute ischemic left ventricular failure in dogs. *Chin Med J* 1992;105:1014–9.

Kamat S. Clinical trial with berberine hydrochloride for the control of diarrhea in acute gastroenteritis. *J Assoc Physicians India* 1967;15:525–9.

Khin UM, Myo K, Nyunt NW, *et al.* Clinical trial of berberine in acute watery diarrhea. *Br Med J* 1985;291:1601–5.

Kholsa PK, Neeraj VI, Gupta SK, Satpathy G. Berberine, a potential drug for trachoma. *Rev Int Trach Pathol Ocul Trop Subtrop Sante Publique* 1992;69:147–65.

Lau CW, Yao XQ, Chen ZY, Ko WH, Huang Y. Cardiovascular actions of berberine. *Cardiovasc Drug Rev* 2001 Fall;19(3):234-44.

Leung, A, Foster S. *Encyclopedia of Common Natural Ingredients Used in Food, Drugs, and Cosmetics*, 2nd ed. New York: John Wiley & Sons, Inc.; 1996:216–9.

Liu C, Xiao P, Liu G. Studies on plant resources, pharmacology and clinical treatment with berberine. *Phytother Res* 1991;5:228–30.

Lloyd JU. *Origin and History of all the Pharmacopeial Vegetable Drugs with Bibliography.* Cincinnatti, OH: Caxton Press; 1929:164–6.

Lloyd JU, Lloyd CG. *Drugs and Medicines of North America. Vol. I – Ranunculaceae.* Cincinati, OH: J.U. and C.G. Lloyd; 1884–5.

Marin-Neto J, Maciel B, Secches A, *et al.* Cardiovascular effects of berberine in patients with severe congestive heart failure. *Clin Cardiol* 1988;11:253–60.

McGuffin M. AHPA Goldenseal Survey Measures Increased Agricultural Production. *HerbalGram* 1999;46:66–7.

McGuffin M, Hobbs C, Upton R, Goldberg A. *American Herbal Products Association's Botanical Safety Handbook: Guidelines for the Safe Use and Labeling for Herbs of Commerce.* Boca Raton: CRC Press; 1997.

Medical Products Agency (MPA). *Naturläkemedel: Authorised Natural Remedies* (as of January 24, 2001). Uppsala, Sweden: Medical Products Agency. 2001a.

Medical Products Agency (MPA). *Läkemedel; Läkemedelsnära Produkter (registrerade homeopatiska produkter).* Uppsala, Sweden: Medical Products Agency. 2001b.

Misik V, Bezakova L, Malekova L, Kostalova D. Lipoxygenase inhibition and antioxidant properties of protoberberine and aporphine alkaloids isolated from *Mahonia aquifolium.* Planta Med 1995;61:372–3.

Moerman D.E. *Native American Ethnobotany.* Portland, OR: Timber Press: 1998; 536–538.

Mohan M, Pant C, Angra S, Mahajan V. Berberine in trachoma (clinical trial). *Indian J Ophthalmol* 1982;30(2):69–75.

Morant J, Ruppanner H (eds.). *Arzneimittel-Kompendium der Schweiz®* 2001/02 *Publikumsausgabe.* Basel, Switzerland: Documed AG. 2001.

MPA. See: Medical Products Agency.

Muller K, Ziereis K. The antisoriatic *Mahonia aquifolium* and its active constituents; I. Pro- and antioxidant properties and inhibition of 5-lipoxygenase. *Planta Med* 1994;60:421–4.

NBJ. See: *Nutrition Business Journal.*

Newall CA, Anderson LA, Phillipson JD. *Herbal Medicines. A Guide for Health-care Professionals.* London, England: The Pharmaceutical Press; 1996:151–2.

Nutrition Business Journal. Top selling U.S. herbs & botanicals in 1999 & 2000. *Nut Bus J* 2001;6(3):9.

Rabbani GH, Butler T, Knight J, *et al.* Randomized controlled trial of berberine sulfate therapy for diarrhea due to enterotoxigenic *E. coli* and *V. cholerae. J Inf Dis* 1987;155:979–84.

Rabbani GH. Mechanism and treatment of diarrhea due to *Vibrio cholerae* and *Escherichia coli*: roles of drugs and prostaglandins. *Dan Med Bull* 1996;43:173–85.

Rehman J, Dillow J, Carter S, Chou J, Le B, Maisel A. Increased production of antigen-specific immunoglogulins G and M following *in vivo* treatment with the medicinal plants *Echinacea angustifolia* and *Hydrastis canadensis. Immunol Lett* 1999;68:391–5.

Reynolds JEF, Parfitt K, Parsons AV, Sweetman SC (eds.). *Martindale The Extra Pharmacopoeia*, 29th Edition. London, UK: The Pharmaceutical Press. 1989.

Riccioppo NF. Electropharmacological effects of berberine on canine cardiac Purkinje fibres and ventricular muscle and atrial muscle of the rabbit. *Br J Pharmacol* 1993;108:534–7.

Roth L, Daunderer M, Kormann K. *Giftpflanzen - Pflanzengifte.Vorkommen - Wirkung - Therapie.* 2. Auflage. Munich, Germany: Ecomed Verlagsgesellschaft AG & Co. KG. 1984.

Ruppanner H, Schaefer U (eds.). *Codex 2000/01 — Die Schweizer Arzneimittel in einem Griff.* Basel, Switzerland: Documed AG. 2000.

Sack R, Froehlich J. Berberine inhibits intestinal secretory response of *Vibrio cholerae* and *Escherichia coli* enterotoxins. *Infect Immun* 1982;35(2):471–5.

Scazzocchio F, Cometa M, Palmery M. Antimicrobial activity of *Hydrastis canadensis* extract and its major isolated alkaloids. *Fitoterapia* 1998;LXIX(suppl. 5):58–9.

Scazzocchio F, Cometa M, Tomassini L, Palmery M. Antibacterial activity of *Hydrastis canadensis* Extract and its Major Isolated Alkaloids. *Planta Med* 2001;67:561–564.

Subbaiah TV, Amin AH. Effect of berberine sulphate on *Entamoeba histolytica. Nature* 1967;215:527–8.

Tierra M. *The Way of Herbs: Fully Updated With the Latest Developments In Herbal Science.* Santa Cruz, CA: Pocket Books, a division of Simon and Schuster;1998.

Tyler VE. Importance of European Phytomedicinals in the American Market: An Overview. In: *Phytomedicines of Europe, Chemistry and Biological Activity.* Lawson L, Bauer R (eds.). Washington DC: American Chemical Society; 1998;6.

United States Congress. 1994. Public Law 103–417: *Dietary Supplement Health and Education Act of 1994.* Washington, DC: 103rd Congress of the United States.

USC. See: United States Congress.

United States Pharmacopeia (USP 25th Revision) - The National Formulary (NF 20th Edition). Rockville, MD: United States Pharmacopeial Convention, Inc. 2002.

Upton, R. (ed.). Goldenseal Root, *Hydrastis canadensis*: Standards of Analysis, Quality Control, and Therapeutics. Soquel, CA: American Herbal Pharmacopoeia and Therapeutic Compendium; 2001.

USP. See: United States Pharmacopeia.

USPF. *Pharmacopeial Forum:* Pharmacopeial Previews: Hydrastis 2000; 26(4). Rockville, MD. US Pharmacopeial Convention.

Watanabe A, Obata T, Nagashima H. Berberine therapy of hypertyraminemia in patients with liver cirrhosis. *Acta Med Okayama* 1982;36(4):277–81.

Wu JF, Liu TP. Effects of berberine on platelet aggregation and plasma levels of TXB2 and 6-keto-PGF1 alpha in rats with reversible middle cerebral artery occlusion. [in Chinese]. *Yao Hsueh Hsueh Pao* 1995;30:98–102.

Zeng XJ, Zeng XH. Relationship between the clinical effects of berberine on severe congestive heart failure and its concentration in plasma studied by HPLC. *Biomedical Chromatography* 1999;13(7):442–4.

Zhang MF, Shen YQ. Antidiarrheal and antiinflammatory effects of berberine. [in Chinese]. *Chung Kuo Yao Li Hsueh Pao* 1989;10:174–6.

Ziablitskii V, Romanovskaia V, Umurzakova R *et al.* Modification to the functional status of the hemostic system with the use of berberine sulfate. *Eksp Klin Farmakol* 1996 Jan–Feb;59(1):37–9.

Clinical Studies on Berberine

Diarrhea

Author/Year	Subject	Design	Duration	Dosage	Preparation	Results/Conclusion
Rabbani et al., 1987	Diarrhea	R, C n=165 adult males with *E. coli* or *Vibrio cholerae* diarrhea	24 hours	400 mg berberine sulfate in a single dose	Berberine sulfate, or berberine sulfate and tetracycline, or tetracycline	In *E. coli* bacterial diarrhea, during 24 hours, berberine demonstrated a 48% reduction in mean stool volumes compared to control (p<0.05). Also reduced liquid diarrheal stools by 42% in treated group and 20% in control. *V. cholerae* diarrhea patients who received berberine alone had significantly reduced stool volume (p< 0.05) over control group. *V. cholerae* patients receiving both berberine and tetracycline did not show a significant decrease in stool volume compared to patients treated with tetracycline alone.
Gupte, 1975	Giardiasis (documented)	C, Cm n=137 children ages 5 months–14 years on berberine vs. 242 patients on metronidazole	5 or 10 days berberine; 5–7 days metronidazole	5 or 10 mg/kg/day of berberine vs. 20 mg/kg/day of metronidazole	Berberine or metronidazole	90% of children who received berberine in the 10 mg/kg/day dose had negative stool specimens after 10 days; 83% remained negative one month later. This compared closely to the effect of metronidazole at 95% after 10 days and 90% after one month. The author concluded berberine is an appropriate choice due to ease of administration and freedom from side effects common with metronidazole.

Ocular Infections

Author/Year	Subject	Design	Duration	Dosage	Preparation	Results/Conclusion
Babbar et al., 1982	Ocular trachoma infections	C n=51	3 weeks, follow-up after 1 year	0.2% berberine chloride eye drops, or 0.2% berberine chloride with 20% sulfacetamide, or 20% sulfacetamide	Berberine chloride or sulfacetamide	Subjects taking only 20% sulfacetamide had slightly better improvement in the areas of conjunctival congestion, pupillary reaction, and follicle number. But subjects still tested positive for *C. trachomatis*. Subjects with 0.2% berberine either by itself or combined with sulfacetamide demonstrated symptom improvement and tested negative for *C. trachomatis*, with no relapse one year later.

Cardiovascular Effect

Author/Year	Subject	Design	Duration	Dosage	Preparation	Results/Conclusion
Marin-Neto et al., 1988	Refractory congestive heart failure	C n=12	30 minutes	0.02 and 0.2 mg/kg per minute	Berberine intravenous infusion	No significant response in lower dose. The dose of 0.2 mg/kg per minute decreased systemic (48%) and pulmonary (41%) vascular resistance, 28% decrease in right atrium, and 32% decrease in left ventricular end-diastolic pressure. Increases were observed in the cardiac index (45%), left ventricular ejection fraction (56%), and stroke index (45%). *Torsades de pointes* observed in 4 patients, concluding more research required before berberine can be recommended in i.v. cardiac therapy.
Huang, 1990b	Ventricular tachyarrhythmias	OB n=100 healthy volunteers	24–48 hours monitoring	Not stated	Berberine, route of administration not stated	65% of patients had 50% or greater, and 38% of patients had 90% or greater suppression of premature ventricular contractions (PVC's). No severe side effects were noted. However, mild gastrointestinal symptoms were reported by some patients.

KEY: C – controlled, **CC** – case-control, **CH** – cohort, **CI** – confidence interval, **Cm** – comparison, **CO** – crossover, **CS** – cross-sectional, **DB** – double-blind, **E** – epidemiological, **LC** – longitudinal cohort, **MA** – meta-analysis, **MC** – multi-center, **n** – number of patients, **O** – open, **OB** – observational, **OL** – open label, **OR** – odds ratio, **P** – prospective, **PB** – patient-blind, **PC** – placebo-controlled, **PG** – parallel group, **PS** – pilot study, **R** – randomized, **RC** – reference-controlled, **RCS** – retrospective cross-sectional, **RS** - retrospective, **S** – surveillance, **SB** – single-blind, **SC** – single-center, **U** – uncontrolled, **UP** – unpublished, **VC** – vehicle-controlled.

Hawthorn

Crataegus monogyna Jacq., *C. laevigata* (Poir.) DC. (syn. *C. oxyacantha* auct)

[Fam. *Rosaceae*]

OVERVIEW

Hawthorn is the name for bushes and small trees in the genus *Crataegus*, of which there are approximately 280 species native to northern temperate zones in East Asia, Europe, and eastern North America. The fruit has been used as food and medicine in Europe for centuries. Hawthorn preparations are among the most popularly prescribed botanical medicines in central Europe, particularly in Germany, Austria, and Switzerland, with the primary approved indication being treatment of declining cardiac performance, according to Stage II New York Heart Association (NYHA) classification. Over the past 20 years, several different commercially available preparations of hawthorn have been investigated in double-blind, placebo-controlled (DB, PC) clinical studies.

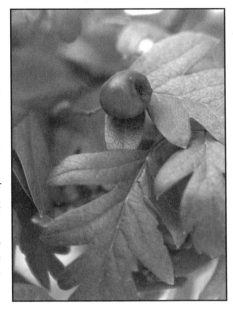

Photo © 2003 stevenfoster.com

PRIMARY USES

• Congestive heart failure, NYHA Stages I and II

NOTE: The NYHA functional classification is most often used to characterize patients' limitations due to failure of the left ventricle. The classification has a strong association with mortality that is independent of left ventricular ejection fraction.

STAGE I: No limitation of physical activity. Ordinary physical activity does not cause undue fatigue or dyspnea.

STAGE II: Slight limitation of physical activity. Comfortable at rest, but ordinary physical activity results in fatigue or dyspnea.

OTHER POTENTIAL USES

• Feeling of pressure and tightness in the cardiac region
• Nervous heart complaints including palpitations, sharp pain in the chest, rapid pulse, or vertigo

PHARMACOLOGICAL ACTIONS

Improves subjective parameters of cardiac insufficiency (as NYHA Stage II); increases cardiac work tolerance; decreases pressure/heart rate product; increases the ejection fraction; raises anaerobic threshold.

DOSAGE AND ADMINISTRATION
Hawthorn leaf with flower (internal)

INFUSION: Pour about 150 ml boiling water over approximately 1.5 g dried herb, steep for 10–15 minutes, squeeze tea bag over cup, 3–4 times daily, during or after meals.

DRY EXTRACT (STANDARDIZED): 160–900 mg, in 2–3 individual doses per day, corresponding to 30–168.7 mg procyanidins, calculated as epicatechin, or 3.5–19.8 mg flavonoids, calculated as hyperoside [4–7:1 (*w/w*) with defined flavonoid or procyanidins content, ethanol 45% (*v/v*) or methanol 70% (*v/v*)].

Hawthorn fruit (internal)

NOTE: According to Kneipp®, a properly prepared tea infusion will yield over 90% into solution of the active principles from the flavonoid and oligomeric procyanidin groups and compares dose for dose with solid-form preparations (Kneipp-Werke, 1996). Other sources report that after a 10-minute infusion, 35% of the *O*-glycoside bound flavonoids, and 40% of the *C*-glycoside bound flavonoids are released into solution (Meyer-Buchtela, 1999).

FLUID EXTRACT: 1:1 (*w/v*) in 25% alcohol (*v/v*), 0.5–1.0 ml, 3 times daily.

TINCTURE: 1:5 (*w/v*), in 45% alcohol (*v/v*), 1–2 ml, 3 times daily.

TINCTURE: 1:3.2 (*w/v*) in 49% alcohol (*v/v*), 30 drops diluted in water, 3 times daily, one-half hour before meals.

TINCTURE: 1:10 (*w/v*), 5–10 drops, 1–3 times daily.

SOLID EXTRACT: 0.25–0.50 teaspoon daily.

SYRUP: 1 teaspoon, 2–3 times daily.

CONTRAINDICATIONS

HAWTHORN LEAF WITH FLOWER: No known restrictions.

HAWTHORN FRUIT: No known restrictions.

PREGNANCY AND LACTATION: No known restrictions, but systematic, scientific safety studies have not yet been conducted.

ADVERSE EFFECTS

HAWTHORN LEAF WITH FLOWER None known.

HAWTHORN FRUIT: None known.

DRUG INTERACTIONS

HAWTHORN LEAF WITH FLOWER: No known interactions, according to German Commission E monograph. Hawthorn may potentiate the effects of digitalis drugs (e.g., digoxin), and it may potentiate the coronary artery dilating effects of theophylline, caffeine, papaverine, sodium nitrate, adenosine, and epinephrine (although these are not considered clinically significant interactions). A healthcare provider should be consulted before combining hawthorn with any heart medications.

HAWTHORN FRUIT: No known interactions.

CLINICAL REVIEW

In fourteen clinical studies on hawthorn conducted on 6,900 participants, all but one showed positive effects for cardiac insufficiency. Eight are DB, PC studies, four are open studies, one is a large multi-center observational study, and one is a DB study comparing hawthorn to standard treatment. Most clinical studies have been conducted using a dry extract of hawthorn leaf with flower standardized to a daily dose of 9 mg or more oligomeric procyanidins. A major international randomized, DB, PC study is currently investigating the influence of the standardized extract of hawthorn leaf with flower on the mortality of patients suffering from congestive heart failure. In this trial (involving approximately 120 investigation centers in seven European countries), up to 2,300 patients with congestive heart failure, NYHA Stage II and III, and markedly impaired left ventricular function will be enrolled and treated over 24 months. The primary outcome variable is the combined end point of cardiac death, nonlethal myocardial infarction, and hospitalization due to progression of heart failure. Secondary outcome variables are total mortality, exercise duration, echocardiographic parameters, and quality of life, as well as pharmacoeconomic parameters. The first patient was enrolled in October 1998. The trial is expected to be completed at the end of 2002.

Hawthorn

Crataegus monogyna Jacq., *C. laevigata* (Poir.) DC. (syn. *C. oxyacantha* auct)
[Fam. *Rosaceae*]

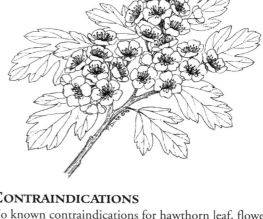

OVERVIEW

Hawthorn fruit has long been used as a food and medicine in Europe; particularly in Germany, Austria, and Switzerland, where it ranks as one of the most popularly used botanical medicines, especially for treating declining heart function. Many clinical studies have been conducted on hawthorn over the past 20 years.

USES

NOTE: Patients should not attempt to self-medicate for suspected or properly diagnosed cardiac conditions, but should seek the advice of a healthcare provider for appropriate treatment.

Congestive heart failure, based on the New York Heart Association (NYHA) functional classification for Stage I, no limitation of physical activity, and Stage II, slight limitation of physical activity, causing fatigue or shortness of breath.

DOSAGE

Hawthorn leaf with flower (internal)

INFUSION: Pour about 150 ml boiling water over approximately 1.5 g dried herb, steep for 10–15 minutes, squeeze tea bag over cup, 3–4 times daily, during or after meals.

DRY EXTRACT (STANDARDIZED): 160–900 mg, in 2–3 individual doses, corresponding to 30–168.7 mg procyanidins, calculated as epicatechin, or 3.5–19.8 mg flavonoids, calculated as hyperoside [4–7:1 (*w/w*) with defined flavonoid or procyanidins content, ethanol 45% (*v/v*) or methanol 70% (*v/v*)].

Hawthorn fruit (internal)

NOTE: Hawthorn fruit products have *not* been tested for effectiveness in recent clinical research. Most of the published studies have been conducted on standardized extracts of hawthorn leaf with flowers.

FLUID EXTRACT: 0.5–1.0 ml , 3 times daily [1:1 (*w/v*) in 25% alcohol (*v/v*)].

TINCTURE: 5–10 drops, 1–3 times daily [1:10 *(w/v)*]

TINCTURE: 1–2 ml, 3 times daily [1:5 (*w/v*), in 45% alcohol (*v/v*)].

CONTRAINDICATIONS

No known contraindications for hawthorn leaf, flower, or fruit.

PREGNANCY AND LACTATION: No known restrictions. Scientific studies are lacking, however, so consult with a healthcare provider before using hawthorn during pregnancy or while breast-feeding.

ADVERSE EFFECTS

No known adverse effects for hawthorn leaf, flower, or fruit.

DRUG INTERACTIONS

HAWTHORN LEAF WITH FLOWER: Hawthorn may increase the effects of the heart drug digoxin and mildly increase the coronary artery dilating effects of substances like caffeine, theophylline in tea, and papaverine in opium-containing products (such as cough medicines). Consult with a healthcare provider before combining hawthorn with any heart medications.

HAWTHORN FRUIT: No known interactions.

AMERICAN BOTANICAL COUNCIL

Hawthorn

Patient Information Sheet

Hawthorn

Crataegus monogyna Jacq., *C. laevigata* (Poir.) DC. (syn. *C. oxyacantha* auct)

[Fam. *Rosaceae*]

OVERVIEW

Hawthorn is a bush or small tree that includes approximately 280 species native to northern temperate zones in East Asia, Europe, and eastern North America (Hobbs and Foster, 1990). The fruit has been used as food and medicine in Europe for centuries. Over the past 20 years, several different commercially available preparations of hawthorn have been investigated in double-blind, placebo-controlled (DB, PC) clinical studies. Hawthorn preparations are among the most popularly prescribed botanical medicines in central Europe, particularly in Germany, Austria, and Switzerland. The primary approved indication is treatment of declining cardiac performance according to Stage II of the New York Heart Association (NYHA) classification. Hawthorn has become increasingly popular as a dietary supplement in the U.S., ranking 20th in sales in mainstream retail stores in 2000 (Blumenthal, 2001). Separate *United States Pharmacopeia-National Formulary* botanical monographs are presently under development for hawthorn leaf with flower and its preparations including extract, powder, and tablet (USP, 2002).

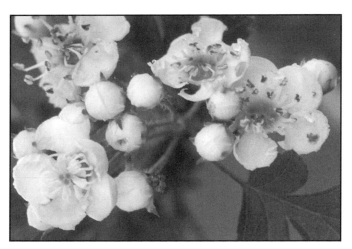

DESCRIPTION

Hawthorn leaf and flower preparations consist of whole or cut, dried, flower-bearing branches of *Crataegus monogyna* Jacq. or *C. laevigata* (Poir) DC. (syn. *C. oxyacantha* auct.), their hybrids, or other *Crataegus* species including *C. piperi* Bitton (syn. *C. columbiana* T.J. Howell var. *piperi* [Britt.] Egglest) and *C. rivularis* Nutt. (syn. *C. douglasii* Lindl. Var. *rivularis* [Nutt.] Sarg.)[Fam. *Rosaceae*]. Various species of hawthorn leaf and flower are recognized as official by different compendia: the *German Pharmacopoeia* recognizes up to five species, and the *Pharmacopoeia Europa* recognizes two. The *American Herbal Pharmacopoeia* (unofficial) recognizes *C. laevigata*

(*C. oxyacantha*) and *C. monogyna*, or their hybrids, and other species (Upton, 1999a, 1999b).

The *Pharmacopoeia Europa* requires that hawthorn preparations contain not less than 1.5% flavonoids, calculated as hyperoside (Ph.Eur., 2001). Both the *Austrian Pharmacopoeia* and the *German Pharmacopoeia,* however, require not less than 0.7% flavonoids (DAB, 1999; ÖAB, 1994). The *Pharmacopoeia Europa* requires a flavonoid content of 1.5% based on a spectrophotometric method, while the 0.7% flavonoid concentration of the *German Pharmacopoeia* is based on a high-performance liquid chromatography method. Thus, the apparent differences in value are based on different analytical methods, not on differences of raw material.

Hawthorn fruit consists of the dried pome of *C. monogyna* Jacq. or *C. laevigata* (Poir) D.C. (syn. *C. oxyacantha* auct.), or hybrids or combinations of these species. The dried fruit contains not less than 1.0% of procyanidins calculated as cyanidin chloride (DAC, 1992; Ph.Eur., 2001).

PRIMARY USES
Hawthorn leaf with flower (internal)

- Congestive heart failure NYHA Stage I and II (Tauchert *et al.,* 1999; Blumenthal, *et al.,* 1998; Loew *et al.,* 1996; Weikl *et al.,* 1996; Bödigheimer and Chase, 1994; Förster *et al.,* 1994; Schmidt *et al.,* 1994; Tauchert *et al.,* 1994; Leuchtgens H, 1993; Weikl and Noh, 1992; Eichstädt *et al.,* 1989; O'Conolly *et al.,* 1986; Hanak and Brückel, 1983; Iwamoto *et al.,* 1981)

  NOTE: NYHA functional classification is most often used to characterize patients' limitation from left ventricular failure. The classification has a strong association with mortality independent of left ventricular ejection fraction.

  STAGE I: No limitation of physical activity. Ordinary physical activity does not cause undue fatigue or dyspnea.

  STAGE II: Slight limitation of physical activity. Comfortable at rest, but ordinary physical activity results in fatigue or dyspnea.

OTHER POTENTIAL USES

- Feeling of pressure and tightness in the cardiac region (Morant and Ruppanner, 2001; Braun *et al.,* 1996)
- Nervous heart complaints such as palpitations, sharp pain in the chest, rapid pulse, or vertigo (Morant and Ruppanner, 2001; Pfister-Hotz, 1997; van Hellemont, 1988; Wichtl, 1997)

DOSAGE
Hawthorn leaf with flower (internal)
Crude Preparations

INFUSION: About 150 ml boiling water poured over approximately 1.5 g dried herb, steeped for 10–15 min., tea bag squeezed over cup, 3–4 times daily, during or after meals (Morant and Ruppanner, 2001; Braun *et al.*, 1996).

NOTE: According to Kneipp®, a properly prepared tea infusion will yield over 90% into solution of the active principles from the flavonoid and oligomeric procyanidin groups and compares dose for dose with solid-form preparations (Kneipp-Werke, 1996). Other sources report that after a 10-minute infusion, 35% of the *O*-glycoside bound flavonoids, and 40% of the *C*-glycoside bound flavonoids are released into solution (Meyer-Buchtela, 1999).

FLUID EXTRACT (DAB, 2000) [1:1 (*w/v*), 45% ethanol (*v/v*), ≥1.0% flavonoids calculated as hyperoside ethanol]: The German Commission E requires that a single- or daily-dose phytoequivalence to the native dry extract dosage must first be confirmed by a clinical-pharmacological experiment or clinical study before a dosage recommendation can be made (Blumenthal *et al.*, 1998).

Standardized Preparations
DRY EXTRACT [4–7:1 (*w/w*) with defined flavonoid or procyanidins content, ethanol 45% (*v/v*) or methanol 70% (*v/v*)]: 160–900 mg, in 2–3 individual doses, corresponding to 30–168.7 mg procyanidins, calculated as epicatechin, or 3.5–19.8 mg flavonoids, calculated as hyperoside, according to Commission E (Blumenthal *et al.*, 1998).

Hawthorn fruit (internal)
Crude Preparations
NOTE: The following doses for hawthorn *fruit* preparations are *not* approved by Commission E and do not correlate to clinical trials summarized in the table in this monograph. These doses are presented as guides for non-official uses of hawthorn fruit preparations that are not documented by recent clinical research but are nevertheless published in the literature as potentially useful in NYHA Stage I and possibly Stage II (Upton, 1999).

FLUID EXTRACT [1:1 (*w/v*) in 25% alcohol (*v/v*)]: 0.5–1.0 ml, 3 times daily (BHP, 1983; Karnick, 1994).

TINCTURE [1:5 (w/v), in 45% alcohol (v/v)]: 1–2 ml, 3 times daily (BHP, 1983).

TINCTURE [1:3.2 (w/v) in 49% alcohol (v/v)]: 30 drops diluted in water, 3 times daily, one-half hour before meals (Morant and Ruppanner, 2001).

TINCTURE [1:10 (w/v)]: 5–10 drops, 1–3 times daily (Hänsel *et al.*, 1992–94).

SOLID EXTRACT: 0.25–0.50 teaspoon daily (Upton *et al.,* 1999a).

SYRUP: 1 teaspoon, 2–3 times daily (Upton *et al.*, 1999a).

DURATION OF ADMINISTRATION
Internal
The Commission E reports that a healthcare provider should be consulted in cases where symptoms continue unchanged for more than six weeks or in case of swelling of the legs. Medical diagnosis is absolutely necessary when pain occurs in the region of the heart, spreading out to the arms, upper abdomen, or the area around the neck, or in cases of respiratory distress (dyspnea) (Blumenthal *et al.*, 1998).

CHEMISTRY
NOTE: Fully validated methods for determining procyanidin content are lacking. Therefore, the findings provided should be taken as relative values (Upton, 1999b).

Hawthorn leaf with flower
Constituents considered most important and primarily responsible for the pharmacological activity of hawthorn include flavonoids and procyanidins. The oligomeric procyanidins with a lower degree of polymerization appear to be more active than those with a higher degree of polymerization. Various concentrations are found in different plant parts and vary from species to species (Upton, 1999b). All species and parts studied contain a wide array of flavonoids (0.5–1.5%). The primary flavonoids are hyperoside (quercetin-3-D-galactoside), vitexin-2"-*O*-rhamnoside, and acetylvitexin-2"-*O*-rhamnoside. The primary flavonoid in the flowers is hyperoside, although in the leaves, vitexin-2"-*O*-rhamnoside and, occasionally, acetylvitexin-2"-*O*-rhamnoside dominate (Rehwald, 1995).

The leaf and flower contain to 1.78% total flavonoids (flavones and flavonols) of which approximately 0.53% are vitexin-2"-*O*-rhamnoside, 0.28% hyperoside, 0.17% rutin, and 0.02% acetylvitexin–2"–*O*–rhamnoside (Hänsel *et al.*, 1992–94; Wagner and Tittel, 1983); 1.0–2.4% oligomeric procyanidins; 0.6% triterpene acids including ursolic, oleanolic, and crataegolic acids; and phenolic acids such as caffeic acid, chlorogenic acid, and related phenolcarboxylic acids (Hänsel *et al.*, 1992–94).

Hawthorn fruit
The fruits contain relatively low levels of flavonoids and consist primarily of oligomeric and polymeric procyanidins (Rehwald, 1995; Tittel and Wagner, 1981). The procyanidins contained in the fruit reportedly have a higher degree of polymerization than the procyanidins in the leaves and flowers. The pulp contains the highest concentration of procyanidins followed by the skin and stalks and procyanidin content is reportedly highest in unripe fruits (decreasing from 6.9% to 0.9% to the end of summer) (Rohr, 1999).

The fruit contains up to 2.96% total procyanidins of which approximately 1.9% are oligomeric procyanidins; 0.42–0.45% triterpene acids including ursolic, oleanolic, and crataegolic acids; and flavonoids (flavone glycosides and C-glycoside flavones), mainly hyperoside (Hänsel *et al.*, 1992–94). A small amount of quercetin derivatives and rutin are also present (Rohr, 1999).

PHARMACOLOGICAL ACTIONS
Hawthorn leaf with flower
Human
The Commission E reported that in cases of cardiac insufficiency classified as NYHA Stage II, hawthorn leaf with flower improves subjective findings, increases cardiac work tolerance, decreases pressure/heart rate product, increases the ejection fraction, and raises the anaerobic threshold (Blumenthal *et al.*, 1998).

Animal
The Commission E reported positive inotropic effect, positive dromotropic effect, negative bathmotropic effect, increases in coronary and myocardial circulatory perfusion, and a reduction in peripheral vascular resistance (Blumenthal *et al.*, 1998). These actions are confirmed in recent reviews (Loew, 1997; Upton, 1999a, 1999b).

In vitro
The extract standardized to procyanidins blocks beta-adrenoceptors (Rácz-Kotilla *et al.*, 1980), and has inotropic effects in isolated heart cells (Bratman and Kroll, 1999), exerts direct positive inotropic *ex vivo* effect in human myocardium taken from patients with congestive heart failure, increases force of contraction in human myocardium 3', 5'-cyclic adenosine

monophosphate (cAMP)-independently (Schwinger *et al.,* 2000) and increases antioxidant activity (Da Silva *et al.,* 2000).

Standardized Preparations

The extract standardized to procyanidins blocks beta-adrenoceptors (Rácz-Kotilla *et al.,* 1980), lowers plasma lipids (Rajendran *et al.,* 1996), and blocks repolarizing potassium currents in ventricular cardiac myocytes (Müller, 1999).

Hawthorn fruit

Human
Cardiotonic (BHP, 1996).

Animal
Alcoholic tincture is a hypolipidemic agent (Rajendran *et al.,* 1996; Shanthi *et al.,* 1994).

NOTE: Since hawthorn fruit contains many of the same procyanidins as the leaf and flower extract, albeit in lower concentrations, the antioxidant effect (and presumably others) are presumed to be similar (Upton, 1999b).

MECHANISM OF ACTION

The mechanism of hawthorn's vasodilating effect remains unclear (Loew, 1997). Based on animal studies, increases in coronary blood flow do not appear to be due to the action of a single group of constituents (e.g., flavonoids) but rather to interactions between various different groups of compounds (Sticher and Meier, 1998). Because the biological activity cannot be attributed to any single substance contained in hawthorn, the entire extract must be viewed as the effective treatment (Reuter, 1994). Hawthorn's hypotensive effect is due to its vasodilating action rather than to an effect via adrenergic, muscarinic, or histaminergic receptors (Abdul-Ghani *et al.,* 1987). The hypotensive effect may be due to procyanidins inhibiting angiotensin-converting enzyme (ACE) (Sticher and Meier, 1998).

Human

- Based on experiments on myocardium taken from terminally failing human hearts (NYHA Class IV), it is suggested that hawthorn leaf with flower extract acts in a way similar to the cAMP-independent positive inotropic action of cardiac glycosides. Additionally, hawthorn improves the force-frequency relation in failing human myocardium (Schwinger *et al.,* 2000).

Animal

- Enhances LDL-receptor activity in rats. The hypocholesterolemic effect caused by the tincture may be due to up-regulation of hepatic LDL receptors (Rajendran *et al.,* 1996).

In vitro

- One study reports that the mechanism of hawthorn's positive inotropic effects remains elusive and the effects are not caused by phosphodiesterase inhibition or a β-sympathomimetic effect. In isolated guinea pig ventricular myocytes, hawthorn extract blocks repolarizing potassium currents in a way that is similar to the action of class III anti-arrhythmic drugs (Müller, 1999).
- Inhibits cAMP phosphodiesterase activity (Schüssler *et al.,* 1991, 1992, 1993, and 1995), which increases cardiac cAMP levels causing a positive inotropic effect (cardiac muscle contractility).
- Inhibits Na^+-/K^+- ATP-ase activity (Brixius *et al.,* 1998; Leukel-Lenz, 1988).

- May inhibit thromboxane (TXA2) synthesis and stimulate prostacyclin (PGI2) (Vibes *et al.,* 1991, 1993, and 1994).
- Antioxidant (Bahorun *et al.,* 1994, 1996; Chatterjee *et al.,* 1997). A good correlation between hawthorn total phenolic content and antioxidant capacity has been shown (Sticher and Meier, 1998).
- Inhibits human neutrophil elastase (Chatterjee *et al.,* 1997).

CONTRAINDICATIONS

Hawthorn leaf with flower
None known (Blumenthal *et al.,* 1998; Braun *et al.,* 1996; ESCOP, 1999).

Hawthorn fruit
None known (Meyer-Buchtela, 1999).

PREGNANCY AND LACTATION: No known restrictions (McGuffin *et al.,* 1997), but further research needs to be conducted to determine safety. The Commission E reports that no experimental data are available concerning embryonic and fetal toxicity, fertility, and postnatal development (Blumenthal *et al.,* 1998). Systematic scientific investigations have not been conducted on pregnant or lactating women. Use during pregnancy or lactation should be decided by a healthcare provider (Morant and Ruppanner, 2001).

ADVERSE EFFECTS

HAWTHORN LEAF WITH FLOWER: None known (Blumenthal *et al.,* 1998; Braun *et al.,* 1996; ESCOP, 1999).

HAWTHORN FRUIT: None known (Meyer-Buchtela, 1999).

DRUG INTERACTIONS

HAWTHORN LEAF WITH FLOWER: No known documented interactions, according to the Commission E monograph of 1994 and later therapeutic reviews, including one by the European Scientific Cooperative on Phytotherapy (Blumenthal *et al.,* 1998; Braun *et al.,* 1996; ESCOP, 1999). Other references suggest that hawthorn preparations may potentiate drugs containing cardiac glycosides (e.g., digoxin) probably resulting from the positive inotropic and coronary vasodilating effects (Brinker, 2001). Earlier research suggested potentiation of digitalis glycosides with hawthorn (Trunzler and Schuler, 1962), and another study suggested that hawthorn preparations may potentiate the coronary artery dilating effects of theophylline, caffeine, papaverine, sodium nitrate, adenosine, and epinephrine (Hahn *et al.,* 1960). Because of the similarity in actions, one reference suggests that hawthorn should not be used with any other heart medications without the advice of a healthcare provider (Newall *et al.,* 1996).

HAWTHORN FRUIT: None known (Meyer-Buchtela, 1999). Depending on dosage the same interactions for leaf and flower may be relevant (Upton, 1999a).

AMERICAN HERBAL PRODUCTS ASSOCIATION (AHPA) SAFETY RATING

CLASS 1: Herbs that can be safely consumed when used appropriately (McGuffin *et al.,* 1997).

REGULATORY STATUS

AUSTRIA: Hawthorn leaf and flower official in the *Austrian Pharmacopoeia* (ÖAB, 1994).

CANADA: Schedule "A" drug not suitable as a non-medicinal ingredient at any level (HPB, 1993). Permitted as a component of OTC Traditional Herbal Medicine (THM) and as a homeo-pathic drug monopreparation in various dilutions, in both cases requiring pre-marketing authorization and application for a Drug Identification Number (DIN) (Health Canada, 2000).

EUROPEAN UNION: Dried false fruit containing not less than 1.0% procyanidins official in the *European Pharmacopoeia*, 3rd ed. Suppl. 1998 (Ph.Eur., 2001) and dried leaf and flower containing not less than 1.5% flavonoids official in Ph.Eur. Suppl. 2001 (Ph.Eur., 2001).

FRANCE: Hawthorn leaf with flower, as well as, homeopathic mother tinctures of hawthorn fresh ripe fruit and of hawthorn fresh flowering twig tips, respectively, are official in the *French Pharmacopeia* (Ph.Fr.X, 1982-1996). Fluid extract and tincture preparations are listed in the *Codex Fr. IX* (ESCOP, 1999; van Hellemont, 1988).

GERMANY: Hawthorn leaf with flower (DAB, 1999) and the fluid extract form (DAB, 2000) official in the *German Pharmacopoeia*. Hawthorn fruit (DAC, 1992) and hawthorn flower (DAC, 1990) are official in the *German Drug Codex* supplement to the DAB. The dry native extract of hawthorn leaf with flower is an approved drug of the Commission E monographs (Blumenthal *et al.*, 1998), and the tea infusion of hawthorn leaf with flower is an approved drug of the *German Standard License* monographs (Braun *et al.*, 1996) with sale limited to pharmacies, without prescription. The mother tincture and liquid dilutions of hawthorn fresh ripe fruit are official preparations of the *German Homoeopathic Pharmacopoeia* (GHP, 1993) and are approved drugs of the Commission D monographs (Hänsel *et al.*, 1992-1994). Thirty-three Hawthorn extract preparations are listed in the German "Rote Liste 1994" (Sticher and Meier, 1998).

ITALY: Dried leaf with flower containing not less than 0.7% flavonoids official in *Italian Pharmacopoeia IX 1985 Supplement 1991* (Ph.Ital., 1991).

SWEDEN: Natural product (DeSmet *et al.*, 1993) As of January 2001, no hawthorn products have been listed in the Medical Products Agency (MPA) "Authorised Natural Remedies" (MPA, 2001).

SWITZERLAND: Hawthorn leaf with flower and standardized dry extract are official in the *Swiss Pharmacopeia* (Ph.Helv.VIII, 1998). Positive classification (List D) by the *Interkantonale Konstrollstelle für Heilmittel* (IKS) and corresponding sales Category D with sale limited to pharmacies and drugstores, without prescription (Morant and Ruppanner, 2001; WHO, 1998). One hawthorn Anthroposophical preparation, 27 hawthorn homoeopathic preparations and 76 hawthorn-containing phytomedicines are listed in the *Swiss Codex 2000/01* (Ruppanner and Schaefer, 2001).

UK: No licensed hawthorn products on the *General Sale List* (GSL) (Newall *et al.*, 1996).

U.S.: Dietary supplement (USC, 1994). The mother tincture 1:10 (*w/v*), 45% ethanol (*v/v*), of the fresh or dried fruit, is an Rx Class C drug official in the *Homoeopathic Pharmacopoeia of the United States* (HPUS, 1990).

CLINICAL REVIEW

Fourteen studies are outlined in the following table, "Clinical Studies on Hawthorn," conducted on 6,900 participants. All but one of the studies (Bödigheimer *et al.*, 1994), demonstrated positive effects for cardiac insufficiency. Eight are DB, PC studies (Bödigheimer and Chase, 1994; Förster *et al.*, 1994; Hanak and

Brückel, 1983; Iwamoto *et al.*, 1981; Leuchtgens, 1993; O'Conolly *et al.*, 1986; Schmidt *et al.*, 1998; Weikl *et al.*, 1996), four are open studies (Eichstädt *et al.*, 1989; Loew *et al.*, 1996; Weikl and Noh, 1992), one is a large multi-center observational study (Tauchert *et al.*, 1999), and one is a DB study comparing hawthorn to standard treatment (Tauchert *et al.*, 1994). NOTE: Most clinical studies have been conducted using a dry extract of hawthorn leaf with flower standardized to a daily dose of 9 mg or more oligomeric procyanidins (Schulz *et al.*, 2000; Hänsel *et al.*, 1992–94).

A major international R, DB, PC study is currently investigating the influence of the standardized extract of hawthorn leaf with flower (WS 1442; Schwabe, Karlsruhe, Germany) on the mortality of patients suffering from congestive heart failure. In this trial (involving approximately 120 investigational centers in seven European countries), up to 2,300 patients with congestive heart failure, NYHA Stage II and III, and markedly impaired left ventricular function will be enrolled and treated over 24 months. The primary outcome variable is the combined end point of cardiac death, nonlethal myocardial infarction, and hospitalization due to progression of heart failure. Secondary outcome variables are total mortality, exercise duration, echocardiographic parameters, and quality of life, as well as pharmacoeconomic parameters. The first patient was enrolled in October 1998. The trial is expected to be completed at the end of 2002 (Holubarsch *et al.*, 2000).

BRANDED PRODUCTS*

Crataegutt® Dragees: Dr. Willmar Schwabe Pharmaceuticals / International Division / Willmar Schwabe Str. 4 / D-76227 Karlsruhe / Germany / Tel: +49-721-4005 ext. 294 / www.schwabepharma.com / Email: melville-eaves@schwabe.de. One tablet contains 30 mg hawthorn flower, fruit and leaf hydroalcoholic dry normalized extract 5:1 (*w/w*), standardized to 5% (50 *mg/g*) oligomeric procyanidins.

Crataegutt® forte Kapseln: Dr. Willmar Schwabe Pharmaceuticals. 1 capsule contains 80 mg hawthorn leaf and flower hydroalcoholic dry normalized extract 5:1 (*w/w*) standardized to 18.75% (187.5 *mg/g*) oligomeric procyanidins (15 mg per capsule).

Crataegutt® novo Filmtabletten: Dr. Willmar Schwabe Pharmaceuticals. One tablet contains 60 mg hawthorn flower, fruit and leaf hydroalcoholic dry normalized extract 5:1 (*w/w*), standardized to 5% (50 *mg/g*) oligomeric procyanidins.

Crataegus Special Extract WS 1442: Dr. Willmar Schwabe Pharmaceuticals. One capsule contains 80 mg hawthorn leaf with flower dry extract 5:1 (*w/w*), standardized to 18.75% oligomeric procyanidins (15 mg per capsule). Solvent: ethanol 45%

Faros® 300 Dragées: Lichtwer Pharma AG / Wallenroder Strasse 8-14 / 13435 Berlin / Germany / Tel: +49-30-40-3700 / Fax: +49-30-40-3704-49 / www.lichtwer.de. One tablet contains 300 mg hawthorn leaf with flower dry native extract 4–7:1 (*w/w*) (average 5.5:1), standardized to 2.25% flavonoid content. Solvent: methanol 70% (*v/v*).

Faros® LI 132 Dragées: Lichtwer Pharma AG. One tablet contains 100 mg hawthorn leaf with flower dry native extract 4–7:1 (*w/w*), standardized to 2.25% flavonoids.

*American equivalents are found in the Product Table beginning on page 398.

REFERENCES

Abdul-Ghani AS, et al. Hypotensive effect of *Crataegus oxyacantha*. *Int J Crude Drug Res* 1987;25:216–20.

Bahorun T, Gressier B, Trotin F, Brunet C, Dine T, et al. Oxygen species scavenging activity of phenolic extracts from hawthorn fresh plant organs and pharmaceutical preparations. *Arzneimittelforshung* 1996;46:1086–9.

Bahorun T, Trotin F, Pommery J, Vasseur J, Pinkas M. Antioxidant activities of *Crataegus monogyna* extracts. *Planta Med* 1994;60:323–8.

BHP. See: *British Herbal Pharmacopoeia*.

Blumenthal M, Busse WR, Goldberg A, Gruenwald J, Hall T, Riggins CW, Rister RS (eds.). Klein S, Rister RS (trans.). *The Complete German Commission E Monographs—Therapeutic Guide to Herbal Medicines*. Austin, TX: American Botanical Council; Boston: Integrative Medicine Communication; 1998;142–4.

Blumenthal M, Goldberg A, Brinckmann J (eds.). *Herbal Medicine: Expanded Commission E Monographs*. Newton, MA: Integrative Medicine Communications; 2000;182–92.

Blumenthal M. Herbs sales down 15% in mainstream market. *HerbalGram* 2001;51:69.

Bödigheimer K, Chase D. Efficay of hawthorne extract in the dosage of 100mg three times daily. Multicentre double-blind study involving 85 patients with congestive heart failure NYHA II. [in German]. *Münch Med Wochenscr* 1994;136(Suppl 1):S7–11.

Bratman S, Kroll D. *Clinical Evaluation of Medicinal Herbs and Other Therapeutic Natural Products*. Roseville, CA: Prima Health; 1999.

Braun R, Surmann P, Wendt R, Wichtl M, Ziegenmeyer J (eds.). *Standard Drug Approval for Prescription Drugs. Text and Commentary*. [in German]. Stuttgart: Deutscher Apotheker Verlag; 1996 Feb;Zulassungsnummer 1349.99.99.

Brinker F. *Herb Contraindications and Drug Interactions*, 3rd ed. Sandy, OR: Eclectic Medical Publications; 2001.

British Herbal Pharmacopoeia (BHP, 2nd edition 1983). Bournemouth, U.K.: British Herbal Medicine Association; 1983;75.

British Herbal Pharmacopoeia (BHP, 4th edition 1996). Exeter, U.K.: British Herbal Medicine Association; 1996;98–101.

Brixius K, Frank K, Muench G, Mueller-Ehmsen J, Schwinger R. WS 1442 (Crataegus-Spezialexrakt) wirkt am insuffizienten menschlichen Myokard Kontraktionskraftsteigernd. *Herz Kreislauf* 1998;30:28–33.

Brown D. Common drugs and their potential interactions with herbs or nutrients. *Health Notes Rev of Complement Integra Med* 1999;6(2):124–41.

Chang Q. Zuo Z, Harrison F, Chow M, Hawthorn. *J Clin Pharmacol* 2002;42:605–12.

Chatterjee S, Koch E, Jaggy H, Krzeminski T. *In-vitro* und *In-vivo* Untersuchungen zur kardioprotektiven Wirkung von oligomeren Procyanidinen in einem Crataegus-Extrakt aus Blättern mit Blüten. *Arzneimittelforshung* 1997;47:821–5.

Da Silva A, Rocha R, Silva C, et al. Antioxidants in medicinal plant extracts. A research study of the antioxidant capacity of *Crataegus*, *Hammamelis*, and *Hydrastis*. *Phytother Res* 2000;14:612–6.

DAB. See: *Deutsches Arzneibuch*.

DAC. See: *Deutscher Arzneimittel-Codex*.

DeSmet P, Keller K, Hänsel R, Chandler RF (eds.). *Adverse effects of Herbal Drugs*, vol. 2. Berlin: Springs-Verlag; 1993. Cited in Upton R (ed.). Hawthorn leaf with flower—*Crataegus* spp.: Analytical, quality control, and therapeutic monograph. In: Upton R (ed.). *American Herbal Pharmacopoeia and Therapeutic Compendium*. Santa Cruz, CA:AHP;1999.

Deutscher Arzneimittel-Codex (DAC 1986: 2. Ergänzung 1990) Band II. Stuttgart, Germany: Deutscher Apotheker Verlag; 1990;W–045:1–6.

Deutscher Arzneimittel-Codex (DAC 1986: 4. Ergänzung 1992) Band II. Stuttgart, Germany: Deutscher Apotheker Verlag; 1992;W–040:1-5.

Deutsches Arzneibuch (DAB Ergänzungslieferung 1999). Stuttgart, Germany: Deutscher Apotheker Verlag; 1999.

Deutsches Arzneibuch (DAB Ergänzungslieferung 2000). Stuttgart, Germany: Deutscher Apotheker Verlag; 2000.

Eichstädt H, Bäder M, Danne O, Kaiser W, Stein U, Felix R. Crataegus-Extrakt hilft dem Patienten mit NYHA II–Herzinsuffizienz. *Therapiewoche* 1989;39:3288–96.

Ellingwood F. *American Materia Medica, Therapeutics and Pharmacognosy*. Portland, OR: Eclectic Medical Publications; 1983 [reprint of 1919 edition].

ESCOP. See: European Scientific Cooperative on Phytotherapy.

European Pharmacopoeia (Ph.Eur. 3rd edition Supplement 2001). Strasbourg, France: Council of Europe; 2001;928–31.

European Scientific Cooperative on Phytotherapy. Crataegi Folium cum Flore. In: *Monographs On The Medicinal Uses of Plant Drugs*. Exeter, U.K.: European Scientific Cooperative on Phytotherapy; Oct 1999.

Farmacopea Ufficiale della Repubblica Italiana (Ph.Ital. IX 1985 Supplement 1991). Rome, Italy:Ministerio della Sanita; 1991.

Förster A, Förster K, Bühring M, Wolfstädter H. *Crataegus* for moderately reduced left ventricular ejection fraction.Double-blind, placebo controlled study investigat-ing the ergospirometry of 72 patients. [in German]. *Münch Med Wschr* 1994;136(Suppl 1):S21–6.

German Homoeopathic Pharmacopoeia (GHP). Translation of the *Deutsches Homöopathisches Arzneibuch* (HAB 1). First edition 1978 with 5 supplements through 1991. Stuttgart, Germany: Deutscher Apotheker Verlag; 1993;355–6.

GHP. See: *German Homoeopathic Pharmacopoeia*.

Hahn F, Klinkhammer F, Oberdorf A. Description and pharmacological investigation of a new therapeutic active agent derived from *Crataegus oxyacantha*. [in German]. *Arzneimittelforshung* 1960;10:825–6. In: Upton R. (ed.). Hawthorn leaf with flower—*Crataegus* spp.: Analytical, quality control, and therapeutic monograph. In: Upton R (ed.). *American Herbal Pharmacopoeia and Therapeutic Compendium*. Santa Cruz, CA:AHP;1999.

Hanack T, Brückel MH. The treatment of mild stable forms of angina pectoris using Crategutt® novo. *Therapiewoche* 1983;33:4331–3.

Hänsel R, Keller K, Rimpler H, Schneider G (eds.). *Hagers Handbuch der Pharmazeutischen Praxis*, 5. Aufl. Drogen A-D. Berlin, Germany: Springer Verlag; 1992–94;1040–62.

Health Canada. *Drug Product Database* (DPD). Ottawa, Ontario: Health Canada Therapeutic Products Programme; 2000.

Health Protection Branch (HPB). *HPB Status Manual*. Ottawa, Ontario: Health Protection Branch; Feb 19, 1993;99.

Hedley C. Humours, hearts and hawthorn. *Euro J Herbal Med* 2000;5(2):27–32.

Hellenbrecht D, Saller R, Rückbeil C, Bühring M. *Eur J Pharmacol* 1990;183:525–6.

Hobbs C, Foster S. Hawthorn: A Literature Review. *HerbalGram* 1990;22:19–33.

Holubarsch C, Colucci W, Meinertz T, Gaus W, Tendera M. Survival and prognosis: investigation of *Crataegus* extract WS 1442 in congestive heart failure (SPICE) – rationale, study design and study protocol. *Eur J Heart Fail* 2000 Dec;2(4):431–7.

Homoeopathic Pharmacopoeia of the United States (HPUS) — Revision Service Official Compendium from July 1, 1992. Falls Church, VA: American Institute of Homeopathy; Dec 1990;2240:CRAT.

HPB. See: Health Protection Branch.

HPUS. See: *Homoeopathic Pharmacopoeia of the United States*.

Iwamoto M, et al. Clinical effect of Craetagutt® on ischemic heart disease with and without hypertensive component. [in German]. *Planta Med* 1981;42:1–16.

Karnick C. Indian Medical Science Series No. 36: *Pharmacopoeial Standards of Herbal Plants*, Vol. I. Delhi, India: Sri Satguru Publications; 1994;109–10.

Kneipp-Werke. Heart and Circulation: Early support of heart and circulation. [in German]. In: *Wegweiser zu den Kneipp® Mitteln*. Würzburg, Germany: Sebastian Kneipp Gesundheitsmittelverlag GmbH; 1996;80–5.

Leuchtgens H. *Crataegus* special extract WS 1442 in NYHA II heart failure. A placebo controlled randomized double-blind study. [in German]. *Fortschr Med* 1993;111:352–4.

Leukel-Lenz A. Pharmacological analysis and investigation of the effect of Crataegus fractions [dissertation]. [in German]. University of Marburg. 1988.

Loew D. *Crataegus* extracts in congestive heart failure. Evidence –based clinical and pharmacological effects. [in German]. *Kassenarzt* 1994;15:43–52.

Loew D. Phytotherapy in heart failure. *Phytomedicine* 1997;4(3):267–71.

McCaleb R, Leigh E, Morien K. *The Encyclopedia of Popular Herbs*. Roseville, CA: Prima Health; 2000.

Loew D, Albrecht M, Podzuweit H. Efficacy and tolerability of a Hawthorn preparation in patients with heart failure stage I and II according to NYHA - a surveillance study. *Phytomedicine* 1996;3(Suppl. 1):92.

McGuffin M, Hobbs C, Upton R, Goldberg A (eds.). *American Herbal Products Association's Botanical Safety Handbook*. Boca Raton, FL: CRC Press; 1997;37.

Medical Products Agency (MPA). Naturläkemedel: Authorised Natural Remedies (as of January 24, 2001). Uppsala, Sweden: Medical Products Agency. 2001.

Meyer-Buchtela E. *Tee-Rezepturen—Ein Handbuch für Apotheker und Ärzte*. Stuttgart, Germany: Deutscher Apotheker Verlag; 1999.

Morant J, Ruppanner H (eds.). Produktinformation u. Patientinformation: Amino Crataegitan® Herztropfen; Bioforce Crataegisan Herztropfen; Medichemie Bioline Faros® 300 Dragées; Schwabe Cardiplant® Tropfen u. Filmtabletten; Sidroga® Weissdorntee; Synpharma Crataegus Synpha® Herztropfen. In: *Arzneimittel—Kompendium der Schweiz®* 2001. Basel, Switzerland: Documed AG.; 2001.

MPA. See: Medical Products Agency.

Müller A, Linke W, Klaus W. *Crataegus* extract blocks potassium currents in guinea pig ventricular cardiac myocytes. *Planta Med* 1999;65(4):335–9.

New York Heart Association (NYHA). 1994. Revisions to Classification of Functional Capacity and Objective Assessment of Patients with Diseases of the Heart.

Newall C, Anderson L, Phillipson J. *Herbal Medicines, A Guide for Health-Care Professionals*. London, U.K.: The Pharmaceutical Press; 1996;157–9.

O'Connolly M, Jansen W, Bernhöft G, Bartsch G. Treatment of decreasing cardiac performance. [in German]. *Fortschr Med* 1986;104(42):805–8.

ÖAB. See: *Österreichisches Arzneibuch*.

Österreichisches Arzneibuch (ÖAB, Vol. I, Suppl 3). Wien, Österreich: Verlag der

Österreichischen Staatsdruckerei; 1994.

Pfister-Hotz G. Phytotherapy in geriatrics. [in German]. *Schweiz Apoth Ztg* 1997;135:118–21.

Ph.Eur. See: *European Pharmacopoeia*.

Ph.Fr. See: *Pharmacopée Française*.

Ph.Helv. See: *Pharmacopoea Helvetica*.

Ph.Ital. See: *Farmacopea Ufficiale della Republica Italiana*.

Pharmacopée Française (Ph.Fr.X). Paris, France: Adrapharm;. 1982–96.

Pharmacopoea Helvetica (Ph.Helv.VIII). Bern, Switzerland: Verlag Eidgenössische Drucksachen und Materialzentrale;. 1998.

Pizzorno JE, Murray MT, editors. *A Textbook of Natural Medicine*, Vol. 1, 2nd ed. New York: Churchill Livingston; 1999.

Rácz-Kotilla E, *et al.* Hypotensive and beta-blocking effect of procyanidins of *Crataegus monogyna*. *Planta Med* 1980;39:239.

Rajendran S, Deepalakshmi P, Parasakthy K, *et al.* Effect of tincture of *Crataegus* on the LDL-receptor activity of hepatic plasma membrane of rats fed an atherogenic diet. *Atherosclerosis* 1996;123:235–41.

Rehwald A. Analytical investigation of *Crataegus* species and *Passiflora incarnata* L. by high performance liquid chromatography [dissertation]. Zurich: Swiss Federal Institute of Technology, 1995. Cited in Upton R (ed.). Hawthorn leaf with flower—*Crataegus* spp.: Analytical, quality control, and therapeutic monograph. In: Upton R (ed.). *American Herbal Pharmacopoeia and Therapeutic Compendium.* Santa Cruz, CA:AHP;1999.

Reuter H. *Crataegus* as a herbal cardiotonic. *Z Phytother* 1994;15(2):73–81.

Rohr G. Analytical investigation on and isolation of procyanidins from *Crataegus* leaves and flowers [dissertation]. Zurich: Swiss Federal Institute of Technology, 1999. In: Upton R (ed.). Hawthorn berry—*Crataegus* spp.: Analytical, quality control, and therapeutic monograph. In: Upton R (ed.). *American Herbal Pharmacopoeia and Therapeutic Compendium.* Santa Cruz, CA:AHP;1999.

Ruppanner H, Schaefer U (eds.). *Codex 2000/01 – Die Schweizer Arzneimittel in einem Griff.* Basel, Switzerland: Documed AG; 2001.

Schmidt U, Albrecht M, Podzuweit H, *et al.* High-dose *Crataegus* therapy in patients suffering from heart failure NYHA class I and II. *Z Phytotherapie* 1998;19:22–30.

Schmidt U, Kuhn U, Ploch M, Hubner W-D. Efficacy of the Hawthorn (Crataegus) preparation LI in 132 in 78 patients with chronic congestive heart failure defined as NYHA functional class II. *Phytomedicine* 1994;1:17–24.

Schulz V, Hansel R, Tyler V. *Rational Phytotherapy: A Physicians' Guide to Herbal Medicine,* 4th ed. Germany Heidelberg,: Berlin: Springer-Verlag' Berlin Heidelberg; 2000.

Schüssler M, Acar D, Cordes A, *et al.* Anti-ischemic effect of flavonoids derived from *Crataegus.* [in German]. *Arch Pharm* 1993; 326:708(P77).

Schüssler M, Fricke U, Hölzl J, Nikolov N. Effects of flavonoids from *Crataegus* species in Langendorff perfused isolated guinea pig hearts. *Planta Med* 1992;58(7):46.

Schüssler M, Fricke U, Nikolov N, Hölzl J. Comparison of the flavonoids occurring in *Crataegus* species and inhibition of 3', 5'-cyclic adenosine monophosphate phosphodiesterase. *Planta Med* 1991;57(Suppl 2):A133.

Schüssler M, Hölzl J, Fricke U. Myocardial effects of flavonoids from *Crataegus* species. *Arzneimittelforschung* 1995;45(8):842–5.

Schwinger R, Pietsch M, Frank K, Brixius K. *Crataegus* Special extract WS 1442 increases force of contraction in human myocardium cAMP-independently. *J Cardio Pharmacol* 2000;35:700–7.

Shanthi S, Parasakthy K, Deepalakshimi P, Devaraj S. Hypolipidemic activity of tincture of *Crataegus* in rats. *Ind J Biochem Biophys* 1994;31:143–6.

Steinman H, Lovell C, Cronin E. Immediate-type hypersensitivity to *Crataegus monogyna* (hawthorn). *Contact Dermatitis* 1984;11:321.

Sticher O, Meier B. Hawthorn (*Crataegus*): Biological Activity and New Strategies for Quality Control. In: Lawson L, Bauer R (eds.). *Phytomedicines of Europe: Chemistry and Biological Activity.* Washington, DC: American Chemical Society; 1998;241–62.

Tauchert M, Gildor A, Lipinski J. High-dose *Crataegus* (Hawthorn) extract WS 1442 for the treatment of NYHA Class II heart failure patients. [in German]. *Herz* 1999;24:465–74.

Tauchert M, Ploch M, Hübner W. Efficacy of Hawthorn extract LI 132 in comparison with Captopril. Double-blind, multicentre study involving 1332 patients with stage II congestive heart failure (NYHA II). [in German]. *Münch Med Wschr* 1994;136(Suppl 1):S27–33.

Tittel G, Wagner H. Analysis and isolation of phenolics from plants by HPLC: Possibilities and limits. *Proc Int Bioflav Symp* 1981:299–310. Cited in Upton R (ed.). Hawthorn berry—*Crataegus* spp.: Analytical, quality control, and therapeutic monograph. In: Upton R (ed.). *American Herbal Pharmacopoeia and Therapeutic Compendium.* Santa Cruz, CA:AHP;1999.

Trunzler V, Schuler E. Comparative investigation of the effect of a *Crataegus* extract , Digotoxin, Digoxin and γ-Strophanthin on isolated heart muscle. [in German]. *Arzneimittelforshung* 1962; 12:198. Cited in: Upton R (ed.). Hawthorn leaf with flower—*Crataegus* spp.: Analytical, quality control, and therapeutic monograph. In: Upton R (ed.). *American Herbal Pharmacopoeia and Therapeutic Compendium.* Santa Cruz, CA:AHP;1999.

United States Congress (USC). Public Law 103–417: Dietary Supplement Health and Education Act of 1994. Washington, DC: 103rd Congress of the United States; 1994.

United States Pharmacopeia (USP 25th Revision) - The National Formulary (NF 20th Edition). Rockville, MD: United States Pharmacopeial Convention, Inc. 2002.

Upton R (ed.). Hawthorn berry—*Crataegus* spp.: Analytical, quality control, and therapeutic monograph. In: Upton R (ed.). *American Herbal Pharmacopoeia and Therapeutic Compendium.* Santa Cruz, CA:AHP;1999a.

Upton R (ed.). Hawthorn leaf with flower—*Crataegus* spp.: Analytical, quality control, and therapeutic monograph. In: Upton R (ed.). *American Herbal Pharmacopoeia and Therapeutic Compendium.* Santa Cruz, CA:AHP;1999b.

USC. See: United States Congress.

USP. See: *United States Pharmacopoeia*.

Van Hellemont J. *Compendium de Phytotherapie.* Bruxelles, Belgique: Association Pharmaceutique Belge; 1986.

Van Hellemont J. *Fytotherapeutisch compendium.* Utrecht, Netherlands: Bohn, Scheltema & Holkema; 1988;179–80.

Vibes J, Lasserre B, Declume C. Effects of a total extract from *Crataegus oxyacantha* blossoms on TXA2 and PGI2 biosynthesis *in vitro* and on TXA2- and PGI2- synthesizing activities of cardiac tissue. *Med Sci Res* 1991;19:143–5.

Vibes J, Lasserre B, Gleye J, Declume C. Inhibition of thromboxane A2 biosynthesis *in vitro* by the main components of *Crataegus oxyacantha* (hawthorn) flower heads. *Prostaglandins Leukot Essent Fatty Acids* 1994;50:173–5.

Vibes J, Lasserre B, Gleye J. Effects of a methanolic extract from *Crataegus oxyacantha* blossoms on TXA2 and PGI2 synthesizing activities of cardiac tissue. *Med Sci Res* 1993;21:435–6.

Wagner H, Tittel G. High-Performance –Liquid-Chromatography (HPLC) as a analytical method to standardize cardiac drugs. [in German]. In: Rietbrock N, Schneiders B, Schuster J (eds.). *Wandlungen in der Therapie der Herzinsuffizienz,* Wiesbaden, Germany: Vieweg; 1983;33–41.

Weikl A, Assmus K, Neukum-Schmidt A, *et al. Crataegus* extract WS 1442. Evidence-based evaluation of its effect on patients with Stage II congestive heart failure (NYHA II). [in German]. *Fortschr Med* 1996;114:291–296.

Weikl A, Noh HS. The effect of *Crataegus* in global congestive heart failure. [in German]. *Herz und Gefäße* 1992;516–24.

WHO. See: World Health Organization.

Wichtl M (ed.). *Teedrogen und Phytopharmaka,* 3rd ed. Stuttgart, Germany: Wissenschaftliche Verlagsgesellschaft; 1997;168–172.

World Health Organization (WHO). *Regulatory Situation of Herbal Medicines: A Worldwide Review.* Geneva, Switzerland: World Health Organization Traditional Medicine Programme; 1998;26–7.

Clinical Studies on Hawthorn (*Crataegus* spp.)

Cardiac Insufficiency

Author/Year	Subject	Design	Duration	Dosage	Preparation	Results/Conclusion
Tauchert et al., 1999	Cardiac insufficiency NYHA Stage II	MC, O n=1,011 patients with cardiac insufficiency	24 weeks	80 mg tablet, 2x/day (160mg extract/day)	Crataegus Special Extract WS 1442	Hawthorn treatment associated with significant improvement in clinical symptoms (exercise tolerance, fatigue, palpitation, and exercise dyspnea); 83% decrease in ankle edema and nocturia; reduction in blood pressure, resting pulse rate, and the difference in the pressure/heart rate product (PHRP); improved ejection fraction and improvements in echocardiography.
Schmidt et al, 1998	Cardiac insufficiency NYHA Stages I and II	O, OL, MC n=3,664 with stable NYHA Stage I or II (average age 66.7 years)	8 weeks	300 mg tablet, 3x/day (900 mg extract/day)	Faros® 300 Dragées	After 8 weeks hawthorn treatment decreased average heart rate (p<0.01) from 79.9 to 75.2 beats per minute. Average pressure-rate product (PRP) scores reduced from 117 mm Hg per minute x 200 to 105.7 mm Hg per minute x 100 (p<0.05). Work tolerance, as determined by bicycle ergometry, increased from 93.5 to 109.7 watts (W) (p<0.001).
Loew et al., 1996	Cardiac insufficiency NYHA Stage I and II	OL, S n=1,476 patients with heart failure of NYHA Stages I and II	Evaluation after 1 month and 2 months	300 mg tablet, 3x/day (900 mg extract/day)	Faros® 300 Dragées	At end of surveillance period, symptom score dropped by a mean of 66.6% with NYHA Stage I patients largely symptom free. A subgroup of patients with borderline hypertension showed decreases in systolic and diastolic pressure (160 to 150 mm Hg and 89 to 85 mm Hg, respectively), a drop in heart rate from 89 to 79 beats per minute, and arrhythmias that were significantly reduced independent of heart failure.
Weikl et al., 1996	Cardiac insufficiency NYHA Stage II	DB, PC, MC n=136 patients with NYHA Stage II cardiac insufficiency (40–80 years)	2 months (after a 2 week run-in phase)	80 mg capsule, 2x/day (160 mg extract daily) vs. placebo	Crataegus Special Extract WS 1442	Hawthorn showed statistically significant superiority (p=0.018, U test, one-sided) in primary target parameter (change in pressure-rate/product [PRP] difference determined by systolic blood pressure x heart rate divided by 100) with a median decrease in PRP of 6.2 compared to +0.1 increase with placebo. Subjective complaints also decreased in hawthorn group (p<0.05).
Bödigheimer and Chase, 1994	Congestive heart failure, NYHA Stage II	R, DB, PC, MC n=85 patients with NYHA Stage II cardiac insufficiency	1 month	100 mg tablet, 3x/day (300 mg extract/day) vs. placebo	Faros® LI 132 Dragées	After 4 weeks there was a statistically insignificant trend towards improvement in clinical symptoms and in ergometric parameters, compared to placebo. The duration of use (only 4 weeks) and the relative low dosage (300 mg/day) may explain these results.
Förster et al., 1994	Congestive heart failure, NYHA Stage II	DB, PC n=72 patients with NYHA Stage II cardiac insufficiency	2 months	300 mg tablet, 3x/day (900 mg extract/day) vs. placebo	Faros® 300 Dragées	Oxygen uptake increased with hawthorn but not with placebo (p<0.05) based on ergospirometry. Time taken to reach anaerobic threshold during exercise increased by 30 seconds in hawthorn group and 2 seconds in placebo group. Hawthorn also showed significant improvements (p<0.001) in subjective complaint scores.
Schmidt et al., 1994	Cardiac insufficiency, NYHA Stage II	R, DB, PC, MC n=78 patients with NYHA Stage II cardiac insufficiency (men and women ages 45–73)	8 weeks with a 1 week washout period	One, 200 mg tablet, 3x/day (600 mg extract/day) vs. placebo	Faros® LI 132 Dragées containing 200mg Crataegus extract LI 132	Statistically significant (p<0.001) increase in exercise tolerance in hawthorn group by 28 watt (W) compared to 5 W in placebo group using ergometer bicycle (12.5 W). Hawthorn group showed significant reductions in systolic blood pressure (p<0.05) and heart rate (p<0.01). Subjective symptoms score also improved significantly (p<0.001).
Tauchert et al., 1994	Congestive heart failure NYHA Stage II	R, DB, MC, Cm n=132 patients with NYHA Stage II cardiac insufficiency	2 months (including a 1 week lower dosage introductory therapy period)	Three, 100 mg tablets, 3x/day (900 mg extract/day) vs. 12.5 mg, 3x/day of ACE inhibitor Captopril (37.5 mg/day)	Faros® LI 132 Dragées vs. captopril	None of the target parameters (ergometry, pressure-rate-product (PRP), score for 5 typical symptoms) showed significant differences between hawthorn and captopril groups. Both showed statistically significant increase (p<0.001) in maximum tolerated exercise performance, 83 to 97 watt (W) in hawthorn group and 83 to 99 W in captopril group. Both treatments reduced PRP and decreased incidence and severity of symptoms (shortness of breath; fatigue after exercise) by 50%.
Leuchtgens, 1993	Cardiac insufficiency, NYHA Stage II	R, DB, PC n=30 patients with NYHA Stage II cardiac insufficiency	2 months	80 mg capsule, 2x/day (160 mg extract/day) vs. placebo	Crataegus Special Extract WS 1442	Hawthorn showed statistically significant (p<0.05) improvements over placebo (hawthorn −11.6, placebo −4.9) in the pressure-rate-product (PRP) during exercise (systolic blood pressure x heart rate/100) using bicycle ergometer, in subjective complaints score (hawthorn −16.5, placebo −4, p<0.05), and in heart rate.

KEY: C – controlled, **CC** – case-control, **CH** – cohort, **CI** – confidence interval, **Cm** – comparison, **CO** – crossover, **CS** – cross-sectional, **DB** – double-blind, **E** – epidemiological, **LC** – longitudinal cohort, **MA** – meta-analysis, **MC** – multi-center, **n** – number of patients, **O** – open, **OB** – observational, **OL** – open label, **OR** – odds ratio, **P** – prospective, **PB** – patient-blind, **PC** – placebo-controlled, **PG** – parallel group, **PS** – pilot study, **R** – randomized, **RC** – reference-controlled, **RCS** – retrospective cross-sectional, **RS** - retrospective, **S** – surveillance, **SB** – single-blind, **SC** – single-center, **U** – uncontrolled, **UP** – unpublished, **VC** – vehicle-controlled.

Cardiac Insufficiency (cont.)

Author/Year	Subject	Design	Duration	Dosage	Preparation	Results/Conclusion
Weikl and Noh, 1992	Congestive heart failure NYHA Stage II	OL n=20 patients with NYHA Stage II cardiac insufficiency and LVEF <55%	1 month	One to two, 80 mg capsules, 3x/day (240–480 mg extract/day)	Crataegutt® forte capsules	480 mg/day increased ejection fraction from 40.18% to 43.5% at rest and 41.51% to 46.56% during exercise using radionuclide angio-cardiography method. Slight decrease in blood pressure during rest and exercise. Treatment of 7 patients with 240 mg/day increased the LVEF from 29.8% to 30.45% based on nuclear resonance scanning method.
Eichstädt et al., 1989	Congestive heart failure, NYHA Stage II LVEF<55%	OL n=20 NYHA Stage II patients	1 month	Two, 80 mg tablet, 3x/day (480 mg extract/day)	Crataegus Special Extract WS 1442 (Crataegutt® forte)	Hawthorn improved exercise tolerance and cardiac performance as well as subjective symptoms using a bicycle ergometer. After 4 weeks, patients maximum exercise tolerance rose from 704 to 772 watts (W) x minute (p<0.05).
O'Conolly et al., 1986	Heart failure, NYHA Stage I or II	R, DB, PC, CO n=36 patients with Stage I or II cardiac insufficiency (average age 74 years)	6 weeks	60 mg tablet, 3x/day (180 mg extract/day)	Crataegutt® novo Filmtabletten	Patients treated with hawthorn had decreased heart rate and improved cardiac output under resting and exercise conditions. Pressure-rate-product (PRP) was significantly reduced and quality of life measurements significantly improved. Significant improvement in psychological assessment including reduction in anxiety (p<0.0001) and sleep behavior.
Hanak and Brückel, 1983	Coronary disease, NYHA Stage I and II	R, DB, PC n=60 patients with stable angina pectoris	3 weeks	60 mg tablet, 3x/day (180 mg extract/day) vs. placebo	Crataegutt® novo Filmtabletten	Electrocardiogram measures improved in hawthorn group, and blood flow and oxygen delivery to the heart muscle rose. Hawthorn patients also exercised for longer periods of time without an angina attack.
Iwamoto et al., 1981	Cardiac insufficiency, NYHA Stage II or III	DB, PC n=80 patients with NYHA Stage II cardiac insufficiency	6 weeks	Weeks 1–2: Two, 30 mg tablets 3x/day after meals (180 mg/day) Weeks 3–6: Two or three, 30 mg tablets 3x/day after meals (180 mg or 270 mg/day)	Crataegutt® Dragées 30 mg of an extract of *Crataegus monogyna* and *C. oxyacantha* per tablet	Compared to placebo, hawthorn group exhibited statistically significant improvement of cardiac function (p<0.001) and of subjective symptoms such as dyspnea and palpitations (p<0.001). No difference in improvements in ECG recordings between hawthorn and placebo groups.

KEY: C – controlled, **CC** – case-control, **CH** – cohort, **CI** – confidence interval, **Cm** – comparison, **CO** – crossover, **CS** – cross-sectional, **DB** – double-blind, **E** – epidemiological, **LC** – longitudinal cohort, **MA** – meta-analysis, **MC** – multi-center, **n** – number of patients, **O** – open, **OB** – observational, **OL** – open label, **OR** – odds ratio, **P** – prospective, **PB** – patient-blind, **PC** – placebo-controlled, **PG** – parallel group, **PS** – pilot study, **R** – randomized, **RC** – reference-controlled, **RCS** – retrospective cross-sectional, **RS** - retrospective, **S** – surveillance, **SB** – single-blind, **SC** – single-center, **U** – uncontrolled, **UP** – unpublished, **VC** – vehicle-controlled.

Hawthorn

Monograph

(This page intentionally left blank.)

Horse Chestnut

Aesculus hippocastanum L.
[Fam. *Hippocastanaceae*]

OVERVIEW

Horse chestnut seed extract (HCSE) is relatively new to the U.S. botanical market. This phytomedicine is gaining popularity due to the high quantity of clinical evidence from Europe documenting its safety and efficacy as a treatment for varicose veins, chronic venous insufficiency (CVI), and related vascular disorders. Europeans have used HCSE for these conditions since the late 16th century. Horse chestnut seeds can be toxic when unprocessed and are unrelated to sweet chestnuts (*Castanea sativa*), which can be eaten without precautions. Standardized and purified preparations of horse chestnut seeds are available.

PRIMARY USES

Internal
- Venous insufficiency (chronic)
- Varicosis, lower veins

External
- Blunt traumas, especially painful hematomas, post-traumatic and postoperative soft tissue swelling
- Injuries with hematomas
- Symptoms associated with varicose veins such as swollen legs (edema), pain and heaviness in the legs, and calf pain

OTHER POTENTIAL USES
- Severe cranio-cerebral trauma
- Prevention and treatment of postoperative edema
- Traumatic head injury, intracranial pressure, and edema
- Hemorrhoids
- Leg ulcers

PHARMACOLOGICAL ACTIONS

Antiedemic; reduces transcapillary filtration; venoactive effect.

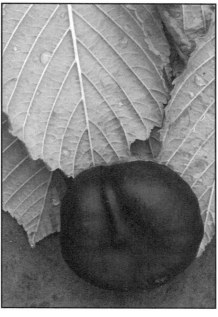

Photo © 2003 stevenfoster.com

DOSAGE AND ADMINISTRATION

Internal

There is little information about the long-term, internal use of horse chestnut. However, in one clinical trial, horse chestnut was given for 56 weeks without adverse effect.

TINCTURE: 20–30 drops (0.5–0.7 ml), with water at mealtimes, 3 times daily [1:2.6 (*w/v*), 65 vol.-% alcohol].

DRY EXTRACT FROM DRIED SEED (standardized): 250–312.5 mg, 2 times daily with meals, in delayed-release form corresponding to 100 mg escin daily [5–8:1 (*w/w*), 16–20% triterpene glycosides].

DRY EXTRACT FROM FRESH SEED (standardized): 2 enteric coated tablets containing 63–90 mg dry native extract each, 3 times daily with water, at mealtimes, corresponding to 120 mg escin daily [5.0–6.1:1 (*w/w*)]. After 1–2 weeks reduce to 1 tablet, 3 times daily.

NOTE: Unprocessed horse chestnut seeds should not be eaten or made into tea because they contain toxins, including esculin, which are removed in processing.

External

There are no external horse chestnut preparations available in the U.S. at this time.

CONTRAINDICATIONS

Internal

Not generally recommended for children or for individuals with chronic renal failure. However, an authoritative clinical review found no clinical basis for contraindications.

External

The gel or ointment should not be applied to broken or ulcerated skin. HCSE is contraindicated in cases of thrombosis or risk of embolism and for application to open wounds or mucous membranes.

PREGNANCY AND LACTATION: There are no known restrictions during pregnancy or lactation. HCSE has been used in some clinical studies involving pregnant women, with some studies excluding those in the third trimester.

ADVERSE EFFECTS

Rare adverse effects include pruritus, nausea, gastric complaints, and irritation of the gastric mucous membranes and reflux. Escin Ib isolated from horse chestnut might partially delay or even inhibit gastric emptying. This potential adverse effect can be minimized by taking the extract in an enteric-coated tablet form with the main meal. Anaphylactic shock, toxic nephropathy, and renal failure have been reported following intravenous administration of isolated escin, but these reactions are not associated with oral ingestion of HCSE preparations. One case of horse chestnut-related contact dermatitis has been reported, but this does not pertain to the oral dosage form.

DRUG INTERACTIONS

Horse chestnut extracts or derivatives, specifically escin, may interfere with the effects of anticoagulants. Escin, the main saponin component in horse chestnut, binds to plasma protein and may affect the binding of other drugs (speculative).

CLINICAL REVIEW

Out of 23 clinical studies on horse chestnut that included a total of 4,339 participants, all of the 20 studies investigating its use in venous disorders demonstrated positive effects. Of the venous disorder studies, 4 were randomized, double-blind, placebo-controlled (R, DB, PC), parallel group (PG) studies, 5 were R, DB, PC, cross-over studies, 4 were R, DB, comparison, PG studies, one was a R, PC, single-blind design, another was a DB, PC, multicenter study, one was an uncontrolled, multicenter study with 71 participants, one was DB design, and three were surveillance studies. The main outcome measure for most studies was reduced leg volume or ankle circumference.

A systematic review of 13 R, DB clinical trials from 1976–1996 involving nearly 1,100 patients using HCSE in the treatment of venous disorders concluded that HCSE was superior to placebo. HCSE was as effective as rutosides (the conventional treatment) in five studies. Adverse effects were mild and infrequent.

A randomized, cross-over study found bioequivalence (phytoequivalence) in two different forms of HCSE. A R, DB, PC study of 70 subjects using HCSE topical gel showed significant reduction in tenderness with experimentally induced hematomas. Subjects with severe cranio-cerebral trauma regained consciousness more quickly and experienced reduced intracranial pressure with purified escin i.v., followed by HCSE tablets, compared to placebo.

Horse Chestnut

Aesculus hippocastanum L.
[Fam. *Hippocastanaceae*]

OVERVIEW

Horse chestnut is relatively new to the U.S. herbal products market. However, it is gaining popularity because of numerous clinical studies showing that it is safe and effective for treating varicose veins, inadequate vein strength, and related disorders.

USES

Venous insufficiency (chronic); varicose veins (legs); symptoms associated with varicose veins such as swollen legs, pain and heaviness in legs, and calf pain; injuries with hematomas (bruises).

DOSAGE

Internal

DRY EXTRACT FROM DRIED SEED (standardized to 16–20% triterpene glycosides): 250–312.5 mg, 2 times daily, equivalent to 100 mg escin daily.

DRY EXTRACT FROM FRESH SEED (standardized): 2 tablets containing 63–90 mg, 3 times daily, equivalent to 120 mg escin daily. After 1–2 weeks reduce to 1 tablet, 3 times daily.

NOTE: Unprocessed horse chestnut seeds should not be eaten or made into tea because they contain toxins, including esculin, which are removed in processing.

External

There are no external horse chestnut preparations available in the U.S. at this time.

CONTRAINDICATIONS

Consult with a healthcare provider before giving oral preparations to children or individuals with chronic kidney failure. The gel or ointment should not be applied to mucous membranes, or broken or ulcerated skin. Consult with a healthcare provider before giving preparations in cases of thrombosis (clots) or risk of embolism.

PREGNANCY AND LACTATION: None known.

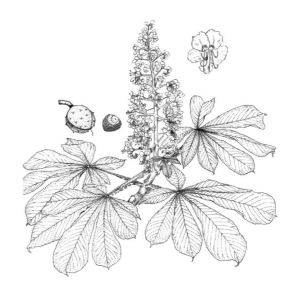

ADVERSE EFFECTS

Rare adverse effects can include pruritus (severe itching), nausea, stomach complaints, irritation of the stomach's lining, and reflux. An isolated horse chestnut seed chemical, escin Ib, might partially delay or even inhibit emptying of the stomach. This possible adverse effect can be minimized by taking the extract in an enteric-coated tablet form with the main meal. In one case report, horse chestnut was linked to contact dermatitis (red, itchy skin), but this did not involve oral preparations (e.g., capsules, tablets).

DRUG INTERACTIONS

The effects of anticoagulant (blood-thinning) drugs may be increased by certain components of horse chestnut, specifically escin.

Comments

When using a dietary supplement, purchase it from a reliable source. For best results, use the same brand of product throughout the period of use. As with all medications and dietary supplements, please inform your healthcare provider of all herbs and medications you are taking. Interactions may occur between medications and herbs or even among different herbs when taken at the same time. Treat your herbal supplement with care by taking it as directed, storing it as advised on the label, and keeping it out of the reach of children and pets. Consult your healthcare provider with any questions.

AMERICAN
BOTANICAL
COUNCIL

The information contained on this sheet has been excerpted from *The ABC Clinical Guide to Herbs* © 2003 by the American Botanical Council (ABC). ABC is an independent member-based educational organization focusing on the medicinal use of herbs. For more detailed information about this herb please consult the healthcare provider who gave you this sheet. To order *The ABC Clinical Guide to Herbs* or become a member of ABC, visit their website at www.herbalgram.org.

Horse Chestnut

Aesculus hippocastanum L.

[Fam. *Hippocastanaceae*]

OVERVIEW

Europeans have used horse chestnut seeds for medicinal purposes since at least the late 16th century when the plant was introduced into Northern Europe from the Near East (Blumenthal *et al.*, 2000; McCaleb *et al.*, 2000). Extracts from horse chestnut seeds were used in France in the early 1800's. Publications from 1896 to 1909 report success in its use for hemorrhoids (Schulz *et al.*, 2000). Although horse chestnut seed extract (HCSE) is relatively new to the U.S. botanical market, it is gaining in popularity due to the significant quantity of clinical evidence from Europe documenting its safety and efficacy as a treatment for varicose veins, chronic venous insufficiency, and related vascular disorders. Horse chestnut seeds can be toxic when unprocessed and are unrelated to sweet chestnuts (*Castanea sativa*), a plant in the family *Fagaceae*, which can be eaten without precautions (McCaleb *et al.*, 2000). Standardized and purified preparations of horse chestnut seeds are available. HCSE is the most widely prescribed oral remedy for venous edema in Germany (Schulz *et al.*, 2000).

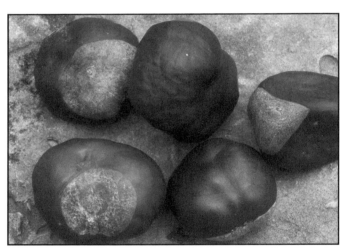

Photo © 2003 stevenfoster.com

DESCRIPTION

Horse chestnut preparations produced from the dried seed of *Aesculus hippocastanum* L. [Fam. *Hippocastanaceae*], containing not less than 3% triterpene glycosides, calculated as anhydrous escin (also spelled aescin), with reference to the dried seed (DAB, 1999). HCSE is a dry extract manufactured from German pharmacopeia-grade horse chestnut seed and is normalized to contain no less than 16%, and no more than 20%, triterpene glycosides, calculated as anhydrous escin (DAB, 1999). The typical drug-to-extract ratio for the native dry extract falls within the range of 5–8:1 (*w/w*), depending on the chemical composition of the starting material, and the subsequent yield of soluble extractive (Blumenthal *et al.*, 2000).

PRIMARY USES

Internal

- Venous insufficiency, chronic (Geissbühler and Degenring, 1999; Shah *et al.*, 1997; Diehm *et al.*, 1996; Rehn *et al.*, 1996; Diehm *et al.*, 1992; Erler, 1991; Pilz, 1990; Steiner, 1990; Steiner and Hillemanns, 1990; Erdlen, 1989; Kalbfleisch and Pfalzgraf, 1989; Rudofsky *et al.*, 1986; Lohr *et al.*, 1986; Bisler *et al.*, 1986)

  NOTE: The German Commission E also approved HCSE for venous insufficiency, usually of the legs, including pain and sensation of heaviness in the legs, nocturnal systremma (cramps in the calves), pruritus, and swelling of the legs (Blumenthal *et al.*, 1998)

- Varicosis, lower veins (Kreysel *et al.*, 1983; Friederich *et al.*, 1978; Neiss and Böhm, 1976)

External

- Blunt traumas, especially painful hematomas, post-traumatic and postoperative soft tissue swelling (Schilcher, 1997)

- Injuries with hematomas (Calabrese and Preston, 1993)

- Symptoms associated with varicose veins, such as swollen legs (edema), pain and heaviness in the legs, and calf pain (Morant and Ruppanner, 2001)

OTHER POTENTIAL USES

- Severe cranio-cerebral trauma (Put, 1979)

- Prevention and treatment of postoperative edema (Reynolds *et al.*, 1989)

- Traumatic head injury, intracranial pressure, and edema (McCaleb *et al.*, 2000)

- Hemorrhoids (Mills and Bone, 2000)

- Leg ulcers (Weiss and Fintelmann, 2000)

DOSAGE

Internal

Crude Preparations

TINCTURE: 1:2.6 (*w/v*), 65 vol.-% alcohol, adult dose 20–30 drops (0.5–0.7 ml), with water at meal times, 3 times daily (Morant and Ruppanner, 2001).

Standardized Preparations

DRY EXTRACT FROM DRIED SEED: 5–8:1 (*w/w*), 16–20% triterpene glycosides: 250–312.5 mg, 2 times daily in delayed-release form, corresponding to 100 mg escin daily. One dose in the morning and another in the evening, with ample liquids during meals (Blumenthal *et al.*, 1998).

DRY EXTRACT FROM FRESH SEED: 5.0–6.1:1 (*w/w*), adult dose: 2 enteric coated tablets containing 63–90 mg dry native extract each, 3 times daily taken with water at mealtimes, corresponding to 120 mg escin daily. After 1–2 weeks reduced to 1 tablet, 3 times daily (Morant and Ruppanner, 2001).

PURIFIED ESCIN (intravenous preparation in the form of sodium escinate): 5.1 mg sodium escinate, 1–2 times daily, maximum adult dose: 20 mg (Reynolds *et al.*, 1989; Weiss, 1988); children 3–10 years: 0.2 mg/kg body weight, infants up to 3 years: 0.1mg/kg body weight (Weiss, 1988) (not available in the U.S.).

NOTE: Unprocessed horse chestnut seeds should not be eaten or made into tea because they contain toxins, including esculin, which are removed in processing (McCaleb *et al*, 2000).

External
Standardized Preparations
GEL: 1 g contains 54–177 mg dry extract standardized to 2% escin. Applied to affected area 2 times daily (Morant and Ruppanner, 2001).

OINTMENT: Contains aqueous extract. Applied to affected area. The type of ointment base contributes to efficacy, as does the use of occlusive dressings (Schilcher, 1997).

Purified Escin Preparation
ESCIN GEL NRF: 23.1 (*Aescini mucilago*), 1% water-soluble escin, a thin layer applied to skin, several times daily as needed. Not for use on open wounds (NRF 3, 1986) (not available in the U.S.).

DURATION OF ADMINISTRATION
Internal
There is little scientific information about the long-term use of horse chestnut; however, one clinical trial administered horse chestnut for 56 weeks without adverse effect (Put, 1979). HCSE is widely used for long-term therapy in German clinical practice, without reports of adverse events (Schulz *et al.*, 2000).

CHEMISTRY
Horse chestnut seed contains 3–6% of a complex mixture of triterpenoid saponins collectively referred to as escin (aescin) (Morgan and Bone, 1998), including the triterpene oligoglycosides escins, Ia, Ib, IIa, IIb, and IIIa (Yoshikawa *et al.*, 1996); the acylated polyhydroxyoleanene triterpene oligoglycosides escins IIIb, IV, V, and VI, and isoaescins Ia, Ib, and V (Yoshikawa *et al.*, 1998); 0.2–0.3 % flavonoids (Wagner, 1967), including flavonol oligosaccharides (Hübner *et al.*, 1999); coumarin derivatives (esculetin and esculin) (Fugmann *et al.*, 1997); sterols (stigmasterol, α-spinasterol, and β-sitosterol); and fatty acids (linolenic, palmitic, and stearic acids) (Leung and Foster, 1996). The sapogenols hippocaesculin and barringtogenol-C are produced by hydrolysis (Konoshima and Lee, 1986).

PHARMACOLOGICAL ACTIONS
Human
Anti-edemic (Geissbühler and Degenring, 1999, Shah *et al.*, 1997, Diehm *et al.*, 1996); reduces transcapillary filtration (Blumenthal *et al.*, 1998; Schilcher, 1997); venoactive (BHP, 1996).

Animal
Anti-edemic (Guillaume and Padioleau, 1994); improved vein compliance; inhibits vasodilation (Guillaume and Padioleau, 1994); anti-inflammatory (Guillaume and Padioleau, 1994; Matsuda *et al.*, 1997; Tsutsumi and Ishizuka, 1967); antioxidant (Bombardelli and Morazzoni, 1996); diminished cutaneous capillary hyperpermeability (Guillaume and Padioleau, 1994); isolated escin demonstrated anti-exudative and vasoconstricting effects (Blumenthal *et al.*, 1998).

In vitro
Antitumor (Konoshima and Lee, 1986); isolated hippocaesculin and barringtogenol-C-21-angelate have antitumor activity (Chandler, 1993; De Meirsman and Rosselle, 1980); isolated escin, and to a lesser extent escinol, inhibits activity of hyaluronidase (Facino *et al.*, 1995); antioxidant (Bombardelli and Morazzoni, 1996); anti-inflammatory and immunomodulatory (Brokos *et al.*, 1999).

MECHANISM OF ACTION
Human
- HCSE reduced lysosomal enzyme activity (Kreysel *et al.*, 1983) elevated in chronic pathological conditions of the veins, thereby preventing breakdown of glycocalyx (mucopolysaccharides) in the region of the capillary wall. Through a reduction of vascular permeability, the filtration of small molecule proteins, electrolytes, and water into the interstitium is inhibited (Blumenthal *et al.*, 1998).
- Inhibited experimentally induced leg edema in patients with chronic venous insufficiency by reducing transcapillary filtration (Pauschinger, 1987).

In vitro
- Decreased free radical generation by granulocytes, thereby indicating potential anti-inflammatory activity (Brokos *et al.*, 1999).
- Inhibited lipid peroxidation *in vitro* (Guillaume and Padioleau, 1994).
- Lowered the rate of lymphocyte proliferation while recruiting lymphocytes to mitotic cycle (Bronkos, 1999).
- Elevated B and NK cells influencing the induction/suppression-balance in the immune system (Bronkos, 1999).

CONTRAINDICATIONS
Internal
Not recommended for children (Morant and Ruppanner, 2001; ESCOP, 1999) or with chronic renal failure (Morant and Ruppanner, 2001). An authoritative clinical review found no clinical basis for contraindications (Schulz *et al.*, 2000).

External
The gel or ointment should not be applied to broken or ulcerated skin (NRF 3, 1986). Contraindicated in cases of thrombosis or risk of embolism and for application to open wounds or mucous membranes (Morant and Ruppanner, 2001).

PREGNANCY AND LACTATION: There are no known restrictions according to the Commission E (Blumenthal *et al.*, 1998). HCSE has been used in some clinical studies involving pregnant women, with some studies excluding those in the third trimester. No adverse effects have been reported (ESCOP, 1999).

ADVERSE EFFECTS
The Commission E noted that in rare cases, pruritus, nausea, and gastric complaints may occur after oral intake (Blumenthal *et al.*, 1998). In rare cases, irritation of the gastric mucous membranes and reflux may occur. Escin Ib isolated from horse chestnut might partially delay or even inhibit gastric emptying. The inhibition of gastric emptying might be mediated by capsaicin-sensitive sensory nerves (CPSN), stimulation of the synthesis and/or release of dopamine, or through the central dopamine2

receptor, which in turn causes the release of prostaglandins (Matsuda and Yoshikawa, 2000). This possible adverse effect can be minimized by taking the extract in an enteric-coated, time-release tablet with the main meal (Morant and Ruppanner, 2001). After *intravenous* administration of *isolated escin*, anaphylactic shock, toxic nephropathy, and renal failure have been reported (Leung and Foster, 1996; Grasso and Corvaglia, 1976), but these reactions are not associated with oral ingestion of the chemically complex HCSE preparations. One case report (Comaish and Kersey, 1980) linking horse chestnut with contact dermatitis has been documented, but this does not pertain to HCSE in internal dosage forms.

DRUG INTERACTIONS

Some sources have theorized that horse chestnut extractives may interfere with the effects of anticoagulants (Ernst, 2000), specifically escin (Madaus AG, 2000). However, another source suggests that this activity pertains to the compound esculetin, found in the *bark*, not the seeds (Brinker, 2001). Escin, the main saponin component in horse chestnut, binds to plasma protein and may affect the binding of other drugs (speculative) (Newall *et al.*, 1996).

AMERICAN HERBAL PRODUCTS ASSOCIATION (AHPA) SAFETY RATING

No rating. NOTE: The herbs evaluated by AHPA in its *Botanical Safety Handbook* were based on an earlier AHPA publication (Foster, 1992) listing the names of approximately 550 of the most commonly-sold herbs in U.S. commerce during the early 1990s (McGuffin *et al.*, 1997). Horse chestnut preparations were not readily available in the U.S. at that time.

REGULATORY STATUS

CANADA: Horse chestnut is listed in Appendix II of the "List of Herbs Unacceptable as Non-medicinal Ingredients in Oral Use Products" (Health Canada, 1995b) and is also listed in Appendix I of the "Herbs that are Restricted or not Accepted as Medicinals in Traditional Herbal Medicines" (Health Canada, 1995a). However, it is permitted as a component of homeopathic drugs (Health Canada, 2000).

FRANCE: Official in the *French Pharmacopoeia* (ESCOP, 1999; Ph.Fr. X, 1982–1996). Nonprescription drug used in self-medication for circulatory stabilization (Goetz, 1999; Noël, 1997).

GERMANY: HCSE is an approved drug in the German Commission E monographs (Blumenthal *et al.*, 1998). Dried seed containing not less than 3.0% triterpene glycosides and HCSE containing 16–20% triterpene glycosides are official in the *German Pharmacopoeia* (DAB, 1999). Escin-Gel is an official preparation in the *German Formulary* (NRF 3, 1986). Fresh-peeled seeds, the mother tincture, and liquid dilutions are official preparations of the *German Homeopathic Pharmacopoeia* (HAB 1, 1978–1985).

SPAIN: Official in the *Spanish Pharmacopeia* (Newall *et al.*, 1996; Reynolds *et al.,* 1989).

SWEDEN: As of January 2001, no horse chestnut products have been listed in the Medical Products Agency (MPA) "Authorised Natural Remedies" (MPA, 2001).

SWITZERLAND: Positive classification (List D) by the *Interkantonale Konstrollstelle für Heilmittel* (IKS) and corresponding sales category D with sale limited to pharmacies and drug-stores, without prescription (Morant and Ruppanner, 2001;

WHO, 1998). One horse chestnut Anthroposophical preparation, 19 phytomedicines preparations, and 5 mainly-botanical combination preparations, are listed in the *Swiss Codex 2000/01* (Ruppanner and Schaefer, 2001).

U.K.: Medicinal product specified in the *General Sale List*, Schedule 1 (subject of full Product License), Table B (external use only) (GSL, 1994).

U.S.: Oral preparations regulated as dietary supplement (USC, 1994).

CLINICAL REVIEW

Twenty-three studies are outlined in the following table, "Clinical Studies on Horse Chestnut," including a total of 4,339 participants. All of the 20 studies that investigated the use of HCSE in venous disorders demonstrated positive effects. Of the 20 studies, four were randomized, double-blind, placebo-controlled, parallel group (R, DB, PC, PG), studies (Diehm *et al.*, 1992; Lohr *et al.*, 1986; Pilz, 1990; Rudofsky *et al.*, 1986), five were R, DB, PC, cross-over (CO) studies (Bisler *et al.*, 1986; Friederich *et al.*, 1978; Neiss and Böhm, 1976; Steiner, 1990; Steiner and Hillemanns, 1990), four were R, DB, comparison, PG design studies (Erdlen, 1989; Erler, 1991; Kalbfleisch and Pfalzgraf, 1989; Rehn *et al.*, 1996), one was a R, PC single-blind design (Diehm *et al.*, 1996), another was a DB, PC, multicenter (MC) study (Shah *et al.*, 1997), one was an uncontrolled, multicenter study with 71 participants (Geissbühler and Degenring, 1999), one was a DB design (Kreysel et al., 1983), three were surveillance studies (Masuhr *et al.*, 1994; Knoche and Knoche, 1978; Rossi *et al.*, 1977). The main outcome measure for most studies was reduced leg volume or ankle circumference. A systematic review of 13 R, DB clinical trials from 1976–1996, using HCSE in the treatment of venous disorders, and involving nearly 1,100 patients, concluded that HCSE was superior to placebo (Pittler and Ernst, 1998). HCSE was as effective as rutosides (the conventional treatment in Europe) in five studies. Adverse effects were mild and infrequent.

A R, CO study found bioequivalence (phytoequivalence) in two different forms of HCSE (Oschmann *et al.*, 1996). A R, DB, PC study of 70 subjects using HCSE topical gel, showed significant reduction in tenderness with experimentally induced hematomas (Calabrese and Preston, 1993). Subjects with severe cranio-cerebral trauma regained consciousness more quickly and experienced reduced intracranial pressure with purified escin i.v., followed by HCSE tablets, compared to placebo (Put, 1979).

BRANDED PRODUCTS*

Aesculaforce® Venen-Gel: Bioforce AG / CH-9325 Roggwil TG / Switzerland / Tel: +41 71 454 61 61 / Fax: +41 71 454 61 62 / www.bioforce.com / Email: info@bioforce.ch. One g of gel contains 54–117 mg dry extract prepared from fresh horse chestnut seed (Hippocastani semen recent extr. Sicc. 5.0–6.1:1) standardized to contain 2% escin.

Aesculaforce® Venen-Tabletten: Bioforce AG. Film-coated tablets (to prevent gastric irritation) contain 63–90 mg dry extract prepared from fresh horse chestnut seed (Hippocastani semen extr. Sicc. 5.0–6.1:1), corresponding to 20 mg escin. Extraction solvent: 60% (*m/m*) ethanol.

Reparil® Dragées: Madaus AG / Ostermerheimer Strasse 198 / Köln / Germany / Tel: +49-22-18-9984-76 / Fax: +49-22-18-9987-21 / Email: b.lindener@madaus.de. One coated tablet contains 20 mg escin amorphosed with adjuvants: polyvidone, magnesium stearate, talc, gum arabic, polyethyl acrylate, methacrylic acid, Macrogol 8000, sodium hydoxide, carmellose sodium, triethyl citrate, dimethicone, titanium dioxide, lactose, colloidal silicon dioxide, sucrose, natural waxes.

Venoplant® retard S: Dr. Willmar Schwabe Pharmaceuticals / International Division / Willmar Schwabe Str. 4 / D-76227 Karlsruhe / Germany / Tel: +49-721-4005 ext. 294 / www.schwabepharma.com / Email: melville-eaves@schwabe.de. Each sustained-release tablet contains 263.2 mg dry extract from horse chestnut seeds (4.5–5.5:1), adjusted to 50 mg triterpene glycosides, calculated as anhydrous aescin; extraction agent: ethanol 50% (w/w).

Venostasin® Retardkapsel: Klinge Pharma GmbH / Postfach 80 10 63 / D-81610 Munich / Germany / Tel: +089 45 44 – 01 / Fax: +089 45 44 - 13 29 / www.klinge.com, www.fujisawa.com. Each 300 mg capsule contains 240–290 mg native dry extract normalized to contain 50 mg triterpene glycosides, calculated as escin. Extract is standardized by diluting with 10–60 mg dextrin.

*American equivalents, if any, are found in the Product Table beginning on page 398.

REFERENCES

BHP. See: *British Herbal Pharmacopoeia.*

Bisler H, Pfeifer R, Kluken N, Pauschinger P. Effects of horse-chestnut seed extract on transcapillary filtration in chronic venous insufficiency. [in German]. *Z Dtsch Med Wschr* 1986;111(35):1321–9.

Blumenthal M, Busse WR, Goldberg A, Gruenwald J, Hall T, Riggins CW, Rister RS (eds.). Klein S, Rister RS (trans.). *The Complete German Commission E Monographs—Therapeutic Guide to Herbal Medicines.* Austin, TX: American Botanical Council; Boston: Integrative Medicine Communication; 1998;148–149.

Blumenthal M, Goldberg A, Brinckmann J (eds.). *Herbal Medicine — Expanded Commission E Monographs.* Newton, MA: Integrative Medicine Communications; 2000:201–4.

Bombardelli E, Morazzoni P. *Aesculus hippocastanum* L. *Fitoterapia* 1996;67(6):483–511.

Brinker F. *Herb Contraindications and Drug Interactions,* 3rd ed. Sandy, OR: Eclectic Medical Publications; 2001:120.

British Herbal Pharmacopoeia (BHP, 4th edition 1996). Exeter, U.K.: British Herbal Medicine Association; 1996;107–8.

Brokos B, Gasiorowski K, Noculak-Palczewska A. *In vitro* anti-inflammatory and immunomodulatory activities of extract and intract from chestnut fruits (*Aesculus hippocastanum* L.). *Herba Polonica* 1999;4:338–44.

Calabrese C, Preston P. Report of the results of a double-blind, randomized, single-dose trial of a topical 2% escin gel versus placebo in the acute treatment of experimentally-induced hematoma in volunteers. *Planta Med* 1993;59(5):394–7.

Chandler R. Herbal medicine: horse chestnut. *Can Pharm J* 1993 July/Aug;126:297–306.

Comaish J, Kersey P. Contact dermatitis to extract of horse chestnut (esculin). *Contact Dermatitis* 1980 Jan;6(2):150.

DAB. See: *Deutsches Arzneibuch.*

De Meirsman R, Rosselle N. *Ars Med* 1980;9(3):247.

de Rossi M, Stumpf H, Trunzler G. The Therapy of Venous Complaints and Related Symptoms Using Venoplant® Retard [in German]. *Der Praktische Arzt* 1977;1624–1628.

Deutsches Arzneibuch (DAB 1999). *Roßkastaniensamen;* Eingestellter Roßkastaniensamentrockenextrakt. In: *Deutsches Arzneibuch.* Stuttgart, Germany: Deutscher Apotheker Verlag; 1999.

Diehm C, Trampisch H, Lange S, Schmidt C. Comparison of leg compression stocking and oral horse-chestnut seed extract therapy in patients with chronic venous insufficiency. *Lancet* 1996;347(8997):292–4.

Diehm C, Vollbrecht D, Amendt K, Comberg H. Medical edema protection—Clinical benefit in patients with chronic deep vein incompetence. A placebo-controlled double-blind study. *Vasa* 1992;21(2):188–92.

Erdlen F. Clinical efficacy of Venostasin® Retard in a double-blind trial. [in German]. *Med Welt* 1989;40:994–6.

Erler M. Horse chestnut extract in the management of peripheral edema: a comparison of clinical treatments.[in German]. *Med Welt* 1991;42:593–6.

Ernst E. Possible interactions between synthetic and herbal medicinal products. Part 1: a systematic review of the indirect evidence. *Perfusion* 2000;13:4–15.

ESCOP. Hippocastani semen, Horse-chestnut seed. In: *Monographs on the Medicinal Uses of Plant Drugs.* Exeter, U.K.: European Scientific Cooperative on Phytotherapy; Oct 1999.

Facino R, Carini M, Stefani R, *et al.* Anti-elastase and anti-hyaluronidase activities of saponins and sapogenins from *Hedera helix, Aesculus hippocastanum,* and *Ruscus aculeatus:* factors contributing to their efficacy in the treatment of venous insufficiency. *Arch Pharm (Weinheim)* 1995;328(10):720–4.

Foster S. *Herbs of Commerce.* Austin, TX: American Herbal Products Assn.; 1992.

Friederich H, Vogelsberg H, Neiss A. A contribution to the evaluation of the clinical efficacy of horse-chestnut. [in German]. *Z Hautkr* 1978;53:369–74.

Fugamm B, Lang Fugmann S, Steglich W (eds.). *Rompp Lorikon Natur stoffo.* Stuttgart, Germany: Georg Thieme Verlag; 1997;183–184.

Geissbühler S, Degenring F. Treatment of chronic venous insufficiency with Aesculaforce® Vein Gel. [in German]. *Schweiz Zschr Ganzheits Med.* 1999;11:82–7.

General Sale List (GSL). Statutory Instrument (S.I.). The Medicines (Products other than Veterinary Drugs). London, UK: Her Majesty's Stationery Office;. 1984; S.I. No. 769, as amended 1985; S.I. No. 1540, 1990; S.I. No. 1129, 1994; S.I. No. 2410.

Goetz P. Phytotherapie in Frankreich. *Z Phytother* 1999;20:320–8.

Grasso A, Corvaglia E. Two cases of suspected toxic tubulonephrosis due to escine. *Gazz Med Ital* 1976;135:581–4.

GSL. See: *General Sales Lis*t.

Guillaume M, Padioleau F. Veinotonic effect, vascular protection, anti-inflammatory and free radical scavenging properties of horse chestnut extract. [in German]. *Arzneimittelforschung* 1994;44(1):25–35.

HAB. See: *Homöopathisches Arzneibuch.*

Health Canada. Appendix I: Herbs that are Restricted or not Accepted as Medicinals in Traditional Herbal Medicines. In: *Drugs Directorate Guideline: Traditional Herbal Medicines and Related Policy on Medicinal Herbs in Traditional Herbal Medicine.* Ottawa, Ontario: Health Canada Drugs Directorate; 1995a.

Health Canada. Appendix II: List of Herbs Unacceptable as Non-medicinal Ingredients in Oral Use Products. In: *Drugs Directorate Policy on Herbals used as Non-medicinal Ingredients in Nonprescription Drugs in Human Use.* Ottawa, Ontario: Health Canada Drugs Directorate; 1995b.

Health Canada. *Drug Product Database* (DPD). Ottawa, Canada: Health Canada Therapeutic Products Programme; 2000.

Homöopathisches Arzneibuch (HAB 1), 1st edition 1978, with supplements through 1985. Stuttgart, Germany: Deutscher Apotheker Verlag; 1978–1985.

Hübner G, Wray V, Nahrstedt A. Flavonol oligosaccharides from the seeds of *Aesculus hippocastanum. Planta Medica* 1999;65:636–42.

Kalbfleisch W, Pfalzgraf H. A critical comparison of the therapeutic dosage of Horse chestnut extract and O-β-hydroxyethylrutoside. [in German]. *Therapiewoche* 1989;39:3703–7.

Knoche HJ, Knoche I. Venoplant retard. Experience report of the varicose system complex. [in German]. *ZFA (Strutgart)* 1978:54(1):47-8.

Konoshima T, Lee K. Antitumor agents, 82. Cytotoxic sapogenols from *Aesculus hippocastanum. J Nat Prod* 1986;49(4):650–6.

Kreysel H, Nissen H, Enghofer E. A possible role of lyosomal enzymes in the pathogenesis of varicosis and the reduction in their serum activity by Venostasin®. *Vasa* 1983;12(4):377–82.

Leung AY, Foster S. *Encyclopedia of Common Natural Ingredients Used in Food, Drugs, and Cosmetics,* 2nd ed. New York: John Wiley & Sons; 1996;304–6.

Lohr E, Garanin G, Jesau P, Fischer H. Therapeutic Approaches in the Management of chronic venous insufficiency with peripheral edema. [in German]. *Munch Med Wochenschr* 1986;128(34):59–81.

Madaus AG. Product data sheet: Reparil® Coated Tablets. Köln, Germany: Madaus AG, 2000.

Masuhr Th, Holscher U, Honold E. Benefit-risk evaluation of Venoplant® retard, a product standardized on aescin and based on the extract of horse chestnut seed, in patients suffering from chronic venous insufficiency. *Top Medizin* 1994;8:21–24.

Matsuda H, Li Y, Murakami T, Ninomiya K, Yamahara J, Yoshikawa M. Effects of escins Ia, Ib, Iia, and Iib from horse chestnut, the seeds of *Aesculus hippocastanum* L., on acute inflammation in animals. *Biol Pharm Bull* 1997;20(10):1092–5.

Matsuda H, Li Y, Yoshikawa M. Possible involvement of dopamine and dopamine 2 receptors in the inhibitions of gastric emptying by escin Ib in mice. *Life Sci* 2000 Nov 3;67(24):2921–7.

McCaleb RM, Leigh E, Morien K. *The Encyclopedia of Popular Herbs.* Roseville, CA: Prima Health; 2000;266–272.

McGuffin M, Hobbs C, Upton R, Goldberg A. *American Herbal Products Association Botanical Safety Handbook: Guidelines for the Safe Use and Labeling for Herbs of Commerce.* Boca Raton, FL: CRC Press; 1997.

Medical Products Agency (MPA). Naturläkemedel: Authorised Natural Remedies (as of January 24, 2001). Uppsala, Sweden: Medical Products Agency; 2001.

Mills SY, Bone B. *Principles and Practice of Phytotherapy.* New York: Churchill Livingstone; 2000;448.

Morant J, Ruppanner H. Patientenin formation: Democal Kreuz-Pflaster D. In: *Arzneimittal-Kompondium der Schweiz* 2001. Basel, Switzerland: Documed AG, 2001.

Morgan M, Bone K. Professional review: horse chestnut. *MediHerb* 1998;(65):1–4.

MPA. See: Medical Products Agency.

Neiss A, Böhm C. Clinical evidence of the efficacy of horse chestnut extract for the symptoms of varicose veins. [in German]. *Munch Med Wochenschr* 1976;118:213–6.

Neues Rezeptur-Formularium (NRF 3. Ergänzung 1986). Stuttgart, Germany: Deutscher Apotheker Verlag; 1986;NRF23.1:1–2.

Newall C, Anderson L, Phillipson J. *Herbal Medicines. A Guide for Health-care Professionals*. London, England: The Pharmaceutical Press; 1996;166–7.

Noël A. Le marché de la phytothérapie reste florisant. *Quotidien du Pharmacien* 29 May 1997;1637.

NRF. See: *Neues Rezeptur-Formularium*.

Oschmann R, Biber A, Lang F, *et al*. Pharmacokinetics of beta-escin after administration of various *Aesculus* extract containing formulation. [in German]. *Pharmazie* 1996 Aug; 51(8):577–81.

Pauschinger K. Clinico-experimental investigations of the effect of horse-chestnut extract on the transcapillary filtration and the intravasal volume in patients with chronic venous insufficiency. *Phlebol Proktol* 1987;2:57–61.

Ph.Fr. See: *Pharmacopée Française*.

Pharmacopée Française (Ph.Fr. X). Paris, France: Adrapharm; 1982-1996.

Pilz E. Ödeme bei Venenerkrankungen. *Med Welt* 1990;40:1143–4.

Pittler M, Ernst E. Horse-chestnut seed extract for chronic venous insufficiency. A criteria-based systematic review. *Arch Dermatol* 1998;134(11):1356–60.

Put T. Advances in the conservative treatment of acute traumatic cerebral edema. Controlled clinical trial with follow-up examination. [in German]. *Munch Med Wochenschr* 1979;121(31):1019–1022.

Rehn D, Unkauf M, Klein P, et al. Comparative clinical efficacy and tolerability of oxerutins and horse chestnut extract in patients with chronic venous insufficiency. [in German]. *Arzneimittelforschung* 1996;46:483–7.

Reynolds J, Parfitt K, Parsons A, Sweetman S (eds.). *Martindale: The Extra Pharmacopoeia*, 29th edition. London, U.K.: The Pharmaceutical Press; 1989;1539–40.

Rudofsky G, Neiß A, Otto K, Seibel K. A double-blind study about the clinical efficacy and reduction of peripheral edema of horse chestnut extract. [in German]. *Phlebol Proktol* 1986;15:47–53.

Ruppanner H, Schaefer U (eds.). *Codex 2000/01 — Die Schweizer Arzneimittel in einem Griff*. Basel, Switzerland: Documed AG; 2001.

Schilcher H. *Phytotherapy in Pediatrics: Handbook for Physicians and Pharmacists*. Stuttgart, Germany: Medpharm Scientific Publishers; 1997;27-28:117–8.

Schulz V, Hansel R, Tyler V. *Rational Phytotherapy, A Physicians' Guide to Herbal Medicine* 4th ed. Germany: Springer-Verlag Berlin Heidelberg; 2000.

Shah D, Bommer S, Degenring F. Aesculaforce® in chronic venous insufficiency. [in German]. *Schweiz Zschr Ganzheits Med* 1997;9(2):86–91.

Steiner M, Hillemanns H. Venostasin® retard in the management of venous problems during pregnancy. *Phlebology* 1990;5:41–4.

Steiner M. Investigations of the prevention and reduction of peripheral edema using a horse chestnut extract. [in German]. *Phlebol Proktol* 1990;19:239–42.

Tsutsumi S, Ishizuka S. Anti-inflammatory effects of the extract *Aesculus hippocastanum* and seed. *Shikwa-Gakutto* 1967;67:1324–8.

United States Congress (USC). Public Law 103-417: Dietary Supplement Health and Education Act of 1994. Washington, DC: 103rd Congress of the United States; 1994.

USC. See: United States Congress.

Wagner J. Über. About the content of horse chestnut extract. Fourth Communication: Investigation of Flavonoles. *ArzneimittelForshung* 1967;17:546–51.

Weiss R. *Herbal Medicine: Translated from Lehrbuch der Phytotherapie*, 6th edition. Beaconsfield, U.K.: Beaconsfield Publishers Ltd.; 1988;188–9.

Weiss RF, Fintelmann V. *Herbal Medicine*, 2nd ed. New York: Thieme; 2000;178–180.

Werbach M, Murray M. *Botanical Influences on Illness*. Tarzana, CA: Third Line Press; 1994;278–9.

WHO. See: World Health Organization.

World Health Organization (WHO). *Regulatory Situation of Herbal Medicines: A Worldwide Review*. Geneva, Switzerland: World Health Organization Traditional Medicine Programme; 1998;26–7.

Yoshikawa M, Murakami T, Matsuda H, *et al*. Bioactive saponins and glycosides. III. Horse chestnut. (1): The structures, inhibitory effects on ethanol absorption, and hypoglycemic activity of escins Ia, Ib, IIa, IIb, and IIIa from the seeds of *Aesculus hippocastanum* L. *Chem Pharm Bull* (Tokyo) 1996;44(8):1454–64.

Yoshikawa M, Murakami T, Yamahara J, Matsuda H. Bioactive saponins and glycosides. XII. Horse chestnut. (2): Structures of escins IIIb, IV, V and VI and isoescins Ia, Ib, and V, acylated polyhydroxyoleanene triterpene oligoglycosides, from the seeds of horse chestnut tree (*Aesculus hippocastanum* L., *Hippocastanaceae*). *Chem Pharm Bull* (Tokyo) *Arzneimittelforschung* 1998;46(11):1764–9.

Clinical Studies on Horse Chestnut (Aesculus hippocastanum L.)

Chronic Venous Insufficiency (CVI)

Author/Year	Subject	Design	Duration	Dosage	Preparation	Results/Conclusion
Geissbühler and Degenring, 1999	Venous insufficiency	U, MC n=71 patients (61 women and 10 men) with chronic venous insufficiency and edema	6 weeks	Morning and evening massage gel into lower leg including ankles and the inner side of the thighs	Aesculaforce® Venen-Gel (1g of gel contains 54–117 mg dry extract standardized to 2% escin)	After 6 weeks of treatment, ankle circumference was reduced significantly (p<0.001) by 0.7 cm compared with baseline. Patients symptoms score also decreased significantly (p<0.001) by 60%. Over 85% of the cases reported good to medium efficacy. [Note: the principal author was employed by the manufacturer.]
Shah et al., 1997	Venous insufficiency	DB, PC, MC n=52 males and females with CVI (mean age test group 54 years; mean age placebo group 56 years)	6 weeks	2 tablets 3x/day (120 mg escin/day)	Aesculaforce® tablet (Each enteric coated tablet contains 63–90 mg native dry extract standardized to 20 mg escin per tablet)	After 2 weeks treatment there was significant (p<0.05) reduction in edema of the ankles and venous filling rate (p=0.03). There was no significant improvement in subjective symptoms. HCSE was well tolerated. [Note: the principal author was employed by the manufacturer.]
Diehm et al., 1996	Venous insufficiency	R, SB, PC, Cm, PG n=240 men and women with CVI (mean age 52 years)	12 weeks preceded by a 2-week placebo run-in	1 capsule 2x/day (100 mg escin/day) vs. mechanical compression with bandages and class II elastic stocking	Venostasin® retard extract capsule (Each capsule contains 240–290 mg native dry extract standardized to 50 mg triterpene glycosides, calculated as escin, with 10–60 mg dextrin)	Lower-leg volumes were significantly reduced in both HCSE (p=0.005) and compression therapy (p=0.002) groups. HCSE decreased lower-leg volume by an average of 43.8 ml compared to 46.7 ml with compression therapy and an increase of 9.8 ml with placebo. HSCE was well-tolerated (98% compliance), whereas compression treatment was reported as uncomfortable, inconvenient and subject to poor (90%) compliance.
Rehn et al., 1996	Grade II CVI	R, DB, Cm, MC, PG n=137 post-menopausal patients with grade II chronic venous insufficiency	12 weeks, preceded by 1 week placebo run-in, follow-up period of 6 weeks without treatment	One 300 mg capsule 2x/day (100 mg escin/day) vs. 1,000 mg/day O- (β-hydrox-yethyl)-ruto-sides for 4 weeks, then 500 mg/day for 8 weeks	HCSE capsules standardized to 50 mg escin each or oxerutin (brand not stated)	Both HCSE and oxerutin significantly reduced leg volume compared to baseline with mean leg volume reduction of 100 ml after 12 weeks. HCSE alleviated subjective symptoms. After 6-week follow-up period both treatments exhibited substantial carry-over effect. Authors concluded that both therapies are effective in treatment of CVI.
Masuhr et al., 1994	Venous insufficiency	S n=4,113 (treated in 842 practices)	87 days	Two, 100 mg tablets per day (100 mg escin/day)	Venoplant® retard, with 100 mg dry extract adjusted to 50 mg escin	In more than 84% of the patients, symptoms either improved or disappeared, with the "good" tolerance in 90% of the cases. The authors concluded that CVI can be successfully treated with a symptom-based therapy using horse chestnut seed extract.
Diehm et al., 1992	Venous insufficiency	R, DB, PC, PG n=39 men and women with venous edema in chronic deep-vein incompetence	6 weeks	One, 300 mg capsule 2x/day (150 mg escin/day)	HCSE capsules standardized to 75 mg escin each (brand not stated)	Compared with baseline, HCSE significantly reduced (p<0.01) leg volume by an average 84 ml compared to 4 ml with placebo. HCSE caused dramatic improvement in feelings of heaviness, tension, fatigue, and paresthesia in the legs. Itching was not helped. Authors conclude that HCSE is a safe and effective adjunct to compression therapy.

KEY: C – controlled, **CC** – case-control, **CH** – cohort, **CI** – confidence interval, **Cm** – comparison, **CO** – crossover, **CS** – cross-sectional, **DB** – double-blind, **E** – epidemiological, **LC** – longitudinal cohort, **MA** – meta-analysis, **MC** – multi-center, **n** – number of patients, **O** – open, **OB** – observational, **OL** – open label, **OR** – odds ratio, **P** – prospective, **PB** – patient-blind, **PC** – placebo-controlled, **PG** – parallel group, **PS** – pilot study, **R** – randomized, **RC** – reference-controlled, **RCS** – retrospective cross-sectional, **RS** - retrospective, **S** – surveillance, **SB** – single-blind, **SC** – single-center, **U** – uncontrolled, **UP** – unpublished, **VC** – vehicle-controlled.

Chronic Venous Insufficiency (CVI) (cont.)

Author/Year	Subject	Design	Duration	Dosage	Preparation	Results/Conclusion
Erler, 1991	Venous insufficiency	R, DB, Cm, PG n=40 patients with CVI and peripheral venous edema	2 months	One, 300 mg capsule 2x/day (150 mg escin/day) vs. 2000 mg/day O-(β-hydrox-yethyl)-ruto-sides	HCSE capsules standardized to 75 mg escin each (brand not stated)	Compared with baseline, HCSE significantly protected calf and ankle from edema provocation. Both HCSE and rutin preparations were comparable in reducing edema, but HCSE had a more pronounced protective effect.
Pilz, 1990	Venous insufficiency	R, DB, PC, PG n=28 patients with CVI	20 days	One, 300 mg capsule 2x/day (100 mg escin/day)	HCSE capsules standardized to 50 mg of escin (brand not stated)	HCSE treatment caused significant reduction ($p<0.05$) of 0.08 cm in leg circumference and decreased edema compared with placebo. Subjective symptoms were also significantly decreased ($p<0.05$).
Steiner, 1990	Venous insufficiency	R, DB, PC, CO n=20 female patients with varicosis during pregnancy	2 weeks	One, 300 mg capsule 2x/day (100 mg escin/day)	Venostasin® Retardkapsel	Compared to placebo, HCSE caused significant reduction ($p=0.009$) of 114 ml in leg volume. Leg circumferences and subjective symptoms were also significantly reduced ($p<0.05$) during HCSE treatment period. HCSE was rated as significantly better than placebo by physicians ($p<0.01$) and patients ($p<0.05$).
Steiner and Hillemanns, 1990	Edema due to venous insufficiency	R, DB, PC, CO n=52 pregnant women with edema due to CVI	20 days	One, 300 mg capsule 2x/day (100 mg escin/day)	Venostasin® Retardkapsel each capsule contains 240–290 mg native dry extract standardized to 50 mg triterpene glycosides, calculated as escin, with 10–60 mg dextrin	Significant reductions ($p<0.01$) in foot volume before and after edema provocation and greater resistance to edema provocation demonstrated in HCSE group compared with placebo. Reductions in foot circumference and less severe subjective symptoms of pain, fatigue, swelling, and itching were also significant in HCSE group.
Erdlen, 1989	Venous insufficiency	R, DB, Cm, PG n=30 patients with CVI	1 month	One, 300 mg capsule 2x/day (100 mg escin/day) or reference medication (type not clearly indicated, presumably rutosides)	HCSE capsules standardized to 50 mg escin each (brand not stated)	HCSE significantly reduced ankle circumference by 0.4 cm and improved subjective symptoms compared with baseline.
Kalbfleisch and Pfalzgraf, 1989	Venous insufficiency	R, DB, Cm, PG n=30 (33) patients with CVI	2 months	One, 300 mg capsule/day (50 mg escin/day) vs. 500 mg O- (β-hydroxyethyl)-rutosides/day	HCSE capsules standardized to 50 mg escin each (brand not stated)	HCSE reduced ankle and calf circumference by 0.2 and 0.18 cm, respectively, compared to baseline. Values were not significantly different from the rutoside.
Rudofsky et al., 1986	Venous insufficiency	R, DB, PC, PG n=39 patients (67% women) with grade I or II chronic venous insufficiency	1 month	One, 300 mg capsule 2x/day (100 mg escin/day)	HCSE capsules standardized to 50 mg escin each (brand not stated)	HCSE treatment resulted in statistically significant ($p<0.001$) reduction by 78 ml in leg volume compared with 34 ml increase with placebo. At 28 days, HCSE caused a significant change in calf and foot circumference ($p<0.01$). Additionally, significant improvement in subjective parameters (pain, tiredness, tension, and pruritus in legs) were reported. No difference with respect to venous capacity or venous drainage when leg was elevated.

KEY: C – controlled, **CC** – case-control, **CH** – cohort, **CI** – confidence interval, **Cm** – comparison, **CO** – crossover, **CS** – cross-sectional, **DB** – double-blind, **E** – epidemiological, **LC** – longitudinal cohort, **MA** – meta-analysis, **MC** – multi-center, **n** – number of patients, **O** – open, **OB** – observational, **OL** – open label, **OR** – odds ratio, **P** – prospective, **PB** – patient-blind, **PC** – placebo-controlled, **PG** – parallel group, **PS** – pilot study, **R** – randomized, **RC** – reference-controlled, **RCS** – retrospective cross-sectional, **RS** - retrospective, **S** – surveillance, **SB** – single-blind, **SC** – single-center, **U** – uncontrolled, **UP** – unpublished, **VC** – vehicle-controlled.

Chronic Venous Insufficiency (CVI) (cont.)

Author/Year	Subject	Design	Duration	Dosage	Preparation	Results/Conclusion
Lohr et al., 1986	Venous insufficiency	R, DB, PC, PG n=74 patients (57 women and 17 men) with CVI	2 months (preceded by a 12-day washout phase with placebo)	One, 300 mg capsule 2x/day (morning and evening) (100 mg escin/day)	Venostasin® Retardkapsel	HCSE treatment resulted in leg volume reduction of 16.5 ml compared to 3.8 ml reduction with placebo. Formation of edema was decreased (− 21.0 ml) with HCSE and increased (+ 0.2) ml with placebo during edema-provoking period. Authors concluded that HCSE therapy showed statistically significant activity in inhibiting progression of edematous disease conditions and was well-tolerated.
Bisler et al., 1986	Venous insufficiency	R, DB, PC, CO n=22 patients with CVI	Single dose of HCSE or placebo followed by 4-week study period	Two, 300 mg capsules/day (100 mg escin/day)	Venostasin® Retardkapsel	Three hours after administration, an acute dose of HCSE had an anti-edematous effect with a statistically significant (p=0.006) decrease (22%) in the capillary filtration coefficient compared with placebo, which caused an increase. Authors conclude that HCSE inhibits edema in CVI of leg by reducing transcapillary filtration.
Kreysel et al., 1983	Varicosis	DB n=15 varicose patients	12 days	One, 300 mg capsule 3x/day (150 mg escin/day)	Venostasin® Retardkapsel	After 12 days of treatment, significant reduction in activity of glycosaminoglycan hydrolase enzymes. Serum activity of 3 lysosomal glycosaminoglycan hydrolases were significantly reduced by 29.1%, 25.7%, and 28.7% respectively, compared to placebo. The authors hypothesize that HCSE acts at the site of enzyme release, exerting a stabilizing effect on the lysosomal membrane.
Friederich et al., 1978	Venous insufficiency or varicosis	R, DB, PC, CO n=95 patients with varicosis or CVI	20 days	One, 300 mg capsule 2x/day (100 mg escin/day)	HCSE capsules standardized to 50 mg escin each (brand not stated)	HCSE caused significant reduction (p<0.05) in CVI-related symptoms including calf spasm, pain, fatigue, and tenseness compared to placebo. No effect on pruritus.
Knoche and Knoche, 1978	Venous complaints	S n=61	9 months	One, 100 mg tablet 2x/day	Venoplant® retard standardized to 50 mg escin and 15 mg milk thistle (*Carduus marianus*) extract	A reduction in lower leg pain was demonstrated as early as 3 days after treatment. Edema formation declined after 7-14 days. Only 3 patients complained of minor side effects, including stomach complaints and dizziness.
de Rossi et al., 1977	Venous complaints (varicosis, thrombophlebitis, phlebothrombosis)	S n=1,236	28 days (average)	One, 100 mg tablet 2x/day	Venoplant® retard tablet containing 100 mg horse chestnut and 15 mg milk thistle (providing 50 mg escin and 7.5 mg silymarin per tablet)	Rapid effect (21% reported improvement by day 4, 52% by day 8, and 70% by day 10) and good gastric tolerance were emphasized by 90% of the physicians.
Neiss and Böhm, 1976	Varicosis	R, DB, PC, CO n=226 (233) predominantly women with varicosis	20 days	One, 300 mg capsule 2x/day (100 mg escin/day)	HCSE capsules standardized to 50 mg escin each (brand not stated)	Compared to placebo, HCSE caused significant (p<0.05) reduction in edema, leg pain, and pruritus.

KEY: C – controlled, **CC** – case-control, **CH** – cohort, **CI** – confidence interval, **Cm** – comparison, **CO** – crossover, **CS** – cross-sectional, **DB** – double-blind, **E** – epidemiological, **LC** – longitudinal cohort, **MA** – meta-analysis, **MC** – multi-center, **n** – number of patients, **O** – open, **OB** – observational, **OL** – open label, **OR** – odds ratio, **P** – prospective, **PB** – patient-blind, **PC** – placebo-controlled, **PG** – parallel group, **PS** – pilot study, **R** – randomized, **RC** – reference-controlled, **RCS** – retrospective cross-sectional, **RS** - retrospective, **S** – surveillance, **SB** – single-blind, **SC** – single-center, **U** – uncontrolled, **UP** – unpublished, **VC** – vehicle-controlled.

Horse Chestnut

Monograph

Other

Author/Year	Subject	Design	Duration	Dosage	Preparation	Results/Conclusion
Oschmann et al., 1996	Bio-equivalence as determined by pharmaco-kinetics	R, CO n=24	3 days each phase with 1-week washout between pases	Single dose of one tablet or one capsule (50 mg escin)	Venoplant® retard 263.2 mg tablet or Venostasin® retard 240–290 mg capsule (providing 50 mg escin per tablet or capsule)	Bioequivalence was established between the 2 dosage forms.
Calabrese and Preston, 1993	Experimentally induced injury with hematomas	R, DB, PC n=70 healthy volunteers	9-hour study period	1 time acute topical application	Topical gel containing HCSE standardized to 2% escin (brand not stated)	Using tonometric sensitivity measurements, escin gel significantly reduced (p<0.001) tenderness to pressure of experimentally induced hematomas. The effect was observed from 1 hour after treatment lasting until the end of the 9-hour study period.
Put, 1979	Severe cranio-cerebral trauma	C, Cm n=142 accident victims with severe cranio-cerebral trauma	Treatment periods varied on an individual basis from 1–56 weeks with follow-ups at 2–3.5 years after accident and treatment	Days 1–5: 20 mg/day escin i.v.; Days 6–9: 10 mg/day escin i.v.; Beginning on day 10: 1 tablet/day vs. corticosteroid i.v. (type not specified)	Purified escin i.v. in the form of sodium escinate (first 10 days) followed by Reparil®-coated tablets	Regaining of consciousness was more rapid in the escin group than the corticosteroid group. Escin was more effective than steroid therapy at reducing intracranial pressure and lowering mortality rates. Follow-up examinations 2–3.5 years after the accident showed significantly higher rehabilitation rate in escin group (49 of 71) compared with steroid group (36 of 71).

KEY: **C** – controlled, **CC** – case-control, **CH** – cohort, **CI** – confidence interval, **Cm** – comparison, **CO** – crossover, **CS** – cross-sectional, **DB** – double-blind, **E** – epidemiological, **LC** – longitudinal cohort, **MA** – meta-analysis, **MC** – multi-center, **n** – number of patients, **O** – open, **OB** – observational, **OL** – open label, **OR** – odds ratio, **P** – prospective, **PB** – patient-blind, **PC** – placebo-controlled, **PG** – parallel group, **PS** – pilot study, **R** – randomized, **RC** – reference-controlled, **RCS** – retrospective cross-sectional, **RS** - retrospective, **S** – surveillance, **SB** – single-blind, **SC** – single-center, **U** – uncontrolled, **UP** – unpublished, **VC** – vehicle-controlled.

Kava

Piper methysticum G. Forst.

[Fam. *Piperaceae*]

OVERVIEW

Kava is traditionally served as a beverage in social or ceremonial rituals in island communities of the South Pacific, where it is revered as the primary cultural and medicinal botanical. While kava use has been popular as a phytomedicine in Europe for decades, it only recently became a top-selling herbal dietary supplement in the U.S., used by consumers mainly for dealing with feelings of anxiety.

Recently, kava has been implicated in some cases of hepatotoxicity in Europe and subsequently in the U.S. As a result, its use has been either limited or banned in such countries as Switzerland, Germany, Canada, Australia, France, and the U.K.

Previous reviews of kava safety did not include evidence suggesting the potential for hepatotoxicity. A toxicological review of kava-associated hepatic adverse event reports (AERs) from Europe and the U.S. concluded that, based on the available data, "there is no clear evidence that the liver damage reported in the U.S. and Europe was caused by the consumption of kava." A detailed review of the chronology of the events related to kava and its alleged association with hepatotoxicity, plus updates on recent developments, is available on the American Botanical Council website (www.herbalgram.org).

PRIMARY USE

Neurology
• Anxiety disorder

OTHER POTENTIAL USES
• Sleep disorder
• Stress and restlessness
• Muscle relaxant

PHARMACOLOGICAL ACTIONS

Anxiolytic; sedative; reduces hot flashes.

DOSAGE AND ADMINISTRATION

The German Commission E monograph published in 1990 recommends a maximum treatment duration of 3 months without medical supervision. This limitation was based not on concerns of potential toxicity of kava (no adverse side effects were noted in the monograph, based on observations at that time), but on the Commission E's desire to ensure that patients using kava for anxiety-related conditions were receiving adequate professional supervision every 3 months. Because some of the recent reports of adverse liver effects are associated with the use of kava for 1 month or less (along with conventional medications or alcohol, in most cases), the American Botanical Council suggested in

December 2001 as a precautionary measure, based on the information available at that time, that use longer than 1 month be monitored by a qualified healthcare professional.

Crude preparations

Daily dosage for cut dried rhizome and other galenical preparations for oral use equivalent to 60–120 mg kavalactones (aka kavapyrones). 60–120 mg of kavapyrones is equivalent to 1.7–3.4g of dried rhizome (based on the *German Drug Codex* quantitative requirement of minimum 3.5% (35 mg/g) kavapyrones).

COLD MACERATE: The fresh or dried rhizome is ground to a powder (traditionally it is masticated to a pulp) and then macerated in cold water. The first filtrate is strained and drunk. The residue is then compressed and the second filtrate can either be mixed with the first or consumed separately. A standard bowl of the traditionally prepared cold macerate beverage contains about 250 mg of kavalactones.

DRIED RHIZOME: 1.5-3 g daily, divided throughout the day, chewed well.

FLUID EXTRACT: (1:2): 3-6 mL daily, divided throughout the day.

Standardized preparations

CAPSULES OR TABLETS: Powdered dry extract (not less than 30% kavalactones) or semisolid (paste) extract (not less than 50% kavalactones) in daily dosage equivalent to 70–280 mg kavalactones. Most controlled clinical trials are based on three 100 mg doses of a dried extract (acetone solvent), standardized to 70 mg (70%) kavalactones, or 210 mg kavalactones per day.

CONTRAINDICATIONS

The Commission E contraindicated the use of kava in cases of endogenous depression. Industry labeling guidelines suggest that it is not for use by persons under 18 years of age. In response to reports of hepatotoxicity that may be associated with use of kava preparations, the FDA, ABC, and various industry trade organizations have advised consumers of the rare but potential risk of severe liver injury associated with the use of kava-containing preparations: Persons who have or have had liver disease or liver problems, persons taking any medication with known or suspected hepatotoxic effects, and persons who frequently use alcoholic beverages should consult a healthcare practitioner before using kava-containing products. Persons who use a kava-containing product and who experience signs of illness associated with liver disease should discontinue use and consult their physician. Symptoms of serious liver disease include jaundice (yellowing of the skin or whites of the eyes) and brown urine. Non-specific symptoms of liver disease can include nausea, vomiting, light-colored stools, unusual tiredness, weakness, stomach or abdominal pain, and loss of appetite.

Kava

Clinical Overview

PREGNANCY AND LACTATION: Kava should not be used during pregnancy or while nursing.

ADVERSE EFFECTS

Adverse effects with recommended doses of kava are relatively rare. Large doses (400 mg kavalactones or more per day for longer than 3 months) may cause a scaly, yellowing skin condition (scaly ichthyosis), which resolves itself when use is discontinued. Kava preparations may be a contributing risk factor for the development of melioidosis, a tropical disease caused by *Burkholderia pseudomallei*. In 2 case reports necrotizing hepatitis occurred after ingestion of an herbal preparation containing kava extract and celandine (*Chelidonium majus*); however, the effects may have resulted from the celandine and/or the combination.

By early 2002, there had been approximately 30 cases of possible hepatoxicity associated with ingestion of kava reported in international literature, with at least 28 cases reported in total (4 in Switzerland; 24 in Germany), prompting regulatory actions by authorities. The hepatic AERs in these cases include cholestatic hepatitis (inflamed liver with obstruction of bile flow), icterus (jaundice), increased liver enzymes, liver cell impairment, severe hepatitis with confluent necrosis, and irreversible liver damage (required transplant in four cases). Additionally, at least 5 cases of liver dysfunction purportedly associated with kava consumption have been reported in the U.S.

Although much of the data on the reported cases of hepatotoxicity is either incomplete or generally unavailable, relatively detailed information has been published for 5 of these cases, including one case of recurring necrotizing hepatitis that was reported in a 39-year old woman who may have consumed an ethanolic-based kava extract. In a 50-year old man a relation between ingestion of kava and fulminant hepatic failure was suggested by the chronology, histological findings, and exclusion of other causes of hepatitis. He reportedly took no other drugs, nor did he consume alcohol; yet his liver function tests showed a 60-fold and 70-fold increase in aspartate aminotransferase (AST) and alanine aminotransferase (ALT) concentrations, respectively.

Kava consumption is considered relatively risk free in its native regions in Polynesia. However, in a population of Australian aboriginal people known to be relatively heavy consumers of alcohol, heavy kava consumption has been associated with increased concentrations of glutamyltransferase, suggesting potential hepatotoxicity with alcohol.

Several reviews of these reports emphasize that in many of these cases other known or suspected liver-toxic medications had been administered concurrently; in most of the other cases the possibility of virus infections or concurrently ingested medications or alcohol could not be ruled out as possible causes. Thus, only a few cases can be conclusively linked to the use of kava. An analysis of the approximately 30 hepatic AERs from Europe and 5 submitted to the U.S. FDA from May 1998 through September 2001 by an American toxicologist concluded that there is "no clear evidence that the liver damage reported in the U.S. and Europe was caused by the consumption of kava" and that those cases in which there is a possible association between the use of a kava extract and liver dysfunction "appear to have been hypersensitivity or idiosyncratic base responses." However, the report's author acknowledged that he did not have adequate medical information on all the case reports to adequately assess them. Two U.S. case reports suggest relative safety of kava. In one case in which 4 prescription drugs plus relatively high levels of kava were used (300 pills or 45,000 mg per day) there was no liver damage observed; in another case, a 13-year old girl consumed 8–10, 500 mg tablets in a suicide attempt, but recovered the following morning. "From a toxicologist perspective, these 2 cases provide some evidence that kava itself is not a direct hepatotoxin even in extremely high concentrations."

DRUG INTERACTIONS

Simultaneous consumption of kava with alcohol, barbiturates, psychopharmacological drugs, or other substances acting on the central nervous system (CNS) may potentiate inebriation or the CNS depressant effect. Kava may potentiate effects of other anxiolytics, and can increase Parkinson symptoms by reducing the effect of levodopa, according to one human case report. There is one case report of "coma" associated with the combined use of kava and the benzodiazepine, alprazolam (Xanax®), cimetidine (Tagamet®), and terazosin (Hytrin®).

CLINICAL REVIEW

Fifteen studies (669 participants) are outlined in the monograph table, "Clinical Studies on Kava." These studies demonstrated kava's positive effects for indications including anxiety, mental function, reaction time, sleep quality, and peri-menopausal symptoms, while 1 study focused on the safety of kava. Six randomized, double-blind, placebo-controlled (R, DB, PC) studies (357 participants) concluded that kava significantly reduced anxiety in several different populations. One R, DB, case-controlled study (172 participants) found a significant reduction in anxiety. Two DB, crossover (CO) trials showed that mental clarity remains intact with kava use. Kava demonstrated a favorable influence on sleep in one PC, CO study. One PC, CO comparison trial showed that kava did not affect reaction time or impair safety, compared to bromazepam and bromazepam combined with kava. A highly significant improvement in peri-menopausal symptoms was demonstrated in a R, DB, PC study. A meta-analysis of seven R, DB, PC trials conducted on various doses of kava confirmed an anxiolytic effect and demonstrated it was significantly superior to placebo as a symptomatic treatment for anxiety. In one PC pilot study (n=13), the preliminary findings suggest that kava might exert a positive effect on reflex vagal control of heart rate in generalized anxiety disorder patients. Another R, DB, PC study by some of these same researchers reviewed the safety profile of kava in 35 subjects. No significant adverse effects were measured between kava and placebo patients on any of the parameters evaluated.

Kava

Piper methysticum G. Forst.
[Fam. *Piperaceae*]

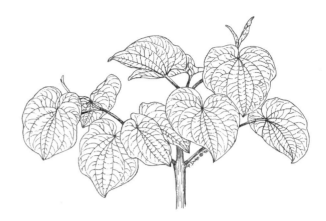

OVERVIEW

Kava is traditionally served as a beverage in social or cere-monial rituals in the South Pacific islands, where it is revered as the primary cultural and medicinal botanical. While kava use has been popular in Europe for decades, it only recently became a top-selling herbal dietary supple-ment in the U.S., used by consumers mainly for dealing with feelings of anxiety.

Recently, kava has been implicated in some cases of hepato-toxicity in Europe and subsequently in the U.S. A detailed review of the chronology of the events related to kava and its alleged association with hepatotoxicity, plus updates on recent developments, is available on the American Botanical Council website (www.herbalgram.org).

USES

Anxiety disorder; sleep disorders; stress and restlessness; muscle relaxant.

DOSAGE

Do not use kava for more than one month without medical supervision.

FLUID EXTRACT (1:2): 3-6 mL daily, divided throughout the day.

CAPSULES OR TABLETS: Powdered dry extract (not less than 30% kavalactones) or semisolid (paste) extract (not less than 50% kavalactones) in daily dosage equivalent to 60–120 mg kavalactones.

CONTRAINDICATIONS

Consult with a healthcare practitioner prior to using kava in cases of depression. Not for use by persons under 18 years of age. Persons who have or have had liver disease or liver problems, persons taking any medication with known or suspected hepatotoxic effects, and persons who frequently use alcoholic beverages should consult a healthcare practitioner before using kava-containing products. Persons who use a kava-containing product and experience signs of illness associated with liver disease should discontinue use and consult their physician. Symptoms of serious liver disease include jaundice (yellowing of the skin or whites of the eyes) and brown urine. Non-specific symptoms of liver disease can include

nausea, vomiting, light-colored stools, unusual tiredness, weakness, stomach or abdominal pain, and loss of appetite.

PREGNANCY AND LACTATION: Kava should not be used during pregnancy or while nursing.

ADVERSE EFFECTS

Adverse effects with recommended doses of kava are relatively rare. Large doses (400 mg kavalactones or more per day for longer than 3 months) may cause a scaly, yel-lowing skin condition (scaly ichthyosis), which resolves itself when use is discontinued. In 2 case reports liver inflammation occurred after ingestion of an herbal prepa-ration containing kava extract and celandine (*Chelidonium majus*); however, the effects may have resulted from the celandine and/or the combination. Current research does not provide clear evidence of any scientific rationale that kava use is associated with liver damage; nevertheless, consumers and patients are advised to heed the above cautions.

DRUG INTERACTIONS

Taking kava along with alcohol, barbiturates, drugs affecting mental activity, or other substances acting on the central nervous system may increase inebriation or the effect of the drug. Kava may also increase the effect of other relaxation-promoting drugs.

Comments

When using a dietary supplement, purchase it from a reliable source. For best results, use the same brand of product throughout the period of use. As with all medications and dietary supplements, please inform your healthcare provider of all herbs and medications you are taking. Interactions may occur between medications and herbs or even among different herbs when taken at the same time. Treat your herbal supple-ment with care by taking it as directed, storing it as advised on the label, and keeping it out of the reach of children and pets. Consult your healthcare provider with any questions.

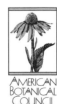

AMERICAN BOTANICAL COUNCIL

The information contained on this sheet has been excerpted from *The ABC Clinical Guide to Herbs* © 2003 by the American Botanical Council (ABC). ABC is an independent member-based educational organization focusing on the medicinal use of herbs. For more detailed information about this herb please consult the healthcare provider who gave you this sheet. To order *The ABC Clinical Guide to Herbs* or become a member of ABC, visit their website at www.herbalgram.org.

Kava

Piper methysticum G. Forst.

[Fam. *Piperaceae*]

OVERVIEW

Kava is traditionally served as a beverage in social or ceremonial rituals in island communities of the South Pacific (e.g., Fiji, Vanuatu, Samoa, Tonga), where it is revered as the primary cultural and medicinal botanical (Lebot *et al.*, 1992; Singh, 1992; Singh and Blumenthal, 1997). Its uses were first described in detail by botanist J.G. Forster on the voyage of Captain James Cook in the late 1700s (Forster, 1777). Kava beverage is used as a symbol of welcome and respect to visiting heads of state and other dignitaries (Singh and Blumenthal, 1997).

Kava use has been popular as a phytomedicine in Europe for decades; it was approved in 1990 as a nonprescription drug by the German Commission E for treatment of symptoms of anxiety, stress, and nervous restlessness (Blumenthal *et al.*, 1998). Kava only recently became a top-selling herbal dietary supplement in the U.S., used by consumers mainly for dealing with feelings of anxiety (Singh and Blumenthal, 1997). The herb ranked ninth in retail sales in mainstream markets (e.g., grocery

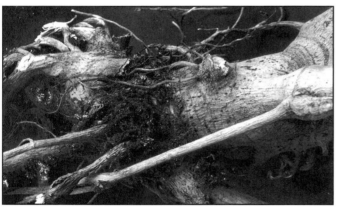

Photo © 2003 stevenfoster.com

stores, drugstores, and mass market retailers) in the U.S. in 2000, with annual sales in this channel totaling about $15 million. (Blumenthal, 2001). Additional sales in health food stores, multilevel marketing organizations, mail order houses, through health professionals, and miscellaneous channels would probably constitute a total estimated market sales of over $40 million.

Recently, kava has been implicated in some cases of hepatotoxicity in Europe (Stoller 2000; Hagemann, 2001) and subsequently in the U.S. (Taylor, 2001; Waller, 2002). The German and Swiss governments have taken regulatory actions based on this preliminary information (Hagemann, 2001; Stoller, 2000), with the Swiss banning the sale of the leading acetone-based kava extract and requiring additional safety data for ethanolic extracts in 2000 (IKS, 2001), and the Germans withdrawing product licenses in 2002 (BfArM, 2002). The French government has banned its sale (Anon., 2002b) and the British government and the dietary supplement industry voluntarily suspended its sale pending resolution of the question of hepatotoxicity (Woodfield, 2001); in early 2003, Kava sales were banned in the UK (MCA, 2002).

Previous reviews of kava safety did not include evidence suggesting the potential for hepatotoxicity. A peer-reviewed assessment of the safety of kava concluded that "when used in normal therapeutic doses, kava appears to offer safe and effective anti-anxiety and muscle relaxant actions without depressing centers of higher thought. The safe use of kava as a dietary supplement in cultures that do not have historical experiences with its use depends on responsible manufacturing, marketing, individual consumption patterns, and education" (Dentali, 1997). One recent meta-analysis of controlled clinical trials found kava to be safe and effective compared to placebo in the treatment of anxiety (Pittler and Ernst, 2002; 2000), and a small clinical study on its adverse effects profile concluded that the herb is relatively safe, not finding significant concerns of hepatotoxicity (Connor *et al.*, 2001). A toxicological review of kava-associated hepatic adverse event reports (AERs) from Europe and the U.S. concluded that based on the available data "there is no clear evidence that the liver damage reported in the U.S. and Europe was caused by the consumption of kava" (Waller, 2002) (see more below at Adverse Effects). A detailed review of the chronology of the events related to kava and its alleged association with hepatotoxicity, plus updates on recent developments, is available on the American Botanical Council website (ABC, 2001; Blumenthal, 2002b).

DESCRIPTION

German pharmacopeial-grade kava consists of the mostly peeled, chopped and dried rhizomes of *Piper methysticum* G. Forst. [Fam. *Piperaceae*], usually freed from the roots, containing not less then 3.5% kavalactones, calculated as kavain (DAC, 1998). There is a *U.S. Pharmacopeia-National Formulary* (USP-NF) kava monograph in development, requiring the dried rhizome, usually peeled and cut in pieces with the roots removed, containing not less than 4.5% of kavalactones (USPC, 2002). Because the peeled skin contains a greater concentration of kavalactones, many extractors use this non-official plant source and/or the unpeeled root and rhizome and occasionally the stems. Commercial kava extracts are commonly standardized to 30–40% kavalactones for dried powdered extracts, and 55–70% for concentrated extracts and pastes.

NOTE: Monographs for two kava preparations are also in process to become official in the USP-NF: (1) Powdered Kava Extract (drug-to-extract ratio 6–20:1, contains not less than 30% kavalactones) and (2) Semisolid Kava Extract (drug-to-extract ratio 13–20:1, contains not less than 50% kavalactones) (USPC, 2000).

PRIMARY USE

Neurology

- Anxiety disorder (Pittler and Ernst, 2002, 2000; Blumenthal *et al.*, 1998; Singh *et al.*, 1998; Volz and Kieser, 1997; Lehmann *et al.*, 1996; Woelk *et al.*, 1993; Warnecke,1991; Kinzler *et al.*, 1991; Lindenberg and Pitule-Schödel, 1990)

OTHER POTENTIAL USES

- Sleep disorder (Emser and Bartylla, 1991)
- Stress and restlessness (Blumenthal *et al.*, 1998)
- Muscle relaxant (Dentali, 1997)

DOSAGE

Daily dosage for cut dried rhizome and other galenical preparations for oral use equivalent to 60–120 mg kavalactones (aka kavapyrones) (Blumenthal *et al.*, 1998; DAC, 1998). 60–120 mg of kavapyrones (kavalactones) is equivalent to 1.7–3.4 g of dried rhizome based on the DAC quantitative requirement of minimum 3.5% (35 mg/g) kavapyrones (kavalactones) (DAC, 1998).

Crude preparations

COLD MACERATE: The fresh or dried rhizome is ground to a powder (traditionally it is masticated to a pulp) and then macerated in cold water. The first filtrate is strained and drunk. The residue is then compressed and the second filtrate can either be mixed with the first or consumed separately (Lebot and Cabalion, 1988). A standard bowl of the traditionally prepared cold macerate beverage contains about 250 mg of kavalactones (Bone, 1993/94).

DRIED RHIZOME: 1.5-3 g daily, divided throughout the day, chewed well (Bone, 1993/94; Burgess, 1998).

FLUID EXTRACT: (1:2): 3-6 mL daily, divided throughout the day (Bone 1993/94; Burgess, 1998).

Standardized preparations

CAPSULES OR TABLETS: Powdered dry extract (not less than 30% kavalactones) or semisolid (paste) extract (not less than 50% kavalactones) in daily dosage equivalent to 70–280 mg kavalactones. Most controlled clinical trials are based on three 100 mg doses of a dried extract (acetone solvent), standardized to 70 mg (70%) kavalactones, or 210 mg kavalactones per day (Pittler and Ernst, 2002, 2000).

DURATION OF ADMINISTRATION

The Commission E monographs published in 1990 recommended that kava not be used for more than three months without medical supervision (Blumenthal *et al.*, 1998). The purpose for this limitation was based not on concerns of potential toxicity of kava (no adverse side effects were noted in the monograph, based on observations at that time), but on the Commission E's desire to ensure that patients using kava for anxiety-related conditions were not doing so on a self-medication basis and were receiving adequate professional supervision every three months, especially since kava was seen as a drug lacking a clear European tradition. Thus, it was considered prudent to monitor the patient after three months (Busse, 2002a).

Because some of the recent reports of adverse liver effects are associated with the use of kava for one month or less (along with conventional medications or alcohol, in some cases), the American Botanical Council suggested in December 2001 as a precautionary measure, based on the information available at that time, that use longer than one month be monitored by a qualified healthcare professional (ABC, 2001; Blumenthal, 2002a, b).

CHEMISTRY

Kava root/rhizome contains 3.5–15% kavalactones (kavapyrones); these include kavain; 5,6–dihydrokavain; methysticin; dihydromethysticin; yangonin; and desmethoxyyangonin or 5,6-dehydrokavain). Kava also contains chalcones (flavokavins A, B, and C); 3.2% minerals (potassium, calcium, magnesium, sodium, aluminum, and iron) and 3.5% amino acids (Pizzorno and Murray, 1999; He *et al.*, 1997; Haberlein *et al.*, 1997; Singh and Blumenthal, 1997; Leung and Foster, 1996; Mack, 1994).

NOTE: There are numerous cultivars of kava containing varying proportions of these compounds. Research by Lebot *et al.* (1992) into the relative proportions of the various lactones in kava has revealed data on the origin of kava and its chemistry which has been modified through native selection of individual plants, where the chemical makeup of the kava, not its morphology, correlated with its ethnobotanical use. Thus, pharmacologically driven selection appears to have created chemical variations of kava far removed from its wild ancestor (Singh and Blumenthal, 1997).

PHARMACOLOGICAL ACTIONS

Human

- Anxiolytic (Pittler and Ernst, 2002, 2000; Boerner, 2001; Malsch and Kieser, 2001; Scherer, 1998; Volz and Kieser, 1997; Lehmann *et al.*, 1996; Woelk *et al.*, 1993; Johnson *et al.*, 1991; Kinzler *et al.*, 1991; Warnecke, 1991; Lindenberg and Pitule-Schödel, 1990);
- sedative (Emser and Bartylla, 1991);
- reduces hot flashes (Warnecke, 1991);
- locally mildly anesthetic (Singh and Blumenthal, 1997);
- improves sleep disorder (Holm *et al.*, 1991; Wheatley, 2001);
- can produce altered vision (Garner and Klinger, 1985).

Animal

- Analgesic (Bruggemann and Meyer, 1963; Hänsel, 1968; Jamieson and Duffield, 1990a);
- antispasmodic (Meyer, 1979);
- anticonvulsant (Klohs *et al.*, 1959; Kretzschmar *et al.*, 1970);
- sedative (Kretzschmar *et al.*, 1970; Gleitz *et al.*, 1996b);
- neuroprotection (Backhauss and Kriegelstein, 1992a,b; Gleitz *et al.*, 1996c).

In vitro

- Muscle-relaxant (without depressing CNS) (Singh, 1983);
- antispasmodic (natural kavain, Martin *et al.*, 2000), (synthetic kavain, Seitz *et al.*, 1997a);
- antithrombotic (Gleitz *et al.*, 1997);
- inhibitor (reversible) of MAO-B in human platelets (Uebelhack *et al.*, 1998).

MECHANISMS OF ACTION

The following mechanisms have been proposed for kava extract and/or specific kavalactones:

- Decreases levels of the excitatory neurotransmitter, glutamate (Meldrum, 1985; Ferger *et al.*, 1998);

Kava

Monograph

- Activation of mesolimbic dopaminergic neuron, causing relaxation and slight euphoria (Baum *et al.*, 1998)
- Binds to GABA receptors in some regions of the brain (Davies *et al.*, 1992; Jussofie, 1993; Jussofie *et al.*, 1994; Boonen and Haberlein, 1998; Boonen *et al.*, 2000)
- Relaxes muscles through direct action on muscle contractility; not by inhibition of neuromuscular transmission (Singh, 1983)
- Increases delta, theta (daydreaming), and slow alpha brain wave activity, and decreases fast alpha and beta (concentrating) activity in a dose-dependent manner (Saletu *et al.*, 1989)
- Interacts with voltage-operated Na+ channels (Gleitz *et al.*, 1996a; Friese and Gleitz, 1998; Magura *et al.*, 1997; Schirrmacher *et al.*, 1999)
- Inhibits [3H]-noradrenaline (norepinephrine) uptake (pyrone-specific), contributing to psychotropic properties (Seitz *et al.*, 1997b)
- Blockade of monoamine uptake resulting in elevation of dopamine and serotonin levels (Seitz *et al.*, 1997a; Boonen *et al.*, 1998; Baum *et al.*, 1998)
- Increases the β/α index in quantitative electroencephalograms, primarily in the β2-region (in dosages up to 600 mg, administered orally to humans); thereby exhibiting anxiolytic action without sedative or hypnotic effects (Johnson *et al.*, 1991)
- Kavalactones demonstrate a profile of cellular actions showing similarity with mood stabilizers (animal) (Grunze *et al.*, 2001)

CONTRAINDICATIONS

The Commission E contraindicated the use of kava in cases of endogenous depression (Blumenthal *et al.*, 1998). Not for use by persons under 18 years of age (AHPA, 2002; CRN, 2002). In response to reports of hepatotoxicity that may be associated with use of kava preparations, the FDA, ABC, and various industry trade organizations have advised consumers of the rare but potential risk of severe liver injury associated with the use of kava-containing preparations: Persons who have or have had liver disease or liver problems, persons taking any medication with known or suspected hepatotoxic effects, and persons who frequently use alcoholic beverages should consult a healthcare practitioner before using kava-containing products. Persons who use a kava-containing product and who experience signs of illness associated with liver disease should discontinue use and consult their physician. Symptoms of serious liver disease include jaundice (yellowing of the skin or whites of the eyes) and brown urine. Non-specific symptoms of liver disease can include nausea, vomiting, light-colored stools, unusual tiredness, weakness, stomach or abdominal pain, and loss of appetite (ABC, 2001; AHPA, 2002; Blumenthal, 2002a, b; CRN, 2002; FDA, 2002).

PREGNANCY AND LACTATION: Kava should not be used during pregnancy or while nursing (Blumenthal *et al.*, 1998; McGuffin *et al.*, 1997).

ADVERSE EFFECTS

Until recently, reports of adverse effects with recommended doses of kava have been relatively rare. Extended consumption of large doses (400 mg kavalactones or more per day for longer than three months) may cause a scaly, yellowing skin condition (scaly

ichthyosis), which resolves itself when use is discontinued (Mathews *et al.*, 1988; Ruze, 1990; McGuffin *et al.*, 1997; Blumenthal *et al.*, 1998). Kava preparations have been reported to be contributing risk factors for the development of melioidosis, a tropical disease caused by *Burkholderia pseudomallei* (BP) and associated with high mortality. In a prospective study, 252 cases of BP were found in Australia over a 10-year period. Consumption of kava was a risk factor in 8% of those cases (Currie *et al.*, 2000). There are two case reports of necrotizing hepatitis after ingestion of an herbal preparation containing kava extract and celandine (*Chelidonium majus*). Glutamic acid pyruvate transaminase (GPT) levels dropped to normal in both cases when the herbs were discontinued, suggesting a possible causal connection. Due to the combination of herbs and lack of confirmed toxicological data on kava and the liver, and direct cause and effect, it is possible that these results are due to the celandine and/or the combination (Strahl *et al.*, 1998).

By early 2002, there had been approximately 30 cases of possible hepatotoxicity associated with ingestion of kava reported in international literature, with at least 28 cases reported in total (Switzerland—4; Germany—24), prompting regulatory actions by authorities (Hagemann, 2001). The hepatic AERs in these cases include cholestatic hepatitis (inflamed liver with obstruction of bile flow), icterus (jaundice), increased liver enzymes (a sign of liver dysfunction), liver cell impairment, severe hepatitis with confluent necrosis, irreversible liver damage (required transplant in four cases), etc. Additionally, at least 5 cases of liver dysfunction purportedly associated with kava consumption have been reported in the U.S. (Waller, 2002).

Although much of the data on the reported cases of hepatotoxicity is either incomplete or generally unavailable, relatively detailed information has been published for 5 of these cases (Kraft *et al.*, 2001; Russmann *et al.*, 2001; Brauer *et al.*, 2000; Escher *et al.*, 2001; Sass *et al.*, 2001; Strahl *et al.*, 1998). In all of these 5 well-documented cases, notes one review, "severe liver damage or liver failure developed within days. This indicates a sudden, strong insult to the organ and contrasts with an often long kava intake...." (Schulze and Siegers, 2002). In the most detailed report, a case of recurring necrotizing hepatitis was reported in a 39-year old woman who may have consumed an ethanolic-based kava extract (Strahl *et al.*, 1998). In a 50-year old man a relation between ingestion of kava and fulminant hepatic failure was suggested by the chronology, histological findings, and exclusion of other causes of hepatitis. He reportedly took no other drugs nor did he consume alcohol, yet his liver function tests showed a 60-fold and 70-fold increase in aspartate aminotransferase (AST) and alanine aminotransferase (ALT) concentrations, respectively (Escher *et al.*, 2001).

Although kava consumption is considered relatively risk free in its native regions in Polynesia, heavy kava consumption has been associated with increased concentrations of glutamyltransferase, suggesting potential hepatotoxicity (in a population known to be relatively heavy consumers of alcohol), according to a report of its use in Australian aboriginal people (Mathews *et al.*, 1988).

In response to the potential for hepatotoxicity, the German Federal Institute for Drugs and Medical Devices (BfArM) called for labeling of such potential risk on package inserts in kava products (BfArM, 2000). Swiss authorities have taken similar measures after four cases were reported (Stoller, 2000). Seen in perspective to total estimated consumption of kava doses, these cases would constitute one case per 10 million daily doses (Busse, 2000).

Several reviews of these reports emphasize that many of these cases noted other known or suspected liver-toxic medications (e.g., diclofenac and others in Europe; docusate, Ogen®, Percocet®, Celexa®, Oxycontin®, Coumadin®, Celebrex®, and others) had been administered concurrently; in most of the other cases the possibility that concurrently ingested medications, alcohol or virus infections could not be ruled out as possible causes (Schmidt, 2001, 2002; Schulz and Siegers, 2002; Waller 2002). Thus, only a few cases can be conclusively linked to the use of kava (e.g., a case in which liver enzyme values were elevated upon re-exposure to kava after an initial presentation of necrotizing hepatitis [Strahl *et al.*, 1998]). One review suggests that the elucidation of possible mechanisms would add evidence of a causal relationship but that the current animal safety data are scarce and indicate a low hepatotoxic potential (Schulze and Siegers, 2002). An analysis of the approximately 30 hepatic AERs from Europe and 5 submitted to the U.S. FDA from May 1998 through September 2001 by an American toxicologist concluded that there is "no clear evidence that the liver damage reported in the U.S. and Europe was caused by the consumption of kava" and that those cases in which there is a possible association between the use of a kava extract and liver dysfunction "appear to have been hypersensitivity or idiosyncratic base responses." (Waller, 2002). However, the report's author acknowledged that he did not have adequate medical information on all the case reports to adequately assess them. Two U.S. case reports suggest relative safety of kava. In one case in which four prescription drugs plus relatively high levels of kava were used (300 pills or 45,000 mg per day) there was no liver damage observed; in another case a 13-year old girl consumed 8–10, 500 mg tablets in a suicide attempt, but recovered the following morning. "From a toxicologist perspective, these two cases provide some evidence that kava itself is not a direct hepatotoxin even in extremely high concentrations." (Waller, 2002).

The report concludes:

> …kava when taken in appropriate doses for reasonable periods of time has no scientifically established potential for causing liver damage. However as with any pharmacologically active agent, there is always the possibility of drug interactions, preexisting disease conditions and idiosyncratic or hypersensitivity reactions, which can exacerbate the toxicity of such an agent. Increased surveillance or reports of adverse effects and judicious use of kava-derived products under the conditions recommended by the natural products industry would be a most prudent approach to confirm its safety and minimize any risk of liver damage. The medical community and the general public should be made aware that concomitant intake of prescription drugs associated with liver damage, excessive alcohol consumption and preexisting liver disease or hepatitis with compromised liver function are conditions which may preclude any kava consumption (Waller, 2002).

A recent pilot study on an American kava extract (KavaPure®, PureWorld, South Hackensack, NJ) assessed the potential adverse effects profile of kava (Connor *et al.*, 2001). The study concluded that there were no significant differences between kava and placebo on any of the parameters evaluated, including withdrawal symptoms, heart rate, blood pressure, laboratory assessments, and sexual function; there were slightly elevated liver enzymes in 3 kava patients (one at baseline) which was not deemed clinically significant by the authors.

DRUG INTERACTIONS

Simultaneous consumption of kava with alcohol, barbiturates, psychopharmacological drugs, or other substances acting on the central nervous system (CNS) may potentiate inebriation or the CNS depressant effect, according to Commission E, based on a variety of evidence, including speculation (Blumenthal *et al.*, 1998). Regarding interactions with alcohol, subjective measures of sedation, cognition, coordination and intoxication were increased in a clinical trial (n=20) in doses of 1gm/kg kava with alcohol (Foo & Lemon, 1997). Despite kava's producing an increase in the hypnotic effect of ethanol in rats (Jamieson and Duffield, 1990b), an 8-day human trial (n=20) using Laitan® (W. Schwabe, Germany) at 300 mg per day did not produce negative additive effects; the kava group even showed increased scores on the concentration test on the 4th day (Herberg, 1993).

Kava may potentiate effects of other anxiolytics, and may increase Parkinson symptoms by reducing the effect of levodopa, possibly due to dopamine antagonism, according to one human case report (Ernst, 2000; Brinker, 2001). There is one case report of "coma" associated with the combined use of kava and the benzodiazepine, alprazolam (Xanax®), cimetidine (Tagamet®), and terazosin (Hytrin®) (Almeida and Grimsley, 1996). There are reports of interactions, some profound, between alprazolam and cimetidine since 1983 (Abernathy *et al.*, 1983). Cimetidine can reduce the hepatic clearance of alprazolam; thus, the simultaneous use of the two drugs increases levels of alprazolam. Terazosin, a hypotensive drug used for benign prostatic hyperplasia, is usually not noted for interactions with other drugs; however, a commonly reported side effect is "dizziness" and "somnolence" (Abbott Labs, 2002), which might help explain the disorientation of the patient. Since this disorientation (despite the title of the report there was no loss of consciousness (in the article the authors refer to a "semicomatose state"), began 3 days after the first use of kava, it is possible that kava may have triggered the adverse event, but the extent that a possible chronic overdose of alprazolam, plus the possible side effect of terazosin, or a combination of both, may have contributed to the "lethargic" state of the patient is not clear (Bergner, 1999).

AMERICAN HERBAL PRODUCTS ASSOCIATION (AHPA) SAFETY RATING

CLASS 2B: Not to be used during pregnancy.

CLASS 2C: Not to be used while nursing.

CLASS 2D: Caution is required when driving or operating other equipment, and simultaneous consumption of kava and alcohol or barbiturates may potentiate inebriation (McGuffin *et al.*, 1997).

REGULATORY STATUS

AUSTRALIA: Schedule 4 to the Customs (Prohibited Imports) Regulations and is listed on Appendix B-"Substances Subject to Import Controls" with annual license and permit required. Importation of kava into the Northern Territory not permitted, and clearance from the State Health authorities required for importation into Western Australia (TGA, 2000a, 2000b). The Australian Therapeutic Goods Administration (TGA) reviewed kava's legal status and invited submissions for consideration (Burgess, 1998). In 2002, the TGA ordered a voluntary recall on the sale of kava based on the prevailing international concerns over potential association with hepatotoxicity (Worth, 2002).

CANADA: Kava is not acceptable as a nonmedicinal ingredient in oral-use products (HPB, 1993; Health Canada 1995a). When identified as a Traditional Herbal Medicine (THM) or a homeopathic drug, kava was formerly regulated as a schedule OTC drug requiring premarket authorization and assignment of a Drug Identification Number (DIN) (Health Canada, 1995b, 2001; WHO, 1998). Health Canada reviewed the safety of kava in light of the recent hepatotoxicity reports (Anon, 2002a) and banned the sale of kava, and issued a product recall in August 2002 (Health Canada, 2002).

FRANCE: No monograph in the *French Pharmacopoeia*. Kava products banned by Ministry of Health in January 2002 due to concerns over potential hepatotoxicity (Anon., 2002b).

GERMANY: Product licenses withdrawn (BfArM, 2002).

SWEDEN: Approved for use as a drug (De Smet *et al.*, 1993).

SWITZERLAND: Dry native extract 10–23:1 (*w/w*) available in solid dosage form (capsule or tablet) is classified by the *Interkantonale Kontrollstelle für Heilmittel* (IKS) as a List D medicinal product, requiring premarketing authorization and product license, with sales limited to pharmacies and drugstores, without prescription (AKS, 2001; Ruppanner and Schaefer, 2001; WHO, 1998). In 2000 the IKS withdrew the license for the acetonic kava product standardized to 70% kavalactones, owing to concerns of possible hepatotoxicity, based on AERs (see Adverse Effects above), despite the fact that most of the serious kava AERs implicated ethanolic extracts. The acetone extract dominates about 80% of the Swiss market, and was thus the first extract to produce AERs. Manufacturers of ethanolic extracts are allowed to maintain their products on the market for three years, during which time they must produce toxicology, pharmacology, and clinical studies on their respective extracts (Busse, 2002b).

U.K.: Kava was formerly an herbal medicine on the *General Sale List*, Schedule I (requiring full Product License), Table A (internal or external use) with maximum single-dose of 625 mg (GSL, 1994). In December 2001 the British Medicines Control Agency (MCA) and the dietary supplement trade organizations agreed to voluntarily suspend the sales of kava until such time as the issue of potential hepatotoxicity was adequately resolved (Woodfield, 2001). In December 2002, MCA announced a ban on Kava effective January 2003 (MCA, 2002).

U.S.: Dietary supplement (USC, 1994). Kava Rhizome, Powdered Kava, Powdered Kava Extract, Semisolid Kava Extract and Kava Tablets are subjects of botanical monographs in development for *United States Pharmacopeia-National Formulary*. Previews of the standards development were published in the *Pharmacopeial Forum* (USPC, 2000; 2002). In March 2001, the FDA issued a public warning on kava in response to concerns about potential hepatotoxicity (FDA, 2002).

CLINICAL REVIEW

Fifteen studies are outlined in the following table, "Clinical Studies on Kava", including 669 participants. These studies demonstrated kava's positive effects for indications including anxiety, mental function, reaction time, sleep quality, and peri-menopausal symptoms, while one study (Connor *et al.*, 2001) focused on the safety of kava. Six randomized, double-blind, placebo-controlled (R, DB, PC) studies have been performed on 357 participants, concluding that kava significantly reduced anxiety in several different populations (Malsch and Kieser, 2001; Singh *et al.*, 1998; Volz and Kieser, 1997; Lehmann *et al.*, 1996; Warnecke *et al.*, 1991; Kinzler *et al.*, 1991). One R, DB,

case-controlled study of 172 participants found a significant reduction in anxiety (Woelk *et al.*, 1993). Two DB, crossover (CO) trials showed that mental clarity remains intact with kava use (Heinze *et al.*, 1994; Munte *et al.*, 1993). Kava demonstrated a favorable influence on sleep in one PC, CO study (Emser and Bartylla, 1991). One PC, CO, comparison trial showed that kava did not affect reaction time or impair safety, compared to bromazepam and bromazepam combined with kava (Herberg, 1996). A highly significant improvement in peri-menopausal symptoms was demonstrated in a R, DB, PC study (Warnecke *et al.*, 1990). A meta-analysis of seven R, DB, PC trials conducted on various doses of kava, confirmed an anxiolytic effect and demonstrated it was significantly superior to placebo as a symptomatic treatment for anxiety (Pittler and Ernst, 2002, 2000). The Cochrane Review has designed a protocol for evaluating R, DB, PC trials of Kava for anxiety, but has not concluded their evaluation (Bent *et al.*, 2001). In one PC pilot study (n=13), the preliminary findings suggest that kava might exert a positive effect on reflex vagal control of heart rate in generalized anxiety disorder patients (Watkins *et al.*, 2001). Another R, DB, PC study by some of these same authors reviewed the safety profile of kava in 35 subjects. No significant differences were found between kava and placebo on any of the parameters evaluated, including withdrawal symptoms, heart rate, blood pressure, laboratory assessments, and sexual function, with slightly elevated liver enzymes in 3 kava patients (one was elevated at baseline) which was not deemed clinically significant (Connor *et al.*, 2001).

BRANDED PRODUCTS*

GITLY kava extract: Produced as 400 mg tablets containing 120 mg kavalactone. Product manufacturer and distributor not identified.

KavaPure®: PureWorld Botanicals Inc. / 375 Huyler St. / South Hackensack, NJ 07606 / U.S.A. / Tel: (201) 440-5000 / Fax: (201) 342-8000 / www.pureworld.com. Powdered extract of kava rhizome standardized to 30% kavalactones.

Kavatrol®: Natrol Inc. / 21411 Prairie Street / Chatsworth, CA 91311 / U.S.A. / Tel: (800) 326-1520 / www.natrol.com. Produced from dried kava roots in a multistage process. Packaged in 200 mg capsules, containing 60 mg kavalactones in each capsule.

Kavosporal®: Polcopharma F Polley & Co. / P.O. Box 100 / Epping / NSW 1710 / Australia / Tel: +61-02-98-7664 / Fax: +61-02-98-6822-6 / Email: sales@polcopharma.com / http://polcopharma.com.au.

Laitan®: Dr. Willmar Schwabe Pharmaceuticals / International Division / Willmar Schwabe Str. 4 / D-76227, Karlsruhe / Germany / Tel: +49-721-4005 ext. 294 / Email: melville-eaves@schwabe.de / www.schwabepharma.com. Standardized to 70% kavalactones.

Laitan® 100: Dr. Willmar Schwabe Pharmaceuticals. Packaged in 100 mg capsules, each standardized to contain 70 mg kavalactones.

WS 1490: Dr. Willmar Schwabe Pharmaceuticals. Standardized to 70% kavalactones.

*American equivalents, if any, are found in the Product Table beginning on page 398.

REFERENCES

Abbott Laboratories. Hytrin website 2002 Feb. Available from: URL: http://www.rxabbott.com/pdf/hytrin.

ABC. See: American Botanical Council.

Abernethy DR, Greenblatt DJ, Divoll M, Moshitto LJ, Harmatz JS, Shader RI. Interaction of cimetidine with the triazolobenzodiazepines alprazolam and triazolam. *Psychopharmacology* 1983;80(3):275–8.

AHPA. See: American Herbal Products Association.

AKS. See: *Arzneimittel-Kompendium der Schweiz*.

Almeida JC, Grimsley EW. Coma from the health food store: interaction between kava and alprazolam. *Ann Intern Med* 1996;125(11):940–1.

American Botanical Council (ABC). American Botanical Council announces new safety information on kava [press release]. Austin (TX): 2001 Dec. 20.

American Herbal Products Association (AHPA). Kava product warning label issued by leading herbal association [press release]. Silver Spring (MD): 2002 Mar 27 [cited 2002 Nov 7]. Available from: URL: http://www.ahpa.org/pr_032702.htm.

Anon. Health Canada issues kava alert. *Toronto Star* 2002 Jan 17.

Anon. Pacific island beverage banned in France after hepatitis scare. *Agence France-Presse* 2002b Jan 9.

Arzneimittel-Kompendium der Schweiz™ (AKS). Produktinformation und Patienteninformation: Kavasol®; Kavasedon®. Basel, Switzerland: Documed AG; 2001.

Backhauss C, Krieglstein J. Extract of kava (*Piper methysticum*) and its methysticin constituents protect brain tissue against ischemic damage in rodents. *Eur J Pharmacol* 1992a;215(2–3):265–9.

Backhauss C, Krieglstein J. Neuroprotective activity of kava extract (*Piper methysticum*) and its methysticin constituents in vivo and in vitro. In: Krieglstein J, Oberpichler-Schwenk H, editors. *Pharmacology of Cerebral Ischemia*. Stuttgart, Germany: Wissenschftliche Verlagsgesllschaft GmBH; 1992b. p. 501–507.

Baum SS, Hill R, Rommelspacher H. Effect of kava extract and individual kavapyrones on neurotransmitter levels in the nucleus accumbens of rats. *Progress Neuro-Psychopharmacology Biol Psych* 1998;22(7):1105–20.

Bent S, Tsourinas C, Romoli M, Linde K. Kava for Anxiety Disorder. In: *The Cochrane Library*. 2001;1.

Bergner P. Piper—A second opinion on herb-drug interaction. *Medical Herbalism* 1999;11(1):16,20.

BfArM. See: Bundesinstitut für Arzneimittel und Medizinprodukte [The German Federal Institute for Drugs and Medical Devices].

Blumenthal M. The Safety of Kava Questioned: Link to possible liver toxicity subject of inquiries. *Texas Pharmacy* 2002a Spring;14–7,20–1,34.

Blumenthal M. Kava safety questioned due to case reports of liver toxicity: expert analyses of case reports say insufficient evidence to make causal connection. *HerbalGram*. 2002b;55:26–32. Also available from: URL: http://www.herbalgram.org/browse.php?content_name=kavaupdate

Blumenthal M. Herb sales down 15% in mainstream market. *HerbalGram* 2001;51:69.

Blumenthal M, Goldberg A, Brinckmann J, editors. *Herbal Medicine: Expanded Commission E Monographs*. Austin (TX): American Botanical Council; Newton (MA): Integrative Medicine Communications; 2000.

Blumenthal M, Busse WR, Goldberg A, Gruenwald J, Hall T, Riggins CW, Rister RS, editors. Klein S, Rister RS (trans.). *The Complete German Commission E Monographs—Therapeutic Guide to Herbal Medicines*. Austin (TX): American Botanical Council; Boston (MA): Integrative Medicine Communication; 1998. p. 156–7.

Boerner RJ. Kava kava in the treatment of generalized anxiety disorder, simple phobia and specific social phobia. *Phytotherapy Research* 2001;15(7):646–7.

Bone K. Kava—A safe herbal treatment for anxiety. *Brit J Phytotherapy* 1993/94;3(4):147–153.

Boonen G, Häberlein H. Influence of genuine kavapyrone enantiomers on the GABA-A binding site. *Planta Medica* 1998;64(6):504–506.

Boonen G, Ferger B, Kuschinsky K, Häberlein H. In vivo effects of the kavapyrones (+)–dihydromethysticin and (+/−)–kavain on dopamine, 3,4–dihydroxyphenylacetic acid, serotonin, and 5–hydroxyindoleacetic acid levels in striatal and cortical brain regions. *Planta Medica* 1998;64(6):507–510.

Boonen G, Pramanik A, Rigler R, Häberlein H. Evidence for specific interactions between kavain and human cortical neurons monitored by fluorescence correlation spectroscopy. *Planta Medica* 2000;66(1):7–10.

Brauer RB, Pfab R, Becker K, et al. Fulminantes Leberversagen nach Einnahme des pflanzlichen Heilmittels Kava-Kava. *Z Gastroenterologie* 2000;39:491.

Brinker F. *Herb Contraindications and Drug Interactions*. 3d ed. Sandy (OR): Eclectic Medical Publications; 2001. p. 125–127.

Bruggemann F, Meyer H. Studies on the analgesic efficacy of the kava constituents dihydrokavain (DHK) and dihydromethysticin (DHM) [in German]. *Arzneimittelforschung* 1963;13:407–9.

Bundesinstitut für Arzneimittel und Medizinprodukte (BfArM) [The German Federal Institute for Drugs and Medical Devices]. BfArM recalls permisisons for kava and kavain products [press release; in German]. 2002 Jun 17 [cited 2002 Jul 15]. Available from: URL: http://www.bfarm.de/de_ver/presse/02_10de.html.

Bundesinstitut für Arzneimittel und Medizinprodukte (BfArM) [The German Federal Institute for Drugs and Medical Devices]. Introduction of a drug safety plan for pharmaceutical products containing kava-kava. (July 24, 2000).

Burgess N. Regulatory issues on *Piper methysticum* (kava). *Aust J Med Herb* 1998;10(1):2–3.

Busse WR. (W. Schwabe Co.). Personal communication to M. Blumenthal. Feb. 25, 2002a.

Busse WR. (W. Schwabe Co.). Personal communication to M. Blumenthal. Jan. 23, 2002b.

Busse WR. (W. Schwabe Co.). Schwabe position on kava extracts and liver toxicity [unpublished]. 2000.

Connor KM, Davidson JRT, Churchill LE. Adverse-effect profile of kava. *CNS Spectrums* 2001;6(10):848–853.

Council for Responsible Nutrition. CRN complements FDA consumer advisory on kava with recommendation for voluntary cautionary labels [press release]. Washington (DC): 2002 Mar 28 [cited 2002 Nov 7]. Available from: URL: http://www.crnusa.org/shellnr032702.html.

CRN. See: Council for Responsible Nutrition.

Currie BJ, Fisher DA, Howard DM, Burrow JN, Lo D, Selva-Nayagam S, et al. Endemic melioidosis in tropical northern Australia: a 10-year prospective study and review of the literature [review]. *Clin Infect Dis* 2000;31(4):981–6.

DAC. See: *Deutscher Arzneimittel-Codex*.

Davies LP, Drew CA, Duffield P, Johnston GA, Jamieson DD. Kava pyrones and resin: studies on GABA-A, GABA-B, and benzodiazepine binding sites in rodent brain. *Pharm Toxicol* 1992;71(2):120–6.

De Smet PAGM, Keller K, Hansel R, Chandler RF, editors. *Adverse Effects of Herbal Drugs 2*. Berlin, Germany: Springer-Verlag; 1993.

Dentali SJ. Herb Safety Review: kava – *Piper methysticum* Forster f. (*Piperaceae*). Silver Spring (MD): Kava Committee of the American Herbal Products Assn.; 1997.

Deutscher Arzneimittel-Codex (DAC). Ergänzungsbuch zum Arzneibuch, Band II. Stuttgart, Germany: Deutscher Apotheker Verlag; 1998;K-155:1–6.

Duffield AM, Jamieson DD, Lidgard RO, Duffield PH, Bourne DJ. Identification of some human urinary metabolites of the intoxicating beverage kava. *J Chromatogr* 1989;475:273–81.

Emser W, Bartylla K. Improvement in quality of sleep: effect of kava extract WS 1490 on the sleep patterns in healthy people. *TW Neurologie Psychiatrie* 1991;5:636–42.

Ernst E. Possible interactions between synthetic and herbal medicinal products. *Perfusion* 2000;13:4–15.

Escher M, Desmeules J, Giostra E, Mentha G. Hepatitis associated with kava, a herbal remedy for anxiety [published erratum appears in *BMJ* 2001;322(7294):1097]. *BMJ* 2001;322(7279):139.

FDA. See United States Food and Drug Administration.

Ferger B, Boonen G, Häberlein H, Kuschinsky K. In vivo microdialysis study of (+/−)-kavain on veratridine–induced glutamate release. *Eur J Pharmacol* 1998;347(2–3):211–4.

Foo H, Lemon J. Acute effects of kava, alone or in combination with alcohol, on subjective measures of impairment and intoxication and on cognitive performance. *Drug Alcohol Rev* 1997;16:147-155. In: Brinker F. *Herb Contraindications and Drug Interactions*. 3d ed. Sandy (OR): Eclectic Medical Publications; 2001. p. 125–127.

Forster G. *A Voyage round the World in his Britannic Majesty's Sloop*, Resolution, *commanded by Capt. James Cook during the years 1772, 3, 4, and 5. vol 2*. London, U.K.: B. White;1777. p. 406–8.

Friese J, Gleitz J. Kavain, dihydrokavain and dihydromethysticin non-competitively inhibit the specific binding of [3H]-batrachotoxinin-A 20-alpha-benzoate to receptor site 2 of voltage-gated Na+ channels. *Planta Med* 1998;64(5):458–9.

Garner LF, Klinger JD. Some visual effects caused by the beverage kava. *J Ethnopharmacol* 1985;13(3):307–11.

General Sale List (GSL). Statutory Instrument 1994 No. 2410; The Medicines (Products Other Than Veterinary Drugs) (*General Sale List*) Amendment Order 1994. London, U.K.: Her Majesty's Stationery Office (HMSO); 1994.

Gleitz J, Beile A, Wilkens P, Ameri A, Peters T. Antithrombotic action of the kava pyrone (+)-kavain prepared from *Piper methysticum* on human platelets. *Planta Medica* 1997;63(1):27–30.

Gleitz J, Friese J, Beile A, Ameri A, Peters T. Anticonvulsive action of (+/−)-kavain estimated from its properties on stimulated synaptosomes and Na+ channel receptor sites. *Eur J Pharmacol* 1996a;315(1):89–97.

Gleitz J, Gottner N, Ameri A, Peters T. Kavain inhibits non–stereospecifically veratridine–activated Na+–channels. *Planta Medica* 1996b;62:580–581.

Gleitz J, Tosch C, Beile A, Peters T. The protective action of tetrodotoxin and (+/-)-kavain on anaerobic glycolysis, ATP content, and intracellular Na+ and Ca2+ of anoxic brain vesicles. *Neuropharmacol* 1996c;35(12):1743–52.

Gleitz J, Beile A, Peters T. (+/-)-Kavain inhibits veratridine-activated voltage-dependent Na+ channels in synaptosomes prepared from rat cerebral cortex. *Neuropharmacol* 1995;34(9):1133–8.

GSL. See: *General Sale List*.

Grunze H, Langosch J, Schirrmacher K, Bingmann D, Von Wegerer J, Walden J. Kava pyrones exert effects on neuronal transmission and transmembraneous cation currents similar to established mood stabilizers—a review. *Prog Neuropsychopharmacol Biol Psychiatry* 2001;25(8):1555–70.

Haberlein H, Boonen G, Beck MA. *Piper methysticum*: enantiomeric separation of kavapyrones by high performance liquid chromatography. *Planta Med* 1997;63:63–5.

Hagemann U. Pharmaceutical products containing kava kava (*Piper methysticum*) and kavain, including homeopathic preparations with a final concentration up to D6 [letter]. Berlin: German Federal Institute for Drugs and Medical Devices (BfArM). Nov. 8, 2001.

Hänsel R. Characterization and physiological activity of some kava constituents. *Pac Sci* 1968;22:293–313.

He X, Lin L, Lian L. Electrospray high performance liquid chromatography-mass spectrometry in phytochemical analysis of kava extract. *Planta Med* 1997;63:70–4.

Health Canada. Health Canada issues a stop-sale order for all products containing kava. 2002 Aug 21 [cited 2002 Nov 11]. Available from: URL: http://www.hc-sc.gc.ca/english/protection/warnings/2002/2002_56e.htm.

Health Canada. *Drug Product Database* (DPD) *Product Information*. Ottawa, Ontario: Health Canada Therapeutic Products Programme; 2001.

Health Canada. *Drugs Directorate Guidelines: Traditional Herbal Medicines*. Ottawa, Ontario: Minister of National Health and Welfare, Canada; 1995b. p. 1–11.

Health Canada. Herbs used as non-medicinal ingredients in nonprescription drugs for human use—Appendix II: list of herbs unacceptable as non-medicinal ingredients in oral use products subject to part B. Ottawa, Ontario: Health Canada Drugs Directorate Bureau of Nonprescription Drugs; 1995a. p. 1–22.

Health Protection Branch. *HPB Status Manual*. Ottawa, Ontario: Health Protection Branch; 1993 Feb 19. p. 111.

Heinze HJ, Münthe TF, Steitz J, Matzke M. Pharmacopsychological effects of oxazepam and kava kava extract in a visual search paradigm assessed with event-related potentials. *Pharmacopsychiatry* 1994;27(6):224–230.

Herberg KW. Safety-related performance after intake of kava-extract, bromazepam and their combination [in German]. *Z Allg Med* 1996;72:973–77.

Herberg KW. Effect of Kava-Special Extract WS 1490 combined with ethyl alcohol on safety-relevant performance parameters [in German]. *Blutalkohol* 1993;30(2):96–105. In: Brinker F. *Herb Contraindications and Drug Interactions*. 3d ed. Sandy (OR): Eclectic Medical Publications; 2001. p. 125–7.

Holm E, Staedt U, Hepp J, Kortsik C, Behne F, Kaske A, et al. The action profile of D,L-kavain: cerebral sites and sleep-wakefulness-rhythm in animals [in German]. *Arzneimittelforschung* 1991;41(7):673–83.

HPB. See: Health Protection Branch.

IKS. See: Interkantonalen Kontrollstelle für Heilmittel.

Interkantonalen Kontrollstelle für Heilmittel (IKS). *Monatsbericht der IKS*. Bern, Switzerland: IKS; 2001 April. p. 220.

Jamieson DD, Duffield PH. The antinociceptive actions of kava components in mice. *Clin Exp Pharm Physiol* 1990a;17(7):495–507.

Jamieson DD, Duffield PH. Positive interaction of ethanol and kava resin in mice. *Clin Exp Pharm Physiol* 1990b;17(7):509–14.

Johnson D, Frauenddorf A, Stecker K, Stein U. Neurophysiological activity profile and tolerability of Kava-Extract WS 1490 [in German]. *Neurol/Psychiat* 1991;5:584–88.

Jussofie A, Schmiz A, Hiemke C. Kavapyrone enriched extract from *Piper methysticum* as modulator of the GABA binding site in different regions of rat brain. *Psychopharmacol* 1994;116(4):469–74.

Jussofie A. Brain area specific differences in the effects of neuroactive steroids on the GABA-A receptor complexes following acute treatment with anaesthetically active steroids. *Acta Endocrinology* 1993;129(5):480–5.

Kilham C. *Kava: Medicine Hunting in Paradise*. Rochester (NY): Inner Traditions; 1996.

Kinzler E, Kromer J, Lehmann E. Effect of a special kava extract in patients with anxiety-, tension-, and excitation states of non-psychotic genesis: double blind study with placebos over 4 weeks [in German]. *Arzneimittelforshung* 1991;41(6):584–8.

Klohs M, et al. A chemical and pharmacological investigation of *Piper methysticum* Forst. *J Med Pharm Chem* 1959;1:95–9.

Kraft M, Spahn TW, Menzel J, Senninger N, Dietl KH, Herbst H, et al. Fulminant liver failure after administration of the herbal anti-depressant kava-kava [in German]. *Dtsch Med Wochenschr* 2001;126(36):970–2.

Kretzschmar R. Kavain psychopharmakon. *München Med Wochenschr 4ème année* 1970;112:154–8.

Lebot V, Cabalion P. Technical Paper No. 195: Kavas of Vanuatu–Cultivars of *Piper methysticum* Forst. Noumea, New Caledonia: South Pacific Commission; 1988. p. 13–15.

Lebot V, Merlin M, Lindstrom L. *Kava: The Pacific Drug*. New Haven (CT): Yale University Press; 1992.

Lehmann E, Kinzler E, Friedemann J. Efficacy of a special Kava extract (*Piper methysticum*) in patients with states of anxiety, tension and excitedness of non-mental origin—a double-blind placebo-controlled study of four weeks treatment. *Phytomedicine* 1996;3(2):113–9.

Leung A, Foster S. *Encyclopedia of Common Natural Ingredients Used in Food, Drugs, and Cosmetics*. 2nd ed. New York (NY): John Wiley and Sons; 1996.

Liberti L, editor. Kava Monograph. *Lawrence Review of Natural Products*. Levittown (PA): Pharmaceutical Information Associates; 1987.

Lindenberg D, Pitule-Schödel H. D,L-kavain in comparison with oxazepam in anxiety disorders. a double-blind study of clinical effectiveness [in German]. *Forschr Med* 1990;108(2):50–4.

Mack R. Kava kava. *Piper methysticum*–a unique economic plant of the Pacific Islands. *J Health Sci* 1994;1(1):43–8.

Magura EI, Kopanitsa MV, Gleitz J, Peters T, Krishtal OA. Kava extract ingredients, (+)-methysticin and (+/-)-kavain inhibit voltage-operated Na+-channels in rat CA 1 hippocampal neurons. *Neuroscience* 1997;81(2):345–51.

Malsch U, Kieser M. Efficacy of kava-kava in the treatment of non-psychotic anxiety, following pretreatment with benzodiazepines. *Psychopharmacol* 2001;157(3):277–83.

Martin HB, Stofer WB, Eichinger MR. Kavain inhibits murine airway smooth muscle contraction. *Planta Medica* 2000;66(7):601–6.

Mathews JD, Riley MD, Fejo L, Munoz E, Milns NR, Gardner ID, et al. Effects of the heavy usage of kava on physical health: summary of a pilot survey in an Aboriginal community. *Med J Aust* 1988;148(11):548–55.

MCA. See: Medicines Control Agency (UK).

McGuffin M, Hobbs C, Upton R, Goldberg A, editors. *American Herbal Products Association's Botanical Safety Handbook*. Boca Raton (FL):CRC Press; 1997.

Medicines Control Agency (UK). MCA investigation of kava kava leads to ban following voluntary withdrawal [press release]. 20 Dec 2002.

Meldrum B. Possible therapeutic applications of antagonists of excitatory amino acid neurotransmitters [review]. *Clin Sci (Lond)* 1985;68(2):113-22.

Meyer HJ. Pharmacology of Kava. In: Efron DH, Holmstedt B, Kline NS, editors. *Ethnopharmacologic Search for Psychoactive Drugs*. New York (NY): Raven Press; 1979. p. 133–40.

Munte TF, Heinze HJ, Matzke M, Steitz J. Effects of oxazepam and an extract of kava roots (*Piper methysticum*) on event-related potentials in a word-recognition task. *Pharmacoelectroencephalog* 1993;27(1):46–53.

Norton S, Ruze P. Kava dermopathy. *J Am Acad Derm* 1994;31(1):89–97.

Pittler MH, Ernst E. Efficacy of kava extract for treating anxiety: systematic review and meta-analysis. *J Clin Psychopharmacol* 2000;20(1):84–9.

Pittler MH, Ernst E. Kava extract for treating anxiety [Cochrane Review]. In: The Cochrane Library; 2002;(2):CD00383.

Pizzorno JE, Murray MT , editors. *Textbook of Natural Medicine, Vol. 1*. 2nd ed. New York (NY): Churchill Livingstone; 1999.

Ruppanner H, Schaefer U (eds.). Kavasedon® Kapseln; Kavasporal® Kapseln; Laitan® Kapseln; Yakona N® Kapseln. In: *Codex 2000/01 — Die Schweizer Arzneimittel in einem Griff*. Basel, Switzerland: Documed AG; 2001. pp. 1208–9, 1244.

Russell P, Bakker D, Singh N. The effects of kava on alerting and speed of access of information from long-term memory. *Bulletin of the Psychonomic Society* 1987;25:236–7.

Russmann S, Lauterburg BH, Helbing A. Kava hepatotoxicity. *Ann Internal Med* 2001;135(1):68–9.

Ruze P. Kava-induced dermopathy: a niacin deficiency? *Lancet* 1990;335(8703):1442–5.

Saletu B, Grunberger J, Linzmayer L, Anderer P. EEG brain-mapping, psychometric and psychophysiological studies on the central effects of kavain—a kava plant derivative. *Human Psychopharmacol* 1989;4:169–90.

Sass M, Schnabel S, Kröger J, et al. Akutes Leberversgaen durch Kava-Kava—eine seltene Indikation zur Lebertransplantation. *Z Gastroenterol* 2001;39:491.

Scherer J. Kava-kava extract in anxiety disorders: an outpatient observational study. *Adv Ther* 1998;15(4):261–9.

Schirrmacher K, Büsselberg D, Langosch JM, Walden J, Winter U, Bingmann D. Effects of (+/−)–kavain on voltage-activated inward currents of dorsal rhizome ganglion cells from neonatal rats. *European Neuropsychopharmacology* 1999;9(1–2):171–6.

Schmidt J. Analysis of kava side effects reports concerning the liver [unpublished]. Lindenmaier M. Brinckmann J (trans). Courtesy American Herbal Products Assn.; 2001, Dec 31.

Schmidt M, Nahrstedt A. Is Kava hepatotoxic? *Deutsche Apotheker Zeitung* 2002;142(9):58–63.

Schulze J, Siegers CP. *Toxicity of kava pyrones—a reappraisal*. *Brit J Pharmacology* 2002 (submitted).

Schulze J, Meng G, Siegers CP. Safety assessment of kavalactone-containing herbal drugs in comparison to other psychotropics [abstract from conference of Swiss Soc. Pharm. and Tox., German Soc. Experimental and Clin. Pharmacol and Tox., Austrian Pharmacol. Soc.—Oct. 1–2, 2001]. *Arch Pharmacol* 2001;364(3):R22.

Seitz U, Ameri A, Pelzer H, Gleitz J, Peters T. Relaxation of evoked contractile activity of isolated guinea-pig ileum by (+/-)–kavain. *Planta Medica* 1997a;63(4):303-306.

Seitz U, Schüle A, Gleitz J. [3H]-Monoamine uptake inhibition properties of kava pyrones. *Planta Med* 1997b;63(6):548–9.

Singh NN, Ellis CR, Singh YN. A double-blind, placebo-controlled study on the effects of kava (Kavatrol®) on daily stress and anxiety in adults. *Alt Ther* 1998;4(2):97–8.

Singh YN. Effects of kava on neuromuscular transmission and muscle contractility. *J Ethnopharmacol* 1983;7(3):267–76.

Singh YN. Kava, an overview [review]. *J Ethnopharmacol* 1992;37(1):13–45.

Singh YN, Blumenthal M. Kava: An overview. *HerbalGram* 1997;39:33–57.

Steiner GG. The correlation between cancer incidence and kava consumption. *Hawaii Med J* 2000;59(11):420–2.

Stoller R. Liver damage and kava extracts. *Schweizerische Ärztezeitung* 2000;81(24):1335–6.

Strahl S, Ehret V, Dahm HH, Maier KP. Necrotizing hepatitis after taking herbal remedies [in German]. *Dtsch Med Wochenschr* 1998;123(47):1410–4.

Taylor CL. Letter to MDs re: possible kava hepatoxicity [letter]. Food and Drug Administration, Dec 19, 2001. Available from: URL: http://www.fda.gov/medwatch/SAFETY/2001/kava.htm.

TGA. See: Therapeutic Goods Administration.

Therapeutic Goods Administration (TGA). Appendix B – Substances Subject to Import Controls (annual license & permit required). Woden, Australia: Therapeutic Goods Administration; 2000a May 29. p. 1–7 .

Therapeutic Goods Administration (TGA). Commonly Asked Questions: Importing Kava and Khat: What are the requirements for the importation of kava? Woden, Australia: Therapeutic Goods Administration; 2000 May 29. p. 1–11.

Uebelhack R, Franke L, Schewe HJ. Inhibition of platelet MAO–B by kava pyrone-enriched extract from *Piper methysticum* Forster (kava–kava). *Pharmacopsychiatry* 1998;31(5):187–92.

United States Congress (USC). Dietary Supplement Health and Education Act of 1994, Pub. L. No. 103–417, 103rd Cong. (1994).

United States Food and Drug Administration, Center for Food Safety and Applied Nutrition. Kava-containing dietary supplements may be associated with severe liver injury [consumer advisory]. 2002 Mar 25 [cited 2002 Nov 7]. Available from: http://www.cfsan.fda.gov/%7Edms/addskava.html.

United States Pharmacopeial Convention (USPC). Pharmacopeial previews. monographs (NF): kava; powdered kava. *Pharmacopeial Forum* 2002 Jan–Feb;28(1).

United States Pharmacopeial Convention (USPC). Pharmacopeial previews. monographs (NF): powdered kava extract; semisolid kava extract. *Pharmacopeial Forum* 2000 May–Jun;26(3):42–50.

USC. See: United States Congress.

USPC. See: United States Pharmacopeial Convention.

Volz H-P, Kieser M. Kava kava extract WS 1490 versus placebo in anxiety disorders — a randomized placebo controlled 25 week outpatient trial. *Pharmacopsychiatr* 1997;30(1):1–5.

Waller DP. Report on Kava and Liver Damage. Silver Spring (MD): American Herbal Products Assn; 2002.

Warnecke G. Psychosomatic dysfunctions in the female climacteric: clinical effectiveness and tolerance of kava extract WS 1490 [in German]. *Fortsch Med* 1991;109(4):119–22.

Warnecke G, Pfaender H, Gerster G, Gracza E. Efficacy of an extract of Kavaroot in patients with climacteric syndrome [in German]. *Zeitschrift für Phytotherapie* 1990;11:81–6.

Watkins LL, Connor KM, Davidson JRT. Effect of kava extract on vagal cardiac control in generalized anxiety disorder: preliminary findings. *J Psychopharmacol* 2001;15(4):283–6.

Wheatley D. Kava and valerian in the treatment of stress-induced insomnia. *Phytother Res* 2001;15(6):549–51.

Woelk H, Kapoula O, Lehrl S, Schröter K, Weinholz P. A comparison of kava special extract WS 1490 and benzodiazepines in patients with anxiety. *Z Allg Med* 1993;69:271–7.

Woodfield R. Safety of Kava-kava products—temporary and voluntary suspension of sale and supply [letter]. London, U.K.: Medicines Control Agency; 2001 Dec 19.

World Health Organization (WHO). *Regulatory Status of Herbal Medicines: A Worldwide Review*. Geneva, Switzerland: World Health Organization Traditional Medicine Programme; 1998. p. 8–9.

Worth T. TGA recalls over the counter medicines containing kava [press release]. 2002 Aug 15.

Kava

Monograph

Clinical Studies on Kava (*Piper methysticum* G. Forst.)

Anxiety

Author/Year	Subject	Design	Duration	Dosage	Preparation	Results/Conclusion
Malsch and Kieser, 2001	Nonpsychotic nervous anxiety, tension, restlessness	R, DB, PC n=40	5 weeks	50 mg/day (week 1) 300 mg/day (after week 1)	WS 1490 (Laitan® 100)	Pretreatment of patients with benzodiazepines was tapered off over 2 weeks. Kava was superior to placebo on HAMA (p=0.01) and subjective well-being scale (p=0.002). Study confirms anxiolytic effects and good tolerance of kava, and shows that further symptom reduction is possible after changeover from benzodiazepine treatment.
Singh et al., 1998	Nonclinical levels of daily stress and anxiety	R, DB, PC, PG n=60	4 weeks	400 mg/day (200 mg 2x/day)	Kavatrol®	Significantly (p<0.0001) decreased daily stress due to interpersonal problems, personal competency, cognitive stressors, environmental hassles, and the sum of these varied stressors. Significantly (p<0.0001) decreased anxiety due to environmental, psychological, and personal circumstances. Significance occurred after one week of treatment with continual decline for subsequent weeks of trial, with no side effects reported.
Volz and Kieser, 1997	Anxiety and agitation caused by unspecified mental disorder	R, DB, PC, MC n=101	25 weeks	100 mg 3x/day (3 × 70 mg of kavalactones per day)	WS 1490 (Laitan® 100)	Significantly (p=0.02) reduced somatic and mental anxiety from eighth week on. Long-term treatment showed greater efficacy (p< 0.001 at week 24) than short-term treatment. Kava was well tolerated; adverse effects were rare; there were no withdrawal symptoms.
Lehmann et al., 1996	Anxiety, tension, and excitedness of nonmental origin	R, DB, PC n=58	4 weeks	100 mg 3x/day (3 × 70 mg of kavalactones per day)	WS 1490 (Laitan® 100)	Showed anxiolytic efficacy and significantly (p< 0.02) reduced total anxiety after one week of treatment. Efficacy increased over subsequent weeks. Did not produce any adverse reactions.
Woelk et al., 1993	Anxiety, tension, agitation of nonpsychotic origin	R, DB, MC, CC n=172	6 weeks	100 mg 3x/day (3 × 70 mg of kavalactones per day)	WS 1490 (Laitan® 100)	Showed equal anxiolytic efficacy as the benzodiazepines (oxazepam and bromazepam). Authors concluded WS 1490 should be included in the therapeutic possibilities to consider in conditions of anxiety, tension, and agitation of nonpsychotic origin.
Warnecke, 1991	Anxiety and depression associated with menopause and post-menopause	R, DB, PC n=40	8 weeks	100 mg 3x/day (3 × 70 mg of kavalactones per day)	WS 1490 (Laitan® 100)	Significantly reduced HAMA overall score of anxiety by an average of 50% by first week, with a continual reduction through week 4 (p<0.001). Therapeutic index for use-risk evaluation was comparable to placebo.
Kinzler et al., 1991	Anxiety syndrome of nonpsychotic origin	R, DB, PC n=58	4 weeks	100 mg 3x/day (3 × 70 mg of kavalactones per day)	WS 1490 (Laitan® 100)	Significantly reduced anxiety symptoms after one week of treatment, and difference between groups increased over course of study. At each checkpoint (7, 14, and 28 days) the treatment group vs. placebo had significantly lowered HAMA scores (p<0.01). Kava caused no adverse experiences.

Mental Function

Author/Year	Subject	Design	Duration	Dosage	Preparation	Results/Conclusion
Herberg, 1996	Reaction time and safety performance	PC, CO, Cm n=18	14 days	400 mg (120 kavalactone) tablet 2x daily of kava extract alone; bromazepam alone (2 × 4.5 mg/day); kava and bromazepam combined	GITLY kava extract or bromazepam	Performance was impaired after treatment with bromazepam and the combination, but remained at the baseline level after treatment with the kava extract. The least impairment of well-being occurred with kava and the greatest with the combination.

KEY: **C** – controlled, **CC** – case-control, **CH** – cohort, **CI** – confidence interval, **Cm** – comparison, **CO** – crossover, **CS** – cross-sectional, **DB** – double-blind, **E** – epidemiological, **LC** – longitudinal cohort, **MA** – meta-analysis, **MC** – multi-center, **n** – number of patients, **O** – open, **OB** – observational, **OL** – open label, **OR** – odds ratio, **P** – prospective, **PB** – patient-blind, **PC** – placebo-controlled, **PG** – parallel group, **PS** – pilot study, **R** – randomized, **RC** – reference-controlled, **RCS** – retrospective cross-sectional, **RS** - retrospective, **S** – surveillance, **SB** – single-blind, **SC** – single-center, **U** – uncontrolled, **UP** – unpublished, **VC** – vehicle-controlled.

Clinical Studies on Kava (*Piper methysticum* G. Forst.)   (cont.)

Mental Function   (cont.)

Author/Year	Subject	Design	Duration	Dosage	Preparation	Results/Conclusion
Heinze et al., 1994	Behavior, mental performance	DB, R, CO, Cm n=12 young healthy males, 24–37 years	5 days	200 mg 3x/day (6 x 70 mg kavalactones per day)	WS 1490 (Laitan® 100) vs. oxazepam	Kava did not alter behavior in psychometric tests, as did oxazepam. May slightly enhance mental performance associated with focal attention and processing capacity.
Munte et al., 1993	Behavior, mental performance	DB, CO, Cm n=12 healthy volunteers 24–37 years	5 days	600 mg/day (200 mg 3x/day); oxazepam (10 mg/day before testing and 75 mg on morning of study); or placebo	WS 1490 (Laitan® 100) vs. oxazepam vs. placebo	Study showed nonsignificant trend toward improved cognitive function with kava. Suggests enhanced memory performance under kava. No adverse effects reported. Oxazepam produced significant decrease in quality and speed of response.
Russell et al., 1987	Reaction time	Cm n=18	6 days	250 ml/day or 500 ml/day	Cold macerate of 30 g root powder	No effect on reaction time or errors with traditional or excess dosages. Consumption did not alter speed of activation of verbal information in long-term memory or reaction to warning signal.

Other

Author/Year	Subject	Design	Duration	Dosage	Preparation	Results/Conclusion
Connor et al., 2001	Safety profile	R, DB, PC n=35 adults with a 1+ month history of generalized anxiety disorder and HAMA score >16 (31–75 years of age)	6 weeks: Week 1: placebo only; Weeks 2–5: kava or placebo Week 6: No treatment, no placebo	Week 2: 140 mg kavalactones/ day or placebo Weeks 3–5: 280 mg kavalactones/ day or placebo	KavaPure® (standardized to 70 mg kavalactones)	No statistically significant differences were seen between kava and placebo groups for blood or urine studies, ECG assessments, blood pressure, heart rate, sexual function, or incidence of adverse events. No withdrawal symptoms were observed 1 week after abrupt cessation of treatment. Authors conclude kava was well-tolerated even though dosage used was higher than used in most other studies, but further studies of long term kava use are needed.
Watkins et al., 2001	Vagal cardia control measured by baroreflex control of heart rate (BRC) and respiratory sinus arrhythmia (RSA)	P, DB, PC n=13 adults with a 1+ month history of generalized anxiety disorder and HAMA score >16 (35–74 years of age)	4 weeks, with assessment 1 day prior to and 4 weeks after beginning treatment	280 mg kava/day or placebo	KavaPure® (standardized to 30% kavalactones)	Kava group showed statistically significantly improved BRC vs placebo group (p<0.05). Degree of BRC improvement correlated significantly with clinical improvement (p<0.05). No change in RSA was observed in either group.
Emser and Bartylla, 1991	Sleep	PC, CO n=12 healthy people 20–31 years	4 days	150 mg/day, 50 mg 3x/day; 300mg/day, 100 mg 3x/day; or placebo	WS 1490 (Laitan®)	Kava favorably influenced sleep. Increased sleep spindle densities and duration of slow wave (deep) sleep. No effects on duration of REM sleep. Tended to decrease sleep stage 1 (falling asleep) and sleep latency (waking stage).
Warnecke et al., 1990	Peri-menopausal symptoms	R, DB, PC n=20	12 weeks	One 150 mg tablet kava extract (30 mg kavalactones) 2x daily for 4 weeks, followed by 1 tablet, 1x daily starting week 5	Kavosporal®	After 4 weeks, the kava group demonstrated a highly significant (p=0.001) reduction in peri-menopausal symptoms. At 12 weeks, statistical sampling was not possible due to a dropout in the number of placebo-group patients.

KEY: C – controlled, **CC** – case-control, **CH** – cohort, **CI** – confidence interval, **Cm** – comparison, **CO** – crossover, **CS** – cross-sectional, **DB** – double-blind, **E** – epidemiological, **LC** – longitudinal cohort, **MA** – meta-analysis, **MC** – multi-center, **n** – number of patients, **O** – open, **OB** – observational, **OL** – open label, **OR** – odds ratio, **P** – prospective, **PB** – patient-blind, **PC** – placebo-controlled, **PG** – parallel group, **PS** – pilot study, **R** – randomized, **RC** – reference-controlled, **RCS** – retrospective cross-sectional, **RS** - retrospective, **S** – surveillance, **SB** – single-blind, **SC** – single-center, **U** – uncontrolled, **UP** – unpublished, **VC** – vehicle-controlled.

Kava

Monograph

(This page intentionally left blank.)

Licorice

Glycyrrhiza spp.

Glycyrrhiza glabra L. (syn. G. *glandulifera* Walst. & Kit.), G. *uralensis* Fisch. Ex DC.
[Fam. *Fabaceae*]

OVERVIEW

Licorice root is one of the most widely used medicinal herbs worldwide and is the single most used herb in Chinese medicine today. In a recent survey of Western medical herbalists, licorice ranked as the 10th most important herb used in clinical practice. While licorice root is commonly taken in combinations for treatment of catarrhs of the respiratory tract, cough and sore throat, as well as for dyspepsia, a few clinical studies have investigated its effects on aphthous, duodenal, and gastric ulcers.

PRIMARY USES

Crude Preparations
• Catarrh of upper respiratory tract

Deglycyrrhized Licorice Extract Preparations
• Aphthous, stomatitis (oral ulcers)
• Gastric ulcers
• Duodenal ulcer

NOTE: The Commission E also approved licorice preparations containing glycyrrhizin for gastric and duodenal ulcers.

OTHER POTENTIAL USES
• Prevention of radiation complications in lungs during radiotherapy
• Chronic hepatitis
• Sore throat
• Cough with viscid expectoration
• Dyspepsia

Purified Licorice Derivatives
• Hepatic failure, subacute
• Reduced risk of liver carcinogenesis in hepatitis C patients

Uses in Traditional Chinese Medicine (TCM)
• Bronchitis, pharyngitis, laryngitis, bronchial asthma, chronic hypocorticoidism

PHARMACOLOGICAL ACTIONS

Anti-inflammatory; expectorant; demulcent; adrenocorticotropic; antioxidant; protection of LDL against lipid peroxidation; accelerates healing of gastric ulcers.

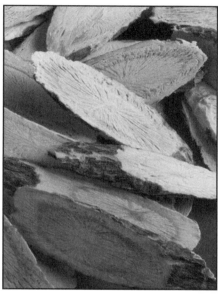

Photo © 2003 stevenfoster.com

DOSAGE AND ADMINISTRATION

Licorice should not be ingested for longer than 4 to 6 weeks without medical advice, although licorice root may be used as a flavoring agent up to a maximum daily dosage equivalent to 100 mg glycyrrhizin. A diet rich in potassium (eg., bananas) is recommended during the period of treatment with licorice.

Crude Preparations

DECOCTION: 1.0–1.5 g licorice root placed in approximately 150–250 ml cold water. Boiled, simmered for 10–15 minutes, then strained; 2–3 times daily.

INFUSION: Approximately 150 ml boiling water poured over 4.5 g licorice root and steeped 10–15 minutes; 2–3 times daily.

FLUID EXTRACT: 2–5 ml, 3 times daily.

POWDERED ROOT: Approximately 5–15 g root daily; equivalent to 200–600 mg glycyrrhizin, 2–4 g single dose.

Deglycyrrhized Licorice (DGL) Preparations

DGL NATIVE DRY EXTRACT: 0.4–1.6 g, 3 times daily.

DGL CHEWABLE TABLETS: For acute cases of gastric or duodenal ulcers; 2–4 tablets chewed before each meal. For chronic cases, 1 to 2 tablets chewed before each meal.

Standardized Preparations

FLUID EXTRACT: 5–15 ml daily, (or 2–5 ml, 3 times daily) corresponding to German Commission E dosage of 5–15 g of root daily.

NATIVE DRY EXTRACT: 0.33–0.8 g, 3 times daily, after meals.

CONTRAINDICATIONS

Patients with cholestatic liver disorders, liver cirrhosis, hypertension, hypokalemia, severe kidney insufficiency, and possibly diabetes (unconfirmed contraindication) should consult a healthcare provider before using licorice.

PREGNANCY AND LACTATION: Not recommended during pregnancy. Heavy exposure to glycyrrhizin (<500 mg/wk) did not affect birth weight, but did double the risk of birth before 38 weeks. No known restrictions during lactation.

ADVERSE EFFECTS

No adverse effects have been associated with licorice when used appropriately. Prolonged use (longer than six weeks) and higher doses (greater than 50 g/day) may lead to sodium and water retention, and to potassium loss accompanied by hypertension, edema, hypokalemia, and, in rare cases, myoglobinuria. Side effects are less likely with aqueous licorice root extract than with isolated glycyrrhizin. In two separate cases, pulmonary edema and life-threatening ventricular tachycardia due to hypokalemia occurred as a result of overdoses of black licorice-flavored candy.

DRUG INTERACTIONS

Licorice may potentiate the side effects of potassium-depleting thiazide diuretics (eg., chlorothiazide, chlorthalidone, hydrochlorothiazide, and metolazone). With potassium loss, sensitivity to digitalis glycosides increases. Licorice should not be combined with corticoid treatment.

CLINICAL REVIEW

Ten studies that included a total of 2,544 participants had variable research designs and evaluated a wide cross-section of therapeutic uses. Eight showed positive effects for indications including the effects of licorice or its active constituents on pulmonary metabolism, pseudohyperaldosteronism, aphthous ulcer, benign gastric ulcer, chronic duodenal ulceration, LDL cholesterol, subacute hepatic failure, and chemoprevention. Three studies were conducted on licorice root extract, four studies on DGL extract, and two on isolated glycyrrhizin preparations. One study on birth outcome found that licorice did not affect birth weight but did double the risk of birth before 38 weeks.

Licorice

Glycyrrhiza spp.

Glycyrrhiza glabra L. (syn. *G. glandulifera Walst.* & Kit.), *G. uralensis* Fisch. Ex DC.

[Fam. *Fabaceae*]

OVERVIEW

Licorice root is one of the most widely used medicinal herbs worldwide and is the single most used herb in Chinese medicine today. In a recent survey of Western medical herbalists, licorice ranked as the 10th most important herb used in clinical practice. While licorice root is commonly taken in combinations for treatment of catarrhs of the respiratory tract, cough, sore throat, and dyspepsia, a few clinical studies have investigated its effects on aphthous, duodenal, and gastric ulcers.

PRIMARY USES

Catarrh of the upper respiratory tract; oral ulcers; gastric and duodenal ulcers.

OTHER USES

Sore throat; cough with viscid expectoration; dyspepsia; prevention of lung complications during radiation therapy; reduction of risk of liver cancer in hepatitis C; chronic hepatitis.

TRADITIONAL CHINESE MEDICINE USES

Bronchitis; pharyngitis; laryngitis; bronchial asthma; chronic hypocorticoidism.

DOSAGE

Licorice should not be ingested for more than 4 to 6 weeks without medical advice. Licorice root may be used as a flavoring agent up to a maximum daily dosage equal to 100 mg glycyrrhizin. A diet high in potassium-rich foods such as bananas is recommended while being treated with licorice.

Crude Preparations

DECOCTION: 1.0–1.5 g licorice root placed in approximately 150–250 ml cold water. Boiled, simmered for 10–15 minutes, then strained; 2–3 times daily.

FLUID EXTRACT: 2–5 ml, 3 times daily.

POWDERED ROOT: Approximately 5–15 g root daily, equivalent to 200–600 mg glycyrrhizin, 2–4 g single dose.

Comments

When using a dietary supplement, purchase it from a reliable source. For best results, use the same brand of product throughout the period of use. As with all medications and dietary supplements, please inform your healthcare provider of all herbs and medications you are taking. Interactions may occur between medications and herbs or even among different herbs when taken at the same time. Treat your herbal supplement with care by taking it as directed, storing it as advised on the label, and keeping it out of the reach of children and pets. Consult your healthcare provider with any questions.

Deglycyrrhized Licorice (DGL) Preparations

DGL NATIVE DRY EXTRACT: 0.4–1.6 g, 3 times daily.

DGL CHEWABLE TABLETS: For acute cases of gastric or duodenal ulcers; 2–4 tablets chewed before each meal. For chronic cases, 1 to 2 tablets chewed before each meal.

Standardized Preparations

FLUID EXTRACT: 2 to 5 ml, 3 times daily [standardized minimum 7% glycyrrhizin].

NATIVE DRY EXTRACT: 0.33–0.8 g, after meals, 3 times daily [standardized minimum 20% glycyrrhizin].

CONTRAINDICATIONS

Patients with cholestatic liver disorders, liver cirrhosis, high blood pressure, hypokalemia, severe kidney insufficiency, and possibly diabetes (unconfirmed contraindication) should consult a healthcare provider before using licorice.

PREGNANCY AND LACTATION: Not recommended for use during pregnancy. No known restrictions during lactation.

ADVERSE EFFECTS

No adverse effects have been associated with licorice when used appropriately. The prolonged use of licorice in high doses (greater than 50 g/day) and for more than six weeks may lead to sodium and water retention, and to potassium loss accompanied by high blood pressure, water retention, and potential cardiac complications. Aqueous licorice root extracts are less likely than isolated glycyrrhizin to produce side effects.

DRUG INTERACTIONS

Licorice may increase the side effects of potassium-depleting thiazide diuretics, including chlorothiazide, chlorthalidone, hydrochlorothiazide, and metolazone. With the loss of potassium, sensitivity to digitalis glycosides (heart medications) increases. Licorice should not be combined with corticosteroid drug treatment.

AMERICAN BOTANICAL COUNCIL

The information contained on this sheet has been excerpted from *The ABC Clinical Guide to Herbs* © 2003 by the American Botanical Council (ABC). ABC is an independent member-based educational organization focusing on the medicinal use of herbs. For more detailed information about this herb please consult the healthcare provider who gave you this sheet. To order *The ABC Clinical Guide to Herbs* or become a member of ABC, visit their website at www.herbalgram.org.

Licorice

Glycyrrhiza spp.

Glycyrrhiza glabra L. (syn. G. *glandulifera* Walst. & Kit.), G. *uralensis* Fisch. Ex DC.
[Fam. *Fabaceae*]

OVERVIEW

Licorice root is presently one of the most widely used medicinal herbs, and has been used therapeutically for several thousand years in Western and Eastern medicine (Gibson, 1978; Leung and Foster, 1996; Wang *et al.,* 2000). Licorice ranks as the 10th most important herb for Western medical herbalists and in Unani traditional medicine clinics in Pakistan (Bergner, 1994; American Institute of Unani Medicine, 1999). In Traditional Chinese Medicine (TCM), licorice root is the most commonly-used herb, though it is almost always used in combination with other herbs (Leung, 1999).

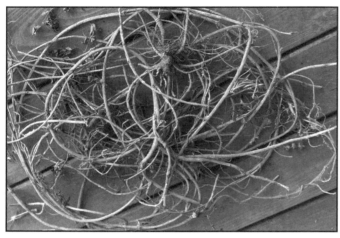

Photo © 2003 stevenfoster.com

DESCRIPTION

Licorice root consists of the dried roots and rhizomes of *Glycyrrhiza glabra* L. (syn. G. *glandulifera* Walst. & Kit.) and its varieties or G. *uralensis* (WHO, 1999; McGuffin *et al.,* 2001), or other species of *Glycyrrhiza* (US FDA, 1998), and contains no less than 4% glycyrrhizic acid (syn. glycyrrhizin) (Ph.Eur., 2001). Peeled roots contain no less than 20% water-soluble extractive, and unpeeled roots contain no less than 25% water-soluble extract (Blumenthal *et al.,* 1998), and no less than 25% dilute ethanol-soluble extract (JP XII, 1991; JSHM, 1993).

PRIMARY USES

Crude Preparations
- Catarrh of the upper respiratory tract (Blumenthal *et al.,* 1998)

Deglycyrrhized Licorice Extract (DGL) Preparations
- Aphthous, stomatitis (oral ulcers) (Das *et al.,* 1989)
- Gastric ulcers (Morgan *et al.,* 1985)
- Duodenal ulcer (Kassir, 1985; Larkworthy and Holgate, 1975)

NOTE: The German Commission E also approved licorice preparations containing glycyrrhizin for gastric and duodenal ulcers.

OTHER POTENTIAL USES

Miscellaneous Preparations
- Prevention of radiation complications in lungs during radiotherapy (Palagina *et al.,* 1999) [extract]
- Chronic hepatitis (Chang and But, 1986; Huang, 1999) [decoction]
- Sore throat, as a demulcent (IP, 1996; WHO, 1999) [form not specified]
- Cough with viscid expectoration (Schilcher, 1997) [extract, tea, or juice]
- Dyspepsia (WHO, 1999) [form not specified]

Purified Licorice Derivatives
- Hepatic failure, subacute (Acharya *et al.,* 1993) [NOTE: i.v. preparation]
- Reduced risk of liver carcinogenesis in hepatitis C patients (Arase *et al.,* 1997)

Uses in TCM
- Bronchitis, pharyngitis, laryngitis, bronchial asthma, chronic hypocorticoidism (PPRC, 1992)

Combination Preparations
- Infantile colic—with chamomile flower (*Matricaria* spp.), fennel seed (*Foeniculum vulgare*), vervain herb (*Verbena hastata*), and lemon balm leaf (*Melissa officinalis*) (Weizman *et al.,* 1993; Zand *et al.,* 1994)
- Productive cough in children—with marshmallow root (*Althaea officinalis*), anise seed (*Pimpinella anisum*), and cowslip flower (*Primula veris*) (Schilcher, 1997)

DOSAGE

Internal

Crude Preparations

DECOCTION: 1.0–1.5 g licorice root placed in approximately 150–250 ml cold water. Boiled, simmered for 10–15 minutes, then strained, 2–3 times daily (Meyer-Buchtela, 1999; ÖAB, 1991; Wichtl and Bisset, 1994).

INFUSION: Approximately 150 ml boiling water poured over 4.5 g licorice root and steeped 10–15 minutes; 2–3 times daily (Braun *et al.,* 1997).

FLUID EXTRACT BP [1:1 (g/ml), 16–20% ethanol (v/v)]: 2–5 ml, 3 times daily (BP, 1980; Bradley, 1992).

POWDERED ROOT: Approximately 5–15 g root daily, equivalent to 200–600 mg glycyrrhizin (Blumenthal *et al.,* 1998), 2–4 g single dose (API, 1989). NOTE: After decocting for 10 minutes, approximately 50% of the available glycyrrhizin, and approximately 45% of the liquiritin are released into the tea. After

30 minutes, approximately 80% of the glycyrrhizin, and 75% of the liquiritin are released, respectively (Meyer-Buchtela, 1999).

Deglycyrrhized Licorice (DGL) Preparations
DGL NATIVE DRY EXTRACT BP [0.5–2.0% total flavonoids, calculated as liquiritigenin]: 0.4–1.6 g, 3 times daily (BP, 1986; Bradley, 1992).

DGL CHEWABLE TABLETS [380 mg DGL 4:1]: For acute cases of gastric or duodenal ulcers; 2–4 tablets chewed before each meal. For chronic cases, 1–2 tablets chewed before each meal (Pizzorno and Murray, 1999).

Standardized Preparations
FLUID EXTRACT DAB [2.0–4.0% glycyrrhizin, 52–65% ethanol (v/v)]: 5–15 ml daily, (or 2–5 ml, 3 times daily) corresponding to Commission E dosage of 5–15 g of root daily (Blumenthal et al., 1998).

FLUID EXTRACT PPRC [minimum 7.0% glycyrrhizin, 20–25% ethanol (v/v)]: 2–5 ml, 3 times daily (PPRC, 1992).

NATIVE DRY EXTRACT [4–5:1 (w/w), minimum 20% glycyrrhizin]: 0.33–0.8 g, after meals 3 times daily.

DURATION OF ADMINISTRATION
No longer than four to six weeks internally without medical advice. There is no objection to using licorice root as a flavoring agent up to a maximum daily dosage equivalent to 100 mg glycyrrhizin (Blumenthal et al., 1998). A diet rich in potassium (e.g., bananas) is recommended during treatment period (Bruneton, 1999).

CHEMISTRY
Licorice root contains triterpenoid saponins, mainly glycyrrhizin (glycyrrhizic acid, glycyrrhizinic acid) (Tang and Eisenbrand, 1992; Ph. Eur. minimum 4%) with the sapogenin glycyrrhetic acid (glycyrrhetin, glycyrrhetinic acid). Glycyrrhetic acid is a triterpene with an oleanan skeleton (Tang and Eisenbrand, 1992). Licorice also contains approximately 1% flavonoids, mainly flavanones (e.g., liquiritin), chalcones (e.g. isoliquiritin), and isoflavonoids (e.g., formononetin); polysaccharides (arabinogalactans); and sterols (β-sitosterol, stigmasterol) (Bradley, 1992; Tang and Eisenbrand, 1992).

PHARMACOLOGICAL ACTIONS
Human
Crude Preparations
Anti-inflammatory; expectorant; demulcent; adrenocorticotropic (Bradley, 1992); reduces serum testosterone in men (Armanini et al., 1999); antioxidant (Fuhrman et al., 1997).

Deglycyrrhized Licorice (DGL) Preparations
Protects LDL against lipid peroxidation (Fuhrman et al., 1997).

Purified Licorice Derivatives
Accelerates the healing of gastric ulcers in controlled clinical studies of glycyrrhizic acid and the aglycone of glycyrrhizic acid (Blumenthal et al., 1998).

Animal
Secretolytic and expectorant effects in rabbits; antispasmodic action in isolated rabbit ileum has been observed (Blumenthal et al., 1998); antioxidant and oxygen radical-scavenging in rats (Yokozawa et al., 2000); may have cancer chemopreventive effects (Wang et al., 2000); induces liver microsomal cytochrome P450 in mice (Hu et al., 1999); inhibits decline in immune complex (IC) clearance in carrageenan-injected mice (Matsumato et al., 1996); prevents gastric mucosal damage in rats (Goso et al.,

1996); protects mitochondrial function against oxidative stresses (Haraguchi et al., 2000); anti-arrhythmic action of total licorice flavonoids (e.g. liquiritigenin and isoliquiritigenin) in mice and guinea pigs (Hu et al., 1999); protects liver (Nose et al., 1994; Shim et al., 2000); inhibits generation of suppressor T-cells in thermally injured mice (Kobayashi et al., 1993). Phytosterols, beta-sitosterol, and stigmasterol are estrogenic in castrated mice (Van Hulle, 1970).

In vitro
Binds estrogen receptors (Zava et al., 1998); antimicrobial (Li et al., 1998; Okada et al., 1989); antioxidant (Okada et al., 1989); decreases arylamine N-acetyltransferase (NAT) activity in Helicobacter pylori cultures from peptic ulcer patients (Chung, 1998); anti-tumor necrosis factor (TNF) activity (Yoshikawa et al., 1997).

MECHANISM OF ACTION
- Glycyrrhizin is metabolized to its aglycone 18-β-glycyrrhetinic acid in the intestine by human intestinal bacteria, which is then absorbed into the blood
- Protects liver through 18-β-glycyrrhetinic acid and glycyrrhizin (Shim et al., 2000)
- Relieves gastric inflammation, possibly by inhibiting prostaglandin synthesis and lipoxygenase (Inoue et al., 1986; Tamura et al., 1979)
- Antigastric ulcer activity is due to the FM 100 fraction (licorione), which lowers gastric acidity, reduces pepsin activity, and inhibits gastric secretion (Huang, 1999)
- Inhibits human 11-β-hydroxysteroid dehydrogenase, the enzyme that catalyzes the conversion of cortisol to cortisone, and bacterial 3-alpha, 20-beta-hydroxysteroid dehydrogenase (Duax et al., 2000)
- Inhibits 11-β-hydroxysteroid dehydrogenase, which minimizes the binding of cortisol to mineralocorticoid receptors, creating a mineralocorticoid-like effect (Farese et al., 1991)
- Inhibits peripheral metabolism of corticol, which binds to mineralocorticoid receptors in the same way as aldosterone (Heikens et al., 1995)
- May also inhibit both 17-β-hydroxysteroid dehydrogenase and 17,20-lyase, which catalyzes conversion of 17-hydroxy-progesterone to androstenedione (Armanini et al., 1999)
- Modulates the cell-mediated immune system, which may be due to glycyrrhizin stimulating the induction of contrasuppressor cells (Kobayashi et al., 1993)
- Demulcent and expectorant actions due to stimulating tracheal mucous secretion (Hikino, 1985)
- Antioxidant action may be related to absorption and binding of licorice's flavonoids (e.g., glabridin) to the LDL particle, thereby protecting the LDL from oxidation (Fuhrman et al., 1997)

CONTRAINDICATIONS
The German Commission E states that licorice is contraindicated in cholestatic liver disorders, liver cirrhosis, hypertension, hypokalemia, and severe kidney insufficiency (Blumenthal et al., 1998). Licorice is also contraindicated in diabetes by the Belgian Pharmaceutical Association (Van Hellemont, 1986), although this was not confirmed in a subsequent monograph by the World Health Organization (WHO, 1999).

PREGNANCY AND LACTATION: Not recommended during pregnancy (Braun *et al.,* 1997; McGuffin *et al.,* 1997; WHO, 1999). The effect of glycyrrhizin was studied on 1,049 Finnish women and their infants. Heavy exposure to glycyrrhizin (<500 mg/wk) did not affect birth weight, but did double the risk of birth before 38 weeks (Strandberg *et al.,* 2001). No known restrictions during lactation.

ADVERSE EFFECTS

No adverse effects have been associated with licorice used within proper dosage and treatment period limits (Schulz *et al.,* 1998; WHO, 1999). With prolonged use (longer than six weeks), and higher doses (greater than 50 g/day), sodium and water retention and a loss of potassium may occur, accompanied by hypertension, edema, hypokalemia, and in rare cases, myoglobinuria (Blumenthal *et al.,* 1998; WHO, 1999). With short-term treatment for cough, these mineralocorticoid effects did not develop (Schilcher, 1997). Within several weeks of discontinuing use, any symptoms of hyperaldosteronism should disappear (Mantero, 1981). Side effects are less likely with aqueous licorice root extract than with isolated glycyrrhizin, due to lower intestinal absorption when consumed as a component of the total extract (Cantelli-Forti *et al.,* 1994). There has been one case report of pulmonary edema following an acute overdose (approximately 1,020 g, containing ~3.6 g glycorrhizic acid in three days) of Hershey Twizzlers® black licorice-flavored candy (Chamberlain and Abolnik, 1997). There is one case report of life-threatening ventricular tachycardia due to hypokalemia induced by overdose (approximately 40–70g daily for four months) of a licorice candy (Eriksson *et al.,* 1999), though the brand of the candy, and the actual quantity of licorice or licorice derivatives contained in the candy are missing from the report.

DRUG INTERACTIONS

Licorice may potentiate the side effects of potassium depleting thiazide diuretics (e.g., chlorothiazide, chlorthalidone, hydrochlorothiazide, and metolazone) (Austin *et al.,* 2000; Blumenthal *et al.,* 1998; Shintani *et al.,* 1992). With potassium loss, sensitivity to digitalis glycosides increases (Blumenthal *et al.,* 1998; Van Hellemont, 1986). The 1998 French Explanatory Note warns not to combine with corticoid treatment (Bruneton, 1999). When decocted in combination with toxic herbs such as prepared aconite root (*Aconitum carmichaelii* Debeaux), a detoxified preparation used in TCM, the yield of anti-arrhythmic licorice flavonoids is significantly higher than when decocted alone. This mitigated the toxic effects (e.g., arrhythmia) induced by aconitine (Hu *et al.,* 1999; Leung, 1999) in mice and guinea pigs.

AMERICAN HERBAL PRODUCTS ASSOCIATION (AHPA) SAFETY RATING

CLASS 2B: Not to be used during pregnancy (McGuffin *et al.,* 1997).

CLASS 2D: Not for prolonged use or in high doses except under supervision of a qualified health practitioner (McGuffin *et al.,* 1997).

REGULATORY STATUS

AUSTRIA: Unpeeled dried root is official in the *Austrian Pharmacopoeia* (Meyer-Buchtela, 1999; Wichtl, 1997).

BELGIUM: Traditional Herbal Medicine (THM) permitted for specific indications (Bradley, 1992; WHO, 1998).

CANADA: Approved active ingredient in THM products and in Homeopathic products, both requiring pre-marketing authorization with Drug Identification Number (DIN) assigned (Health Canada, 2001). Food if no claim statement is made.

CHINA: Dried root and rhizome, prepared (stir-fried with honey) root and rhizome, alcoholic fluid extract and dry aqueous native extract, containing not less than (NLT) 20.0% glycyrrhetic acid, are official drugs of the *Pharmacopoeia of the People's Republic of China* (PPRC, 1997).

EUROPEAN UNION: Dried unpeeled or peeled, root and stolons containing NLT 4.0% glycyrrhizic acid and standardized ethanolic fluid extract containing NLT 3.0% and NMT 5.0% glycyrrhizic acid are official in *European Pharmacopoeia* (Ph.Eur. 2001).

FRANCE: THM permitted for specific indications, internal or locally (mouth and throat). Official in *French Pharmacopoeia* (Bradley, 1992; Bruneton, 1999; WHO, 1998).

GERMANY: Dried root or dry extract for infusion, decoction, liquid or solid dosage forms, are approved non-prescription drugs in the Commission E monographs (Blumenthal *et al.,* 1998). Licorice root tea is approved as an over-the-counter (OTC) drug in the *German Standard License* monographs (Braun *et al.,* 1997). Peeled dried root containing NLT 4.0% glycyrrhizic acid, and standardized ethanolic fluid extract containing NLT 5.0% and NMT 7.0% glycyrrhizic acid are official in *German Drug Codex* supplement to *German Pharmacopoeia* (DAC, 1990 & 1995). Standardized ethanolic fluid extract containing NLT 2.0% and NMT 4.0% glycyrrhizic acid are official in *German Pharmacopoeia* (DAB, 1999).

INDIA: Dried unpeeled roots and stolons containing NLT 4.0% glycyrrhizinic acid are official in *Indian Pharmacopoeia* (IP, 1996). Dried unpeeled stolon and root are official in the Government of India *Ayurvedic Pharmacopoeia of India* (API, 1989). Prepared mature root (min. 4 years) is an official single-drug and/or component of multiple-ingredient drugs dispensed in Unani system of medicine (CCRUM, 1986 & 1997). A monograph for dried root occurs in the *Indian Herbal Pharmacopoeia* (IHP I, 1998).

ITALY: Listed in the *Italian Pharmacopoeia* (Newall *et al.,* 1996).

JAPAN: Traditional Kampo medicine. Dried peeled or unpeeled root and stolon are official in the *Japanese Pharmacopoeia* (JSHM, 1993).

RUSSIAN FEDERATION: Official in the *State Pharmacopoeia of the Union of Soviet Socialist Republics*, Ph.USSR X (Bradley, 1992; Newall *et al.,* 1996).

SWEDEN: Classified as foodstuff. As of January 2001, no licorice products are listed in the Medical Products Agency (MPA) "Authorised Natural Remedies" (MPA, 2001).

SWITZERLAND: Official in *Swiss Pharmacopoeia*, Ph.Helv.VII (Bradley, 1992; WHO, 1998; Wichtl, 1997). Licorice is an approved component of multi-ingredient phytomedicines listed in the *Swiss Codex* 2001/02 available in juice, syrup, tea infusion, and tincture dosage forms (Ruppanner and Schaefer, 2000) with positive classification (List D) by *Interkantonale Kontrollstelle für Heilmittel* (IKS) and corresponding sales Category D with sale limited to pharmacies and drugstores, without prescription (Morant and Ruppaner, 2001).

U.K.: Herbal medicine on the *General Sale List*, Schedule 1 (requires full Product License), Table A (internal or external use) (GSL, 1994). Dried unpeeled roots and stolons containing NLT

4.0% glycyrrhizinic acid, ethanolic fluid extract, and DGL dry aqueous extract containing 0.5~2.0% total flavonoids, calculated as liquiritigenin, are official in the *British Pharmacopoeia* (BP, 1986).

U.S.: Dietary supplement or food depending on label claim statement (USC, 1994). Licorice root and derivatives are affirmed as Generally Recognized as Safe (GRAS) for use as a flavoring agent or flavor enhancer in vitamin or mineral dietary supplements, herb and seasoning products and nonalcoholic beverages, including tea (US FDA, 1998). Dried roots, rhizome and stolons, powdered root, and powdered dry extract are subjects of botanical monographs in development for the *US National Formulary*. Previews of the standards development were published in *Pharmacopeial Forum* (USP, 2002).

CLINICAL REVIEW

Ten studies are outlined in the following table, "Clinical Studies on Licorice," including a total of 2,544 participants. Eight studies including a total of 1,505 participants. All but one of these studies (Armanini *et al.*, 1999) demonstrated positive effects for indications such as treatment of various types of ulcers, chemoprevention, and use as an antioxidant. Three studies were conducted on licorice root extract (Armanini *et al.*, 1999; Armanini *et al.*, 1996; Palagina *et al.*, 1999), four studies were on DGL extract (Fuhrman *et al.*, 1997; Das *et al.*, 1989; Kassir, 1985; Morgan *et al.*, 1985), and two studies were conducted on isolated glycyrrhizin preparations (Arase *et al.*, 1997; Acharya *et al.*, 1993). These include an open (O) study on the effects of licorice root tablets on gonadal function (Armanini *et al.*, 1999), a comparison (Cm) study on pulmonary metabolism during radiotherapy (Palagina *et al.*, 1999), an O study on pseudohyperaldosteronism (Armanini *et al.*, 1996), a placebo-controlled (PC) study on LDL cholesterol (Fuhrman *et al.*, 1997), an O, uncontrolled study on aphthous ulcer (Das *et al.*, 1989), a Cm, randomized (R) study on chronic duodenal ulceration (Kassir, 1985), and a single-blind, controlled, R study on benign gastric ulcers (Morgan *et al.*, 1985). Isolated glycyrrhizin has been investigated as a chemopreventive in one retrospective Cm (Arase *et al.*, 1997) and one O study on the treatment of subacute hepatic failure (Acharya *et al.*, 1993). One study on birth outcome found that licorice did not affect birth weight but did double the risk of birth before 38 weeks (Strandberg *et al.*, 2001).

BRANDED PRODUCTS

Caved-S®: Tillots Pharma AG / Hauptstrasse 27 / CH–4417 Zeifen / Switzerland / Tel: +41-61-935-2626 / Fax: +41-61-935-2625. Each tablet contains 380 mg deglycerized licorice extract. This product is no longer available.

Saila Licorice Root Tablets: Saila S.p.A. / 83 Viale Garibladi / Silvi Marina, Teramo / Italy. One tablet contains 500 mg glycyrrhizin.

Stronger Neo Minophagen-C (SNMC); Minophagen Pharmaceutical Co. / No. 3 Tomizawa Bldg. / 2-7, Yotsuya 3-chome / Shinjuku, Tokyo 160 / Japan / Tel: +81-3-3355-6561 / Fax: +81-3-3355-6565. Standardized to contain 0.2% glycyrrhizin, 0.1% cysteine, and 2.0% glycine in physiologic saline, intravenous. This product is no longer available.

REFERENCES

Acharya S, Dasarathy S, Tandon A, Joshi Y, Tandon B. A preliminary open trial on interferon stimulator (SNMC) derived from *Glycyrrhiza glabra* in the treatment of subacute hepatic failure. *Indian J Med Res* 1993;98:69–74.

American Institute of Unani Medicine. Most popular botanicals in Unani traditional medicine [report]. Endicott, NY: American Institute of Unani Medicine; 1999.

API. See: *Ayurvedic Pharmacopoeia of India.*

Arase Y, Ikeda K, Murashima N, *et al.* The long-term efficacy of glycyrrhizin in chronic hepatitis C patients. *Cancer* 1997;79:1494–1500.

Armanini D, Bonanni G, Palermo M. Reduction of serum testosterone in men by licorice [letter]. *New Engl J Med* 1999;341:1158.

Armanini D, Lewicka S, Pratesi C, *et al.* Further studies on the mechanism of the mineralocorticoid action of licorice in humans. *J Endocrinol Invest* 1996;19(9):624–9.

Ayurvedic Pharmacopoeia of India (API), Part I, Vol. I, 1st edition. New Delhi, India: Government of India Ministry of Health and Family Welfare, Department of Health; 1989;127–8.

Austin S, Batz F, Yarnell E, Brown D. Common drugs and their potential interactions with herbs or nutrients. *Healthnotes Rev of Comp and Integrative Med* 2000;7(1):77–8.

Baker M, Fanestil D. Liquorice as a regulator of steroid and prostaglandin metabolism. *Lancet* 1991;337:428–9.

Bensky D, Gamble A, Kaptchuk T. *Chinese Herbal Medicine: Materia Medica*, 2nd edition. Seattle, WA: Eastland Press, Inc.; 1993; 323–5.

Bergner P. The top 25 herbs. *Medical Herbalism* 1994 Spring;6(1).

Blumenthal M, Busse WR, Goldberg A, Gruenwald J, Hall T, Riggins CW, Rister RS (eds.). Klein S, Rister RS (trans.). *The Complete German Commission E Monographs—Therapeutic Guide to Herbal Medicines.* Austin, TX: American Botanical Council; Boston: Integrative Medicine Communication; 1998; 161–2.

BP. See: *British Pharmacopoeia.*

Bradley P (ed.). *British Herbal Compendium*, Vol. 1. Dorset, UK: British Herbal Medicine Association; 1992;145–8.

Braun R, Surmann R, Wendt R, Wichtl M, Ziegenmeyer J. *Standardzulassungen für Fertigarzneimittel: Text und Kommentar.* Stuttgart, Germany: Deutscher Apotheker Verlag; 1997.

British Pharmacopoeia (BP 1980, Addendum 1986). London, UK: Her Majesty's Stationery Office; 1986;417–8, 480–1.

British Pharmacopoeia (BP 1980). London, UK: Her Majesty's Stationery Office; 1980;563.

Bruneton J. Pharmacognosy Phytochemistry Medicinal Plants, 2nd edition. Paris, France: Lavoisier Publishing; 1999;688–94.

Cantelli-Forti G, Maffei F, Hrelia P, *et al.* Interaction of licorice on glycyrrhizin pharmacokinetics. *Environ Health Perspectives* 1994;102:65–8.

CCRUM. See: Central Council for Research in Unani Medicine.

Central Council for Research in Unani Medicine (CCRUM). *Standardisation of Single Drugs of Unani Medicine,* Part III, 1st edition. New Delhi, India: Ministry of Health and Family Welfare, Government of India; 1997;272–4.

Central Council for Research in Unani Medicine (CCRUM). *A Handbook of Common Remedies in Unani System of Medicine,* 2nd edition. New Delhi, India: Ministry of Health and Family Welfare, Government of India; 1986.

Chamberlain J, Abolnik I. Letter to the Editor: Pulmonary edema following a licorice binge. *Western J Med* 1997;167(3):184–5.

Chandler R. *Glycyrrhiza glabra.* In: De Smet P, Keller K, Hänsel R, Chandler R. (eds.). *Adverse Effects of Herbal Drugs*, Vol. 3. New York: Springer Verlag; 1997.

Chang H, But P (eds.). *Pharmacology and Applications of Chinese Materia Medica*, Vol. 1. Philadelphia, PA: World Scientific; 1986;304–16.

Chung J. Inhibitory actions of glycyrrhizic acid on arylamine N-acetyltransferase activity in strains of *Helicobacter pylori* from peptic ulcer patients. *Drug Chem Toxicol* 1998;21:35–70.

DAB. 1999. See: *Deutsches Arzneibuch.*

DAC. See: *Deutscher Arzneimittel-Codex.*

Das S, Das V, Gulati A, Singh V. Deglycyrrhizinated liquorice in aphthous ulcers. *J Assoc Physicians India*1989;37(10):647.

Deutsches Arzneibuch (DAB Ergänzungslieferung 1999). Stuttgart, Germany: Deutscher Apotheker Verlag; 1999.

Deutscher Arzneimittel-Codex (DAC 1986, 7. Ergänzung 1995). Stuttgart, Germany: Deutscher Apotheker Verlag. 1995;S-207:1-3.

Deutscher Arzneimittel-Codex (DAC 1986, 2. Ergänzung 1990). Stuttgart, Germany: Deutscher Apotheker Verlag. 1990;S-210:1-6.

Duax W, Ghosh D, Pletnev V. Steroid dehydrogenase structures, mechanism of action, and disease. *Vitam Horm* 2000;58:121–48.

Eriksson J, Carlberg B, Hillörn V. Life-threatening ventricular tachycardia due to liquorice-induced hypokalaemia. *J Int Med* 1999;245:307–10.

Europäisches Arzneibuch (Ph.Eur. 3, Nachtrag 1998). Stuttgart, Germany: Deutscher Apotheker Verlag; 1998;622–23.

European Pharmacopoeia (Ph.Eur. 3rd edition Supplement 2001). Strasbourg, France: Council of Europe. 2001;1061-1064.

Farese R Jr, Biglieri E, Shackleton C, Irony I, Gomez-Fontes R. Licorice-induced hypermineralocorticoidism. *N Engl J Med* 1991;325:1223–7.

Feldman H, Gilat T. A trial of deglycyrrhizinated liquorice in the treatment of duodenal ulcer. *Gut* 1971;12:499–510.

Fuhrman B, Buch S, Vaya J, et al. Licorice extract and its major polyphenol glabridin protect low-density lipoprotein against lipid peroxidation: *In vitro* and *ex vivo* studies in humans in and in atherosclerotic lipoprotein E-deficient mice. *Am J Clin Nutr* 1997;66:267–75.

General Sales List (GSL). Statutory Instrument (S.I.). The Medicines (Products other than Veterinary Drugs). London, UK: Her Majesty's Stationery Office. 1984; S.I. No. 769, as amended 1985; S.I. No. 1540, 1990; S.I. No. 1129, 1994; S.I. No. 2410.

Gibson M. Glycyrrhiza in old and new perspectives. *Lloydia* 1978;41(4):348–54.

Glick L. Deglycyrrhizinated liquorice for peptic ulcer. *Lancet* 1982 Oct 9;ii:817.

Goso Y, Ogata Y, Ishihara K, Hotta K. Effects of traditional herbal medicine on gastric mucin against ethanol-induced gastric injury in rats. *Comp Biochem Physiol C Pharmacol Toxicol Endocrinol* 1996;113(1):17–21.

GSL. See: *General Sale List.*

Haraguchi H, Yoshida N, Ishikawa H, et al. Protection of mitochondrial functions against oxidative stresses by isoflavans from *Glycyrrhiza glabra. J Pharm Pharmacol* 2000;52(2):219–23.

Health Canada. *Glycyrrhiza glabra.* In: *Drug Product Database (DPD).* Ottawa, Ontario: Health Canada Therapeutic Products Programme. 2001.

Heikens J, Fliers E, Endert E, Ackermans M, van Montfrans G. Liquorice-induced hypertension—a new understanding of an old disease: case report and brief review. *Neth J Med* 1995;47(5):230–4.

Hikino H. Recent research on oriental medicinal plants. In: Wagner H, Hikino H, Farnsworth N (eds.). *Economic and Medicinal Plant Research*, Vol. 1. London, UK: Academic Press; 1985;53–85.

Hu W, Li Y, Hou Y, et al. The induction of liver microsomal cytochrome P450 by Glycyrrhiza uralensis and glycyrrhetinic acid in mice. *Biomed Environ Sci* 1999;12(1):10–4.

Hu X, et al. Anti-arrhythmic effects of total flavonoids of licorice. [in Chinese]. *Zhongcaoya* 1996;27(12):733–5.

Huang K. *The Pharmacology of Chinese Herbs*, 2nd edition. Boca Raton, FL: CRC Press; 1999;363–9.

IHP. See: *Indian Herbal Pharmacopoeia.*

Indian Herbal Pharmacopoeia (IHP Volume I). Jammu-Tawi, India: Regional Research Laboratory, Council of Scientific & Industrial Research (CSIR). 1998;89-98.

Indian Pharmacopoeia (IP), Vol. I (A-O). Delhi, India: Controller of Publications, Government of India, Ministry of Health & Family Welfare; 1996;440–2.

Inoue H, Saito K, Koshihara Y, Murota S. Inhibitory effect of glycyrrhetinic acid derivatives of lipoxygenase and prostaglandin synthetase. *Chem Pharm Bull* 1986;34:897.

IP. See: *Indian Pharmacopoeia.*

Japanese Standards for Herbal Medicine. 1993. Tokyo, Japan: Yakuji Nippo, Ltd.; 1993;130–3.

JP XII. See: *Pharmacopoeia of Japan XII.*

JSHM. See: *Japanese Standards for Herbal Medicines.*

Kapoor L. *CRC Handbook of Ayurvedic Medicinal Plants.* Boca Raton, FL: CRC Press, Inc.; 1990;194–5.

Kassir Z. Endoscopic controlled trial of four drug regimens in the treatment of chronic duodenal ulceration. *Irish Med J* 1985;78:153–6.

Kobayashi M, Schmitt D, et al. Inhibition of burn-associated suppressor cell generation by glycyrrhizin through the induction of contrasuppressor T-cells. *Immunol Cell Cio*1993;71:181–9.

Larkworthy W, Holgate P. Deglycyrrhizinized liquorice in the treatment of chronic duodenal ulcer. A retrospective endoscopic survey of 32 patients. *Practitioner* 1975;215(1290):787–92.

Leung A. Licorice as "mitigator" of harsh drugs. *Leung's Chinese Herb News* 1999;23:3.

Leung A, Foster S. *Encyclopedia of Common Natural Ingredients Used in Food, Drugs, and Cosmetics*, 2nd ed. New York, NY: John Wiley & Sons, Inc.; 1996;346–9.

Li W, Asada Y, Yoshikawa T. Antimicrobial flavonoids from *Glycyrrhiza glabra* hairy root cultures. *Planta Med* 1998;64:746–7.

Mantero F. Exogenous mineralocorticoid-like disorders. *Clin Endocrinol Metab* 1981;10(3): 465–78.

Matsumoto T, Tanaka M, Yamada H, Cyong J. Effect of licorice roots on carrageenan-induced decrease in immune complex clearance in mice. *J Ethnopharmacol* 1996;53:1–4.

McGuffin M, Hobbs C, Upton R, Goldberg A (eds.). *American Herbal Product Association's Botanical Safety Handbook.* Boca Raton, FL: CRC Press; 1997;58.

McGuffin M, Kartesz J, Leung A, Tucker A (eds.). *Herbs of Commerce* 2nd ed. Silver Spring, MD: American Herbal Products Assn; 2001.

Medical Products Agency (MPA). *Naturläkemedel: Authorised Natural Remedies (as of January 24, 2001).* Uppsala, Sweden: Medical Products Agency. 2001.

MediHerb. Licorice—the universal herb. *MediHerb Newsletter* 1989.

Meyer-Buchtela E. *Tee-Rezepturen: Ein Handbuch für Apotheker und Ärzte.* Stuttgart, Germany: Deutscher Apotheker Verlag; 1999.

Morant J, Ruppanner H (eds.). *Arzneimittel-Kompendium der Schweiz®* 2001 *Publikumsausgabe.* Basel, Switzerland: Documed AG. 2001.

Morgan A, Pacsoo C, McAdam W. Maintenance therapy: a two-year comparison between Caved-S® and Cimetidine treatment in prevention of symptomatic gastric ulcer recurrence. *Gut* 1985;26:599–602.

Morgan A, McAdam W, Pacsoo C, Darnborough A. Comparison between cimetidine and Caved-S® in the treatment of gastric ulceration, and subsequent maintenance therapy. *Gut* 1982;23(6):545–51.

MPA. See: Medical Products Agency.

Murray M, Pizzorno J. *Encyclopedia of Natural Medicine.* Rocklin, CA: Prima Publishing; 1998;817.

Newall CA, Anderson LA, Phillipson JD. *Herbal Medicines: A Guide for Health-care Professionals.* London, U.K.: The Pharmaceutical Press. 1996;183-186.

Nose M, Ito M, et al. A comparison of the antihepatotoxic activity between glycyrrhizin and glycyrrhetinic acid. *Planta Med* 1994;60:136–9.

ÖAB. See: *Österreichisches Arzneibuch.*

Okada K, Tamura Y, Yamamoto M, et al. Identification of antimicrobial and antioxidant constituents from licorice of Russian and Xinjiang origin. *Chem Pharm Bull* 1989;37(9):2528–30.

Österreichisches Arzneibuch. (ÖAB 1991 mit 2. Nachtrag). Wien, Österreich: Verlag der Österreichischen Staatsdruckerei; 1991.

Palagina M, Khasina M, Klimkina T, Luchaninova V, Shvets O. State of pulmonary metabolism during radiotherapy of thoracic neoformations and possibilities of its correction. [in Russian]. *Ter Arkh* 1999;71(3):45–8.

Pharmacopoeia of Japan (JP XII 1991). Tokyo, Japan: The Society of Japanese Pharmacopoeia; 1991.

Pharmacopoeia of the People's Republic of China (PPRC English Edition 1997 Volume I). Beijing, China: Chemical Industry Press. 1997;153-154, 274-275.

Pharmacopoeia of the People's Republic of China (PPRC English Edition 1992). Guangzhou, China: Guangdong Science and Technology Press; 1992;165–6, 277–1.

Ph.Eur. See: *European Pharmacopoeia.*

Ph.Eur. 1998. See: *Europäisches Arzneibuch.*

Pizzorno JE, Murray MT, editors. *Textbook of Natural Medicine*, Vol. 1., 2nd ed. New York: Churchill Ligingstone; 1999;767–73.

PPRC. See: *Pharmacopoeia of the People's Republic of China.*

Rosenblat M, Belinky P, Vaya J. Macrophage enrichment with the isoflavan glabridin inhibits NADPH oxidase-induced cell-mediated oxidation of low-density lipoprotein. *J Biol Chem* 1999;274(20):13790–9.

Ruppanner H, Schaefer U (eds.). *Codex 2000/01 — Die Schweizer Arzneimittel in einem Griff.* Basel, Switzerland: Documed AG. 2000.

Schilcher H. *Phytotherapy in Paediatrics: Handbook for Physicians and Pharmacists.* Stuttgart, Germany: Medpharm Scientific Publishers; 1997;36–40.

Schulz V, Hänsel R, Tyler V. *Rational Phytotherapy: A Physicians' Guide to Herbal Medicine.* Berlin, Germany: Springer Verlag; 1998;154, 160–1, 184–6.

Shim S, Kim N, Kim D. ß-Glucuronidase inhibitory activity and hepatoprotective effect of 18ß-glycyrrhetinic acid from the rhizomes of *Glycyrrhiza uralensis. Planta Med* 2000;66(1):40–3.

Shintani S, Murase H, Tsukagoshi H, Shiigai T. Glycyrrhizin (licorice)-induced hypokalemic myopathy. Report of two cases and review of the literature. *Eur Neurol* 1992;32:44–51.

Strandberg TD, Javenpaa A-L, Vanhanen H, McKeigue PM. Birth Outcome in Relation to Licorice Consumption during Pregnancy. *American Journal of Epidemiology* 2001;153(11):1085–1088.

Tamura Y, Nishikawa T, Yamada K, Yamamoto M, Kumagai A. Effects of glycyrrhetinic acid and its derivatives on −5 *alpha*- and 5 *beta*-reductase in rat liver. *Arzneimittelforshung* 1979;29:647.

Tang W, Eisenbrand G. *Chinese Drugs of Plant Origin: Chemistry, Pharmacology, and Use in Traditional and Modern Medicine.* Berlin:Springer-Verlag;1992;567–88.

Tsarong T. *Handbook of Traditional Tibetan Drugs: Their Nomenclature, Composition, Use, and Dosage.* Kalimpong, India: Tibetan Medical Publications; 1986.

Tsumura & Co. Kampo ingredients kept in imperial storehouse for 1200 years retain their efficacy. *Kampo Today* 1997 Feb;2(1).

United States Congress (USC). Public Law 103–417: Dietary Supplement Health and Education Act of 1994. Washington, DC: 103rd Congress of the United States; 1994.

United States Food and Drug Administration (US FDA). Licorice and licorice derivatives. In: *Code of Federal Regulations* (21 CFR) Part 184 – Direct Food Substances Affirmed As Generally Recognized as Safe. Washington, DC: Office of the Federal Register National Archives and Records Administration; 1998;427–33.

United States Pharmacopeia (USP 25th Revision) - The National Formulary (NF 20th Edition). Rockville, MD: United States Pharmacopeial Convention, Inc. 2002.

USC. See: United States Congress.

US FDA. See: United States Food and Drug Administration.

USP. See: United States Pharmacopeial Convention.

Van Hellemont J. *Compendium de Phytotherapie.* Bruxelles, Belgique: Association Pharmaceutique Belge; 1986.

Van Hulle C. Über die östrogene Wirkung der Süßholzwurzel. *Die Pharmazie* 1970;25(10):620–1.

Wang Z, Athar M, Bickers D. Licorice in foods and herbal drugs: chemistry, pharmacology, toxicology and uses. In: Mazza G, Oomah BD (eds.). *Herbs, Botanicals & Teas.* Lancaster, PA: Technomic Publishing Co., Inc.; 2000;321–53.

Weizman Z, Alkrinawi S, Goldfarb D, Bitran C. Efficacy of herbal tea preparation in infantile colic. *J Pediatr* 1993;122(4):650–2.

Werbach M, Murray M. *Botanical Influences on Illness: A Sourcebook of Clinical Research*, 2nd edition. Tarzana, CA: Third Line Press, Inc.; 2000;264–5.

Wichtl M (ed.). *Teedrogen und Phytopharmaka*, 3. Auflage: Ein Handbuch für die Praxis auf wissenschaftlicher Grundlage. Stuttgart, Germany: Wissenschaftliche Verlagsgesellschaft mbH. 1997;351-355.

Wichtl M, Bisset NG (eds.). *Herbal Drugs and Phytopharmaceuticals: A Handbook for Practice on a Scientific Basis.* Stuttgart, Germany: Medpharm Scientific Publishers; 1994;301–4.

WHO. See: World Health Organization.

World Health Organization (WHO). *WHO Monographs on Selected Medicinal Plants*, Vol. 1. Geneva, Switzerland; 1999;183–94.

World Health Organization (WHO). *Regulatory Status of Herbal Medicines: A Worldwide Review.* Geneva, Switzerland: World Health Organization Traditional Medicine Programme; 1998;14, 17, 25–6, 30.

Yokozawa T, Liu Z, Chen C. Protective effects of Glycyrrhizae radix extract and its compounds in a renal hypoxia (ischemia)-reoxygenation (reperfusion) model. *Phytomedicine* 2000;6(6):439–45.

Yoshikawa M, Matsui Y, Kawamoto H, *et al.* Effects of glycyrrhizin on immune mediated cytotoxicity. *J Gastroenterol Hepatol* 1997;12:243–8.

Zand J, Walton R, Rountree B. *Smart Medicine for a Healthier Child: A Practical A-to-Z Reference to Natural and Conventional Treatments for Infants & Children.* Garden City Park, NY: Avery Publishing Group; 1994;161.

Zava D, Dollbaum C, Blen M. Estrogen and progestin bioactivity of foods, herbs, and spices. *Proc Soc Exp Biol Med* 1998;217:369–78.

Clinical Studies on Licorice (*Glycyrrhiza* spp.)

Ulcers

Author/Year	Subject	Design	Duration	Dosage	Preparation	Results/Conclusion
Das *et al.*, 1989	Aphthous ulcer	O, U n=20	2 weeks	Mouthwash with 200 mg DGL extract solution, 4x/day	DGL powdered extract dissolved in 200 ml warm water (brand not stated)	15 of 20 (75%) experienced 50–75% improvement within 1 day followed by complete healing of ulcers by 3rd day.
Kassir, 1985	Chronic duodenal ulceration	Cm, R n=874 (169 in Caved-S® group)	3 months	380 mg tablet 3x/day	Caved-S® tablet (380 mg DGL extract) vs. antacid (AL-Mg hydroxide equivalent) vs. cimetidine vs. Gefarnate	At 6 weeks a highly significant difference (p<0.01) in favor of antacid, but at 12 weeks no significant difference (p>0.05) among the 4 groups. There were fewer relapses in the DGL group compared to the 3 other treatments.
Morgan *et al.*, 1985	Benign gastric ulcer	SB, C, R, Cm n=82	3 months healing study continued as 2–year maintenance study	Two, 380 mg DGL extract tablets plus antacid combination chewed between meals 3x/day vs. cimetidine (200 mg 3x daily and 400 mg at bedtime)	Caved-S® containing 380 mg DGL extract per tablet vs. cimetidine	No significant difference between 2 drug regimens. After ulcer healing, drug dosage was reduced. After one year of maintenance therapy, there were 4 ulcer recurrences in each group. After second year, recurrence rate was 29% in Caved-S® group and 25% in cimetidine group. Authors conclude that long-term maintenance therapy is safe and reasonably effective.

Other

Author/Year	Subject	Design	Duration	Dosage	Preparation	Results/Conclusion
Strandberg *et al.*, 2001	Birth effects	O n=1,049 questionairres distributed in the hospital and review of maternity records	9 months	Glycyrrhizin levels from licorice consumption grouped into 3 levels: low (<250 mg/week; n=751), moderate (250–499 mg/week; n=145) and heavy (≥500 mg/wk; n=110)	Brand not stated	Heavy exposure to glycyrrhizin (<500 mg/wk) did not affect birth weight, but did double the risk of birth before 38 weeks.
Armanini *et al.*, 1999	Gonadal function	O n=7 healthy men (ages 22–24 years)	1 week treatment followed by 4 days of no treatment	7 g licorice root extract/day (500 mg glycyrrhizin)	Saila licorice root tablets	Serum testosterone concentrations decreased and serum 17-hydroxy-progesterone concentrations increased during treatment period. Authors concluded that men with decreased libido or other sexual dysfunction should be cautioned about licorice ingestion.
Palagina *et al.*, 1999	Pulmonary metabolism during radiotherapy in women ages 20–40 years with breast cancer Stage I–II	Cm n=25 women with breast cancer Stage I–II	2 weeks	Not available	Ural licorice extract (brand not stated)	Administration of licorice promoted inactivation of lipid peroxidation and maintenance of most biochemical parameters on baseline level. It is speculated that this effect is due to licorice components with antioxidant and lung surfactant synthesis stimulant actions. Authors conclude that licorice extract is promising for prevention of radiation complications in lungs during radiotherapy in chest area.

KEY: C – controlled, **CC** – case-control, **CH** – cohort, **CI** – confidence interval, **Cm** – comparison, **CO** – crossover, **CS** – cross-sectional, **DB** – double-blind, **E** – epidemiological, **LC** – longitudinal cohort, **MA** – meta-analysis, **MC** – multi-center, **n** – number of patients, **O** – open, **OB** – observational, **OL** – open label, **OR** – odds ratio, **P** – prospective, **PB** – patient-blind, **PC** – placebo-controlled, **PG** – parallel group, **PS** – pilot study, **R** – randomized, **RC** – reference-controlled, **RCS** – retrospective cross-sectional, **RS** - retrospective, **S** – surveillance, **SB** – single-blind, **SC** – single-center, **U** – uncontrolled, **UP** – unpublished, **VC** – vehicle-controlled.

Clinical Studies on Licorice (*Glycyrrhiza* spp.)   (cont.)

Other (cont.)

Author/Year	Subject	Design	Duration	Dosage	Preparation	Results/Conclusion
Arase et al., 1997	Chemo-prevention	RS, Cm n=453 patients with hepatitis C (84 in SNMC group)	16 years (median, 10.1 years)	100 ml/day intravenous first 8 weeks, followed by 2–7x/week for 2–16 years	Stronger Neo-Minophagen-C (SNMC) providing 0.2% glycyrrhizin, 0.1% cysteine, and 2.0% glycine in physiologic saline	After 10 years, cumulative incidence of hepatocellular carcinoma (HCC) was 7% in SNMC group and 12% for non-treatment group. After 15 years, cumulative incidences were 12% and 25%, respectively. Statistically significant reduction in serum alanine aminotransferase (ALT) levels was reported in 34 of 84 patients (35.7%) in treatment group. HCC in 30 patients with normal ALT levels was slightly lower than the 54 remaining patients with higher ALT scores (p=0.08). An increase in blood pressure was noted in 3 of 84 patients. Authors concluded that long-term administration of SNMC in patients with chronic HCC is effective in reducing risk of liver carcinogenesis.
Fuhrman et al., 1997	Antioxidant action	PC (ex vivo assay) n=20 healthy male volunteers	2 weeks	100 mg DGL extract/day	DGL extract in softgel capsule (brand not stated)	In licorice group, 44% reduction in lipid peroxides formed per mg of LDL cholesterol after exposure of plasma to copper sulfate ex vivo, and 36% reduction after exposure to water-soluble free radical generator, vs. no significant changes observed in plasma of placebo group.
Armanini et al., 1996	Pseudohyper-aldosteronism	O n=6 male volunteers	1 week	7g licorice root extract/day (500 mg glycyrrhizin)	Saila licorice root tablets	Pseudohyperaldosteronism occurred during treatment period. Ratio of tetrahydrocortisol + allo tetrahydrocortisol to tetrahydroscortisone in urine increased in 5 cases after 3 days without increase of plasma mineralocorticoid activity. Authors concluded that pseudohyperaldosteronism is due to decreased activity of 11-ß-hydroxysteroid-dehydrogenase and in some cases a direct effect on mineralocorticoid receptors.
Acharya et al., 1993	Subacute hepatic failure	O n=18	3 months	40 or 100 ml/day intravenous first 30 days, followed by 3x/week for 8 weeks	Stronger Neo-Minophagen-C (SNMC) providing 0.2% glycyrrhizin, 0.1% cysteine, and 2.0% glycine in physiologic saline	Survival rate was 72.2% compared to reported rate of 31.1% in 98 patients who received supportive therapy (p<0.01). Authors concluded that further studies are necessary to standardize the dose and duration of therapy with SNMC in subacute hepatic failure.

KEY: C – controlled, **CC** – case-control, **CH** – cohort, **CI** – confidence interval, **Cm** – comparison, **CO** – crossover, **CS** – cross-sectional, **DB** – double-blind, **E** – epidemiological, **LC** – longitudinal cohort, **MA** – meta-analysis, **MC** – multi-center, **n** – number of patients, **O** – open, **OB** – observational, **OL** – open label, **OR** – odds ratio, **P** – prospective, **PB** – patient-blind, **PC** – placebo-controlled, **PG** – parallel group, **PS** – pilot study, **R** – randomized, **RC** – reference-controlled, **RCS** – retrospective cross-sectional, **RS** – retrospective, **S** – surveillance, **SB** – single-blind, **SC** – single-center, **U** – uncontrolled, **UP** – unpublished, **VC** – vehicle-controlled.

Licorice

Monograph

(This page intentionally left blank.)

Milk Thistle

Silybum marianum (L.) Gaertn.

[Fam. *Asteraceae*]

OVERVIEW

Milk thistle preparations have been used in European medicine for over 2,000 years to treat liver and biliary tract diseases. In 1998, $180 million was spent on milk thistle preparations in Germany alone. In the U.S. in 2000, milk thistle ranked 11th in sales of all herbal products sold in food, drug, and mass market outlets, reaching about $9 million in retail sales. With an estimated 50 clinical studies involving over 2,400 patients carried out using a proprietary milk thistle preparation from Germany, it is perhaps the best documented therapeutic agent available to treat various types of liver intoxication.

PRIMARY USES

- Liver disease, alcoholic
- Liver cirrhosis, alcoholic
- Infectious hepatitis
- Drug-induced hepatitis

OTHER POTENTIAL USES

- Liver disease secondary to diabetes mellitus
- To decrease toxicity of narcotics used in cholecystectomy surgery (gallbladder removal)
- *Amanita* mushroom poisoning (i.v. drip of purified compound silybinin)

PHARMACOLOGICAL ACTIONS

Hepatoprotective; reduces serum gamma glutamyl transpeptidase (GGT) and transaminases (ALT, AST); reduces triglyceride in serum; normalizes serum-bilirubin and BSP retention; reduces malondialdehyde concentration in serum; increases superoxide dismutase (SOD) activity in erythrocytes and lymphocytes; reduces cytotoxic lymphocytes in blood; reduces procollagen-III peptide in serum.

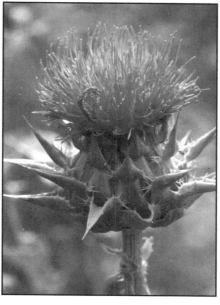

Photo © 2003 stevenfoster.com

DOSAGE AND ADMINISTRATION

For chronic conditions, milk thistle must be taken over an extended period for efficacy. For acute conditions that last longer than a week or recur periodically, patients are encouraged to seek a healthcare provider's advice. The duration of use for standardized preparations depends on the severity and chronic nature of the condition. Research has suggested that standardized extracts may be used continuously for as long as 24 months.

NOTE: The crude and infusion forms are indicated only for mild dyspeptic complaints, whereas high dosage and/or standardized extract forms are required for serious liver diseases. Due to the poor water solubility of silymarin, only a small fraction (<10%) of silymarin is released into an aqueous infusion.

DRY EXTRACT (STANDARDIZED): 40–70:1 (*w/w*), 70–80% silymarin, daily equivalent to 200–400 mg of silymarin, calculated as silibinin in divided doses. Many clinical trials have used a daily dose equivalent to 420 mg of silymarin, delivered in three divided doses. The dose of 140 mg must be swallowed with sufficient amounts of fluid.

NOTE: Most clinical studies on milk thistle have employed the concentrated, standardized extract.

CONTRAINDICATIONS

None known.

PREGNANCY AND LACTATION: No known restrictions.

ADVERSE EFFECTS

Crude Preparations

None known.

Standardized Preparations

A mild laxative effect has been observed occasionally. In one case report, a more severe gastrointestinal reaction to a milk thistle product occurred, but the link to the standardized extract is unclear.

DRUG INTERACTIONS

None known. Concomitant use of the purified silymarin fraction with butyrophenones or phenothiazines has resulted in the reduction of lipid peroxidation damage of the liver.

CLINICAL REVIEW

In 21 clinical studies on milk thistle that included a total of 2,430 participants, all but two studies demonstrated positive effects for indications including cirrhosis and alcoholic liver disease, hepatitis, and psychotropic drug-induced liver damage. Eight double-blind, placebo-controlled (DB, PC) studies investigated cirrhosis and alcoholic liver disease, involving over 600 patients. The most recent DB, PC study did not result in statistically significant findings on liver cirrhosis. Two randomized (R), DB, PC trials investigated milk thistle extract as a treatment for acute viral hepatitis A and B (HBV) and chronic active hepatitis due to HBV and/or hepatitis C (HCV). One observational study on 998 patients showed that milk thistle extract reduces collagen fibrogenesis in patients with toxic livers. Treatment of psychotropic drug-induced hepatic damage with purified silymarin is the subject of another R, DB, PC study and one multi-center study involving 220 patients over four years, which found that intravenous purified silibin complemented standard treatment, lowering mortality rates in cases of acute *Amanita* mushroom poisoning. A recent systematic review and meta-analysis funded by the National Institutes of Health (NIH) concluded that (1) the available evidence suggests that milk thistle extract is relatively safe, associated with few, generally minor, adverse events; (2) despite substantial *in vitro* and animal research, the mechanism of action is not fully defined and may be mulitfactorial; and (3) clinical efficacy is not clearly established because interpretation of the evidence is hampered by poor study methods and/or poor quality of reporting in publications. Other problems noted by NIH researchers included heterogeneity in etiology and extent of liver disease, small sample sizes, variation in formulation (for products other than Legalon®), dosing, and duration of therapy. Possible benefits have been shown most frequently for improvement in aminotransferases and liver function tests.

Milk Thistle

Silybum marianum (L.) Gaertn.
[Fam. *Asteraceae*]

OVERVIEW

Milk thistle preparations have been used in European medicine for over 2,000 years for the treatment of liver diseases. In the U.S. in 2000, milk thistle ranked 11th in sales of all herbal products sold in food, drug, and mass market outlets, reaching about $9 million in retail sales. With numerous clinical studies involving over 2,400 patients, it is perhaps the best documented therapy available for treating liver intoxication.

USES

Alcoholic liver disease; alcoholic liver cirrhosis; infectious hepatitis; drug-induced hepatitis.

DOSAGE

For chronic conditions, milk thistle must be taken over an extended period for efficacy. For acute conditions that last longer than a week or recur periodically, patients are encouraged to seek a healthcare provider's advice.

DRY EXTRACT (STANDARDIZED): 40–70:1 (*w/w*), 70–80% silymarin, daily equivalent to 200–400 mg of silymarin, calculated as silibinin in divided doses. Many clinical trials have used a daily dose equal to 420 mg of silymarin divided into three doses. The dose of 140 mg should be swallowed with sufficient amounts of fluid.

CONTRAINDICATIONS

No known contraindications.

PREGNANCY AND LACTATION: No known restrictions.

ADVERSE EFFECTS

The standardized preparation has occasionally caused a mild laxative effect.

DRUG INTERACTIONS

None known. Ingesting silymarin at the same time as psychopharmaceutical drugs, butyrophenones, or phenothiazines has produced the benefit of decreased lipid peroxidation damage of the liver.

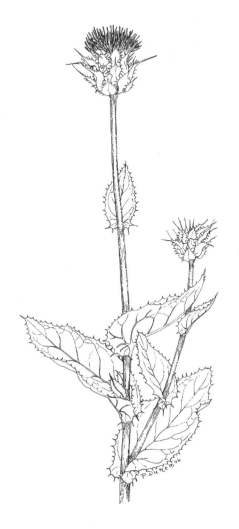

Comments

When using a dietary supplement, purchase it from a reliable source. For best results, use the same brand of product throughout the period of use. As with all medications and dietary supplements, please inform your healthcare provider of all herbs and medications you are taking. Interactions may occur between medications and herbs or even among different herbs when taken at the same time. Treat your herbal supplement with care by taking it as directed, storing it as advised on the label, and keeping it out of the reach of children and pets. Consult your healthcare provider with any questions.

AMERICAN
BOTANICAL
COUNCIL

The information contained on this sheet has been excerpted from *The ABC Clinical Guide to Herbs* © 2003 by the American Botanical Council (ABC). ABC is an independent member-based educational organization focusing on the medicinal use of herbs. For more detailed information about this herb please consult the healthcare provider who gave you this sheet. To order *The ABC Clinical Guide to Herbs* or become a member of ABC, visit their website at www.herbalgram.org.

Milk Thistle

Silybum marianum (L.) Gaertn.

[Fam. *Asteraceae*]

OVERVIEW

Milk thistle preparations have been used in European medicine for over 2,000 years to treat liver and biliary tract diseases (Der Marderosian and Liberti, 1997; Flora *et al.*, 1998; Foster, 1991). In 1998, $180 million was spent on milk thistle preparations in Germany alone (McCaleb *et al.*, 2000). In the U.S. in 2000, milk thistle ranked 11th in sales of all herbal products sold in food, drug, and mass market outlets, reaching about $9 million in retail sales (Blumenthal, 2001). With an estimated 50 clinical studies involving over 2,400 patients carried out using a proprietary milk thistle preparation from Germany (Blumenthal *et al.*, 2000), it is perhaps the best documented therapeutic agent available to treat various types of liver intoxication (Morazzoni and Bombardelli, 1995).

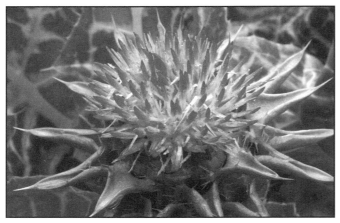

Photo © 2003 stevenfoster.com

DESCRIPTION

Milk thistle preparations consist of the dried fruits (also known as achenes) of *Silybum marianum* (L.) Gaertn. [Fam. *Asteraceae*], freed from the pappus. The U.S. *National Formulary* requires that milk thistle preparations contain no less than 20% silymarin, calculated as silybin (USP, 2002). Silymarin is the collective name for the flavonolignans silibinin (silybin), silydianin, and silychristin. The *German Pharmacopoeia* requires that preparations made of the crude milk thistle fruits, contain at least 1.5% silymarin (DAB, 1999). The semi-purified standardized dry extract, which has been the subject of numerous clinical studies, has a drug-to-extract ratio range of 40–70:1 (*w/w*) and contains no less than 70% silymarin (Blumenthal *et al.*, 1998).

PRIMARY USES

Liver Disorders

- Liver disease, alcoholic (Bunout *et al.*, 1992; Deák *et al.*, 1990; Müzes *et al.*, 1990; Fehér *et al.*, 1989; Salmi and Sarna, 1982; Fintelmann and Albert, 1980)

- Liver cirrhosis, alcoholic (Ferenci *et al.*, 1989; DiMario *et al.*, 1981)
- Infectious hepatitis (Buzzelli *et al.*, 1993; Magliulo *et al.*, 1978; Hammerl *et al.*, 1971; Poser, 1971; Sarre, 1971)
- Drug-induced hepatitis (Palasciano *et al*, 1994; Kurz-Dimitrowa, 1971)

OTHER POTENTIAL USES

- Liver disease secondary to diabetes mellitus (Velussi *et al.*, 1997)
- To decrease toxicity of narcotics used in cholecystectomy surgery (gallbladder removal) (Fintelmann, 1973)
- *Amanita* mushroom poisoning (Hruby *et al.*, 1984; Serne *et al.*, 1996)

Combinations

- The German Commission E has approved a fixed combination of milk thistle seed (crude), peppermint leaf (*Mentha* x *piperita*), and wormwood (*Artemisia absinthium*) for treatment of dyspeptic discomfort, especially functional disorders of the biliary tract (Blumenthal *et al.*, 1998)

DOSAGE

Internal

Crude Preparations

POWDERED SEED: 12–15 g daily for making infusions and other oral galenical preparations (Blumenthal *et al.,* 1998).

DECOCTION: 3–4 times daily, 3 g seed is placed in 150 ml cold water, boiled, simmered for 20–30 minutes, and strained (Wichtl and Bisset, 1994).

INFUSION: 150 ml boiling water is poured over 3.5 g crushed seed and steeped for 10–15 minutes, 3 to 4 times per day, one-half hour before meals, for mild digestive disorders (Braun *et al.*, 1996). A small amount of peppermint leaf may be added to improve efficacy and flavor (Weiss and Fintelmann, 2000).

NOTE: The infusion form is indicated only for mild dyspeptic complaints, whereas high dosage and/or standardized extract forms are required for serious liver diseases. Due to the poor water solubility of silymarin, only a small fraction (<10%) of silymarin is released into an aqueous infusion (Foster and Tyler, 1999; Meyer-Buchtela, 1999; Wichtl, 1989).

Standardized Preparations

DRY EXTRACT: 40–70:1 (*w/w*), 70–80% silymarin, daily equivalent to 200–400 mg of silymarin, calculated as silibinin (Blumenthal *et al.*, 1998) in divided doses. Many clinical trials have used a daily dose equivalent to 420 mg of silymarin, delivered in three divided doses. The dose of 140 mg is swallowed with sufficient amounts of fluid (Blumenthal *et al.,* 2000). NOTE: Most clinical studies on milk thistle have employed the extract concentrated and standardized to 70% silymarin.

DURATION OF ADMINISTRATION

Crude Preparations

For chronic conditions, milk thistle must be taken over an extended period for efficacy. For acute conditions that last longer than one week or recur periodically, consult a healthcare provider (Braun *et al*, 1996).

Standardized Preparations

The duration of use depends on the severity and chronic nature of the condition. Research has suggested that standardized extracts may be used continuously for as long as 24 months (Ferenci *et al.*, 1989; Parés, 1998), although longer periods are possible.

CHEMISTRY

Milk thistle seed contains 1.5–3.0% flavonolignans including silybin, silydianin, and silychristin collectively referred to as silymarin; 20–30% fixed oil, of which approximately 50–60% is linoleic acid, approximately 30% is oleic acid, and approximately 9% is palmitic acid; 25–30% protein; 0.038% tocopherol; 0.63% sterols, including cholesterol, campesterol, stigmasterol, and sitosterol; and some mucilage (Morazzoni and Bombardelli, 1995; Wichtl and Bissett, 1994).

PHARMACOLOGICAL ACTIONS

Internal
Human
Standardized Preparations

Hepatoprotective (BHP, 1996). Reduces serum gamma glutamyl transpeptidase (GGT), alanine transaminase (ALT), and aspartate transaminase (AST), reduces triglyceride in serum, normalizes serum-bilirubin and BSP retention, reduces malondialdehyde concentration in serum, increases superoxide dismutase (SOD) activity in erythrocytes and lymphocytes, reduces cytotoxic lymphocytes in blood, and reduces procollagen-III peptide in serum (Leng-Peschlow 1996a, 1996b).

Animal

Isolated silymarin has anti-inflammatory and anti-arthritic actions (Gupta *et al.*, 1999); increases bile flow and bile salt secretion (Crocenzi *et al.*, 2000); increases secretion of bile into duodenum and exerts gastroprotective effect to prevent ischemic mucosal injury (Alarcon de la Lastra *et al.*, 1995); is prophylactic and antidotal for *Amanita*/deathcap mushroom poisoning (Desplaces *et al.*, 1975; Schriewer *et al.*, 1975; Vogel *et al.*, 1984); protects against sawfly (*Arge pullata*) larvae-induced ruminant hepatotoxicosis (Thamsborg *et al.*, 1996); reduces activity level of GGT, ALT, and AST (Wang *et al.*, 1996); increases glutathione level (Vatenzuela *et al.*, 1989); inhibits synthesis of liver lecithin (Montanini *et al.*, 1977); and protects against thioacetamide damage (Schriewer *et al.*, 1973).

In vitro

Isolated silymarin is hepatoprotective (Farghali *et al.*, 2000; Mereish and Solow, 1990); antioxidant (Müzes *et al.*, 1991); inhibits alpha-amanitin uptake in hepatocyte membrane (Tongiani *et al.*, 1977); stimulates RNA-polymerase I (Morazzoni and Bombardelli, 1995); enhances human polymorphonuclear leukocyte (PMN) motility (Kalmar *et al.*, 1990); and has anticarcinogenic effects in human prostate carcinoma DU145 cells (Zi *et al.*, 1998).

External
Animal

Isolated silymarin inhibits benzoyl peroxide-induced tumor promotion, oxidative stress and inflammatory responses in skin (Zhao *et al.*, 2000); reduces skin tumor (Katiyar *et al.*, 1997).

MECHANISM OF ACTION

Milk thistle's hepatoprotective mechanism of action is not clearly understood, though it can be attributed mainly to its flavonolignan content (Der Manderosian and Liberti, 1997). Isolated silymarin acts as an antagonist in preventing liver-damage: phalloidin and amanitin (death-cap toxins), lanthanides, carbon tetrachloride, galactosantine, thioacetamide, and the hepatotoxic virus FV3 of cold-blooded vertebrates (Blumenthal *et al.*, 1998).

- Anti-inflammatory: Anti-inflammatory and anti-arthritic actions may be due to silymarin's inhibition of 5-lipoxygenase (Gupta *et al.*, 1999).

- Antioxidant: Silymarin scavenges pro-oxidant free radicals, increases glutathione production by the liver, intestines and stomach; increases intracellular concentration of glutathione in rats (Valenzuela *et al.*, 1989; Valenzuela and Garrido, 1994). Semi-purified extract of milk thistle increases activity of SOD and glutathione peroxidase in human erythrocytes *in vitro*, which may explain its protective effect against free radicals and its stabilizing effect on red blood cell membrane (Altorjay *et al.*, 1992).

- Cholagogic and choleretic: Silymarin may increase biliary excretion and endogenous pool of bile salts by stimulating synthesis of hepatoprotective bile salts such as beta-muricholate and ursodeoxycholate (Crocenzi *et al.*, 2000).

- Regenerative: Silymarin stimulates the action of nucleolar polymerase A, resulting in an increase in ribosomal protein synthesis, thereby stimulating regenerative ability of the liver and formation of new hepatocytes (Blumenthal *et al.*, 1998). Based on molecular modeling, silibinin appears to initiate a steroid hormone by binding competitively to RNA-polymerase I, resulting in enzyme activity stimulation (Sonnenbichler *et al.*, 1998).

- Protective and regulatory: Silymarin alters the structure of the outer cell membrane of the hepatocytes in such a way as to prevent penetration of the liver toxin into the interior of the cell (Blumenthal *et al.*, 1998; Leng-Peschlow, 1996b). Stabilizes cell membranes by decreasing phospholipid turnover rate and blocking penetration of liver toxins (such as phalloidin, alpha-amanitin) into the cell (Montanini *et al.*, 1977). Isolated silibinin selectively inhibits leukotriene formation by Kupffer cells of the liver (Dehmlow *et al.*, 1996). Isolated silychristin (silymarin II) inhibits peroxidase and lipoxygenase (Fugmarm *et al.*, 1997). Hepatoprotective effect may be due to silymarin's inhibition of lipid peroxidation and modulation of hepatocyte Ca(2+)(i) (Farghali *et al.*, 2000).

- Anti-fibrotic actions: Animal research (Boigk *et al.*, 1997) and a human clinical trial (Shuppan *et al.*, 1999) have suggested that the hepatoprotective properties of silymarin may include anti-fibrotic activity, thereby interfering with the process that occurs in the hepatocytes secondary to inflammation when collagen invades the normal structure of the hepatocyte, which frequently is a result of alcohol abuse or chronic active viral hepatitis. The ability of silymarin to block fibrosis in the liver was first shown in studies with rats subjected to complete bile duct occlusion (Boigk *et al.*, 1997). This action was later demonstrated in an open-label, uncontrolled study with 998 patients with liver disease resulting from a variety of factors including alcohol abuse, chronic active hepatitis B or C, drugs, and chemical exposure in the workplace (Schuppan *et al.*, 1998). Treatment with 140 mg of silymarin (equivalent to approximately 60 mg of silibinin) three times daily for three months led to a significant reduction in amino terminal procollagen III peptide (PIIINP), a marker of fibrosis, in 19% of the patients. This measure had dropped to the normal range expected for a healthy person at three months.

CONTRAINDICATIONS
None known (Blumenthal *et al.*, 1998; Braun *et al.*, 1996; Brinker, 2001).

PREGNANCY AND LACTATION: No known restrictions (Blumenthal *et al.*, 1998).

ADVERSE EFFECTS
Crude Preparations
None known (Blumenthal *et al.*, 1998; Braun *et al.*, 1996).

Standardized Preparations
A mild laxative effect has been observed occasionally (Blumenthal *et al.*, 1998). There is one case report of a more severe gastrointestinal reaction to a milk thistle product (Adverse Drug Reactions Advisory Committee, 1999); the link to the standardized extract is unclear.

DRUG INTERACTIONS
None known, according to the Commission E (Blumenthal *et al.*, 1998) and other authoritative German pharmaceutical literature (Braun *et al.*, 1996). Concomitant use of purified silymarin and butyrophenones or phenothiazines has resulted in the reduction of lipid peroxidation damage of the liver. In a clinical study where milk thistle was tested for its potential benefit in reducing the hepatotoxicity of these psychopharmaceutical agents (Palasciano *et al.*, 1994). One case report suggests possible protection from dilantin-induced hepatotoxicity (Brinker, 2001).

AMERICAN HERBAL PRODUCTS ASSOCIATION (AHPA) SAFETY RATING
CLASS 1: Can be safely consumed when used appropriately (McGuffin *et al.*, 1997).

REGULATORY STATUS
AUSTRALIA: Approved as a Therapeutic Good (Medicine) by the Therapeutic Goods Administration (TGA).

CANADA: Permitted as a component of OTC Traditional Herbal Medicine (THM) products and as an OTC 1X homeopathic drug, in both cases requiring pre-marketing authorization and application for a Drug Identification Number (DIN) (Health Canada, 2000).

FRANCE: Approved as a nonprescription drug.

GERMANY: Crude and standardized milk thistle preparations are approved nonprescription drugs of the Commission E monographs (Blumenthal *et al.*, 1998) and the tea infusion form is a non-prescription drug of the *German Standard License* monographs, with sales limited to pharmacies and drugstores (Braun *et al.*, 1996). The ripe fruit, freed from pappus, containing not less than 1.5% silymarin is official in the *German Pharmacopoeia* (DAB, 1999). The mother tincture and the ethanolic decoction of the ripe dried fruit are official preparations of the *German Homeopathic Pharmacopoeia* (GHP, 1993).

ITALY: Approved as a prescription drug.

SWEDEN: No milk thistle-containing products are presently registered in the Medical Products Agency's (MPA) "Authorized Natural Remedies," "Homeopathic Remedies" or "Drugs" listings (MPA, 2001).

SWITZERLAND: Positive classification (List D) by *Interkantonale Kontrollstelle für Heilmittel* (IKS) and corresponding sales category D with sale limited to pharmacies and drugstores, without prescription (Morant and Ruppanner, 2001; WHO, 1998). 11 milk thistle-containing phytomedicines and 21 homeopathic preparations are listed in the *Swiss Codex 2000/01* (Ruppanner and Schaefer, 2001).

U.K.: Not entered in the *General Sale List* (GSL).

U.S.: Dietary supplement (USC, 1994). Milk thistle seed and milk thistle seed powder have official monographs in the U.S. *National Formulary*, 20th edition (USP, 2002). The mother tincture 1:10 (*w/v*), 65% ethanol (*v/v*), of the fresh or dried seeds, is an OTC Class C drug official in the *Homoeopathic Pharmacopoeia of the United States* (HPUS, 1990).

CLINICAL REVIEW
Twenty-one studies are outlined in the following table, "Clinical Studies on Milk Thistle," including a total of 2,370 participants. All but two of these studies (Parés *et al.*, 1998; Bunout *et al.*, 1992) demonstrate positive effects for indications including cirrhosis and alcoholic liver disease, hepatitis, and psychotropic drug-induced liver damage. Eight double-blind, placebo-controlled (DB, PC) studies investigated cirrhosis and alcoholic liver disease, involving over 600 patients (Deák *et al.*, 1990; DiMario *et al.*, 1981; Fehér *et al.*, 1989; Ferenci *et al.*, 1989; Fintelmann and Albert, 1980; Müzes *et al.*, 1990; Parés *et al.*, 1998; Salmi and Sarna, 1982). The most recent DB, PC study did not result in statistically significant findings on liver cirrhosis (Parés *et al.*, 1998). Two randomized (R), DB, PC trials investigated milk thistle extract as a treatment for acute viral hepatitis A and B (HBV) (Magliulo *et al.*, 1978) and chronic active hepatitis due to HBV and/or hepatitis C (HCV) (Buzzelli *et al.*, 1993). One observational study on 998 patients showed that milk thistle extract reduces collagen fibrogenesis in patients with toxic livers (Schuppan *et al.*, 1998). Treatment of psychotropic drug-induced hepatic damage with purified silymarin was the subject of another R, DB, PC study (Palasciano *et al.*, 1994), and one multi-center study involving 220 patients over four years found intravenous purified silibin complemented standard treatment, lowering mortality rates in cases of acute *Amanita* mushroom poisoning (Hruby *et al.*, 1984). A recent systematic review and meta-analysis (Mulrow *et al.*, 2000) funded by the National Institutes of Health's Agency for Healthcare Research and Quality concluded that (1) the available evidence suggests that milk thistle extract is relatively safe, associated with few, generally minor, adverse events; (2) despite substantial *in vitro* and animal research, the mechanism of action is not fully defined and may be mulitfactorial; and (3) clinical efficacy is not clearly established because interpretation of the evidence is hampered by poor study methods and/or poor quality of reporting in publications; other problems include heterogeneity in etiology and extent of liver disease, small sample sizes, variation in formulation (for products other than Legalon®, the leading standardized preparation), dosing, and duration of therapy. Possible benefits have been shown most frequently for improvement in aminotransferases and liver function tests.

BRANDED PRODUCTS

IdB 1016 Silipide: Indena S.p.A. / Viale Ortles 12 / 20139 Milano, Italy / Tel: +39-02-57-4961 / Fax: +39-02-57-4046-20 / Email: indenami@tin.it. One capsule contains 150 mg purified dry extract of milk thistle seed standardized to 80% silymarin (120 mg).

Legalon® 35 Dragées: Madaus AG / Ostermerheimer Strasse 198 / Köln / Germany / Tel: +49-22-18-9984-76 / Fax: +49-22-18-9987-21 / Email: b.lindener@madaus.de. One tablet contains 43.25 mg–46.6 dry extract from milk thistle fruits standardized to 35 mg silymarin, calculated as silibinin. (Introduced in 1966.)

Legalon® 70: Madaus AG. One capsule contains 86.5–93.3 mg dry extract from milk thistle fruits (36–44:1) standardized to 70 mg silymarin, calculated as silibinin (extractant: ethyl acetate > 96.7%). (Introduced in 1974.)

Legalon® 140: Madaus AG. One capsule contains 173.0–186.7 mg dry extract from milk thistle fruits (36–44:1) standardized to 140 mg silymarin, calculated as silibinin (extractant: ethyl acetate > 96.7%). (Introduced in 1990.)

American equivalents, if any, are found in the Product Table beginning on page 398.

REFERENCES

Adverse Drug Reactions Advisory Committee. An adverse reaction to the herbal medication milk thistle (*Silybum marianum*). *MJA* 1999;170:218–9.

Alarcon de la Lastra AC, Martin MJ, Motilva V, *et al*. Gastroprotection induced by silymarin, the hepatoprotective principle of *Silybum marianum* in ischemia-reperfusion mucosal injury: role of neutrophils. *Planta Med* 1995;61(2):116–9.

Allain H, Schuck S, Lebreton S, *et al*. Aminotransferase levels and silymarin in *de novo* Tacrine-treated patients with Alzheimer's Disease. *Dement Geriatr Cogn Disord* 1999;10:181–5.

Alshuler L. Milk Thistle: Goals and Objectives. *Int J Integrative Med* 1999;1(1):29–34.

Altorjay I, Dalmi L, Sari B, *et al*. The effect of silibinin (Legalon®) on the free radical scavenger mechanisms of human erythrocytes *in vitro*. *Acta Physiol Hung* 1992;80(1–4):375–80.

Angulo P, Patel T, Jorgensen RA *et al*. Silymarin in the treatment of patients with primary biliary cirrhosis with a suboptimal response to ursodeoxycholic acid. *Hepatology* 2000;32(5):897–900.

Anon. 1989. *Legalon*®. Cologne, Germany: Madaus AG.

Australian Department of Health and Aged Care. Australian Hepatitis C (HCV) Research Register. Project No: 115. Sidney, Australia: Australian Population Health Division, Commonwealth Department of Health and Aged Care. 14. December 1998.

BHP. See: *British Herbal Pharmacopoeia*.

Blumenthal M. Herb sales down 15% in mainstream market. *HerbalGram* 2001;51:69.

Blumenthal M, Busse WR, Goldberg A, Gruenwald J, Hall T, Riggins CW, Rister RS (eds.). Klein S, Rister RS (trans.). *The Complete German Commission E Monographs—Therapeutic Guide to Herbal Medicines*. Austin, TX: American Botanical Council; Boston: Integrative Medicine Communication; 1998;11, 169–70, 278.

Blumenthal M, Goldberg A, Brinckmann J (eds.). Milk Thistle Fruit. In: *Herbal Medicine: Expanded Commission E Monographs*. Newton, MA: Integrative Medicine Communications. 2000;257–63.

Boigk G, Stroedter L, Herbst H, *et al*. Silymarin retards collagen accumulation in early and advanced biliary fibrosis secondary to complete bile duct obliteration in rats. *Hepatology* 1997;26(3):643–9.

Braun R, Surmann P, Wendt R, Wichtl M, Ziegenmeyer J (eds.). Mariendistelfrüchte. In: *Standardzulassungen für Fertigarzneimittel—Text und Kommentar*, 11. Ergänzungslieferung. Stuttgart, Germany: Deutscher Apotheker Verlag, February 1996; Zulassungsnummer 1589.99.99;1–2.

Brinker F. *Herb Contraindications and Drug Interactions*, 3rd ed. Sandy, OR: Eclectic Medical Publications. 2001.

British Herbal Pharmacopoeia (BHP, 4th ed. 1996). Exeter, U.K.: British Herbal Medicine Association. 1996;134–5.

Bunout D, Hirsch S, Petermann M, *et al*. Controlled study on the effect of silimarin in alcoholic liver disease. [in Spanish]. *Rev Med Chile* 1992;120:1370–5.

Buzzelli G, Moscarella S, Giusti A, *et al*. A pilot study on the liver protective effect of

silybin phosphatidylcholine complex (IdB1016) in chronic active hepatitis. *Int J Clin Pharmacol Ther Toxicol* 1993;31(9):456–60.

Crocenzi FA, Pellegrino JM, Sanchez Pozzi EJ, *et al*. Effect of silymarin on biliary bile salt secretion in rat. *Biochem Pharmacol* 2000;59(8):1015–1022.

DAB. See: *Deutsches Arzneibuch*.

Deák G, Müzes G, Läng I, Niederland V, *et al*. Immunomodulator effect of silymarin therapy in chronic alcoholic liver diseases. [in Hungarian]. *Orv Hetil* 1990 Jun 17;131(24):1291–2, 1295–6.

Dehmlow C, Erhard J, de Groot H. Inhibition of Kupffer cell functions as an explanation for the hepatoprotective properties of silibinin. *Hepatology* 1996;23(4):749–54.

Der Marderosian A, Liberti L. *Milk Thistle. The Review of Natural Products*. St. Louis, MO: Facts and Comparisons. Jan 1997.

Desplaces A, Choppin J, Vogel G, Trost W, The effects of silymarin on experimental phalloidine poisoning. *Arzneimittelforschung* 1975;25(1):89–96.

Deutsches Arzneibuch (DAB Ergänzungslieferung 1999). Stuttgart, Germany: Deutscher Apotheker Verlag. 1999; Mariendistelfrüchte:1–5.

DiMario F, Farini R, Okolicsanyi L, Naccarato R. The Effects of Silymarin on the Liver Function Parameters of Patients with Alcohol-Induced Liver Disease: A Double Blind Study. In: de Ritis F, Csomos G, Braatz R (eds.). *Der Toxischmetabolische Leberschaden*. Lübeck, Germany: Hans. Verl.-Kontor. 1981;54–8.

Farghali H, Kamenikova L, Hynie S, Kmonickova E. Silymarin effects on intracellular calcium and cytotoxicity: a study in perfused rat hepatocytes after oxidative stress injury. *Pharmacol Res* 2000;41(2):231–7.

Fehér J, Deák G, Müzes G, *et al*. Hepatoprotective activity of silymarin therapy in patients with chronic alcoholic liver disease. [in Hungarian]. *Orv Hetil* 1989;130(51):2723–7.

Ferenci P, Dragosics B, Dittrich H, *et al*. Randomized controlled trial of silymarin treatment in patients with cirrhosis of the liver. *J Hepatol* 1989; 9(1):105–13.

Fintelmann V. Serumcholinesterase and other liver enzymes in postsurgical conditions. [in German]. *Med Klin* 1973;68:809–15.

Fintelmann V, Albert A. The therapeutic activity of Legalon® in toxic hepatic disorders demonstrated in a double-blind trial. [in German]. *Therapiewoche* 1980;30:5589–94.

Floersheim, G.L., O. Weber, P. Tschumi, M. Ulbrich. Poisoning by the deathcap fungus (*Amanita phalloides*): Prognostic factors and therapeutic measures. [in German]. *Schweiz Med Wochenschr* 1982;112(34):1164–77.

Flora K, Hahn M, Rosen H, Benner K. Milk thistle (*Silybum marianum*) for the therapy of liver disease. *Am J Gastroenterol* 1998; 93(2):139–43.

Foster S. Milk Thistle – *Silybum marianum*. Austin, TX: American Botanical Council. No. 305, 1991.

Foster S, Tyler VA. *Tyler's Honest Herbal: A Sensible Guide to the Use of Herbs and Related Remedies*, 4th ed. New York, NY: Haworth Herbal Press, 1999.

Fugmann B, Lang-Fugmann S, Steglich W (eds.). Silybin. In: *Rompp Lexikon: Naturstoffe*. Stuttgart, Germany: Georg Thieme Verlag. 1997;590.

German Homoeopathic Pharmacopoeia (GHP). Translation of the *Deutsches Homöopathisches Arzneibuch* (HAB 1). First edition 1978 with 5 supplements through 1991. Stuttgart, Germany: Deutscher Apotheker Verlag. 1993;821–7

GHP. See: *German Homeopathic Pharmacopoeia*.

Gupta OP, Sing S, Bani S, *et al*. Anti-inflammatory and anti-arthritic activities of silymarin acting through inhibition of 5-lipoxygenase. *Phytomedicine* 1999;7(1):21–4.

Hammerl H, Pichler O, Studlar M. The effect of silymarin on liver diseases. [in German]. *Med Klin* 1971;66(36):1204–8.

Health Canada. Drug Product Database (DPD). Ottawa, Canada: Health Canada Therapeutic Products Programme. 2000.

Hikino H, Kiso Y. Natural Products for Liver Disease. In: Wagner H, Hikino H, Farnsworth NR. *Economic and Medicinal Plant Research*, Vol. 2. New York, NY: Academic Press. 1988.

Homeopathic Pharmacopoeia of the United States (HPUS) Revision Service Official Compendium from July 1, 1992. Falls Church, VA: American Institute of Homeopathy. June 1990;2276-CDMR.

HPUS. See: *Homeopathic Pharmacopoeia of the United States*.

Hruby, C. Silibinin in the treatment of deathcap fungus poisoning. *Forum* 1984;6:23–6.

Kalmar L, Kadar J, Somogyi A, *et al*. Silibinin (Legalon® 70) enhances the motility of human neutrophils immobilized by formyl-tripeptide, calcium ionophore, lymphokine and by normal human serum. *Agents Actions* 1990;29(3–4):239–46.

Katiyar SK, *et al*. Protective effects of silymarin against photocarcinogenesis in a mouse skin model. *J Nat Cancer Inst* 1997;89:556–65.

Kelly GS. Insulin resistance: lifestyle and nutritional interventions. *Altern Med Rev* 2000;5(2):109–32.

Kurz-Dimitrowa D. Preservation of liver function in psychiatric patients receiving long-term treatment with psychopharmaceuticals. [in German]. *Z Präklin Geriatr* 1971;9:275.

Leng-Peschlow E. Alcohol-related liver diseases-use of Legalon® for therapy. *Quart*

Rev Nat Med 1996a; summer:103–11.

Leng-Peschlow E. Properties and medical use of flavonolignans (silymarin) from *Silybum marianum. Phytother Res* 1996b;10(supl):S25–6.

Magliulo E, Gagliardi B, Fiori GP. Results of a double blind study on the effect of silymarin in the treatment of acute viral hepatitis, carried out at two medical centers. [in German]. *Med Klin* 1978;73(28–29):1060–5.

McCaleb RS, Leigh E, Morien K. *The Encyclopedia of Popular Herbs.* Boulder, CO: Herb Research Foundation; Roseville, CA: Prima Publishing, 2000.

McGuffin M, Hobbs C, Upton R, Goldberg A (eds.). *American Herbal Products Association's Botanical Safety Handbook.* Boca Raton, FL: CRC Press, 1997;107.

Medical Products Agency (MPA). *Läkemedel; Läkemedelsnära Produkter (registrerade homeopatiska produkter); Naturläkemedel (Authorised Natural Remedies).* Uppsala, Sweden: Medical Products Agency. 2001.

Mereish K, Solow R. Effect of antihepatotoxic agents against microcystin–LR toxicity in cultured rat hepatocytes. *Pharm Res* 1990 Mar;7(3):256–9.

Meyer-Buchtela, E. Milk thistle fruits. [in German]. In: *Tee-Rezepturen—Ein Handbuch für Apotheker und Ärzte,* 1. Ergänzungslieferung. Stuttgart, Germany: Deutscher Apotheker Verlag, 1999.

Mingrino F, Tosti U, Anania S, *et al.* A Clinical investigation into the therapeutic effects of silymarin in acute infective hepatitis in children. *Min Ped* 1979;31:451–60.

Montanini I, Castigli E, Arienti UG, Porcellati G. The Effects of silybin on liver phospholipid synthesis in the rat in vivo. *Farmaco (Sci)* 1997 Feb;32(2):141–6.

Morant J, Ruppanner H (eds.). Bioforce Boldocynara N. In: *Arzneimittel-Kompendium der Schweiz®* 2001. Basel, Switzerland: Documed AG. 2001.

Morazzoni P, Bombardelli E. *Silybum marianum (Carduus marianus). Fitoterapia* 1995;66(1):3–42.

MPA. See: Medical Products Agency.

Mulrow C, Lawrence V, Jacobs B *et al.* Milk thistle: Effects on liver disease and cirrhosis and clinical adverse effects. Evidence Report/Technology Assessment, #21. Agency for Healthcare Research and Quality, 2000.

Müzes G, Deák G, Láng I, *et al.* Effect of silymarin (Legalon®) therapy on the antioxidant defense mechanism and lipid peroxidation in alcoholic liver disease: double blind protocol. [in Hungarian]. *Orv Hetil* 1990;131(16):863–6.

Müzes G, Deák G, Láng I, *et al.* Effect of the bioflavonoid silymarin on the *in vitro* activity and expression of superoxide dismutase (SOD) enzyme. [in Hungarian]. *Acta Physiol Hungar* 1991;78(1):3–9.

Palasciano G, Portinacasa P, Palmieri V, *et al.* The effect of silymarin on plasma levels of malondialdehyde in patients receiving long-term treatment with psychotropic drugs. *Curr Therapeut Res* 1994; 55(5):537–45.

Par A, Roth E, Rumi G Jr, *et al.* Oxidative stress and antioxidant defense in alcoholic liver disease and chronic hepatitis C. [in Hungarian]. *Orv Hetil* 2000;141(30):1655–9.

Parés A, Planas R, Torres M, *et al.* Effects of silymarin in alcoholic patients with cirrhosis of the liver: results of a controlled, double blind, randomized and multicenter trial. *J Hepatol* 1998;28(4):615–21.

Poser G. Experience in the treatment of chronic hepatopathies with silymarin. [in German]. *Arzneimittelforschung* 1971;21(8):1209–12.

Ruppanner H, Schaefer U (eds.). *Codex 2000/01 — Die Schweizer Arzneimittel in einem Griff.* Basel, Switzerland: Documed AG. 2001.

Salmi HA, Sarna S. Effect of silymarin on chemical, functional, and morphological alterations of the liver. A double blind controlled study. *Scand J Gastroenterol* 1982;17(4):517–21.

Sarre H. The clinical experience regarding Silymarin in the treatment of chronic liver diseases. [in German]. *Arneimittelforschung* 1971;21(8):1209–12.

Schriewer H, Kastrup W, Wiemann W, Rauen HM. The antihepatotoxic effect of silymarin on lipid metabolism in the rat disturbed by phalloidine intoxication. [in German]. *Arzneimittelforschung* 1975;25(2):188–94.

Schuppan D, Strösser W, Burkard G, *et al.* Legalon® lessens fibrosing activity in patients with chronic liver diseases. [in German]. *Z Allgemeinmed* 1998;74:577–84.

Serne EH, Toorians AWFT, Gietema JA, *et al. Amanita phalloides,* a potentially lethal mushroom: Its clinical presentation and therapeutic options. *Netherlands J Med* 1996;49:19–23.

Sonnenbichler J, Sonnenbichler I, Scalera F. Influence of the Flavonolignan Silibinin of Milk Thistle on Hepatocytes and Kidney Cells. In: Lawson LD, Bauer R (eds.). *Phytomedicines of Europe: Chemistry and Biological Activity.* Washington, DC: American Chemical Society, 1998;263–77.

Thamsborg SM, Jorgensen, Brummerstedt E, Bjerregard J. Putative effect of silymarin on sawfly (*Arge pullata*)-induced hepatotoxicosis in sheep. *Vet Hum Toxicol* 1996;38(2):89–91.

Tongiani R, Malvaldi G, Bertelli A. Effects of dibensothioline and silymarin on the dry weight of isolated hepatocytes of rats acutely poisoned with phalloidin and alpha-amanitin. *Curr Probl Clin Biochem* 1977;7:87–101.

United States Congress (USC). Public Law 103–417: Dietary Supplement Health and Education Act of 1994. Washington, DC: 103rd Congress of the United States. 1994.

United States Pharmacopeia (USP 25th Revision) *National Formulary* (NF 20th Edition). Rockville, MD: United States Pharmacopeial Convention, Inc., 1999;2481–2.

USC. See: United States Congress.

USP. See: *United States Pharmacopeia.*

Valenzuela A, Aspillaga M, Vial S, Guerra R. Selectivity of silymarin on the increase of the glutathione content in different tissues of the rat. *Planta Med* 1989;55(5):420–2.

Valenzuela A, Garrido A. Biochemical bases of the pharmacological action of the flavonoid silymarin and of its structural isomer silibinin. *Biol Res* 1994;27(2):105–12.

Velussi M, Cernigoi AM, DeMonte A, *et al.* Long-term (12 months) treatment with an anti-oxidant drug (silymarin) is effective on hyperinsulinemia, exogenous insulin need, and malondialdehyde levels in cirrhotic diabetic patients. *J Hepatol* 1997;26(4):871–9.

Vogel G, Tuchweber B, Trost W, Mengs U. Protection by silibinin against *Amanita phalloides* intoxication in beagles. *Toxicol Appl Pharmacol* 1984;73:355–62.

Wang M, LaGrange L, Tao J. Hepatoprotective properties of *Silybum marianum* herbal preparation on ethanol-induced liver damage. *Fitoterapia* 1996;LXVII(2):166–71.

Weiss RF, Fintelmann V. *Herbal Medicine,* 2d ed. New York: Thieme, 2000.

WHO. See: World Health Organization.

Wichtl M. Milk thistle fruits. [in German]. In: *Teedrogen,* 2. Auflage. Stuttgart, Germany: Wissenschaftliche Verlagsgesellschaft. 1989.

Wichtl M, Bisset NG (eds.). *Herbal Drugs and Phytopharmaceuticals.* Stuttgart, Germany: Medpharm Scientific Publishers, 1994;121–3.

World Health Organization (WHO). *Regulatory Situation of Herbal Medicines: A Worldwide Review.* Geneva, Switzerland: World Health Organization Traditional Medicine Programme. 1998;26–7.

Zhao J, Lahiri-Chatterjee M, Sharma Y, Agarwal R. Inhibitory effect of a flavonoid antioxidant silymarin on benzoyl peroxide-induced tumor promotion, oxidative stress and inflammatory response in SENCAR mouse skin. *Carcinogenesis* 2000;21(4):811–6.

Zi X, Grasso AW, Kung HJ, *et al.* A flavonoid antioxidant, silymarin, inhibits activation of erbB1 signaling and induces cyclin-dependent kinase inhibitors, G1 arrest, and anticarcinogenic effects in human prostate carcinoma DU145 cells. *Cancer Res* 1998;58:1920–9.

Clinical Studies on Milk Thistle (*Silybum marianum* [L.] Gaertner)

Cirrhosis and Alcohol Liver Disease

Author/Year	Subject	Design	Duration	Dosage	Preparation	Results/Conclusion
Parés et al., 1998	Cirrhosis of the liver	DB, PC, R, MC n=125 alcoholic patients with cirrhosis of liver	2 years	1 capsule, 3x/day (420 mg silymarin/day) vs. placebo	Brand not stated	Compared to placebo, milk thistle extract had no significant effect on the course of disease after 2 years of treatment. Milk thistle did not improve survival rates, liver function tests, or histological parameters in patients with severe and acute alcohol-induced cirrhosis of the liver. No significant side effects were observed.
Bunout et al., 1992	Alcoholic liver disease	PC, R n=59 patients with chronic alcoholic liver disease	15 months	1 capsule, 2x/day (280 mg silymarin/day) vs. placebo	Brand not stated	Compared to placebo, milk thistle did not change the evolution of mortality of alcoholic liver disease within 15 months. 10 patients died during follow-up (5 milk thistle and 5 placebo). In milk thistle group 58% continued to drink alcohol during trial and follow-up; 65% in control group continued to drink alcohol. Authors note higher dose used in other studies gave positive results.
Deak et al., 1990	Alcoholic liver disease	DB, PC (n=not available) Patients had chronic alcoholic liver disease	6 months	Silymarin (dose not available) vs. placebo	Legalon® 70	Compared with placebo, milk thistle significantly enhanced lectin-induced proliferative activity of lymphocytes, normalized the originally low T-cell percentage and originally high CD8+ cell percentage, and decreased antibody-dependent and natural cytotoxicity of lymphocytes. There were no significant changes in placebo group with the exception of moderate elevation of T-cell percentage.
Müzes et al., 1990	Alcoholic liver disease	DB, PC (n=12) patients with chronic alcoholic liver disease (mean age 37±9 years)	6 months	420 mg silymarin/day vs. placebo	Legalon® 70	Milk thistle extract significantly enhanced low superoxide dismutase (SOD) expression on lymphocytes as determined by flow-cytoflourimetry. Milk thistle markedly increased glutathione activity but decreased serum malondialdehyde concentration. No significant changes reported in placebo group.
Fehér et al., 1989	Alcoholic liver disease	DB, PC n=36 chronic alcoholic patients with hepatic fibromatosis or micro-nodular cirrhosis	6 months	2 capsules, 3x/day (420 mg silymarin/day) vs. palcebo	Legalon® 70	Compared to baseline and placebo, milk thistle significantly normalized serum bilirubin, aspartate aminotransferase (AST), and alanine-aminotransferase (ALT) values. Histological alterations improved in milk thistle group and remained unchanged in placebo group. The authors concluded a significant decrease in serum procollagen-III peptide levels combined with improved histological changes confirmed that milk thistle can be recommended as supportive therapy in chronic alcohol disease.
Ferenci et al., 1987	Alcohol and non-alcohol-induced cirrhosis	R, DB, PC n=170 patients with cirrhosis (92 alcoholic; 78 non-alcoholic)	2–6 years, mean observation period 41 months (Patients were treated with silymarin for only 2 years)	2 capsules, 3x/day (420 mg silymarin/day) vs. placebo	Legalon® 70	No significant change in biochemical parameters at 2 years. However, 2-year survival rate was 82% in milk thistle group vs. 68% placebo; 4-year survival rate was 58± 9% with milk thistle and 39± 9% with placebo (p=0.036). Survival rate was higher in subgroup of patients with alcoholic cirrhosis (p=0.01) and in Child's A group classification of portal hypertension, though treatment was ineffective in Child's B and C group hypertension. No adverse effects observed.
Salmi and Sarna, 1982	Alcohol liver disease	R, DB, PC n=97 patients with slight acute and subacute liver disease	4 weeks with 3 additional re-examinations 1, 2, and 3 weeks after start of the trial (alcohol abstinence required during the trial)	2 capsules, 3x/day (420 mg silymarin/day) vs. placebo	Legalon® 70	After 4 weeks, milk thistle caused a highly significant (30%) decrease in mean serum AST levels compared to a 5% increase in placebo group. ALT levels decreased by 41% in milk thistle group and increased 3% with placebo. Histological changes normalized more significantly in milk thistle group. Milk thistle decreased serum total and conjugated bilirubin more than placebo, but not at a statistically significant level.
DiMario et al., 1981	Fatty liver, alcoholic hepatitis, hepatic cirrhosis	DB, PC n=43 patients with alcohol-induced liver disease	1–2 months	420 mg silymarin/day vs. placebo	Legalon® 70	Significantly improved markers of liver function (AST (p<0.05); ALT (p<0.01); bilirubin (p<0.05, and prothrombin (p<0.05). Significantly improved clinical symptoms of weakness, anorexia, and nausea.

KEY: C – controlled, **CC** – case-control, **CH** – cohort, **CI** – confidence interval, **Cm** – comparison, **CO** – crossover, **CS** – cross-sectional, **DB** – double-blind, **E** – epidemiological, **LC** – longitudinal cohort, **MA** – meta-analysis, **MC** – multi-center, **n** – number of patients, **O** – open, **OB** – observational, **OL** – open label, **OR** – odds ratio, **P** – prospective, **PB** – patient-blind, **PC** – placebo-controlled, **PG** – parallel group, **PS** – pilot study, **R** – randomized, **RC** – reference-controlled, **RCS** – retrospective cross-sectional, **RS** - retrospective, **S** – surveillance, **SB** – single-blind, **SC** – single-center, **U** – uncontrolled, **UP** – unpublished, **VC** – vehicle-controlled.

Milk Thistle

Monograph

Cirrhosis and Alcohol Liver Disease (cont.)

Author/Year	Subject	Design	Duration	Dosage	Preparation	Results/Conclusion
Fintelmann and Albert, 1980	Alcohol liver disease	R, DB, PC n=66 patients with acute alcoholic hepatitis	1 month	2 capsules, 3x/day (420 mg silymarin/day) vs. placebo	Legalon® 70	Treatment with milk thistle caused mean AST, ALT, and GGT levels to normalize significantly and much sooner (13 vs. 24 days) than placebo. More patients in milk thistle group experienced normalization of all 3 parameters vs. placebo. Significant differences were evident after 1 week.

Hepatitis

Author/Year	Subject	Design	Duration	Dosage	Preparation	Results/Conclusion
Buzzelli et al., 1993	Chronic active hepatitis due to HBV and/or HCV	R, DB, PC n=20 patients with HBV- and/or HCV-related chronic active hepatitis	1 week	2 capsules, 2x/day (2 hours before breakfast and dinner) (480 mg silymarin/day) vs. placebo	IdB 1016 Silipide 1 capsule contains 150 mg purified dry extract equivalent to 120 mg silymarin.	Milk thistle significantly reduced mean serum concentrations of AST and ALT (p<0.01), total bilirubin (p<0.05), and gamma-glutamyltranspeptidase (GGT) (p<0.02). However, there were no significant changes in malonaldehyde, copper, or zinc serum concentrations. Milk thistle improved hepatic function, mainly by reducing transaminases and other indices (GGT and total bilirubin) related to liver cell necrosis and/or hepatocyte membrane permeability.
Magliulo et al., 1978	Acute viral hepatitis A and B	R, DB, PC, MC n=57 patients with acute viral hepatitis (14–66 years)	21–28 days (average 24.9 days)	2 tablets, 3x/day (420 mg silymarin/day) vs. placebo	Legalon® 70	After 5 days, mean levels of AST, ALT, and total bilirubin were significantly lower in milk thistle group compared to placebo. At 3 weeks, milk thistle group showed significant normalization of bilirubin (40% vs. 11%) and AST (82% vs. 52%) compared to placebo. Milk thistle did not influence the course of the immune reaction in hepatitis B surface antigen (HbsAg). Milk thistle extract caused accelerated regression of pathological markers, and authors concluded that it can be indicated for use in the treatment of acute viral hepatitis.
Hammerl et al., 1971	Chronic hepatitis, cirrhosis and toxic damage to liver	O, U n=43 (14 chronic hepatitis, 22 cirrhosis, 7 toxico-metabolic liver damage)	more than 1 year	First 3 weeks: 3 tablets, 3x/day (315 mg silymarin/day) reduced to 2 tablets, 3x/day (210 mg silymarin/day)	Legalon® 35	Milk thistle showed significant changes in all test parameters including bromsulphalein test (liver excretion function), albumin/globulin quotient (mesenchymal reaction), serum, bilirubin, transaminase, and serum triglycerides (metabolic performance of liver) and a preponderant trend towards normalization. Authors concluded that milk thistle has a protective and curative action on liver.
Poser, 1971	Chronic liver disease	O, U n=67 out-patients with toxic metabolic liver damage, chronic hepatitis, and cholangitis (4–64 years)	3 months	3–5 tablets, 3x/day (315–525 mg silymarin/day) depending on severity of condition	Legalon® 35	Milk thistle significantly improved SGOT, SGPT, and glutamate-dehydrogenase (GLDH), but there was no statistically significant difference in bilirubin level. After 3 months, chronic-persisting hepatitis was bioptically cured and conditions associated with bile duct inflammation improved. Patients with cholangitic hepatopathies (bile duct inflammation) responded especially well to milk thistle treatment.
Sarre, 1971	Chronic persisting hepatitis and other hepatopathies	E n=67	3 months	3–5 tablets, 3x/day (315–525 mg silymarin/day) depending on severity of condition	Legalon® 35 Dragées	Significantly decreased SGOT, SGPT, and GLDH. No effect on bilirubin levels. Bioptically cured chronic-persisting hepatitis. Toxic-metabolic and cholangitic hepatopathies responded well to silymarin treatment. Effective in treating both young (4 years) and old (64 years) patients without adverse side effects.

KEY: C – controlled, **CC** – case-control, **CH** – cohort, **CI** – confidence interval, **Cm** – comparison, **CO** – crossover, **CS** – cross-sectional, **DB** – double-blind, **E** – epidemiological, **LC** – longitudinal cohort, **MA** – meta-analysis, **MC** – multi-center, **n** – number of patients, **O** – open, **OB** – observational, **OL** – open label, **OR** – odds ratio, **P** – prospective, **PB** – patient-blind, **PC** – placebo-controlled, **PG** – parallel group, **PS** – pilot study, **R** – randomized, **RC** – reference-controlled, **RCS** – retrospective cross-sectional, **RS** - retrospective, **S** – surveillance, **SB** – single-blind, **SC** – single-center, **U** – uncontrolled, **UP** – unpublished, **VC** – vehicle-controlled.

Clinical Studies on Milk Thistle *(Silybum marianum* [L.] Gaertner) (cont.)

Psychotropic Drug-Induced Liver Damage

Author/Year	Subject	Design	Duration	Dosage	Preparation	Results/Conclusion
Palasciano et al., 1994	Hepatic damage caused by psychotropic drugs (variety of xenobiotic compounds)	DB, PC, R n=60 female psychiatric patients receiving chronic psychotropic drug therapy (40–60 years)	90 days, examined at baseline, days 15, 30, 60, and 90, and again at 30 days after completion	Group 1A & B: psychotropic drugs with either 400 mg silymarin, 2x/day or placebo Group 2A & B: suspension of psychotropic drugs with either 400 mg silymarin, 2x/day or placebo	Purified silymarin (brand not stated)	Silymarin reduced lipoperoxidative hepatic damage resulting from treatment with butyrophenones and phenothiazines. Effect of silymarin was greater when treatment with psychotropic drugs was suspended. Serum levels of malondialdehyde decreased, and indices of hepatocellular damage improved with silymarin. Using ANOVA test for repeated measures, a significant treatment-time interaction was observed for silymarin (p=0.005). Study suggests that silymarin treatment for lipoperoxidative hepatic damage may be beneficial in cases of long-term psychotropic drug treatment.
Kurz-Dimitrowa, 1971	Psychoactive or anti-convulsant drug therapy	n=66 psychiatric patients	61 days	1–3 tablets, 3x/day (105–315 mg silymarin/day)	Legalon® 35	Normalized bromsulphalein levels in 54% of patients, normalized or improved GOT levels in 68% of patients, and improved vitality and mood in patients receiving psychoactive drugs.

Other

Author/Year	Subject	Design	Duration	Dosage	Preparation	Results/Conclusion
Schuppen et al., 1999	Fibrosis in chronic liver disease	OL (drug monitoring study) n=874 men and women (average age 55)	3 months	140 mg, 3x/day	Legalon®	Primary test parameter was amino terminal procollagen-III peptide (PIIINP) readings, as an indicator of fibrogenesis, with this factor dropping to normal range in 19% of patients. Total score of symptom scale showed definite and a clinically relevant decrease in subjective symptoms during treatment (e.g., lack of appetite, nausea, upper abdominal pressure). Of the subjects, 98% confirmed that Legalon® was well-tolerated; 2% reported moderate or poor tolerability (e.g., diarrhea, flatulence, gastrointestinal fullness, gastrointestinal pain).
Allain et al., 1999	Aminotransferase levels in tacrine-induced liver transaminase elevation	R, DB, PC n=217 patients with mild to moderate Alzheimer's dementia	12 weeks	420 mg/day silymarin, and 40 mg/day tacrine for 6 weeks, then increase to 80 mg/day tacrine or tacrine (same dose), and placebo	Legalon® (silymarin) Cognex® (tacrine)	Silymarin does not prevent tacrine-induced ALAT elevation but does reduce rate of gastrointestinal and cholinergic side effects without impact on cognitive status. Silymarin can be used to improve tolerability of tacrine in initial phases of Alzheimer's treatment.
Velussi et al., 1997	Diabetic patients with cirrhosis	R, O, C, Cm n=60 cirrhotic patients	1 year	2 capsules, 3x/day (420 mg silymarin/day) plus standard therapy vs. standard therapy	Legalon® 70	After 4 months, milk thistle significantly decreased (p<0.01) fasting blood glucose levels, mean daily blood glucose levels, daily glucosuria and HbA1c levels. Authors conclude that treatment with milk thistle may reduce lipoperoxidation of cell membranes and insulin resistance, significantly decreasing endogenous insulin overproduction and need for exogenous insulin administration.
Fintelmann, 1973	Narcotic use in cholecystectomy surgery	C, Cm n=83 patients undergoing cholecystectomy	12 days (2–4 days pre-operative; 1–8 days post-operative)	2 tablets, 3x/day (210 mg silymarin/day) or 4 tablets, 3x/day (420 mg silymarin/day)	Legalon®	Pre- and post-operative administration of 4 tablets, 3x/day appeared to decrease toxicity of narcotics used in cholecystectomy surgery. Compared to control, milk thistle did not have a significant effect on enzyme parameters. Authors caution that their study is inconclusive due to a small patient population, a duration of pre-operative dosing that was too short, and research conditions that were not optimal.

Amanita Mushroom Poisoning

Author/Year	Subject	Design	Duration	Dosage	Preparation	Results/Conclusion
Hurby et al., 1984	Acute *Amanita* poisoning	U, MC n=220 patients with *Amanita* poisoning	4 years (1979–82)	20 mg/kg weight i.v.	Purified silibin i.v. infusion (brand not stated)	Mortality rate of 12.8% in silybin group. Authors conclude that use of silybin i.v. as an adjunct to standard treatment methods lowers mortality rates below previously known levels.

KEY: **C** – controlled, **CC** – case-control, **CH** – cohort, **CI** – confidence interval, **Cm** – comparison, **CO** – crossover, **CS** – cross-sectional, **DB** – double-blind, **E** – epidemiological, **LC** – longitudinal cohort, **MA** – meta-analysis, **MC** – multi-center, **n** – number of patients, **O** – open, **OB** – observational, **OL** – open label, **OR** – odds ratio, **P** – prospective, **PB** – patient-blind, **PC** – placebo-controlled, **PG** – parallel group, **PS** – pilot study, **R** – randomized, **RC** – reference-controlled, **RCS** – retrospective cross-sectional, **RS** - retrospective, **S** – surveillance, **SB** – single-blind, **SC** – single-center, **U** – uncontrolled, **UP** – unpublished, **VC** – vehicle-controlled.

Milk Thistle

Monograph

(This page intentionally left blank.)

Peppermint

Mentha x *piperita* L.

[Fam. *Lamiaceae*]

OVERVIEW

Peppermint is one of the most popular herbs for use in teas, flavorings, and candies. Both peppermint leaf and peppermint oil are official in the U.S. *National Formulary,* while peppermint water and peppermint spirit have official monographs in the *United States Pharmacopeia*. The U.S. is the world's leading producer of peppermint oil, supplying more than 4,000 metric tons of oil annually. Three peppermint products are ranked among the top ten best-selling single-herb teas. Although the traditional use of peppermint is primarily as a tea to improve digestion, most clinical studies have investigated the actions of peppermint oil in enteric-coated capsules used internally to treat irritable bowel syndrome and externally to treat tension headache.

PRIMARY USES

Internal
Gastrointestinal
Crude Preparations
- Indigestion and relief of bloating due to excess gas production
- Spastic complaints of the gastro-intestinal tract, gallbladder, and bile ducts

Essential Oil
- Non-ulcer or functional dyspepsia
- Irritable bowel syndrome

External
Neurology
Essential Oil
- Tension headaches (solutions rubbed on forehead and temples)

OTHER POTENTIAL USES

Internal
Essential Oil
- Catarrh of the respiratory tract and inflammation of the oral mucosa
- Colonic spasm during barium enema
- Colonic spasm during colonoscopy

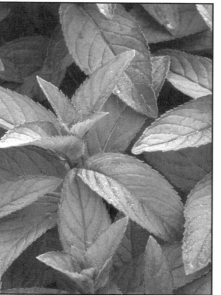
Photo © 2003 stevenfoster.com

External
Essential Oil
- Myalgia and neuralgia
- Fecal odor in patients with colostomies

PHARMACOLOGICAL ACTIONS
Internal
CRUDE PREPARATIONS: Antispasmodic action on the smooth muscles of the digestive tract; choleretic; carminative.

ESSENTIAL OIL: Antispasmodic; carminative; cholagogic; antibacterial; secretolytic/mucolytic; relaxes smooth muscle; relieves colonic spasms; carminative on lower esophageal sphincter.

External
ESSENTIAL OIL: Analgesic in tension headache; menthol vapors stimulate cold receptors in nose.

DOSAGE AND ADMINISTRATION
The Health Canada labeling standard warns patients not to take peppermint internally for more than two weeks, or if symptoms recur when treating indigestion, unless directed by a healthcare provider. [EDITORS' NOTE: In Canada, all non-prescription drugs are given a duration use related to the indicated condition. This is based on the reasoning that the patient should be checked by a healthcare practitioner to look for underlying causes if the symptoms have not cleared up in the specified time.] The German Standard License monograph warns that for acute gastrointestinal complaints that last for more than one week or recur periodically, the patient should see a healthcare provider.

Internal
Crude Preparations
DRIED LEAF: 1–4 g, 3 times daily after meals for flatulent digestive pains.

INFUSION: Approximately 150 ml of boiled water poured over 1.5 g of dried leaf, steeped for 5–10 minutes in a covered vessel, tea bag squeezed over the cup, can be administered 2–5 times daily on an empty stomach to relieve upset stomach.

TINCTURE: 2–5 ml, 3 times daily [1:5 (*g/ml*), 45% ethanol].

Essential Oil

ESSENTIAL OIL: 6–12 drops total daily dose [EDITORS' NOTE: Caution: Peppermint oil is highly concentrated; therefore, divide into 3 doses and dilute in water or juice.]; 0.05–0.2 ml 3 times daily.

ESSENTIAL OIL IN ENTERIC-COATED CAPSULE: 0.2 ml oil (187 mg), 3 times daily with water before meals, for irritable colon.

INHALANT: 3–4 drops of essential oil added to hot water and the steam vapor inhaled deeply.

Combination Preparations

ESSENTIAL OIL: 90 mg peppermint oil and 50 mg caraway oil, 1 enteric-coated capsule, 3 times daily, before meals, for non-ulcer dyspepsia.

External

Essential Oil

ESSENTIAL OIL: Drops, diluted with lukewarm water or vegetable oil, rubbed in the affected skin areas.

ESSENTIAL OIL: 10 g in ethanol 90% solution, spread across forehead and temples. Repeated application after 15–30 minutes for tension headache.

NASAL OINTMENT: Semi-solid preparation containing 1–5% essential oil.

TINCTURE: Aqueous-alcoholic preparation containing 5–10% essential oil for local application.

CONTRAINDICATIONS

CRUDE HERB: Gallstones, esophageal reflux.

ESSENTIAL OIL: Achlorhydria (absence of free hydrochloric acid in gastric juice), obstruction of bile ducts, gallbladder inflammation, and severe liver damage. A healthcare provider should be consulted before using peppermint oil in cases of gallstones. Peppermint oil should not be used on the faces (particularly the noses) of infants and small children. Peppermint oil is contraindicated for infants and small children due to the potential risk of spasms of the tongue or respiratory arrest.

PREGNANCY AND LACTATION: No known restrictions.

ADVERSE EFFECTS

Twelve cases of oral-contact sensitivity to peppermint oil and/or menthol have been reported in patients with intra-oral symptoms in association with burning-mouth syndrome, recurrent oral ulceration, or a lichenoid reaction.

DRUG INTERACTIONS

Menthol-containing preparations may interfere with gastrointestinal-stimulant drugs (e.g., cisapride) used to treat nighttime heartburn due to the reflux of stomach acid into the esophagus. Concurrent administration of peppermint oil with antacids or ingestion during meals can cause the oil to be released from capsules prematurely, resulting in a loss of effectiveness.

CLINICAL REVIEW

In twenty-three clinical studies on peppermint conducted on a total of 1,186 participants, all but one demonstrated positive results for various gastrointestinal and neurological conditions. These include 14 double-blind (DB) studies investigating the treatment of non-ulcer or functional dyspepsia, irritable bowel syndrome, spasm during barium enema, and tension headaches. In 1998, a meta-analysis of DB, placebo-controlled trials concluded that peppermint oil could provide symptomatic relief of irritable bowel syndrome, though the authors cited methodological flaws in most of the studies. In 2000, a systematic review of randomized, controlled trials concluded that using peppermint oil to treat irritable bowel syndrome requires further study.

Peppermint

Mentha x piperita L.
[Fam. *Lamiaceae*]

OVERVIEW

Peppermint is one of the most popular herbs in teas, candies, and chewing gums. The U.S. is the world's leading producer of peppermint oil, making an average of 4,117 tons annually. Although the traditional use is as a tea to improve digestion, most clinical trials have studied the oil in enteric-coated capsules used internally to treat irritable bowel syndrome and externally to treat tension headache.

USES

INTERNAL: Peppermint leaf: General indigestion and non-ulcer dyspepsia. Peppermint oil: Irritable bowel syndrome (enteric-coated capsules); colonic spasm during barium enema and during colonoscopy; catarrh of upper respiratory tract and inflammation of mucous linings of the mouth.

EXTERNAL: Peppermint oil: Tension headaches (oil solution rubbed on forehead and temples; use extreme caution with undiluted peppermint oil); for muscle and nerve pain (usually in the form of liniments).

DOSAGE
Internal
CONCENTRATED PEPPERMINT WATER: 0.25–1.0 ml.

DRIED LEAF: 1–4 g, 3 times daily after meals for flatulent digestive pains.

INFUSION (TEA): Pour about 150 ml of boiled water over 1.5 g of dried leaf, steep for 5–10 minutes in a covered vessel, squeeze tea bag over the cup, and take 2–5 times daily on an empty stomach to relieve upset stomach.

PEPPERMINT SPIRIT: 20 drops (1 ml) with water.

TINCTURE: 2–5 ml; 3 times daily [1:5 (*g/ml*), 45% ethanol].

ESSENTIAL OIL: 6–12 drops total daily dose [EDITOR'S NOTE: Caution: Peppermint oil is highly concentrated; therefore, divide into 3 doses and dilute in water or juice.]; 0.05–0.2 ml 3 times daily.

ESSENTIAL OIL IN ENTERIC-COATED CAPSULE: 0.2 ml oil (187 mg), 3 times daily with water before meals for irritable colon.

INHALANT: 3–4 drops of essential oil added to hot water and the steam vapor inhaled deeply.

Combination Preparations
ESSENTIAL OIL: 90 mg peppermint oil and 50 mg caraway oil, 1 enteric-coated capsule, 3 times daily, before meals, for non-ulcer dyspepsia.

External
ESSENTIAL OIL: Spread on forehead and temples. Repeat after 15–30 minutes for tension headache.

ESSENTIAL OIL: Drops rubbed in the affected skin areas, should be diluted with lukewarm water or vegetable oil.

NASAL OINTMENT: Semi-solid preparation containing 1–5% essential oil.

TINCTURE: Aqueous-alcoholic preparation containing 5–10% essential oil for local application.

CONTRAINDICATIONS

CRUDE HERB: Gallstones, esophageal reflux.

ESSENTIAL OIL: Achlorhydria (absence of free hydrochloric acid in gastric juice), obstruction of bile ducts, gallbladder inflammation, and severe liver damage. Consult with a healthcare provider before using peppermint oil in cases of gallstones.

Peppermint oil should not be used on the faces (particularly the noses) of infants and small children. Peppermint oil is contraindicated for infants and small children because of the potential risk of spasms of the tongue or respiratory arrest.

PREGNANCY AND LACTATION: No known restrictions.

ADVERSE EFFECTS

No adverse effects are known. Oral-contact sensitivity to peppermint oil and/or menthol has caused side effects of burning-mouth syndrome, recurrent oral ulceration, or a skin condition known as lichenoid reaction.

DRUG INTERACTIONS

Peppermint preparations may interfere with gastrointestinal-stimulant drugs (e.g., cisapride) used to treat nighttime heartburn. Use of peppermint oil capsules with antacids or during meals can cause the oil to be released prematurely, resulting in a loss of effectiveness.

Comments

When using a dietary supplement, purchase it from a reliable source. For best results, use the same brand of product throughout the period of use. As with all medications and dietary supplements, please inform your healthcare provider of all herbs and medications you are taking. Interactions may occur between medications and herbs or even among different herbs when taken at the same time. Treat your herbal supplement with care by taking it as directed, storing it as advised on the label, and keeping it out of the reach of children and pets. Consult your healthcare provider with any questions.

AMERICAN BOTANICAL COUNCIL

Peppermint

Mentha x piperita L.

[Fam. *Lamiaceae*]

OVERVIEW

Peppermint is one of the most popular herbs for use in teas, flavorings, and confections (e.g., chewing gum and candies). Both peppermint leaf and peppermint oil are official in the U.S. *National Formulary,* while peppermint water and peppermint spirit have official monographs in the *United States Pharmacopeia* (USP, 2002). The U.S. is the world's leading producer of peppermint oil (Fugmann *et al.,* 1997), supplying more than 4,000 metric tons of oil annually (NASS/USDA, 2000). Three peppermint products are ranked in the top ten list of best selling single-herb teas (SPINS, 2000). Although most traditional uses of peppermint are based on teas used as a digestive aid, most clinical studies have investigated the actions of peppermint oil in enteric-coated capsules used internally to treat irritable bowel syndrome (IBS) and externally to treat tension headache.

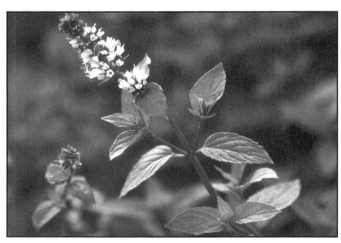

Photo © 2003 stevenfoster.com

DESCRIPTION

Peppermint leaf preparations consist of the fresh or dried leaf of *Mentha* x *piperita* L. [Fam. *Lamiaceae*]. The whole, dried leaf must contain not less than 1.2% (ml/g), and the cut leaf must contain not less than 0.9% volatile oil (Ph.Eur., 1997). Peppermint oil consists of the essential oil, obtained by steam-distilling freshly harvested, flowering sprigs (Blumenthal *et al.,* 1998), and is neither partially, nor wholly dementholized (USP, 2002).

PRIMARY USES

Internal
Gastrointestinal
Crude Preparations

- Indigestion and relief of bloating due to excess gas production (Health Canada, 1996)
- Spastic complaints of gastrointestinal tract, gallbladder, and bile ducts (Blumenthal *et al.,* 1998; Braun *et al.,* 1996)

Essential Oil

- Non-ulcer or functional dyspepsia (Freise and Köhler, 1999; Madisch *et al.,* 1999; May *et al.,* 1996, 2000)
- Irritable bowel syndrome (IBS) (Liu *et al.,* 1997; Carling *et al.,* 1989; Lawson *et al.,* 1988; Nash *et al.,* 1986; Dew *et al.,* 1984; Rees *et al.,* 1979; Pittler and Ernst, 1998)

External
Neurology
Essential Oil

- Tension headaches (Göbel *et al.,* 1994, 1996)

OTHER POTENTIAL USES

Internal
Essential Oil

- Catarrh of the respiratory tract and inflammation of the oral mucosa (Blumenthal *et al.,* 1998)
- Colonic spasm during barium enema (Sparks *et al.,* 1995; Jarvis *et al.,* 1992)
- Colonic spasm during colonoscopy (Duthie, 1981; Leicester and Hunt, 1982)
- Fecal odor in patients with colostomies (McKenzie and Gallacher, 1989)

External
Essential Oil

- Myalgia and neuralgia (Blumenthal *et al.,* 1998)

DOSAGE

Crude Preparations
Internal

CONCENTRATED PEPPERMINT WATER (BP): 0.25–1.0 ml (BP, 1980; Karnick, 1994).

DRIED LEAF: 3–6 g (Blumenthal *et al.,* 1998); 2–3 g, 3 times daily after meals for flatulent digestive pains (Bradley, 1992) 2–4 g, 3 times daily (Health Canada, 1996).

INFUSION: Approximately 150 ml of boiled water poured over 1.5 g of dried leaf, steeped for 5–10 minutes in a covered vessel, tea bag squeezed over the cup, can be administered 2–5 times daily (Morant and Ruppanner, 2001; Braun *et al.,* 1996; Hänsel *et al.,* 1992–1994; Meyer-Buchtela, 1999), on an empty stomach to relieve upset stomach (Robbers and Tyler, 1999).

NOTE: Peppermint tea infusion yields ca. 21% of total available essential oil (Duband *et al.,* 1992). At 10 minutes of steeping time, the maximum amount of volatile oil is obtained including ca. 24% of the menthol and 19.5% of the menthone (Hänsel *et al.,* 1992–1994; Meyer-Buchtela, 1999). Steeping time limited to 5 minutes maximizes yield of menthol and menthone, as they volatilize rapidly (Niesel, 1992). After 5 minutes of steeping, 42–55% of the available rosmarinic acid is released, depending on the leaf particle size or surface area (Carius, 1990; Meyer-Buchtela, 1999).

PEPPERMINT SPIRIT USP: 20 drops (1 ml) with water (Robbers and Tyler, 1999).

TINCTURE [1:5 (*g/ml*), 45% ethanol]: 5–15 ml (Blumenthal *et al.*, 1998; Erg.B.6, 1953); 2–3 ml, 3 times daily (Bradley, 1992; Health Canada, 1996).

Essential Oil
Internal
ESSENTIAL OIL: 6–12 drops total daily dose, according to German Commission E (Blumenthal *et al.*, 1998) [EDITORS' NOTE: Caution: Peppermint oil is highly concentrated; therefore, divide into 3 doses and dilute in water or juice.]; 0.05–0.2 ml 3 times daily (Health Canada, 1996).

ESSENTIAL OIL IN ENTERIC-COATED CAPSULE: 0.2 ml oil (187 mg), 3 times daily with water before meals, for irritable colon (Morant and Ruppanner, 2001; Blumenthal *et al.*, 1998; Krogh, 1989; Liu *et al.*, 1997).

External
ESSENTIAL OIL: Drops rubbed in the affected skin areas, should be diluted with lukewarm water or vegetable oil (Blumenthal *et al.*, 1998). 10 g in ethanol 90% solution, spread across forehead and temples. Repeated application after 15–30 minutes for tension headache (Göbel *et al.*, 1996).

INHALANT: 3–4 drops of essential oil added to hot water and the steam vapor inhaled deeply (Blumenthal *et al.*, 1998).

NASAL OINTMENT: Semi-solid preparation containing 1–5% essential oil (Blumenthal *et al.*, 1998).

TINCTURE: Aqueous-alcoholic preparation containing 5–10% essential oil for local application (Blumenthal *et al.*, 1998).

Combination Preparations
Internal
ESSENTIAL OIL: 90 mg peppermint oil, 50 mg caraway oil, in enteric-coated capsule, 1 capsule 3 times daily, with water before meals, for non-ulcer dyspepsia (Freise and Köhler, 1999; Madisch *et al.*, 1999).

DURATION OF ADMINISTRATION
The Health Canada labeling standard warns patients not to take peppermint internally for more than two weeks, or if symptoms recur when treating indigestion, unless directed by a healthcare provider (Health Canada, 1996). [EDITORS' NOTE: In Canada, all non-prescription drugs are given a duration use related to the indicated condition. This is based on the reasoning that the patient should be checked by a healthcare practitioner to look for underlying causes if the symptoms have not cleared up in the specified time.] The German Standard License monograph warns that for acute gastrointestinal complaints that last for more than one week or periodically recur, see a doctor (Braun *et al.*, 1996).

CHEMISTRY
Peppermint leaf contains up to 7% phenolic acids (caffeic, chlorogenic, and rosmarinic) (Bruneton, 1999); 3.5–4.5% labiate tannins; 0.5–4.0% terpene rich volatile oil, and flavonoids (glycosides of apigenin, diosmetin, and luteolin) (Hänsel *et al.*, 1992–1994; Meyer-Buchtela, 1999). Peppermint oil (European pharmacopeial grade) must contain 30–55% menthol, 14–32% menthone, 2.8–10.0% menthyl acetate, 3.5–14.0% cineole, 1.5–10.0% isomenthone, 1–9% menthofuran, 1–5% limonene, and no more than 4% pulegone or 1% carvone (Ph.Eur., 1997).

PHARMACOLOGICAL ACTIONS
Internal
Human
CRUDE PREPARATIONS: Antispasmodic action on the smooth muscles of the digestive tract, choleretic, carminative (Blumenthal *et al.*, 1998; Bradley, 1992).

ESSENTIAL OIL: Antispasmodic, carminative, cholagogic, antibacterial, secretolytic/mucolytic (Blumenthal *et al.*, 1998); relaxes smooth muscle (Micklefield *et al.*, 2000); relieves colonic spasms (Leicester and Hunt, 1982); carminative on lower esophageal sphincter (Sigmund and McNally, 1969).

External
Human
ESSENTIAL OIL: Analgesic in tension headache (Göbel *et al.*, 1994, 1996); menthol vapors stimulate cold receptors in nose (Burrow *et al.*, 1983).

Internal
Animal
Peppermint tea increases bile secretion (Steinmetzer, 1926); peppermint oil applied locally suppresses free acid flow (Necheles and Meyer, 1935); peppermint oil shortens emptying time of stomach by 46% (Sapoznik *et al.*, 1935); and inhibits serum cholinesterase (Caujolle *et al.*, 1944); flavonoids are choleretic (Pasechnik, 1966; Pasechnik and Gella, 1966); aqueous extract acts as a sedative and diuretic (Della Loggia *et al.*, 1990).

In vitro
Oil is bacteriostatic against *Candida albicans*, *Escherichia coli*, *Staphylococcus aureus*, and *Pseudomonas aeruginosa* (Koscik, 1955); and bactericidal against *Bacillus anthracis* and swine erysipelas bacteria (Abdullin, 1962) and isolated human coli (Taylor *et al.*, 1984b). Leaf extract is antiviral against Newcastle disease (NDV), herpes simplex, vaccinia, Semliki Forest, and West Nile viruses (Herrmann and Kucera, 1967); flavonoids inhibit ileum muscular contractions and relax gastrointestinal smooth muscle (Lallement-Guilbert and Bézanger-Beauquesne, 1970; Hill and Aaronson, 1991); alcoholic extract is antispasmodic (Forster *et al.*, 1980; Forster, 1983); and inhibits colonic motility (Taylor *et al.*, 1984a).

MECHANISM OF ACTION
- The pharmacological actions are due partly to the volatile oil (Harries *et al.*, 1978), to flavonoids and phenolic acids (Bruneton, 1999; Steinegger and Hänsel, 1988), and to the labiate tannins (Schilcher, 1997).
- Some studies have proposed that the mechanism for the carminative action is peppermint's ability to reduce the tonus of the esophageal sphincter, releasing entrapped air (Demling and Steger, 1969; Giachetti *et al.*, 1988).
- Based on *in vitro* experiments, the antispasmodic effect of the volatile oil is due to the inhibition of smooth muscle contractions through blocking calcium influx into muscle cells (Hawthorne *et al.*, 1988; Hills and Aaronson, 1991; Taylor *et al.*, 1984b).
- Peppermint inhibits enterocyte glucose uptake by direct action at the brush border membrane. In serous membranes, it inhibits the response to acetylcholine without reducing the effect of mucosal glucose. This is consistent with a reduced availability of calcium, which causes a relaxing effect on the intestinal smooth muscle (Beesley *et al.*, 1996).

- After ingestion of an enteric-coated capsule, the menthol is not metabolized in the small or large intestine, but it reaches the colon. A third of the menthol is reabsorbed, and the rest acts locally on the smooth muscle. About 35% of the applied menthol is found in the urine after 24 hours (Morant and Ruppanner, 2001).

CONTRAINDICATIONS

CRUDE HERB: Gallstones (Blumenthal *et al.,* 1998; Braun *et al.,* 1996); esophageal reflux (Sigmund and McNally, 1969).

ESSENTIAL OIL: Achlorhydria (absence of free hydrochloric acid in gastric juice) (Morant and Ruppanner, 2001; Rees *et al.,* 1979); obstruction of bile ducts, gallbladder inflammation, and severe liver damage. In case of gallstones, to be used only after consultation with a healthcare provider. Peppermint oil should not be used on the faces (particularly the noses) of infants and small children (Blumenthal *et al.,* 1998). Peppermint oil is contraindicated for infants and small children due to the potential risk of spasms of the tongue or respiratory arrest (Schulz *et al.,* 1998).

PREGNANCY AND LACTATION: No known restrictions (Blumenthal *et al.,* 1998; McGuffin *et al.,* 1997).

ADVERSE EFFECTS

None known according to Commission E (Blumenthal *et al.,* 1998; Braun *et al.,* 1996). Twelve cases of oral-contact sensitivity to peppermint oil and/or menthol have been reported in patients with intra-oral symptoms in association with burning-mouth syndrome, recurrent oral ulceration, or a lichenoid reaction (Morton *et al.,* 1995).

DRUG INTERACTIONS

None known (Braun *et al.,* 1996; Blumenthal *et al.,* 1998; ESCOP, 1997). Menthol-containing preparations may interfere with gastrointestinal-stimulant drugs (e.g., cisapride) used to treat nighttime heartburn due to the reflux of stomach acid into the esophagus (Austin *et al.,* 2000). Concurrent administration of peppermint oil with antacids or ingestion during meals can cause the oil to be released from capsules prematurely resulting in a loss of effectiveness (Morant and Ruppanner, 2001).

AMERICAN HERBAL PRODUCTS ASSOCIATION (AHPA) SAFETY RATING

CLASS 1: Herb that can be consumed safely when used appropriately (McGuffin *et al.,* 1997).

REGULATORY STATUS

AUSTRIA: Dried leaf official in *Austrian Pharmacopoeia,* ÖAB 1990–1996 (Meyer-Buchtela, 1999; Reynolds *et al.,* 1993; Wichtl, 1997*).*

BELGIUM: Permitted as Traditional Herbal Medicine (THM) digestive aid (Bradley, 1992; WHO, 1998).

CANADA: Peppermint Leaf Labeling Standard: Schedule OTC Traditional Herbal Medicine as an aid to digestion (Health Canada, 1996). Also permitted as a homeopathic drug. In both cases requires premarket authorization and assignment of a Drug Identification Number (DIN) (Health Canada, 2001). Food ingredient without claim (Health Canada, 1997).

EUROPEAN UNION: Whole, dried leaf containing no less than 1.2% essential oil; cut, dried leaf containing not less than 0.9% essential oil; and steam-distilled oil from fresh, flowering, aerial parts are official in the *European Pharmacopoeia* (Ph.Eur., 1997).

FRANCE: Dried leaf official in *French Pharmacopoeia,* Ph.Fr. X (Bradley, 1992; Reynolds *et al.,* 1993). Traditional Herbal Medicine for internal and external use with specific indications listed in the French Expl. Note, 1998. (Bradley, 1992; Bruneton, 1999; WHO, 1998). Oil is aromatherapy drug (Goetz, 1999).

GERMANY: Peppermint leaf and oil are approved drugs of the Commission E monographs (Blumenthal *et al.,* 1998). Peppermint leaf tea is an approved drug in the German Standard License monographs (Braun *et al.,* 1996).

ITALY: Dried leaf official in *Italian Pharmacopoeia* (Reynolds *et al.,* 1993).

RUSSIAN FEDERATION: Dried leaf official in the *State Pharmacopoeia of the Union of Soviet Socialist Republics,* Ph.USSR X (Bradley, 1992; Reynolds *et al.,* 1993).

SWEDEN: Classified as a natural remedy intended for self-medication, requiring premarketing authorization. A monograph for a peppermint-containing muliple-herb product, Uva-E tablet, is published in the Medical Products Agency (MPA) "Authorised Natural Remedies" (MPA, 1998, 2001; WHO, 1998).

SWITZERLAND: Dried leaf official in *Swiss Pharmacopoeia* Ph.Helv.VII (Reynolds *et al.,* 1993; Wichtl, 1997). Peppermint oil is a Category C nonprescription drug with sale limited to pharmacies. Peppermint tea is a Category D nonprescription drug with sale limited to pharmacies and drugstores (Morant and Ruppanner, 2001; WHO, 1998).

U.K.: Herbal medicine for oral use. *General Sale List,* Schedule 1, Table A (Bradley, 1992; Wichtl and Bisset, 1994). Peppermint leaf and oil official in the *British Pharmacopoeia,* BP 1993 (Health Canada, 1996).

U.S.: Generally Recognized as Safe (GRAS) (US FDA, 1998). Dietary supplement or conventional food depending on label claim statement (USC, 1994). Peppermint leaf and oil have official monographs in the *National Formulary.* Peppermint water and peppermint spirit have official monographs in the *United States Pharmacopeia* (USP, 2002).

CLINICAL REVIEW

Twenty-three studies (1,185 total participants) are outlined in the following table, "Clinical Studies on Peppermint." All but one of these studies (Nash, *et al.,* 1986) demonstrated positive results for various gastrointestinal and neurological conditions. Included are 14 double-blind (DB) studies investigating treatment of non-ulcer or functional dyspepsia (Freise and Köhler, 1999; Madisch *et al.,* 1999; May *et al.,* 1996, 2000), IBS (Liu *et al.,* 1997; Carling *et al.,* 1989; Lawson *et al.,* 1988; Nash *et al.,* 1986; Dew *et al.,* 1984; Rees *et al.,* 1979); spasm during barium enema (Sparks *et al.,* 1995); and tension headaches (Göbel *et al.,* 1994, 1996). In 1998, a meta-analysis of DB, placebo-controlled trials indicated that peppermint oil could provide symptomatic relief of IBS, though the authors cited methodological flaws in most of the studies (Pittler and Ernst, 1998). In 2000, a systematic review of randomized, controlled trials concluded that peppermint oil for irritable bowel syndrome requires further study (Jailwala *et al.,* 2000).

BRANDED PRODUCTS*

Colpermin®: Tillotts Pharma AG / Hauptstrasse 27 / CH–4417 Zeifen / Switzerland / Tel: +41–61–935–2626 / Fax: +41–61–935–2625. Enteric-coated capsules containing 187 mg (0.2 ml) peppermint leaf oil with 368 mg excipients per capsule, and E 132 coloring agent.

Enteroplant®: Dr. Willmar Schwabe Pharmaceuticals / International Division / Willmar Schwabe Str. 4 / D-76227 Karlsruhe / Germany / Tel: +49-721-4005 ext. 294 / www.schwabepharma.com / Email: melville–eaves@schwabe.de. Enteric-coated capsules containing 90 mg peppermint leaf oil and 50 mg caraway seed oil.

Euminz®: Lichtwer Pharma AG / Wallenroder Strasse 8-14 / 13435 Berlin / Germany / Tel: +49-30-40-3700 / Fax: +49-30-40-3704-49 / www.lichtwer.de. Liquid preparation containing 10 g of peppermint leaf oil and ethanol (90%).

Peppermint oil BP: Manufacturer information unavailable.

*American equivalents, if any, are found in the Product Table beginning on page 398.

REFERENCES

Abdullin K. Bactericidal effect of essential oils. *Uch Zap Kazansk Vet Inst* 1962;84:75–9.

Austin S, Batz F, Yarnell E, Brown D. Common drugs and their potential interactions with herbs or nutrients. *Healthnotes Rev Complement Integrat Med* 2000;7(2):164.

Beesley A, Hardcastle J, Hardcastle P, Taylor C. Influence of peppermint oil on absorptive and secretory processes in rat small intestine. *Gut* 1996;39(2):214–9.

Blumenthal M, Busse WR, Goldberg A, Gruenwald J, Hall T, Riggins CW, Rister RS (eds.). Klein S, Rister RS (trans.). *The Complete German Commission E Monographs—Therapeutic Guide to Herbal Medicines*. Austin, TX: American Botanical Council; Boston: Integrative Medicine Communication; 1998; 180-2.

BP. See: *British Pharmacopoeia*.

Bradley P (ed.). *British Herbal Compendium*, Vol. 1. Dorset, UK: British Herbal Medicine Association 1992;174–6.

Braun R, Surmann R, Wendt R, Wichtl M, Ziegenmeyer J (eds.). *Standardzulassungen für Fertigarzneimittel: Text und Kommentar*, 11. Ergänzungslieferung. Stuttgart, Germany: Deutscher Apotheker Verlag; 1996 Feb;1499.99.99.

Briggs C. Peppermint: medicinal herb and flavouring agent. *CPJ/RPC* 1993 Mar;89–92.

British Pharmacopoeia (BP), Vol I. London, UK: Her Majesty's Stationery Office; 1980;333–5, 560, 719–20.

Bruneton J. *Pharmacognosy Phytochemistry Medicinal Plants*, 2nd ed. Paris, France: Lavoisier Publishing; 1999;532–7.

Burrow A, Eccles R, Jones A. The effects of camphor, eucalyptus and menthol vapour on nasal resistance to airflow and nasal sensation. *Acta Otolaryngol (Stockh)* 1983;96(1–2):157–61.

Carius W. Effect of pressurized extraction process on the release of active ingredients from tea derived remedies [dissertation]. [in German]. Saarbrücken: Mathematisch-Naturwissenschaftliche Fakultät der Universität des Saarlandes; 1990.

Carling L, Svedberg Le, Hulten S. Short-term treatment of the irritable bowel syndrome: a placebo-controlled trial of peppermint oil against hyoscyamine. *Opuscula Medica* 1989;34:55–7.

Caujolle F, Vincent D, Franck C. Action of essential oils on serum cholinesterase. *Compt Rend Soc Biol* 1944;138:556–8.

Della Loggia R, Tubaro A, Lunder T. Evaluation of some pharmacological activities of a peppermint extract. *Fitoterapia* 1990;61:215–21.

Demling L, Steger W. About the rationale of folk medicine: peppermint and onion. [in German]. *Fortschr Med* 1969;37:1305–6.

Dew M, Evans B, Rhodes J. Peppermint oil for the irritable bowel syndrome: a multicentre trial. *Br J Clin Pract* 1984;38(11–12):394, 398.

Duband F, Carnat A, Carnat A, *et al*. Composition aromatique et polyphenolique de l'infuse dementhe, *Mentha x piperita* L. *Ann Pharm Fr* 1992;50:146–55.

Duthie H. The effect of peppermint oil on colonic motility in man. *Br J Surg* 1981;68:820.

Ergänzungsbuch zum Deutschen Arzneibuch 6. Ausgabe (Erg.B.6. 1953). Stuttgart: Deutscher Apotheker Verlag; 1953.

Erg.B.6. See: *Ergänzungsbuch zum Deutschen Arzneibuch*.

ESCOP. See: European Scientific Cooperative on Phytotherapy.

Europäisches Arzneibuch (Ph.Eur. 3). Stuttgart, Germany: Deutscher Apotheker Verlag; 1997;1466–1468.

European Pharmacopoeia (Ph.Eur.) (3rd ed. 1997). Strasbourg, France: Council of Europe. 1997.

European Scientific Cooperative on Phytotherapy. *Menthae piperitae folium and Menthae piperitae aetheroleum. In: Monographs on the Medicinal Uses of Plant Drugs*. Exeter, U.K.: European Scientific Cooperative on Phytotherapy; 1997.

Evans B, Levine D, Hayberry J, *et al*. Multicentre trial of peppermint oil capsules in irritable bowel syndrome. *Gastroenterology World Congress*; 1982;50.

Feng X. Effect of peppermint oil hot compresses in preventing abdominal distension in postoperative gynecological patients. [in Chinese]. *Chung Hua Hu Li Tsa Chih* 1997;21(10):577–8.

Fernández F. *Menta piperita* en el tratamiento de syndrome de colon irritable. *Invest Med Inter* 1990;17:42–6.

Forster H. Spasmolytische Wirkung pflanzlicher Carminativa. *Z Allg Med* 1983;59:1327–33.

Forster H, Niklas H, Lutz S. Antispasmodic effects of some medicinal plants. *Planta Med* 1980; 40:309–19.

Freise J, Köhler S. Peppermint oil-caraway oil fixed combination in non-ulcer dyspepsia comparison of the effects of two Galenical preparations. [in German]. *Pharmazie* 1999;54(3):210–215.

Fugmann B, Lang-Fugmann S, Steglich W. Pfefferminzöle. In: *Römpp-Lexikon Naturstoffe*. Stuttgart, Germany: Georg Thieme Verlag; 1997;478–9.

General Sale List (GSL). Statutory Instrument (S.I.). The Medicines (Products other than Veterinary Drugs). London, UK: Her Majesty's Stationery Office; 1984; S.I. No. 769, as amended 1985; S.I. No. 1540, 1990; S.I. No. 1129, 1994; S.I. No. 2410.

Giachetti D, Taddei E, Taddei I. Pharmacological activity of essential oils on Oddi's sphincter. *Planta Med* 1988;54(5):389–92.

Göbel H, Fresenius J, Heinze A, Dworschak M, Soyka D. Effectiveness of Oleum *Menthae piperitae* and paracetamol in therapy of tension headache. [in German]. *Nervenarzt* 1996;67(8):672–81.

Göbel H, Schmidt G, Soyka D. Effect of peppermint and eucalyptus oil preparations on neurophysiological and experimental algesimetric headache parameters. *Cephalalgia* 1994;14(3):229–34; discussion 182.

Goetz P. Phytotherapie in Frankreich. *Z Phytother* 1999;20:320–8.

GSL. See: *General Sale List*.

Hänsel R, Keller K, Rimpler H, Schneider G (eds.). *Hager's Handbuch der Pharmazeutischen Praxis*, Drogen E-O, 5th ed. Berlin, Germany: Springer-Verlag; 1992–1994;828–39.

Harries N, James K, Pugh W. Antifoaming and carminative actions of volatile oils. *J Clin Pharmacy* 1978;2:171–7.

Hawthorne M, Ferrante J, Luchowski E, *et al*. The actions of peppermint oil and menthol on calcium channel dependent processes in intestinal, neuronal, and cardiac preparations. *J Aliment Pharmacol Therap* 1988;2:101–8.

Health Canada. *Drug Product Database (DPD)*. Ottawa, Ontario: Health Canada Therapeutic Products Programme. 2001.

Health Canada. *Labelling Standard: Peppermint*. Ottawa, Canada: Health Canada Therapeutic Products Programme; 17 May 1996;1–4.

Health Canada. Peppermint Essence, Peppermint Extract or Peppermint Flavour. In: *The Food and Drugs Act and Regulations* 1997. Ottawa, Canada: Minister of Public Works and Government Services Canada; 1997;50. B10.019[S].

Herrmann E, Kucera L. Antiviral substances in plants of the mint family (*Labiatae*). III. Peppermint (*Mentha piperita*) and other mint plants. *Proc Soc Exp Biol Med* 1967;124(3):874–8.

Hills J, Aaronson P. The mechanism of action of peppermint oil in gastrointestinal smooth muscle. *Gastroenterolgy* 1991;101:55–65.

Jailwala J, Imperiale T, Kroenke K. Pharmacologic treatment of the irritable bowel syndrome: a systematic review of randomized, controlled trials. *Ann Intern Med* 2000;133(2):136–47.

Jarvis L, Hogg J, Houghton C. Topical peppermint oil for the relief of spasm at barium enema. *Clin Radiol* 1992;46:A435.

Karnick C. *Pharmacopoeial Standards of Herbal Plants*, Vol. 1. Delhi, India: Sri Satguru Publications; 1994;243–4.

Koch TR Peppermint oil and irritable bowel syndrome. *Am J Gastroenterol* 1998;93(11):2304–5.

Koscik A. [Antibiotic properties of vegetable oils]. *Roczniki Akad Med Bialymstoku* 1955;1:227–36.

Krogh CME (ed.). *Compendium of Pharmaceuticals and Specialties*. Ottawa, Canada: Canadian Pharmaceutical Association; 1989;454–5.

Lallement-Guilbert N, Bézanger-Beauquesne L. Recherches sur les flavonoids de quelques Labiées médicinales (romarin, mentha poivrée, sauge officinale). *Plant Méd Phytothér* 1970;4:92–107.

Lawson M, Knight R, Tran K, Walker G, Robers-Thomson I. Failure of enteric-coated peppermint oil in the irritable bowel syndrome: a randomized double-blind crossover study. *J Gastroent Hepatol* 1988;3:235–8.

Lech Y, Olesen K, Hey H, *et al*. Treatment of irritable bowel syndrome with peppermint oil. A double-blind study with a placebo. [in Danish]. *Ugeskr Laeger* 1988;150(40):2388–9.

Leicester R, Hunt R. Peppermint oil to reduce colonic spasm during endoscopy. *Lancet* 1982;2(8305):989.

Leung A, Foster S. *Encyclopedia of Common Natural Ingredients Used in Food, Drugs, and Cosmetics*, 2nd ed. New York, NY: John Wiley & Sons, Inc; 1996;368–72.

Liu J, Chen G, Yeh H, Huang C, Poon S. Enteric-coated peppermint-oil capsules in the treatment of irritable bowel syndrome: a prospective randomized trial. *J Gastroenterol* 1997;32(6):765–8.

Madisch A, Heydenreich C, Wieland V, Hufnagel R, Hotz J. Treatment of functional dyspepsia with a fixed peppermint oil and caraway oil combination preparation as compared to cisapride. A multicentre, reference-controlled double-blind equivalence study. *Arzneimittelforschung* 1999;49(11);925–32.

May B, Kuntz H, Kieser M, Kohler S. Efficacy of a fixed peppermint oil/caraway oil combination in non-ulcer dyspepsia. *Arzneimittelforschung* 1996;46(12):1149–53.

May B, Kohler S, Schneider B. Efficacy and tolerability of a fixed combination of peppermint oil and caraway oil in patients suffering from functional dyspepsia. *Aliment Pharmacol The* 2000 Dec 27;14(12):1671–7.

McGuffin M, Hobbs C, Upton R, Goldberg A (eds.). *American Herbal Product Association's Botanical Safety Handbook*. Boca Raton, FL: CRC Press; 1997;75.

McKenzie J, Gallacher M. A sweet smelling success: use of peppermint oil in helping patients accept their colostomies. *Nurs Time* 1989;85(27):48–9.

Medical Products Agency (MPA). Naturläkemedel: Authorised Natural Remedies (as of January 24, 2001). Uppsala, Sweden: Medical Products Agency. 2001.

Medical Products Agency (MPA). Naturläkemedelsmonografi: Uva-E. Uppsala, Sweden: Medical Products Agency. 1998.

Meyer-Buchtela E. *Tee-Rezepturen: Ein Handbuch für Apotheker und Ärzte*. Stuttgart, Germany: Deutscher Apotheker Verlag; 1999.

Micklefield G, Greving I, May B. Effects of peppermint oil and caraway oil on gastroduodenal motility. *Phytother Res* 2000;24(1):20–3.

Morant J, Ruppanner H (eds.). *Arzneimittel-Kompendium der Schweiz®* 2001. Basel, Switzerland: Documed AG; 2001.

Morton C, Garioch J, Todd P, Lamey P, Forsyth A. Contact sensitivity to menthol and peppermint in patients with intra-oral symptoms. *Contact Dermatitis* 1995;32(5):281–4.

MPA. See: Medical Products Agency.

Nash P, Gould S, Barnardo D. Peppermint oil does not relieve the pain of irritable bowel syndrome. *Br J Clin Pract* 1986;40:292–293.

NASS/USDA. See: National Agricultural Statistics Service U.S. Department of Agriculture.

National Agricultural Statistics Service U.S. Department of Agriculture (NASS/USDA). *United States: Area, Production, and Yields of Mint Oils* [report]. Washington, DC: U.S. Department of Agriculture; 2000.

Necheles H, Meyer J. The inhibition of gastric secretion by oil of peppermint. *Am J Physiol* 1935;110:686–91.

Niesel S. Investigation about the release and to the stability of selected plant contents materials under special consideration of modern phytochemical procedures [dissertation]. [in German]. Berlin, Germany: Fachbereich Pharmazie der Freien Universität Berlin; 1992.

Pasechnik I. Study of choleretic properties specific to flavonoids from *Menthae piperita* leaves. [in Russian]. *Farmakol Toksikol* 1966;29(6):735–7.

Pasechnik I, Gella E. Choleretic preparation from peppermint. [in Russian]. *Farm Zh (Kiev).* 1966; 21(5):49–53.

Ph.Eur. 3. See: *Europäisches Arzneibuch*.

Ph.Eur. See: *European Pharmacopoeia*.

Pittler M, Ernst E. Peppermint oil for irritable bowel syndrome: a critical review and meta-analysis. *Am J Gastroenterol* 1998;93(7):1131–5.

Pizzorno JE, Murray MT, editors. *Textbook of Natural Medicine*, Vol 1, 2nd ed. New York: Churchill Livingstone. 1999;827–30.

Rees WDW, Evans BK, Rhodes J. Treating irritable bowel syndrome with peppermint oil. *Br Med J* 1979;6:835–836.

Reynolds JEF, Pafitt K, Parsons AV, Sweetman SC (eds.). *Martindale: The Extra Pharmacopoeia*, 30th edition. London, U.K.: The Pharmaceutical Press. 1993;899.

Robbers J, Tyler V. *Herbs of Choice: The Therapeutic Use of Phytomedicinals*. New York, NY: Haworth Herbal Press 1999;66–8.

Robson N. Carminative properties of peppermint in magnesium trisilicate, BP (let-ter). *Anaesthesia* 1987;42(7):776–7.

Sapoznik H, Arens R, Meyer J, Necheles H. The effect of oil of peppermint on the emptying time of the stomach. *JAMA* 1935;104:1792–4.

Shaw G, Srivastava E, Sadlier M, *et al.* Stress management for irritable bowel syndrome: a controlled trial. *Digestion* 1991;50(1):36–42.

Schilcher H. *Phytotherapy in Paediatrics: Handbook for Physicians and Pharmacists*. Stuttgart, Germany: Medpharm Scientific Publishers; 1997; 46–8, 56.

Schulz V, Hänsel R, Tyler V. *Rational Phytotherapy: A Physicians' Guide to Herbal Medicine*. Berlin, Germany: Springer Verlag; 1998.

Sigmund C, McNally E. The action of a carminative on the lower esophageal sphincter. *Gastroenterol* 1969;56:13–8.

Somerville K, Richmond C, Bell G. Delayed release peppermint oil capsules (Colpermin®) for the spastic colon syndrome: a pharmacokinetics study. *Br J Clin Pharmacol* 1984;18(4):638–40.

Sparks M, O'Sullivan P, Herrington A, Morcos S. Does peppermint oil relieve spasm during barium enema? *Br J Radiol* 1995;68(812):841–3.

Spence Information Services (SPINS). Top Ten Items – Natural Products Supermarkets – Medicinal Single Teas – Ranked by Dollar Sales – Total US. April 2000. San Francisco, CA: SPINS; 2000.

SPINS. See: Spence Information Services.

Steinegger E, Hänsel R. *Lehrbuch der Pharmakognosie und Phytopharmazie*. Berlin, Germany: Springer Verlag; 1988.

Steinmetzer K. Experimental investigation of Cholagoga. [in German]. *Wiener Klin Wschr* 1926;39:1418–22; 1455–7.

Sullivan T, Warm J, Schefft B, *et al.* Effects of olfactory stimulation on the vigilance performance of individuals with brain injury. *J Clin Exp Neuropsychol* 1998;20(2):227–36.

Tate S. Peppermint oil: a treatment for postoperative nausea. *J Adv Nurs* 1997;26(3):543–9.

Taylor B, Duthie H, Oliveira R, Rhodes J. Ultrasound used to measure the response of colonic motility to essential oils. *Gastrointest Motil Proc Int Symp, 9th 1983*. 1984a;441–8.

Taylor B, Luscombe D, Duthie H. Inhibitory effects of peppermint oil and menthol on isolated human coli. *Gut* 1984b;25:A1168–9.

Tyler V, Brady L, Robbers J. *Pharmacognosy*, 9th ed. Philadelphia, PA: Lea & Febiger; 1988;113–9.

United States Congress (USC). Public Law 103–417: Dietary Supplement Health and Education Act of 1994. Washington, DC: 103rd Congress of the United States; 1994.

United States Food and Drug Administration (US FDA). *Code of Federal Regulations* (21 CFR) Part 182 – Substances Generally Recognized as Safe. Washington, DC: Office of the Federal Register National Archives and Records Administration; 1998;427–33.

United States Pharmacopeia (USP 25th Revision) - The National Formulary (NF 20th Edition). Rockville, MD: United States Pharmacopeial Convention, Inc. 2002.

USC. See: United States Congress.

US FDA. See: United States Food and Drug Administration.

USP. See: *United States Pharmacopeia*.

Warm J, Dember W, Parasuraman R. Effects of olfactory stimulation on performance and stress in a visual sustained attention task. *J Soc Cosmet Chem* 1991;42:199–210.

WHO. See: World Health Organization.

Wichtl M, Bisset N (eds.). *Herbal Drugs and Phytopharmaceuticals: A Handbook for Practice on a Scientific Basis*. Stuttgart, Germany: Medpharm Scientific Publishers; 1994.

Wichtl M (ed.). *Teedrogen und Phytopharmaka, 3. Auflage: Ein Handbuch für die Praxis auf wissenschaftlicher Grundlage*. Stuttgart, Germany: Wissenschaftliche Verlagsgesellschaft mbH. 1997;391–4.

World Health Organization (WHO). *Regulatory Status of Herbal Medicines: A Worldwide Review*. Geneva, Switzerland: World Health Organization Traditional Medicine Programme; 1998;17;26–7.

Clinical Studies on Peppermint (Mentha x piperita L.)

Gastrointestinal

Author/Year	Subject	Design	Duration	Dosage	Preparation	Results/Conclusion
Tate, 1997	Postoperative nausea	R, PC, Cm n=18 patients undergoing major gynecological surgery	3 days (day of operation and 2 postoperative days)	Essential peppermint oil vs. peppermint essence (placebo) vs. no treatment	Peppermint oil vs. peppermint essence (placebo) vs. no treatment	Statistically significant differences were demonstrated on day of operation using Kruskal-Wallis test (p=0.0487). Using Mann-Whitney U-test, a difference between placebo and experimental groups was shown (U=3; p=0.02). Experimental group required less conventional antiemetics and received more opioid analgesia postoperatively. Author concludes that peppermint oil may improve postoperative nausea in gynecological patients.
Liu et al., 1997	Irritable bowel syndrome (IBS)	P, R, DB, PC n=110	4 weeks	1 capsule, 3–4x/day, 15–30 minutes before meals vs. placebo	Colpermin® enteric-coated capsule containing 187 mg peppermint oil vs. placebo	Using Mann-Whitney U-test, symptom improvement in peppermint oil group was significantly better (p<0.05) compared to placebo. In peppermint group 79% experienced alleviation of severity of abdominal pain (29 were pain-free); 83% had less abdominal distension, 83% had reduced stool frequency; 73% had fewer borborygmi; 79% had less flatulence. Colpermin® peppermint leaf oil was effective and well-tolerated.
Sparks et al., 1995	Spasm during barium enema	R, DB, C n=141 mean age=60 years	3 days bowel preparation before 1 day treatment and examination	Barium suspension with added peppermint oil, 1x/day vs. standard barium sulfate	Barium suspension with 370 ml water and 30 ml peppermint preparation (16 ml peppermint oil BP and 0.4 ml polysorbate) plus 10 ml peppermint preparation added to enema tubing	Significant decrease in spasm was observed in treatment group (60%) compared with control group (35%) (p<0.001). Fewer in peppermint group required intravenous buscopan (5 vs. 9) or exhibited spasm (23 vs. 39). Authors concluded that addition of peppermint oil to barium suspension appears to reduce incidence of colonic spasm during examination. Technique is simple, safe and economical and may lessen the need for intravenous administration of spasmolytic agents.
Shaw et al., 1991	Irritable bowel syndrome (IBS)	R, C n=35	Average of 6, 40-minute sessions with physiotherapist over 6 months	40 minutes of stress management with physiotherapist vs. Colpermin® 3x/day	Stress management program vs. treatment with Colpermin® enteric-coated capsule containing 187 mg peppermint oil vs. conventional management	Two-thirds of patients enrolled in the stress management program found it effective in relieving symptoms (p<0.002) and experienced fewer attacks (p<0.004), of less severity, with benefit maintained for at least 12 months compared to the Colpermin® group.
Fernández, 1990	Irritable bowel syndrome (IBS)	O, MC n=50	4 weeks	1 capsule, 3x/day 30 minutes before meals	Capsule containing 0.2 ml peppermint oil	Evaluation of all signs and symptoms, both pre-treatment and post-treatment, confirmed statistically significant decrease of symptoms.
McKenzie and Gallacher, 1989	Trial 1: Fecal odor in colostomy bags; Trial 2: Effect on colostomy acceptance	O, U Trial 1: n=10 patients, Trial 2: n=20 patients	Trial 1: 1 day Trial 2: 3 days starting on third postoperative day	1 capsule, 3x/day	Enteric-coated capsule containing peppermint oil in a thixotropic paste (brand not stated)	Trial 1: Contents of colostomy bags were checked for intact or partially digested capsules and for smell of peppermint. Only one patient passed capsule unchanged. Trial 2: 14 of 20 patients found odor improved and 1 found it worse. 15 found their colostomies more acceptable and wished to continue taking peppermint. Consistency of feces and frequency of bag-changing appeared to improve.
Carling et al., 1989	Irritable bowel syndrome (IBS)	R, DB, CO n=40	2 weeks		Enteric-coated capsule containing 0.2 ml peppermint oil vs. 0.2 mg hyoscyamine or placebo	Peppermint oil treatment tended to have more pronounced effect on symptoms than placebo or hyoscyamine but was not statistically significant. Findings favor the short-term use of enteric-coated peppermint oil as an antispasmodic for IBS.

KEY: **C** – controlled, **CC** – case-control, **CH** – cohort, **CI** – confidence interval, **Cm** – comparison, **CO** – crossover, **CS** – cross-sectional, **DB** – double-blind, **E** – epidemiological, **LC** – longitudinal cohort, **MA** – meta-analysis, **MC** – multi-center, **n** – number of patients, **O** – open, **OB** – observational, **OL** – open label, **OR** – odds ratio, **P** – prospective, **PB** – patient-blind, **PC** – placebo-controlled, **PG** – parallel group, **PS** – pilot study, **R** – randomized, **RC** – reference-controlled, **RCS** – retrospective cross-sectional, **RS** - retrospective, **S** – surveillance, **SB** – single-blind, **SC** – single-center, **U** – uncontrolled, **UP** – unpublished, **VC** – vehicle-controlled.

Gastrointestinal (cont.)

Author/Year	Subject	Design	Duration	Dosage	Preparation	Results/Conclusion
Lawson et al., 1988	Irritable bowel syndrome (IBS)	R, DB, CO n=18	4 weeks	3 capsules, 3x/day	Enteric-coated capsule containing 0.2 ml peppermint oil (brand not stated)	Peppermint group had small, but statistically significant increase in frequency of defecation but no significant change in scores for global severity of symptoms or scores for specific symptoms of pain, bloating, urgent defecation, and sensation of incomplete evacuation.
Nash et al., 1986	Irritable bowel syndrome (IBS)	R, DB, PC, CO n=34	4 weeks	2 capsules, 3x/day	Capsule containing 0.2 ml peppermint oil vs. placebo Colpermin®	In terms of overall symptoms, patients' assessments at end of 2 and 4 weeks of treatment showed no significant difference between peppermint oil and placebo.
Dew et al., 1984	Irritable bowel syndrome (IBS)	R, DB, PC, CO, MC n=29 mean age 42 years	2 weeks	1–2 capsules, 3x/day depending on severity of symptoms	Elanco LOK gelatin capsules containing 0.2 ml peppermint oil coated with cellulose acetate phthalate vs. placebo capsules containing 0.2 ml of arachis oil.	Patients in peppermint group were relieved of symptoms, while the number of their daily bowel movements was unaffected. Patients felt significantly better while taking peppermint compared with placebo (p<0.001) and considered peppermint better than placebo in relieving abdominal symptoms (p<0.001). Study suggested beneficial effect of peppermint for treatment of IBS based on patient data.
Somerville et al., 1984	Pharmacokinetics of peppermint oil in spastic colon syndrome	Cm, U n=12 6 healthy volunteers (17–37 years) and 6 ileostomy patients (22–49 years)	24 hours	2 capsules, 3x/day	Colpermin® enteric-coated capsule containing 187 mg peppermint oil vs. peppermint oil in soft-gel capsules	Total 24-hour urinary excretion of menthol was similar in both preparations, but peak menthol excretion levels were lower and were delayed with enteric-coated capsule vs. soft gelatin capsules. Menthol excretion was reduced in ileostomy patients taking enteric-coated capsules, and moderate amounts of unmetabolized menthol were recovered from ileostomy effluent. Enteric-coated capsules can deliver unmetabolized oil directly to the colon.
Leicester and Hunt, 1982	Colonic spasm during endoscopy	U n=20	1 day	Peppermint oil injected along the biopsy channel of colonoscope into lumen of colon, 1x	Peppermint oil BP	Peppermint oil caused a relaxant effect on gastrointestinal tract that relieved colonic spasms within 30 seconds after injection in all 20 patients, allowing easier passage of the instrument or assisting in polypectomy.
Duthie, 1981	Colonic motility	R, PC, CO n=6	1 day	Peppermint oil injected into the lumen of the colon, 1x	Peppermint oil 0.2 ml in 50 ml of 0.9% sodium chloride with 1 in 10,000 polysorbate as suspending agent vs. vehicle alone (placebo)	Period of inhibition of all motor activity in all 6 subjects began within 2 minutes of peppermint oil administration lasting 7–23 minutes (mean 12 minutes). Decrease in percentage activity and motility index seen in all 6 subjects during first 10 minutes after introducing oil. Differences were statistically significant (actual statistics not stated). Decrease in motility index 10–20 minutes after oil was also statistically significant.
Rees et al., 1979	Irritable bowel syndrome (IBS)	DB, PC, CO n=16	6 weeks (3 weeks each)	1–2 capsules, 3x/day depending on severity of symptoms	Elanco LOK gelatin capsules containing 0.2 ml peppermint oil coated with cellulose acetate phthalate vs. placebo capsules containing 0.2 ml of arachis oil	Overall assessment showed that patients felt significantly better (p<0.01) during peppermint treatment period compared to placebo and considered peppermint oil more effective than placebo in relieving abdominal symptoms (p<0.005).

KEY: C – controlled, **CC** – case-control, **CH** – cohort, **CI** – confidence interval, **Cm** – comparison, **CO** – crossover, **CS** – cross-sectional, **DB** – double-blind, **E** – epidemiological, **LC** – longitudinal cohort, **MA** – meta-analysis, **MC** – multi-center, **n** – number of patients, **O** – open, **OB** – observational, **OL** – open label, **OR** – odds ratio, **P** – prospective, **PB** – patient-blind, **PC** – placebo-controlled, **PG** – parallel group, **PS** – pilot study, **R** – randomized, **RC** – reference-controlled, **RCS** – retrospective cross-sectional, **RS** - retrospective, **S** – surveillance, **SB** – single-blind, **SC** – single-center, **U** – uncontrolled, **UP** – unpublished, **VC** – vehicle-controlled.

Gastrointestinal

Combination Preparations

Author/Year	Subject	Design	Duration	Dosage	Preparation	Results/Conclusion
Micklefield et al., 2000	Gastro-duodenal motility	P, C, Cm, CO n=6 healthy volunteers (24–40 years)	1 day	1 capsule/day	Enteroplant® enteric-coated capsule; 90 mg peppermint oil and 50 mg caraway oil vs. non-enteric-coated capsule of peppermint-caraway oil combination	Both enteric-coated and non-enteric-coated preparations have effects on migrating motor complex (MMC), primarily a decrease in the number of contractions and contraction amplitudes. Non-enteric-coated preparation shows effect mainly during first MMC after administration, and enteric-coated preparation has a temporarily delayed effect during the second MMC after administration. Authors conclude that both preparations are safe, acting locally to cause smooth muscle relaxation. No adverse effects were noted.
Freise and Köhler, 1999	Non-ulcer dyspepsia	P, Cm, R, DB, C, MC n=223	29 days plus a 1-week washout phase before study	1 capsule, 3x/day with water before meals	Enteroplant® enteric-coated capsule; 90 mg peppermint oil and 50 mg caraway seed oil vs. enteric-soluble formulation containing 36 mg peppermint oil and 20 mg caraway oil	Statistically significant decline in pain intensity observed in both groups. Equivalent efficacy of both preparations was demonstrated (p<0.001). Concomitant variable results were similar in both groups. Test preparation significantly better (p= 0.04) in pain frequency. Authors conclude that the enteric-coated capsule provides an advantage over the acid-soluble formulation because it not only reduces pain intensity, it also potentially decreases the number of side effects, including nausea and eructation, with peppermint taste.
Madisch et al., 1999	Functional dyspepsia	Cm, R, DB, C, MC n=118	4 weeks plus a 1-week washout phase before study	1 capsule, 2x/day with water, morning and noon, plus 1 placebo capsule/day in evening vs. 10 mg cisapride, 3x/day before meals	Enteroplant® enteric-coated capsule; 90 mg peppermint oil and 50 mg caraway seed oil vs. prokinetic agent Propulsid® cisapride	Reduction in visual analogue scale (VAS) pain intensity scores was comparable with drop of 4.62 points in peppermint/caraway group and 4.60 points in cisapride group (p=0.021). Reduction in frequency of VAS pain scores was equivalent by week 4 (p=0.0034). Flatulence decreased in peppermint group by 71.8% and 65.7% in cisapride group. Treating physicians concluded that 78.6% of peppermint group were very much or much improved compared to 70.9% in cisapride group. Peppermint/caraway oil preparation provides comparable effect to cisapride, is well-tolerated, is only one quarter the cost of cisapride therapy, and has fewer potential side effects.
May et al., 1996	Non-ulcer dyspepsia for at least 14 days	R, DB, PC, PG, MC n=45 mean age Enteroplant group=42 years, mean age placebo=47 years	4 weeks	1 capsule, 3x/day with water before meals	Enteroplant® enteric-coated capsule; 90 mg peppermint oil and 50 mg caraway seed oil vs. placebo	Clinical Global Impression (CGI) values were improved in 94.7% of treatment group vs. 55% placebo group (p=0.004). In treatment group, 63.2% were pain-free compared to only 25% in placebo group (p=0.005). Improvement in pain intensity was 89.5% in treatment group vs. 45% in placebo group (p=0.015). Authors conclude that treatment was equally successful for patients diagnosed with IBS and dyspepsia and that Enteroplant® has a risk-to-benefit ratio more favorable than standard treatment with synthetic chemical medicaments.
May et al., 2000	Functional dyspepsia	R, DB, PC n=96	4 weeks	1 capsule, 2x/day with water before meals	Enteroplant® (PCC) enteric-coated capsule; 90 mg peppermint oil and 50 mg caraway seed oil vs. placebo	Primary efficacy variables were the intra-individual change in (1) pain intensity, and (2) sensation of pressure, heaviness, and fullness between days 1 and 29, and the investigators' rating of (3) global improvement (Clinical Global Impressions [CGI] item 2) on day 29. The average intensity of pain was reduced by 40% vs. baseline in the PCC group and by 22% in the placebo group. Regarding pressure, heaviness, and fullness, a 43% reduction was observed for PCC vs. 22% for placebo. In CGI item 2, 67% (PCC) vs. 21% (placebo) of patients were described as much or very much improved. In all three target parameters, the superiority of PCC over a placebo was statistically significant.

KEY: C – controlled, **CC** – case-control, **CH** – cohort, **CI** – confidence interval, **Cm** – comparison, **CO** – crossover, **CS** – cross-sectional, **DB** – double-blind, **E** – epidemiological, **LC** – longitudinal cohort, **MA** – meta-analysis, **MC** – multi-center, **n** – number of patients, **O** – open, **OB** – observational, **OL** – open label, **OR** – odds ratio, **P** – prospective, **PB** – patient-blind, **PC** – placebo-controlled, **PG** – parallel group, **PS** – pilot study, **R** – randomized, **RC** – reference-controlled, **RCS** – retrospective cross-sectional, **RS** - retrospective, **S** – surveillance, **SB** – single-blind, **SC** – single-center, **U** – uncontrolled, **UP** – unpublished, **VC** – vehicle-controlled.

Neurology, Psychiatry

Author/Year	Subject	Design	Duration	Dosage	Preparation	Results/Conclusion
Sullivan et al., 1998	Effects on vigilance performance in brain injury	R, C n=40 patients with brain injury	30-minute vigilance task	Periodic whiffs of peppermint-scented air delivered by pumps that force air through plastic tubing into a glass reservoir	Peppermint-scented air vs. unscented air	Under fragrance conditions, controls reduced frequency of commissive errors (false alarms) over course of vigil, an adaptive strategy given the low probability of signals employed. False alarm rate of observers with brain injury increased precipitously toward end of vigil in unscented air condition. Exposure to scent of peppermint rendered false alarm scores of observers with brain injury similar to controls, a result that is consistent with evidence that olfactory stimulation activates brain areas vital for planning and judgement.
Göbel et al., 1996	Tension headaches	R, DB, PC, Cm, CO n=41 male and female patients (18–65 years)	Four headache episodes per patient	Topical application of peppermint oil or placebo solution to forehead and temples, repeated 1x after 15 or 30 minutes vs. oral 1,000 mg acetaminophen or 1,000 mg placebo vs. simultaneous application of 1,000 mg acetaminophen and 10% peppermint oil in ethanol solution	Euminz® (containing 10 g peppermint oil with ethanol 90%) vs. Paracetamol® (500 mg acetaminophen) vs. 90% ethanol solution with traces of peppermint oil for blinding purposes	Study involved analyses of 164 headache attacks of patients suffering from tension headaches. Compared to placebo, peppermint leaf oil significantly reduced clinical headache intensity within 15 minutes ($p<0.01$) with a continuing effect over the one hour observation period. No significant difference between acetaminophen and peppermint. Simultaneous acetaminophen and peppermint use did not result in significant additive effect. Authors conclude that peppermint oil efficiently alleviates tension-type headaches as well as acetaminophen. It is well-tolerated and a cost-effective alternative to conventional therapies.
Göbel et al., 1994	Neuro-physiological, psychological, and experimental algesimetric parameters	Cm, CO, R, DB, PC n=32 healthy subjects	1 day	Oil and ethanol mixture applied to forehead and temples with small sponge	Peppermint oil and ethanol vs. peppermint oil with eucalyptus oil and ethanol vs. placebo (brands not stated)	Peppermint oil demonstrated significant analgesic effect with reduction in sensitivity to headache. Peppermint oil with eucalyptus oil had little influence on pain sensitivity but increased cognitive performance and had a muscle-relaxing and mentally relaxing effect.
Warm et al., 1991	Effects on signal detectability in tasks demanding sustained attention	R, C n=36 college students (men and women with normal or corrected-to-normal vision)	40 minutes divided into 4 consecutive 10-minute periods	Repeated exposure time of 150 milli-seconds per 10-minute period	Peppermint-scented air vs. muguet-scented air (International Flavors and Fragrances, Inc.) vs. unscented air	A statistical difference was found between groups exposed to air scented with fragrance of peppermint ($p<0.05$) or muguet ($p<0.05$) vs. placebo. Authors concluded that this scented air can enhance rate of signal detections in a vigilance task without a concomitant increase in errors of commission vs. placebo. It is suggested that exposure to fragrance may serve as an effective form of ancillary stimulation in tasks demanding close attention for prolonged periods.

KEY: C – controlled, **CC** – case-control, **CH** – cohort, **CI** – confidence interval, **Cm** – comparison, **CO** – crossover, **CS** – cross-sectional, **DB** – double-blind, **E** – epidemiological, **LC** – longitudinal cohort, **MA** – meta-analysis, **MC** – multi-center, **n** – number of patients, **O** – open, **OB** – observational, **OL** – open label, **OR** – odds ratio, **P** – prospective, **PB** – patient-blind, **PC** – placebo-controlled, **PG** – parallel group, **PS** – pilot study, **R** – randomized, **RC** – reference-controlled, **RCS** – retrospective cross-sectional, **RS** - retrospective, **S** – surveillance, **SB** – single-blind, **SC** – single-center, **U** – uncontrolled, **UP** – unpublished, **VC** – vehicle-controlled.

Saw Palmetto

Serenoa repens (W. Bartram) Small (syn. *Sabal serrulata* [Michx.] Nutt. ex Schult. & Schult. f.;
Serenoa serrulata (Michx.) G. Nichols.)

[Fam. *Arecaceae*]

OVERVIEW

Since the mid-1990s, saw palmetto has been one of the 10 top-selling herbs in the U.S. Total sales in mainstream retail stores in 2000 in the U.S. were over $43 million, ranking saw palmetto sixth in total herb sales. In Europe, saw palmetto extract is the most commonly used phytotherapeutic agent for benign prostatic hyperplasia (BPH) and it is one of the most frequently prescribed botanical preparations in Germany. Saw palmetto berry was commonly recommended for various prostatic conditions by healthcare professionals in the early part of the 20th century. It was an official drug, listed in the *United States Pharmacopeia* from 1906 to 1916 and in the *National Formulary* from 1926 to 1950. In the 20th century, the *United States Dispensatory*, 23rd edition, included saw palmetto as a treatment for enlargement of the prostate gland.

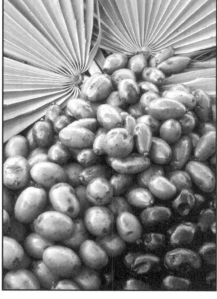

Photo © 2003 stevenfoster.com

PRIMARY USES

• Benign prostatic hyperplasia (BPH), Stages I and II

PHARMACOLOGICAL ACTIONS

Anti-estrogenic activity; increases urinary flow rate; decreases residual urine; decreases painful urination; decreases nocturia.

DOSAGE AND ADMINISTRATION

Research suggests that 4–6 weeks are needed for therapeutic effect to manifest.

CUT FRUIT AND OTHER EQUIVALENT GALENICAL PREPARATIONS: 1–2 g.

CRUDE BERRIES: 10 g, twice daily.

FLUID EXTRACT: 1–2 ml twice daily [1:1 (*g/ml*)]; 2–4 ml twice daily [1:2 (*g/ml*)].

SOFT NATIVE EXTRACT: 160 mg twice daily or 320 mg once daily [10:1–14:1 (*w/w*), containing approximately 85–95% fatty acids].

DRY NORMALIZED EXTRACT: 400 mg twice daily [4:1 (*w/w*) contains ca. 25% fatty acids].

TEA: Not effective because the lipophilic active constituents are insoluble in water.

NOTE: Most clinical studies have been conducted with native extract.

CONTRAINDICATIONS

Saw palmetto is contraindicated in advanced BPH with severe urinary retention. It should not be used without first ruling out prostate cancer.

PREGNANCY AND LACTATION: Due to potential hormonal activity, saw palmetto is not recommended for pregnant or lactating women, although the herb is seldom used by women.

ADVERSE EFFECTS

Gastrointestinal disturbance occurs rarely. Ingestion of large amounts of saw palmetto berries may cause diarrhea, while ingestion of saw palmetto on an empty stomach may cause nausea. Hypertension was reported in 3.1% of patients taking the saw palmetto extract Permixon® (a proprietary saw palmetto extract from France) although this effect is not usually observed in other trials or case studies on saw palmetto. The general safety profile of saw palmetto is superior to that of finasteride. Sexual dysfunction was less common with saw palmetto and the herb has not been associated with erectile dysfunction, ejaculatory disturbance, or altered libido. Gastrointestinal disturbances, urinary tract infections, ejaculation problems, and impotence were reported in 2% of patients taking saw palmetto in a three-year trial.

DRUG INTERACTIONS

There are no confirmed interactions with saw palmetto. Most clinical trials excluded men taking diuretics, alpha blockers, and anticoagulants; thus, the potential for drug-herb interaction cannot be dismissed. A review of the literature does not reveal evidence of adverse drug interactions between saw palmetto and conventional drugs.

CLINICAL REVIEW

In nineteen studies that included 7,210 participants, all but two demonstrated positive effects for benign prostatic hyperplasia (BPH). Numerous studies revealed that saw palmetto improved symptoms of BPH including one randomized, single-blind, placebo-controlled, parallel group multicenter study (R, SB, PC, PG, MC), two open-label (OL), MC studies, a R, double-blind (DB), controlled study, a R, comparative study, a prospective MC study, and a R, PC study. Two OL studies found positive results, but another OL study failed to find significant improvement in objective measures of bladder outlet obstruction. Similarly, one DB, C study found no difference between saw palmetto and placebo. Several clinical trials have shown that serum levels of testosterone, dihydrotestosterone (DHT), and PSA are not changed significantly. One PC study looked at hormone levels, found no changes in testosterone, luteinizing hormone (LH), or follicle stimulating hormone (FSH) levels.

It is well accepted that at least 30–50% of BPH patients report an improvement of their symptoms after treatment with placebo. This percentage is about the same after simple monitoring. Two meta-analyses of 18 R, PC studies concluded that saw palmetto treatment for at least 30 days improved urologic symptoms and flow measures. Adverse effects were mild and infrequent. The authors concluded that further research is needed using standardized preparations to determine saw palmetto's long-term effectiveness and ability to prevent BPH complications. Another meta-analysis focused on 11 R clinical trials and 2 OL trials using saw palmetto extract on men with BPH. The analysis concluded that saw palmetto, compared to placebo, provided a significant improvement in peak urinary flow rate and reduction in nocturia.

Some anecdotal reports have stated that saw palmetto can mask prostate cancer by lowering PSA levels. However, several large studies totaling 1,256 patients did not show this effect.

A meta-analysis of recent PC trials included 7 clinical studies. All trials lasted 3 months and indicated a decrease in nocturia frequency (0.5 times per night) and an increase in peak urinary flow rate by 1.5 ml/sec over placebo. A 6-month, DB, PC, R study comparing Permixon® and finasteride (Proscar®) included 1,809 patients with BPH, and showed equally improved symptom score in both groups (37% with Permixon® vs. 39% with finasteride), and equally improved peak urinary flow rate. One of the first trials conducted in the U.S. reported symptomatic, but not urodynamic, improvement in 46 men treated for 6 months with a saw palmetto berry extract.

Five studies focused on the use of the combination of saw palmetto and nettles to treat the symptoms of BPH. Originally, it was thought that saw palmetto relieved the symptoms associated with an enlarged prostate without reducing the enlargement. However, one R, DB, PC study on the Nutralite® product examined the use of a saw palmetto, nettles, lemon bioflavonoid extract, and vitamin A combination and found significant improvement in prostate epithelial contraction without adverse effects. Further studies are needed to confirm the finding. Another trial on the same saw palmetto combination product suggested a significant reduction in prostate tissue DHT levels, as determined by needle biopsy. Four well-designed studies on the fixed combination, PRO 160/120®, ranged from 12 weeks to one year, and found good efficacy and tolerance.

Saw Palmetto

Serenoa repens (W. Bartram) Small
[Fam. *Arecaceae*]

OVERVIEW

Saw palmetto berries were first used by Native Americans as a diuretic and sexual tonic, as well as for stomachache and dysentery. Since the mid-1990s, saw palmetto has been one of the 10 top-selling herbs in the U.S. Total sales in mainstream retail stores in 2000 were over $43 million, ranking saw palmetto sixth in herb sales.

USES

Mild to moderate benign prostatic hyperplasia (BPH); enlarged prostate, Stages I and II.

DOSAGE

4–6 weeks are needed for effectiveness.

CRUDE BERRIES: 10 g, twice daily.

FLUID EXTRACT: 1–2 ml, twice daily [1:1 (*g/ml*)]; 2–4 ml, twice daily [1:2 (*g/ml*)].

SOFT NATIVE EXTRACT: 160 mg, twice daily or 320 mg once daily [10:1–14:1 (*w/w*), contains approximately 85–95% fatty acids].

DRY NORMALIZED EXTRACT: 400 mg, twice daily [4:1 (*w/w*) contains ca. 25% fatty acids].

NOTE: Most clinical studies have been conducted with the native extract standardized to approx. 85–95% fatty acids.

CONTRAINDICATIONS

Saw palmetto should not be used by individuals with advanced BPH and severe urinary retention without first consulting with a healthcare provider to rule out prostate cancer.

PREGNANCY AND LACTATION: Due to potential hormonal activity, saw palmetto is not recommended for pregnant or breast-feeding women, although the herb is seldom used by women.

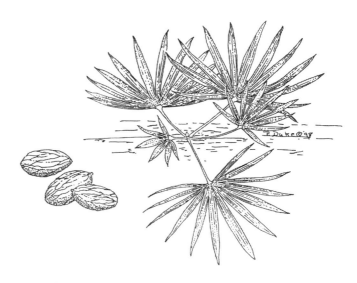

ADVERSE EFFECTS

Gastrointestinal disturbance occurs rarely. Ingesting large amounts of saw palmetto berries may cause diarrhea while ingesting saw palmetto on an empty stomach may cause nausea. High blood pressure occurred in only 3% of patients who took saw palmetto extract in a large clinical trial of 951 men although this effect is not normally associated with the use of saw palmetto. Compared to finasteride, the leading prescription drug for BPH, saw palmetto extracts have a better general safety profile and produce less frequent sexual complaints. Saw palmetto has not been associated with erectile dysfunction, ejaculatory disturbance, or altered libido, as can occur with some men using prescription medications for BPH.

DRUG INTERACTIONS

There are no known interactions between saw palmetto and conventional drugs.

Comments

When using a dietary supplement, purchase it from a reliable source. For best results, use the same brand of product throughout the period of use. As with all medications and dietary supplements, please inform your healthcare provider of all herbs and medications you are taking. Interactions may occur between medications and herbs or even among different herbs when taken at the same time. Treat your herbal supplement with care by taking it as directed, storing it as advised on the label, and keeping it out of the reach of children and pets. Consult your healthcare provider with any questions.

AMERICAN
BOTANICAL
COUNCIL

The information contained on this sheet has been excerpted from *The ABC Clinical Guide to Herbs* © 2003 by the American Botanical Council (ABC). ABC is an independent member-based educational organization focusing on the medicinal use of herbs. For more detailed information about this herb please consult the healthcare provider who gave you this sheet. To order *The ABC Clinical Guide to Herbs* or become a member of ABC, visit their website at www.herbalgram.org.

Saw Palmetto

Serenoa repens (W. Bartram) Small (syn. *Sabal serrulata* [Michx.] Nutt. ex Schult. & Schult. f.;
Serenoa serrulata (Michx.) G. Nichols.

[Fam. *Arecaceae*]

OVERVIEW

Saw palmetto is a small, low-growing, dwarf-palm tree, native to southeastern North America, particularly Florida. The berries were a staple food and medicine of the indigenous Floridians before the Europeans' arrival (Duke, 1985; Vogel, 1970). Indigenous Americans prepared an aqueous infusion of the berries to treat stomachache and dysentery (Duke, 1985). They also used the fruit as a diuretic and sexual tonic (Duke, 1985). Since the mid-1990s, saw palmetto has been one of the ten top-selling herbs in the U.S. (Blumenthal *et al.*, 1998; Blumenthal, 2001). Total sales in mainstream retail stores in 2000 in the U.S. were over $43 million, ranking saw palmetto sixth in total herb sales (Blumenthal, 2001). In Europe saw palmetto extract is the most commonly used phytotherapeutic agent for benign prostatic hyperplasia (BPH) (Di Silverio *et al.*, 1993), and in Germany it is one of the most frequently prescribed botanical preparations (Blumenthal *et al.*, 1998). Saw palmetto berry was commonly recommended for various prostatic conditions by healthcare professionals in the early part of the 20th century. It was an official drug, listed in the *United States Pharmacopeia* (USP) from 1906 to 1916 and in the *National Formulary* (NF) from 1926 to 1950 (Boyle, 1991) before its use as a therapeutic option for urinary tract disorders by the medical community declined in the U.S. (Tyler, 1994). In the 20th century, the *United States Dispensatory*, 23rd edition, included saw palmetto with an indication for treatment of enlargement of the prostate gland (Wood and Osol, 1943).

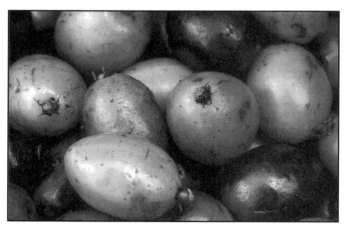

Photo © 2003 stevenfoster.com

DESCRIPTION

Saw palmetto preparations consist of the berry (fruit) of *Serenoa repens* (W. Bartram) Small (syn. *Sabal serrulata*) [Fam. *Arecaceae*] or its extracts.

PRIMARY USES

Prostate

Benign prostatic hyperplasia (BPH) (Marks *et al.*, 2001, 2000; Ziegler, 1998; Redecker, 1998; Di Silverio *et al.*, 1998; Braeckman *et al.*, 1997; Bach and Ebeling, 1996; Kondás *et al.*, 1996; Carraro *et al.*, 1996; Braeckman, 1994; Casarosa *et al.*, 1988; Champault *et al.*, 1984). The German Commission E approved the use of saw palmetto for mild to moderate BPH stages I and II (Blumenthal *et al.*, 1998).

DOSAGE

Internal

Crude Preparations

CUT FRUIT AND OTHER EQUIVALENT GALENICAL PREPARATIONS: 1–2 g (Blumenthal *et al.*, 1998).

CRUDE BERRIES: 10 g twice daily (Pizzorno and Murray, 1999).

FLUID EXTRACT: 1:1 (*g/ml*), 1–2 ml twice daily; 1:2 (*g/ml*) 2–4 ml twice daily (Blumenthal *et al.*, 2000).

SOFT NATIVE EXTRACT: 10:1–14:1 (*w/w*), contains approximately 85–95% fatty acids, 160 mg twice daily (Blumenthal *et al.*, 2000) or 320 mg once daily (Braeckman *et al.*, 1997).

DRY NORMALIZED EXTRACT: 4:1 (*w/w*) contains approximately 25% fatty acids, 400 mg twice daily (Blumenthal *et al.*, 2000).

TEA: Not effective because the lipophilic-active constituents are insoluble in water (Bratman and Kroll, 1999).

NOTE: Most clinical trials have been conducted with native extract.

DURATION OF ADMINISTRATION

Research suggests that, four to six weeks of treatment are needed for a therapeutic effect (Braeckman, 1994; Champault *et al.*, 1984).

CHEMISTRY

The main constituents of saw palmetto include carbohydrates (inert sugar, mannitol, high-molecular-weight polysaccharides with galactose, arabinose, and uronic acid), fixed oils (free fatty acids and their glycerides), steroids, flavonoids, resin, pigment, tannin, and volatile oil (Newall *et al.*, 1996). The fruits and seeds are rich in triacylglycerol-containing oil (50% of the fatty acids contain 14 or less carbons) (Bruneton, 1999). The liposterolic fraction is the primary active component. A recent systematic review described the chemistry of saw palmetto fruit and related species at different dates of maturity, dosage forms and commercial products, and fruit samples from other species of palm in order to help control the quality of commercial products (Peng *et al.*, 2002).

PHARMACOLOGICAL ACTIONS
Human
Anti-estrogenic activity (Di Silverio *et al.,* 1992); increases urinary flow rate (Redecker, 1998; Ziegler and Holscher, 1998; Braeckman *et al.,* 1997); decreases residual urine (Redecker, 1998; Ziegler and Holscher, 1998; Braeckman *et al.,* 1997); decreases painful urination (Champault *et al.,* 1984); decreases nocturia (Boyle *et al.,* 2000; Ziegler and Holscher, 1998; Vahlensieck *et al.,* 1993a, 1993b); anti-inflammatory (Ziegler and Holscher, 1998); anti-exudative (Ziegler and Holscher, 1998).

Animal
Anti-androgenic in rats (Carilla *et al.,* 1984); relaxes smooth muscle in rats (Gutierrez *et al.,* 1996); anti-edemic (Stenger *et al.,* 1982).

In vitro
Anti-inflammatory (Breu *et al.,* 1992).

MECHANISM OF ACTION
Human
- Lowers DHT levels in prostate tissue (Marks *et al.,* 2001).

Animal
- Suppresses prostatic epithelium through a nonhormonal mechanism (Epstein *et al.,* 1999).
- Reduces dihydrotestosterone (DHT) in prostate tissue, which has been implicated as a causative factor of BPH *in vivo* (Koch and Biber; 1994).
- Competes with endogenous estrogen for receptor sites (Di Silverio *et al.,* 1992).
- Induces apoptosis and inhibits cell proliferation in prostate epithelium and stroma (Vacherot *et al.,* 2000).

In vitro
The following mechanisms are based on results from *in vitro* studies using supraphysiologic dosages.
- Inhibits action of 5α-reductase, which catalyzes the metabolism of testosterone to DHT (Bayne *et al.,* 2000; Chavez and Chavez, 1998; Marks *et al.,* 2000; Sultan *et al.,* 1984), due to the free fatty acid content of the fruit's lipophilic extracts (Niederprüm *et al.,* 1994; Weisser *et al.,* 1996).
- Inhibits receptor binding of androgens (Chavez and Chavez, 1998; Sultan *et al.,* 1984).
- Inhibits noncompetitively human α1-adrenoreceptors *in vitro* (Goepel *et al.,* 1999).
- Inhibits both the cyclooxygenase and lipoxygenase pathways *in vitro* (Breu *et al.,* 1992).
- Inhibits growth factors *in vitro* (Plosker and Brogden, 1996).
- Binds selectively to and increases apoptic index for prostate cells *in vitro* (Bayne *et al.,* 2000).

CONTRAINDICATIONS
Saw palmetto is not indicated for advanced BPH with severe urinary retention. It should not be used without first ruling out prostate cancer (Bratman and Kroll, 1999). For this reason, the German Commission E clarifies that saw palmetto relieves only the symptoms associated with BPH and recommends consulting a healthcare provider at regular intervals (Blumenthal *et al.,* 1998).

PREGNANCY AND LACTATION: No known restrictions (Blumenthal *et al.,* 2000), although saw palmetto is seldom used by women. Due to potential hormonal activity, saw palmetto is not recommended for pregnant or lactating women, though this has not been confirmed by scientific studies (Blumenthal and Riggins, 1997; Newall *et al.,* 1996; Elghamry and Hänsel, 1969).

ADVERSE EFFECTS
Rare cases of gastrointestinal disturbance have been reported (Blumenthal *et al.,* 1998). Ingestion on an empty stomach may cause nausea (Bruneton, 1999). Hypertension was reported in 3.1% of patients taking the saw palmetto extract Permixon® (a proprietary form of saw palmetto) (Carraro *et al.,* 1996), although hypertension is not a generally reported effect associated with the use of saw palmetto, either from clinical trials or case reports. The general safety profile of saw palmetto extracts has been shown to be better than finasteride (Wilt *et al.,* 1998). Sexual dysfunction was less common with saw palmetto (p<0.001), and the herb has not been associated with erectile dysfunction, ejaculatory disturbance, or altered libido (Wilt *et al.,* 1998). Gastrointestinal disturbances, urinary tract infections, ejaculation problems, and impotence were reported in 2% of patients taking saw palmetto in a clinical trial on 315 men with BPH stage II or III over three years (Brach and Ebeling, 1996). Other trials have noted mild GI upset in a small percentage (1.3%) of patients (Wilt *et al.,* 1998).

DRUG INTERACTIONS
There are no known interactions associated with saw palmetto (Brinker, 2001). Most clinical trials excluded men taking diuretics, alpha blockers, and anticoagulants; thus, the potential for drug-herb interactions cannot be dismissed, though none have been reported by patients or healthcare providers. A review of the literature does not reveal evidence of adverse drug interactions between saw palmetto and conventional drugs. *In vitro*, saw palmetto potentially inhibits the binding of α1-adrenoceptor antagonists (e.g., tamsulosin and prozacin) and calcium mobilization; the clinical relevance has not been confirmed (Brinker, 2001).

AMERICAN HERBAL PRODUCTS ASSOCIATION (AHPA) SAFETY RATING
CLASS 1: Herbs that can be safely consumed when used appropriately. The editors note that rare cases of stomach problems have been recorded and that the German Commission E suggests regular consultation with a healthcare provider when using saw palmetto for treatment of enlarged prostate, based on the assumption that it treats only the symptoms without eliminating hypertrophic concern (McGuffin *et al.,* 1997).

REGULATORY STATUS
CANADA: Approved active ingredient in over 45 licensed products including some Traditional Herbal Medicines (THMs). Natural Health Products (NHPs) and homeopathic medicines (Health Canada, 2002).

FRANCE: Authorized as a prescription drug reimbursable by the national health insurance (Chauvarie, 2001).

GERMANY: Dried fruit and other galenical preparations or lipophilic extracts are approved by the Commission E as non-prescription drugs (Blumenthal *et al.,* 1998). Fresh ripe fruit for preparation of mother tincture and liquid dilutions are official in *German Homeopathic Pharmacopoeia* (GHP, 1993).

BELGIUM: Approved as a prescription adjuvant in BPH treatment.

ITALY: Authorized as a registered drug only (Ris, 2001).

SWEDEN: Classified as Natural Remedy for self-medication requiring premarketing authorization. Two combination products, Curbicin® with pumpkin seed (*Curcubita pepo*) and Prostakan® with nettle root (*Urtica dioica*), are registered in the Medical Products Agency (MPA) "Authorised Natural Remedies" with the approved indication: "Traditionally used in case of micturition problems caused by benign prostatic hyperplasia, e.g. frequent need to urinate and nocturia. Prior to treatment other serious conditions should have been ruled out by doctor" (MPA, 2001). A product monograph for Curbicin® and a document discussing the risk for an anticoagulation effect are included (MPA, 2000, 1999).

SWITZERLAND: Herbal medicine with positive classification (List D) by the *Interkantonale Konstrollstelle für Heilmittel* (IKS) and corresponding sales Category D with sale limited to pharmacies and drugstores, without prescription (Morant and Rupanner, 2001; Ruppanner and Schaefer, 2000). Three saw palmetto monopreparation phytomedicines, six polypreparations (i.e., multi-ingredient products), and 12 saw palmetto homeopathic preparations are listed in the *Swiss Codex 2000/01* (Ruppanner and Schaefer, 2000).

U.K.: Herbal Medicine on the *General Sale List*, Table A (internal or external use), Schedule 1 (requires full Product License) (MCA, 2002).

U.S.: Dietary supplement (USC, 1994). In view of the levels of evidence in clinical trials of "moderate scientific quality" indicating that commercial extracts of saw palmetto are more effective than placebo to treat symptoms of BPH, the *United States Pharmacopeia* (USP) moved saw palmetto preparations from *National Formulary* (NF) status to inclusion into the USP. This is the first time this has been done for an herb formerly classed only as a dietary supplement. This USP status is designated only for articles that are either approved by the Food and Drug Administration and/or have a USP-accepted use (USP, 2002). The mother tincture 1:10 (*w/v*), 65% alcohol (*v/v*), of ripe fruit, is an OTC Class C drug official in *Homeopathic Pharmacopoeia of the United States* (HPUS, 1992).

CLINICAL REVIEW

Nineteen studies are outlined in the following table, "Clinical Studies on Saw Palmetto," including 7,210 participants. All but two (Gerber *et al.*, 1998; Champault *et al.*, 1984), demonstrated positive effects for BPH. Numerous studies concluded that saw palmetto improves symptoms of BPH including one randomized, single-blind, placebo controlled, parallel group multi-center study (R, SB, PC, PG, MC) (Braeckman *et al.*, 1997), two open-label (OL), MC studies, (Braeckman, 1994; Ziegler and Holscher, 1998), an R, DB, controlled study (Carraro *et al.*, 1996), a R, comparative study (Di Silverio *et al.*, 1998), a prospective MC study (Bach and Ebeling, 1996), a R, PC study (Champault *et al.*, 1984), and two observational studies (Vahlensieck *et al.*, 1993a and 1993b). Two OL studies found positive results (Kondás *et al.*, 1996; Redecker, 1998), but another OL study failed to find significant improvement in objective measures of bladder outlet obstruction (Gerber *et al.*, 1998). Similarly, one DB, C study found no difference between saw palmetto and placebo (Reece *et al.*, 1986). Several clinical trials (Carraro *et al.*, 1996; Rhodes *et al*, 1993; Strauch *et al.*, 1994) have shown that serum levels of testosterone, dihydrotestosterone,

and prostate-specific-antigen (PSA) are not changed significantly. One PC study looked at hormone levels, finding no changes in testosterone, luteinizing hormone (LH), or follicle stimulating hormone (FSH) levels (Casarosa *et al.*, 1988).

It is well-accepted that at least 30–50% of BPH patients report an improvement in their symptoms after treatment with placebo (Bruneton, 1999). This percentage is about the same after simple monitoring (Chapple, 1993). Two meta-analyses of 18 R, PC trials concluded that saw palmetto treatment for at least 30 days improves urologic symptoms and flow measures (Wilt *et al.*, 1998, 2000). Adverse effects were mild and infrequent. The authors concluded that further research is needed using standardized preparations to determine saw palmetto's long-term effectiveness and ability to prevent BPH complications. Another meta-analysis (Boyle *et al.*, 2000) focused on 11 R clinical trials and two OL trials using saw palmetto extract on men with BPH. The analysis concluded that saw palmetto compared to placebo provided significant improvement in the peak urinary flow rate and a reduction in nocturia.

Some anecdotal reports state that saw palmetto can mask prostate cancer by lowering PSA levels. However, several large studies including a total of 1,256 patients did not show this effect (Carraro *et al.*, 1996; Braeckman, 1994). Originally, it was thought that saw palmetto relieves the symptoms associated with an enlarged prostate without reducing the enlargement (Blumenthal *et al.*, 1998). However, a recent study has detected shrinkage of the epithelial tissue in the transition zone of the gland (Marks *et al.*, 2000; Marks and Tyler, 1999). Further studies are needed to confirm the finding.

A meta-analysis of recent PC trials included seven clinical studies (Boyle *et al.*, 2000). All trials lasted three months, and indicated a decrease in nocturia frequency (0.5 times per night) and an increase in the peak rate of urinary flow rate by 1.5 ml/second over placebo. A six-month, R, DB, PC study (Carraro *et al.*, 1996) comparing Permixon® and finasteride (Proscar®) included 951 patients with BPH, and showed an equally improved symptom score in both groups (37% with Permixon® vs. 39% with finasteride), and equally improved peak urinary flow rates. One of the first U.S. trials (Gerber *et al.*, 1998) reported symptomatic, but not urodynamic, improvement in 46 men treated for six months with a saw palmetto berry extract.

Five studies focused on a saw palmetto and nettle combination for BPH symptoms. One R, DB, PC study on the Nutralite® product examined use of a saw palmetto, nettles, lemon bioflavonoid extract, and vitamin A combination, and found significant improvement in prostate epithelial contraction without adverse effects (Marks *et al.*, 2000). The same combination produced a 32% reduction in dihydrotestosterone levels compared to baseline in six months in prostate tissue extracted via needle biopsy (Marks *et al.*, 2001). Four well-designed studies on the fixed combination, PRO 160/120®, ranging from 12 weeks to one year, found good efficacy and tolerance (Sökeland, 2000; Sökeland and Albrecht, 1997; Metzher *et al.*, 1996; Schneider *et al.*, 1995).

BRANDED PRODUCTS*

IDS 89: Strathmann AG & Co. / Sellhpsweg 1 / 22459 / Hamburg / Germany / Tel: +49-401-55-9050 / Fax: +49-40-55-9051-00 / www.strathmann.de / Email: info@strathmann.de.

LG 166/S: Laboratori Guidotti S.p.A, Via Trieste 40 56126 Pisa, Italy / Tel: +39-05-05-0521-1 / Fax: +39-05-04-0250 / Email: a.viti@giofil.it / www.giofil.it. 160 mg liposterolic extract.

Nutrilite® Saw Palmetto with Nettle Root: Nutrilite® / 5600 Beach Blvd. / Buena Park, CA 90622 / U.S.A. / Tel: (714) 562-6200 / www.nutrilite.com. One tablet contains 106 mg saw palmetto lipoidal extract and 80 mg nettle root extract.

Permixon®: Pierre Fabre Médicament / 45, Place Abel-Gance / 92654 Boulogne / France / Tel: +33-01-49-10-8000 / Fax: +33-01-49-10-9712 / www.dermaweb.com. Liposterolic hexane extract of saw palmetto berries, comprised of free (90%) and esterified (7%) fatty acids, sterols, polyprenic compounds, and flavonoids. This extract was the template for current liposterolic extracts manufactured using either ethanol or carbon dioxide extraction.

PRO 160/120®: Dr. Willmar Schwabe Pharmaceuticals / International Division / Willmar Schwabe Str. 4 / D-76227, Karlsruhe / Germany / Tel: +49-721-4005 ext. 294 / www.schwabepharma.com / Email: melville-eaves@schwabe.de. Fixed combination of 160 mg of saw palmetto extract (WS 1473), 10–14.3:1, and 120 mg of stinging nettle root (*Urtica dioica*) dry extract (WS 1031), 8.3–12.5:1.

Prostagutt® (a.k.a. WS 1473): Dr. Wilmar Schwabe Pharmaceuticals. Liposterolic extract made from alcohol extraction.

Prostagutt® forte: Dr. Willmar Schwabe Pharmaceuticals. Fixed combination of 160 mg of saw palmetto extract (WS 1473), 10–14.3:1, and 120 mg of stinging nettle root (*Urtica dioica*) dry extract (WS 1031), 8.3–12.5:1.

Prostaserene®: Therabel Research / Egide Van Ophemstraat 110 / 1180 / Bruxelles / Belgium / Tel: +32-02-370-4611 / Fax: +32-02-370-4690. Liposterolic extract of saw palmetto berries.

Solaray® Saw Palmetto: Nutraceutical Corporation / 1400 Kearns Blvd / Park City, Utah 84060 / U.S.A. / Tel: 800-669-8877 / www.nutraceutical.com. Each 160-mg gelcap contains 85%-95% (approximately 136 mg) essential fatty acids and steroids.

Strogen forte®: Strathmann AG & Co. The liposterolic extract is produced through carbon dioxide extraction. Sabal extract IDS 89 is a constituent of Strogen® forte.

Strogen® S: Strathmann AG & Co. Sabal extract IDS 89 is a constituent of Strogen® S.

Talso®: Sanofi Synthelabo GmbH / 174 avenue de France / 75013 Paris / France / Tel: +331 53 77 4000 / www.sanofi-synthelabo.fr.

*American equivalents, if any, are found in the Product Table beginning on page 398.

REFERENCES

Bach D, Ebeling L. Long-term drug treatment of benign prostatic hyperplasia — results of a prospective 3-year multicenter study using *Sabal* extract IDS 89. *Phytomedicine* 1996;3(2):105–11.

Bayne CW, Ross M, Donnelly F, Habib FK. The selectivity and specificity of the actions of the lipido-sterolic extract of *Serenoa repens* (Permixon®) on the prostate. *J Urol* 2000 Sep;164:876–81.

Blumenthal M. Herb sales down 15% in mass market. *HerbalGram* 2001;451:69.

Blumenthal M, Goldberg A, Brinckmann J. *Herbal Medicine–Expanded Commission E Monographs.* Newton, MA: Integrative Medicine Communications; 2000; 335–40.

Blumenthal M, Busse WR, Goldberg A, Gruenwald J, Hall T, Riggins CW, Rister RS (eds.). Klein S, Rister RS (trans.). *The Complete German Commission E Monographs—Therapeutic Guide to Herbal Medicines.* Austin, TX: American Botanical Council; Boston: Integrative Medicine Communication; 1998; 201.

Blumenthal M and Riggins C. *Popular Herbs in the U.S. Market: Therapeutic Monographs.* Austin, TX; American Botanical Council; 1997.

Boyle P, Robertson C, Lowe F, Roehrborn C. Meta-analysis of clinical trials of Permixon® in the treatment of symptomatic benign prostatic hyperplasia. *Urology* 2000;55:533–9.

Boyle W. *Official Herbs: Botanical Substances in the United States Pharmacopeias 1820–1990.* East Palestine, OH: Buckeye Naturopathic Press; 1991.

Braeckman J, Bruhwyler J, Vandekerckhove K, Geczy J. Efficacy and safety of the extract of *Serenoa repens* in the treatment of benign prostatic hyperplasia: Therapeutic equivalence between twice and once daily dosage forms. *Phytother Res* 1997; 11:558–63.

Braeckman J. The extract of *Serenoa repens* in the treatment of benign prostatic hyperplasia: A multicenter open study. *Curr Therapeut Res* 1994;55:776–85.

Bratman S, Kroll D. *The Natural Pharmacist. Clinical Evaluation of Medicinal Herbs and Other Therapeutic Natural Products.* Rocklin, CA:Prima Publishing; 1999.

Breu W, Hagenlocher M, Redl K, *et al.* Anti-inflammatory activity of *Sabal* fruit extracts prepared with supercritical carbon dioxide. *In vitro* antagonists of cyclooxygenase and 5-lipoxygenase metabolism. [in German]. *Arzneimittelforschung* 1992;42(4):547–51.

Brinker F. *Herb Contraindications and Drug Interactions.* 3d ed. Sandy, OR, Eclectic Medical Publications; 2001;103–7.

Brown D. Phytotherapy review and commentary: One-a-day saw palmetto extract for BPH. *Townsend Lett Doc Patients* 1998;Oct:146–7.

Brown D. Comparing saw palmetto extract and finasteride for BPH. *Quart Rev Nat Med* 1997a;Spring:13–4.

Brown D. Saw palmetto for BPH—the beat goes on! *Quart Rev Nat Med* 1997b; Summer:101–2.

Bruneton, J. *Pharmacognosy, Phytochemistry, Medicinal Plants.* Paris: Lavoisier Publishing; 1999:162–6.

Carilla E, Briley M, Fauran F, Sultan C, Duvilliers C. Binding of Permixon®, a new treatment for prostatic benign hyperplasia, to the cytosolic androgen receptor in the rat prostate. *J Steroid Biochem* 1984;20(1):521–3.

Carraro J, Raynaud J, Koch G *et al.* Comparison of phytotherapy (Permixon®) with finasteride in the treatment of benign prostate hyperplasia: a randomized international study of 1,098 patients. *Prostate* 1996;29(4):231–40.

Casarosa C, di Coscio M, Fratta M. Lack of effects of lyposterolic estract of *Serenoa repens* on plasma levels of testosterone, follicle-stimulating hormone, and luteinizing hormone. *Clin Ther* 1988;10(5):585–8.

Champault G, Bonnard A, Cauquil J, Patel J. The medical treatment of prostatic adenoma. A controlled study: PA-109 versus placebo in 110 patients. [in French]. *Ann Urol* (Paris) 1984;18(6):407–10.

Chapple C. Correlation of symptomatology, urodynamics, morphology, and size of the prostate in benign prostatic hyperplasia. *Curr Opinion Urol* 1993;3:5–9.

Chauvarie J. Personal communication to M. Blumenthal. Dec 5, 2001.

Chavez M, Chavez P. Saw palmetto. *Hospital Pharm* 1998;33(11):1335–61.

Denis U. Editorial review of "Comparison of phytotherapy – Permixon® – with finasteride in the treatment of benign prostatic hyperplasia: a randomized international study of 1089 patients." *Prostate* 1996;29:241–2.

Di Silverio F, Monti S, Sciarra A, *et al.* Effects of long-term treatment with *Serenoa repens* (Permixon®) on the concentration and regional distribution of androgens and epidermal growth factor in benign prostatic hyperplasia. *Prostate* 1998;37(2):77–83.

Di Silverio F, Flammia G, Sciarra A., *et al.* Plant extracts in BPH. *Minerva Urol Nefrol* 1993;45(4):143–9.

Di Silverio F, D'Eramo G, Lubrano C, *et al.* Evidence that *Serenoa repens* extract displays an antiestrogenic activity in prostatic tissue of benign prostatic hypertrophy patients. *Eur Urol* 1992;21(4):309–14.

Duke J. *Handbook of Medicinal Herbs.* Boca Raton: CRC Press; 1985.

Elghamry H, Hänsel R. Activity and isolated phytoestrogen of shrub palmetto fruits (*Serenoa repens* Small), a new estrogenic plant. *Experientia* 1969; 25:828–9.

Epstein J, Partin A, Simon I, *et al.* Prostate tissue effects of saw palmetto extract in men with symptomatic BPH. *Am Urol Assoc Ann Meeting* 1999;May.

Foster S, Tyler VE. *Tyler's Honest Herbal: A Sensible Guide to the Use of Herbs and Related Remedies,* 4th ed. New York: The Haworth Herbal Press; 1999;343–5, 415.

Gerber G. Saw palmetto for the treatment of men with lower urinary tract symptoms. *J Urol* 2000 May;163:1408–12.

Gerber G. Zagaja G, Bales G, *et al.* Saw palmetto (*Serenoa repens*) in men with lower urinary tract symptoms: effects on urodynamic parameters and voiding symptoms. *Urology* 1998;51(6):1003–7.

German Homeopathic Pharmacopoeia (GHP), 5th Supplement 1991 to the first edition 1978. Translation of the *German Homöopathisches Arzneibuch* (HAB 1), 5. Nachtrag 1991, Amtliche Ausgabe." Stuttgart, Germany: Deutscher Apotheker Verlag. 1993;349–50.

GHP. See: *German Homeopathic Pharmacopoeia.*

Goepel M, Hecker U, Krege S, Rubben H, Michel M. Saw palmetto extracts potently and noncompetitively inhibit human α1-adrenoceptors *in vitro. Prostate* 1999 Feb;38(3):208–15.

Gutierrez M, Garcia de Boto M, Cantabrana B, Hidalgo A. Mechanisms involved in the spasmolytic effect of extracts from *Sabal serrulata* fruit on smooth muscle. *Gen*

Pharmacol 1996;27(1):171–6.

Health Canada. Drug Product Database (DPD). Ottawa, Ontario: Health Canada Therapeutic Products Programme. 2002. Available at: http://www.hc-sc.gc.ca/hpb/drugs-dpd/.

Homeopathic Pharmacopoeia of the United States (HPUS) — Revision Service Official Compendium from July 1, 1992. Falls Church, VA: American Institute of Homeopathy. December 1992;8012;SABL.

HPUS. See: *Homeopathic Pharmacopoeia of the United States.*

Koch E, Biber A. Pharmacological effects of *Sabal* and *Urtica* extracts as a basis for a rational medication of benign prostatic hyperplasia. *Urologe* 1994;34:3–8.

Kondás J, Philipp V, Diószeghy G. *Sabal serrulata* extract (Strogen forte®) in the treatment of symptomatic benign prostatic hyperplasia. *Inter Urol Nephrol* 1996;28(6):767–72.

Lowe F, Robertson C., Roehrborn C. *et al.* Meta-analysis of clinical trials of Permixon®. *J Urol* 1998;159:257. Abstract 986.

Marks L, Hess D, Dorey F. *et al.* Tissue effects of saw palmetto and finasteride: use of biopsy cores for *in situ* quantification of prostatic androgens. *Urology* 2001; 57:999–1005.

Marks L, Partin A, Epstein J, *et al.* Effects of a saw palmetto herbal blend in men with symptomatic benign prostatic hyperplasia. *J Urol* 2000 May; 163(5):1451–6.

Marks L, Tyler V. Saw palmetto extract: newest (and oldest) treatment alternative for men with symptomatic benign prostatic hyperplasia. *Urology* 1999;53(3):457–61.

MCA. See: Medicines Control Agency.

McGuffin M, Hobbs C, Upton R, Goldberg A. *American Herbal Products Association's Botanical Safety Handbook.* Boca Raton: CRC Press; 1997.

McPartland J, Pruitt P. Benign prostatic hyperplasia treated with saw palmetto: a literature search and an experimental case study. *J Am Osteopath Assoc* 2000;100(2):89–96.

Medical Products Agency (MPA). *Naturläkemedel: Authorised Natural Remedies* (as of January 24, 2001). Uppsala, Sweden: Medical Products Agency. 2001.

Medical Products Agency (MPA). *Naturläkemedlet Curbicin® och risk för antikoagulationseffekt – möjligen relaterat till E vitamininnehållet.* Uppsala, Sweden: Medical Products Agency. 2000.

Medical Products Agency (MPA). *Naturläkemedelsmonografi: Pharbio Medical International AB Curbicin® Tabletter.* Uppsala, Sweden: Medical Products Agency. 1999.

Medicines Control Agency (MCA). Consolidated List of Substances Which are Present in Authorised Medicines for General Sale. London, U.K.: Medicines Control Agency. February 2002. Available at: http://www.mca.gov.uk/.

Metzker H, Kieser M, Hölscher U. Efficacy of a combined Sabal-Urtica preparation in the treatment of benign prostatic hyperplasia (BPH): A double-blind, placebo-controlled, long-term study. *Urologe* 1996;36:292–300.

Morant J, Ruppanner H (eds.). Bioforce Prostasan N; Madaus Prosta–Urgenin®; Pharmaton Prostatonin®; Phytomed Prostatatropfen/Prostatatabletten; PMI Pharma ProstaRen®; Robapharm Permixon®; SB Consumer Healthcare Prosta–Caps Fink®; Schwabe Prostagutt®–F. In: *Arzneimittel–Kompendium der Schweiz®* 2001. Basel, Switzerland: Documed AG. 2001;1943, 1970, 2082–3.

MPA. See: Medical Products Agency.

Newall S, Anderson L, Phillipson J. *Herbal Medicines. A guide for health-care professionals.* London, England: The Pharmaceutical Press; 1996:296.

Niederprüm H, Schweikert H, Zänker K. Testosterone 5α-reductase inhibition by free fatty acids from *Sabal serrulata* fruits. *Phytomedicine* 1994;1:127–33.

Peng T, Popin W, Huffman M. Quality Management of Saw Palmetto Products. In: Ho C-T, Zheng QY (eds.). *Quality Management of Nutraceuticals.* Washington, DC: ACS Symposium Series; American Chemical Society; 2002.

Pizzorno JE, Murray MT, editors. *Serenoa repens* (saw palmetto). *Textbook of Natural Medicine.* New York: Churchill Livingstone; 1999;943–946.

Plosker G, Brogden R. *Serenoa repens* (Permixon®): a review of its pharmacology and therapeutic efficacy in benign prostrate hyperplasia. *Drugs Aging* 1996;9:379–95.

Reece Smith H, Memon A, Smart C, Dewbury K. The value of Permixon® in benign prostatic hypertrophy. *Br J Urol* 1986;58(1):36–40.

Redecker K. Sabal extract WS 1473 in benign prostatic hyperplasia. *Extracta Urol* 1998;21(3):23–5.

Rhodes L, Primka R, Berman C, *et al.* Comparison of finasteride (Proscar®), a 5 alpha reductase inhibitor, and various commercial plant extracts in *in vitro* and *in vivo* 5 alpha reductase inhibition. *Prostate* 1993;22(1):43–51.

Ris G. Personal communication to M. Blumenthal. Dec 17, 2001.

Ruppanner H, Schaefer U (eds.). *Codex 2000/01 — Die Schweizer Arzneimittel in einem Griff.* Basel, Switzerland: Documed AG. 2000;755–757, 762–6.

Schneider HJ, Honold E, Masuhr Th. Treatment of benign prostatic hyperplasia: Results of a surveillance study in the practices of urological specialists using a combined plant-based preparation (Sabal extract WS 1473 and Urtica extract WS 1031). *Fortschr Med* 1995;113(3):37–40.

Sökeland J. Combined sabal and urtica extract compared with finasteride in men with benign prostatic hyperplasia: analysis of prostate volume and therapeutic outcome. *BJU International* 2000;86:439–442.

Sökeland J, Albrecht J. A combination of Sabal and Urtica extracts vs. Finasteride in BPH (Stage I and II acc. To Alken): a comparison of therapeutic efficacy in a one-year double blind study. *Urologe* 1997;36:327–333.

Stenger A, Tarayre J, Carilla E, *et al.* Pharmacological and biochemical study of the hexanoic extract of *Serenoa repens* B (PA 109). [in German]. *Gax Med de France* 1982;89:2041–8.

Strauch G, Perles P, Vergult G, *et al.* Comparison of finasteride (Proscar®) and *Serenoa repens* (Permixon®) in the inhibition of 5-alpha reductase in health male volunteers. *Eur Urol* 1994;26(3):247–52.

Sultan C, Terraza A, Devillier C, Carilla E, Briley M, Loire C, Descomps B. Inhibition of androgen metabolism and binding by a liposterolic extract of "Serenoa Repens B" in human foreskin fibroblasts. *J Steroid Biochem* 1984;20(10):515–9.

Tenaglia R, Di Silverio F. Ruolo della *Serenoa repens* nell'ipertrofia prostatica. *Excerpta Med* 1986;145–50.

Tyler VE. *Herbs of Choice: The Therapeutic Use of Phytomedicinals.* Binghamton (NY): Hawthorn Press; 1994. p. 82–4.

United States Congress (USC). Public Law 103–417: Dietary Supplement Health and Education Act of 1994. Washington, DC: 103rd Congress of the United States. 1994.

United States Pharmacopeia (USP 25th Revision) – *The National Formulary* (NF 20th Edition). Rockville, MD: United States Pharmacopeial Convention, Inc. 2002.

United States Pharmacopeia. Saw Palmetto and other dosage forms derived from it moved from *NF* to *USP. Pharmacopeial Forum;* May–Jun 2000;26(3).

USC. See: United States Congress.

USP. See: *United States Pharmacopeia.*

Vacherot F, Azzouz M, Gil-Diez-De-Medina S, *et al.* Induction of apoptosis and inhibition of cell proliferation by the lipo-sterolic extract of *Serenoa repens* (LSESr, Permixon®) in benign prostatic hyperplasia. *Prostate* 2000 Nov;45(3):259–266.

Vahlensieck W, Volp A, Kuntze M, Lubos W. Changes in Micturition in Patients with Benign Prostate Hyperplasia Treated with an Extract of Sabal Fruit [in German]. *Urologe* 1993a; 33:380–383.

Vahlensieck W, Volp A, Lubos W, Kuntze M. Benign Prostate Hyperplasia–Treatment with Sabal Fruit Extract [in German]. *Fortschr Med* 1993b;111:323–326.

Vogel V. *American Indian Medicine.* Norman, OK: University of Oklahoma Press; 1970; 365–366.

Weisser H, Tunn S, Behnke B, Krieg M. Effects of the *Sabal serrulata* extract IDS 89 and its subfractions on 5 alpha-reductase activity in human benign prostatic hyperplasia. *Prostate* 1996 May;28(5):300–6.

Wilt T, Ishani A, Stark G, *et al.* Saw palmetto extracts for treatment of benign prostatic hyperplasia: a systematic review. *JAMA* 1998;280(18):1604–9.

Wilt T, Ishani A, Stark G, *et al.* Serenoa repens for benign prostatic hyperplasia. *Cochrane Database Syst Rev* 2000;2:CD001423.

Wood H, Osol A. *United States Dispensatory,* 23rd ed. Philadelphia, PA: J.B. Lippincott; 1943;971–2.

Ziegler H, Holscher U. Efficacy of palmetto fruit special extract WS 1473 in patients with Alken stage I–II benign prostatic hyperplasia—open mulitcentre study. *Jatros Uro* 1998;14(3):34–43.

Clinical Studies on Saw Palmetto (*Serenoa repens* [W. Bartram] Small)

Benign Prostatic Hyperplasia (BPH)

Author/Year	Subject	Design	Duration	Dosage	Preparation	Results/Conclusion
Ziegler and Holscher, 1998	BPH	O, MC n=109 men with BPH in Stages I and II	3 months	160 mg; 2x/day	Prostagutt® (WS 1473)	Saw palmetto caused a significant (p<0.001) improvement in subjective assessment. Therapy was well-tolerated. Significant improvement in mean flow rate (p<0.0001), micturition time (p<0.0001), and time to peak flow rate (p<0.0001) with intent-to-treat analysis. No significant change in micturition volume. Significant decrease in residual volume (p<0.0001), significant decline in daytime micturition (p<0.0001) and in nocturia (p<0.0001).
Redecker, 1998	BPH	O n=50 men with BPH in Stages I and II	3 months	160 mg; 2x/day	Prostagutt® (WS 1473)	Saw palmetto caused a significant increase in maximum urinary flow rate (p<0.001), a reduction in residual urine volume, and reduction of micturition frequency (26 ml to 15 ml).
Di Silverio, 1998	BPH	R, C n=25 men with BPH	3 months	160 mg; 2x/day or no treatment	Permixon®	Compared to control, those receiving saw palmetto had a significant reduction in prostatic DHT (p<0.001) and epidermal growth factor (EGF) (p<0.01). They had a significant increase in testosterone levels (p<0.001). Highest values were in peri-urethral area.
Braeckman, 1997	BPH	R, SB, PC, P MC n=132 men with BPH	1 year	160 mg; 2x/day, or 320 mg, 1x/day	Prostaserene®	Both doses of saw palmetto extract significantly improved International Prostate Symptom Score (p<0.0001), quality of life score (p<0.0001), prostatic volume (p<0.0001), maximum flow rate (p<0.0001), mean flow rate (p<0.01), and residual urinary volume. The two doses were not significantly different. The extract was found to be safe.
Bach and Ebeling, 1996	BPH	P, MC n=315 men with BPH Stage II or III	3 years	160 mg; 2x/day	Strogen® S (IDS 89)	For 80% of patients, clinical status and quality of life improved markedly. 50% of patients had an improvement in residual urine, flow time, and flow rate. Adverse side effects (e.g., gastrointestinal disturbances, urinary tract infections, ejaculation problems, impotence) were experienced by 2% of patients.
Kondás et al., 1996	BPH	O n=38 men with moderate BPH Stages II–III (Vahlensieck)	12 months	320 mg/day	Strogen forte® (IDS 89)	Of patients participating, 74% had an improvement on International Prostate Symptom Score. Greatest improvement rates were noted for sensation of residue, interruption of micturition, and force of urinary stream. Subjective reports of improvement did not depend on size of hyperplastic prostate. Significant increase in average peak flow rate (p<0.001). Decrease in residual volume (p<0.001). Decrease in average volume of prostate (p<0.02). No adverse reactions.
Carraro, 1996	BPH	R, DB, C n=951 men with moderate BPH	6 months	160 mg, 2x/day Permixon® or 5 mg/day finasteride	Permixon® and finasteride	Both treatments equally decreased symptoms of BPH. Saw palmetto had minimal effect on prostate volume and no effect on PSA concentration. Saw palmetto was more effective than finasteride in reducing lower urinary tract symptoms in men with smaller prostate size. Significant results in favor of finasteride for urinary flow rate and prostate volume. Significant decrease in PSA levels with finasteride. Significantly more subjects withdrew from study with finasteride.
Braeckman, 1994	BPH	O, MC n=305 men with mild to moderate BPH	3 months	160 mg, 2x/day	Prostaserene®	After 45 days of treatment there was significant (p<0.0001) improvement in International Prostate Symptom Score, quality of life, urinary flow rate, residual urinary volume, and prostate size. Serum PSA concentration was not modified by saw palmetto extract, decreasing the risk of possible development of prostate cancer during treatment. Only 5% of patients reported side effects.

KEY: C – controlled, **CC** – case-control, **CH** – cohort, **CI** – confidence interval, **Cm** – comparison, **CO** – crossover, **CS** – cross-sectional, **DB** – double-blind, **E** – epidemiological, **LC** – longitudinal cohort, **MA** – meta-analysis, **MC** – multi-center, **n** – number of patients, **O** – open, **OB** – observational, **OR** – odds ratio, **P** – prospective, **PB** – patient-blind, **PC** – placebo-controlled, **PG** – parallel group, **PS** – pilot study, **R** – randomized, **RC** – reference-controlled, **RCS** – retrospective cross-sectional, **RS** - retrospective, **S** – surveillance, **SB** – single-blind, **SC** – single-center, **U** – uncontrolled, **UP** – unpublished, **VC** – vehicle-controlled.

Saw Palmetto

Monograph

Benign Prostatic Hyperplasia (BPH) (cont.)

Author/Year	Subject	Design	Duration	Dosage	Preparation	Results/Conclusion
Vahlensieck et al., 1993a	BPH	OB n=578 (BPH Stages II and III)	8 months; 12 weeks of treatment	160 mg, 2x/day	Talso®	Clear clinical improvements were seen in symptoms, including urine flow, urine retention, nocturia, and daytime micturition. The residue urine volume was reduced by approximately half after 12 weeks, with 30% reduction after 4 weeks. The physicians evaluated efficacy as good or very good in over 80% of the subjects with over 95% of the subjects demonstrating good or very good tolerability.
Vahlensieck et al., 1993b	BPH	OB n=1,334	8 months	160 mg, 2x/day	Talso®	The study was based on symptom treatment and patient evaluations. During the treatment period, pollakiuria was reduced by 37%, nocturia by 54%, and the volume of residual urine was reduced by 50%. The number of patients with dysuria was reduced from 75% to 37%. 80% of the patients rated good or very good efficacy at 80% and good or very good tolerability at 95%.
Casarosa, 1988	BPH	PC n=20 men with BPH and normal levels of testosterone, LH, and FSH. (50–70 years)	30 days	160 mg, 2x/day or placebo	LG 166/S	One month of treatment with saw palmetto extract did not alter testoterone, LH, or FSH levels. These findings are in contrast to those of Tenaglia and DiSilverio (1986) who found increases in the hormone levels. The authors have no explanation for the discrepancy.
Champault, 1984	BPH	R, PC n=110 men (ages 47–92), with BPH, not needing surgery	28 days	160 mg, 2x/day or placebo	Saw palmetto extract (PA 109)	Patients taking saw palmetto had significant decrease in nocturnal micturitions (p<0.001), dysuria (painful urination), and rate of micturition as compared to placebo. No adverse effects reported. Significant increase in urinary flow with saw palmetto extract (p<0.001).

Combination Preparations

Author/Year	Subject	Design	Duration	Dosage	Preparation	Results/Conclusion
Marks et al., 2001	BPH	R, PC, Cm n=40 (saw palmetto vs. placebo), n=22 (finasteride vs. control), measuring prostate tissue androgen levels using needle biopsies	6 months	318 mg saw palmetto extract/day; 1 tablet, 3x/day with meals, or placebo	Nutrilite® Saw Palmetto with Nettle Root (containing saw palmetto extract 106 mg, nettle root extract 80 mg, lemon bioflavonoid extract 33 mg, and vitamin A, 190 IU)	In the saw palmetto group, tissue DHT levels were reduced by 32% from 6.49 ng/g to 4.40 ng/g (p<0.005). The effect of chronic finasteride therapy was statistically significant (p<0.01) in lowering prostate tissue DHT levels (80%) compared to levels of testosterone. No significant change in tissue DHT levels was observed with the placebo.
Marks et al., 2000	BPH	R, DB, PC n=41 men with symptomatic BPH. OL extension after 6 months	6 months	318 mg saw palmetto extract/day, 1 tablet, 3x/day with meals, or placebo	Nutrilite® Saw Palmetto with Nettle Root (containing saw palmetto extract 106 mg, nettle root extract 80 mg, lemon bioflavonoid extract 33 mg, and vitamin A, 190 IU)	Saw palmetto blend group had non-statistically significant improvement vs. placebo in clinical parameters (e.g., International Prostate Symptom Score, uroflowmetry, residual urine volume, prostate volume). After 6 months, saw palmetto blend was associated with prostate epithelial contraction, notably in transition zone (p<0.01), suggesting possible mechanism for clinical significance found by other studies. No serious adverse effects were associated with saw palmetto blend.

KEY: C – controlled, **CC** – case-control, **CH** – cohort, **CI** – confidence interval, **Cm** – comparison, **CO** – crossover, **CS** – cross-sectional, **DB** – double-blind, **E** – epidemiological, **LC** – longitudinal cohort, **MA** – meta-analysis, **MC** – multi-center, **n** – number of patients, **O** – open, **OB** – observational, **OL** – open label, **OR** – odds ratio, **P** – prospective, **PB** – patient-blind, **PC** – placebo-controlled, **PG** – parallel group, **PS** – pilot study, **R** – randomized, **RC** – reference-controlled, **RCS** – retrospective cross-sectional, **RS** - retrospective, **S** – surveillance, **SB** – single-blind, **SC** – single-center, **U** – uncontrolled, **UP** – unpublished, **VC** – vehicle-controlled.

Benign Prostatic Hyperplasia (BPH)

Combination Preparations (cont.)

Author/Year	Subject	Design	Duration	Dosage	Preparation	Results/Conclusion
Sökeland, 2000	BPH	R, MC, DB n=431	48 weeks	2 capsules PRO 160/120®/day vs. finasteride (5 mg/day) vs. placebo	PRO 160/120® (Prostagutt forte™, fixed combination of 160 mg of saw palmetto extract [WS 1473] and 120 mg of stinging nettle dry extract [WS 1031]) or finasteride	The efficacy of both PRO 160/120® and finasteride were shown to be equivalent in the International Prostate Symptom Score with tolerability significantly better with PRO 160/120®. 96 adverse events were recorded in 54 patients using finasteride compared with 74 in 52 patients taking PRO 160/120®.
Sökeland and Albrecht, 1997	BPH (Stages I and II)	R, RC, MC, DB, PG n=543	48 weeks	2 capsules PRO 160/120®/day vs. finasteride (5 mg/day) vs. placebo or one capsule of 5 mg of finasteride per day	PRO 160/120® (Prostagutt forte™, fixed combination of 160 mg of saw palmetto extract [WS 1473] and 120 mg of stinging nettle dry extract [WS 1031]) or finasteride	International-Prostate-Symptom-Score (I-PSS) value improved by a total of 4.8 points with the PRO 160/120®. The study found equivalent efficacy between the two groups. Less adverse events, including diminished ejaculation volume, erectile dysfunction and headache, were reported in the PRO 160/120® group. The study recommended that patients should receive finasteride only after the use of the combination for at least 3 months was unsuccessful.
Metzker et al., 1996	BPH (Stages I and II)	DB, PC n=40	350 days	2 capsules PRO 160/120®/day vs. finasteride (5 mg/day) vs. placebo	Prostagutt forte™ (fixed combination of 160 mg of saw palmetto extract [WS 1473] and 120 mg of stinging nettle dry extract [WS 1031])	The study concluded good efficacy and tolerance in the administration of PRO 160/120® for approximately one year of therapy. After 24 weeks, maximum urine volume per second by 3.3 ml/s had occurred with the combination compared to only a slight improvement of 0.55 ml/s with placebo. Subjective reports corresponding to the I-PSS found a highly significant (p<0.001) advantage with the combination vs. placebo.
Schneider et al., 1995	BPH (Stages I and II)	S n=2,080	12 weeks	2 capsules PRO 160/120®/day vs. finasteride (5 mg/day) vs. placebo	Prostagutt forte™ (fixed combination of 160 mg of saw palmetto extract [WS 1473] and 120 mg of stinging nettle dry extract [WS 1031])	Treatment with the combination was found to be an effective method to avoid surgery or not to make it necessary as soon. Physician and patient assessment confirmed the efficacy and tolerance of PRO 160/120®.

Lower Urinary Tract Symptoms

Author/Year	Subject	Design	Duration	Dosage	Preparation	Results/Conclusion
Gerber et al., 1998	Lower urinary tract symptoms	O n=46 men with lower urinary tract symptoms secondary to BPH	6 months	160 mg, 2x/day	Solaray® Saw Palmetto	The International Prostate Symptom Score significantly improved (p<0.001) after 2 months of treatment. No significant change in peak urinary flow rate, post void residual urine volume, or detrusor pressure at peak flow. No significant improvement in objective measures of bladder outlet obstruction. Saw palmetto was well-tolerated.

KEY: C – controlled, **CC** – case-control, **CH** – cohort, **CI** – confidence interval, **Cm** – comparison, **CO** – crossover, **CS** – cross-sectional, **DB** – double-blind, **E** – epidemiological, **LC** – longitudinal cohort, **MA** – meta-analysis, **MC** – multi-center, **n** – number of patients, **O** – open, **OB** – observational, **OL** – open label, **OR** – odds ratio, **P** – prospective, **PB** – patient-blind, **PC** – placebo-controlled, **PG** – parallel group, **PS** – pilot study, **R** – randomized, **RC** – reference-controlled, **RCS** – retrospective cross-sectional, **RS** - retrospective, **S** – surveillance, **SB** – single-blind, **SC** – single-center, **U** – uncontrolled, **UP** – unpublished, **VC** – vehicle-controlled.

(This page intentionally left blank.)

St. John's Wort

Hypericum perforatum L.
[Fam. *Clusiaceae*]

OVERVIEW

In the fifth century B.C.E., the Greek physician Hippocrates was one of the first to document therapeutic uses of St. John's wort (SJW). It rose from virtual obscurity in the U.S. to become the fifth best-selling dietary supplement in mainstream retail stores in the U.S. after major media coverage of clinical research documenting its relative safety and efficacy for treating mild to moderate depression. The National Institutes of Health's (NIH) National Center for Complementary and Alternative Medicine (NCCAM) recently sponsored a three-year, multi-center trial comparing the effects of a standardized extract of SJW and the selective serotonin reuptake inhibitor (SSRI), sertraline (Zoloft®). Since 1979, there have been more than 35 controlled clinical studies of SJW extracts for the treatment of mild to moderate depression. Several meta-analyses have documented the relative safety and probable efficacy of this phytomedicine. SJW is prescribed frequently by healthcare providers in Germany, where approximately 130 million preparations containing SJW were prescribed in 1999.

PRIMARY USES

Internal
- Depression, mild to moderate

External
- Healing wounds (acute and contused injuries)
- First-degree burns
- Myalgia (muscle pain)

OTHER POTENTIAL USES
- Seasonal Affective Disorder (SAD)
- Obsessive-Compulsive Disorder (OCD)
- Menopause
- Fatigue
- Pediatric nocturnal incontinence
- Premenstrual Syndrome (PMS)

PHARMACOLOGICAL ACTIONS

Antidepressant, relaxant, improves mental performance, does not change alertness or have sedative effect; may have relaxing effect and improve concentration, memory, and receptivity.

DOSAGE AND ADMINISTRATION

For depression, the onset of response to SJW is similar to that for conventional antidepressants, requiring 2–4 weeks, or as long as 6 weeks. To prevent relapse, antidepressant should be continued at full therapeutic doses for at least 6 months after remission.

Internal
Crude Preparations
FLUID EXTRACT: 1:1 (*g/ml*), 2 ml, twice daily.

Standardized Preparations
DRY EXTRACT: 5–7:1, 300 mg, 3 times daily.
EXTRACT: Standardized to 0.3% hypericin, 900 mg daily in 3 divided doses; standardized to 2–4.5% hyperforin, 900 mg daily in 3 divided doses.

External
OILY MACERATE (OLEUM HYPERICI): Fresh-flowering tops in olive oil or wheatgerm oil are macerated for several weeks, stirred often, strained through a cloth and the pulp pressed. To be applied directly to affected areas.

CONTRAINDICATIONS

None known, according to the German Commission E (1984, 1990 revision)

PREGNANCY AND LACTATION: No known restrictions.

ADVERSE EFFECTS

In general, SJW produces few adverse side effects. Between October 1991 and December 1999, over 8 million patients are estimated to have been treated with Germany's leading SJW preparation with only 95 reports of side effects. These included "allergic" skin reactions (27), increased Quick Values (prothrombin time) (16), gastrointestinal complaints (9), breakthrough bleeding (birth control pill) (8), plasma cyclosporin reductions (7), and others. Photosensitization, depicted by erythema (redness of the skin) with exposure to sunlight or other ultraviolet radiation, is possible, but relatively rare and is sometimes reported in fair-skinned individuals taking excessive dosages (1,800 mg/day). A recent review of SJW adverse reactions suggests this precaution should not constitute a general contraindication, since photosensitization is so rare and because sunlight can promote recovery from depression.

DRUG INTERACTIONS

Potential drug interactions with SJW have become the primary area of concern with this popular phytomedicine. However, some of these concerns may not be supported by clinical experience. In a review of drug interactions reportedly associated with SJW, calculations show one interaction per 300,000 treatments with the leading German SJW product.

SJW should not be taken in combination with any pharmaceutical antidepressants without professional guidance. SJW is believed to interact with oral contraceptives and anticoagulants (e.g., warfarin). Preliminary findings suggest that SJW does not interact with the effects of alcohol; however, patients with depression should avoid alcohol. An uncontrolled study on 13 subjects taking SJW at normal doses (900 mg standardized extract/day) resulted in significant increases in urinary 6–beta–hydroxycortisol/cortisol ratio, suggesting that SJW is an inducer of CYP3A4, since cortisol is metabolized primarily by CYP3A4. A recent study revealed that constituents of SJW extract, especially hyperforin, are potent ligands (K(i) = 27 nM) for the pregnane X receptor, an orphan nuclear receptor that regulates expression of the cytochrome P450 (CYP) 3A4 monooxygenase. Treatment of primary human hepatocytes with SJW extracts, or hyperforin, results in a marked induction of CYP3A4 expression. CYP3A4 is involved in the oxidative metabolism of more than 50% of all drugs and can cause a decrease in the therapeutic activity and concentration of such drugs, including contraceptives and theophylline. SJW also may increase clearance from the bloodstream of the protease inhibitor Indinavir, and the anti-rejection drug cyclosporine and may also interfere with the absorption of digoxin. A recent study found that SJW induces intestinal P-glycoprotein/MDR1 (in rats and humans), and induces intestinal and hepatic CYP3A4 (in humans), thereby decreasing plasma levels of cyclosporine, Indinavir, and digoxin. However, a review of SJW drug interactions questions the clinical relevance of interactions based solely on pharmacokinetic measurements, with digoxin, theophylline, and amitriptyline needing to be examined critically, since reduced plasma levels are not the same as reduced active levels at the receptors. To-date there are no reported cases suggesting clinically significant weakening in effect of the three drugs cited. One 14-day study on 10 patients, using the anti-seizure drug carbamazepine (Tegretol®), found that 300 mg SJW extract, three times daily, did not increase the clearance of the drug. Sudden discontinuation of SJW after prolonged use may lead to higher plasma levels of these drugs if used simultaneously, with the risk of adverse effects.

CLINICAL REVIEW

Of 23 studies outlined in the table of clinical studies on SJW (2,745 total participants), all but two studies demonstrate positive effects of SJW on depression. Five randomized, double-blind, placebo-controlled (R, DB, PC) studies (626 participants) concluded that SJW significantly benefits patients with depression without significant side effects. Five R, DB, multicenter (MC) trials (1,191 participants) found equal effectiveness to tricyclic antidepressant drugs (amitriptyline, imipramine, malprotiline) with greater tolerability, and that SJW was safer for the heart.

Three small pilot studies (60 total patients) show promising findings for fatigue and SAD, and one small open-label study (12 patients) indicated potential benefits for OCD. One small pilot study of SJW for the treatment of premenstrual syndrome suggests that SJW might reduce the severity and duration of premenstrual symptoms, warranting a larger R, DB trial. A drug-monitoring study on menopausal symptoms suggests that SJW is useful for treatment of associated symptoms and increasing the sense of sexuality in middle-age women.

In a review of 17 studies on SJW and 9 studies on fluoxetine (Prozac®), researchers showed that SJW was as effective as fluoxetine in the treatment of subthreshold and mild depression.

Researchers concluded that SJW may be a viable approach to avoiding the risk that mild depression becomes a full-blown disorder.

A review and meta-analysis of 23 clinical studies on SJW showed that the standardized extract was more effective than placebo in treating mild to moderate depression. A follow-up meta-analysis (27 trials; 2,291 patients) concluded that SJW was significantly superior to placebo and that short term use of SJW might be valuable in less severe forms of depression as an alternative to watchful waiting or low doses of tricyclic antidepressants with fewer short term adverse side effects. A recent trial comparing SJW with the conventional antidepressant imipramine is the largest comparison trial to date and the first to compare the two agents at the normal daily dose of imipramine (150 mg). (Previous trials used 75 mg imipramine to reduce adverse side effects and maintain patient compliance.) This study concluded that SJW is equivalent to imipramine in efficacy, and is better-tolerated by patients. A newer, larger trial (n=240) comparing SJW directly with fluoxetine concluded that SJW was equivalent to fluoxetine in efficacy, particularly in depressive patients suffering from anxiety, and was better tolerated for safety. A total of 11 studies have compared SJW preparations with conventional antidepressants (7 tricyclic; 4 SSRI) concluding that SJW is effective for mild to moderate depression with a low side effect profile.

A recently published systematic review of 8 well-controlled R, DB, controlled (C), trials suggested that SJW is more effective than placebo in the treatment of mild to moderate depression. The absolute increased response rate with SJW ranged from 23% to 55% higher than with placebo, but ranged from 6% to 18% lower compared with tricyclic antidepressants. Treatment with SJW and fluoxetine was compared in patients with mild to moderate depression. Results showed that SJW and fluoxetine are equipotent with respect to all main parameters used to investigate antidepressants in this population. Although SJW may be superior in improving the responder rate, the main difference between the two treatments is safety. SJW was superior to fluoxetine in overall incidence of side effects, number of patients with side effects, and the types of side effects reported. A previous review of 15 C clinical trials (12 PC) reported that the only substantial documentation for the use of SJW in mild to moderate depression is for the products Jarsin® 300 (Lichtwer Pharma) and Psychotonin-M® (Steigerwald). The review concluded that SJW should not be taken for more than 6 weeks, since most trials showing efficacy have been conducted over a shorter period of time. A recent study received considerable media attention due to its negative findings on patients with severe depression; however, the study lacked an active control (no active drug was used to measure the response rate of severely depressed patients vs. SJW and placebo). The first study funded by the NIH's NCCAM (R, DB, PC, MC, 340 participants) found that neither sertraline nor SJW were effective compared to placebo for moderately severe major depressive disorder. Critics emphasize that the initial design included patients with major depression of only mild to moderate severity (HAMD score $\geq$ 15) but was later changed to include patients with moderate to severe depression (HAMD score $\geq$ 20).

St. John's wort

Hypericum perforatum
[Fam. *Clusiaceae*]

OVERVIEW

St. John's wort (SJW) rose from virtual obscurity in the U.S. to become the fifth best-selling dietary supplement in mainstream retail stores. Its rise to fame came after the national media reported clinical research showing that SJW is safe and effective for treating mild to moderate depression. The Greek physician Hippocrates (ca. 460-377 B.C.E.) was one of the first to speak of the health benefits of SJW. Preparations include teas, alcoholic tinctures, and tablets using either the plant in its crude form or standardized preparation. SJW is typically standardized to contain a consistent level of hypericin (0.3%), or hyperforin (3-5%), two naturally occurring chemicals found in the plant.

USES

Internal
Depression (mild to moderate).

External
Wound healing; first-degree burns; muscle pain (myalgia).

OTHER POTENTIAL USES

Seasonal Affective Disorder (SAD: mental depression related to certain seasons, especially winter); obsessive-compulsive disorder (OCD); menopause; fatigue; pediatric nocturnal incontinence; premenstral syndrome (PMS).

DOSAGE

FLUID EXTRACT: 1:1 (*g/ml*), 2 ml, twice daily.

DRY EXTRACT: 5–7:1, 300 mg, 3 times daily.

EXTRACT (STANDARDIZED): standardized to 0.3% hypericin or 2–4.5% hyperforin; 900 mg daily in 3 divided doses.

CONTRAINDICATIONS

No known contraindications.

PREGNANCY AND LACTATION: No known restrictions.

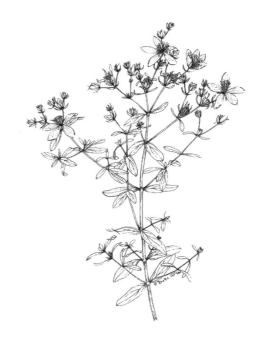

ADVERSE EFFECTS

Photosensitization (redness of the skin caused by exposure to sunlight or other ultraviolet radiation), especially in fair-skinned individuals, may occur with excessive dosages (1,800 mg/day), but this reaction is relatively rare.

DRUG INTERACTIONS

SJW should not be taken in combination with any pharmaceutical antidepressants unless under professional guidance. SJW may interact with oral contraceptives, anticoagulant drugs like warfarin, the asthma drug theophylline, the anti-HIV drug Indinavir, the immunosuppressant drug cyclosporine, and the cardiac medication digoxin. Abruptly stopping SJW after prolonged use may increase the concentration of drugs like carbamazepine (Tegretol®). Patients with depression should avoid alcohol. Because SJW has been shown to potentially act with these and possibly other drugs, consumers and patients are advised to consult with a properly qualified healthcare professional before using SJW with any other over-the-counter or prescription medications.

Comments

When using a dietary supplement, purchase it from a reliable source. For best results, use the same brand of product throughout the period of use. As with all medications and dietary supplements, please inform your healthcare provider of all herbs and medications you are taking. Interactions may occur between medications and herbs or even among different herbs when taken at the same time. Treat your herbal supplement with care by taking it as directed, storing it as advised on the label, and keeping it out of the reach of children and pets. Consult your healthcare provider with any questions.

AMERICAN BOTANICAL COUNCIL

The information contained on this sheet has been excerpted from *The ABC Clinical Guide to Herbs* © 2003 by the American Botanical Council (ABC). ABC is an independent member-based educational organization focusing on the medicinal use of herbs. For more detailed information about this herb please consult the healthcare provider who gave you this sheet. To order *The ABC Clinical Guide to Herbs* or become a member of ABC, visit their website at www.herbalgram.org.

St. John's Wort

Hypericum perforatum L.

[Fam. *Clusiaceae*]

OVERVIEW

St. John's wort (SJW) has been used for various ailments since the ancient Greeks; the Greek physician Hippocrates (ca.400 B.C.E.) was one of the first to document its therapeutic use. Since the time of the Swiss physician Paracelsus (ca. 1540 C.E.) it was used to treat mental disorders (Blumenthal *et al.*, 2000; Hobbs, 1988/89). SJW rose from virtual obscurity in the U.S. to become the fifth best-selling dietary supplement in mainstream retail stores in 2000 (Blumenthal, 2001) following major media coverage of clinical research documenting its relative safety and efficacy for treating mild to moderate depression. In 1998 and 1999 it had risen to second place in mainstream sales (Brevoort, 1998), but fell to fifth place due, in part, to some adverse publicity regarding reports of its interactions with several classes of prescription drugs (Blumenthal, 2001). The

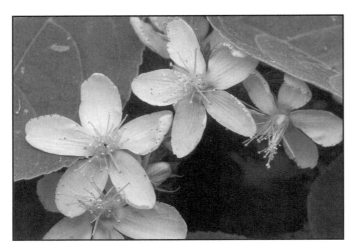

Photo © 2003 stevenfoster.com

National Institutes of Health's (NIH) National Center for Complementary and Alternative Medicine (NCCAM) recently sponsored a three-year, multi-center trial comparing the effects of a standardized extract of SJW and the selective serotonin reuptake inhibitor (SSRI) sertraline (Hypericum Depression Trial Study Group, 2002). Since 1979, there have been more than 35 controlled clinical studies of SJW extracts for the treatment of mild to moderate depression (Blumenthal *et al.*, 2000). Two meta-analyses have documented the relative safety and suggested probable efficacy of this phytomedicine (Linde and Mulrow, 2001; Linde *et al.*, 1996). SJW is prescribed frequently by healthcare providers in Germany, where approximately 130 million daily doses containing hypericum were prescribed in 1999 (Schulz, 2001). SJW preparations have also been used in traditional European herbal medicine for topical antimicrobial and skin healing purposes (Reichling *et al.*, 2001).

DESCRIPTION

St. John's wort (*Hypericum perforatum* L., Fam. *Clusiaceae*) preparations consist of dried above-ground parts (flowers and stems), gathered during the flowering season. Preparations include aqueous extracts (teas), standardized extracts, alcoholic tinctures, dry extracts in capsules or tablets, and oil infusions (topical) (Blumenthal *et al.*, 2000). Standardization is typically to 0.3% hypericin, or 2–4.5% hyperforin (Bruneton, 1999). *In vitro* research suggests that hyperforin may be the main antidepressive constituent (Muller *et al.*, 1998). However, flavonoids and other fractions have also shown antidepressant activity, suggesting "additive or synergistic actions of different single compounds may be responsible for the antidepressant efficacy of SJW" (Butterweck *et al.*, 2002b). The *German Drug Codex* formerly required that SJW preparations be standardized to hypericins content; this is no longer a required chemical marker (Bühler, 1995). The U.S. *National Formulary* requires not less than 0.04% total hypericins, calculated as hypericin (USP, 2002).

PRIMARY USES

Internal
Depression
- Mild to moderate (Harrer *et al.*, 1994; Harrer and Sommer, 1994; Laakmann *et al.*, 1998a; Lenoir *et al.*, 1999; Linde *et al.*, 1996; Linde and Mulrow, 2001; Philipp *et al.*, 1999; Wheatley, 1997; WHO, 2002; Woelk, 2000)

External
- Healing wounds (acute and contused injuries) according to the German Commission E (Blumenthal *et al.*, 1998)
- First-degree burns (Blumenthal *et al.*, 1998)
- Relieving myalgia (muscle pain) (Blumenthal *et al.*, 1998)

OTHER POTENTIAL USES
(Based mainly on pilot studies)
- Seasonal Affective Disorder (SAD) (Kasper, 1997; Martinez *et al.*, 1994)
- Obsessive-Compulsive Disorder (OCD) (Taylor and Kobak, 2000)
- Premenstrual syndrome (Stevinson and Ernst, 2000)
- Menopause (Grube *et al.*, 1999)
- Fatigue (according to a pilot study) (Stevinson *et al.*, 1998)
- Pediatric nocturnal incontinence (clinical experience) (Weiss and Fintelmann, 2000)

DOSAGE
Internal
Crude Preparations
FLUID EXTRACT: 1:1 (*g/ml*), 2 ml, twice daily.

DRY EXTRACT: 5–7:1, 300 mg, 3 times daily (Blumenthal *et al.*, 2000).

Standardized Preparations

EXTRACT: Standardized to 0.3% hypericin, 900 mg daily in 3 doses of 300 mg each; or products standardized to 2–4.5% hyperforin, 900 mg/day in 3 doses (Bruneton, 1999).

External

OILY MACERATE (OLEUM HYPERICI): Fresh-flowering tops in olive oil or wheatgerm oil are macerated for several weeks, stirred often, strained through a cloth and the pulp pressed. To be applied directly to affected areas (Blumenthal et al., 2000).

DURATION OF ADMINISTRATION

For depression, the onset of response to SJW is similar to that for conventional antidepressants, requiring 2–4 weeks, or as long as 6 weeks. To prevent relapse, antidepressant should be continued at full therapeutic doses for at least 6 months after remission (AHCPR, 1999).

CHEMISTRY

SJW contains 6.5–15% catechin-type tannins and condensed-type proanthocyanidins (catechin, epicatechin, leucocyanidin); 2–5% flavonoids, mostly 0.5–2% hyperoside, 0.3–1.6% rutin, 0.3% quercitrin, 0.3% isoquercitrin, quercetin, and kaempferol; bioflavonoids (about 0.26% biapigenin), phloroglucinol derivatives (up to 4% hyperforin); phenolic acids (caffeic, chlorogenic, ferulic); 0.05–1.0% volatile oils, mainly higher n-alkanes, 0.05–0.15% naphthodianthrones (hypericin and pseudohypericin); sterols (sitosterol); vitamins C and A, up to 10 ppm xanthones; and choline (Bruneton, 1999; ESCOP, 1996; Leung and Foster, 1996; Newall et al., 1996; Upton, 1997; Wichtl and Bisset, 1994).

PHARMACOLOGICAL ACTIONS

Standardized Preparations
Human

The primary action of SJW is antidepressant (Phillipp et al., 1999; Lenoir et al., 1999; Leakmann et al., 1998a, 1998b; Wheatley, 1997; Linde et al., 1996). Some references refer to relaxant effects in relation to the Commission E approval for anxiety and nervous unrest, but this may only be in the context of the overall antidepressant activity (Schulz et al., 2000) or in small studies on sleep continuity (Schulz et al., 1995) or resting EEG (Johnson et al., 1994). Other actions include improved mental performance possibly resulting from improvement of depressed states (Lehrl et al., 1993). SJW does not appear to change alertness or have sedative effects; there may be some additional central nervous system effects, again related to improvement of depression including improvement of concentration, memory, and receptivity (Schulz et al., 2000; Schulz et al., 1994; Johnson et al., 1994; Lehrl, 1993).

Animal

Many animal studies have been published on SJW demonstrating a variety of actions, including the following, suggesting antidepressant activity: SJW potentiates dopaminergic behavioral responses (alcoholic extracts), and serotoninergic effects (carbon dioxide extracts) (Bhattacharya, 1998); reduces alcohol intake in rats (Rezvani et al., 1999); SJW extract and hypericin given daily for 8 weeks significantly increased 5-HT (serotonin) levels in rat hypothalamus (Butterweck et al., 2002a); and flavonoids from SJW showed antidepressant activity in rats in the forced swimming test (Butterweck et al., 2000).

In vitro

There has been confusion about the potential monoamine oxidase (MAO) inhibiting effect of SJW. Earlier research suggested that SJW possibly inhibits MAO, using 80% pure hypericin (Suzuki et al., 1984). However, a more recent study suggests that 95% pure hypericin does not inhibit MAO, but a crude ethanolic extract (Herb Pharm, Williams, OR) does, at 2 mcg/ml (Cott, 1995). MAOI activity has not been reported in vivo in animals or in humans (Cott, 1997). SJW unspecifically inhibits biogenic amine and amino acid neurotransmitter uptake (serotonin, dopamine, noradrenaline, GABA, L-glutamate) (Chatterjee et al., 1998; Butterweck et al., 1997); inhibits serotonin reuptake (Perovic and Müller, 1995; Müller and Rossol, 1994; Holzl, 1989); is antiretroviral (using purified hypericin) (Lavie et al., 1990; Meruelo et al., 1988); modulates interleukin-1x (hypericin) (Panossian et al., 1996) and interleukin-6 (SJW) (Thiele et al., 1994); is antiviral (influenza and herpes simplex type 1) (Serkedjieva et al., 1990), and is antimicrobial (primarily hyperforin) toward methicillin-resistant *Staphylococcus aureus* but not against gram-negative bacteria or *Candida albicans* (Reichling et al., 2001). Isolated hypericin from SJW extracts showed highest phototoxicity in vitro, but this was controlled by the flavonoid fraction, particularly quercitrin (Wilhelm et al., 2001).

MECHANISM OF ACTION

- Components of a hydro-ethanolic SJW extract bound with high affinity at $GABA_A$, $GABA_B$, adenosine, benzodiazepine, inositol, triphosphate, and MAO-A and MAO-B receptors (Cott, 1997).

- May inhibit uptake of several neurotransmitters (Müller and Rossol, 1994; Perovic and Müller, 1995; Holzl, 1989; Chatterjee et al., 1998; Raffa, 1998; Butterweck et al., 1997).

- May inhibit uptake of neuropeptides and neurosteroids (Perovic and Müller, 1995; Holzl et al., 1989; Chatterjee et al., 1998; Raffa, 1998; Butterweck et al., 1997).

- SJW may inhibit 5-hydroxytryptamine (5HT, serotonin) receptor expression resulting in inhibition of 5HT reuptake (Müller and Rossol, 1994).

- One indirect study based on changes in hormone levels suggests that antidepressant effects might be mediated mainly through changes in serotonin and dopamine neurotransmission but not noradrenaline (in humans) (Franklin and Cowen, 2001).

- May act on information substances (shared components of immune and nervous systems) such as leukotriene B4 and interleukin-1a inhibiting release of arachidonic acid, leukotriene B4, production of IL–1α, and activating NO synthesis (Panossian et al., 1996; Thiele et al., 1994).

- Hyperforin, but not hypericin, in SJW induces CYP3A4 expression in human hepatocytes and activates the steroid X receptor, possibly suggesting a mechanism for drug interactions (Moore et al., 2000; Wentworth et al., 2000).

- Hyperforin from SJW leads to elevation of Na^+, thus explaining its apparent effect on serotonin uptake inhibition into platelets and synaptosomes and the non-selective profile on many neurotransmitter transport systems which are driven by Na^+ gradient membranes (Müller et al., 2001).

CONTRAINDICATIONS

The Commission E stated "none known" in 1984 and in the 1990 monograph revision (Blumenthal *et al.*, 1998). Recent drug interaction reports suggest professional guidance when certain conventional pharmaceuticals may be simultaneously administered (see Drug Interactions).

PREGNANCY AND LACTATION: No known restrictions. Animal reproductive studies did not produce mutagenicity at relatively high doses (Upton *et al.*, 1997). Due to lack of available data, the WHO monograph recommends that SJW not be administered during pregnancy or nursing without advice of a healthcare provider (WHO, 2002).

ADVERSE EFFECTS

In general, SJW produces few adverse side effects. Between October 1991 and December 1999, over 8 million patients are estimated to have been treated with Germany's leading SJW preparation (Jarsin® or Jarsin®300); during this period only 95 reports of side effects were received by the German Adverse Drug Reaction Recording System. These included "allergic" skin reactions (27 reports), increased Quick Values (prothrombin time) (16), gastrointestinal complaints (9), breakthrough bleeding (birth control pill) (8), plasma cyclosporin reductions (7), and others (Schulz, 2001). Photosensitization, depicted by erythema (redness of the skin) with exposure to sunlight or other ultraviolet radiation is possible, although this is relatively rare and is sometimes reported in fair-skinned individuals taking excessive dosages (1,800 mg/day) (Brockmuller, 1997; Blumenthal *et al.*, 1998). A recent review of SJW adverse reactions suggests that this precaution should not constitute a general contraindication, since the incidence of photosensitization is so rare and because sunlight can promote recovery from depression (Schulz, 2001).

DRUG INTERACTIONS

Potential drug interactions with SJW have become the primary area of concern with this popular phytomedicine. However, one source suggests that some of these concerns may not be borne out by clinical experience. In a review of drug interactions reportedly associate with SJW, the author calculates one interaction per 300,000 treatments with the leading German SJW product (Jarsin®, Schulz, 2001).

SJW should not be taken in combination with any pharmaceutical antidepressants (Gordon, 1998; Prost *et al.*, 2000), unless under professional guidance. SJW is believed to interact with oral contraceptives and anticoagulants (e.g., warfarin) (TGA, 2000; Di Carlo *et al.*, 2001; Lantz *et al.*, 1999; McGuffin *et al.*, 1997). Preliminary findings suggest that SJW does not interact with the effects of alcohol; however, patients with depression should avoid alcohol (Schmidt, 1993). An uncontrolled study on 13 subjects taking SJW at normal doses (900 mg of the standardized extract/day), resulted in significant increases in urinary 6–beta–hydroxycortisol/cortisol ratio, suggesting that SJW is an inducer of CYP3A4, since cortisol is metabolized primarily by CYP3A4 (Roby *et al.*, 2000). A recent study (Moore, 2000) revealed that constituents of SJW extract, especially hyperforin, are a potent ligand (K(i) = 27 nM) for the pregnane X receptor, an orphan nuclear receptor that regulates expression of the cytochrome P450 (CYP) 3A4 monooxygenase. Treatment of primary human hepatocytes with SJW extracts, or hyperforin, results in a marked induction of CYP3A4 expression. CYP3A4 is involved in the oxidative metabolism of more than 50% of all

drugs, and can cause a decrease in the therapeutic activity and concentration of such drugs, including contraceptives (Moore, 2000) and possibly theophylline (Baede-van Dijk *et al.*, 2000). SJW also may increase clearance from the bloodstream of the protease inhibitor indinavir, and the anti-rejection drug cyclosporine (Piscitelli *et al.*, 2000; Ruschitzka *et al.*, 2000), and may also interfere with the absorption of digoxin (Tatro, 2000). A recent study found that SJW induces intestinal P-glycoprotein/MDR1 (in rats and humans), and induces intestinal and hepatic CYP3A4 (in humans), thereby decreasing plasma levels of cyclosporine, indinavir, and digoxin (Dürr *et al.*, 2000). However, a review of SJW drug interactions questions the clinical relevance of interactions that are postulated solely on the basis of pharmacokinetic measurements, with digoxin, theophylline, and amitriptyline needing to be examined critically, since reduced plasma levels are not the same as reduced active levels at the receptors. The author states that to-date there are no reported cases suggestive of a clinically significant weakening in effect of the three drugs cited (Schulz, 2001). One 14-day study on 10 patients, using the antiseizure drug carbamazepine (Tegretol®), found that 300 mg St. John's wort extract, three times daily, did not increase the clearance of the drug (Burstein *et al.*, 2000). Sudden discontinuation of SJW after prolonged use may lead to higher plasma levels of these drugs if used simultaneously, with the risk of adverse effects (Baede-van Dijk *et al.*, 2000).

AMERICAN HERBAL PRODUCTS ASSOCIATION (AHPA) SAFETY RATING

CLASS 2D: Based on earlier *in vitro* research and the Commission E monograph, AHPA cautioned that SJW may potentiate pharmaceutical MAO-inhibitors (McGuffin *et al.*, 1997), although there are no animal or human data to support this.

REGULATORY STATUS

AUSTRALIA: Complementary medicine available without prescription from pharmacies, health food shops, supermarkets, and complementary medicine practitioners (TGA, 2000). Required label warning: "St. John's wort affects the way some prescription medicines work. Consult your doctor." (Trickey, 2000).

CANADA: Nonprescription drug for internal or external use classified as either "Schedule OTC Herbs and Natural Products" or "Schedule Homeopathic Products," in either case requiring premarketing authorization and assignment of Drug Identification Number (DIN) by the Therapeutic Products Programme (TPP) (Health Canada, 2001a). In January 2001, added to "Drugs of Current Interest (DOCI) List" maintained by the Canadian Adverse Drug Reaction Monitoring Program (Health Canada, 2001b). Potential drug-interaction warning statement required.

EUROPEAN UNION: Whole or cut, dried, flowering tops harvested during flowering time, containing no less than 0.08% total hypericins, official in the *European Pharmacopoeia* (Ph.Eur., 2001).

FRANCE: Dried flowering top or aerial part official in *French Pharmacopoeia* approved only for external use but not prior to sun exposure (Bruneton, 1999; ESCOP, 1996).

GERMANY: Approved by Commission E as a nonprescription drug for internal and external use (Blumenthal *et al.*, 1998). Whole or cut aerial parts, collected just before or during the flowering period, official for internal or external use in the *German Drug Codex* supplement to the *German Pharmacopoeia* (DAC, 1998). Whole, fresh, flowering plant for preparation of mother tincture is official in German Commission D monographs and corresponding *German Homeopathic Pharmacopoeia* (BAnz, 1985; GHP, 1993).

SWEDEN: Classified as Natural Remedy, requiring premarket authorization. As of January 2001, nine SJW-containing products are listed in the Medical Products Agency (MPA) "Authorised Natural Remedies," and a monograph is published with the approved indication: "Traditionally used in case of slight mood lowering and for minor nervous tension" (MPA, 1999; 2001a; Tunón, 1999). St. John's wort homeopathic preparations are also registered drugs (MPA, 2001b).

SWITZERLAND: Official in *Swiss Pharmacopoeia* (Upton *et al.*, 1997; Wichtl, 1997). Herbal medicine with positive classification (List D) by the *Interkantonale Kontrollstelle für Heilmittel* (IKS) and corresponding sales Category D with sale limited to pharmacies and drugstores, without prescription (Morant and Ruppanner, 2001; Ruppanner and Schaefer, 2000). Numerous SJW phytomedicines and homeopathic preparations are listed in the *Swiss Codex 2000/01* (Ruppanner and Schaefer, 2000).

U.K.: Licensed product for internal use; *General Sale List* (GSL), Table B (external use only), Schedule 1 (requires full product license) (GSL, 1994). A recent article reviewed the benefits and risks of SJW and their regulatory implications in the U.K. (McIntyre, 2000).

U.S.: Dietary supplement (USC, 1994). Dried, flowering tops gathered shortly before or during flowering, containing no less than 0.04% total hypericins, official in U.S. *National Formulary*, 19th edition (USP, 2002).

CLINICAL REVIEW

Twenty-three studies are outlined in the following table, "Clinical Studies on St. John's Wort", including a total of 2,745 participants. All but three of these studies (Lenoir *et al.*, 1999; Shelton *et al.*, 2001; Hypericum Depression Trial Study Group, 2002) demonstrate positive effects of SJW on depression. Five randomized, double-blind, placebo-controlled (R, DB, PC) studies have been performed on 626 participants, concluding that SJW significantly benefits patients with depression without significant side effects (Philipp *et al.*, 1999; Laakmann *et al.*, 1998a, 1998b; Harrer and Sommer 1994; Hübner *et al.*, 1994; Hänsgen *et al.*, 1994). Five R, DB multicenter (MC) trials, with 1,191 participants, found equal effectiveness to tricyclic antidepressant drugs (amitriptyline, imipramine, malprotiline) with greater tolerability for SJW (Wheatley, 1997; Vorbach *et al.*, 1994; Harrer *et al.*, 1994), and that SJW was safer for the heart than tricyclic antidepressants (Czekalla *et al.*, 1997).

Three small pilot studies on a total of 60 patients show promising findings for the conditions of fatigue and SAD (Stevinson *et al.*, 1998; Kasper, 1997; Matinez *et al.*, 1994), and one small open-label (OL) study on 12 patients indicated the potential benefits of SJW for OCD (Taylor and Kobak, 2000). One small pilot study of SJW for the treatment of PMS suggests that SJW might improve the severity and duration of premenstrual symptoms, warranting a larger R, DB trial (Stevinson and Ernst, 2000). A drug-monitoring study on menopausal symptoms suggests that SJW is useful for treatment of associated symptoms, and increasing the sense of sexuality in middle-age women (Grube *et al.*, 1999).

In a review of 17 studies on SJW and 9 studies on fluoxetine (Prozac®), researchers showed that SJW was as effective as fluoxetine in the treatment of subthreshold and mild depression (Volz,

2000). Researchers concluded that SJW is effective in subthreshold depression exhibiting very few or no side effects, easy availability, and may be a viable approach to avoiding the risk that mild depression becomes a full-blown disorder.

A review and meta-analysis of 23 clinical studies on SJW showed that the extract was more effective than placebo in treating mild to moderate depression (Linde *et al.*, 1996). Based on the evidence available at the time, the same review concluded that further studies were needed to establish whether SJW is as effective as conventional antidepressant drugs (Linde *et al.*, 1996). A follow-up meta-analysis by the Cochrane Center of 27 trials with 2,291 patients concluded that SJW was significantly superior to placebo (Linde and Mulrow, 2001). The review concluded that the short term use of SJW might be valuable in less severe forms of depression as an alternative to watchful waiting or the commonly used approach to low doses of tricyclic antidepressants and that SJW has less short term adverse side effects than tricyclics. A recent trial comparing SJW with the conventional antidepressant imipramine is the first to compare the two agents at the normal daily dose of imipramine (150 mg) (Woelk, 2000). Previous trials used only 75 mg imipramine in order to reduce adverse side effects and maintain patient compliance. This study is the largest comparison trial to date and concluded that the SJW extract used in the study (Remotiv® marketed by Bayer in Germany) is equivalent to imipramine in efficacy, and is more well-tolerated by patients. A newer, larger trial (n=240) comparing SJW (Ze 117) directly with fluoxetine concluded that SJW was of equivalent efficacy as fluoxetine, particularly in depressive patients suffering from anxiety, and was better tolerated for safety than the SSRI (Friede *et al.*, 2001). A total of 11 studies have compared SJW preparations with conventional antidepressants (7 tricyclic; 4 SSRI) concluding that SJW is effective for mild to moderate depression with a low side effect profile (Kasper, 2001).

A recently published systematic review of R, C, DB trials selected, and assessed for methodological quality, eight well-controlled studies (Gaster and Holroyd, 2000). The results suggest that SJW is more effective than placebo in the treatment of mild to moderate depression. The absolute increased response rate with the use of SJW ranged from 23% to 55% higher than with placebo, but ranged from 6% to 18% lower compared with tricyclic antidepressants. The treatment with SJW and the commonly used SSRI fluoxetine (Prozac®), was compared in patients with mild to moderate depression. The results showed that SJW and fluoxetine are equipotent with respect to all main parameters used to investigate antidepressants in this population. Although SJW may be superior in improving the responder rate, the main difference between the two treatments is safety. SJW was superior to fluoxetine in overall incidence of side effects, number of patients with side effects, and the type of side effect reported (Schrader, 2000). A previous review of 15 controlled clinical trials (12 PC) reported that the only substantial documentation for the use of SJW in mild to moderate depression is for the products Jarsin® 300 (Lichtwer Pharma) and Psychotonin-M® (Steigerwald) (Volz, 1997). The review concluded that SJW should not be taken for more than 6 weeks, since most trials showing efficacy have been conducted over a shorter period of time. A recent study by Shelton *et al.* (2001) received considerable media attention due to its negative findings on patients with severe depression. The study was noted for its lack of an active control (no SSRI or other active drug was used to measure the response rate of severely depressed patients vs. SJW and placebo) (Cott *et al.*, 2001).

Results were recently published for the first study funded by the NIH's NCCAM. This long awaited and much publicized R, DB, PC, MC, 3-arm study (340 participants) found that neither sertraline (Zoloft®) nor SJW were effective compared to placebo for moderately severe major depressive disorder. Critics emphasize that the initial design included patients with major depression of only mild to moderate severity (HAMD score ≥ 15) but was later changed to include patients with moderate to severe depression (HAMD score ≥ 20). Widespread publicity on this trial focused on the failure of SJW without equally noting the failure of sertraline which was given a slight edge over SJW because of sertraline's better performance on a secondary measure (a Clinical Global Impression scale that included partial responders). (Outcomes on secondary measurements are not considered appropriate measures for ascribing success or failure.) The authors of this study acknowledged that 35% of clinical trials on known antidepressant drugs failed. More than 50% of trials with investigational antidepressant drugs fail (Robinson and Rickels, 2000).

BRANDED PRODUCTS*

Hyperiforce®: Bioforce AG / CH-9325 Roggwil TG / Switzerland / Tel: +41 71 454 61 61 / Fax: +41 71 454 61 62 / www.bioforce.com / Email: info@bioforce.ch. 275 mg/tablet of a 1:9.0 ethanol/water extract of fresh tips of shoots. One tablet 3 times/day after meals provides 1 mg hypericin/day.

Jarsin® 300: Lichtwer Pharma AG / Wallenroder Strasse 8-14 / 13435 Berlin / Germany / Tel: +49-30-40-3700 / Fax: +49-30-40-3704-49 / www.lichtwer.de. 300 mg St. John's wort extract/capsule in coated tablets standardized to 0.3% total hypericins.

Kira®: Lichtwer Pharma AG, c/o ABKIT, INC. / 207 East 94th Street / New York, NY 10128 / U.S.A. / Tel: 800-226-6227 / Fax: 212-860-8323 / www.abkit.com / Email: info@abkit.com. 300 mg dried methanolic extract produced from leaves, stems, and flowers standardized to 300 mcg total hypericin.

LI 160: Lichtwer Pharma AG. 300 mg St. John's wort extract/capsule in coated tablets standardized to 0.3% total hypericins.

Remotiv®: Bayer Vital GmbH & Co. KG / Consumer Care / Welser Strasse 5 – 7 / 51149 Köln / Germany / Tel: + 49-01-30-82-6301 / www.bayer-ag.de. Each 250 mg film-coated tablet of St. John's wort extracted in 50% alcohol, standardized to 2% hypericins.

STEI 300: Steiner Arzneimittel / Postfach 450520 / 12175 Berlin / Germany / Tel: +49-03-07-1094-0 / Fax: +49-03-07-1250-12 / www.steinerarznei-berlin.de. Each 350 mg capsule contains 0.2%–0.3% hypericin, and 2%–3% hyperforin.

WS 5570: Dr. Willmar Schwabe Pharmaceuticals / International Division / Willmar Schwabe Str. 4 / D-76227, Karlsruhe / Germany / Tel: +49-721-4005 ext. 294 / ·Email: melville-eaves@schwabe.de / www.schwabepharma.com. An 80% v/v hydroalcoholic extract of St. John's wort, drug to extract ratio 3–7.1.

WS 5572: Dr. Willmar Schwabe Pharmaceuticals. St. John's wort extract standardized to 5% hyperforin.

WS 5573: Dr. Wilmar Schwabe Phramaceuticals. Each 300 mg capsule contains dry SJW extract standardized to 0.5% hyperforin.

Ze 117: Zeller AG / Seeblickstrasse 4 / CH-8590 Romanshorn 1 / Switzerland / www.zellerag.ch. St. John's wort extracted in 50% alcohol, standardized to 2% hypericins in a 250 mg tablet, drug to extract ratio 4–7:1.

*American equivalents are found in the Product Table beginning on page 398.

REFERENCES

Agency for Health Care Policy and Research. *Treatment of Depression–Newer Pharmacotherapies*. Summary, Evidence report/Technology Assessment: Number 7, March 1999.

AHCPR. See: Agency for Health Care Policy and Research.

Baede-van Dijk P, van Galen E, Lekkerkerker J. Drug interactions of *Hypericum perforatum* (St. John's wort) are potentially hazardous. *Ned Tijdschr Geneeskd* 2000 Apr 22;144(17):811–2.

BAnz. See: Bundesanzeiger.

Bhattacharya S, Chakrabarti A, Chatterjee S. Activity profiles of two hyperforin-containing Hypericum extracts in behavioral models. *Pharmacopsychiatry* 1998;31 (suppl. 1):22–9.

Bladt S, Wagner H. Inhibition of MAO by fractions and constituents of Hypericum extract. *J Geriatr Psychiat Neurol* 1994; 7(1):557–9.

Blumenthal M. Herb sales down 15% in mainstream market. *HerbalGram* 2001;51:69.

Blumenthal M, Busse WR, Goldberg A, Gruenwald J, Hall T, Riggins CW, Rister RS (eds.). Klein S, Rister RS (trans.). *The Complete German Commission E Monographs—Therapeutic Guide to Herbal Medicines*. Austin, TX: American Botanical Council; Boston: Integrative Medicine Communication; 1998.

Blumenthal M, Goldberg A, Brinckmann J, eds. *Herbal Medicine: Expanded Commission E Monographs*. Austin TX: American Botanical Council; Newton MA; Integrative Medicine Communications; 2000.

Brenner R, Azbel V, Madhusoodanan S, Pawlowska, M. Comparison of an Extract of Hypericum (LI 160) and Sertraline in the Treatment of Depression: A Double-Blind, Randomized Pilot Study. *Clinical Therapeutics* 2000; 22(4).

Brevoort P. The booming U.S. botanical market: an overview. *HerbalGram* 1998;44:33–40.

Brinker F. *Herb Contraindications and Drug Interactions*, 3d ed. Sandy, OR: Eclectic Medicinal Publications; 2001:178–84.

Brockmuller J, Reum T, Bauer S, *et al*. Roots I: Hypericin and pseudohypericin: pharmacokinetics and effects on photosensitivity in humans. *Pharmacopsychiatry* 1997; 30 (suppl. 2):94–101.

Bruneton, J. *Pharmacognosy, Phytochemistry, Medicinal Plants*, 2nd ed. Paris, France: Lavoisier Publishing; 1999.

Bühler. Communication from BfarM (German Federal Institute for Drugs and Medical Devices) to German Non-prescription Drug Association (BAH), Sept. 11, 1999.

Bundesanzeiger (BAnz). *Monographien der Kommission D*. Cologne, Germany: BAnz. 10.10.1985;Nr.190a.

Burstein A, Horton R, Dunn T *et al*. Lack of effect of St. John's wort on carbamazepine pharmacokinetics in healthy volunteers. *Clin Pharm & Ther* 2000 Dec;68(6):605–12.

Butterweck V, Bockers T, Korte B, Wittkowski W, Winterhoff H. Long-term effects of St. John's wort and hypericin on monoamine levels in rat hypothalamus and hippocampus. *Brain Res* 2002a Mar 15;930(1-2):21-9.

Butterweck V, Jurgenliemk G, Nahrstedt A, Winterhoff H. Flavonoids from Hypericum perforatum show antidepressant activity in the forced swimming test. *Planta Med* 2000 Feb;66(1):3-6.

Butterweck V, Nahrstedt A, Evans J, Hufeisen S, Rauser L, Savage J, *et al*. In vitro receptor screening of pure constituents of St. John's wort reveals novel interactions with a number of GPCRs. *Psychopharmacol* (Berl) 2002b Jul;162(2):193-202.

Butterweck V, Wall A, Lieflander-Wulf U, *et al*. Effects of the total extract and fractions of *Hypericum perforatum* in animal assays for antidepressant activity. *Pharmacopsychiatry* 1997;30(2):117–24.

Chatterjee, S, Noldner M, Koch E, Erdelmeier C. Antidepressant activity of *Hypericum perforatum* and hyperforin: the neglected possibility. *Pharmacopsychiatry* 1998;31 (suppl. 1):7–15.

Cott J. *In vitro* receptor binding and enzyme inhibition by *Hypericum perforatum* extract. *Pharmacopsychiatry* 1997; 30 (suppl. 2):108–12.

Cott J. Medicinal plants and dietary supplements: sources for innovative treatments or adjuncts: an introduction. *Psychopharm Bulletin* 1995; 31(1):131–7.

Cott J, Fugh-Berman A. Is St. John's wort (*Hypericum perforatum*) an effective antidepressant? *J Nerv Ment Dis* 1998;186(8):500–1.

Cott J, Rosenthal N, Blumenthal M. St. John's wort and major depression. *JAMA* 2001;286(1):42.

Czekalla J, Gastpar M, Hübner W et al. The effect of hypericum extract on cardiac conduction as seen in the electrocardiogram compared to that of imipramine. *Pharmacopsychiatry* 1997; 30:86–8.

DAC. See: *Deutscher Arzneimittel-Codex.*

De Smet P, Nolen W. St. John's wort as an antidepressant. *BMJ* 1996; 313(7052):241–2.

Deutscher Arzneimittel-Codex (DAC 1998 Ergänzungsbuch zum Arzneibuch, Band II). Stuttgart, Germany: Deutscher Apotheker Verlag. 1998;J–010;1–5.

Di Carlo G, Borrelli F, Ernst E, Izzo AA. St. John's wort: Prozac from the plant kingdom. *Trends Pharm Sci* 2001;22(6):292–6.

Dürr D, Steiger B, Gerd A, Kullak-Ublick G et al. St. John's Wort induces intestinal P-glycoprotein/MDR1 and intestinal and hepatic CYP3A4. *Clin Pharm & Ther* 2000 Dec;68(6):598–604.

ESCOP. See: European Scientific Cooperative on Phytotherapy.

European Pharmacopoeia (Ph.Eur. 3rd ed. 1997 Supple. 2001). Strasbourg, France: Council of Europe. 2001;972–3.

European Scientific Cooperative on Phytotherapy (ESCOP). Hyperici Herba — St. John's Wort. In: *ESCOP Monographs on the Medicinal Uses of Plant Drugs.* Exeter, U.K.: ESCOP. March 1996.

Felter HW, Lloyd JU. 1983. *King's American Dispensatory*, 18th ed., 3rd rev. Portland, OR: Eclectic Medical Publications; [reprint of 1898 original], 1083–9.

Franklin M, Cowen PJ. Researching the antidepressant actions of *Hypericum perforatum* (St. John's wort) in animals and man. *Pharmacopsychiatry* 2001;34 Suppl.1:S29–37.

Friede M, Henneicke von Zepelin H-H, Freudenstein. Differential therapy of mild to moderate depressive episodes (ICD–10 F 32.1) with St. John's wort. *Pharmacopsychiatry* 2001;34 Suppl. 1:S38–41.

Fugh-Berman A and Cott J. Dietary supplements and natural products as psychotherapeutic agents. *Psychosom Med* 1999 Sept/Oct;61(5):712–28.

Gaster B, Holroyd J. St John's wort for depression: a systematic review. *Arch Intern Med* 2000 Jan 24;160(2):152–6.

General Sale List (GSL). Statutory Instrument 1994 No. 2410; The Medicines (Products Other Than Veterinary Drugs) (*General Sale List*) Amendment Order 1994. London, U.K.: Her Majesty's Stationery Office (HMSO). 1994.

German Homeopathic Pharmacopoeia (GHP), 1st ed. 1978 with supplements through 1991. Translation of the German "*Homöopathisches Arzneibuch* (HAB 1), Amtliche Ausgabe." Stuttgart, Germany: Deutscher Apotheker Verlag. 1993.

GHP. See: *German Homeopathic Pharmacopoeia.*

GSL. See: *General Sale List.*

Gordon JB. SSRI's and St. John's wort possible toxicology. *Am Fam Physician* 1998; 57(5):950, 953.

Grube B, Walper A, Wheatley D. St. John's wort extract: efficacy for menopausal symptoms of psychological origin. *Advances in Ther* 1999 Jul/Aug;16(4):177–86.

Hänsgen K, Vesper J, Ploch M. Multicenter double-blind study examining the antidepressant effectiveness of the Hypericum extract LI 160. *J Geriatr Psychiatr Neurol* 1994;7(suppl. 1):S15–8.

Harrer G, Schmidt U, Kuhn U, Biller A. A comparison of equivalence between St. John's wort extract Lottyp-57 and fluoxetine. *Arzneimittelforschung* 1999;49:289–96.

Harrer G, Sommer H. Treatment of mild/moderate depressions with Hypericum. *Phytomedicine* 1994;1:3–8.

Harrer G, Hübner W, Podzuweit H. Effectiveness and tolerance of the Hypericum extract LI 160 compared to maprotiline: a multicenter double-blind study. *J Geriatr Psychiatry Neurol* 1994; 7(suppl.):S24–8.

Health Canada. *Hypericum perforatum.* In: *Drug Product Database* (DPD). Ottawa, Ontario: Health Canada Therapeutic Products Programme. 2001a.

Health Canada. *Hypericum perforatum.* In: Drugs of Current Interest (DOCI) List. Ottawa, Ontario: Health Canada Therapeutic Products Programme. January 2001b.

Hobbs C. St. John's wort, *Hypericum perforatum.* *HerbalGram* 1988/1989;18/19:24–33.

Holzl J. Investigations about antidepressant and mood changing effects of *Hypericum perforatum.* *Planta Med* 1989; 55:601–2.

Hübner W, Lande S, Podzuweit H. Hypericum treatment of mild depressions with somatic symptoms. *J Geriatr Psychiatr Neurol* 1994;7(suppl.):S12–4.

Hypericum Depression Trial Study Group. Effect of *Hypericum perforatum* (St John's Wort) in major depressive disorder—A randomized controlled trial. *JAMA* 2002;287:1807–14.

Jakovljevic V, Popovic M, Mimica-Dukic, N, Sabo A, Gvozdenovic Lj. Pharmacodynamic study of *Hypericum perforatum* L. *Phytomedicine* 2000;7(6):449–53.

Johnson D, Ksciuk H, Woelk H, Sauerwein-Giese E, Frauendorf A. Effects of Hypericum extract LI 160 compared with maprotiline on resting EEG and evoked potentials in 24 volunteers. *J Geriatr Psychiatr Neurol* 1994;7(suppl 1):S44–S46.

Karnick C. *Pharmacopoeial Standards of Herbal Plants*, Vols. 1–2. Delhi: Sri Satguru

Publications; (1):189–192;(2):125, 1994.

Kasper S. *Hypericum perforatum–* Review of clinical studies. *Pharmacopsychiatry* 2001;34 Suppl. 1:S51–5.

Kasper S. Treatment of seasonal affective disorder (SAD) with Hypericum extract. *Pharmacopsychiatry* 1997; 30:S89–93.

Laakmann, G, Schüle C, Baghai T, Kieser M. St. John's wort in mild to moderate depression: the relevance of hyperforin for the clinical efficacy. *Pharmacopsychiatry* 1998a; 31(suppl. 1):54–9.

Laakmann, G, Deniel A, Kieser M. Clinical significance of hyperforin for the efficacy of Hypericum extracts on depressive disorders of different severities. *Phytomedicine* 1998b; 5(6):435–42.

Lantz M, Buchalter E, Giambanco V. St. John's wort and antidepressant drug interactions in the elderly. *J Geriatr Psychiatry Neurol* 1999; 12:7–10.

Lavie G, Mazur Y, Lavie D, et al. Hypericin as an antiretroviral agent. *Annals NY Acad Sci* 1990; 616:556–62.

Lehrl S, et al. Results from measurements of the cognitive capacity in patients during treatment with Hypericum extract. *Nervenheilkunde* 1993; 12:268–366.

Lenoir S, Degenring F, Saller R. A double-blind randomized trial to investigate three different concentrations of a standardized fresh plant extract obtained from the shoot tips of *Hypericum perforatum* L. *Phytomedicine* 1999; 6(3):141–6.

Leung A and Foster S. *Encyclopedia of Common Natural Ingredients Used in Food, Drugs and Cosmetics*, 2nd ed. New York: John Wiley & Sons, Inc; 1996;310–2.

Linde K, Mulrow C. St. John's wort for depression (*Cochrane Review*). In: The Cochrane Library, 1, 2001. Oxford; Update Software.

Linde K, Ramirez G, Mulrow C, Pauls A, Weidenhammer W, Melchart D . St. John's wort for depression—an overview and meta-analysis of randomized clinical trials. *BMJ* 1996; 313(7052):253–8.

Martinez B, Kasper S, Ruhrmann S, Moller HJ. Hypericum in the treatment of seasonal affective disorders. *J Geriatr Psychiatry Neurol* 1994 Oct; 7(suppl. 1):S29–33.

McCaleb R, Leigh E, Morien K. *The Encyclopedia of Popular Herbs: Your complete guide to the leading medicinal plants.* Boulder CO: The Herb Research Foundation; Roseville CA: PrimaHealth Publishing; 2000.

McGuffin M, Hobbs C, Upton R, Goldberg A. *American Herbal Product Association's Botanical Safety Handbook.* Boca Raton: CRC Press; 1997.

McIntyre M. A review of the benefits, adverse events, drug interactions, and safety of St. John's wort (*Hypericum perforatum*): the implications with regard to the regulation of herbal medicines (editorial). *J Alt Compl Med* 2000;6(2):115–24.

Medical Products Agency (MPA). *Naturläkemedel: Authorised Natural Remedies* (as of January 24, 2001). Uppsala, Sweden: Medical Products Agency.

Medical Products Agency (MPA). *Homeopatika: Företag med registrerade homeopatika* (updated 2001–02–-26). Uppsala, Sweden: Medical Products Agency. 2001b.

Medical Products Agency (MPA). *Naturläkemedelsmonografi: Johannesört.* Uppsala, Sweden: Medical Products Agency. 1999.

Meruelo D, Lavie G, Lavie D. Therapeutic agents with dramatic antiretroviral activity and little toxicity at effective doses: aromatic polycyclic diones hypericin and pseudohypericin. *PNAS* 1988; 85:5230–4.

Moore LB, Goodwin B, Jones SA, et al. St. John's wort induces hepatic drug metabolism through activation of the pregnane X receptor. *Proc Natl Acad Sci USA* 2000 Jun 20;97(13):7500–2.

Morant J, Ruppanner H (eds.). *Arzneimittel-Kompendium der Schweiz®* 2001. Basel, Switzerland: Documed AG. 2001.

MPA. See: Medical Products Agency.

Müller W, Rossol R. Effects of Hypericum extract on the expression of serotonin receptors. *J Geriatr Psychiat Neurol* 1994; 7(suppl. 1):S63–4.

Müller W, Singer A, Wonnemann M. Hyperforin–Antidepressant activity by a novel mechanism of action. *Pharmacopsychiatry* 2001;34 Suppl. 1:S98–102.

Müller W, Singer A, Wonneman M., et al. Hyperforin represents the neurotransmitter reuptake inhibiting constituent of hypericum extract. *Pharmacopsychiatry* 1998; 31:16–21.

Newall C, Anderson L, Phillipson J. *Herbal Medicines: A Guide for Health-Care Professionals.* London: The Pharmaceutical Press; 1996.

Obach R. Inhibition of human cytochrome P450 enzymes by constituents of St. John's wort, an herbal preparation used in the treatment of depression. *J Pharmacol Exp Ther* 2000 Jul;294(1):88–95.

Panossian A, Gabrielian E, Manvelian V, et al. Immunosuppressive effects of hypericin on stimulated human leukocytes: inhibition of the arachidonic acid release, leukotriene B4 and interleukin-1a production, and activation of nitric oxide formation. *Phytomedicine* 1996;3(1):19–28.

Perovic S, Müller W. Pharmacological profile of Hypericum extract; effect on serotonin uptake by postsynaptic receptors. *Arzneimittelforschung* 1995; 45(11):1145–8.

Ph.Eur. See: *European Pharmacopoeia.*

Philipp M, Kohnen R, O'Hiller K. Hypericum extract versus imipramine or placebo in patients with moderate depression: randomized multicentre study of treatment for eight weeks. *BMJ* 1999; 319:1534–8.

Piscitelli S, Burstein A, Chaitt D, *et al.* Indinavir concentrations and St John's wort. *Lancet* 2000; 355:547–8.

Prost N, Tichadou F, Rodor F, *et al.* St. John's wort-venlafaxine interaction. *Presse Med* 2000; 29(23):1285–6.

Raffa R. Screen of receptor and uptake-site activity of hypericin component of St. John's wort reveals sigma receptor binding. *Life Sci* 1998;62(16):PL265–70.

Reichling J, Weseler A, Saller R. A current review of the antimicrobial activity of *Hypericum perforatum* L. *Pharmacopsychiatry* 2001;34 Suppl.1:S116–8.

Rezvani A, Overstreet D, Yang Y, *et al.* Attenuation of alcohol intake by extract of *Hypericum perforatum* in two different strains of alcohol-preferring rats. *Alcohol and Alcoholism* 1999; 34(5):699–705.

Robinson DS, Rickels K. Concerns about clinical drug trials [editorial]. *J Clin Psychopharmacol* 2000 Dec;20(6):593–6.

Roby CA, Anderson GD, Kantor E *et al.* St. John's wort: effect on CYP3A4 activity. *Clin Pharm Ther* 2000;67(5):451–7.

Ruppanner H, Schaefer U (eds.). *Codex 2000/01 — Die Schweizer Arzneimittel in einem Griff.* Basel, Switzerland: Documed AG. 2000.

Ruschitzka F, Meier P, Turina M, *et al.* Acute heart transplant rejection due to Saint John's wort. *Lancet* 2000; 355:548–9.

Schempp, CM, Muller K, Winghofer B, Shulte-Monting J, Simon JC. Single-dose and steady-state administration of *Hypericum perforatum* (St. John's wort) does not influence skin sensitivity to UV radiation, visible light, and solar-simulated radiation. [letter]. *Arch Dermatol* 2001 Apr;137(4):512–3.

Schilcher H. *Phytotherapy in Paediatrics—Handbook for Physicians and Pharmacists.* Stuttgart: Medpharm Scientific Publishers; 1997;61–2.

Schmidt U, Harrer G, Kuhn U, *et al.* Wechselwirkungen von Hypericum-Extrakt mit Alkohol. *Nervenheilkunde* 1993;12:314–9.

Schrader E. Equivalence of St John's wort extract (Ze 117) and fluoxetine: a randomized, controlled study in mild-moderate depression. *Int Clin Psychopharmacol* 2000 Mar;15(2):61–8

Schrader E, Meier B, Brattström A. Hypericum treatment of mild-moderate depression in a placebo-controlled study. A prospective, double-blind, randomized, placebo-controlled, multicentre study. *Hum Psychopharmacol* 1998;13:163–169.

Schüle C, Baghai T, Ferrera A, Laackmann G. Neuroendocrine effects of *Hypericum perforatum* extract WS 5570 in 12 healthy male volunteers. *Pharmacopsychiatry* 2001;34 Suppl.1:S127–133.

Schulz V. Incidence and clinical relevance of the interactions and side effects of *Hypericum* preparations. *Phytomedicine* 2001;8(2):152-160.

Schulz H, Jobert M. Effects of hypericum extract on the sleep EEG in older volunteers. *J Geriatr Psych Neurol* 1994; 7(suppl. 1): S39–43.

Schulz V, Hänsel R, Tyler VE. *Rational Phytotherapy: A Physicians' Guide to Herbal Medicine* 4th ed. New York: Springer; 2000;57–77.

Serkedjieva J, Manolova N, Zgorniak-Nowosielska I, *et al.* Antiviral activity of the infusion (SHS–174) from flowers of *Sambucus nigra* L., aerial parts of *Hypericum perforatum* L., and roots of *Saponaria officinalis* L. against influenza and herpes simplex viruses. *Phytother Res* 1990; 4(3):97–100.

Shelton RC, Keller MB, Gelenberg A, *et al.* Effectiveness of St. John's wort in major depression: a randomized controlled trial. *JAMA* 2001;285:1978-1986.

Staffeldt, B *et al.* Pharmacokinetic of hypericin and pseudohypericin after oral ingestion of St.John's wort extract LI 160 in healthy subjects. [in German]. *Nervenheilkunde* 1993;12:331–8.

Stevinson C, Dixon M, Ernst E. *Hypericum* for fatigue-a pilot study. *Phytomedicine* 1998; 5(6):443–7.

Stevinson C, Ernst E. A pilot study of *Hypericum perforatum* for the treatment of premenstrual syndrome. *BJOG* 2000 Jul;107(7):870–6.

Suzuki O *et al.* Inhibition of monoamine oxidase by hypericin. *Planta Med* 1984;272–4.

Tatro DS. Drug interactions with St.John's wort. *Druglink* 2000 May;34–8.

Taylor L, Kobak K. An open-label trial of St. John's wort (*Hypericum perforatum*) in obsessive-compulsive disorder. *J Clin Psy* 2000 Aug;61(8)575–8.

TGA. See. Therapeutic Goods Administration.

Therapeutic Goods Administration (TGA). Australia government Adverse Drug Reactions Unit. Media Release; 2000.

Therapeutic Goods Administration (TGA). Media Release: TGA alert to doctors and pharmacists and complementary health practitioners. Woden, Australia: Therapeutic Goods Administration. 13. March 2000;1–4.

Thiele B, Brink I, Ploch M. Modulation of cytokine expression by Hypericum extract. *J Geriatr Psychiatry Neurol* 1994; 7(suppl. l):S60–2.

Trickey R. Hypericum labelling. *Access: National Herbalists Association of Australia.* September 2000;22:1.

Tunón H. Phtyotherapie in Schweden. *Z Phytother* 1999;20:268–77.

United States Congress (USC). Public Law 103–417: Dietary Supplement Health and Education Act of 1994. Washington, DC: 103rd Congress of the United States. 1994.

United States Pharmacopeia (USP 25th Revision) – *The National Formulary* (NF 20th Edition). Rockville, MD: United States Pharmacopeial Convention, Inc. 1999;2509–10.

Upton R (ed.). St. John's Wort: *Hypericum perforatum.* *HerbalGram* 1997 Jul;40:(suppl.)1–32.

USC. See: United States Congress.

USP. See: *United States Pharmacopeia.*

Volz, H.P. Controlled clinical trials of Hypericum extracts in depressed patients: an overview. *Pharmacopsychiatry* 1997; 30:72–6.

Volz HP, Laux P. Potential treatment for subthreshold and mild depression: a comparison of St. John's wort extracts and fluoxetine. *Compr Psychiatry* 2000;41(2 Suppl. 1):133–7.

Vorbach E Hübner W, Arnoldt K. Effectiveness and tolerance of the Hypericum extract LI 160 in comparison with imipramine: randomized double-blind study with 135 outpatients. *J Geriatr Psychiatry Neurol* 1994; 7(suppl. 1): S19–23.

Wentworth JM, Agostini M, Love J, *et al.* St John's wort, a herbal antidepressant, activates the steroid X receptor. *J Endocrinol* 2000;166:R11–R16.

Weiss R, Fintelmann V. *Herbal Medicine,* 2nd ed. New York: Thieme; 2000; 235.

Wheatley D. LI 160, an extract of St.John's wort, versus amitriptyline in mildly to moderately depressed outpatients-a controlled 6 week clinical trial. *Pharmacopsychiatry* 1997; 30(suppl.):77–80.

WHO. See: World Health Organization.

Wichtl M (ed.). *Teedrogen und Phytopharmaka, 3. Auflage: Ein Handbuch für die Praxis auf wissenschaftlicher Grundlage.* Stuttgart, Germany: Wissenschaftliche Verlagsgesellschaft mbH. 1997;309–12.

Wichtl M, Bisset N (eds.). *Herbal Drugs and Phytopharmaceuticals.* Stuttgart: Medpharm Scientific Publishers; 1994;273–5.

Wilhelm K-P, Biel S, Siegers C-P. Role of flavonoids in controlling phototoxicity of *Hypericum perforatum* extracts. *Phytomed* 2001;8(4):306–309.

Woelk H. Comparison of St. John's wort and imipramine for treating depression: randomized controlled trial. *BMJ* 2000 Sep;321:536–9.

World Health Organization. *WHO monographs on selected medicinal plants* Vol. 2, Herba Hyperici. Geneva, Switzerland: WHO Publications; 2002.

Wichtl M, Bisset N (eds.). *Herbal Drugs and Phytopharmaceuticals.* Stuttgart: Medpharm Scientific Publishers; 1994;273–5.

Clinical Studies on St. John's wort (*Hypericum perforatum L.*)

Depression

Author/Year	Subject	Design	Duration	Dosage	Preparation	Results/Conclusion
Hypericum Depression Trial Study Group, 2002	Major depression	R, DB, PC, MC n=340 adults with baseline total HAMD score ≥ 20	8–18 weeks	900–1,500 mg SJW/day or 50–100 mg sertraline/day or placebo; divided into 3 doses/day	LI 160 SJW extract standardized to between 0.12% and 0.28% hypericin; sertraline (Zoloft®)	Initial treatment phase = 8 weeks. Patients responding positively were given respective treatments for additional 18 weeks. On the 2 primary outcome measures neither sertraline nor SJW performed significantly differently from placebo, based on HAMD or CGI scale. Full response occurred in 31.9% placebo group, 24.8% sertraline group (p=0.26), and 23.9% SJW group (p=0.21). Sertraline was better than placebo on a secondary measure: a CGI improvement scale that included partial responders (p=0.02). Authors concluded that the study does not support the efficacy of SJW in moderately severe major depression, acknowledging the low assay sensitivity of this trial, and the fact that 35% of trials on known antidepressants result in failure.
Friede et al., 2001	Mild to moderate depression	R, DB, MC n=240 (HAMD scores 16–24)	6 weeks	500 mg/day Ze 117 vs. 20 mg/day fluoxetine	Ze 117 vs. fluoxetine	SJW extract is equivalent in efficacy (p=0.09) to fluoxetine for both overall depressive symptoms and the main symptoms of depressive disorders. SJW is particularly effective in depressive patients suffering from anxiety symptoms. Tolerability for SJW revealed better safety (p<0.001) than for fluoxetine.
Shelton et al., 2001	Severe depression	R, DB, PC, MC n=200 patients with baseline HAMD ≥ 20	SJW for 4 weeks (n=98) or placebo (n=102) for 8 weeks	900 mg/day increased to 1200 mg/day or placebo	SJW standardized extract (LI 160) or placebo	The number of patients with a remission of depression was significantly higher with SJW than placebo (p=0.2), but they had low rates 14.3% with SJW vs. 4.9% for placebo in the full intention-to-treat analysis. SJW was well tolerated, with the only adverse effect being headaches (41% vs. 25%). The random analyses for the HAMD, HAMA, CGI-S, and CGI-I showed significant effects for time but not for treatment or time-by-treatment interaction. The study concluded that SJW was not effective in treating major depression (no active control used).
Brenner et al., 2000	Mild to moderate depression; comparison of SJW and selective serotonin reuptake inhibitors (SSRIs)	R, DB, C n=30	7 weeks	600 mg per day of standardized SJW extract or 50 mg per day of sertraline for 1 week, followed by 900 mg per day of SJW or 75 mg per day of sertraline	LI 160 vs. sertraline	Severity of symptoms, as measured by HAMD and the Clinical Gobal Impression scale was significantly reduced in both treatment groups (p<0.01). The difference in clinical response, based on reduction in HAMD for each group, was not statistically significant. SJW extract was found to be at least as effective as sertraline in treating mild to moderate depression.
Woelk, 2000	Mild to moderate depression without suicidal ideation (ICD-10)	R, DB, PG, MC (40 centers) n=324 HAMD scale >18. Mean HAMD 22.4 (SJW); 22.1 (imipramine) (ages >18 years)	6 weeks	250 mg SJW extract, 2x/day; 75 mg imipramine, 2x/day	Remotiv® (Ze 117) vs. imipramine	157 subjects on SJW had HAMD scores drop from mean or 22.4 at baseline to 12.00 at 12 weeks end, compared to 167 imipramine patients' scores of 22.1 dropping to 12.75 (no statistical difference between groups). CGI scores at end were mean of 2.22 of 7 for SJW group and 2.42 for imipramine group (no statistical difference between groups). In self-assessment, mean scores were 2.44 for SJW and 2.60 for imipramine (no statistical difference between groups). Tolerability scores were better for SJW (1.65) than drug (2.35); (no statistical difference between groups). Researchers concluded that SJW is therapeutically equal to imipramine for mild to moderate depression and tolerated better. This is largest trial on SJW comparing it to imipramine at standard dose (150 mg/day).
Philipp et al., 1999	Moderate depression	R, DB, MC, PG, PC, Cm n=262	2 months	1050 mg/day SJW , 350 mg, 3x/day vs. daily dosing of 50 mg, 25 mg, then 25 mg (100 mg total/day) imipramine	STEI 300 vs. imipramine	SJW was more effective than placebo and as effective as 100 mg/day imipramine in the treatment of depression as measured by HAMD, HAMA, and Clinical Global Impression scales. Improved quality of life also demonstrated in Zung self-rating depression scale. Proven safe with less adverse effects than imipramine.

KEY: C – controlled, **CC** – case-control, **CGI** – clinical global impression scale, **CGI-I** – clinical global improvement impression scale, **CGI-S** – clinical global severity impression scale, **CH** – cohort, **CI** – confidence interval, **Cm** – comparison, **CO** – crossover, **CS** - cross-sectional, **DB** – double-blind, **D-S** – von Zerssen depression severity scale, **DSM** – Diagnostic and Statistical Manual of Mental Disorders, **E** – epidemiological, **HAMA** – Hamilton Anxiety Scale, **HAMD** – Hamilton Depression Scale, **ICD** – International Classification of Disease, **LC** – longitudinal cohort, **MA** – meta-analysis, **MC** – multi-center, n – number of patients, **O** – open, **OB** – observational, **OL** – open label, **OR** – odds ratio, **P** – prospective, **PB** – patient-blind, **PC** – placebo-controlled, **PG** – parallel group, **PS** – pilot study, **R** – randomized, **RC** – reference-controlled, **RCS** – retrospective cross-sectional, **RS** - retrospective, **S** – surveillance, **SB** – single-blind, **SC** – single-center, **U** – uncontrolled, **UP** – unpublished, **VC** – vehicle-controlled.

Depression (cont.)

Author/Year	Subject	Design	Duration	Dosage	Preparation	Results/Conclusion
Lenoir et al., 1999	Mild to moderate depression (ICD-10)	R, DB, PG, Cm, MC n =260 (over 20 years old)	6 weeks	1 tablet 3x/day (1 mg total hypericin/day or 33 mg total hypericin/day or 17 mg total hypericin/day)	Hyperiforce® tablets containing approximately 60 mg SJW extract (4–5:1) of shoot tips standardized to 0.33 mg total hypericin content/tablet (controls standardized to 0.11 mg or 0.055 mg total hypericin/tablet)	At the end of the treatment period, a reduction of about 50% in Hamilton Depression scores was observed in all groups. No significant differences between dosages. SJW was determined to be effective in all 3 doses and is well tolerated.
Laakmann et al., 1998a	Mild to moderate depression	R, DB, PC, MC, PG n=145 (mean age, 51 years placebo; 48.7 years W5573 group; 47.3 years SJW group)	7 weeks	900 mg/day (300 mg, 3x/day)	WS 5573 (0.5% hyperforin) or WS 5572 (5% hyperforin) or placebo	Study demonstrated relationship between hyperforin dose and antidepressant efficacy. 5% hyperforin SJW product enhanced patients' quality of life by producing appreciable relief from symptoms compared to 0.5% (p=0.017) and placebo (p=0.004). No statistical difference between 0.5% and placebo. Study suggests hyperforin is a therapeutically active constituent with antidepressant activity.
Wheatley, 1997	Mild to moderate depression (DSM-IV)	R, DB, PG, MC n=156 (HAMD score between 17–24, mean score SJW=20.6 amitriptylline=20.8) (ages 20–65 years)	6 weeks	900 mg/day SJW extract (300 mg, 3x/day) or amitriptyline (3x25 mg in a fixed dose manner)	LI 160 vs. amitriptyline	Comparable efficacy to amitriptyline with clear tolerability advantage. No statistically significant difference in response rate was shown between SJW and amitriptyline (p=0.064). In the CGI item "side-effects of drugs," greater tolerability for SJW was apparent (p<0.001 at week 2, p<0.05 at weeks 4 and 6).
Schrader et al., 1998	Mild to moderate depression	R, P, DB, PC, MC n=159	6 weeks	One, 250 mg tablets SJW extract 2x daily (1 mg hypericin daily)	Ze 117 SJW extract standardized to 0.5 mg hypericin/tablet	Of SJW patients, 56% were deemed responsive to treatment compared to 15% on placebo. There were few adverse effects: 5 placebo, 6 SJW (mostly minor gastrointestinal upsets in SJW group). Researchers noted that the good tolerability profile contributed to the high compliance of the SJW group.
Vorbach et al., 1994	Typical depression with single episode, recurrent episode, neurotic depression, and adjustment disorder with depressed mood (DSM-III-R).	R, DB, Cm, MC n=130 (mean HAMD score: 20.2 SJW group; 19.4 imipramine group) (ages 18–75 years)	6 weeks	900 mg/day SJW extract (300 mg, 3x/day) vs. imipramine (3x25mg daily)	LI 160 vs. imipramine	SJW showed equal effectiveness to and better tolerability than imipramine. Improved HAMD total score by 56% on SJW and 45% on imipramine. SJW caused less frequent and less severe side effects than imipramine.
Harrer et al., 1994	Depression (ICD-10)	R, DB, Cm, MC n=102 (HAMD score >16) (ages 25–65 years)	4 weeks	900 mg/day SJW extract (300 mg, 3x/day), maprotiline, (25 mg 3x/day)	LI 160 vs. maprotiline	Showed roughly equal efficacy to maprotiline. No significant difference between groups on HAMD, D-S, and CGI scores (HAMD score >16). 25% in SJW group and 35% in maprotiline group reported adverse drug effects.

KEY: **C** – controlled, **CC** – case-control, **CGI** – clinical global impression scale, **CGI-I** – clinical global improvement impression scale, **CGI-S** – clinical global severity impression scale, **CH** – cohort, **CI** – confidence interval, **Cm** – comparison, **CO** – crossover, **CS** - cross-sectional, **DB** – double-blind, **D-S** – von Zerssen depression severity scale, **DSM** – Diagnostic and Statistical Manual of Mental Disorders, **E** – epidemiological, **HAMA** – Hamilton Anxiety Scale, **HAMD** – Hamilton Depression Scale, **ICD** – International Classification of Disease, **LC** – longitudinal cohort, **MA** – meta-analysis, **MC** – multi-center, **n** – number of patients, **O** – open, **OB** – observational, **OL** – open label, **OR** – odds ratio, **P** – prospective, **PB** – patient-blind, **PC** – placebo-controlled, **PG** – parallel group, **PS** – pilot study, **R** – randomized, **RC** – reference-controlled, **RCS** – retrospective cross-sectional, **RS** - retrospective, **S** – surveillance, **SB** – single-blind, **SC** – single-center, **U** – uncontrolled, **UP** – unpublished, **VC** – vehicle-controlled.

Clinical Studies on St. John's wort (*Hypericum perforatum* L.) (cont.)

Depression (cont.)

Author/Year	Subject	Design	Duration	Dosage	Preparation	Results/Conclusion
Harrer and Sommer, 1994	Mild to moderate depression (ICD-9)	R, DB, PC, MC n=89 (HAMD score <20) (ages 20–64 years)	1 month	900 mg/day (300 mg, 3x/day)	LI 160 vs. placebo	Significantly (p<0.05) reduced depressive symptoms after 2 weeks and even further after 4 weeks (p<0.01) compared to placebo. No notable side effects were reported.
Hübner et al., 1994	Mild depression and somatic symptoms (ICD-09)	R, DB, PC n=39 (Mean HAMD score 12.55 SJW group, 12.37 placebo group) (ages 20–64 years)	4 weeks	900 mg/day (300 mg, 3x/day)	LI 160 vs. placebo	Significant reduction in HAMD score in SJW group compared to placebo (p<0.01). Final score=7.17. Significant reduction in falling asleep compared to placebo (p<0.01). Benefited patients with good tolerability and high compliance (p<0.05). By week 4, 5% statistical difference level in HAMD between placebo and SJW groups. No adverse effects reported.
Hänsgen et al., 1994	Major depression and temporary depressive neurosis (DSM-III-R)	R, DB, PC, MC n=72 (HAMD score >16) (ages 18–70 years)	6 weeks	900 mg/day (300 mg, 3x/day)	LI 160 vs. placebo	Significantly improved all 4 psychometric tests vs. placebo, with no serious side effects reported: Hamilton depression scale (p<0.001), depression scale of von Zerssen (p<0.001), complaint inventory, Clinical Global Impression Scale.

Fatigue and Seasonal Affective Disorder

Author/Year	Subject	Design	Duration	Dosage	Preparation	Results/Conclusion
Stevinson et al., 1998	Fatigue	O, U, pilot n=20 (mean age, 44.4 years)	6 weeks	900 mcg/day hypericin (300 mcg 3x/day)	Kira®	Significantly lowered perceived fatigue after 2 weeks (p<0.05) and reduced significantly more after 6 weeks (p<0.01). Significantly (p<0.05) reduced mean scores of depression and anxiety.
Martinez et al., 1994	Seasonal affective disorder (SAD) (DSM-III-R) HAMD scale>16	R, SB n=20 (ages 29–63 years)	4 weeks	900 mg/day (300 mg, 3x/day)	LI 160 with bright light (3000 lux) vs. LI 160 with dim light (<300 lux)	Significant improvement in symptoms over time with SJW and bright light (p=0.001). No adverse drug reactions reported.

Other

Author/Year	Subject	Design	Duration	Dosage	Preparation	Results/Conclusion
Shüle et al, 2001	Effect of SJW on cortisol, growth hormone, and prolactin	R, PC, CO n=12 healthy males between 20 and 35 years old	5 hours	300 mg WS 5570, 600 mg WS 5570, or placebo	WS 5570 SJW extract or placebo	No prolactin stimulation was observed (p>0.05) in SJW or placebo. A small but statistically significant (p<0.05) increase in growth hormone occurred after 300 mg SJW. After 600 mg SJW, cortisol stimulation was clearly observed (p<0.05) from 30 to 90 minutes after application.
Schempp et al., 2001	Phototoxicity of SJW in treatment of depression (UV-B, UV-A, visible light, solar-simulated radiation)	R, P n=72	Single-dose or steady-state 7 days	Single dose: 6 or 12 coated tablets, 3x daily (containing 5400 or 10,800 mcg total hypericins). Steady-state trial: initial dose of 6 tablets (1800 mcg hypericins) followed by 3 x 1 tablets (2700 mcg) per day for 7 days	LI 160	No significant changes were observed (erythema and melanin index) in either the single or multiple doses administered, with the exception of a slight, (p=0.50) influence on UV-B-induced pigmentation. The authors concluded that this study did not indicate phototoxic potential in the oral administration of higher than therapeutic doses (2–4 times) of SJW for depression.

KEY: C – controlled, **CC** – case-control, **CGI** – clinical global impression scale, **CGI-I** – clinical global improvement impression scale, **CGI-S** – clinical global severity impression scale, **CH** – cohort, **CI** – confidence interval, **Cm** – comparison, **CO** – crossover, **CS** - cross-sectional, **DB** – double-blind, **D-S** – von Zerssen depression severity scale, **DSM** – Diagnostic and Statistical Manual of Mental Disorders, **E** – epidemiological, **HAMA** – Hamilton Anxiety Scale, **HAMD** – Hamilton Depression Scale, **ICD** – International Classification of Disease, **LC** – longitudinal cohort, **MA** – meta-analysis, **MC** – multi-center, **n** – number of patients, **O** – open, **OB** – observational, **OL** – open label, **OR** – odds ratio, **P** – prospective, **PB** – patient-blind, **PC** – placebo-controlled, **PG** – parallel group, **PS** – pilot study, **R** – randomized, **RC** – reference-controlled, **RCS** – retrospective cross-sectional, **RS** - retrospective, **S** – surveillance, **SB** – single-blind, **SC** – single-center, **U** – uncontrolled, **UP** – unpublished, **VC** – vehicle-controlled.

Other (cont.)

Author/Year	Subject	Design	Duration	Dosage	Preparation	Results/Conclusion
Burnstein et al., 2000	SJW effects on steady state carbamazepine and carbamazepine-10,11-epoxide pharmacokinetics	U n=8	21 days	100 mg 2x/day for 3 days, then 200 mg, 2x/day for 3 days, then 400 mg 1x/day for 14 days; then 300 mg SJW with carbamazepine, 3x/day for 14 days	St. John's wort (0.3% standardized tablet) or carbamazepine (brand not stated)	The study concluded that SJW did not increase clearance of carbamazepine.
Taylor and Kobak, 2000	Obsessive-compulsive disorder (OCD)	O n=12 patients with 12 months diagnosis of OCD (DSM-IV)	12 weeks	450 mg SJW extract, 2x/day	450 mg SJW extract standardized to 0.3% hypericin (brand not stated)	Significant change from baseline, with mean change in Yale-Brown Obsessive-Compulsive Scale of 7.4 points (p=0.01). At end of trial, 5 patients were rated much or very much improved on clinician CGI, 6 were minimally improved, and 1 had no change. Side effects included diarrhea (3 subjects) and restless sleep (2 subjects). Improvements noted in first week. Results warrant placebo-controlled study of SJW for OCD.
Grube et al., 1999	Menopausal symptoms	O Drug monitoring study n=106 women 43–65 years old with symptoms characteristic of pre- and post-menopause	12 weeks	One, 300 mg tablet, 3x/day	Kira®	Self-assessment by Menopause Rating Scale for assessing sexuality and CGI. Psychological, psychosomatic, and vasomotor symptoms recorded at baseline, 5, 8, and 12 weeks. Significant improvement in psychological and psychosomatic symptoms. Menopausal symptoms reduced or disappeared in majority (76.4% by patient assessment; 79.2% by physician assessment). About 80% of women considered sexuality was improved with SJW
Czekalla et al., 1997	Electrocardiogram effects in patients with depression	R, DB, Cm, MC n=209	6 weeks	1,800 mg/day or 150 mg/ day imipramine	Jarsin® 300 vs. imipramine	SJW did not delay conduction through the atria or depolarization and repolarization in the ventricles. Imipramine increased heart rate and can cause pathological repolarization. High-dose SJW extract (i.e., 2x normal daily dose) produced fewer cardiac conduction defects than tricyclic antidepressants for treating elderly patients or patients with a pre-existing conductive dysfunction, and should be considered safer than tricyclic antidepressants, especially in patients with pre-existing conduction disorders.

KEY: **C** – controlled, **CC** – case-control, **CGI** – clinical global impression scale, **CGI-I** – clinical global improvement impression scale, **CGI-S** – clinical global severity impression scale, **CH** – cohort, **CI** – confidence interval, **Cm** – comparison, **CO** – crossover, **CS** - cross-sectional, **DB** – double-blind, **D-S** – von Zerssen depression severity scale, **DSM** – Diagnostic and Statistical Manual of Mental Disorders, **E** – epidemiological, **HAMA** – Hamilton Anxiety Scale, **HAMD** – Hamilton Depression Scale, **ICD** – International Classification of Disease, **LC** – longitudinal cohort, **MA** – meta-analysis, **MC** – multi-center, n – number of patients, **O** – open, **OB** – observational, **OL** – open label, **OR** – odds ratio, **P** – prospective, **PB** – patient-blind, **PC** – placebo-controlled, **PG** – parallel group, **PS** – pilot study, **R** – randomized, **RC** – reference-controlled, **RCS** – retrospective cross-sectional, **RS** - retrospective, **S** – surveillance, **SB** – single-blind, **SC** – single-center, **U** – uncontrolled, **UP** – unpublished, **VC** – vehicle-controlled.

Tea, Black/Green

Camellia sinensis (L.) Kuntze (syn. C. *sinensis* L.)

[Fam. *Theaceae*]

OVERVIEW

The use of tea as a beverage in China dates back to 2700 B.C.E. Next to water, tea is the most widely consumed beverage in the world. In addition, it is used widely in the traditional medicine systems of China, Hong Kong, Japan, and Korea. Green tea and black tea, although derived from the leaves of the same plant, have different concentrations of the active constituents. The immediate processing of harvested leaves used for green tea limits enzymatic changes, whereas leaves used for black tea are fermented before preparation, triggering the enzymatic process. Thus, green tea contains higher concentrations of the active catechin constituents compared to black tea. According to the United Nations Food and Agriculture Organization, scientific evidence increasingly shows that both black and green tea can contribute significantly to a healthy lifestyle.

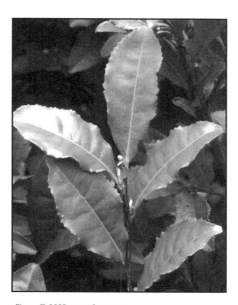

Photo © 2003 stevenfoster.com

PRIMARY USES

Cardiovascular

- Reduced risk of atherosclerosis
- Reduced risk of cardiovascular disease
- Reduced risk of myocardial infarction
- Modulation of plasma antioxidant capacity
- Decreased serum lipid concentration

OTHER POTENTIAL USES

Oncology

- Prevention of colon cancer
- Reduced incidence of oral mucosal leukoplakia
- Decreased recurrence of Stage I and II breast cancer
- Reduced risk and incidence of pancreatic cancer
- Reduced risk and incidence of squamous cell lung cancer
- Reduced risk and incidence of esophageal cancer

Miscellaneous

- Symptomatic treatment of mild diarrhea
- Reduced risk of osteoporosis
- Promotes diuresis

- Digestive aid
- Dysuria; edema
- Weight loss
- Functional asthenia
- CNS stimulant
- Headache

PHARMACOLOGICAL ACTIONS

BLACK TEA: Protects against ischemic heart disease.

GREEN TEA: Increases plasma antioxidant capacity; decreases serum concentrations of total cholesterol, triglyceride and atherogenic index; inhibits endogenous formation of nitrosoproline. *Standardized Preparations:* Activate thermogenesis and fat oxidation.

BLACK AND GREEN TEA: Increase plasma antioxidant capacity; inhibit endogenous formation of nitrosoproline.

DOSAGE AND ADMINISTRATION

Clinical studies reveal that the regular long-term daily ingestion of tea is safe and contributes significantly to the prevention of some serious diseases.

GREEN TEA INFUSION: 150–250 ml boiling water poured over 1.0–2.5 g finely cut dried leaf, steeped 3–5 min. for use as a stimulant (alkaloids extract rapidly). Steeped at least 10 min. for use in treatment of diarrhea (catechins take longer to extract). Drunk several times daily. Tea should be steeped for 15–20 min. in order to maximize the yield of catechins, though this will make the tea taste bitter. At least 1 cup drunk daily for antioxidant effect.

GREEN TEA POWDER: 8 capsules (250 mg each) daily with meals to treat obesity.

BLACK TEA INFUSION: 150–250 ml boiling water poured over 2.5 g finely cut dried leaf, steeped 2–5 min. for use as a stimulant (alkaloids extract rapidly). Steeped at least 10 min. for use in treatment of diarrhea (catechins take longer to extract), 2–3 times daily. Drunk 3–4 times daily for protection against atherosclerosis; 1 or more times daily to reduce risk of myocardial infarction.

DRY ETHANOLIC GREEN TEA EXTRACT: two, 250 mg capsules, 3 times daily with meals for weight control [standardized to 25% catechins].

The ABC Clinical Guide to Herbs | 335

NOTE: Stimulant action of tea is strongest when allowed to steep for only 2–5 min. as caffeine dissolves quickly in hot water. Longer steeping times (10–20 min.) will increase the yield of catechins, which decreases the stimulant effect because the polyphenols bind the caffeine. Catechins from black and green tea are rapidly absorbed and milk does not impair their bioavailability, despite earlier studies reporting that adding milk results in the complexation of tea polyphenols by milk proteins, thereby completely inhibiting their antioxidant effects.

CONTRAINDICATIONS

There are a few contraindications known. Individuals with weakened cardiovascular systems, renal diseases, thyroid hyperfunction, elevated susceptibility to spasm, and certain psychic disorders (eg., panicky states of anxiety) should use tea with caution.

PREGNANCY AND LACTATION: No known restrictions during pregnancy or lactation. One reference recommends that pregnant women should not ingest more than 5 cups daily (approximately 300 mg caffeine daily). Tea ingestion while nursing may cause sleep disorders in infants.

ADVERSE EFFECTS

The side effects of tea and other nervous system stimulants may include nervousness, anxiety, heart irregularities, headaches, tremors, hypertension, restlessness, insomnia, daytime irritability, irritation of the gastric mucosa, and diuresis. These effects are generally for relatively high dosages and are not associated with the ingestion of reasonable amounts of tea (e.g., 1–10 cups per day).

DRUG INTERACTIONS

Xanthine (e.g., caffeine, theophylline) derivatives from black tea can diminish the effects of coronary vasodilator drugs such as dipyridamole and should not be taken concurrently. Green tea has possible synergistic effects when taken in combination with sulindac and/or tamoxifen and may reduce their adverse effects. Green tea is a source of vitamin K and one case report suggested probable antagonism of warfarin by green tea. Herbs high in tannins may impair the absorption of theophylline, a bronchodilator drug used to treat people with asthma. Tannins in tea can also interfere with intestinal absorption of nutrients and vitamins. In infants, tannins can bind iron and reduce its absorption contributing to the development of microcytic anemia. Resorption of alkaline medications can be delayed due to chemical bonding with tea tannins. Large amounts of caffeine may increase activity and the side effects of theophylline. Limiting the intake of caffeine-containing beverages to small amounts will prevent this potential interaction, as well as those associated with numerous other drugs that are affected by caffeine consumption.

CLINICAL REVIEW

Of 29 selected clinical studies on tea leaf that included a total of 68,242 subjects, all but three demonstrated positive effects for indications including cardiovascular health, cancer, osteoporosis, obesity, and bowel conditions. Most of the studies were large-population epidemiological studies on the influence of black and/or green tea consumption on disease prevention. They include 15 cardiovascular studies investigating a range of potential applications, including two crossover studies on plasma antioxidant activity, a randomized, placebo-controlled (R, PC) study on energy expenditure and fat oxidation, a PC study on the protective effect of tea against ischemic heart disease, a multi-center, case-controlled study on the protective effect of tea against myocardial infarction, and studies on its effects on serum lipid concentrations and resistance of LDL to oxidation. At least 13 large-population, case-control cancer studies have been published. Five recent case-control cancer studies evaluated the consumption of tea and its protective effect against development of pancreatic and colorectal cancer, stomach cancer, lung cancer, esophageal cancer, and various other cancers. Other studies investigated the use of tea in protecting against osteoporosis in older women and its effect on fecal flora in nursing home residents. One DB, PC study investigated its use in the treatment of severe obesity.

Tea, Black/Green

Camellia sinensis (L.) Kuntze (syn. *C. sinensis* L.)
[Fam. *Theaceae*]

OVERVIEW

The use of tea as a beverage in China dates back to 2700 B.C.E. Currently, it is widely used in the traditional medical systems of China, Hong Kong, Japan, and Korea. Next to water, tea is the most widely consumed beverage in the world today. Green and black tea, though from the same plant, are processed differently and contain varying strengths of chemical compounds.

USES

To reduce risk of atherosclerosis, cardiovascular disease, and myocardial infarction; in cases of elevated cholesterol (to help lower); possible prevention of certain cancers (breast, pancreatic, colon, lung, and esophageal); mild stimulant; possible aid in weight loss; diuretic action; possible reduced risk of osteoporosis.

DOSAGE

GREEN TEA INFUSION (TEA): Pour 150–250 ml boiling water over 1.0–2.5 g finely cut dried leaf, steep 3–5 minutes for use as a stimulant. Steep 15–20 minutes and drink several times daily for diarrhea. Drink at least 1 cup daily for antioxidant effect.

GREEN TEA POWDER: 8 capsules (250 mg each) daily with meals to help treat obesity.

BLACK TEA INFUSION (TEA): Pour 150–250 ml boiling water over 2.5 g finely cut dried leaf, steep 2–5 minutes for use as a stimulant (alkaloids extract rapidly). Steep at least 10 minutes for use in treatment of diarrhea (catehcins take longer to extract), 2–3 times daily. Drink 3–4 times daily for protection against atherosclerosis, 1 or more times daily to reduce risk of myocardial infarction (heart attack).

DRY ALCOHOLIC GREEN TEA EXTRACT: 2 capsules (250 mg each), 3 times daily with meals for weight control [standardized to 25% catechins].

CONTRAINDICATIONS

Use with caution in weakened cardiovascular systems, kidney diseases, thyroid hyperfunction (hyperthyroid), increased susceptibility to muscle spasm, and panicky states of anxiety.

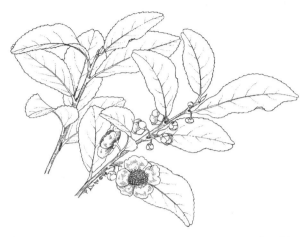

PREGNANCY AND LACTATION: Pregnant women should not ingest more than 5 cups daily (300 mg caffeine daily). Drinking tea while nursing may cause sleep disorders in infants.

ADVERSE EFFECTS

Nervousness, anxiety, heart irregularities, headaches, tremors, hypertension, restlessness, insomnia, daytime irritability, irritation of the stomach lining, and increased urination are possible adverse effects that can occur with use/overuse of central nervous system stimulants like the caffeine found in tea. However, these effects rarely occur with use of normal amounts.

DRUG INTERACTIONS

Compounds in black tea may reduce the effects of coronary vasodilator drugs, such as dipyridamole, if taken simultaneously. Green tea has possible synergistic effects when combined with sulindac and/or tamoxifen and may reduce their adverse effects. Green tea may also interact with drugs such as the blood-thinning drug warfarin (reducing its effects), and large amounts of caffeine may increase activity and side effects of the asthma drug theophylline. Tannins in tea can also interfere with intestinal absorption of nutrients and vitamins, and may lead to microcytic anemia in children.

Comments

When using a dietary supplement, purchase it from a reliable source. For best results, use the same brand of product throughout the period of use. As with all medications and dietary supplements, please inform your healthcare provider of all herbs and medications you are taking. Interactions may occur between medications and herbs or even among different herbs when taken at the same time. Treat your herbal supplement with care by taking it as directed, storing it as advised on the label, and keeping it out of the reach of children and pets. Consult your healthcare provider with any questions.

AMERICAN BOTANICAL COUNCIL

Tea, Black/Green

Camellia sinensis (L.) Kuntze (syn. *C. sinensis* L.)

[Fam. *Theaceae*]

OVERVIEW

The use of tea as a beverage in China dates back to at least 2700 B.C.E. (Huang, 1999). Tea continues to be used in the traditional medicine systems of China, Hong Kong, Japan, and Korea (But *et al.*, 1997). Next to water, tea is the most widely consumed beverage in the world (Bushman, 1998; Graham, 1992). International tea production is projected to increase from the 1993–95 average of 1.97 million tons to 2.7 million (UN FAO, 1999). In 1999, the U.S. imported 16,961,460 pounds of green tea, 187,765,660 pounds of black tea, and 7,777,542 pounds of instant tea (USDA, 2000). According to the United Nations Food and Agriculture Organization, there is an increasing body of scientific evidence that both green and black tea can contribute significantly to a healthy lifestyle, and their regular use should be promoted internationally (UN FAO, 1999). Most of the scientific evidence focuses on the cardiovascular and potentially cancer-preventive activity of tea polyphenols and other tea compounds (Gutman and Ryu, 1996; Dufresne and Farnworth, 2001).

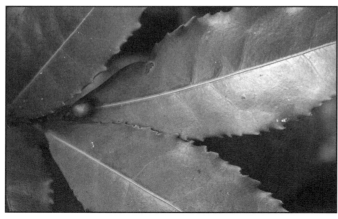

Photo © 2003 stevenfoster.com

DESCRIPTION

Green tea and black tea, although they are derived from the leaves of the same plant *Camellia sinensis* (L.) Kuntz [Fam. *Theaceae*], have different concentrations of active constituents. The immediate processing of harvested leaves used for green tea limits enzymatic changes, whereas leaves used for black tea are fermented before preparation, which triggers the enzymatic process. Thus, green tea contains higher concentrations of the active constituents, catechins, compared to black tea.

Green tea is the young leaf of *C. sinensis* and its cultivated varieties. It is unfermented and subjected to rapid desiccation with applied heat. It contains no less than 2% caffeine (Bruneton, 1999; Ph.Fr.X, 1982–96). It must contain not less than 33% water-soluble extractive on a dry basis, and no less than 4%, or more than 7%, total ash (Health Canada, 1997).

Black tea is the young leaf of *C. sinensis* and its cultivated varieties, fully fermented, and subjected to rapid desiccation with applied heat. It contains no less than 2.5% caffeine (Bruneton, 1999; Ph.Fr.X, 1982–96), and must contain no less than 25% water-soluble extractive on a dry basis (Health Canada, 1997).

The U.S. Department of Agriculture (USDA) evaluates flavor characteristics of prepared tea using Standard A-2 of the Tea Association of the United States (USDA, 1995). Uniform standards of tea purity, quality, and fitness for consumption are established by the U.S. Secretary of Health and Human Services in accordance with section 3 of the Tea Importation Act (USCS, 1995; 1998). The International Organization for Standardization (ISO) has published standard methods for the classification of grades of tea (ISO, 1997; Willson and Clifford, 1992).

PRIMARY USES

Cardiovascular

- Reduced risk of atherosclerosis (Geleijnse *et al.*, 1999)
- Reduced risk of cardiovascular disease (Imai and Nakachi, 1995; Stensvold *et al.*, 1992)
- Reduced risk of myocardial infarction (Sesso *et al.*, 1999; Hertog *et al.*, 1993, 1995; Hertog, 1994; Knekt *et al.*, 1996; Stensvold *et al.*, 1992)
- Modulation of plasma antioxidant capacity (Leenen *et al.*, 2000; van het Hof *et al.*, 1999; Princen *et al.*, 1998; Ishikawa *et al.*, 1997)
- Decreased serum lipid concentration (Kono *et al.*, 1992, 1996)

OTHER POTENTIAL USES

Oncology

- Prevention of colon cancer (August *et al.*, 1999; Ji *et al.*, 1997)
- Reduced incidence of oral mucosal leukoplakia (Li *et al.*, 1999)
- Decreased recurrence of Stage I and II breast cancer (Nakachi *et al.*, 1998)
- Reduced risk and incidence of pancreatic cancer (Ji *et al.*, 1997)
- Reduced risk and incidence of squamous cell lung cancer (Ohno *et al.*, 1995)
- Reduced risk and incidence of esophageal cancer (Gao *et al.*, 1994)

Miscellaneous

- Symptomatic treatment of mild diarrhea (Bruneton, 1999; But *et al.*, 1997; Meyer-Buchtela, 1999)
- Reduced risk of osteoporosis (Hegarty *et al.*, 2000)
- Promotes diuresis (Bruneton, 1999; Shih-Chen, 1973)

- Digestive aid (Shih-Chen, 1973)
- Dysuria; edema (But *et al.*, 1997)
- Weight loss (Bruneton, 1999; Wichtl and Bisset, 1994)
- Functional asthenia (Bruneton, 1999)
- CNS stimulant (Leung and Foster, 1996; Meyer-Buchtela, 1999)
- Headache (But *et al.*, 1997; Leung and Foster, 1996)

DOSAGE
Internal
Crude Preparations
GREEN TEA INFUSION: 150–250 ml boiling water is poured over 1.0–2.5 g fine cut dried leaf, and steeped 3–5 minutes for use as a stimulant (alkaloids extract rapidly). Steeped at least 10 minutes for use in treatment of diarrhea (catechins take longer to extract). Drunk several times daily (Meyer-Buchtela, 1999). Tea should be steeped for 15–20 minutes to maximize the yield of catechins, though this will make the tea taste bitter (Schulz *et al.*, 1998). At least 1 cup daily for antioxidant effect (Leenen *et al.*, 2000).

GREEN TEA POWDER: 8 capsules (250 mg each) are taken daily, with meals, to treat obesity (Lecomte, 1985).

BLACK TEA INFUSION: 150–250 ml boiling water is poured over 2.5 g fine cut, dried leaf, and steeped 2–5 minutes for use as a stimulant (alkaloids extract rapidly). Steeped at least 10 minutes to treat diarrhea (catechins take longer to extract), 2–3 times daily (Meyer-Buchtela, 1999; Wichtl and Bisset, 1994). Drunk 3–4 times daily for protection against atherosclerosis (Geleijnse *et al.*, 1999), 1 or more times daily to reduce risk of myocardial infarction (Sesso *et al.*, 1999).

Standardized Preparations
DRY ETHANOLIC GREEN TEA EXTRACT: 25% catechins, 2 capsules (250 mg each), 3 times daily with meals for weight control (Dulloo *et al.,* 1999).

NOTE: Stimulant action of tea is strongest when allowed to steep for 2–5 minutes as caffeine dissolves quickly in hot water. Longer steeping (10–20 minutes) increases the catechin yield, and decreases the stimulant effect because the polyphenols bind the caffeine (Wichtl and Bisset, 1994). Green and black tea catechins are rapidly absorbed, and milk does not impair their bioavailability (Hollman *et al.*, 2001; Leenen *et al.,* 2000; van het Hof *et al.*, 1998). Earlier studies reported that adding milk results in complexation of tea polyphenols by milk proteins, completely inhibiting their antioxidant effects (Serafini *et al.*, 1996).

DURATION OF ADMINISTRATION
Internal
Most human studies conclude that the regular, long-term, daily use of tea is safe and contributes significantly to prevention (or at least some reduction of incidence) of some serious diseases.

CHEMISTRY
Green Tea
Green tea leaf contains 1–5% xanthine alkaloids (caffeine, theobromine, theophylline, xanthine) (Huang, 1999); 20–30% flavonols; 3–4% flavonols and flavone-glycosides; about 5% phenolic acids; 2–3% proanthocyanidins, 0.59–3.97% free amino acids; and minerals including significant amounts of aluminum, manganese, fluoride, and potassium (Meyer-Buchtela, 1999; Scholz and Bertram, 1995). Tea leaf polyphenols such as catechins, include (+)-catechin (C), (+)-gallocatechin (GC),

(–)-epicatechin (EC), (–)-epigallocatechin (EGC), (–)-epicatechin gallate (ECG), and (–)-epigallocatechin gallate (EGCG) (Miketova *et al.*, 1998). Components of prepared green tea infusion, measured in weight percentage of extracted solids include 30–42% catechins, 5–10% flavonols, 2–4% other flavonoids, 7–9% xanthine alkaloids, 6–8% minerals, 4–6% amino acids, 4–6% organic acids, and 1–2% ascorbic acid (Graham, 1992).

Black Tea
Black tea leaf contains polyphenols, such as catechins EGC, EC, EGCG, ECG (Bronner and Beecher, 1998); xanthine alkaloids (2.6–3.5% caffeine, 0.16–0.2% theobromine, 0.02–0.04% theophylline); 1–3% flavanols; 2–3% flavonols and flavone-glycosides; 2–4% phenolic acids; about 2% theaflavine; 6–30% thearubigins; 0.66–2.82% free amino acids; and minerals including significant amounts of aluminum, manganese, fluoride, and potassium (Meyer-Buchtela, 1999; Scholz and Bertram, 1995). After fermentation from green tea to black tea, about 15% of the catechins remain unchanged and the rest convert into theaflavines and thearubigins. The components of prepared black tea infusion measured in weight % of extracted solids include 3–10% catechins, 12–18% thearubigins, 3–6% theaflavines, 6–8% flavonols, 10–12% phenolic acids and depsides, 8–11% xanthine alkaloids, 13–15% amino acids, and about 10% minerals (Graham, 1992).

PHARMACOLOGICAL ACTIONS
Human
Crude Preparations
BLACK TEA: Protects against ischemic heart disease (Geleijnse *et al.*, 1999).

GREEN TEA: Increases plasma antioxidant capacity (Nakagawa *et al.*, 1999); decreases serum concentrations of total cholesterol, triglycerides, and atherogenic index (Imai and Nakachi, 1995); inhibits endogenous formation of nitrosoproline (Xu *et al.*, 1993).

BLACK AND GREEN TEA: Increase plasma antioxidant capacity (Leenen *et al.*, 2000); inhibit endogenous formation of nitrosoproline (Wang and Wu, 1991).

UNSPECIFIED: Inhibits alpha-amylase activity and lowers pH in digestive tract (Hara, 1997); inhibits endogenous formation of nitrosoproline (Stich, 1992).

Standardized Preparations
GREEN TEA: Activates thermogenesis and fat oxidation (Dulloo *et al.*, 1999).

UNSPECIFIED: Reduces fecal moisture, pH, ammonia, and sulfide, and potentially reduces oxidation (Goto *et al.*, 1999).

Animal
GREEN TEA: Inhibits angiogenesis (Cao and Cao, 1999); hypolipidemic (Chan *et al.*, 1999); inhibits unwanted fecal microbes (Isogai *et al.*, 1998); inhibits activity of nitrosamines, polycyclic aromatic hydrocarbons, and heterocyclic amines (Bu-Abbas *et al.*, 1994, 1995); inhibits the formation and growth of solid tumors (Hirose *et al.*, 1994; Mukhtar *et al.*, 1994; Yin *et al.,* 1994); increases the activity of antioxidant and detoxifying enzymes (glutathione reductase, glutathione peroxidase, glutathione S-transferase (GST), catalase, and quinone reductase) in lungs, liver, and small intestine (Khan *et al.*, 1992); has an antimutagenic effect on compounds that induce gastrointestinal epithelial cancers (Yamane *et al.*, 1991); lowers cholesterol (Muramatsu *et al.*, 1986; Yamaguchi *et al.* 1991).

BLACK AND GREEN TEA: Extracts of both green and black tea exhibit cancer chemopreventive action (Heber *et al.*, 1999); are anti-mutagenic and inhibit colon carcinogenesis (Hernaez *et al.*, 1998); inhibit activity of nitrosamines, polycyclic aromatic hydrocarbons, and heterocyclic amines (Weisburger *et al.*, 1994); inhibit formation and growth of solid tumors (Wang *et al.*, 1994).

UNSPECIFIED: Inhibits unwanted fecal microbes (Toda *et al.*, 1991). Green tea, but not its isolated catechins, has growth-promoting effects on mammary gland development (Sayama *et al.*, 1996); lowers cholesterol (Chisaka *et al.*, 1988).

In vitro
GREEN TEA: Inhibits enzyme urokinase (Jankun *et al.*, 1997); is antioxidant (Frankel, 1997); inhibits low density lipoprotein (LDL) cholesterol oxidation (Luo *et al.*, 1997); has inhibitory effect on growth of mammary cancer cell lines by inhibiting interaction of estrogen with its receptors (Komori *et al.*, 1993).

UNSPECIFIED: Exhibits radical-scavenging activity (Nanjo *et al.*, 1999); inhibits growth of human lung cancer cell line (Fujiki *et al.*, 1998); is antioxidant (Plumb *et al.*, 1999); inhibits enzyme catechol-*O*-methyl-transferase (COMT) (Borchardt and Huber, 1975).

MECHANISM OF ACTION
Anti-carcinogenesis
- Tea catechins are absorbed through the oral mucosa, which may assist in preventing oral and esophageal cancers. Levels of EGCG are higher in saliva than in blood after ingestion of a single cup of tea. Drinking tea slowly delivers high concentrations of catechins to the oral cavity and then the esophagus, whereas tea extract in solid dosage forms results in no detectable salivary catechin level (Yang *et al.*, 1999).
- Evidence (*in vitro*) suggests that the synergy of total catechins in whole green tea leaf infusion is more effective as a cancer preventive than isolated EGCG (Suganuma *et al.*, 1999).
- The mechanism of green tea's anti-carcinogenic effects against digestive tract cancers is unclear (Cao and Cao, 1999; Ji *et al.*, 1997).
- Green and black teas inhibit human carcinogens possibly due to antioxidative and antiproliferative effects of polyphenolic fraction (Katiyar, 1992; Yang and Wang, 1993).
- Polyphenols may inhibit carcinogenesis by blocking endogenous formation of nitrosamines, polycyclic aromatic hydrocarbons, and heterocyclic amines (Bu-Abbas *et al.*, 1994, 1995; Weisburger *et al.*, 1994).
- Green and black tea have comparable antioxidant effects that may diminish the formation of oxidized metabolites of DNA, with an associated lower risk of cancers (Weisburger, 1999).
- Green tea may alter gut flora. Its effects on reduction of dysbiosis suggest a mechanism for prevention of colon cancer (Yarnell, 1999).
- Tea catechins inhibit alpha-amylase activity in the small intestine, and some are absorbed into the portal vein. By lowering the pH in the digestive tract, tea catechins decrease putrefactive products and increase organic acids (Hara, 1997).

Antioxidant
- Green and black tea have comparable antioxidant effects that may play a role in lowering the oxidation of LDL cholesterol, with a consequent decreased risk of heart disease (Weisburger, 1999).
- Flavonoids in green or black tea may reduce the risk of myocardial infarction by inhibiting the oxidation of LDL cholesterol (Rimm *et al.*, 1996; van het Hof *et al.*, 1999), reducing platelet aggregation (Ho *et al.*, 1992), or reducing ischemic damage (Laughton *et al.*, 1991).
- Green tea contributes to the prevention of cardiovascular disease by increasing the antioxidant capacity of plasma (Nakagawa *et al.*, 1999).
- Proposed mechanisms of tea flavonoid antioxidant activity include its hydrogen-donating ability, delocalization of electrons, and metal ion chelation. Tea beverage has greater *in vitro* antioxidant capacity than most fruits and vegetables per serving and is more potent than vitamins C and E and the carotenoids. Tea and its flavonoids protect LDL cholesterol from oxidation following co-incubation *in vitro* (Najemnik *et al.*, 1999).

Central nervous system stimulant
- Tea contains water-soluble xanthine alkaloids such as caffeine, which stimulate the central nervous system and adrenal glands, increasing synthesis and release of specific neurotransmitters and hormones. Caffeine increases secretion of the neurotransmitter norepinephrine and the adrenal hormone epinephrine, while blocking central adenosine receptors (Gawin, 1988; Gilman *et al.*, 1985).

Thermogenesis
- By inhibiting catechol *O*-methyltransferase (COMT), the enzyme that degrades norepinephrine, tea catechins prolong the life of norepinephrine in the synaptic cleft, while tea alkaloids inhibit phosphodiesterases, which prolongs the life of cAMP in the cell, resulting in an increased, and more sustained effect, of norepinephrine on thermogenesis (Dulloo *et al.*, 1999).
- Epigallocatechin gallate (EGCG) can attenuate peroxide production in glial cells by either inhibiting the deamination of monoamines or acting as a free radical scavenger, thereby reducing oxidative neuronal damage associated with various neurodegenerative diseases (Mazzio, 1998).

CONTRAINDICATIONS
None known (Meyer-Buchtela, 1999). Persons with weakened cardiovascular systems, renal diseases, thyroid hyperfunction, elevated susceptibility to spasm, and certain psychic disorders (e.g., panicky states of anxiety) should use tea with caution (Fleming *et al.*, 2000).

PREGNANCY AND LACTATION: No known restrictions during pregnancy or lactation (McGuffin *et al.*, 1997), though pregnant women should typically not ingest more than five cups daily (about 300 mg caffeine daily) and ingestion of tea while nursing may cause sleep disorders in some infants (Fleming *et al.*, 2000).

ADVERSE EFFECTS
Side effects of nervous system stimulants may include nervousness, anxiety, heart irregularities, headaches, tremors, hypertension, restlessness, insomnia, daytime irritability, irritation of the gastric mucosa, and diuresis (McGuffin *et al.*, 1997).

These effects are generally for high dosages of caffeine-containing herbs and are not associated with the ingestion of reasonable amounts of tea (e.g., 1–10 cups per day).

DRUG INTERACTIONS

Xanthine (e.g., caffeine, theophylline) derivatives from black tea can diminish effects of coronary vasodilator drugs such as dipyridamole and should not be taken concurrently (Morant and Ruppanner, 2001). Green tea has a possible synergistic effect when taken with sulindac and/or tamoxifen and may reduce their adverse effects (Suganuma et al., 1999). Green tea is a source of vitamin K; one case report suggests that green tea is a probable antagonist of warfarin (Taylor and Wilt, 1999). Herbs high in tannins may impair absorption of theophylline, a bronchodilator drug used to treat asthmatics (Austin, 1999; Brinker, 2001). Tea tannins can also interfere with intestinal absorption of nutrients and vitamins (Huang, 1999). In infants, tannins can bind iron and reduce its absorption, contributing to the development of microcytic anemia (Merhav, 1985). Resorption of alkaline medications can be delayed due to chemical bonding with tea tannins (Fleming et al., 2000). In vitro, black tea constituents can cause precipitation of amitriptyline, fluphenazine, haloperidol, and Imipramine (Lasswell et al., 1984; Kulhanek, 1981). Large amounts of caffeine may increase activity and side effects of theophylline. Limiting intake of caffeine-containing beverages to small amounts will avoid this potential interaction (Austin, 1999; Threlkeld, 1991), and those associated with numerous other drugs affected by caffeine consumption (Brinker, 2001).

AMERICAN HERBAL PRODUCTS ASSOCIATION (AHPA) SAFETY RATING

CLASS 2D: Black teas are not recommended for excessive or long-term use (McGuffin et al., 1997). (EDITORS' NOTE: It is unclear why AHPA has given a Class 2d safety rating to black tea and not to green tea. Both black and green tea are, in fact, recommended for long-term use for health benefits.)

REGULATORY STATUS

BELGIUM: Permitted as a traditional herbal diuretic (De Smet et al., 1993).

CANADA: Food (Health Canada, 1997). Substantiated health claims will be permitted with premarket authorization after Natural Health Product (NHP) regulations become final in 2001 or 2002.

FRANCE: Traditional Herbal Medicine listed in Annex I of the 1998 French Explanatory Note with four approved oral use indications and two topical use indications. Green and black tea are official in the French Pharmacopoeia, Ph.Fr. X (Bruneton, 1999).

GERMANY: Food. Not reviewed by the German Commission E. No monograph in the German Pharmacopoeia.

ITALY: Food.

SWEDEN: Classified as a foodstuff and natural product (De Smet et al., 1993). No products containing tea leaf are presently registered in the Medical Products Agency's (MPA) "Authorized Natural Remedies," "Homeopathic Remedies" or "Drugs" listings (MPA, 2001).

SWITZERLAND: One multiple-ingredient digestive aid instant tea (Drosana® Verdauungs und Magentee) containing tea leaf dry extract is listed in the Swiss Codex 2000/01 (Ruppanner and Schaefer, 2000). No monograph in the Swiss Pharmacopoeia.

U.K.: Food. Not entered in the General Sale List (GSL). No monograph in the British Pharmacopoeia.

U.S.: Generally Recognized as Safe (GRAS) (US FDA, 1998). Dietary supplement or food depending on label claim statement (USC, 1994). No monograph in the USP-NF.

CLINICAL REVIEW

Twenty-nine studies are outlined in the following table, "Clinical Studies on Tea Leaf," including a total of 68,242 subjects. All but three of these studies (Princen et al., 1998; Nakachi et al., 1998; Hartman et al., 1998) demonstrated positive effects for indications in the areas of cardiovascular health, cancer, osteoporosis, obesity, and bowel conditions. Most of the studies are large-population epidemiological studies on the influence of black and/or green tea consumption on disease prevention. The table includes 15 cardiovascular studies investigating a range of potential applications, including two cross-over studies on plasma antioxidant activity (Leenen et al., 2000; van het Hof et al., 1999); a randomized, placebo-controlled (R, PC) study on energy expenditure and fat oxidation (Dulloo et al., 1999); a PC study on tea's protective effect against ischemic heart disease (Geleijnse et al., 1999); a multi-center, case-controlled (MC, CC) study on tea's protective effect against myocardial infarction (Sesso et al., 1999); and tea's effects on serum lipid concentrations and resistance of LDL cholesterol to oxidation (Ishikawa et al., 1997; Kono et al., 1992, 1996; van het Hof et al., 1997). At least 13 large-population, CC cancer studies have been published. Five recent CC cancer studies listed in the table evaluated the consumption of tea and its protective effect against development of pancreatic and colorectal cancers (Ji et al., 1997); various cancers (Imai et al., 1997); stomach cancer (Yu et al., 1995); lung cancer (Ohno et al., 1995); and esophageal cancer (Gao et al., 1994). Other studies investigated tea's use in protecting older women against osteoporosis (Hegerty et al., 2000), and tea's effect on fecal flora in nursing home residents (Goto et al., 1998, 1999). One DB, PC study investigated tea's use in the treatment of severe obesity and found significant weight loss after 30 days (Lecomte, 1985). A recent meta-analysis examined the effect of tea on stroke, myocardial infarction, and all coronary heart disease. The estimated effects of tea on stroke and coronary heart disease were too heterogeneous to assess. The study found an estimated 11% decrease in the incidence rate of myocardial infarction (fixed-effects relative risk estimate = 0.89, 95% confidence interval: 0.79, 1.01).

BRANDED PRODUCTS

Arkocaps/Phytotrim®: Arkopharma Laboratories / BP 28-06511 / Carros Cedex / France / Tel: +33-49-32-91-128 / Email: info@arkopharma.com. Capsules contain 250 mg powdered green tea leaf.

Exolise®: Arkopharma Laboratories. Capsules contain 250 mg alcoholic green tea leaf dry extract standardized to 25% (250 mg/g) total catechins and 10% (100 mg/g) caffeine.

Lipton "Brisk" Tea® (black tea): Unilever Bestfoods North America / 800 Sylvan Ave. / Englewood Cliffs, NJ 07632 / U.S.A. / Tel: (800) 697-7887 / (888) LIPTON-T / Email: letters.liptontusa@unilever.com / www.liptont.com. 2.21 g tea leaf per single serve bag providing 46.9 mg total catechins (8.6 mg epicatechin, 14.2 mg epicatechin gallate, 7.0 mg epigallocatechin, 17.1 mg epigallocatechin gallate), 11.9 mg total theafavines, 10.7 mg flavonols, 151.2 mg thearubigins and 220.7 mg total polyphenols.

Lipton® Green Tea: Unilever Bestfoods North America. 2.27 g tea leaf per single serve bag providing 186.3 mg total catechins (26.7 mg epicatechin, 30.3 mg epicatechin gallate, 50.6 mg epigallocatechin, 78.7 mg epigallocatechin gallate), 0.2 mg total theafavines, 12.0 mg flavonols, and 198.5 mg total polyphenols.

Twinings® Darjeeling Tea (black): Twinings London / 216 The Strand / London / U.K. / www.twinings.com. Each dose of 2.2 g leaf provides 7.6 mg epicatechin, 20.2 mg epigallocatechin, 43 mg epigallocatechin gallate, 2.2 mg theaflavin, 1.4 mg theaflavin monogallate, and 0.8 mg theaflavin digallate.

REFERENCES

August D, Landau J, Caputo D, et al. Ingestion of green tea rapidly decreases prostaglandin E2 levels in rectal mucosa in humans. *Cancer Epidemiol Biomarkers Prev* 1999;8(8):709–13.

Austin S. Common drugs and their potential interactions with herbs or nutrients. *Healthnotes Rev Comp Integr Med* 1999;6(3):221.

Borchardt R, Huber J. Catechol-*O*-methyltransferase: structure activity relationships for inhibition by flavonoids. *J Med Chem* 1975;18:120–2.

Brinker, F. Interactions of pharmaceutical and botanical medicines. *J Naturopathic Med* 1997;7(2):14–20.

Brinker F. *Herb Contraindications and Drug Interactions*, 3rd edition. Sandy, OR: Eclectic Medical Publications; 2001;187-190.

Bronner W, Beecher G. Method for determining the content of catechins in tea infusions by high-performance liquid chromatography. *J Chromatog* 1998;805:137–2.

Bruneton J. *Pharmacognosy Phytochemistry Medicinal Plants*, 2nd edition. Paris, France: Lavoisier Publishing; 1999;1072–8.

Bu-Abbas A, Clifford M, Ioannides C, Walker R. Stimulation of rat hepatic UDP-glucuronosyl transferase activity following treatment with green tea. *Food Chem Toxicol* 1995;33:27–30.

Bu-Abbas A, Clifford M, Walker R, Ioannides C. Marked antimutagenic potential of aqueous green tea extracts: mechanism of action. *Mutagenesis* 1994;9:325–31.

Bushman J. Green tea and cancer in humans: a review of the literature. *Nutr and Cancer* 1998;31(3):151–9.

But P, et al (eds.). *International Collation of Traditional and Folk Medicine*, Vol. 2., Northeast Asia Part II. Singapore: World Scientific Publishing; 1997;57–8.

Cao Y, Cao R. Angiogenesis inhibited by drinking tea. *Nature* 1999;398:381.

Chan P, Fong W, Cheung Y, et al. Jasmine Green Tea epicatechins are hypolipidemic in hamsters (*Mesocricetus auratus*) fed a high fat diet. *J Nutr* 1999;129(6):1094–101.

Chisaka T, Matsuda H, Kubomura Y, et al. The effect of crude drugs on experimental hypercholesteremia: mode of action of (–)-epigallocatechin gallate in tea leaves. *Chem Pharm Bull* 1988;36:227–33.

De Smet P, Keller K, Hänsel R, Chandler RF (eds.). *Adverse Effects of Herbal Drugs 2*. Berlin, Germany: Springer Verlag; 1993;26.

Dufresne CJ, Farnworth ER. A review of latest research findings on the health promotion properties of tea. *J Nutr Biochem* 2001;12:404-421.

Dulloo A, Duret C, Rohrer D, et al. Efficacy of a green tea extract rich in catechin polyphenols and caffeine in increasing 24-h energy expenditure and fat oxidation in humans. *Am J Clin Nutr* 1999;70(6):1040–5.

Fleming T, Gruenwald J, Brendler T, Jaenicke C. et al (eds.). *Physicians' Desk Reference for Herbal Medicines*, 2nd ed. Montvale, NJ: Medical Economics Company, Inc;2000;369–72.

Frankel E. *Natural Antioxidants in Foods and Biological Systems*. Davis, CA: University of California Department of Food Science & Technology; 1997.

Fujiki H, Suganuma M, Okabe S. Cancer inhibition by green tea. *Mutation Res* 1998;402:307–10.

Gao Y, McLaughlin J, Blot W, et al. Reduced risk of esophageal cancer associated with green tea consumption. *J Natl Cancer Inst* 1994;86:855–8.

Gawin F. Cocaine and other stimulants: actions, abuse and treatment. *New Eng J Med* 1988;318:1127.

Geleijnse J, Launer L, Hofman A, Pols H, Witteman J. Tea flavonoids may protect against atherosclerosis. *Arch Intern Med* 1999;159(18):2170–4.

Gilman A et al. *Goodman and Gilman's The Pharmacological Basis of Therapeutics*, 7th ed. New York, NY: Macmillan Publishing Company; 1985.

Goto K, Kanaya S, Nishikawa T, et al. The influence of tea catechins on fecal flora of elderly residents in long-term care facilities. *Ann Long-Term Care* 1998;6:1–7.

Goto K, Kanaya S, Ishigami T, Hara Y. The effects of tea catechins on fecal conditions

of elderly residents in a long-term care facility. *J Nutr Sci Vitaminol (Tokyo)* 1999;45(1):135–41.

Graham H. Green tea composition, consumption, and polyphenol chemistry. *Prev Med* 1992;21:334–50.

Gutman RL, Ryu, B-H. Rediscovering Tea. *HerbalGram* 1996;37:34–41.

Hara Y. Influence of tea catechins on the digestive tract. *J Cell Biochem Suppl* 1997;27:52–8.

Hartman T, Tangrea J, Pietinen P, et al. Tea and coffee consumption and the risk of colon and rectal cancer in middle-aged Finnish men. *Nutr Cancer* 1998;31(1):41–8.

Heber D, Blackburn G, Go V (eds.). *Nutritional Oncology*. San Diego, CA: Academic Press; 1999;349–51.

Health Canada. Tea regulations. In: *The Food and Drugs Act and Regulations* 1997, Division 20, Sections B.20.001-B-20.005. Ottawa, Canada: Minister of Public Works and Government Services Canada; 1997;B71.

Hegarty V, May H, Khaw K. Tea drinking and bone mineral density in older women. *Am J Clin Nutr* 2000;71(4):1003–7.

Hernaez J, Xu M, Dashwood R. Antimutagenic activity of tea towards 2-hydroxyamino-3-methylimidazo[4,5-f]quinoline: effect of tea concentration and brew time on electrophile scavenging. *Mutat Res* 1998;402(1–2):299–306.

Hertog M, Kromhout D, Aravanis C, et al. Flavonoid intake and long-term risk of coronary heart disease and cancer in the Seven Countries Study. *Arch Intern Med* 1995;155:381–6.

Hertog M, Feskens E, Hollman P, Katan M, Kromhout D. Dietary antioxidant flavonoids and risk of coronary heart disease: The Zutphen Elderly Study. *Lancet* 1993;342:1007–11.

Hertog M. *Flavinols and flavones in foods and their relation with cancer and coronary heart disease risk*. The Hague, Netherlands: DIP-data Koninklijke Bibliotheek; 1994.

Hirose M, Hoshiya T, Akagi K, Futakuchi M, Ito N. Inhibition of mammary gland carcinogenesis by green tea catechins and other naturally occurring antioxidants in female Sprague-Dawley rats pretreated with 7,12–dimethylbenz[alpha]anthracene. *Cancer Lett* 1994;83:149–56.

Ho C, Chen Q, Shi H, et al. Antioxidative effect of polyphenol extract prepared from various Chinese teas. *Prev Med* 1992;21:520–5.

Hodgson J, Puddey I, Croft K, et al. Acute effects of ingestion of black and green tea on lipoprotein oxidation. *Am J Clin Nutr* 2000;71(5):1103–7.

Hodgson J, Puddey I, Burke V, Beilin L, Jordan N. Effects on blood pressure of drinking green and black tea. *J Hypertens* 1999;17(4):457–63.

Hollman PC, Van Het Hof KH, Tijburg LB, Katan MB. Addition of milk does not affect the absorption of flavanols from tea in man. *Free Radic Res* 2001 Mar; 34(3):297-300.

Huang K. *The Pharmacology of Chinese Herbs*, 2nd edition. Boca Raton, FL: CRC Press; 1999;209–13.

Imai K et al. Cancer-preventive effects of drinking green tea among a Japanese population. *Prev Med* 1997;26:769–75.

Imai K, Nakachi K. Cross sectional study of effects of drinking green tea on cardiovascular and liver diseases. *BMJ* 1995;310:693–6.

International Organization for Standardization (ISO). International Standard ISO 11286: *Tea—Classification of grades by particle size analysis*. Geneva, Switzerland. ISO Technical Committee ISO/TC 34, Agricultural food products, Subcommittee SC 8, Tea; 1997.

Ishikawa T, Suzukawa M, Ito T, et al. Effect of tea flavonoid supplementation on the susceptibility of low-density lipoprotein to oxidative modification. *Am J Clin Nutr* 1997;66:261–6.

ISO. See: International Organization for Standardization.

Isogai E, Isogai H, Takeshi K, Nishikawa T. Protective effect of Japanese green tea extract on gnotobiotic mice infected with an *Escherichia coli* O157:H7 strain. *Microbiol Immunol* 1998;42:125–8.

Jankun J, Selman S, Swiercz R, Skrzypczak-Jankun E. Why drinking green tea could prevent cancer. *Nature* 1997;387:561.

Ji B, Chow W, Hsing A, et al. Green tea consumption and the risk of pancreatic and colorectal cancers. *Int J Cancer* 1997;70:255–8.

Ji B, Chow W, Yang G, et al. The influence of cigarette smoking, alcohol, and green tea consumption on the risk of carcinoma of the cardia and distal stomach in Shanghai, China. *Cancer* 1996;77:2449–57.

Katiiyar S, Agarwal R, Mukhtar H. Green tea in chemoprevention of cancer. *Comprehen Ther* 1992;18:3–8.

Khan S, Katiyar S, Agarwal R, Mukhtar H. Enhancement of antioxidant and phase II enzymes by oral feeding of green tea polyphenols in drinking water to SKH-1 hairless mice: possible role in cancer chemoprevention. *Cancer Res* 1992;52:4050–2.

Knekt P, Jarvinen R, Reunanen A, et al. Flavonoid intake and coronary mortality in Finland: a cohort study. *BMJ* 1996;312:478–81.

Komori A, Yatsunami J, Okabe S, et al. Anticarcinogenic activity of green tea polyphenols. *Jpn J Clin Oncol* 1993;23:186–90.

Kono S, Shinchi K, Wakabayashi K, *et al.* Relation of green tea consumption to serum lipids and lipoproteins in Japanese men. *J Epidemiol* 1996;6(3):128–33.

Kono S, Shinchi K, Ikeda N, Yanai F, Imanishi K. Green tea consumption and serum lipid profiles: a cross-sectional study in northern Kyushu, Japan. *Prev Med* 1992;21(4):526–31.

Kulhanek F, Linde O. Coffee and tea influence pharmacokinetics of antipsychotic drugs [letter]. *Lancet* 1981 Aug 15;2(8242):359–60.

Lasswell W Jr, Weber S, Wilkins J. *In vitro* interaction of neuroleptics and tricylic anti-depressants with coffee, tea, and gallotannic acid. *J Pharm Sci* 1984 Aug;73(8):1056–8.

Laughton M, Evans P, Moroney M, *et al.* Inhibition of mammalian 5-lipoxygenase and cyclo-oxygenase by flavonoids and phenolic dietary additives. Relationship to antioxidant activity and to iron ion-reducing ability. *Biochem Pharmacol* 1991;42:1673–81.

Lecomte A. Green tea 'Arkocaps'/Phytotrim® double-blind trial clinical results. *Revue de l'Assoc Mondiale de Phytother* 1985;1:36–40.

Leung A, Foster S. *Encyclopedia of Common Natural Ingredients Used in Food, Drugs, and Cosmetics*, 2nd ed. New York, NY: John Wiley & Sons; 1996;489–92.

Leenen R, Roodenburg A, Tijburg L, Wiseman S. A single dose of tea with or without milk increases plasma antioxidant activity in humans. *Eur J Clin Nutr* 2000;54(1):87–92.

Li N, Sun Z, Han C, Chen J. The chemopreventive effects of tea on human oral pre-cancerous mucosa lesions. *Proc Soc Exp Biol Med* 1999;220(4):218–24.

Li N, Sun Z, Liu Z, Han C. Study on the preventive effect of tea on DNA damage of the buccal mucosa cells in oral leukoplakias induced by cigarette smoking. [in Chinese]. *Wei Sheng Yen Chiu* 1998;27(3):173–4.

Luo M, Kannar K, Wahlqvist M, O'Brien R. Inhibition of LDL oxidation by green tea extract. *Lancet* 1997;349:360–1.

Mazzio E, Harris N, Soliman K. Food constituents attenuate monoamine oxidase activity and peroxide levels in C6 astrocyte cells. *Planta Med* 1998 Oct;64(7):603–6.

McGuffin M, Hobbs C, Upton R, Goldberg A (eds.). *American Herbal Product Association's Botanical Safety Handbook.* Boca Raton, FL: CRC Press; 1997.

Medical Products Agency (MPA). *Läkemedel; Läkemedelsnära Produkter* (registrerade homeopatiska produkter); *Naturläkemedel* (Authorised Natural Remedies). Uppsala, Sweden: Medical Products Agency. 2001.

Merhav H, Amitai Y, Palti H, Godfrey S. Tea drinking and microcytic anemia in infants. *Am J Clin Nutr* 1985 Jun;41(6):1210–3.

Meyer-Buchtela E. *Tee-Rezepturen: Ein Handbuch für Apotheker und Ärzte.* Stuttgart, Germany: Deutscher Apotheker Verlag; 1999.

Miketova P, Schram K, Whitney J, *et al.* Mass spectrometry of selected components of biological interest in green tea extracts. *J Nat Prod* 1998;61(4):461–7.

Morant J, Ruppanner H (eds.). *Arzneimittel-Kompendium der Schweiz®* 2001. Basel, Switzerland: Documed AG; 2001.

MPA. See: Medical Products Agency.

Mukhtar H, Katiyar S, Agarwal R. Cancer chemoprevention by green tea components. *Adv Exp Med Biol* 1994;354:123–34.

Muramatsu K, Fukuyo M, Hara Y. Effect of green tea catechins on plasma cholesterol level in cholesterol-fed rats. *J Nutr Sci Vitaminol* 1986;32:613–22.

Najemnik C, Sinzinger H, Kritz H. [Tea — a potent agent to prevent disease?] *Wiener klinische Wochenschrift* 1999;111(7):259–61.

Nakachi K, Suemasu K, Suga K, *et al.* Influence of drinking green tea on breast cancer malignancy among Japanese patients. *Jpn J Cancer Res* 1998;89(3):254–61.

Nakagawa K, Ninomiya M, Okubo T, *et al.* Tea catechin supplementation increases antioxidant capacity and prevents phospholipid hydroperoxidation in plasma of humans. *J Agric Food Chem* 1999;47(10):3967–73.

Nanjo F, Mori M, Goto K, Hara Y. Radical scavenging activity of tea catechins and their related compounds. *Biosci Biotechnol Biochem* 1999;63(9):1621–3.

Ohno Y, Wakai K, Genka K, *et al.* Tea consumption and lung cancer risk: a case-control study in Okinawa, Japan. *Jpn J Canc Res* 1995;86:1027–34.

Ooshima T, Minami T, Aono W, *et al.* Reduction of dental plaque deposition in humans by oolong tea extract. *Caries Res* 1994;28:146–9.

Peters U, Poole C, Arab L. Does Tea Affect Cardiovascular Disease? A Meta–Analysis. *American Journal of Epidemiology* 2001;154(6):495–503.

Pharmacopée Française (Ph.Fr.Xe Édition). Paris, France: Adrapharm; 1982–1996.

Ph.Fr.X. See: *Pharmacopée Française.*

Plumb G, Price K, Williamson G. Antioxidant properties of flavonol glycosides from tea. *Redox Report* 1999;4(1/2):13–6.

Princen H, van Duyvenvoorde W, Buytenhek R, *et al.* No effect of consumption of green and black tea on plasma lipid and antioxidant levels and on LDL oxidation in smokers. *Arterioscler Thromb Vasc Biol* 1998;18(5):833–41.

Rimm E, Katan M, Ascherio A, *et al.* Relation between intake of flavonoids and risk for coronary heart disease in male health professionals. *Ann Intern Med* 1996;125:384–9.

Ruppanner H, Schaefer U (eds.). *Codex 2000/01 — Die Schweizer Arzneimittel in*

einem Griff. Basel, Switzerland: Documed AG. 2000.

Sayama K, Ozeki K, Taguchi M, Oguni I. Effects of green tea and tea catechins on the development of mammary gland. *Biosci Biotechnol Biochem* 1996;60(1):169–70.

Scholz E, Bertram B. *Camellia sinensis* (L.) O. Kuntze – Der Teestrauch. *Z Phytother* 1995;16:235–50.

Schulz V, Hänsel R, Tyler VE. *Rational Phytotherapy: A Physicians' Guide to Herbal Medicine.* Berlin, Germany: Springer Verlag; 1998;192–3.

Serafini M, Ghiselli A, Ferro-Luzzi A. *In vivo* antioxidant effect of green and black tea in man. *Euro J Clin Nutr* 1996;50:28–32.

Sesso H, Gaziano J, Buring J, Hennekens C. Coffee and tea intake and the risk of myocardial infarction. *Am J Epidemiol* 1999;149(2):162–7.

Shih-Chen L. *Chinese Medicinal Herbs.* San Francisco, CA: Georgetown Press; 1973;81–7.

Snow J. *Camellia sinensis* (L.) Kuntze (*Theaceae*). *Protocol J Bot Med* 1995;1(2):47–51.

Stensvold I, Tverdal A, Solvoll K, Foss O. Tea consumption, relationship to cholesterol, blood pressure, and coronary and total mortality. *Prev Med* 1992;21(4):546–53.

Stich H. Teas and tea components as inhibitors of carcinogen formation in model systems and man. *Prev Med* 1992;21:377–84.

Suganuma M, Okabe S, Kai Y, *et al.* Synergistic effects of (–)-epigallocatechin gallate with (–)-epicatechin, sulindac, or tamoxifen on cancer-preventive activity in the human lung cancer cell line PC-9. *Cancer Res* 1999;59(1):44–7.

Taylor J, Wilt V. Probable antagonism of warfarin by green tea. *Annals of Pharmacother* 1999;33:426–8.

Threlkeld D. Respiratory drugs, bronchodilators, xanthine derivatives. In: *Facts and Comparisons Drug Information.* St. Louis, MO: Facts and Comparisons; 1991 Feb;178–9a.

Toda M, Okubo S, Hara Y, Shimamura T. Antibacterial and bactericidal activities of tea extracts and catechins against methicillin resistant Staphylococcus aureus. [in Japanese]. *Jpn J Bacteriol* 1991;46(5):839–45.

UN FAO. See: United Nations Food and Agriculture Organization.

United Nations Food and Agriculture Organization (UN FAO). *FAO promoting international tea trade mark at intergovernmental tea meeting* [press release]. Rome, Italy: Intergovernmental group on tea UN FAO; 1999.

United Nations Food and Agriculture Organization (UN FAO). *Market Developments in 1997/98 and its Short-Term Prospects* [report]. Rome, Italy: Intergovernmental group on tea UN FAO; 1998 July.

United States Congress (USC). Public Law 103–417: Dietary Supplement Health and Education Act of 1994. Washington, DC: 103rd Congress of the United States; 1994.

United States Customs Service (USCS). *Code of Federal Regulations* (21 CFR) Part 1220 – Regulations Under the Tea Importation Act. Washington, DC: Office of the Federal Register National Archives and Records Administration; 1998;614–23.

United States Customs Service (USCS). Tea Importation Act: 21 U.S.C. 41–50, 19 CFR 12.33 – Food and Drugs, Chapter 2 – Teas. Washington, DC: Office of the Federal Register National Archives and Records Administration; 1995.

United States Department of Agriculture. (USDA). Tropical Products: World Markets and Trade — U.S. Tea Trade. Washington, DC: USDA Foreign Agriculture Service; 2000 March;Circular Series FTROP 1–00.

United States Department of Agriculture. (USDA). *Commercial Item Description: Tea, Black (Bags or Loose).* Washington, DC: USDA; 1995 Sept 27;A-A-20033B.

United States Food and Drug Administration (US FDA). *Code of Federal Regulations* (21 CFR) Part 182 – Substances Generally Recognized as Safe. Washington, DC: Office of the Federal Register National Archives and Records Administration; 1998;427–33.

USC. See: United States Congress.

USCS. See: United States Customs Service.

USDS. See: United States Department of Agriculture.

US FDA. See: United States Food and Drug Administration.

van het Hof K, Wiseman S, Yang C, Tijburg L. Plasma and lipoprotein levels of tea catechins following repeated tea consumption. *Proc Soc Exp Biol Med* 1999;220(4):203–9.

van het Hof K, Kivits G, Weststrate J, Tijburg L. Bioavailability of catechins from tea: the effect of milk. *Eur J Clin Nutr* 1998;52(5):356–9.

van het Hof K, de Boer H, Wiseman S, *et al.* Consumption of green or black tea does not increase resistance of low-density lipoprotein to oxidation in humans. *Am J Clin Nutr* 1997;66:1125–32.

Wang H, Wu Y. Inhibitory effect of Chinese tea on N-nitrosation *in vitro* and *in vivo*. IARC Scientific Publications; 1991;546–9.

Wang Z, Huang M, Lou Y, *et al.* Inhibitory effects of black tea, green tea, decaffeinated black tea, and decaffeinated green tea on ultraviolet B light-induced skin carcinogenesis in 7,12-dimethylbenz[a]anthracene-initiated SKH-1 mice. *Cancer Res* 1994;54:3428–35.

Weisburger J. Tea and health: the underlying mechanisms. *Proc Soc Exp Biol Med*

1999;220(4):271–5.

Weisburger J, Nagao M, Wakabayashi K, Oguri A. Prevention of heterocyclic amine formation by tea and tea polyphenols. *Cancer Lett* 1994;83:143–7.

Wichtl M, Bisset N (eds.). *Herbal Drugs and Phytopharmaceuticals: A Handbook for Practice on a Scientific Basis.* Stuttgart, Germany: Medpharm Scientific Publishers; 1994;490–2.

Willson K, Clifford M (eds.). *Tea: Cultivation to Consumption.* London, UK: Chapman & Hall; 1992;659–705.

Xu G, Song P, Reed P. Effects of fruit juices, processed vegetable juice, orange peel and green tea on endogenous formation of N-nitrosoproline in subjects from a high-risk area for gastric cancer in Moping County, China. *Eur J Canc Prev* 1993;2:327–35.

Yamaguchi Y, Hayashi M, Yamazoe H, Kunitomo M. Preventive effects of green tea extract on lipid abnormalities in serum, liver and aorta of mice fed an atherogenic diet. *Nippon Yakurigaku Zasshi* 1991;97:329–37.

Yamane T, Hagiwara N, *et al.* Inhibition of azoxymethane-induced colon carcinogenesis in rats by green tea polyphenol fraction. *Jpn J Cancer Res* 1991;82:1336–9.

Yang C, Lee M, Chen L. Human salivary tea catechin levels and catechin esterase activities: implication in human cancer prevention studies. *Cancer Epidemiol Biomarkers Prev* 1999;8(1):83–9.

Yang C, Wang Z. Tea and cancer. *J Nat Canc Inst* 1993;85:1038–49.

Yarnell E. Green tea catechins improve gut flora. *Health Notes Review* 1999;6(1):12–13.

Yin P, Zhao J, Cheng S, *et al.* Experimental studies of the inhibitory effects of green tea catechin on mice large intestinal cancers induced by 1,2-dimethylhydrazine. *Cancer Lett* 1994;79:33–8.

Yu G, Hsieh C, Wang L, *et al.* Green tea consumption and risk of stomach cancer: a population-based case-control study in Shanghai, China. *Cancer Causes & Control* 1995;6:532–8.

Clinical Studies on Tea Leaf (*Camellia sinensis* [L.] Kuntze)

Cardiovascular

Author/Year	Subject	Design	Duration	Dosage	Preparation	Results/Conclusion
Leenen et al., 2000	Plasma antioxidant activity	C, R, CO n=21 healthy volunteers, 10 male, 11 female	1 day (tests at baseline and several times up to 2 hours post-tea drinking)	300 ml black or green tea	Aqueous infusion of black or green tea. 2 g dried leaf in 300 ml boiled water, with or without milk (brands not stated) vs. water	Consumption of a single dose of black or green tea induced a significant rise in plasma antioxidant activity (p<0.001). Plasma was analyzed for total catechins and antioxidant activity using the ferric-reducing ability of plasma (FRAP) assay. Addition of milk did not interfere with the increase. A larger increase was observed for green tea vs. black tea.
Hodgson et al., 2000	Lipoprotein oxidation	C, R, Cm n=20 healthy males	90 minutes	400 ml black or green tea/day	Aqueous infusion of black tea or sencha (Japanese green tea). 1.9 g dried leaf in 400 ml boiled water for 4 minutes (brands not stated) vs. water control with matched caffeine content	Significant increases in urinary 4–O–methylgallic acid for black and green tea (p<0.0001) were observed. Caffeine did not significantly influence lipoprotein oxidation. Only black tea had a mild acute effect on *ex vivo* lipoprotein oxidation in human serum, but effect was short-lived and of borderline significance.
Dulloo et al., 1999	Energy expenditure and fat oxidation	R, PC n=10 healthy males	24 hours on 3 occasions	Two, 250 mg capsules 3x/day, green tea extract (150 mg caffeine, 375 mg catechins)	Exolise® green tea leaf alcoholic dry extract vs. 150 mg caffeine/day vs. placebo (cellulose)	Compared to placebo, tea extract resulted in a significant increase in 24-hour energy expenditure (4%; p< 0.01) and significant decrease in 24-hour respiratory quotient (from 0.88 to 0.85; p< 0.001) with no change in urinary nitrogen. Urinary norepinephrine excretion was higher in tea group than placebo (40%, p< 0.05). Authors concluded that tea has thermogenic properties and promotes fat oxidation.
Geleijnse et al., 1999	Aortic athero-sclerosis	P n=3,454 men and women, free of cardiovascular disease at baseline	2–3 years after baseline assessment; medium duration of follow-up was 1.9 years	125 ml black tea 3.0–3.5x/day	Aqueous infusion of black tea leaf (brands not stated)	Multivariable analyses showed a significant inverse association of tea intake with severe aortic atherosclerosis. Odds ratios (OR) decreased from 0.54 (95% confidence interval [CI], 0.32–0.92) for drinking 125~250 ml (1~2 cups) of tea per day to 0.31 (CI, 0.16–0.59) for drinking more than 500 ml/day (4 cups per day). Associations were stronger in women than men. Association of tea intake with mild and moderate atherosclerosis was not statistically significant. Authors concluded that drinking tea provides a protective effect against ischemic heart disease. (Often called the Rotterdam Study.)
Hodgson et al., 1999	Blood pressure	C, R, Cm, CO n=20 healthy males	21 days; 7 days each intervention	400 ml black or green tea 4x/day	Aqueous infusion of black tea or sencha (Japanese green tea). 1.9 g dried leaf in 400 ml boiled water for 4 minutes (brands not stated) vs. water control with matched caffeine content	Black (and not green) tea produced a transient (within the first 30 minutes) increase in blood pressure relative to that produced by caffeine. Consumption over 7 days of either black or green tea had no effect on ambulatory blood pressure.

KEY: **C** – controlled, **CC** – case-control, **CH** – cohort, **CI** – confidence interval, **Cm** – comparison, **CO** – crossover, **CS** – cross-sectional, **DB** – double-blind, **E** – epidemiological, **LC** – longitudinal cohort, **MA** – meta-analysis, **MC** – multi-center, **n** – number of patients, **O** – open, **OB** – observational, **OL** – open label, **OR** – odds ratio, **P** – prospective, **PB** – patient-blind, **PC** – placebo-controlled, **PG** – parallel group, **PS** – pilot study, **R** – randomized, **RC** – reference-controlled, **RCS** – retrospective cross-sectional, **RS** - retrospective, **S** – surveillance, **SB** – single-blind, **SC** – single-center, **U** – uncontrolled, **UP** – unpublished, **VC** – vehicle-controlled.

Cardiovascular (cont.)

Author/Year	Subject	Design	Duration	Dosage	Preparation	Results/Conclusion
Sesso et al., 1999	Myocardial infarction	MC, CC n=340 case-control pairs, white men and women, no prior history of myocardial infarction or angina pectoris (<76 years)	Home interviews conducted 10 weeks after hospital discharge	0 to ≥ 1 cup/day green tea	Aqueous infusion of black tea leaf (brands not stated) vs. coffee and decaffeinated coffee	Only tea was inversely associated with risk of myocardial infarction. 24.9% of cases and 32.0% of controls drank >1 cup/day. Regular tea drinkers had a significantly lower risk of myocardial infarction compared to non-tea drinkers (OR=0.55, 95%, CI, 0.36–0.85), independent of coronary risk factors and lipids. The heaviest tea drinkers had more favorable HDL cholesterol levels.
van het Hof et al., 1999	Plasma antioxidant activity	CO n=18 healthy adults	3 days	1 cup green tea, black tea, or black tea with milk 8x/day (1 cup every 2 hours)	Aqueous infusion of black tea leaf or green tea leaf (brands not stated) with or without milk vs. water	Catechin levels in blood rapidly increased upon repeated tea consumption. Addition of milk did not affect any parameters measured. Accumulation of catechins in LDL particles was not sufficient to improve intrinsic resistance of LDL to oxidation ex vivo.
Princen et al., 1998	Plasma antioxidant activity	R, SB, PC n=29 healthy smokers, 13 male, 16 female	1 month	One, 150 ml cup black or green tea 6x/day, or 3.6 g isolated green tea polyphenols/day	Aqueous infusion of black tea leaf or green tea leaf (brands not stated) vs. isolated green tea polyphenols vs. placebo	Authors concluded that black or green tea at 6 cups/day had no effect on plasma lipids and no sparing effect on plasma antioxidant vitamins, and that intake of a high dose of isolated green tea polyphenols decreases plasma vitamin E. No effect was found on LDL cholesterol oxidation ex vivo after consumption of green or black tea or intake of green tea polyphenol isolate.
Ishikawa et al., 1997	Antioxidant activity; susceptibility of LDL cholesterol to oxidation	R, Cm n=22 normo-lipidemic healthy male volunteers	2 months (4 weeks no tea, 4 weeks tea; control group, 8 weeks water)	150 ml black tea 5x/day	Aqueous infusion of 2.2 g Twinings® Darjeeling black tea leaf vs. water	After 4-week treatment period, lag time before initiation of LDL cholesterol oxidation was significantly (p<0.01) prolonged from 54 to 62 minutes. LDL cholesterol exposed to tea had reduced oxidizability. 1 and 2 hours after tea ingestion, levels of EGCG and ECG in plasma increased significantly (p<0.05). Authors speculated that tea may ameliorate atherosclerosis by suppressing oxidation of LDL cholesterol.
van het Hof et al., 1997	Antioxidant activity, resistance of LDL cholesterol to oxidation	PG, Cm n=45 healthy non-smoking volunteers	One month (2 weeks mineral water, 2 weeks tea) control group, 4 weeks water	150 ml, 6x/day black tea or green tea prepared from freeze-dried, water-soluble extractive	Aqueous infusions of 0.5 g Lipton® freeze-dried black tea leaf extract and 0.5 g Lipton green tea leaf extract vs. mineral water control	Significant increase in total antioxidant activity of plasma occurred after 4 weeks of green tea, or alter serum lipid concentrations. This tea preparation, dosage and duration of use had no effect on variables of oxidative stress to lipids or serum lipid concentrations or resistance of LDL cholesterol to oxidation ex vivo.
Kono et al., 1996	Hypocholes-terolemia	E, MC n=2,062 Japanese male self-defense officials	2 years (1991–92)	Average 1 cup, 3x/day green tea	Aqueous infusion of green tea leaf (brands not stated)	Green tea consumption was inversely associated with serum levels of total cholesterol (TC), and LDL cholesterol, but not with either high-density lipoprotein (HDL) cholesterol or triglycerides. 10 cups/day of green tea was associated with differences of 6.2 mg/dl in TC (95% CI, 0.4–12.1) and 6.2 mg/dl in LDL cholesterol (95% CI, 0.7–11.7). These findings of association of green tea with blood cholesterol suggest a possible causal relationship.
Imai and Nakachi, 1995	Cardio-vascular disease and liver disorders	E, P, CS n=1,371 Japanese men (>40 years)	5 years (1986–90)	≤ 3 cups/day to ≥ 10 cups/day green tea	Aqueous infusion of green tea leaf (brands not stated)	As daily green tea intake increased from less than 3 to 4–9, and more than 10 cups, researchers observed significantly increased serum HDL and decreased LDL lipoprotein levels. Additionally, increased green tea consumption was associated with significantly improved liver profiles in which aspartate aminotransferase and alanine aminotransferase levels dropped. An inverse association between green tea ingestion and various serum markers shows that green tea may act protectively against cardiovascular disease and disorders of the liver.

KEY: C – controlled, **CC** – case-control, **CH** – cohort, **CI** – confidence interval, **Cm** – comparison, **CO** – crossover, **CS** – cross-sectional, **DB** – double-blind, **E** – epidemiological, **LC** – longitudinal cohort, **MA** – meta-analysis, **MC** – multi-center, **n** – number of patients, **O** – open, **OB** – observational, **OL** – open label, **OR** – odds ratio, **P** – prospective, **PB** – patient-blind, **PC** – placebo-controlled, **PG** – parallel group, **PS** – pilot study, **R** – randomized, **RC** – reference-controlled, **RCS** – retrospective cross-sectional, **RS** - retrospective, **S** – surveillance, **SB** – single-blind, **SC** – single-center, **U** – uncontrolled, **UP** – unpublished, **VC** – vehicle-controlled.

Cardiovascular (cont.)

Author/Year	Subject	Design	Duration	Dosage	Preparation	Results/Conclusion
Hertog et al., 1993	Coronary heart disease	P n=805 elderly Dutch men	30 years (1960–1990)	I cup, 2–4x/day black tea	Aqueous infusion of black tea leaf (brands not stated)	Black tea consumption contributed about 70% to daily flavonoid intake. Authors concluded that flavonoids in regularly consumed foods and beverages, such as black tea, may reduce the risk of death from coronary heart disease in elderly men.
Kono et al., 1992	Serum lipid concentrations and athero-sclerosis	E, CS n=I 306 male Japanese self-defense officials (49–56 years)	27 months (October 1986–December 1988)	0 to ≥ 9 cups/day green tea	Aqueous infusion of green tea leaf (brands not stated)	Increased green tea consumption, especially more than 9 cups/day, is associated with decreased total serum cholesterol and decreased LDL cholesterol, very low density lipoproteins and triglycerides, increased HDL, and reduced atherogenic index. Adjusted mean concentrations of total cholesterol were 8 mg/dl lower in men drinking 9 cups or more/day than those drinking zero to 2 cups/day.
Stensvold et al., 1992	Coronary heart disease	CS, P n=20,089 Norwegian men and women (9,856 men, 10,233 women with-out history of cardiovascular disease or diabetes)	12 years (1976–1988)	0 to ≥ 5 cups/day black tea	Aqueous infusion of black tea leaf (brands not stated)	Men and women who drank 5 or more cups of black tea per day had lower cholesterol levels than non-tea drinkers. Tea drinkers were less likely to die from heart attack, and systolic blood pressure was inversely related to tea consumption. The mean serum cholesterol decreased with increasing tea consumption; the linear trend coefficient corresponded to a difference of 0.24 mmol/l (9.3 mg/dl) in men and 0.15 mmol/l (5.8 mg/dl) in women between drinkers of less than I cup and those of 5 or more cups/day.

Cancer

Author/Year	Subject	Design	Duration	Dosage	Preparation	Results/Conclusion
August et al., 1999	Colon cancer	Phase I/II study n=14 normal volunteers	24 hours	0.6, 1.2, or 1.8 green tea solids	Green tea solids dissolved in warm water (brand not stated)	Blood samples taken 2, 4, 8, and 24 hours after tea ingestion. Rectal biopsies at 4, 8, and 24 hours. 71% of subjects responded to green tea with at least a 50% inhibition of prostaglandin E2 (PGE2) levels at 4 hours, indicating possible chemoprevention of colorectal cancer.
Li et al., 1999	Oral mucosa leukoplakia	R, DB, PC n=59 oral mucosa leukoplakia patients	6 months	Two, 380 mg mixed tea extract cap-sules 4x/day, plus topical application of 10% mixed tea in glycerol smeared on mucosa lesion 3x/day	External: 10% mixed tea extract in glycerol vs. placebo and glycerin. Internal: 380 mg capsule of mixed tea extract composed of 66.7% green tea aqueous dry native extract, 16.7% green tea polyphenols, and 16.7% tea pigments (theaflavins, thearubigins, and theabromine)	After 6 months, size of oral lesion decreased in 37.9% of 29 treated patients and increased in 3.4% compared to decrease in 10% of 30 control patients and increase of 6.7%. Incidence of micronucleated exfoliated oral mucosa cells in treatment group was lower than in control group (p<0.01). Significant differences (p<0.05) in number and total volume of silver-stained Nucleolar Organizer Regions (AgNOR) and proliferating index of Proliferation Cell Nuclear Antigen (PCNA) indicating decrease of cell proliferation in treatment group. Overall results provide some direct evidence on protective effects of tea on oral cancer.
Nakachi et al., 1998	Stage I, II, and III breast cancer	E n=472 patients with Stage I, II, and III breast cancer	7 years	≤ 4 cups/day vs. ≥ 5 cups/day green tea	Aqueous infusion of green tea leaf (brands not stated)	Increased consumption of green tea was correlated with decreased recurrence of Stage I and Stage II breast cancer (p<0.05 for crude disease-free survival). No improvement in prognosis was observed in Stage III breast cancer.

KEY: **C** – controlled, **CC** – case-control, **CH** – cohort, **CI** – confidence interval, **Cm** – comparison, **CO** – crossover, **CS** – cross-sectional, **DB** – double-blind, **E** – epidemiological, **LC** – longitudinal cohort, **MA** – meta-analysis, **MC** – multi-center, **n** – number of patients, **O** – open, **OB** – observational, **OL** – open label, **OR** – odds ratio, **P** – prospective, **PB** – patient-blind, **PC** – placebo-controlled, **PG** – parallel group, **PS** – pilot study, **R** – randomized, **RC** – reference-controlled, **RCS** – retrospective cross-sectional, **RS** - retrospective, **S** – surveillance, **SB** – single-blind, **SC** – single-center, **U** – uncontrolled, **UP** – unpublished, **VC** – vehicle-controlled.

Tea, Black/Green

Monograph

Cancer (cont.)

Author/Year	Subject	Design	Duration	Dosage	Preparation	Results/Conclusion
Hartman et al., 1998	Rectal and colon cancer	E, CH n=27,111 male smokers (50–69 years)	8 years	0 cups/day vs. < 1 cup/day vs. ≥ 1 cup/day green tea	Aqueous infusion of black tea leaf. No standard preparation (brands not stated)	This study does not support the hypothesis that coffee and tea protect against colorectal cancer risk. Tea had little effect on incidence of rectal cancer. A positive association was seen for increased consumption of tea and colon cancer.
Ji et al., 1997	Pancreatic and colorectal cancers	E, CC n=2,266 Chinese patients with newly diagnosed cancers: 931 colon, 884 rectum, 451 pancreas, 1,1552 controls	33 months (October 1990– June 1993)	1–199g/month to ≥ 300g/month green tea leaves	Aqueous infusion of green tea leaf (brands not stated)	Significant inverse association with each cancer was observed with increasing green tea dosage. Women with highest tea consumption had 33% reduced risk of colon cancer, 43% reduced risk of rectal cancer, and 47% reduced risk of pancreatic cancer (p=0.07, 0.001, and 0.008 respectively). For men, 18% reduced risk of colon cancer, 43% reduction risk of rectal cancer, and 47% reduced risk of pancreatic cancer (p=0.38, 0.04 and 0.04, respectively).
Imai et al., 1997	Cancer prevention (type not stated)	P, CH n=8,552 Japanese men and women	10 years	Range extending to > 10 cups/day green tea	Aqueous infusion of green tea leaf (brands not stated)	Green tea consumption delayed onset of cancer incidence, especially in females drinking more than 10 cups/day. Preventive effects were not statistically significant in males. Relative risk of cancer incidence (females RR = 0.57, 95%, CI = 0.33-0.98; males RR = 0.68, 95%, CI = 0.39-1.21) was lowest among those with highest consumption levels.
Yu et al., 1995	Stomach cancer	CC, MC n=1,422 Chinese patients, 711 matched controls (<80 years)	27 months (October 1991– December 1993)	Varied	Aqueous infusion of green tea leaf (brands not stated)	Protective effect against stomach cancer from green tea (OR=0.71; 95% CI, 0.54–0.93). Adjusted OR decreased as consumption increased (p=0.006).
Ohno et al., 1995	Lung cancer	CC n=999 333 Japanese male and female patients	4 years (1988–1991)	1–4 cups/day to ≥ 10 cups/day green tea	Aqueous infusion of green tea leaf (brands not stated)	Odds ratios in females: 1–4 cups/day 0.77 (0.28–3.13), 5–9 cups/day 0.77 (0.26–2.25), 10 or more cups/day 0.57 (0.31–1.06). Corresponding numbers for males: 0.85 (0.46–1.55), 0.85 (0.46–1.56), 0.57 (0.31–1.06). Risk reduction was detected mainly in squamous cell carcinoma.
Gao et al., 1994	Esophageal cancer	E, RS, CC, MC n=734 Chinese patients, 1,552 controls (30–74 years)	28 months (October 1990– January 1993)	0 to ≥ 200 g /month green tea leaves	Aqueous infusion of green tea leaf (brands not stated)	Protective effect of green tea on esophageal cancer was observed among women (OR=0.50, 95% CI=0.30–0.83). Risk decreased significantly with increased consumption (p=0.05) in women, but not in men.

KEY: C – controlled, **CC** – case-control, **CH** – cohort, **CI** – confidence interval, **Cm** – comparison, **CO** – crossover, **CS** – cross-sectional, **DB** – double-blind, **E** – epidemiological, **LC** – longitudinal cohort, **MA** – meta-analysis, **MC** – multi-center, **n** – number of patients, **O** – open, **OB** – observational, **OL** – open label, **OR** – odds ratio, **P** – prospective, **PB** – patient-blind, **PC** – placebo-controlled, **PG** – parallel group, **PS** – pilot study, **R** – randomized, **RC** – reference-controlled, **RCS** – retrospective cross-sectional, **RS** - retrospective, **S** – surveillance, **SB** – single-blind, **SC** – single-center, **U** – uncontrolled, **UP** – unpublished, **VC** – vehicle-controlled.

Clinical Studies on Tea Leaf (*Camellia sinensis* [L.] Kuntze) (cont.)

Other

Author/Year	Subject	Design	Duration	Dosage	Preparation	Results/Conclusion
Hegarty et al., 2000	Osteoporosis	CS n=1,256 post-menopausal women (65–76 years old) tea group n=1,134 non-tea group n=122	1 day (BMD measured and questionnaires filled out)	≥ 1 cup/day black or green tea	Aqueous infusions of green tea leaf and black tea leaf with or without milk (brands not stated)	Compared with non-tea drinkers, tea drinkers had significantly greater (~5%) mean bone mineral density (BMD) measurements, adjusted for age and body mass index, at lumbar spine (0.033 g/cm2; p=0.02). Differences at femoral neck (0.013 g/cm2) were not significant. Authors concluded that nutrients in tea, such as flavonoids, may influence BMD and tea may protect against osteoporosis in older women.
Goto et al., 1999	Effect on fecal flora	O n=35 residents in long-term care facility fed same diet of rice gruel and minced food	6 weeks	Green tea extract, 3x/day with meals (300 mg total catechins/day)	Green tea leaf extract (brand not stated)	Compared to baseline, all fecal parameters decreased significantly during tea extract administration including moisture content, pH, ammonia, sulfide, and oxidation-reduction potential (ORP). These reductions indicated favorable improvements of subject's bowel conditions.
Goto et al., 1998	Effect on fecal flora	O n=15 male and female nursing home residents fed by nasogastric or gastric tube	3 weeks	161.3 mg, 3x/day green tea extract (300 mg total catechins/day)	Green tea leaf extract, 62.5% total catechins (30.5% EGCG, 18.5% EGC, 7.0% ECG, 6.5% EC) (brand not stated)	Compared to baseline, lactobacilli and bifidobacteria levels increased significantly (p<0.01–0.05). Levels of enterobacteriaceae, bacteroidaceae, eubacteria, and total bacteria decreased significantly compared to baseline (p<0.01–0.05). Levels of unwanted bacterial metabolites decreased significantly at 21 days (p<0.01–0.05). Fecal pH lowered significantly (p<0.05). After 7 days of discontinuance, all levels returned to pretrial levels.
van het Hof et al., 1998	Bioavailability of catechins	R, C, CO n=12 healthy male (5) and female (7) adults	3 weeks (crossover at 1-week intervals)	1 single dose (3 g tea solids) green tea, black tea, or black tea with milk	Aqueous infusions of 3 g green tea leaf (900 mg catechins) and 3 g black tea leaf (300 mg catechins), with and without milk	Consumption of green tea or black tea resulted in a rapid increase of catechin levels in blood. Maximum changes were reached after 2.3 hours for green and 2.2 hours for black tea. Addition of milk did not impair tea catechin bioavailability.
Lecomte, 1985	Obesity	R, DB, PC n=60 obese women (30–45 years)	1 month (follow-ups at 15 and 30 days treatment)	Eight, 250 mg capsules/day green tea leaf powder with meals (2 breakfast, 3 lunch, 3 dinner)	Arkocaps/ Phytotrim® green tea leaf powder (250 mg powdered leaf per capsule) vs. placebo	Significant average weight loss of 1.7 kg at day 15 and 2.9 kg at day 30 in green tea group. Significant decrease in waist measurement after 30 days. Significant reductions in total cholesterol and blood triglycerides but no reduction in HDL cholesterol. Author concluded that green tea powder caused significant weight loss compared to placebo and demonstrates utility in treatment of obesity.

KEY: **C** – controlled, **CC** – case-control, **CH** – cohort, **CI** – confidence interval, **Cm** – comparison, **CO** – crossover, **CS** – cross-sectional, **DB** – double-blind, **E** – epidemiological, **LC** – longitudinal cohort, **MA** – meta-analysis, **MC** – multi-center, **n** – number of patients, **O** – open, **OB** – observational, **OL** – open label, **OR** – odds ratio, **P** – prospective, **PB** – patient-blind, **PC** – placebo-controlled, **PG** – parallel group, **PS** – pilot study, **R** – randomized, **RC** – reference-controlled, **RCS** – retrospective cross-sectional, **RS** - retrospective, **S** – surveillance, **SB** – single-blind, **SC** – single-center, **U** – uncontrolled, **UP** – unpublished, **VC** – vehicle-controlled.

Tea, Black/Green

Monograph

(This page intentionally left blank.)

Valerian

Valeriana officinalis L. (syn. *V. exaltata* J.C. Mikan)

[Fam. *Valerianaceae*]

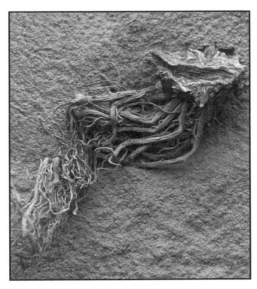

Photo © 2003 stevenfoster.com

OVERVIEW

Valerian has a long history of use in western Europe as a sedative and sleep aid, with medicinal uses dating to Hippocrates' time (ca. 460-377 B.C.E.). In the U.S., valerian root is widely used in sleep aids and sedatives in alcoholic tincture, aqueous infusions, and crude root powdered and dried extracts in capsules and tablets. Valerian is often combined with other herbs traditionally known to promote sleep (e.g., hops, passionflower, lemon balm, lavender, and chamomile). Three such combination products have been clinically studied and are described in the proprietary products section of this book. Valerian ranked 8th in total sales in mainstream retail outlets in the U.S. in 2000, with sales totaling approximately $17 million.

PRIMARY USES

- Anxiety
- Insomnia
- Sleep disorders
- Restlessness based on nervous disorders

OTHER POTENTIAL USES

- Increased mood related to enhanced sleep
- Fibromyalgia (in baths)

PHARMACOLOGICAL ACTIONS

Improvement of mild-to-moderate sleeping disorders without adverse effects on REM sleep, and without significant hangover effects.

DOSAGE AND ADMINISTRATION

No time limit has been set for the use of valerian by many authoritative sources. However, long term clinical trials (>30days) have not been conducted.

Internal

INFUSIONS: 2–3 g of fresh or dried root per cup, once to several times daily.

TINCTURE: 1/2–1 tsp. (1–3 ml), once to several times daily.

EXTRACTS: Amount equivalent to 2–3 g of crude herb, once to several times daily

TEA OR DRY EXTRACT (sleep aid): Single dose 1/2 to 1 hour before bedtime, with earlier dose in evening if necessary. Adult: Proportion dose according to body weight, as tea infusion or dry extract. Children 3–12 years old: With medical supervision only.

External

BATH: 100 g for 1 full bath; equivalent preparations.

CONTRAINDICATIONS

The World Health Organization (WHO) contraindicates the use of valerian for children under 12 years without medical supervision. However, German authorities note clinical use of valerian in pediatrics is permissible at age 3 and up, as long as valepotriate and baldrinal-free preparations are used.

PREGNANCY AND LACTATION: WHO contraindicates the use of valerian during pregnancy because safety during pregnancy has not been established clinically. WHO also contraindicates valerian during lactation due to the lack of research in this area.

ADVERSE EFFECTS

Unlike benzodiazepines, valerian appears to cause no residual morning sleepiness; however, it may slightly impair judgment and driving ability for 2–3 hours after intake. Chronic use of high doses of valerian (530 mg to 2 gm per dose, 5 times per day) over many years raises the possibility of withdrawal symptoms if the herb is abruptly discontinued. Rare adverse effects of valerian have included headache and stomach upset.

DRUG INTERACTIONS

Although many authors have speculated on potential interactions between valerian, alcohol, barbiturates, and benzodiazepines in humans, such interactions have not been documented. Experimental animal data shows valerian potentiation of benzodiazepines.

CLINICAL REVIEW

In 29 clinical studies on valerian (5,201 participants), all studies demonstrated positive effects for indications including anxiety, sleep disorders, and mood. The majority of clinical trials have consistently demonstrated that valerian is significantly more effective than placebo in improving sleep in persons with sleep disturbances. Modern human studies have investigated its use in combination with hops, as an alternative to benzodiazepine to treat nonchronic and nonpsychiatric sleep disorders; its use in combination with hops as a sedative to treat disturbed sleep; its effects in combination with hops (*Humulus lupulus*) on driving safety; its use in combination with St. John's wort (*Hypericum perforatum*) as an alternative to diazepam to treat symptoms of anxiety; and its use in combination with camphor, night-blooming cereus (*Selenicereus grandiflorus*), and hawthorn (*Crataegus* spp.) to treat functional cardiovascular disorders, hypotension, or meteorosensitivity. Two double-blind, placebo-controlled (DB, PC) studies concluded that valerian in combination with lemon balm (*Melissa officinalis*) improved sleep quality for insomniacs,

and a third concluded it did not impair driving or operating heavy machinery. One randomized (R), DB, PC cross-over study found a valerian, hops, and lemon balm combination effective for individuals experiencing sleep difficulties. One R, DB, controlled study concluded that valerian did not adversely influence alertness, reaction time, or concentration. The approved modern therapeutic applications for valerian appear to be supported by its history of use in well established systems of traditional and conventional medicine, many supporting *in vitro* and *in vivo* pharmacological experiments in animals, extensive phytochemical investigations, and human clinical studies—all of which tend to show CNS depressant activities.

Valerian

Valeriana officinalis L. (syn. *V. exaltata* J.C. Mikan)
[Fam. *Valerianaceae*]

OVERVIEW

Valerian has a long history of use in western Europe as a sedative and sleep aid, with medicinal uses dating back to Hippocrates' time (ca. 460-377 B.C.E.). In the U.S., valerian root is widely used in sleep aids and sedatives in various forms including teas, tablets, and capsules. Often, valerian is combined with other herbs traditionally known to promote sleep including hops, passionflower, lemon balm, chamomile, and lavender.

USES

Anxiety; insomnia; sleep disorders; restlessness linked to nervous disorders; enhanced mood based on improved sleep.

DOSAGE

No duration limit has been set for the use of valerian.

INFUSION (tea): 2–3 g of fresh or dried root per cup, once to several times daily.

TINCTURE: 1/2–1 tsp. (1–3 ml), once to several times daily.

EXTRACTS: Amount equivalent to 2–3 g of crude herb, once to several times daily.

TEA OR DRY EXTRACT (sleep aid): Single dose 1/2 to 1 hour before bedtime, with earlier dose in evening if necessary. Adults: Proportion dose according to body weight, as tea infusion or dry extract; Children 3–12 years old: With professional supervision only.

CONTRAINDICATIONS

Consult with a healthcare provider before using in children under 12 years. German pediatric authorities claim that valerian may be used in children age 3 and up, provided the preparations are free of the active compounds valepotriates and baldrinal.

PREGNANCY AND LACTATION: Valerian should not be taken during pregnancy because its safety during pregnancy has not been established clinically. Valerian is contraindicated during breast-feeding because of the lack of research in this area. However, experimental animal data suggest safety of valerian extracts; no adverse effects on fertility or fetotoxicity have been observed.

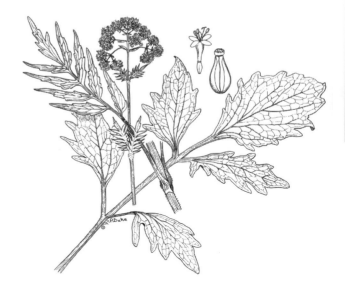

ADVERSE EFFECTS

Valerian is considered generally safe. Unlike benzodiazepines, valerian appears to cause little or no residual morning sleepiness. However, it may slightly impair judgment and driving ability for 2–3 hours after intake. Adverse effects may include headache and stomach upset, but these effects are rare.

DRUG INTERACTIONS

Valerian may potentially interact with alcohol, barbiturates, and benzodiazepines, but these interactions have not been clinically proven in humans.

Comments

When using a dietary supplement, purchase it from a reliable source. For best results, use the same brand of product throughout the period of use. As with all medications and dietary supplements, please inform your healthcare provider of all herbs and medications you are taking. Interactions may occur between medications and herbs or even among different herbs when taken at the same time. Treat your herbal supplement with care by taking it as directed, storing it as advised on the label, and keeping it out of the reach of children and pets. Consult your healthcare provider with any questions.

AMERICAN
BOTANICAL
COUNCIL

The information contained on this sheet has been excerpted from *The ABC Clinical Guide to Herbs* © 2003 by the American Botanical Council (ABC). ABC is an independent member-based educational organization focusing on the medicinal use of herbs. For more detailed information about this herb please consult the healthcare provider who gave you this sheet. To order *The ABC Clinical Guide to Herbs* or become a member of ABC, visit their website at www.herbalgram.org.

Valerian

Valeriana officinalis L. (syn. *V. exaltata* J.C. Mikan)

[Fam. *Valerianaceae*]

OVERVIEW

Valerian has a long history of use in Western Europe as a sedative and sleep aid, with medicinal use dating to Hippocrates (ca. 460–377 B.C.E.) (Blumenthal *et al.*, 2000). Valerian is used in countless preparations worldwide. In the U.S., for example, valerian root is known extensively as a dietary supplement in the form of alcoholic tinctures, aqueous infusions (teas), and as a crude-root, powdered and dried extract in capsules and tablets. Often, valerian is combined with other herbs traditionally known to promote sedation or sleep, e.g., hops (*Humulus lupulus*), passion flower (*Passiflora incarnata*), and lemon balm (*Melissa officinalis*) (Blumenthal *et al.*, 1998). Three such combination products have been clinically studied and are described in the section of this book dealing with proprietary products. Valerian ranked eighth in total sales in mainstream retail outlets in the U.S. in 2000, with sales totaling approximately $17 million (Blumenthal, 2001).

Valerian root and two of its preparations, valerian root powder and valerian extract, are official in the *United States Pharmacopeia* (USP) 25th edition, and *National Formulary* (NF) 20th edition. Crude valerian root, fluid extract, alcoholic tincture, and ammoniated tincture were formerly official in the USP from 1820 through 1930 (Boyle, 1991; Lloyd, 1929) and the NF (Grieve, 1979; Leung and Foster, 1996). Valerian root is official in the national pharmacopeias of Austria, France, Great Britain, Hungary, Russia, and Switzerland, among others (Blumenthal *et al.*, 2000). In Germany, valerian is official in the *German Pharmacopoeia,* and approved in the Commission E monographs for its sedative and sleep-promoting activity (Blumenthal, *et al.*, 1998).

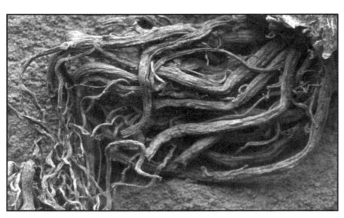

Photo © 2003 stevenfoster.com

DESCRIPTION

Valerian root extract consists of the fresh or carefully dried (below 40°C) subterranean parts of *Valeriana officinalis* L. (syn. *V. exaltata* J.C. Mikan) [Fam. *Valerianaceae*] (Blumenthal *et al.*, 1998),

including the rhizome, roots, and stolons. The whole dried root contains no less than 0.5% (*v/m*) volatile oil, and the cut dried root contains no less than 0.3% (*v/m*) volatile oil. The dried root contains no less than 0.17% of sesquiterpenic acids expressed as valerenic acid, calculated with reference to the dried drug (Ph. Eur. 2001). The NF requires dried valerian root to contain no less than 0.5% volatile oil, and not less than 0.05% valerenic acid (USP-NF, 1999). Valerian root dry extract consists of the native extractive yielded from comminuted valerian root, extracted in 70% alcohol, manufactured according to the *German Pharamacopoeia* monograph. The drug-to-extract ratio ranges from 3:1 to 6:1 (*w/v*) (DAB, 1999). The NF requires that the dry extract contain no less than 0.3% of valerenic acid, with a drug-to-extract ratio between 4:1 and 7:1 (USP, 2002).

PRIMARY USES

Neurology

- Anxiety: The World Health Organization (WHO) lists uses supported by clinical data, including as a mild sedative and sleep-promoting agent; a milder alternative or possible substitute for stronger synthetic sedatives (e.g., benzodiazepines); and for treatment of nervous excitation and sleep disturbances induced by anxiety (WHO, 1999). This indication is supported by numerous clinical trials (Bourin *et al.*, 1997; Sousa *et al.*, 1992; Kohnen and Oswald, 1988; Panijel, 1985; Boeters, 1969).

- Insomnia: The German Commission E approved the use of valerian for sleep disorders, insomnia, and restlessness based on nervous disorders (Blumenthal *et al.*, 1998). The European Scientific Cooperative on Phytotherapy (ESCOP) notes that valerian is used for "tenseness, restlessness, and irritability, with difficulty in falling asleep" (ESCOP, 1997). These approved indications are supported by numerous clinical trials of varying size, design, and duration for various types of valerian preparations (i.e., valerian only, valerian with other sedative herbs, and valepotriate-only preparations) (Dominguez *et al.*, 2000; Dorn, 2000; Donath *et al.*, 2000; Cerny and Schmid, 1999; Rodenbeck *et al.*, 1998; Schmitz and Jackel, 1998; Dressing *et al.*, 1996; Orth-Wagner, 1995; Schultz *et al.*, 1994; Dressing and Reimann, 1992; Lindahl and Lindwall, 1989; Balderer and Borberly, 1985; Leatherwood and Chauffard, 1985; Gessner and Klasser, 1984; Leatherwood *et al.*, 1982).

OTHER POTENTIAL USES

- Increased mood related to enhanced sleep (Vorbach *et al.*, 1996; Kamm-Kohl *et al.*, 1984)
- Fibromyalgia (as bath) (Ammer and Melnizky, 1999)

DOSAGE
Internal
INFUSIONS: 2–3 g of fresh or dried root per cup, one to several times daily (Blumenthal et al., 1998).

TINCTURE: 1/2–1 teaspoon (1–3 ml), one to several times daily (Blumenthal et al., 1998).

EXTRACTS: Amount equivalent to 2–3 g of crude herb, one to several times daily (Blumenthal, et al., 1998).

TEA OR DRY EXTRACT (sleep aid): Single dose 1/2 to 1 hour before bedtime, with an earlier dose in the evening, if necessary (ESCOP, 1997). For adults, the dose should be in proportion to body weight; use as a tea infusion or dry extract. Children from 3–12 years old should use valerian only under medical supervision (ESCOP, 1997).

External
BATH: 100 g for one full bath; equivalent preparations (Blumenthal et al., 1998).

INFUSION: 2–3 g, in 150 ml water (Blumenthal, et al., 1998).

DURATION OF ADMINISTRATION
Many authoritative sources have set no time limit for the use of valerian (Blumenthal et al., 1998; ESCOP, 1997; WHO, 1999; Upton, 1999). Although long-term valerian use in European clinical practice indicates relative safety, clinical trials of longer than 30 days have not been conducted.

CHEMISTRY
Valerian contains over 150 chemical constituents, many of which are physiologically active. The primary active constituents can be divided into four categories: the essential oils and their sesquiterpenes (e.g., valerenic acid), the iridoids (iridoid esters: valepotriates, valtrate, isovaltrate, acevaltrate, dihydrovaltrate, and isovaleroxyhydroxydihydrovaltrate [IVHD] and their degradation products [baldrinal and derivatives]), amino acids (arginine, GABA, glutamine, tyrosine), and alkaloids (Upton, 1999; Bruneton, 1999; Leung and Foster, 1996). The iridoids are chemically unstable and degrade in moisture, heat (above 40°C), or acidity (pH<3) to baldrinal and isopropylbaldrinal (Bruneton, 1999) and, therefore, are not found in most commercial preparations (Blumenthal et al., 1998). Other constituents include caffeic acid, chlorogenic acid, β-sitosterol, methyl 2-pyrrolketone, choline, tannins, gum, alkaloids, and resin (Bradley, 1992; ESCOP, 1997; Newall et al., 1996).

PHARMACOLOGICAL ACTIONS
Human
Coronary artery dilating and anti-arrhythmic effects. Valerian is included in a German heart tonic to maintain neuro-cardiac stability (Mowrey, 1986). In an open, multi-center trial of 2,243 patients with a variety of functional cardiac disorders, an herbal combination (valerian, hawthorn [Crataegus spp.], night-blooming cereus [Selenicereus grandiflorus], and camphor [Cinnamomum camphora]) was associated with improvement (Bussany-Caspari, 1986). No controlled trials have evaluated valerian's effects in patients with specific cardiovascular disorders.

Sedative-hypnotic. Case series and randomized controlled trials have demonstrated valerian extract is effective in treating mild-to-moderate sleeping disorders without adverse effects on REM sleep, and without significant hangover effects (See the table, "Clinical Studies on Valerian," at the end of this monograph).

Animal
Coronary artery dilating and anti-arrhythmic effects. Valepotriates prevented the appearance of acute coronary insufficiency, abolished vasopressin-induced arrhythmia, provoked a short-lived increase in coronary blood flow, and had moderate positive inotropic and negative chronotropic effects (Petkov, 1979). In mice, valeranone, found in small quantities in valerian and in larger amounts in its relative, Nardostachys jatamansii, exerted weak hypotensive effects (Morazzoni and Bombardelli, 1995). In cats, intravenous injection of valerian extracts produced a significant increase in coronary blood flow, a transient fall in blood pressure, and a decrease in heart rate (Zhang et al., 1982).

Spasmolytic. In guinea pig ileum, valerenic acid, valtrate, and valeranone exert a spasmolytic action through direct effects on smooth muscle (Hazelhoff et al., 1982; Wagner and Jurcic, 1979).

Sedative-hypnotic. In mice, intraperitoneal injections of valerenic acid, valerenal, and whole herb extracts produced significant sedation, ataxia, and anti-convulsant effects (Hendriks et al., 1981; Veith et al., 1986). Intraperitoneal injections of 100 mg/kg had sedative effects as strong as barbiturates, doses of 400 mg/kg led to death (Hendriks et al., 1985). In comparison with diazepam and chlorpromazine, valerian extract had weak anti-convulsive properties (Leuschner et al., 1993). Valerian root extract (Valdispert®) reduced motility and increased thiopental-induced and pentobarbital-induced sleeping time (Capasso et al., 1996; Hiller, 1996; Leuschner et al., 1993). The aroma of valerian root exerted sedative effects in mice (Buchbauer et al., 1992). In rats, valerian had sedative effects on electroencephalogram (EEG) activity (Fink and Hoelzl, 1984). Valerian extract, but not its individual chemical constituents, significantly decreased glucose metabolism in the brain (Grusla et al., 1986). Valepotriates suppressed symptoms associated with diazepam withdrawal in rats (Andreatini and Leite, 1994). This has led some authors and clinicians to propose that valerian may be useful in treating benzodiazepine withdrawal syndrome in humans (Brinker, 2001; Rasmussen, 1997). Cats given 10 mg/kg of a valerian extract by gastric lavage had a significant decrease in restless, fearful, and aggressive behaviors (vonEickstedt, 1969). Unlike diazepam, valerian did not affect spontaneous ambulation, rearing, or approach-avoidance conflict in mice in a water-lick conflict test. However, valerian and imipramine significantly inhibited immobility induced by a forced swimming test in rats, and significantly reversed reserpine-induced hypothermia in mice, leading researchers to conclude that valerian may be a useful antidepressant (Sakamoto et al., 1992).

In vitro
Valerian extracts containing amino acids and valerenic acid bind weakly with the GABA (A) receptor in rat brain assays (Ferreira et al., 1996; Holzl and Godau, 1989; Mennini et al., 1993). In rat brain cortex, aqueous extract of valerian inhibited the uptake and stimulated the release of GABA, leading to increased concentrations of GABA in synaptic clefts (Santos et al., 1994a; 1994b; 1994c); these effects may be due in part to the presence of GABA in valerian root extracts (Cavadas et al., 1995), or may be due to valerenic acid's ability to inhibit GABA breakdown (Riedel et al., 1982; Wichtl and Bisset, 1994; Hendriks et al., 1981).

MECHANISM OF ACTION

Although the sedative effects of valerian have been demonstrated in human clinical studies, scientists have struggled to agree upon the single chemical compound responsible for valerian's activity. Valerian's effects on the central nervous system (CNS) have been attributed variously to valepotriates, their breakdown products (baldrinals), valerenic acid, valerenal, and valeranone, and other constituents in the essential oil (Wichtl and Bisset, 1994; Bradley, 1992; Houghton, 1988; Hendriks, et al., 1981, 1985; Hendriks, 1977; Holzl, 1998; Wagner, 1980). Multiple compounds may work together synergistically to produce a sedative effect (Upton et al., 1999; Houghton 1999; Weiss and Fintelmann, 2000). Animal studies show that valerenic acid may inhibit enzymes that break down GABA, thus increasing GABA levels and producing a CNS-depressing effect (Newall et al., 1996). An in vitro study to elucidate the sedative activity of valerian demonstrated that valerian extract LI 156 acted upon the melatonin receptor in a dose-dependent manner. This effect was not associated with valerenic acid (Fauteck et al., 1996).

CONTRAINDICATIONS

As a general precaution, the WHO contraindicates the use of valerian during pregnancy and lactation, and for children younger than 12 years without medical supervision (WHO, 1999). ESCOP also mentions these same precautions, but contraindicates valerian in children less than three years old. However, German authorities note that the clinical use of valerian in pediatrics is permissible beginning at age three, as long as valepotriate- and baldrinal-free preparations are used (Schilcher, 1997).

PREGNANCY AND LACTATION: ESCOP and the WHO contraindicate valerian during pregnancy due to fact that its safety during pregnancy has not been established clinically (ESCOP, 1997; WHO, 1999). However, in pregnant rats given valepotriates for 30 days, there was no impact on fertility, no fetotoxicity, and no other adverse effect on mother or offspring (Tufik et al., 1994). Research on potential mutagenicity and carcinogenicity of valerian preparations has shown that official valerian preparations are extremely low in valepotriates and that these compounds are mostly destroyed in the extraction process (Bos et al., 1998; WHO, 1999).

ADVERSE EFFECTS

Unlike benzodiazepines, valerian appears to cause no residual morning sleepiness; however, it may slightly impair judgment and driving ability for two to three hours after intake (Gerhard et al., 1996). Chronic use of high doses of valerian (530 mg to 2 gm per dose, five times per day) for many years raised the possibility that withdrawal symptoms may occur if the herb is discontinued abruptly as documented in a case report of a 58 year-old man who had been taking valerian with numerous conventional drugs (Garges et al., 1998). An authoritative German pharmaceutical text (Hobbs, 1979), suggests that continued use may cause minor side effects e.g., headaches, excitability, and insomnia, but subsequent review by the German Commission E did not find sufficient basis to include this side effect in its official monograph on valerian originally published in 1985 and revised in 1990. Cytotoxic effects have been reported in vitro, but the compounds responsible for these effects (valepotriates) decompose rapidly during storage and following oral administration (Bos et al., 1998; Bounthanh et al., 1981). In a study of 23 patients taking a nonprescription valerian extract preparation (doses from 0.5 to 12.0 grams), no acute or subclinical evidence of liver damage was observed (Chan, 1998; Chan et al., 1995). The adverse effects of valerian include rare cases of headache and upset stomach (Leathwood and Chauffard, 1982; Leathwood et al., 1982; Schulz et al., 2001). However, an intentional overdose as high as 20 grams, 20 times the normal daily dose of powdered root in capsules (40–50 capsules at 470 mg per capsule), was not associated with significant morbidity. The patient was released from the hospital within 24 hours of admission (Willey et al., 1995). In one report of intentional abuse, a young adult drug user attempted to induce a psychoactive effect by injecting an alcoholic solution of valerian; he became ill, but recovered over the next three days (Mullins and Horowitz, 1998).

DRUG INTERACTIONS

Animal studies suggest that valerian may potentiate the sedative effects of barbiturates (Brinker, 2001; Hendriks et al., 1981; Hiller, 1996; Leuschner et al., 1993; Sakamoto et al., 1992). Although some authors have speculated on potential interactions between valerian, alcohol, barbiturates, and benzodiazepines in humans, no such interactions have been documented (Braeckow et al., 1972; Brinker, 2001; Miller, 1998). One study found no potentiating effects of valerian on alcohol's impact on concentration, attentiveness, reaction time, or driving performance (Albrecht, 1995).

AMERICAN HERBAL PRODUCTS ASSOCIATION (AHPA) SAFETY RATING

CLASS 1: Herbs that can be safely consumed when used appropriately (McGuffin et al., 1997).

REGULATORY STATUS

AUSTRIA: Official in Austrian Pharmacopoeia (Meyer-Buchtela, 1999; Upton, 1999).

BELGIUM: Oral use as Traditional Herbal Medicine (THM), accepted for specific indications (Bradley, 1992).

CANADA: Dried root in tablet, capsule, powder, extract, tincture, or tea bags labeled as THM indicated as sleep aid or sedative; requires premarket authorization and assignment of a Drug Identification Number (DIN) and conformance with the Valerian Labeling Standard (Health Canada, 1996).

EUROPEAN UNION: "Whole," dried, underground parts containing no less than (NLT) 0.5% volatile oil, and "cut," dried, underground parts (NLT 0.3% volatile oil; NLT 0.17% sesquiterpenic acids), official in European Pharmacopoeia (Ph. Eur., 2001).

FRANCE: Oral use as THM accepted for specified indications (Bradley, 1992). Dried root (NLT 0.5% volatile oil), official in French Pharmacopoeia (Upton, 1999).

GERMANY: Dried root, for preparation of tea infusion, tincture, or extract is an approved nonprescription drug of the German Commission E Monographs (Blumenthal et al., 1998). Tea infusion and hydro-alcoholic tincture forms are approved nonprescription drugs of the German Standard License monographs (Braun et al., 1986 and 1996). Extract or volatile oil for balneotherapy (bath therapy) is approved in the German Commission B8 Monographs (Wichtl and Bisset, 1994). Dry native extract, 3–6:1 (w/w), is official in German Pharmacopoeia (DAB, 1999). The mother tincture (and liquid dilutions) of dried root are official preparations of the German Homeopathic Pharmacopoeia (GHP, 1993)

ITALY: Dried root (NLT 0.5% volatile oil) official in *Italian Pharmacopoeia* (Ph. Ital. 1991).

RUSSIAN FEDERATION: Official in *State Pharmacopoeia of the Union of Soviet Socialist Republics* (Bradley, 1992; Newall *et al.*, 1996).

SWEDEN: Classified as Natural Remedy for self-medication requiring advance application for marketing authorization. A valerian monograph is published in the Medical Products Agency (MPA) "Authorised Natural Remedies," which lists four registered monopreparations, and 10 multiple-herb (with passionflower, lemon balm, or hops) preparations (MPA, 1997 and 2001; Tunón, 1999). Two valerian products (Baldrian-Dispert and Neurol) are regulated as *Pharmaceutical Specialties*, or conventional over-the-counter (OTC) drugs (Tunón, 1999).

SWITZERLAND: Herbal medicine with positive classification (List D) by the *Interkantonale Kontrollstelle für Heilmittel* (IKS) and corresponding sales category D with sale limited to pharmacies and drugstores, without prescription (Morant and Ruppanner, 2001; Ruppanner and Schaefer, 2000). There are 62 valerian phytomedicines and 11 homeopathic preparations listed in the *Swiss Codex 2000/01* (Ruppanner and Schaefer, 2000). Dried root official in *Swiss Pharmacopoeia* 1997 (Meyer-Buchtela, 1999; Upton, 1999).

U.K.: *General Sale List* (GSL), Schedule 1, Table A (Bradley, 1992). Dried root (NLT 0.5% volatile oil) and powdered dried root (NLT 0.3% volatile oil) official in *British Pharmacopoeia* (Health Canada, 1996; Upton, 1999).

U.S.: Generally Recognized as Safe (GRAS) (US FDA, 1998). Dietary supplement (USC, 1994). Application for OTC approval for use as a nighttime sleep aid is pending (Pinco and Israelsen, 1994). Valerian root (NLT 0.5% volatile oil; NLT 0.05% valerenic acid) and powdered valerian (NLT 0.3% volatile oil; NLT 0.04% valerenic acid) are official in *U.S. National Formulary* (USP, 2002). Powdered valerian extract, 4–7:1 (*w/w*) (NLT 0.3% valerenic acid) added to NF 19 1st Supplement (USP, 2000). The mother tincture 1:10 (*w/v*), 55% alcohol (*v/v*), of fresh or dried root, is an OTC Class C drug official in *Homeopathic Pharmacopoeia of the United States* (HPUS, 1993).

CLINICAL REVIEW

Twenty-nine studies are outlined in the following table, "Clinical Studies on Valerian," including more than 5,200 participants. All studies found positive effects for indications including anxiety, sleep disorders, and mood. Five studies (480 participants) report on the effectiveness of valerian for anxiety (Bourin *et al.*, 1997; Sousa *et al.*, 1992; Kohnen and Oswald, 1988; Panijel, 1985; Boeters, 1969). The majority of clinical trials have consistently demonstrated that valerian is significantly more effective than a placebo in improving sleep in persons with sleep disturbances (Balderer and Borbely, 1985; Chauffard *et al.*, 1982; Dressing *et al.*, 1996; Donath *et al.*, 2000; Dorn, 2000; Dressing and Riemann, 1992; Gessner and Klasser, 1984; Jansen, 1977; Kamm-Kohl *et al.*, 1984; Leathwood and Chauffard, 1982, 1985; Leathwood *et al.*, 1982; Lindahl and Lindwall, 1989; Orth-Wagner *et al.*, 1995; Rodenbeck *et al.*, 1998; Schellenberg *et al.*, 1994; Schmidt-Voigt, 1986; Schmitz and Jackel, 1998; Schulz *et al.*, 1994; Vorbach *et al.*, 1996). Modern human studies have investigated the use of valerian in combination with hops, as an alternative to benzodiazepine to treat nonchronic and nonpsychiatric sleep disorders (Schmitz and Jackel, 1998); its use in combination with hops as a sedative to treat disturbed sleep

(Fussel *et al.*, 2000; Vonderheid-Guth *et al.*, 2000; Lataster *et al.*, 1996; Vorbach *et al.*, 1996; Kammerer, 1993); its effects in combination with hops on driving safety (Gerhard *et al.*, 1996; Kammerer *et al.*, 1996); its use in combination with St. John's wort (*Hypericum perforatum*) as an alternative to diazepam to treat symptoms of anxiety (Panijel, 1985); and its use in combination with camphor, night-blooming cereus (*Selenicereus grandiflorus*), and hawthorn (*Crataegus* spp.) to treat functional cardiovascular disorders, hypotension, or meteorosensitivity (Busanny-Caspari, 1986). Three double-blind, placebo-controlled (DB, PC) studies concluded that valerian in combination with lemon balm (*Melissa officinalis*) improved sleep quality for insomniacs (Dressing *et al.*, 1996; Dressing and Reimann, 1992), and did not impair driving or operating heavy machinery (Albrecht *et al.*, 1995). A randomized (R), DB, PC, crossover study found a combination of valerian, hops, and lemon balm helpful for individuals experiencing sleep difficulties (Lindahl and Lindwall, 1989). A recent R, DB, controlled study concluded that valerian did not adversely influence alertness, reaction time, or concentration (Kuhlmann *et al.*, 1999).

The approved modern therapeutic applications for valerian appear to be supported by its history of use in well-established systems of traditional and conventional medicine, *in vitro* and *in vivo* pharmacological experiments on animals, extensive phytochemical investigations, and human clinical studies, all of which tend to show valerian's central nervous system-depressant activities (Blumenthal *et al.*, 2000).

BRANDED PRODUCTS*

Alluna™: GlaxoSmithKline / One Franklin Plaza / Philadelphia, PA 19102 / U.S.A. / Tel: 888-825-5249 / www.gsk.com. Each tablet contains 500 mg valerian extract (4-6:1) with 120 mg hops extract (5-7:1).

Euphytose®: Roche Nicholas SA / 33 rue de l'Industrie / 74240 Gaillard / France / Tel: +33-04-50-87-7070. Six herbs, including *Crataegus, Ballota, Passiflora, Valeriana, Cola*, and *Paullinia*.

Euvegal® forte: Dr. Willmar Schwabe Pharmaceuticals / International Division / Willmar Schwabe Str. 4, D-76227 / Karlsruhe / Germany / Tel: +49-721-4005 ext. 294 / www.schwabepharma.com / Email: melville-eaves@schwabe.de. Each tablet contains 160 mg valerian root extract 4.5:1 and 80 mg lemon balm leaf extract 5.5:1.

Harmonicum Much®: Prof. Dr. Much AG. Information on manufacturer and current product status unavailable.

Hova®: Gebro Pharma GmbH / A-6391 Fieberbrunn / Austria / Tel: +43-53-54-5300-0 / Fax: +43-53-54-5300-0 / www.gebro.com / E-mail: pharma@gebro.com. Each tablet contains 60 mg valerian and 30 mg hop flower extract.

Ivel®: Kanoldt Arzneimittel GmbH / c/o Knoll AG / Knollstrasse 50 / 67008 Ludwigshafen / Germany / Tel: +49-06-21-5890 / Fax: +49-06-21-5892-896 / www.knoll.de / Email: info@knoll.de. Each tablet contains 500 mg valerian extract (4-6:1) with 120 mg hops extract (5-7:1).

LI 156: Lichtwer Pharma AG / Wallenroder Strasse 8-14 / 13435 / Berlin / Germany / Tel: +49-30-40-3700 / Fax: +49-30-40-3704-49 / www.lichtwer.de. Each tablet contains 300 mg dry extract of valerian with a drug/extract ratio of 5:1.

Nature's Way® Valerian Root capsules: Nature's Way Products, Inc. / 10 Mountain Spring Parkway / Springville, UT 84663 / U.S.A. / Tel: (801) 489-1500 / www.naturesway.com. Each capsule contains 530 mg valerian root with a guaranteed natural potency of 0.1% valerenic acids.

Novo-Baldriparan®: Novo-Nordisk A/S / Novo Allé / 2880 Bagsværd / Denmark / Tel: +45-4444-8888 / Fax: +45-4449-0555 / E-mail: webmaster@novonordisk.com. This product is no longer available.

ReDormin®: Zeller AG / Seeblickstrasse 4 / CH-8590 Romanshorn 1 / Switzerland / www.zellerag.ch. Contains valerian extract ZE91019.

Sedariston® Konzentrat: Steiner Arzneimittel / Postfach 450520 / 12175 Berlin / Germany / Tel: +49-03-07-1094-0 / Fax: +49-03-07-1250-12 / www.steinerarznei-berlin.de. Tablets each contain 50 mg of valerian and 100 mg of St. John's wort.

Sedonium®: Lichtwer Pharma AG. Contains valerian extract LI 156.

Songha Night®: Pharmaton Natural Health Products / P.O. Box 368 / Ridgefield, CT 06877 / U.S.A. / Tel: 800-451-6688 / Fax: 203-798-5771 / www.pharmaton.com / Email: askpharmaton@rdg.boehringer-ingelheim.com. Each coated tablet contains 120 mg valerian extract and 80 mg lemon balm extract.

Valdispert®: Solvay Arzneimittel GmbH / Hans-Bockler-Allee 20 / Hannover 30173 / Germany / Tel: +49-511-8-5724e +006 / Fax: +49-511-8-57312e +006 / www.solvay.com. Unable to verify dosage or manufacturing status.

Valdispert® forte: Solvay Arzneimittel GmbH. Each tablet contains 45 mg *Valeriana officinalis* radix dry aqueous alkaline extract (5–6:1), corresponding to 225–270 mg of dried root, standardized to contain 0.05 mg valerenic acid and acetoxyvalerenic acid.

Valerina Natt®: Pharbio Medical International AB / c/o Cederroth International AB / Box 715 / S-19427 Upplands Väsby / Sweden / Tel: +46-85-90-9630-0 / Fax: +46-85-90-9647-1 / Email: info@cederroth.com / www.pharbio.cederroth.com. Contains 100 mg valerian extract (4:1), corresponding to 400 mg dried root; 45 mg hops (*Humulus lupulus*) extract (8.5:1), corresponding to 382 mg dried strobile; 25 mg lemon balm (*Melissa officinalis*) leaf extract (6.5:1), corresponding to 162 mg dried leaf; and 275 mg of excipient materials.

Valmane®: Lyssia GmbH / c/o Solvay Arzneimittel GmbH. Each tablet contains 50 mg of a valepotriate mixture. Unable to verify current availability of product.

Valverde®: Ciba-Geigy AG / Novartis Consumer Health AG / Route de l'Etraz / CH 1260 Nyon 1 / Switzerland / www.consumer-health.novartis.com. This product is no longer available.

Ze91019: Zeller AG / Seeblickstrasse 4 / CH-8590 Romanshorn 1 / Switzerland / www.zellerag.ch. Extract used in Alluna™ Sleep, Ivel®, and ReDormin®.

* American equivalents, if any, are found in the Product Table beginning on page 398.

REFERENCES

Albrecht M. Psychopharmaceuticals and safety in traffic. *Z Allg Med* 1995;71:1215–21.

Albrecht M, Bergner W, Laux P, Martin C. Psychopharmaceuticals and traffic safety: The influence of Euvegal® forte sugar-coated tablets on driving ability and combination effects with alcohol. *Zeitschrift fur Allgemein Medizin* 1995;71:1215–1225.

Ammer K, Melnizky P. Medicinal baths for treatment of generalized fibromyalgia. [in German]. *Forsch Komplementarmed* 1999;6:80–5.

Andreatini R, Leite J. Effect of valepotriates on the behavior of rats in the elevated plus-maze during diazepam withdrawal. *Eur J Pharmacol* 1994;260:233–5.

Anon. Herb sales in the mainstream market –1998 vs. 1997. Information Resources Inc.; 1999.

Balderer G, Borbely A. Effect of valerian on human sleep. *Psychopharmacology* 1985;87:406–9.

BHP. *British Herbal Pharmacopoeia (BHP)*. Exeter: British Herbal Medicine Association; 1996.

Blumenthal M. Herb sales down 15% in mainstream market. *HerbalGram* 2001;51:69.

Blumenthal M, Busse WR, Goldberg A, Gruenwald J, Hall T, Riggins CW, Rister RS (eds.). Klein S, Rister RS (trans.). *The Complete German Commission E Monographs—Therapeutic Guide to Herbal Medicines*. Austin, TX: American Botanical Council; Boston: Integrative Medicine Communication; 1998; 226–7.

Blumenthal M, Goldberg A, Brinckmann J. *Herbal Medicine: Expanded Commission E Monographs*. Newton, MA: Integrative Medicine Communications; 2000;394–7.

Boeters U. Treatment of control disorders of the autonomic nervous system with valepotriate (Valmane®). *Munch Med Wochenschr* 1969;111:1873–6.

Bos R, Hendriks H, Scheffer J, Woerdenbag H. Cytotoxic potential of valerian constituents and valerian tinctures. *Phytomedicine* 1998;5:219–25.

Bos R, Woerdenbag HJ, DeSmet PAGM, Scheffer JJC. *Valeriana* species. In: *Adverse Effects of Herbal Drugs* Vol. 3. DeSmet PAGM, Keller K, Hänsel R, Chandler RF. New York: Springer-Verlag, 1997;165–80.

Bounthanh C, Bergmann C, Beck J, Haag-Berrurier M, Anton R. Valepotriates, a new class of cytotoxic and antitumor agents. *Planta Med* 1981;41:21–8.

Bourin M, Bougerol T, Guitton B, Broutin E. A combination of plant extracts in the treatment of outpatients with adjustment disorder with anxious mood: controlled study versus placebo. *Fundamental & Clin Pharmacol* 1997;11:127–32.

Boyle W. *Official Herbs: Botanical Substances in the United States Pharmacopeia–1820–1990*. East Palestine, OH: Buckeye Naturopathic Press, 1991.

BP. *British Pharmacopoeia* (BP). London: Her Majesty's Stationery Office; 1988.

Bradley P (ed.). *British Herbal Compendium — A Handbook of Scientific Information on Widely Used Plant Drugs*, Volume I. Exeter, U.K.: British Herbal Medicine Association (BHMA); 1992;214–8.

Braeckow R, Eickstedt K, Kuhne U. Effects of chlorpromazine and valtratum on ethanol anesthesia and ethanol blood level. *Arzneimittelforschung* 1972;22:1977–80.

Braun R, Surmann P, Wendt R, Wichtl M, Ziegenmeyer J (eds.). Baldrianwurzerl. In: *Standardzulassungen für Fertigarzneimittel–Text und Kommentar*, 11. Ergänzungslieferung. Stuttgart, Germany: Deutscher Apotheker Verlag; Zulassungsnummer; 1996 Feb;6199.99.99.

Braun R, *et al.* (eds.). Baldriantinktur. In: *Standardzulassungen für Fertigarzneimittel–Text und Kommentar*. Stuttgart, Germany: Deutscher Apotheker Verlag; Zulassungsnummer; 1986;6099.99.99.

Braeckow R, Eickstedt K, Kuhne U. Effects of chlorpromazine and valtratum on ethanol anesthesia and ethanol blood level. [in German]. *Arzneimittelforschung* 1972;22:1977–80.

Brinker F. *Herb Contraindications and Drug Interactions*, 3d ed. Sandy, OR: Eclectic Institute; 2001:196–7.

Brown D. *Herbal Prescriptions for Better Health,* 2nd ed. Rocklin, CA: Prima Publishing; 2000.

Bruneton, J. *Pharmacognosy, Phytochemistry, Medicinal Plants*. Paris: Lavoisier Publishing; 1999;595–600.

Buchbauer G, Jager W, Jirovetz L, Meyer F, Dietrich H. Effects of valerian root oil, borneol, isoborneol, bornyl acetate and isobornyl acetate on the motility of laboratory animals (mice) after inhalation. [in German]. *Pharmazie* 1992;47:620–2.

Busanny-Caspari Eea. Indications: Functional heart complaints, hypotension and weather sensitivity. [in German]. *Therapiewoche* 1986;36:2545–50.

Capasso A, DeFeo V, DeSimone F, Sorrentino L. Pharmacological effects of aqueous extract from *Valeriana*. *Phytother Res* 1996;10:309–12.

Cavadas C, Araujo I, Cotrim M, *et al. In vitro* study on the interaction of *Valeriana officinalis* L. extracts and their amino acids on GABA-A receptor in rat brain. [in German]. *Arzneimittelforschung* 1995;45:753–5.

Cerny A, Schmid K. Tolerability and efficacy of valerian/lemon balm in healthy volunteers (a double-blind, placebo-controlled, multicentre study). *Fitoterapia* 1999;70(3):221–8.

Chan T. An assessment of the delayed effects associated with valerian overdose [letter]. *Int J Clin Pharmacol Ther* 1998;36:569.

Chan T, Tang C, Critchley J. Poisoning due to an over-the-counter hypnotic sleep-Qik (hyoscine, cyproheptadine, valerian). *Postgrad Med J* 1995;71:227–8.

Chauffard F, Heck E, Leathwood P. Detection of mild sedative effects: Valerian and sleep in man. *Experientia* 1982;37:622.

DAB. See: *Deutsches Azneibuch*.

Deutsches Arzneibuch (DAB Ergänzungsbuch 1999). Stuttgart, Germany: Deutscher Apotheker Verlag. 1999.

Dominguez R, Bravo-Valverde R, Kaplowitz B, Cott J. Valerian as a hypnotic for Hispanic patients. *Cultur Divers Ethni Minor Psychol* 2000 Feb;6(1):84–92.

Donath F, Quispes S, Diefenbach K, *et al.* Critical evaluation of the effect of valerian extract on sleep structure and sleep quality. *Pharmacopsychiatry* 2000;33:47–53.

Dorn M. Efficacy and tolerability of Baldrian versus oxazepam in non-organic and non-psychiatric insomniacs: a randomized, double-blind, clinical, comparative study. [in German]. *Forsch Komplementarmed Klass Naturheilkd* 2000, Apr;7(2):79–84.

Dressing H, Kohler S, Muller W. Improvement in sleep quality with a high dose valerian-melissa preparation. *Psychopharmacotherapy* 1996;3:123–30.

Dressing H, Riemann D. Insomnia: are *Valeriana/Melissa* combinations of equal value to benzodiazepine? [in German]. *Therapiewoche* 1992;42:726–36.

Drozdov D. Use of aminazine with valerian in hypertensive disease. *Vrach Delo* 1975;48–50.

ESCOP. Valeriana radix. Monographs on the medicinal uses of plants. Exeter: European Scientific Cooperative on Phytotherapy; 1997.

Europäisches Arzneibuch, 3rd ed. Stuttgart: Deutscher Apotheker Verlag; 1997.

European Pharmacopoeia (Ph. Eur.) (3rd edition 1997, Supplement 2001). Strasbourg, France: Council of Europe; 2001;1575–7.

Farmacopea Ufficiale della Repubblica Italiana (Ph.Ital. IX 1985 suppl. 1991). Rome, Italy:Ministero della Sanita; 1991.

Fauteck J–D, Pietz B, Winteroff H, Wittkowski W. Interaction of *Valerian officinalis* with melatonin receptors: A possible explanation of its biological action. [Abstract]. 2nd International Congress on Phytomedicine. Munich, Germany, September 11–14,1996.

Ferreira F, Santos M, Faro C, *et al.* Effect of extracts of *Valeriana officinalis* on [3H] GABA. *Revista Portuguesa de Farmacia* 1996;46:74–7.

Fink C, Hoelzl J. Wirkungen vonvaltrat auf das EEG des isoliert perfundierten ratenhirns. *Arzneimittelforshung* 1984;34:170–4.

Flynn R, Roest M. *Your guide to standardized herbal products.* Prescott, AZ: One World Press; 1995.

Fugh-Berman A, Cott J. Dietary supplements and natural products as psychotherapeutic agents. *Psychosom Med* 1999;61:712–28.

Fussel A, Wolf A, Brattström A. Effect of a Fixed Valerian-Hop Extract Combination (Ze 9109) on Sleep Polygraphy in Patients with Non-organic Insomnia: A Pilot Study. *Eur J Med Res* 2000;5:385-390.

Garges H, Varia I, Doraiswamy P. Cardiac complications and delirium associated with valerian root withdrawal [letter]. *JAMA* 1998;280:1566–7.

Gerhard U, Linnenbrink N, Georghiadou C, Hobi V. Vigilance-decreasing effects of 2 plant-derived sedatives. *Schweiz Rundsch Med Prax* 1996 April;85(15):473–81.

German Homeopathic Pharmacopoeia (GHP), 1st ed. 1978 with supplements through 1991. Translation of the German "*Homöopathisches Arzneibuch* (HAB 1), Amtliche Ausgabe." Stuttgart, Germany: Deutscher Apotheker Verlag; 1993;893–5.

Gessner B, Klasser M. Studies on the effect of Harmonicum Much® on sleep using polygraphic EEG recordings. *EEG EMG Z Elektroenzephalogr Verwandte Geb* 1984;15:45–51.

GHP. See: *German Homeopathic Pharmacopoeia.*

Grieve M. *A Modern Herbal.* New York: Dover Publishers; 1979;824 –8.

Grusla D, Holzl J, Kriegelstein J. Activity of valerian in the rat brain. [in German]. *Deutsche Apotheker Zeitung* 1986;126:2249–53.

Hazelhoff B, Malingre T, Meijer D. Antispasmodic effects of valeriana compounds: an *in-vivo* and *in-vitro* study on the guinea-pig ileum. *Archives Internationales de Pharmacodynamie et de Ther* 1982;257:274–87.

Health Canada. *Valerian Labelling Standard.* Ottawa, Ontario: Health Canada Therapeutic Products Programme. 17. May 1996.1-6.

Hendriks H. Eugenyl isovalerate and isoeugenyl isovalerate in the essential oil of valerian root. *Phytochemistry* 1977;16:1853–4.

Hendriks H, Bos R, Allersma D, Malingre T, Koster A. Pharmacological screening of valerenal and some other components of essential oil of *Valeriana officinalis. Planta Med* 1981;42:62–8.

Hendriks H, Bos R, Woerdenbag H, Koster A. Central nervous depressant activity of valerenic acid in the mouse. *Planta Med* 1985;1:28–31.

Hiller K. Neuropharmacological studies on ethanol extracts of *Valeriana officinalis* L: Behavioral and anticonvulsant properties. *Phytother Res* 1996;10:145–51.

Hobbs C. Valerian: A literature review. *HerbalGram* 1989;21:19–34.

Hobbs H. *Hagers Handbuk der Pharmazeutischen,* Praxis; 1979. p. 25. cited in Morazzoni and Bombardelli, 1995.

Hoffmann D. *The Complete Illustrated Holistic Herbal.* Rockport, MA: Element Books Inc.; 1996.

Holzl J. Valerian–*Valeriana officinalis.* [in German]. *Z Phytother* 1998;19:47–54.

Holzl J, Godau P. Receptor binding studies with *Valeriana officinalis* on the benzodiazepine receptor. *Planta Med* 1989;55.

Homeopathic Pharmacopoeia of the United States (HPUS) — Revision Service Official

Compendium from July 1, 1992. Falls Church, VA: American Institute of Homeopathy; 1993 Dec;9413:VLRN.

Houghton PJ. The biological activity of valerian and related plants. *J Ethnopharmacol* 1988;22:121–42.

Houghton PJ. The scientific basis for the reputed activity of valerian. *J Pharm Pharmacol* 1999;51:505–12.

HPUS. See: *Homeopathic Pharmacopoeia of the United States.*

Jansen W. Double-blind study with baldrisedon. [in German]. *Therapiewoche* 1977;27:2779–86.

Kamm-Kohl A, Jansen W, Brockmann P. Moderne baldriantherapie gegen nervose storungen im senium. *Med Welt* 1984;35:1450–4.

Kammerer E. Phytogenic sedatives-hypnotics—does a combination of valerian and hops have a value in the modern drug repertoire? [in German]. *Z Arztl Fortbild (Jena)* 1993;87:401–6.

Kammerer E, Brattstöm A, Herberg K-W. Effects of a hop-valerian combination on fitness and driving safety. *Der Bay Int* 1996;16(3):32-36.

Kohnen·R, Oswald W. The effects of valerian, propranolol, and their combination on activation, performance, and mood of healthy volunteers under social stress conditions. *Pharmacopsychiatry* 1988;21:447–8.

Kuhlmann J, Berger W, Podzuweit H, Schmidt U. The influence of valerian treatment on "reaction time, alertness and concentration" in volunteers. *Pharmacopsyciatry* 1999;32:235–41.

Lataster MJ, Brattström A. The treatment of patients with sleep disorders: efficacy of tolerance of valerian-hop tablets. *Notabene Medici* 1996;4:182-185.

Leathwood P, Chauffard F. Aqueous extract of valerian reduces latency to fall asleep in man. *Planta Med* 1985;144–8.

Leathwood P, Chauffard F. Quantifying the effects of mild sedatives [review]. *J Psych Res* 1982;17:115–22.

Leathwood P, Chauffard F, Heck E, Munoz-Box R. Aqueous extract of valerian root (*Valeriana officinalis* L.) improves sleep quality in man. *Pharmacol Biochem Behav* 1982;17:65–71.

Leung A, Foster S. *Encyclopedia of Common Natural Ingredients Used in Food, Drugs and Cosmetics,* 2nd ed. New York: John Wiley & Sons, Inc.; 1996.

Leuschner J, Mueller J, Rudmann M. Characterization of the central nervous depressant activity of a commercially available valerian root extract. [in German]. *Arzneimittelforschung* 1993;43:638–41.

Lindahl O, Lindwall L. Double blind study of a valerian preparation. *Pharmacol Biochem Behav* 1989;32:1065–6.

Lloyd JU. *Origin and History of All the Pharmacopoeial Vegetable Drugs.* Cincinnati, OH: Caxton Press, 1929.

Mayer B, Springer E. Psychoexperimental studies on the effect of a valepotriate combination as well as the combined effects of valtratum and alcohol. [in German]. *Arzneimittelforschung* 1974;24:2066–70.

McGuffin M, Hobbs C, Upton R, Goldberg A. *American Herbal Products Association's Botanical Safety Handbook: Guidelines for the Safe Use and Labeling for Herbs of Commerce.* Boca Raton: CRC Press; 1997.

Medical Products Agency (MPA). Naturläkemedel: Authorised Natural Remedies (as of January 24, 2001). Uppsala, Sweden: Medical Products Agency. 2001.

Medical Products Agency (MPA). Naturläkemedelsmonografi: Valeriana. Uppsala, Sweden: Medical Products Agency. 1997.

Mennini T, Bernasconi P, Bombardelli E, Morazzoni P. *In vitro* study on the interaction of extracts and pure compounds from *Valeriana officinalis* roots with GABA, benzodiazepine and barbiturate receptors in rat brain. *Fitoterapia* 1993;64:291–300.

Meyer-Buchtela E. *Tee-Rezepturen: Ein Handbuch für Apotheker und Ärzte.* Stuttgart, Germany: Deutscher Apotheker Verlag. 1999;Baldrianwurzel.

Miller L. Herbal medicinals: selected clinical considerations focusing on known or potential drug-herb interactions. *Arch Intern Med* 1998;158:2200–11.

Morant J, Ruppanner H (eds.). *Arzneimittel-Kompendium der Schweiz® 2001.* Basel, Switzerland: Documed AG. 2001.

Morazzoni P, Bombardelli E. *Valeriana officinalis*: traditional use and recent evaluation of activity. *Fitoterapia* 1995;66:99–112.

Mowrey D. *The Scientific Validation of Herbal Medicine.* New Canaan, Conn.: Keats Pub; 1986; 316.

MPA. See: Medical Products Agency.

Mullins M, Horowitz B. The case of the salad shooters: intravenous injection of wild lettuce extract. *Vet & Human Toxicol* 1998;40:290–1.

Newall C, Anderson L, Phillipson J. *Herbal Medicines: A Guide for Health-Care Professionals.* London: Pharmaceutical Press; 1996;260–2.

Orth-Wagner S, Ressin W, Friederich I. Phytosedative for sleeping disorders containing extracts from valerian root, hop grains and balm leaves. [in German]. *Z Phytother* 1995;16:147–52, 155–6.

Panijel M. Treatment of moderately severe anxiety states. [in German]. *Therapiewoche* 1985;35:4659–68.

Petkov V. Plants and hypotensive, antiatheromatous and coronarodilating action.

Amer J Chinese Med 1979;7:197–236.

Ph. Eur. See: *European Pharmacopoeia.*

Ph. Ital. See: *Farmacopea Ufficiale della Repubblica Italiana.*

Pinco RG, Israelsen LD. European-American Phytomedicines Coalition Citizen Petition to Amend FDA's Monograph on Nighttime Sleep-aid Drug Products for Over-the-Counter ("OTC") Human Use to Include Valerian; 1994.

Rasmussen P. A role for phytotherapy in the treatment of benzodiazepine and opiate drug withdrawal. *Eur J Herb Med* 1997;3:11–21.

Riedel E, Hansel R, Ehrke G. Inhibition of gamma-aminobutyric acid catabolism by valerenic acid derivatives. *Planta Med* 1982;48:219–20.

Rodenbeck A, Simen S, Cohrs S, et al. Alterations of the sleep stage structure as a feature of GABAergic effects of a valerian-hop preparation in patients with psychophysiological insomnia. *Somnologie* 1998;2:26–31.

Ruppanner H, Schaefer U (eds.). *Codex 2000/01 — Die Schweizer Arzneimittel in einem Griff.* Basel, Switzerland: Documed AG. 2000.

Sakamoto T, Mitani Y, Nakajima K. Psychotropic effects of Japanese valerian root extract. *Chem & Pharm Bull* 1992;40:758–61.

Santos M, Ferreira F, Cunha A, et al. An aqueous extract of valerian influences the transport of GABA in synaptosomes. *Planta Med* 1994a;60:278–279.

Santos M, Ferreira F, Cunha A, et al. Synaptosomal GABA release as influenced by valerian root extract: Involvement of the GABA carrier. *Archives Internationales de Pharmacodynamie et de Therapie.* 1994b;327:220–31.

Santos M, Ferreira F, Faro C, et al. The amount of GABA present in aqueous extracts of valerian is sufficient to account for [3H]GABA release in synaptosomes [letter]. *Planta Med* 1994c;60:475–6.

Schellenberg R, Schwartz A, Schellenberg V, Jahing L. Quantitative EEG-monitoring and psychometric evaluation of the therapeutic efficacy of Biral N in psychosomatic diseases. *Naturamed* 1994;4:9.

Schilcher H. *Phytotherapy in Pediatrics: Handbook for Physicians and Pharmacists,* 2nd ed. Stuttgart: Medpharm Scientific Publishers; 1997;58–61,181.

Schmidt-Voigt J. Treatment of nervous sleep disorders and unrest with a sedative of purely vegetable origin. [in German]. *Therapiewoche* 1986;36:663–7.

Schmitz M, Jackel M. Comparative study for assessing quality of life of patients with exogenous sleep disorders (temporary sleep onset and sleep interruption disorders) treated with a hops-valerian preparation and a benzodiazepine drug. [in German]. *Wien Med Wochenscr* 1998;148:291–8.

Schulz H, Stolz C, Mueller J. The effect of valerian extract on sleep polygraphy in poor sleepers: A pilot study. *Pharmacopsychiatry* 1994;27:147–51.

Schulz V, Hänsel R, Tyler VE. *Rational Phytotherapy: A Physicians' Guide to Herbal Medicine,* 4th ed. Berlin: Springer; 2001:87–97.

Sousa M, Pacheco P, Roldao V. Double-blind comparative study of the efficacy and safety of Valdispert® vs. clobazapam. *KaliChemie Medical Research and Information.* 1992.

Straube G. The importance of valerian roots in therapy. *Ther Ggw* 1968;107:555–62.

Tufik S, Fujita K, Seabra M, Lobo L. Effects of a prolonged administration of valepotriates in rats on the mothers and their offspring. *J Ethnopharmacol* 1994;41:39–44.

Tunón H. Phtyotherapie in Schweden. [in German]. *Z Phytother* 1999;20:268–77.

United States Congress (USC). Public Law 103–417: Dietary Supplement Health and Education Act of 1994. Washington, DC: 103rd Congress of the United States. 1994.

United States Food and Drug Administration (U.S. FDA). *Code of Federal Regulations,* Title 21, Part 182 – Substances Generally Recognized as Safe. Washington, DC: Office of the Federal Register National Archives and Records Administration; 1998;427–433.

United States Pharmacopeia (USP 24th Revision) *The National Formulary* (NF 19th Edition). Rockville, MD: United States Pharmacopeial Convention, Inc.; 1999;2533–2534.

United States Pharmacopeia (USP 25th Revision) *The National Formulary* (NF 20th Edition) Rockville, MD: United States Pharmacopeial Convention, Inc.; 2002.

Upton R (ed.). Valerian Root: *Valeriana officinalis.* Analytical, Quality Control, and Therapeutic Monograph. *American Herbal Pharmacopoeia and Therapeutic Compendium.* Santa Cruz, CA, USA: American Herbal Pharmacopoeia; 1999.

US FDA. See: United States Food and Drug Administration.

USC. See: United States Congress.

USP. See: *United States Pharmacopeia.*

Veith J, Schneider G, Lemmer B, Willems M. The effect of degradation products of valepotriates on the motor activity of light-dark synchronized mice. *Planta Med* 1986;179–83.

Vonderheid-Guth B, Todorova A, Brattstöm A, Dimpfel W. Pharmacodynamic effects of valerian and hops extract combination (Ze 9109) on the quantitative-topographical EEG in healthy volunteers. *Eur J Med Res* 2000;5:139-144.

vonEickstedt K. Modification of the alcohol effect by valepotriate. [in German]. *Arzneimittelforschung* 1969;19:995–7.

Vorbach E, Gortelmayer R, Bruning J. Treatment of insomnia: efficacy and tolerance of a valerian extract. [in German]. *Psychopharmakother* 1996;3:109–15.

Wagner H. Comparative studies on the sedative action of *Valeriana* extracts, valepotriates and their degradation products. *Planta Med* 1980;39:358–65.

Wagner H, Jurcic K. On the spasmolytic activity of *Valeriana* extracts. *Planta Med* 1979;37:84–6.

Weiss RF, Fintelmann V. *Herbal Medicine,* 2d ed. New York:Thieme. 2000;261–4.

WHO. *WHO Monographs on Selected Medicinal Plants Vol. I.* Geneva: World Health Organization. 1999.

Wichtl M (ed.). *Teedrogen und Phytopharmaka, 3. Auflage: Ein Handbuch für die Praxis auf wissenschaftlicher Grundlage.* Stuttgart, Germany: Wissenschaftliche Verlagsgesellschaft mbH. 1997;603–7.

Wichtl M, Bissett N. *Herbal Drugs and Phytopharmaceuticals,* 2nd ed. Stuttgart: MedPharm CRC Press; 1994;566.

Willey L, Mady S, Cobaugh D, Wax P. Valerian overdose: A case report. *Vet Human Toxicol* 1995;37:364–5.

Zhang B, Meng H, Wang T, et al. Effects of *Valeriana officinalis* L extract on cardiovascular system. [in Chinese]. *Yao Hsueh Hsueh Pao - Acta Pharmaceutica Sinica* 1982;17:382–4.

Clinical Studies on Valerian (*Valeriana officinalis* L.)

Valerian

Monograph

Anxiety

Author/Year	Subject	Design	Duration	Dosage	Preparation	Results/Conclusion
Sousa, 1992	Anxiety	R, DB, C n=80 adult patients with various anxiety syndromes		270 mg/day or 30 mg clobazam/day	Valdispert® or clobazam 30 mg/day	The valerian preparation was as effective and well-tolerated as clobazam, according to the Hamilton Anxiety Rating Scale and the Leeds anxiety questionnaire.
Kohnen and Oswald, 1988	Anxiety	DB n=48 adults placed in an experimental situation of social stress	24 hours	100 mg valerian or 20 mg propranolol or a combination of the 2	Valerian extract (brand not stated)	The valerian preparation reduced subjective sensations of anxiety, but the study did not demonstrate any difference between groups.
Boeters, 1969	Anxiety	O n=70 hospitalized patients with dysregulation of the autonomic nervous system due to various etiologies	7 days to 3 months	150–300 mg/day valepotriate mixture	Valmane®	Functional cardiac disorders, tachycardia, hypertension, sweating, restless legs, and other dysregulations were influenced positively by Valmane®. The preparation produced mildly sedative effects and was effective in treatment of restlessness and tension. Apart from mild daytime fatigue, no evidence of somatic adverse effects or psychotropic effects was observed.

Combination Preparations

Author/Year	Subject	Design	Duration	Dosage	Preparation	Results/Conclusion
Bourin et al, 1997	Anxiety	R, PC n=182 patients diagnosed with adjustment disorder and anxious mood	4 weeks	2 tablets 3x/day	Euphytose® (six herbs including *Crataegus, Ballota, Passiflora, Valeriana, Cola,* and *Paullinia*)	Significant improvement in Hamilton anxiety scores comparing combination product to placebo (p=0.012).
Panijel, 1985	Anxiety	DB, C n=100 adults suffering from anxiety disorders	2 weeks	1 tablet/day (50 mg of valerian and 100 mg of St. John's wort /day) or 2 mg diazepam 2x/day	Sedariston® Konzentrat (providing 50 mg of valerian and 100 mg of St. John's wort)	The herbal combination was reportedly effective in 78% vs. only 54% of the diazepam group (p<0.01). Side effects were reported by only 4% of those taking the herbs vs. 14% of those taking diazepam.

KEY: C – controlled, **CC** – case-control, **CH** – cohort, **CI** – confidence interval, **Cm** – comparison, **CO** – crossover, **CS** – cross-sectional, **DB** – double-blind, **E** – epidemiological, **LC** – longitudinal cohort, **MA** – meta-analysis, **MC** – multi-center, **n** – number of patients, **O** – open, **OB** – observational, **OL** – open label, **OR** – odds ratio, **P** – prospective, **PB** – patient-blind, **PC** – placebo-controlled, **PG** – parallel group, **PS** – pilot study, **R** – randomized, **RC** – reference-controlled, **RCS** – retrospective cross-sectional, **RS** - retrospective, **S** – surveillance, **SB** – single-blind, **SC** – single-center, **U** – uncontrolled, **UP** – unpublished, **VC** – vehicle-controlled.

The ABC Clinical Guide to Herbs | 361

Clinical Studies on Valerian (*Valeriana officinalis* L.) (cont.)

Sleep

Author/Year	Subject	Design	Duration	Dosage	Preparation	Results/Conclusion
Dominguez et al., 2000	Sleep	O, case study n=20 sleep questionnaires	2 weeks	1–3, 470 mg capsules before bed	Nature's Way® valerian root capsules	Global improvement at Week 2 was significantly better than at Week 1 (Wilcoxon ranks test, p=0.005), perhaps reflecting a time-dependent or dose-response relationship. This case study suggests that valerian can be an agent for improving insomnia in a symptomatic population.
Donath et al., 2000	Sleep	R, PC, DB, CO n=16 men and women with previously established psychophysiological insomnia (ICSD-code I.A.1.) (mean age 49)	Single dose and 14 days vs. placebo with 13 day washout between	Two, 300 mg capsules dry extract of valerian 1 hour before bedtime vs. placebo	Sedonium® and placebo	No effects on sleep structure and subject sleep assessment were observed after a single dose of valerian. Sleep efficiency increased significantly after multi-dose treatment for both valerian and placebo, compared to baseline polysomnography. However, slow-wave sleep (SWS) latency was reduced after multi-dose treatment with valerian compared with placebo (13.5 vs. 21.3 min., p<0.05). Compared to baseline, SWS percentage of time in bed was increased with valerian (8.1% vs. 9.8%, p<0.05). An extremely low number of adverse events were observed during the valerian treatment period compared with the placebo period (3 vs. 18). Because valerian showed positive effects on sleep structure and sleep perception of insomnia patients, the authors suggest valerian can be recommended for treatment of patients with mild psychophysiological insomnia.
Dorn, 2000	Insomnia	R, DB, Cm n=70	4 weeks	Two, 300 mg tablets 30 minutes before bedtime or 5 mg oxazepam tablet	LI 156 300 mg valerian dried extract tablets; oxazepam 5 mg	In both groups, sleep quality improved significantly (p<0.001), but no statistically significant difference could be found between groups (p=0.70). Effect varied between groups and was between 0.02 and 0.25, with a more favorable adverse effect profile of valerian compared to oxazepam. Primary outcome was measured by the factor "sleep quality". Secondary outcomes were other sleep characteristics including well-being and anxiety (HAMA).
Vorbach, 1996	Sleep quality	C n=121 patients with non-organic sleep disturbances for at least 4 weeks	4 weeks	Two, 300 mg tablets/day	Sedonium® (LI 156)	Four standard rating scales were employed. Significant improvement in sleep quality, feeling of refreshment after sleep, and well-being during the day; no significant side effects reported. Results were observed after 2–4 weeks of use, with no acute effects during first days of study.
Schulz et al., 1994	Sleep	DB, PC n=14 elderly poor sleepers	1 week	405 mg 3x/day	Valdispert® forte	Subjects in valerian group had increase in slow-wave sleep and decrease in Stage 1 sleep. There was no effect on self-reported sleep quality, sleep onset time, REM sleep time, or time awake after onset of sleep.
Balderer and Borberly, 1985	Sleep	DB, PC n=18 healthy subjects with a history of sleep disturbances	3 weeks	450 or 900 mg extract 30 minutes before bed	Aqueous valerian extract (brand not stated)	Valerian extract had mild sleep-promoting action without significant residual or "hangover" effect.
Leathwood and Chauffard, 1985	Sleep	R, PC, DB n=8 mild insomnia	1 night	450 mg and 900 mg	Aqueous valerian root extract (brand not stated)	Significantly decreased sleep latency; there was no further improvement with doubling the dose.
Gessner and Klasser, 1984	Sleep	R, DB n=11 adults	2 nights	1 or 2 capsules (60 or 120 mg)	Harmonicum Much® valepotriate preparation	Both dosages showed a decrease in sleep Stage 4 and a slight reduction of REM sleep, and slight increase of sleep Stage awake, 1, 2, and 3. Changes or Beta-intensity of EEG during REM sleep show stronger hypnotic effect for 120 mg dosage than for 60 mg dosage. Maximum effect was observed between 2 and 3 hours after medication.
Kamm-Kohl et al., 1984	Mood and sleep	PC n=80 hospitalized geriatric patients	2 weeks	6 tablets/day (482 mg valerian extract/day)	Valdispert® forte	Significant improvements in mood and behavioral disturbances, as well as sleep.

KEY: C – controlled, **CC** – case-control, **CH** – cohort, **CI** – confidence interval, **Cm** – comparison, **CO** – crossover, **CS** – cross-sectional, **DB** – double-blind, **E** – epidemiological, **LC** – longitudinal cohort, **MA** – meta-analysis, **MC** – multi-center, **n** – number of patients, **O** – open, **OB** – observational, **OL** – open label, **OR** – odds ratio, **P** – prospective, **PB** – patient-blind, **PC** – placebo-controlled, **PG** – parallel group, **PS** – pilot study, **R** – randomized, **RC** – reference-controlled, **RCS** – retrospective cross-sectional, **RS** - retrospective, **S** – surveillance, **SB** – single-blind, **SC** – single-center, **U** – uncontrolled, **UP** – unpublished, **VC** – vehicle-controlled.

Clinical Studies on Valerian (*Valeriana officinalis* L.) (cont.)

Sleep (cont.)

Combination Preparations

Author/Year	Subject	Design	Duration	Dosage	Preparation	Results/Conclusion
Fussel et al., 2000	Sleep	PS n=30 patients with mild to moderate, non-organic insomnia	2 weeks	2 tablets in the evening (total of 500 mg valerian extract and 120 mg hops extract per day)	Ze91019 Alluna™ (US) Ivel® (Germany) ReDormin® (Switzerland)	Polysomnography data were recorded on baseline and after 2 weeks. Sleep latency was reduced statistically significantly while sleep efficiency increased. An increase in slow wave sleep was recorded. In a self-assessment, patients reported an improvement of feeling refreshed in the morning after 2 weeks. No adverse events were recorded.
Vonderheid-Guth et al., 2000	Sleep	R, SB, CO 2 studies n=12	1, 2, and 4 hours after application in each study, studies spaced 3 months apart	1st dosage: 1 tablet (500 mg valerian and 120 mg hops) vs. placebo; 2nd dosage: 3 tablets (total 1,500 mg valerian and 360 mg hops) vs. placebo	Ze91019 Alluna™ (US) Ivel® (Germany) ReDormin® (Switzerland)	The study concluded that pharmacodynamic responses could be repeated. The quantitative topographical EEG demonstrated a visible effect on the CNS, especially after intake of the high dosage of the valerian-hops combination.
Cerny and Schmid, 1999	Sleep	R, PC, DB, PG, MC n=95 healthy volunteers (58 women, 40 men)	30 days	3 tablets (total 360 mg valerian and 240 mg lemon balm [*Melissa officinalis*] combination) or placebo	Songha Night® coated tablets and placebo	Valerian/lemon balm group had significantly higher quality of sleep (33%) compared to placebo group (9%) (p=0.04).
Rodenbeck et al., 1998	Insomnia	PC n=15	4 weeks	500 mg valerian with 120 mg hops	Ivel® valerian and hops extract vs. placebo	There was a significant decrease in slow-wave sleep and an increase in Stage II sleep among those assigned to the herbal preparation.
Schmitz and Jackel, 1998	Sleep disorders	R, DB, C n= 46 patients with sleep disorders according to the DSM-IV criteria	2 weeks	Two, tablets (total 200 mg valerian extract with 45.5 mg hops extract) vs. 3 mg benzodiazapine	Hova® compared to benzodiazapine	Patients' state of health improved during therapy with both agents and deterioration after cessation was reported for both groups. Withdrawal symptoms were reported only in benzodiazepine groups.
Dressing et al., 1996	Insomnia	DB, PC n=57 adults with insomnia	2 weeks	Two, tablets 160 mg valerian extract with 80 mg lemon balm extract each), 2x/day	Euvegal® forte valerian and lemon balm tablet vs. placebo	Sleep quality improved in valerian/lemon balm combination compared to placebo (p=0.02) and remained in effect one week after medication was discontinued (p=0.12).
Lataster et al., 1996	Sleep	MC, OL n=3,447	4–6 weeks	Dosage not stated	Valerian and hops extract (each tablet contains 500 mg valerian, 60 mg hops)	The efficacy of the combination was evaluated as good to very good by 75% of the physicians. The number of patients who slept through the night rose from 24.4% to 77.4%. The self-efficacy report of feeling rested upon awakening rose from 26.5% to 64.9%.
Orth-Wagner, 1995	Sleep	O n=225 patients with sleep difficulties	2 weeks	Two, tablets 1–3 times daily	Novo-Baldriparan®	89% noted improvements in ability to fall asleep, and 80% reported improvements in ability to sleep through the night; most also reported an improvement in overall well-being.

KEY: C – controlled, **CC** – case-control, **CH** – cohort, **CI** – confidence interval, **Cm** – comparison, **CO** – crossover, **CS** – cross-sectional, **DB** – double-blind, **E** – epidemiological, **LC** – longitudinal cohort, **MA** – meta-analysis, **MC** – multi-center, **n** – number of patients, **O** – open, **OB** – observational, **OL** – open label, **OR** – odds ratio, **P** – prospective, **PB** – patient-blind, **PC** – placebo-controlled, **PG** – parallel group, **PS** – pilot study, **R** – randomized, **RC** – reference-controlled, **RCS** – retrospective cross-sectional, **RS** - retrospective, **S** – surveillance, **SB** – single-blind, **SC** – single-center, **U** – uncontrolled, **UP** – unpublished, **VC** – vehicle-controlled.

Sleep (cont.)

Combination Preparations (cont.)

Author/Year	Subject	Design	Duration	Dosage	Preparation	Results/Conclusion
Dressing and Reimann, 1992	Insomnia	DB, PC n=20 adults with insomnia	9 days	1 tablet (160 mg valerian with 80 mg lemon balm) or 0.125 mg Halcion®	Euvegal® forte valerian and lemon balm tablet vs. placebo	Both active treatments were equivalent and significantly better than placebo. The herbs caused less daytime sedation and impairment of mental functions.
Lindahl and Lindwall, 1989	Sleep difficulties	R, DB, PC, CO n=27 insomniacs	2 nights	400 mg/night	Valerina Natt®	Of the 27 patients, 21 rated valerian-containing mixture as significantly more effective (p<0.001) than the control preparation for sleep quality; 24 of 27 patients (89%) reported "improved sleep" and 12 of these patients (44%) reported "perfect sleep" after taking valerian-containing preparation. No adverse effects were observed.
Leathwood et al, 1982	Sleep	R, DB, PC, CO n=128	9 nights	400 mg	Hova®, or aqueous valerian extract, or placebo	Subjects had statistically significant (p<0.05) decrease in subjective sleep latency and significant improvement in sleep quality. Improvement was most notable among people who were poor or irregular sleepers, and smokers. No detectable hangover effect was noted in the morning.

Hazards in Driving and Operating Machinery

Author/Year	Subject	Design	Duration	Dosage	Preparation	Results/Conclusion
Kuhlmann et al., 1999	Alertness, reaction time, and concentration	R, C, DB n=99 males and females in first segment and 91 in second segment	Single night plus 2 weeks of nighttime administration	600 mg LI 156 or flunitrazepam (1 mg) and placebo	LI 156 vs. flunitrazepam and placebo	Neither single nor repeated nighttime administration of valerian had adverse impact on reaction time, alertness, and concentration the morning after intake. Valerian subjects showed better improvement in psychometric performance than those on placebo, and significantly (p=0.4481) better than those on drug.
Mayer and Springer, 1974	Assess potential hazards in driving	R, DB, PC n=24 healthy volunteers	Acute	200 mg, 400 mg, or 150–200 mg	Valmane® (valepotriates with alcohol) and placebo	Demonstrated a dose-dependent increase in concentration abilities in volunteers; when given in combination with alcohol, the preparation did not affect blood alcohol levels, have sedative effects, and/or affect driving performance.

Combination Preparations

Author/Year	Subject	Design	Duration	Dosage	Preparation	Results/Conclusion
Gerhard et al., 1996	Assess potential hazards in driving or operating machinery	C, Cm n=80 healthy adults	One night (single oral administration with observation on the following morning)	1.5 g dried extract or 4 g fluid extract	2 Valverde® herbal combinations (containing valerian and hops) and a syrup of valerian were compared to flunitrazepam and placebo (brands not stated)	Objectively measurable impairment of performance on morning after medication occurred only in flunitrazepam group. In addition, 50% of the volunteers in flunitrazepam group reported mild side effects, compared with only 10% from other groups. Examination of acute effects of plant remedies 1–2 hours after administration revealed very slight, but statistically significant impairment of vigilance and retardation in the processing of complex information.
Kammerer et al., 1996	Driving safety	R, DB, CO n=18	21 days	2 tablets after dinner (total of 1,000 mg valerian extract and 120 mg hops extract per day), or placebo	Valerian and hops extract (each tablet contains 500 mg valerian, 60 mg hops)	The study concluded that the combination did not produce significant adverse effects and did not impair psychometrically measured fitness and subjective state of health. In addition, no significant interaction with alcohol is to be expected.
Albrecht et al., 1995	Driving ability and combination with alcohol	R, DB, PC n=54	3 weeks	2 tablets 2x/day or placebo	Euvegal® forte (each tablet contains 160 mg valerian root extract and 80 mg lemon balm leaf extract)	Traffic safety was evaluated using psychometric tests. The treatment group showed no difference in driving ability compared to placebo, and treatment did not potentiate the effect of alcohol consumption. The study concluded that Euvegal® does not cause impairment of the operation of machinery or the driving of vehicles.

KEY: C – controlled, **CC** – case-control, **CH** – cohort, **CI** – confidence interval, **Cm** – comparison, **CO** – crossover, **CS** – cross-sectional, **DB** – double-blind, **E** – epidemiological, **LC** – longitudinal cohort, **MA** – meta-analysis, **MC** – multi-center, **n** – number of patients, **O** – open, **OB** – observational, **OL** – open label, **OR** – odds ratio, **P** – prospective, **PB** – patient-blind, **PC** – placebo-controlled, **PG** – parallel group, **PS** – pilot study, **R** – randomized, **RC** – reference-controlled, **RCS** – retrospective cross-sectional, **RS** – retrospective, **S** – surveillance, **SB** – single-blind, **SC** – single-center, **U** – uncontrolled, **UP** – unpublished, **VC** – vehicle-controlled.

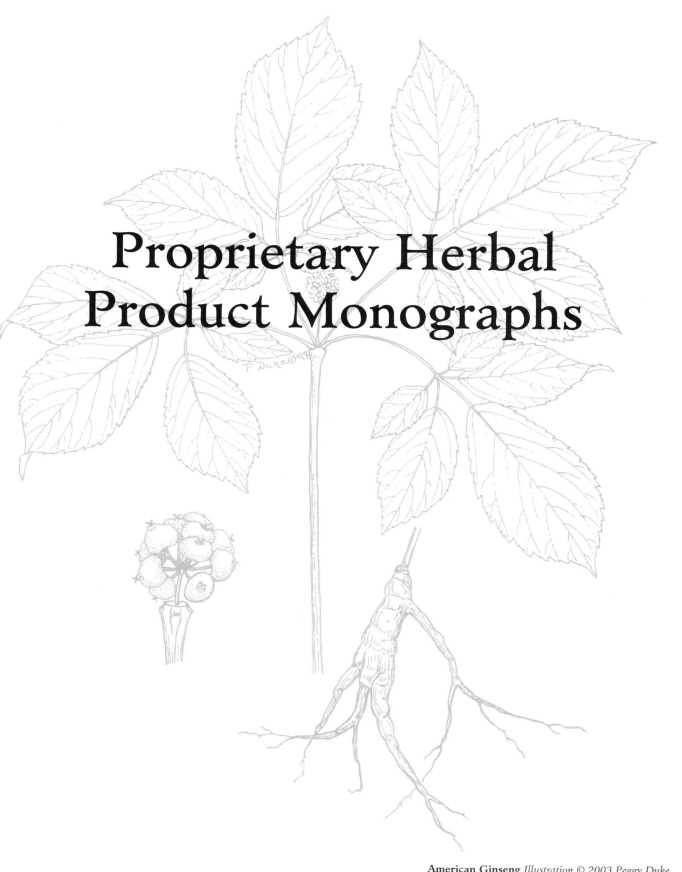

Proprietary Herbal Product Monographs

American Ginseng *Illustration © 2003 Peggy Duke*

INTRODUCTION

MONOPREPARATIONS

The main section of this book is comprised of monographs on monopreparations, i.e., commercial preparations containing one herb or herbal extract. Most of the clinical studies on these monopreparations have been conducted in Western Europe, particularly Germany, where phytotherapy usually is based on the use of single herbal products. Proprietary monopreparations may be products made by a patented extraction process or products with a specific chemical profile resulting from the standardization of specific constituents. These techniques frequently attempt to provide the consumer with a product of consistent quality, often containing uniform levels of one or more marker compounds that in many cases are also the primary active ingredients. This tends to create a product of consistent activity and efficacy. This proprietary product section includes one monopreparation called Pycnogenol®. Two tables beginning on page 398 list the proprietary herbal products mentioned in this book, both monopreparations and multi-herb products, upon which clinical research has been conducted.

MULTI-HERB PRODUCTS

In European countries, as well as in the traditional herbal medicine systems of India (Ayurveda), China (traditional Chinese medicine, TCM), and Japan (Kampo), multi-herb products are used frequently instead of monopreparations. In fact, in Asia the use of multi-herb products is the rule, not the exception. The majority of herbal products used in Germany prior to 1990 were products containing fixed combinations of herbs (Schilcher, 1997). Many multi-herb products contain similar, sometimes identical combinations based on extensive traditional use or clinical evidence, whereas other preparations are absolutely unique. The level of clinical evidence supporting specific multi-herb products varies widely. For several multi-herb products it has been shown that the therapeutic effect of the combination is greater than the sum of the individual constituents' activities, and may result in better results compared to those of herbal monopreparations or of synthetic drugs. This section includes only multi-herb products with at least two human studies supporting their use. Multi-herb products with only one clinical study are listed in the combination section of the table of clinical studies and in the Branded Products section of the respective single herb monographs (e.g., echinacea, valerian). Please note that this review contains several specific multi-herb products but does not include all products upon which clinical research has been conducted. *Inclusion of specific proprietary products in this section and else where in this book is not meant to serve as an endorsement of particular products, but only as an acknowledgement of the extent of clinical studies associated with the respective product.*

EUROPEAN MULTI-HERB PRODUCTS AND COMMISSION E FIXED COMBINATIONS

The German Commission E approved the use of 66 "fixed combinations"—herbal formulas that represent various commercial herbal products sold as nonprescription medicines in German pharmacies (Blumenthal *et al.*, 1998). Of the combination formulas approved by Commission E, 35 are intended for digestive complaints, while 21 deal with colds, flus, and catarrhal

conditions of the upper respiratory tract (with or without viscous phlegm), dry or spastic cough, and related conditions. The next largest category of combinations is intended to treat unrest and insomnia due to nervousness.

The Commission E approved the use of combination formulas only if each herb in the formula "makes a positive contribution to the evaluation of the total preparation" i.e., contributes directly to the overall safety and efficacy of the formula. In approving such formulas, each herb must also have an individual monograph that is the result of an evaluation of the available literature on that botanical. The evaluation must focus on safety primarily and then efficacy according to a "doctrine of reasonable certainty" (Blumenthal *et al.*, 1998). In addition, the herbs in each formula must be found in "dosages appropriate for effectiveness." Thus, the rationale for the use of herbs in combinations in Commission E-approved formulas is significantly different from the way herbs are used in complex formulas in Asian traditional medicine, where individual herbs are not required to contribute directly to the intended application of the formula, as stipulated by Commission E, but their inclusion in the formula is based on a variety of rationale, as noted below.

The most frequently prescribed nonprescription drug in Germany is a proprietary, multi-herb product named Sinupret®, used for sinusitis and inflammatory conditions of the respiratory tract (see Sinupret® monograph below). In 1997, Sinupret® ranked 12th in number of prescriptions among all drug products, with 3.4 million prescriptions (Schulz *et al.*, 2001). The following multi-herb products from the European market are also included in this chapter: Alluna™, Esberitox®, Euvegal®, Mastodynon®, Phytodolor®, and Prostagutt® forte.

CHINESE MULTI-HERB PRODUCTS

China contains one of the world's oldest systems of traditional herbal medicine that has been documented in writing, with early texts dating back as far as 170 B.C.E. (Dharmananda, 2002). Chinese herbal medicine is based primarily on the combination of numerous herbs into simple or relatively complex formulas. In TCM, multi-herb products are based on a sophisticated system of "energetics" in which the herbs are employed based on their empirically observed properties. Thus, the formulas usually rely on one "superior" herb to dictate the therapeutic focus of the formula, and then are primarily based on the "heating" or "cooling" properties of each herb and the five characteristic flavors (sweet, bitter, spicy, salty, and sour), which correspond to particular pharmacological activities (Hsu, 1986). While a thorough explanation of the intricacies of the TCM system of herbal medicine is not possible here, suffice it to say that many combinations have become standardized, often employed in modern TCM using the same formulations as found in classic texts for centuries, while sometimes being slightly modified, based on the professional judgement of the practitioner. However, from a Western perspective, few controlled clinical trials have been published in Western medical journals on TCM herbal formulas. A notable exception was a recent trial on a Chinese herbal formula to treat irritable bowel syndrome (IBS), published in a special complementary and alternative medicine edition of the *Journal of the American Medical Association* (Bensoussan *et al.*, 1998). In this three-arm trial, patients received either a standardized formula, a customized formula prepared for each subject based on the concept of differential diagnosis, or placebo. The results suggested that the Chinese herbs were significantly better than placebo in providing relief from the symptoms of IBS, as measured in the trial.

INDIAN (AYURVEDIC) MULTI-HERB PRODUCTS

Ayurveda is the ancient system of traditional medicine in India, owing its origins to medical writings found in the RigVeda, a sacred Sanskrit text that is believed to have been written from 4500 to 1600 B.C.E. (Kapoor, 1990). In Ayurvedic herbal formulas, the inclusion of multiple herbs is based on a rationale that is similar to TCM (some authors consider Ayurveda to be the older, philosophical basis for TCM) but distinctly different from the European system of herbal medicine. The primary governing concept in Ayurveda is that the proper combination of herbs can greatly enhance their respective healing abilities. Ayurvedic herbal formulas begin with an individual herb that encompasses the primary action considered most appropriate for the individual's particular condition. Additional herbs with similar primary actions are included to support the activity of the formula. For example, in a diaphoretic formula, used to induce perspiration and treat a common cold, additional herbs may be added to help enhance mucous discharge from the throat or lungs. Further, herbs with potential actions that contradict the activity of the main herbs might be added to balance the formula or prevent it from exhibiting an excessive or one-sided action. They can also help reduce potential adverse side effects of some of the main herbs. Stimulant herbs such as black pepper (*Piper nigrum*), long pepper (*P. longum*), ginger (*Zingiber officinale*), and cayenne pepper (*Capsicum* spp.) may also be included to enhance absorption (Lad and Frawley, 1986). The rationality of this long-used empirical practice is validated by modern research demonstrating that the compound piperine in long pepper and black pepper increases activity of dietary supplements and conventional pharmaceutical drugs by enhancing the serum concentration, extent of absorption and bioavailability by inhibiting drug metabolism (i.e., breakdown) (Badmaev *et al.*, 2000; Khajuria *et al.*, 1998; Bano *et al.*, 1991; Atal *et al.*, 1985, 1981).

Liv.52® is an example of an Ayurvedic multi-herb product and is used for liver dysfunction. In total sales volume, including statistics for the entire pharmaceutical industry (both nonprescription and prescription drugs), Liv.52® is the leading brand in India (ORG-MARG Private Limited, 2001).

JAPANESE (KAMPO) MULTI-HERB PRODUCTS

Kampo, Japan's traditional herbal medicine, is playing an increasingly important role in Japanese healthcare and represents a $1 billion segment of annual drug sales in Japan (Matsumoto *et al.*, 1999). In a recent survey, 96% of responding physicians indicated that they practice Kampo (Watanabe *et al.*, 2001), and Japan's Ministry of Health and Welfare approves 148 Kampo prescription drugs for reimbursement under the national health insurance (Tsumura, 1999).

Kampo is based on TCM, which developed a sophisticated understanding of the effectiveness and safety of combinations of herbs derived from long practical experience. Following the introduction of Chinese medicine to Japan in the fourth century, Japanese practitioners gradually altered the original formulas. Particularly, after the 17th century, the original formulas were validated through clinical experience, and the foundation was laid for uniquely Japanese Kampo medicine. Thus, although Kampo has its roots in China, it is also a product of Japanese culture and experience.

Like other forms of Asian traditional medicine, Kampo takes a holistic approach to health, seeking to enhance the body's natural harmony and recuperative power. Chronic conditions such as allergies, asthma, menopausal symptoms, disorders of the elderly, autonomic imbalance, and other non-specific complaints, and rheumatism are often treated with Kampo, due to the gentle action and multiple active substances of Kampo formulations. Kampo is also recommended for patients who respond poorly or have adverse reactions to Western medicine, as well as for common complaints like colds and gastritis.

Hochu-ekki-to® is a well-known Kampo formula originally described in the Chinese medical classic *Nei Wai Shang Bian Huo Lun* (*Nai-gai-sho-ben-waku-ron* in Japanese) by Li Dong Yuan (1247 C.E.). This formulation was traditionally prescribed for patients showing a decline of digestive function and marked fatigability of extremities. Since inclusion in the above-mentioned text, Hochu-ekki-to® has undergone more than 700 years of use by healers in the traditional systems of medicine of China, Japan, and other East Asian countries. Moreover, like many other Kampo formulations, since it was approved as a prescription drug by Japan's Ministry of Health & Welfare in the 1970's, the extract form, which is produced according to pharmaceutical GMP standards, has accumulated more than 20 years of clinical experience as used by conventional physicians as a component of the modern medical system in Japan. Hochu-ekki-to® is the second-leading Kampo formulation, with annual sales of $52.3 million (U.S. dollars) in 1998 (Japan Kampo-Medicine Manufacturers Association, 2001).

TIBETAN FORMULAS

Tibetan medicine has been used for centuries and dates back to 300 B.C.E. Owing to Tibet's geographical location, its medicine was deeply influenced by both the Indian Ayurvedic and the Chinese medical systems, as well as Persian medicine (which also incorporated tenets of ancient Greek medicine). The primary text upon which traditional Tibetan medicine is based is called the *Gyu-zhi* (*The Four Tantras*), an Ayurvedic text written in Sanskrit and translated to Tibetan in the eight century C.E. (Fallarino, 1994). Like Ayurvedic and Chinese formulas, Tibetan herbal combinations usually contain a large number of herbs (8–25) intended to restore balance to the body. The classification of herbal properties in Tibetan medicine includes six tastes (sweet, sour, salty, bitter, acrid, astringent), eight properties (heavy, smooth, cool, soft, light, rough, acrid, sharp) and 17 effects (hot, cold, warm, cool, thick, thin, moist, rough, light, heavy, steady, motive, blunt, tender, dry, soft). Herbs with the opposite effects of the disease are chosen for each combination. For example, a lung infection is considered a hot disease, and is therefore treated with a combination containing *Rhodiola rosea*, an herb with cooling properties. Practitioners use a combination of herbs to treat the condition because the cause of disease is thought to originate from a combination of disturbances in the body (Khangkar, 1986).

Padma 28® is a product from Tibetan tradition. This chapter reviews seven clinical studies supporting its possible use for intermittent claudication, plus one preliminary study suggesting its use for each of the following conditions: angina pectoris, hypercholesterolemia and hypertriglyceridemia, and childhood respiratory tract infections.

PROPRIETARY MONOGRAPHS

With the exception of the monograph on Pycnogenol®, the monographs in this section cover specific proprietary herbal combination products and contain information taken primarily from product packages and other sources. In the cases of some of the combinations sold in Europe and non-European countries, where they are frequently licensed as nonprescription drugs, the Primary Uses section includes uses usually approved by the appropriate agencies of foreign governments. Additional information (Dosage, Duration of Administration, Action, Contraindications, Pregnancy and Lactation, Adverse Effects, Drug Interactions, etc.) in these monographs is also derived from product package labels and/or package inserts, often reflecting the labeling as approved or required by the government agencies.

The DSHEA Structure-Function Claim section refers to the claim made on the U.S. label, as authorized by Section 6 of the Dietary Supplement Health and Education Act of 1994 (DSHEA). Under this law, manufacturers are authorized to make "statements of nutritional support" regarding dietary supplement products, including how a supplement can affect the structure or function of the human body. Such claims are not required to be pre-approved by the Food and Drug Administration (FDA). The claims must meet the following criteria: (1) they must be truthful and nonmisleading; (2) the company must possess scientific information to document the statement; (3) the company must notify the FDA that it intends to market the product with this claim within 30 days of introducing the product claim to the market (post-market notification); (4) the product must be labeled as a "dietary supplement"; (5) the claims may not make any therapeutic claims, i.e., they cannot claim to prevent, treat, or cure a disease; and (6) the product must carry the disclaimer: "This statement has not been evaluated by the Food and Drug Administration. This product is not intended to diagnose, treat, cure or prevent any disease." (DSHEA, 1994). FDA regulations also prohibit the use of any name of a pathology or disease in a claim, but do allow manufacturers to make claims that have been previously allowed for nonprescription drugs *if* the claim does not deal with a disease state (e.g., antacid, antigas, digestive aid, laxative, nighttime sleep aid, etc.) (FDA, 2000; Israelsen and Blumenthal, 2000).

EDITORS' NOTE: The monographs presented in the section on specific proprietary herbal combination products are presented as some of the best examples of multi-herbal formulas that have been subjected to various types of human clinical trials. By including these products in this book, the editors are neither endorsing the products nor the manufacturers; these products are included as concrete examples of formulas from various herbal traditions that have been tested in published clinical trials. Thus, the editors and publisher are merely acknowledging the research on them as a means to provide healthcare professionals with examples of complex formulas with potential use in self-care and healthcare.

References for this proprietary herbal product section begin on page 390.

Pycnogenol®
(French Maritime Pine Bark Extract)
Pinus pinaster Aiton subsp. *atlantica*
[Fam. *Pinaceae*]

OVERVIEW

French maritime pine bark extract, sold under the trade name Pycnogenol® (manufactured by Horphag Research, Geneva, Switzerland) was ranked 15th among the top-selling herbal dietary supplements in the U.S. in mainstream retail outlets (food, drug, and mass market stores) with total sales in this channel of trade exceeding $3 million in 2000 (Blumenthal, 2001). Sales in natural food store, multi-level marketing, and mail order channels are presumably much higher, but accurate statistics for aggregate sales in these markets are not available. Traditionally, North American pine bark has been used by Native American Indians to treat colds and rheumatism, and for wound healing (Moerman, 1998; Chandler *et al.*, 1979).

Recent research suggests significant antioxidant activity for this extract, based primarily on its proanthocyanidin content. Currently, Pycnogenol® is used primarily to help prevent edema formation of the lower legs (Gulati, 1999) and capillary bleeding, especially in cases of retinopathy (Spadea and Balestrazzi, 2001). Pycnogenol® has been shown to prevent platelet aggregation in smokers (Pütter *et al.*, 1999) and in cardiovascular patients (Wang *et al.*, 1999). It has been used in reducing pain associated with menstrual disorders (Kohama and Suzuki, 1999) and has demonstrated improved lung function and symptom scores in asthmatics (Hosseini *et al.*, 2001b), normalized blood pressure in mild hypertensives (Hosseini *et al.*, 2001a), and improved symptoms in patients with systemic lupus erythematosus (SLE) (Stefanescu *et al.*, 2001).

DESCRIPTION

French maritime pine bark extract is made by extraction of the outer bark of *Pinus pinaster* Ait. subsp. *atlantica*. The French subspecies *atlantica* of *P. pinaster* differs from the Iberian (Spanish) and Moroccan subspecies by its resistance against salt (Saur *et al.*, 1993) and in the profile of its phytochemical constituents (Bahrman *et al.*, 1994).

The fresh bark is powdered and extracted with ethanol and water in patented equipment allowing an automated continuous process (Rohdewald, 2002). After purification of the raw extract, the aqueous solution of the extracted constituents is spray-dried. The resulting fine brownish powder is stable if stored in a dry, dark environment. The extract is standardized to a procyanidin content of 70 ±5%, primarily catechins and epicatechins.

PRIMARY USES
Cardiovascular
- Venous insufficiency, chronic (Arcangeli, 2000; Petrassi *et al.*, 2000; Schmidtke and Schoop, 1995; Sirnelli-Walter and Weil-Masson, 1988; Doucet *et al.*, 1987; Schmidtke and Schoop, 1984; Feine-Haake, 1975)

OTHER POTENTIAL USES
- Abdominal and menstrual pain (Kohama and Suzuki, 1999)
- Asthma (Hosseini *et al.*, 2001b)
- Endometriosis (Kohama and Suzuki, 1999)
- Enhanced sperm quality in case of man diagnosed with malformed sperm (Roseff and Gulati, 1999)
- Mild hypertension (Hosseini *et al.*, 2001a)
- Prevention of platelet aggregation (Pütter *et al.*, 1999)
- Retinal disorder, vascular (Spadea and Balestrazzi, 2001)
- Retinopathy, diabetic (Magnard *et al.*, 1970)
- Systemic lupus erythematosus (SLE), second line therapy (Stefanescu *et al.*, 2001)

DOSAGE
- For prevention and treatment of chronic venous disorders: daily doses ranging from 100–300 mg per day were effective in controlled clinical trials (Gulati, 1999).
- For prevention and treatment of retinal vascular disorders: doses from 40–150 mg have been used in clinical trials (Spadea and Balestrazzi, 2001; Magnard *et al.*, 1970).
- For treatment of endometriosis and menstrual disorders: 30–60 mg have been found to be effective (Kohama and Suzuki, 1999).
- To normalize platelet function doses of 150–200 mg are needed (Pütter *et al.*, 1999).
- To normalize blood pressure 200 mg were given (Hosseini *et al.*, 2001a).
- To reduce asthma symptoms, 1 mg/lb body weight were taken (Hosseini *et al.*, 2001b).

DURATION OF ADMINISTRATION

Clinical experience demonstrated that beneficial effects can be substantiated after 4 weeks of treatment with Pycnogenol® in cases of chronic venous disorders and retinal vascular disorders. However, results improved significantly when the treatment period was extended to 2 months (Gulati, 1999).

Blood pressure in mild hypertensive patients was normalized following treatment period of 8 weeks (Hosseini *et al.*, 2001a).

For prevention of menstrual disorders treatment periods will vary from individual to individual; however, one study noted beneficial effects after 14–30 days (Kohama and Suzuki, 1999).

Asthma symptoms were improved after 4 weeks treatment (Hosseini *et al.*, 2001b).

For improvement of sperm quality, treatment period was 9 months (Roseff and Gulati, 1999).

Continuous intake of Pycnogenol® as a dietary supplement can be recommended to protect the cardiovascular system from the development of atherosclerosis and thrombus formation in moderate doses from 50–100 mg. (This effect is the result of Pycnogenol®'s ability to normalize platelet aggregation and thromboxane levels, to antagonize vasoconstriction induced by adrenaline, to inactivate free radicals, and the anti-oxidative effect influencing the oxidation of lipids.)

CHEMISTRY

Pycnogenol® is prepared from the bark of French maritime pine trees (*P. pinaster*) by a standardized process. The trees are cultivated as a monoculture exclusively in one narrow area in Southwest France and the bark is harvested from 30-year old trees; therefore, chemical studies indicate that there is little variation in the composition of the extract over the years.

French maritime pine bark extract contains procyanidins, catechin, epicatechin, taxifolin, phenolic acids, and glucosides or glucose esters of its constituents.

Procyanidins

The procyanidins consist of units of catechin and epicatechin. The chain length of the procyanidins in Pycnogenol® range from dimers up to octamers. The dimers had been identified as the isomeric forms B1, B3, B6, and B7. A trimer C2, consisting of catechin-epicatechin-catechin is also identified (Rohdewald, 2002). The presence of tetramers to octamers was demonstrated by mass spectrometry (MALDI-TOF) (Rohdewald, 1998). The total amount of procyanidins in Pycnogenol® is standardized to 70 ±5%. Catechin, epicatechin, and taxifolin represent the so-called "monomeric" procyanidins. Taxifolin was found as its glycoside and in its free form (Rohdewald, 1998).

Phenolic acids

Phenolic acids, also called fruit acids, in French maritime pine bark extract are derivates from benzoic acid (p-hydroxybenzoic acid, protocatechic acid, gallic acid, vanillic acid) and from cinnamic acid (caffeic acid, ferulic acid, p-cumaric acid).

Additionally, the glucose ester of ferulic acid and p-cumaric acid were identified and the glucoside of vanillic acid (Rohdewald, 1998).

Other constituents

Free glucose is present in small amounts, rhamnose, xylose, and arabinose could be detected, but not quantified. Vanillin is also found in very small quantities (Rüve, 1996).

PHARMACOLOGICAL ACTIONS

Humans

Symptoms of chronic venous insufficiency including edema of the lower legs, feeling of heaviness in the lower legs, cramps, and pain were significantly reduced (Arcangeli, 2000; Petrassi *et al.*, 2000; Schmidtke and Schoop, 1995, 1984); vision was improved in cases of retinal vascular disorder (Spadea and Balestrazzi, 2001; Magnard *et al*, 1970); smoking-induced platelet aggregation was prevented (Pütter *et al.*, 1999); in patients with cardiovascular diseases, platelet aggregation was reduced (Wang *et al.*, 1999); mild hypertension was reduced to normal (Hosseini *et al.,* 2001a); asthma symptoms and lung function were improved (Hosseini *et al.,* 2001b); reduction of menstrual cramps and pain have been reported (Kohama and Suzuki, 1999); and malformation of human sperm have been normalized (Roseff and Gulati, 1999).

Animal

Increased capillary resistance (Gábor *et al.*, 1993); anti-inflammatory (Blazsó *et al.*, 1997); anti-hypertensive (Blaszó *et al.*, 1996); immunomodulation (Liu *et al.*, 1998; Cheshier *et al.*, 1996); improvement of cognitive function (Liu *et al.*, 1999); UV-protection (Blazsó *et al.*, 1995); spasmolytic activity of ferulic acid on rat uterus (Ozaki and Ma, 1990).

In vitro

Radical scavenging activity (Packer *et al.*, 1999; Rohdewald, 1998; Elstner and Kleber, 1990); protection of DNA (Nelson *et al.*, 1998); increased production of superoxide dismutase (SOD), catalase, and glutathione (Wei *et al.*, 1997); protection of brain cells against amyloid-β-protein toxicity (Rohdewald, 1998) and glutamate-induced toxicity (Kobayashi, 2000; Rohdewald, 1998); inhibition of adrenalin-induced platelet aggregation (Rüve, 1996); inhibition of angiotensin-converting enzyme (ACE) (Blaszó *et al.*, 1996); inhibition of adrenalin-induced vasoconstriction (Fitzpatrick *et al.*, 1998); UV-protection (Guochang, 1993); apoptosis of human mammary cancer cells (Huynh and Teel, 2000); and spasmolytic action of constituents of Pycnogenol®, caffeic, and protocatechic acid on smooth muscles (de Urbina *et al.*, 1990). Pycnogenol® has been shown to exhibit anticalgranulin activity in human keratinocytes (*in vitro*), suggesting potential use for treatment of psoriasis and various dermatoses (Rihn *et al.*, 2001). Pycnogenol® increases human growth hormone secretion (Buz'Zard *et al.,* 2002).

MECHANISM OF ACTION

- High affinity to proteins (Packer *et al.*, 1999) decreases capillary permeability thereby reducing microbleeding and preventing edema formation (Gabór *et al.*, 1993).

- Stimulates production of the endothelium-derived factor (nitric oxide, NO) causing vasorelaxation (Fitzpatrick *et al.*, 1998) leading to increased microcirculation (Wang *et al.*, 1999). Pycnogenol®, in addition to its antioxidant activity, stimulates constitutive endothelial NO synthase activity to increase NO levels, which could counteract the vasoconstrictor effects of epinephrine (E) and norepinephrine (NE) (Fitzpatrick *et al.*, 1998). Furthermore, additional protective effects could result from the well-established properties of NO to decrease platelet aggregation and adhesion, as well as to inhibit low-density lipoprotein (LDL) cholesterol oxidation, all of which could protect against atherogenesis and thrombus formation. Pycnogenol® stimulates NO production (Fitzpatrick *et al.*, 1998) and inhibits thromboxane formation (Watson, 1999), both effects leading to reduced platelet-aggregation (Pütter *et al.*, 1999).

- Antioxidant activity is closely related to anti-inflammatory effects (Blázso *et al.*, 1995). [Because anti-inflammatory processes generate free radicals, the inhibition of the superoxide radical by fractions of Pycnogenol® *in vitro* is closely related to the anti-inflammatory activity of the same fractions *in vivo*. In addition to the inhibition of prostaglandins and leukotrienes (Hosseini *et al.,* 2001b), the scavenging of free radicals is a contributing factor to an anti-inflammatory activity].

- Phenolic acids possess spasmolytic activity on uterine muscles *in vivo* (Ozaki and Ma, 1990; de Urbina *et al.*, 1990).

CONTRAINDICATIONS

None known.

PREGNANCY AND LACTATION: As a general precaution, Pycnogenol® should not be taken during the first 3 months of pregnancy. Safety pharmacology demonstrated absence of mutagenic and teratogenic effects, no perinatal toxicity, and no negative effects on fertility (Rohdewald, 2002).

ADVERSE EFFECTS

Gastric upset, diarrhea, constipation. To avoid these small side effects, Pycnogenol® should be taken with meals. The average frequency of minor adverse effects including headache and dizziness is 1.6 %. Adverse effects are not related to dose or total duration of treatment. Data are based on documentation of reports on 2000 patients (Rohdewald, 2002).

DRUG INTERACTIONS

None known.

Because of its mechanism of action of inhibiting platelet aggregation, Pycnogenol® should not be added to treatment with antiplatelet drugs; however, this interaction is theoretical and has not been demonstrated in clinical experience.

AMERICAN HERBAL PRODUCTS ASSOCIATION (AHPA) SAFETY RATING

There is no listing for *P. pinaster*, Pycnogenol®, or French maritime pine bark extract in the *American Herbal Products Association's Botanical Safety Handbook* (McGuffin *et al.*, 1997), probably due to the fact that most of the herbs rated for safety in this volume are based on those herbs previously listed in the AHPA *Herbs of Commerce* (Foster, 1992). At that time, pine bark extract was only beginning to be marketed in the U.S.

REGULATORY STATUS

CANADA: Decision pending.

FRANCE: A French maritime pine bark extract is approved as a non-prescription herbal drug for treatment of venous disorders.

GERMANY: Not reviewed by the German Commission E (Blumenthal *et al.*, 1998).

GREECE: Non-prescription herbal drug for treatment and prevention of chronic venous insufficiency.

JAPAN: Food supplement; also approved as cosmetic ingredient.

PEOPLE'S REPUBLIC OF CHINA & HONG KONG: Health food.

SWEDEN: No pine bark extract products are presently registered in the Medical Products Agency's (MPA) "Authorised Natural Remedies" listings (MPA, 2001).

SWITZERLAND: Non-prescription herbal drug for treatment and prevention of chronic venous insufficiency. One purified pine bark extract product is listed in the *Codex 2000/01* (Ruppanner and Schaefer, 2000).

U.K.: Food supplement. For adults only. Not to be used by children or pregnant women (FAC, 2000; Crates, 2000). (This is consistent with the labelling of other food supplements in the UK).

U.S.: Dietary supplement (USC, 1994).

CLINICAL REVIEW

Fourteen clinical studies are included in the following table, "Clinical Studies on Pycnogenol® (French Maritime Pine Bark Extract)." Nine double-blind, placebo-controlled studies (DB, PC) have been conducted on a total of 244 patients. Four DB, PC studies (Arcangeli, 2000; Petrassi *et al.*, 2000; Schmidtke and Schoop, 1995, 1984) focused on chronic venous insufficiency and confirmed results of three open studies with 255 patients in total (Sirnelli-Walter and Weil-Masson, 1988; Doucet *et al.*, 1987; Feine-Haake, 1975). One DB, PC study conducted by Spadea and Balestrazzi (2001) confirmed preliminary findings of a previous open study (Magnard *et al.*, 1970) on the effects of retinopathy. One PC study demonstrated complete inhibition of smoking-induced platelet aggregation (Pütter *et al.*, 1999), and a DB, PC study with cardiovascular patients showed a significant decrease in platelet aggregation and improved microcirculation (Wang *et al.*, 1999). A DB, PC, crossover (CO) study showed reduction of asthma symptoms and improvement of lung function (Hosseini *et al.*, 2001b). Blood pressure of mild hypertensives was normalized in a DB, PC, CO study (Hosseini *et al.*, 2001a). Pycnogenol® supplementation contributed to improvement of symptoms of SLE in a DB, PC pilot study (Stefanescu *et al.*, 2001).

Clinical Studies on Pycnogenol®, French Maritime Pine Bark extract (*Pinus pinaster* Aiton subsp *atlantica*)

Chronic venous insufficiency

Author/Year	Subject	Design	Duration	Dosage	Preparation	Results/Conclusion
Arcangeli, 2000	Chronic venous insufficiency	R,DB,PC n=40	3 months	300 mg (1 capsule 3x/day)	100 mg capsules	Reduction of heaviness, swelling, and pain were 54%, 64%, and 64% respectively. The elimination of these symptoms was in the order of 33%, 63%, and 58%, respectively.
Petrassi et al., 2000	Chronic venous insufficiency	R,DB,PC n=40	3 months	300 mg (1 capsule 3x/day)	100 mg capsules	Reduction of heaviness and swelling were 60% and 74%, respectively. Elimination of these symptoms was in the order of 33% and 88%, respectively.
Schmidtke and Schoop, 1995	Hydrostatic edema of the lower limbs	DB,PC,R n=40 22 men, 18 women	6 days	360 mg/day vs. placebo (no compression therapy during the course of treatment)	20 mg tablets	After 6 day treatment, leg volume increased from maintaining sitting position for 1 and 2 hours respectively, was significantly reduced (p<0.001) in active group and not in the placebo group. Authors concluded, based on objective and subjective effects, that Pycnogenol® is an effective and well-tolerated remedy that can be recommended in the treatment of venous disorders.
Sirnelli-Walter and Weil-Masson, 1988	Chronic venous insufficiency, PMS	O n=80	3 months	80 mg (2 tablets 2x/day)	20 mg tablets	Elimination of symptoms: 89% edema, 85% swelling, 83% heaviness of legs, 77% night cramps, 75% hemorrhoids, 73% pruritis, 69% pain, 44% ecchymoses, and 39% varicose vein. Mammary tension and abdominal pain eliminated in 61.58% and 44% cases, respectively. In menopausal disorders, nocturnal sweating and hot flashes eliminated in 77% and 62% cases, respectively.
Doucet et al., 1987	Chronic venous insufficiency	O n=65	2 months	80 mg (4 tablets daily), for 20 days each month after end of menstruation	20 mg tablets	Improvement of 100% pruritus, 89% night cramps, 79% sensation of swelling, 59% edema, and 62.5% heaviness of legs.
Schmidtke and Schoop, 1984	Chronic venous insufficiency	PC n=29	4 days	120 mg (2 tablets 3x/day)	20 mg tablets	Significantly less increase in leg volume (p<0.01).
Feine-Haake, 1975	Chronic venous insufficiency	O n=110	4–12 weeks	2 tablets 3x daily for 1st week (90 mg/day); 1 tablet 3x/day (45 mg/day) thereafter for 3–12 weeks)	15 mg tablets	Efficacy rate was 70% to 83% for reduction of cramps, pain, and swelling of legs.

Retinal Vascular Disorders

Author/Year	Subject	Design	Duration	Dosage	Preparation	Results/Conclusion
Spadea and Balestrazzi, 2001	Retinal vascular disorders	R,DB,PC n=40	2 months	150 mg	50 mg capsules	The deterioration of vision was not only prevented, but even improved significantly. Retinal vascularization improved. Electroretinogram confirmed beneficial effects of Pycnogenol®.
Magnard et al., 1970	Diabetic retinopathy	O n=40	1–6 months	Initial dose: 80–120 mg (2–3 tablets 2x/day 1st week); Maintenance dose: 40–80 mg (1–2 tablets/day)	20 mg tablets	Improvement Score was good to excellent in 36 subjects, moderate in 3, and no effect in 1.

KEY: C – controlled, **CC** – case-control, **CH** – cohort, **CI** – confidence interval, **Cm** – comparison, **CO** – crossover, **CS** – cross-sectional, **DB** – double-blind, **E** – epidemiological, **LC** – longitudinal cohort, **MA** – meta-analysis, **MC** – multi-center, **n** – number of patients, **O** – open, **OB** – observational, **OL** – open label, **OR** – odds ratio, **P** – prospective, **PB** – patient-blind, **PC** – placebo-controlled, **PG** – parallel group, **PS** – pilot study, **R** – randomized, **RC** – reference-controlled, **RCS** – retrospective cross-sectional, **RS** - retrospective, **S** – surveillance, **SB** – single-blind, **SC** – single-center, **U** – uncontrolled, **UP** – unpublished, **VC** – vehicle-controlled.

Clinical Studies on Pycnogenol®, French Maritime Pine Bark extract *(Pinus pinaster Aiton subsp atlantica)* (cont.)

Platelet Aggregation

Author/Year	Subject	Design	Duration	Dosage	Preparation	Results/Conclusion
Pütter et al., 1999	Smoking-induced platelet aggregation	PC n=38	Single dose	25–200 mg (single doses)	25 mg tablets	Complete prevention of smoking-induced platelet aggregation.
Wang et al., 1999	Platelet aggregation in cardiovascular patients	R,DB,PC n=40	4 weeks	450 mg (3 tablets 3x/day)	50 mg tablets	Significant reduction of platelet aggregation (p<0.05), increased microcirculation.

Other

Author/Year	Subject	Design	Duration	Dosage	Preparation	Results/Conclusion
Hosseini et al., 2001a	Mild hypertension (140–159 mmHG)	R,DB,PC,CO n=11	16 weeks	200 mg (2 capsules 2x/day)	50 mg capsules	Significant decrease of systolic blood pressure (p<0.05) compared to placebo. Decrease of diastolic blood pressure did not reach significance. Thromboxane levels decreased significantly (p<0.05).
Hosseini et al., 2001b	Asthma	R,DB,PC,CO n=22	8 weeks	1 mg/lb/day, max 200 mg/day	20 mg capsules	Lung function (FEV1/FVC) was significantly improved (p< 0.003) compared to placebo. Asthma Symptom Scores improved. Leukotriene levels decreased significantly (p< 0.003) compared to placebo.
Stefanescu et al., 2001	Systemic lupus erythematosus (SLE), second line therapy beside standard medication	DB,PC,PS n=11 10 women, 1 man	2 months	120 mg/day for 30 days, thereafter 60 mg for 30 days	20 mg tablets	Index for SLE was significantly decreased compared to placebo (p< 0.018). Non-significant improvement shown by reduction of reactive oxygen species production. Spontaneous apoptosis, p56[lck] specific activity in peripheral blood lymphocytes, and erythrocyte sedimentation rate.
Kohama and Suzuki, 1999	Endometriosis, menstrual pain, chronic abdominal pain	O n=39	14–30 days	30–60 mg (2 capsules/day for 2–4 wks; 4 capsules on demand)	15 mg capsules	Improvement of cramps 70%, abdominal pain 80–90%.

KEY: **C** – controlled, **CC** – case-control, **CH** – cohort, **CI** – confidence interval, **Cm** – comparison, **CO** – crossover, **CS** – cross-sectional, **DB** – double-blind, **E** – epidemiological, **LC** – longitudinal cohort, **MA** – meta-analysis, **MC** – multi-center, **n** – number of patients, **O** – open, **OB** – observational, **OL** – open label, **OR** – odds ratio, **P** – prospective, **PB** – patient-blind, **PC** – placebo-controlled, **PG** – parallel group, **PS** – pilot study, **R** – randomized, **RC** – reference-controlled, **RCS** – retrospective cross-sectional, **RS** - retrospective, **S** – surveillance, **SB** – single-blind, **SC** – single-center, **U** – uncontrolled, **UP** – unpublished, **VC** – vehicle-controlled.

MULTI-HERB PROPRIETARY PRODUCT MONOGRAPHS
(Alphabetized by Product Name)

Alluna™ Sleep

MANUFACTURER: GlaxoSmithKline; Pittsburgh, PA. (Other brand names for this product, if any, may be found in the table on page 404.)

CONTENTS: Extracts of valerian root (*Valeriana officinalis*) (500mg) and hops (*Humulus lupulus*) (120 mg) [extract strength not declared].

PRIMARY USES: Sleep, insomnia.

DSHEA STRUCTURE-FUNCTION CLAIM: "Promotes a Healthy Natural Sleep Pattern."

DOSAGE: 2 tablets.

DURATION OF ADMINISTRATION: 1 month.

ACTIONS: Mild sedative and sleep promoting agent.

CONTRAINDICATIONS: None listed.

PREGNANCY AND LACTATION: None listed.

ADVERSE EFFECTS: None listed.

DRUG INTERACTIONS: None listed.

EDITORS' NOTE: Product is labeled as an "Herbal Supplement"; tablets are blister packed, each tablet individually sealed. "Not a drug" printed on front panel.

NOTE: This information was derived from the label of the manufacturer and consideration of additional safety information is advised. Please consult Brinker, 2001; McGuffin *et al.*, 1997, and the single herb monograph for valerian in this book for more information on the safety of each of the herbs listed in this multi-herb product. In some cases, potential toxicity may be reduced or otherwise altered through the combination of herbs into one product.

Clinical Studies on Alluna™ Sleep

Sleep

Author/Year	Subject	Design	Duration	Dosage	Preparation	Results/Conclusion
Fussel *et al.*, 2000	Sleep	PS n=30	2 wks	2 tablets in the evening (1000 mg valerian extract and 240 mg hops extract per day)	Ze 91019 Alluna™ (US) Ivel® (Germany) Redormin® (Switzerland) (500 mg valerian extract and 120 mg hops extract)	Polysomnography data on patients with mild to moderate, non-organic insomnia were recorded on baseline and after 2 weeks. Sleep latency was reduced statistical significantly while sleep efficiency increased. An increase in slow wave sleep was recorded. In a self-assessment patients reported an improvement of feeling refreshed in the morning after 2 weeks. No adverse events were recorded.
Vonderheid-Guth *et al.*, 2000	Sleep	R, SB, CO 2 studies n=12	1, 2, and 4 hours after application in each study, studies spaced 3 months apart	1st dosage: 1 tablet vs. placebo; 2nd dosage: 3 tablets (1500 mg valerian extract and 360 mg hops extract per day) vs. placebo	Ze 91019 Alluna™ (US) Ivel® (Germany) Redormin® (Switzerland) (500 mg valerian extract and 120 mg hops extract)	The study concluded that pharmaco-dynamic responses could be repeated. The quantitative topo-graphical EEG demonstrated a visible effect on the CNS, especially after intake of the high dosage of the valerian-hops combination.
Kammer *et al.*, 1996	Sleep	R, DB, CO n=18	21 days	2 tablets in the evening, or placebo	Ze 91019 Alluna™ (US) Ivel® (Germany) Redormin® (Switzerland)	The study concluded that the combination did not produce significant adverse effects and did not impair psychometrically measured fitness and subjective state of health. In addition, no significant interaction with alcohol is to be expected.
Lataster and Brattström, 1996	Sleep	MC, OL n=3447	4–6 wks	2 tablets in the evening	Ze 91019 Alluna™ (US) Ivel® (Germany) Redormin® (Switzerland)	The efficacy of the combination was evaluated as good to very good by 75% of the physicians. The number of patients who slept through the night rose from 24.4% to 77.4%. The self-efficacy report of feeling rested upon awakening rose from 26.5% to 64.9%.

KEY: **C** – controlled, **CC** – case-control, **CH** – cohort, **CI** – confidence interval, **Cm** – comparison, **CO** – crossover, **CS** – cross-sectional, **DB** – double-blind, **E** – epidemiological, **LC** – longitudinal cohort, **MA** – meta-analysis, **MC** – multi-center, **n** – number of patients, **O** – open, **OB** – observational, **OL** – open label, **OR** – odds ratio, **P** – prospective, **PB** – patient-blind, **PC** – placebo-controlled, **PG** – parallel group, **PS** – pilot study, **R** – randomized, **RC** – reference-controlled, **RCS** – retrospective cross-sectional, **RS** - retrospective, **S** – surveillance, **SB** – single-blind, **SC** – single-center, **U** – uncontrolled, **UP** – unpublished, **VC** – vehicle-controlled.

Esberitox®

MANUFACTURER: Schaper & Brümmer; Salzgitter, Germany. (Other brand names for this product, if any, may be found in the table on page 404.)

CONTENTS: Esberitox® (prior to 1985): 5 mg of *E. purpurea* and *E. angustifolia* root (1:1), 2 mg of *Thuja occidentalis* herb, and 10 mg *Baptisia tinctoria* root plus homeopathic preparations (dilutions) made from additional herbs.

Esberitox® N1 Tablets (since 1985): 7.5 mg of *E. purpurea* and *E. angustifolia* root extract (1:1), 2 mg of *Thuja occidentalis* herb, and 10 mg *Baptisia tinctoria* root (without homeopathic dilutions) (Melchart *et al.*, 1994).

Esberitox® N2 Tablets (since 1990): 7.5 mg of *E. purpurea* root extract (1:1), 2 mg of *Thuja occidentalis* herb, and 10 mg *Baptisia tinctoria* root (changed echinacea material; *E. angustifolia* no longer used) (Melchart *et al.*, 1994).

Esberitox®N Tablets (since 1993): 7.5 mg of *E. purpurea* root and *E. pallida* root (1:1).

PRIMARY USES: Acute and chronic infections of the respiratory tract (viral or bacterial); accompanying antibiotics in case of severe bacterial infections such as bronchitis, angina, pharyngitis, otitis media, sinusitis; temporarily weakened immune system with recurring infections; herpes simplex labialis (cold sores); bacterial skin infections; leukopenias after radiation or cytostatic treatment.

DSHEA STRUCTURE-FUNCTION CLAIM: Immunomodulator for strengthening the body's immune system.

DOSAGE: Adults: 3 tablets, 3 times daily; Infants: 1 tablet, 3 times daily; Children up to 6 years: 1–2 tablets, 3 times daily; Children up to 12 years: 2 tablets, 3 times daily.

DURATION OF ADMINISTRATION: Not longer than eight weeks.

ACTIONS: Immunostimulation.

CONTRAINDICATIONS: Known hypersensitivity to one of the active or inactive ingredients or against composite flowers; for principle reasons not for use in case of progressive systemic diseases such as tuberculosis, leukosis, collagenosis, multiple scleroses, AIDS, HIV infection, and other autoimmune diseases.

PREGNANCY AND LACTATION: None listed.

ADVERSE EFFECTS: In individual cases, reactions due to a hypersensitivity may occur.

DRUG INTERACTIONS: None listed.

NOTE: This information was derived from the label of the manufacturer and consideration of additional safety information is advised. Please consult Brinker, 2001; McGuffin *et al.*, 1997, and the single herb monograph for echinacea in this book for more information on the safety of each of the herbs listed in this multi-herb product. In some cases, potential toxicity may be reduced or otherwise altered through the combination of herbs into one product.

Clinical Studies on Esberitox®

Upper Respiratory Tract Infections

Author/Year	Subject	Design	Duration	Dosage	Preparation	Results/Conclusion
Henneicke-von Zepelin *et al.*, 1999	Common cold (acute viral URTI)	R,DB,PC, MC (15 centers) n=238 patients (ages 18–70 years)	7–9 days once identified as having a common cold	Three, 20 mg tablets 3x/day	Esberitox® N2	The echinacea combination product was significantly better than the placebo (p=0.0497), with statically significant results in overall well being (p=0.0048), rhinitis (p=0.0581), and bronchitis scores (p=0.1031). This study suggests this to be a safe and effective treatment, and notes the greatest benefits are experienced when beginning the treatment as soon after the onset as possible.
Reitz, 1990	URTI symptoms and signs	R, DB, PC n=150	8 weeks initially with monitoring for an additional year	One 22.5 mg tablet 3x/day	Esberitox® N1	Majority of symptoms and signs at 7 and 14 days were significantly better than placebo, nasal symptoms most predominant. No difference in result from blood work was reported.
Vorberg, 1984	URTI symptoms and signs in patients suffering from common cold	R, DB, PC n=100	10 days	One 15 mg tablet 3x/day	Esberitox® tablet	Echinacea combination group reported significant superiority compared to placebo group in all examined parameters of common cold (p<0.001) including fatigue, reduced performance, runny nose, and sore throat.
Forth and Beuscher, 1981	URTI prevention	R, PC n=95 (not fully double blinded)	16 weeks (Nov–Feb)	25 drops liquid, 3x/day or 1 tablet 3x/day or placebo	Esberitox®	Patients had relative risk reduction of 49% overall even though no apparent difference for the other 7 symptoms were observed in all groups compared to placebo. However, improvements of nasal symptoms were significant.

KEY: **C** – controlled, **CC** – case-control, **CH** – cohort, **CI** – confidence interval, **Cm** – comparison, **CO** – crossover, **CS** – cross-sectional, **DB** – double-blind, **E** – epidemiological, **LC** – longitudinal cohort, **MA** – meta-analysis, **MC** – multi-center, **n** – number of patients, **O** – open, **OB** – observational, **OL** – open label, **OR** – odds ratio, **P** – prospective, **PB** – patient-blind, **PC** – placebo-controlled, **PG** – parallel group, **PS** – pilot study, **R** – randomized, **RC** – reference-controlled, **RCS** – retrospective cross-sectional, **RS** - retrospective, **S** – surveillance, **SB** – single-blind, **SC** – single-center, **U** – uncontrolled, **UP** – unpublished, **VC** – vehicle-controlled.

Euvegal® forte

MANUFACTURER: Dr. Willmar Schwabe Karlsruhe / Germany. (Other brand names for this product, if any, may be found in the table on page 404.)

CONTENTS: Each tablet contains 160 mg valerian root (*Valeriana officinalis*) extract (4–5:1) and 80 mg lemon balm leaf (*Melissa officinalis*) extract (4–6:1).

PRIMARY USES: Restlessness; sleep-induction disturbances due to nervous conditions.

DSHEA STRUCTURE-FUNCTION CLAIM: Promotes restful sleep (Valerian Nighttime™, NaturesWay).

DOSAGE: Restlessness: 2x2 tablets per day; as sleep aid: 2 tablets half an hour prior to going to bed.

DURATION OF ADMINISTRATION: The product is well tolerated. If the symptoms persist, a physician should be consulted.

ACTIONS: Sedative.

CONTRAINDICATIONS: None listed.

PREGNANCY AND LACTATION: No known risks subsequent to marketing as a nonprescription drug in Europe. However, results from experimental studies are not available, and the product should therefore not be taken during pregnancy and lactation.

ADVERSE EFFECTS: None listed.

DRUG INTERACTIONS: None listed.

NOTE: This information was derived from the label of the manufacturer and consideration of additional safety information is advised. Please consult Brinker, 2001; McGuffin *et al.*, 1997, and the single herb monograph for valerian in this book for more information on the safety of each of the herbs listed in this multi-herb product. However, in some cases, potential toxicity may be reduced or otherwise altered through the combination of herbs into one product.

Clinical Studies on Euvegal® forte

Insomnia

Author/Year	Subject	Design	Duration	Dosage	Preparation	Results/Conclusion
Dressing *et al.*, 1996	Insomnia	DB, PC n=68 adults with insomnia	2 weeks	2 tablets, 160 mg valerian extract with 80 mg lemon balm extract (each), 2x/day	Euvegal® forte valerian and lemon balm tablet vs. placebo	Sleep quality improved in valerian/lemon balm combination compared to placebo (p=0.02) and remained in effect 1 week after medication was discontinued (p=0.10).
Albrecht *et al.*, 1995	Driving ability and combination with alcohol	R, DB, PC n=54	3 weeks	2 tablets, 2x/day or placebo	Euvegal® forte	Traffic safety was evaluated using psychometric tests. The treatment group showed no difference in driving ability compared to placebo, and treatment did not potentiate the effect of alcohol consumption. The study concluded that Euvegal® does not cause impairment of the operation of machinery or the driving of vehicles.
Dressing *et al.*, 1992	Insomnia	DB, PC, CO n=20 adults with insomnia	9 days	160 mg valerian with 80 mg lemon balm or 0.125 mg triazolam (Halcion®)	Euvegal® forte valerian and lemon balm tablet vs. placebo	Both active treatments were equivalent and significantly better than placebo. The herbs caused less daytime sedation and impairment of mental functions.

KEY: **C** – controlled, **CC** – case-control, **CH** – cohort, **CI** – confidence interval, **Cm** – comparison, **CO** – crossover, **CS** – cross-sectional, **DB** – double-blind, **E** – epidemiological, **LC** – longitudinal cohort, **MA** – meta-analysis, **MC** – multi-center, **n** – number of patients, **O** – open, **OB** – observational, **OL** – open label, **OR** – odds ratio, **P** – prospective, **PB** – patient-blind, **PC** – placebo-controlled, **PG** – parallel group, **PS** – pilot study, **R** – randomized, **RC** – reference-controlled, **RCS** – retrospective cross-sectional, **RS** - retrospective, **S** – surveillance, **SB** – single-blind, **SC** – single-center, **U** – uncontrolled, **UP** – unpublished, **VC** – vehicle-controlled.

Hochu-ekki-to®

MANUFACTURER: Tsumura & Co., Tokyo, Japan. (Other brand names for this product, if any, may be found in the table on page 404.)

CONTENTS: Astragalus root JP (*Astragalus membranaceus* (Fisch.) Bge., Fabaceae); Asian ginseng root JP (*Panax ginseng* C.A. Mey., Araliaceae); Atractylodes rhizome JP (*Atractylodes lancea* (Thunb.) DC, Asteraceae); Japanese angelica root JP (*Angelica acutiloba* Kitagawa, Apiaceae); Bupleurum root JP (*Bupleurum falcatum* L., Apiaceae); Jujube fruit JP (*Zyzyphus jujuba* Mill., Rhamnaceae); Citrus unshiu peel JP (*Citrus unshiu* Markovich, Rutaceae); Licorice root JP (*Glycyrrhiza uralensis* Fisch., Fabaceae); Cimicifuga rhizome JP (*Cimicifuga simplex* Wormskjord, Ranunculaceae); Ginger rhizome JP (*Zingiber officinale* Roscoe, Zingiberaceae); [JP = *Japanese Pharmacopeia*].

PRIMARY USES: Hochu-ekki-to® is indicated for the following symptoms/conditions of patients having delicate constitution, reduced digestive functions, and severe fatigability of limbs: Summer emaciation, reinforcement of physical strength after illness, tuberculosis, anorexia, gastroptosis (downward stomach displacement), common cold, hemorrhoids, anal prolapse, uterine prolapse, impotence, hemiplegia (paralysis of one side of body), and hyperhidrosis (excessive perspiration).

DSHEA STRUCTURE-FUNCTION CLAIM: Not sold in the U.S.

DOSAGE: 7.5 g per day.

DURATION OF ADMINISTRATION: Not established. The product could be administered continuously as long as the patient's symptoms/findings are improved. However the patient should be monitored carefully, and if no improvement is observed, continuous administration should be avoided.

OTHER DATA OR SPECIAL INSTRUCTIONS:

1. Herb-drug Interaction: The product should be used carefully when co-administered with preparations containing licorice, glycyrrhizinic acid and/or its salts. Pseudo-aldosteronism, myopathy or hypokalemia is likely to occur (if used with licorice).

2. Use in the elderly: Because elderly patients often have reduced physiological function, careful supervision and measures such as reducing the dose are recommended.

3. Pediatric use: The safety of this product in children has not been established (insufficient clinical data).

4. Other precautions: Eczema, dermatitis, etc. may be aggravated.

(continued on next page)

Clinical Studies on Hochu-ekki-to®

Author/Year	Subject	Design	Duration	Dosage	Preparation	Results/Conclusion
Karibe, 1997	Effect on Methicillin Resistant Staphlococcus Aureus (MRSA) carriers	C n=44	Not stated	Not stated	Hochu-ekki-to® (TJ-41)	Subjects did not receive any other treatment such as vancomycin or other antibiotics, and MRSA readings were negative for 61.6% of the patients receiving Hochu-ekki-to® (61.6%). Hochu-ekki-to® significantly reduced the time necessary to achieve a negative MRSA reading; 47.0 +/- 5.5 days compared to 88.4 +/- 12.8 days for the control group.
Kuratsune et al., 1997	Chronic fatigue syndrome	DB, PC n=9	8 to 12 weeks	7.5 g per day	Hochu-ekki-to® (TJ-41)	On the Performance Status (PS) scale, 34.5% of the patients improved 3 or more levels in the PS scale, to the degree comfortable living became possible. A high level of improvement was reported in symptoms such as fatigue, exhaustion, low-grade fever, muscle pain, and mental alertness.
Niwa et al., 1996	Immune function in post-operative patients with gastrointestinal (GI) cancer	Cm n=25	8 wks	7.5 g per day	Hochu-ekki-to® (TJ-41)	Immune function was measured using blood assays of NK and LAK activity. Significant activity was found regarding NK activity, from 29.9% pre-treatment to 42.2% after 8 weeks. LAK activity did not change. Improvement was observed in appetite, fatigue, and diarrhea.
Igarashi et al., 1995	Effect on anorexia, fatigue, and malaise	MC n=45	4–12 weeks, average of 10.5	5.0–7.5 g per day	Hochu-ekki-to® (TJ-41)	In a subjective evaluation, 88.9% of patients reported improved or markedly improved symptoms. All 25 atonic constitution patients reported their symptoms as improved or better.
Mori et al., 1992	Fatigue accompanying chemotherapy	R, Cm n=43	5 weeks, 1 wk prior to chemotherapy, 4 wks after chemotherapy	2.5 g, 3 times per day before meals or control	Hochu-ekki-to® (TJ-41)	Patients receiving TJ-41 (the Tsumura code this formula) had less fatigue, better appetite, and improved mood without side effects. Results were based upon patient evaluation and records kept by physicians and nurses. TJ-41 did not show any effect on nausea or vomiting compared to control. The study concluded that TJ-41 had a significant effect in the prevention of fatigue in cancer chemotherapy.

KEY: **C** – controlled, **CC** – case-control, **CH** – cohort, **CI** – confidence interval, **Cm** – comparison, **CO** – crossover, **CS** – cross-sectional, **DB** – double-blind, **E** – epidemiological, **LC** – longitudinal cohort, **MA** – meta-analysis, **MC** – multi-center, **n** – number of patients, **O** – open, **OB** – observational, **OL** – open label, **OR** – odds ratio, **P** – prospective, **PB** – patient-blind, **PC** – placebo-controlled, **PG** – parallel group, **PS** – pilot study, **R** – randomized, **RC** – reference-controlled, **RCS** – retrospective cross-sectional, **RS** - retrospective, **S** – surveillance, **SB** – single-blind, **SC** – single-center, **U** – uncontrolled, **UP** – unpublished, **VC** – vehicle-controlled.

Hochu-ekki-to® (cont.)

ACTIONS: Immunostimulant, tonic.

CONTRAINDICATIONS: None listed.

PREGNANCY AND LACTATION: The safety of this product in pregnant women has not been established. Therefore, the product should be used only if the expected therapeutic benefits outweigh the possible risks associated with treatment in pregnant women and women who may possibly be pregnant.

ADVERSE EFFECTS: The incidence rate of adverse reactions of this product has not been investigated yet.

1. Clinically significant adverse reactions

   a. Pseudoaldosteronism: Pseudoaldosteronism such as hypokalemia, increased blood pressure, retention of sodium/body fluid, edema, increased body weight, etc. may occur. The patient should be carefully monitored (measurement of serum potassium level, etc.), and if any abnormality is observed, administration should be discontinued and appropriate measures such as administration of potassium preparations should be taken.

   b. Myopathy: Myopathy may occur as a result of hypokalemia. The patient should be carefully monitored,

and if any abnormality such as weakness, convulsion/paralysis of limbs, etc. are observed, administration should be discontinued and appropriate measures such as administration of potassium preparations should be taken.

2. Other adverse reactions

   a. Hypersensitivity: Rash, urticaria, etc. may occur. If such symptoms are observed, administration should be discontinued.

   b. Hepatic: Increases in AST (GOT), ALT (GPT), Al-P, γ-GTP and bilirubin levels may occur.

   c. Gastrointestinal: Anorexia, epigastric distress, nausea, diarrhea, etc. may occur.

DRUG INTERACTIONS: None listed.

NOTE: This information was derived from the label of the manufacturer and consideration of additional safety information is advised. Please consult Brinker, 2001; McGuffin et al., 1997, and the single herb monographs for ginger and licorice in this book for more information on the safety of each of the herbs listed in this multi-herb product. In some cases, potential toxicity may be reduced or otherwise altered through the combination of herbs into one product.

Hova®

MANUFACTURER: Gebro Broscheck GmbH, Austria. (Other brand names for this product, if any, may be found in the table on page 404.)

CONTENTS: Each tablet contains valerian (*Valeriana officinalis* L.) (60 mg) and hop flower (*Humulus lupulus* L.) extract (30 mg).

PRIMARY USES: Sleep, insomnia.

DSHEA STRUCTURE-FUNCTION CLAIM: "Promotes a Healthy Natural Sleep Pattern".

DOSAGE: 2 tablets.

DURATION OF ADMINISTRATION: 1 month.

ACTIONS: Mild sedative and sleep promoting agent.

CONTRAINDICATIONS: None listed.

PREGNANCY AND LACTATION: None listed.

ADVERSE EFFECTS: None listed.

DRUG INTERACTIONS: None listed.

NOTE: This information was derived from the label of the manufacturer and consideration of additional safety information is advised. Please consult Brinker, 2001; McGuffin et al., 1997, and the single herb monograph for valerian in this book for more information on the safety of each of the herbs listed in this multi-herb product. In some cases, potential toxicity may be reduced or otherwise altered through the combination of herbs into one product.

Clinical Studies on Hova®

Sleep

Author/Year	Subject	Design	Duration	Dosage	Preparation	Results/Conclusion
Schmitz and Jackel, 1998	Sleep disorders	R, DB, C n= 46 patients with sleep disorders according to the DSM-IV criteria	2 weeks	2 tablets (200 mg valerian extract with 45.5 mg hops extract or 3 mg benzodiazapine)	Hova® compared to benzodiazapine	Patients' state of health improved during therapy with both agents and deterioration after cessation was reported for both groups. Withdrawal symptoms were reported only in benzodiazepine groups.
Leathwood et al, 1982	Sleep	R, DB, PC, CO n=128	9 nights	400 mg	Hova®	Subjects had statistically significant (p<0.05) decrease in subjective sleep latency and significant improvement in sleep quality. Improvement was most notable among people who were poor or irregular sleepers, and smokers. No detectable hangover effect was noted in the morning.

KEY: C – controlled, **CC** – case-control, **CH** – cohort, **CI** – confidence interval, **Cm** – comparison, **CO** – crossover, **CS** – cross-sectional, **DB** – double-blind, **E** – epidemiological, **LC** – longitudinal cohort, **MA** – meta-analysis, **MC** – multi-center, **n** – number of patients, **O** – open, **OB** – observational, **OL** – open label, **OR** – odds ratio, **P** – prospective, **PB** – patient-blind, **PC** – placebo-controlled, **PG** – parallel group, **PS** – pilot study, **R** – randomized, **RC** – reference-controlled, **RCS** – retrospective cross-sectional, **RS** - retrospective, **S** – surveillance, **SB** – single-blind, **SC** – single-center, **U** – uncontrolled, **UP** – unpublished, **VC** – vehicle-controlled.

Liv.52®

MANUFACTURER: The Himalaya Drug Company, Bangalore, India. (Other brand names for this product, if any, may be found in the table on page 404.)

CONTENTS: Active ingredients in the proprietary formula: capers (*Capparis spinosa*) (root bark); chicory (*Cichorium intybus*) (seed); black nightshade (*Solanum nigrum*) (whole plant); arjuna (*Terminalia arjuna*) (bark); negro coffee (*Cassia occidentalis*) (seed); yarrow (*Achillea millefolium*) (aerial parts); tamarisk (*Tamarisk gallica*) (whole plant).

PRIMARY USES: Liver dysfunction.

DSHEA STRUCTURE-FUNCTION CLAIM: "Maintenance of optimum liver health" (LiverCare®, Himalaya USA).

DOSAGE: 1 or 2 x 500 mg, two to three times per day. Dosage may be adjusted based on body weight and/or severity of the condition.

DURATION OF ADMINISTRATION: May be used daily for an extended period of time.

ACTIONS: Hepatic stimulant, hepatoprotector.

CONTRAINDICATIONS: None listed.

PREGNANCY AND LACTATION: None listed.

ADVERSE EFFECTS: None listed. No reported Adverse Effects since market entry in 1954.

DRUG INTERACTIONS: Liv.52® has been shown to effectively alleviate the hepatotoxicity of drugs.

NOTE: This information was derived from the label of the manufacturer and consideration of additional safety information is advised. Please consult Brinker, 2001; McGuffin *et al.*, 1997, and the single herb monographs in this book for more information on the safety of each of the herbs listed in this multi-herb product. In some cases, potential toxicity may be reduced or otherwise altered through the combination of herbs into one product.

(Refer to table of Clinical Studies on next page.)

Liver/Hepatitis

Author/Year	Subject	Design	Duration	Dosage	Preparation	Results/Conclusion
Chauhan and Kulkarni, 1991	Alcoholic liver disease	PC n=25	2 weeks	Two, 250 mg tablets, 2 times/day	Liv.52® tablets or placebo	The study was divided into 2 groups. Group A : (8 patients) measured ethanol absorption by comparing blood samples. Liv.52® treatment produced a marked increase in ethanol absorption vs. placebo in moderate drinkers, with no effect on occasional drinkers. Group B measured ethanol metabolism (9 moderate, 8 occasional drinkers), and found that Liv.52® reversed the effect of low blood ethanol and high acetaldehyde seen in heavy alcohol users. The study concluded that improved acetaldehyde elimination from the use of Liv.52® may reduce the harmful effect of ethanol on the liver and potentially the brain.
Mandal and Roy, 1983	Infective hepatitis (Group A), chronic active hepatitis (Group B) and cirrhosis (Group C)	DB, PC n=104 (Group A:30 treatment, 15 control; Group B: 24, 8; Group C: 19, 8)	Group A: 6 weeks; Group B: 12 months; Group C: 24 months	Four, 250 mg tablets, 3 times/day	Liv.52® tablets or placebo	Group A: patients with infective hepatitis showed a marked symptomatic improvement with Liv.52®, with lowered levels of serum bilirubin and alkaline phosphatase twice as quickly compared to control. Group B: patients with chronic active hepatitis demonstrated an immediate, significant drop in serum alkaline phosphatase, from 35 units (King-Armstrong or KA) to less than 10 within 12 months. Control group dropped from 35 to 25 units. Group C: 4 patients with cirrhosis showed clinical improvement in 12 months, 10 patients improved in 24 months compared to no improvement in control. Drop in serum alkaline phosphatase to 14 KA in 24 months vs. increase in control. Greater excretion of BSP in 80% of the treated group versus 20% in the control group. Histopathological examination revealed improvements in 4 cases and no progress in fibrosis in other treated cases versus fibrosis progression in control.
Saxena et al., 1980	Infective hepatitis	PC n=30	5 weeks	15 drops: 0–1 yr 2 tsp syrup: 1–3 yrs 2, 250 mg tablets: above 3 yrs, 3xday	Liv.52® drops, syrup, liquid, or tablets	Significant improvement observed after one week, with a reduction in symptoms compared to placebo at the end of the second week. Liver function tests returned to normal more quickly than with placebo.
Patney and Kumar, 1978	Serum B-hepatitis (Australian Antigen Positive)	PC n=20	6 months	6 tablets/day	Liv.52® tablets	Hematology studies indicated that Liv.52®, combined with steroids and other supportive therapy, significantly improved symptoms and sped up recovery time.
Singh et al., 1977	Infective hepatitis	PC n=50	8 weeks	6 tablets/day	Liv.52® tablets with B-complex and cortico-steroids vs. control of B-complex and cortico-steroids	Subjects with Liv.52® experienced symptom relief in 1/2 the time compared to control. Liver function tests showed improvement in both groups.
Sama et al., 1976	Infective hepatitis	R, DB, PC n=34	6 weeks with a 3-month follow-up	Six, 250 mg tablets/day	Liv.52® tablets	Subjects treated with Liv.52® showed a quicker clinical recovery and a 50% drop in bilrubin. The placebo group had a higher weight loss.

KEY: **C** – controlled, **CC** – case-control, **CH** – cohort, **CI** – confidence interval, **Cm** – comparison, **CO** – crossover, **CS** – cross-sectional, **DB** – double-blind, **E** – epidemiological, **LC** – longitudinal cohort, **MA** – meta-analysis, **MC** – multi-center, **n** – number of patients, **O** – open, **OB** – observational, **OL** – open label, **OR** – odds ratio, **P** – prospective, **PB** – patient-blind, **PC** – placebo-controlled, **PG** – parallel group, **PS** – pilot study, **R** – randomized, **RC** – reference-controlled, **RCS** – retrospective cross-sectional, **RS** - retrospective, **S** – surveillance, **SB** – single-blind, **SC** – single-center, **U** – uncontrolled, **UP** – unpublished, **VC** – vehicle-controlled.

Mastodynon®

MANUFACTURER: Bionorica AG; Neumarkt, Germany. (Other brand names for this product, if any, may be found in the table on page 404.)

CONTENTS: 10 g (10.8 ml) Mastodynon® drops contain as active ingredients 2.0 g *Agnus castus* ø [chaste tree, *Vitex*], 1.0 g *Caulophyllum thalictroides* (HAB 34) Dil. D4 (HAB 1; V.3a), 1.0 g Cyclamen Dil. D4, 1.0 g Ignatia Dil. D6, 2.0 g Iris Dil. D2, 1.0 g *Lilium tigrinum* Dil. D3. Mastodynon® drops contain ethanol 53% v/v.

PRIMARY USES: Disorders associated with premenstrual syndrome (PMS) including: mastodynia (breast pain), psychic lability, constipation, fluid retention/swelling, headache, migraine, and fibrocystic mastopathy.

DSHEA STRUCTURE-FUNCTION CLAIM: "For disorders of the menstrual cycle" (in product literature).

DOSAGE: 30 drops 2x/day (morning and evening) with water.

DURATION OF ADMINISTRATION: 3 months.

ACTIONS: None listed.

CONTRAINDICATIONS: Hypersensitivity to *Agnus castus* (chaste tree) and/or *Caulophyllum thalictroides* and/or Cyclamen and/or Ignatia and/or Iris and/or *Lilium tigrinum*.

PREGNANCY AND LACTATION: None listed.

ADVERSE EFFECTS: Nausea, gastric complaints, slight weight increase, itching exanthemes, acne, or headache.

DRUG INTERACTIONS: None listed.

MANUFACTURER'S NOTE: "Mastodynon® drops contain ethanol. It therefore should not be used, if there is a history of successful withdrawal after alcohol abuse."

NOTE: This information was derived from the label of the manufacturer and consideration of additional safety information is advised. Please consult Brinker, 2001; McGuffin *et al.,* 1997, and the single herb monograph for chaste tree in this book for more information on the safety of each of the herbs listed in this multi-herb product. In some cases, potential toxicity may be reduced or otherwise altered through the combination of herbs into one product.

Clinical Studies on on Mastodynon®

Mastopathy

Author/Year	Subject	Design	Duration	Dosage	Preparation	Results/Conclusion
Halaške *et al.,* 1999	Cyclic mastalgia	R, DB, PC n=97	3 cycles	30 drops, 2x/day	Mastodynon®	Using a visual analog scale (VAS) the mean decrease in pain intensity (mm) after one/two/three cycles was 21.4mm/33.7mm/34.3mm for the Mastodynon® group versus 10.6mm/20.3mm/35.7mm for placebo (p=0.018; p=0.006; p=0.064).
Kubista *et al.,* 1986	Cyclic mastodynia	R, DB, PC (3 treatment groups) n=160	At least 4 cycles	30 drops, 2x/day; or 5 mg, 2x/day gestagen (lynestrenol) from the 16th to the 25th day of the cycle; or placebo	Mastodynon®	74.55 of Mastodynon® group reported a marked improvement in symptoms compared with 82.1% for gestagen group and 36.8% for placebo. Mastodynon® was significantly more effective than placebo (p<0.01).

Infertility

Author/Year	Subject	Design	Duration	Dosage	Preparation	Results/Conclusion
Gerhard *et al.,* 1998	Fertility disorders: secondary amenorrhea, luteal insufficiency, idiopathic infertility	R, DB, PC, P n=96 (with 66 suitable for evaluation)	3 months	30 drops, 2x/day	Mastodynon®	Desired outcome measure (pregnancy or spontaneous menstruation in amenorrhea group; pregnancy or improved luteal hormone concentrations in other groups) was achieved in 57.6% of Mastodynon® participants versus 36.0% of placebo participants (p=0.069). In the amenorrhea and luteal insufficient groups, pregnancy occurred more than twice as often with Mastodynon® compared with placebo.

KEY: **C** – controlled, **CC** – case-control, **CH** – cohort, **CI** – confidence interval, **Cm** – comparison, **CO** – crossover, **CS** – cross-sectional, **DB** – double-blind, **E** – epidemiological, **LC** – longitudinal cohort, **MA** – meta-analysis, **MC** – multi-center, **n** – number of patients, **O** – open, **OB** – observational, **OL** – open label, **OR** – odds ratio, **P** – prospective, **PB** – patient-blind, **PC** – placebo-controlled, **PG** – parallel group, **PS** – pilot study, **R** – randomized, **RC** – reference-controlled, **RCS** – retrospective cross-sectional, **RS** - retrospective, **S** – surveillance, **SB** – single-blind, **SC** – single-center, **U** – uncontrolled, **UP** – unpublished, **VC** – vehicle-controlled.

Nutrilite® Saw Palmetto with Nettle Root

MANUFACTURER: Access Business Group, Buena Park, California. (Other brand names for this product, if any, may be found in the table on page 404.)

CONTENTS: Nutrilite® Saw Palmetto with Nettle Root; Each softgel contains a blend of 106 mg saw palmetto lipoidal extract (*Serenoa repens*), 80 mg nettle root extract (*Urtica dioica*), 160 mg pumpkin seed oil (*Cucurbita pepo*), 33 mg lemon bioflavonoid concentrate, and 100 IU natural β-carotene concentrate.

PRIMARY USES: None listed.

DSHEA STRUCTURE-FUNCTION CLAIM: "Both Saw palmetto and Nettle root help support normal urinary flow".

DOSAGE: 3 softgels/day.

DURATION OF ADMINISTRATION: Continuous.

ACTIONS: Helps support normal prostate health.

CONTRAINDICATIONS: None listed.

PREGNANCY AND LACTATION: None listed.

ADVERSE EFFECTS: None listed.

DRUG INTERACTIONS: None listed.

EDITORS' NOTE: Unlike many other products in this section, this product was developed as a dietary supplement for the U.S., although it may be marketed as a licensed nonprescription drug in selected foreign countries, as required by local regulations. Thus, some of the labeling information found on other products is not listed for this product. However, the 3 ingredients are considered very safe, with few adverse effects (see saw palmetto monograph).

NOTE: This information was derived from the label of the manufacturer and consideration of additional safety information is advised. Please consult Brinker, 2001; McGuffin *et al.*, 1997, and the single herb monograph for saw palmetto in this book for more information on the safety of each of the herbs listed in this multi-herb product. In some cases, potential toxicity may be reduced or otherwise altered through the combination of herbs into one product.

Clinical Studies on Nutrilite® Saw Palmetto with Nettle Root

Prostate

Author/Year	Subject	Design	Duration	Dosage	Preparation	Results/Conclusion
Marks *et al.*, 2001	BPH	R, DB, PC, Cm n=40 (saw palmetto vs. placebo); n=22 (finasteride vs. control), measuring prostate tissue androgen levels using needle biopsies	6 months	One, softgel 3x/day with meals (320 mg/day saw palmetto extract, 240 mg/day nettle root extract, 480 mg/day pumpkin seed oil, 100 mg/day lemon bioflavonoid concentrate, and 300 IU/day natural b-carotene concentrate) or placebo	Nutrilite® Saw Palmetto with Nettle Root; finasteride	No significant change in tissue dihydrotestosterone (DHT) levels was observed with the placebo compared to tissue samples biopsied at baseline. In the saw palmetto blend group, tissue DHT levels were significantly reduced by 32% from 6.49 ng/g to 4.40 ng/g (p<0.005). Chronic finasteride therapy significantly (p<0.01) lowered prostate tissue DHT levels by ~80%.
Marks et al., 2000	BPH	R, DB, PC n=44 men with symptomatic BPH; OL extension after 6 months with 41 men electing to continue therapy	6 months	One, softgel 3x/day with meals (320 mg/day saw palmetto extract, 240 mg/day nettle root extract, 480 mg/day pumpkin seed oil, 100 mg/day lemon bioflavonoid concentrate, and 300 IU/day natural b-carotene concentrate) or placebo	Nutrilite® Saw Palmetto with Nettle Root	Saw palmetto blend group had non-statistically significant improvement vs. placebo in clinical parameters (e.g., International Prostate Symptom Score, uroflowmetry, residual urine volume, prostate volume). After 6 months, saw palmetto blend was associated with significant prostate epithelial contraction, notably in the transition zone (p<0.01), suggesting a possible mechanism for the clinical effects observed in other studies. No serious adverse effects were associated with the saw palmetto blend.

KEY: **C** – controlled, **CC** – case-control, **CH** – cohort, **CI** – confidence interval, **Cm** – comparison, **CO** – crossover, **CS** – cross-sectional, **DB** – double-blind, **E** – epidemiological, **LC** – longitudinal cohort, **MA** – meta-analysis, **MC** – multi-center, **n** – number of patients, **O** – open, **OB** – observational, **OL** – open label, **OR** – odds ratio, **P** – prospective, **PB** – patient-blind, **PC** – placebo-controlled, **PG** – parallel group, **PS** – pilot study, **R** – randomized, **RC** – reference-controlled, **RCS** – retrospective cross-sectional, **RS** - retrospective, **S** – surveillance, **SB** – single-blind, **SC** – single-center, **U** – uncontrolled, **UP** – unpublished, **VC** – vehicle-controlled.

Padma® Basic / Padma®28

MANUFACTURER: Padma Inc., Schwerzenbach, Switzerland. Distributed in the U.S. by EcoNugenics, Inc. (Other brand names for this product, if any, may be found in the table on page 404.)

CONTENTS: The original Padma 28® formula contains dried and powdered herbs (403 mg) in a tablet. Those herbs that comprise 30 mg or more include:

costus root (*Saussurea costus*)

neem fruit (*Azadirachta indica*)

iceland moss (*Cetraria islandica*)

chebulic myrobalan fruit (*Terminalia chebula*)

cardomom fruit (*Elettaria cardamomum*)

red saunders heart wood (*Pterocarpus santalinus*)

Other Herbs: allspice fruit (*Pimenta dioica*), bengal quince fruit (*Aegle marmelos*), columbine aerial parts (*Aquilegiae vulgaris*), licorice root (*Glycyrrhiza glabra*), English plantain aerial parts, (*Plantago lanceolata*), knotweed aerial part (*Polygonum aviculare*), golden cinquefoil aerial part (*Potentilla aurea*), clove flower (*Syzygium aromaticum*), spiked ginger lily rhizome (*Hedychium spicatum*), heartleaf sida aerial parts (*Sida cordifolia*), Valerian root (*Valeriana officinalis*), lettuce leaf (*Lactuca sativa* var. capitata), calendula flower (*Calendula officinalis*), natural camphor (*Cinnamomum camphora*), aconite root (*Aconitum napellus*). Non-herbal ingredient: calcium sulfate.

NOTE: The formulation of Padma® Basic differs from Padma 28® only in the removal of the aconite root (*A. napellus*) in order to meet regulatory requirements for the U.S. and some European countries. However, it is generally well known that most of the aconite used in Asian traditional medicine is processed in a manner to eliminate or reduce potential toxicity.

PRIMARY USES: Peripheral arterial occlusive disease (PAOD) stage II (Intermittent claudication) (Drabaek *et al.*, 1993; Mehlsen *et al.*, 1993; Sallon *et al.*, 1998; Samochowiec *et al.*, 1987; Schrader *et al.*, 1985; Smulski and Wójcicki, 1995; Winther *et al.*, 1994). Recurrent respiratory tract infections in children (Jankowski *et al.*, 1991). In Switzerland, the registered indications are the early symptoms of PAOD such as tingling, feeling of heaviness and tension in arms and legs, numbness of hands and feet, cramps in the calf (IOCM, 1999). Other uses include hypercholesterolemia, hypertriglyceridemia (Samochowiec *et al.*, 1992), and angina pectoris (Wójcicki and Samochowiec, 1986).

DSHEA STRUCTURE-FUNCTION CLAIM: "Supports the immune system," "Promotes healthy circulation," "Supports with antioxidant activity" (Padma Ad, 2000).

DOSAGE: Two tablets (403 mg), twice daily.*

DURATION OF ADMINISTRATION: 4–6 months (per clinical studies).

ACTIONS: Preliminary results have found anti-inflammatory (Matzner and Sallon, 1995; Winther *et al.*, 1994), and antioxidative actions (Fishman, 1994; Ginsburg *et al.*, 1999; Suter and Richter, 2000).

Clinical research has also shown the promotion of fibrinolysis (Winther *et al.*, 1994) and the lowering of cholesterol and triglyceride levels (Samochowiec *et al.*, 1992; Samochowiec and Wójcicki, 1987; Wójcicki *et al.*, 1989b; Wójcicki *et al.*, 1988). Experimental research has found effects on the formation of atherosclerosis (Gieldanowski, 1992; Winther, 1994; Wójcicki *et al.*, 1988) and potential hepatoprotective effect in cases of alcohol abuse (Wójcicki *et al.*, 1989a; Nefyodov *et al.*, 2000). In cases of toxic liver injury in rats, Padma 28® has been shown to normalize the formation of amino acids and related compounds (Nefyodov *et al.*, 2000).

The mechanism of action is still unclear, though the anti-inflammatory action has been linked to the *in vitro* inhibition of inducible nitric oxide synthesis in macrophage cell line (Moeslinger *et al.*, 2000), the inhibition of the oxidative burst response in neutrophils (Ginsburg *et al.*, 1999, Matzner and Sallon, 1995), the inhibition of neutrophil elastase, and to antioxidant as well as Fe(II)-chelating properties (Ginsburg *et al.*, 1999; Suter and Richter, 2000).

CONTRAINDICATIONS: None listed.

PREGNANCY AND LACTATION: None listed. However, a healthcare professional should be consulted before using this product during pregnancy or nursing.

ADVERSE EFFECTS: Rarely, minor gastric upsets have been reported. In this case, the tablets can be taken along with a meal.

DRUG INTERACTIONS: Patients should wait 1 1/2 to 2 hours between taking the herb tablets and any medication. This will help ensure that the herbal ingredients do not interfere with the usual absorption of the medication.

OTHER DATA OR SPECIAL INSTRUCTIONS: Tablets are best taken on an empty stomach, 1/2 hour before mealtime with a glass of warm water. Patients who have difficulty swallowing tablets, may let them dissolve in a glass of warm water before swallowing the mixture.

The tablets are lactose- and gluten-free. They are suitable for diabetics.

* The commercially available products, Padma 28® and Padma® Basic have consistently contained the same 403 mg dosage: In order to successfully blind the taste and smell in placebo-controlled, clinical studies, the dosage in studies has varied between 340 mg, 380 mg, and 403 mg.

NOTE: This information was derived from the label of the manufacturer and consideration of additional safety information is advised. Please consult Brinker, 2001; McGuffin *et al.*, 1997, and the single herb monographs for licorice and valerian in this book for more information on the safety of each of the herbs listed in this multi-herb product. In some cases, potential toxicity may be reduced or otherwise altered through the combination of herbs into one product.

(Refer to table of Clinical Studies on next page.)

Clinical Studies on Padma® 28

Intermittent Claudication

Author/Year	Subject	Design	Duration	Dosage	Preparation	Results/Conclusion
Sallon et al., 1998	Intermittent claudication	R, PC, DB n=83	6 months	2 capsules, twice daily or placebo	Padma® 28	Padma® 28 improved pain-free walking distance (58%), changes in ankle systolic pressure (mean of 12.5%) and its recovery time (0.8 min.) compared to pre-treatment values. Study concluded that Padma® 28 may be an effective treatment option for intermittent claudication.
Mehlsen et al., 1995	Intermittent claudication	R, DB, PC n=86	4 months	2 capsules, twice daily or placebo	Padma® 28	After 1 month and throughout the study, the treated patients obtained improvements in pain-free and maximum walking distance (115 m to 227 m; p<0.001) compared to placebo.
Smulski and Wojcicki, 1995	Intermittent claudication	R, DB, PC n=100	4 months	2 capsules, twice daily or placebo	Padma® 28	Patients showed a significant (p<0.01) increase of maximum walking distance from 87.5 to 187.5 meters in treatment group compared to a nonsignificant increase of 12.5 meters in placebo group. The formula was found to be significantly more effective at increasing walking distance after 12 weeks (p<0.01) and 16 weeks (p<0.01) compared to placebo, without side effects.
Winther et al., 1994	Intermittent claudication	R, DB, PC n=36	4 months	Two, 340 mg tablets, twice daily	Padma® 28	The treatment group showed an oxidative burst response of monocytes after stimulation with zymozan decreased. Neither group demonstrated a significant change in platelet aggregation in vitro. Padma® 28 increased fibrinolytic activity, measured by a more than 40% shortening of the ECLT and a drop in the level of PAI-1.
Drabaek et al., 1993	Intermittent claudication	R, DB, PC 2 groups of 18 patients each n=36	4 months	2 capsules, twice daily or placebo	Padma® 28	The maximum distance walked (115m–227m) and the distance walked without pain (52m–86m) was significantly longer (p<0.05) with Padma® 28 without side effects.
Samochowiec et al., 1987	Intermittent claudication (PAOD stage II)	R, DB, PC n=100	4 months	2 capsules, twice daily or placebo	Padma® 28	The treatment group showed an increase in walking distance of 78 meters (98%; p<0.001) and a significant reduction (p<0.5 or more) in levels of cholesterol, triglycerides, total lipids (-10%), and betalipoproteins (-18%).
Schrader et al., 1985	Intermittent claudication	R, PC, DB n=43	4 months	3 capsules twice daily or placebo	Padma® 28	Padma® 28 increased the distance walked (>100 vs. 27 meters) compared to placebo. The distance walked without pain was greater with Padma® 28 but not statistically significant. No side effects were observed.

Other

Author/Year	Subject	Design	Duration	Dosage	Preparation	Results/Conclusion
Samochowiec et al., 1992	Hypercholesterolaemia and hypertriglyceridemia	C n=52	16 weeks	Two, 380 mg capsules, twice daily	Padma® 28	Padma® 28 demonstrated a statistically significant effect in both groups. The triglycerides decreased from 284 mg/dL to 160 mg/dL in the hypertriglyceriemia group, and the cholesterol was lowered from 271 mg/dL to 210 mg/dL in the hypercholesterolemia group.
Jankowski et al., 1991	Respiratory Tract Infections (recurring)	C n=19 (ages 2 to 4)	2 months	1 tablet, three times daily	Padma® 28	In 12 children (63.1%), Padma® 28 significantly increased (85%) the spontaneous bactericidal activity of blood serum against 3 bacterial strains; Salmonella typhimurium 568, and Escherichia coli strains 044 and 055. In 4 children, the activity increased slightly (21%) and 3 children (15.7%) showed no effect.
Wojcicki and Samochowiec, 1986	Angina Pectoris	C, DB, PC n=50	2 weeks	2 capsules, twice daily or placebo	Padma® 28	80% of the patients obtained a good or excellent clinical response. The mean number of anginal attacks was reduced from 37.5 to 11.5 during treatment with Padma® 28 (p<0.001), and treatment significantly reduced (p<0.001) the amount of nitroglycerin tablets used. The platelet aggregation threshold increased by 125% and exercise tolerance improved significantly (p<0.001).

KEY: C – controlled, **CC** – case-control, **CH** – cohort, **CI** – confidence interval, **Cm** – comparison, **CO** – crossover, **CS** – cross-sectional, **DB** – double-blind, **E** – epidemiological, **LC** – longitudinal cohort, **MA** – meta-analysis, **MC** – multi-center, **n** – number of patients, **O** – open, **OB** – observational, **OL** – open label, **OR** – odds ratio, **P** – prospective, **PB** – patient-blind, **PC** – placebo-controlled, **PG** – parallel group, **PS** – pilot study, **R** – randomized, **RC** – reference-controlled, **RCS** – retrospective cross-sectional, **RS** - retrospective, **S** – surveillance, **SB** – single-blind, **SC** – single-center, **U** – uncontrolled, **UP** – unpublished, **VC** – vehicle-controlled.

Phytodolor®

MANUFACTURER: Steigerwald, Darmstadt, Germany. (Other brand names for this product, if any, may be found in the table on page 404.)

CONTENTS: 100 ml liquid extract contains: 60 ml (4.5:1) aspen leaves and bark (*Populus tremula*), 20 ml (4.5:1) common ash bark (*Fraxinus excelsior*), 20 ml (4.8:1) European goldenrod aerial parts (*Solidago virgaurea*).

PRIMARY USES: Rheumatoid arthritis.

DSHEA STRUCTURE-FUNCTION CLAIM: "Provides nutritional support for optimal muscle and joint function."

DOSAGE: 20 drops (1 ml) mixed in water or other drink, administered 3–4 times daily.

DURATION OF ADMINISTRATION: While results may be achieved in two weeks, for best results use for a minimum of 4 weeks.

ACTIONS: Anti-inflammatory.

CONTRAINDICATIONS: In rare cases, due to salicin and salicylic alcohol content, individuals with a known allergy to salicylates may have an allergic reaction. Due to 45.6% alcohol content, the product should be avoided by pregnant women, children, or anyone with a disease or condition for which alcohol is contraindicated.

PREGNANCY AND LACTATION: Not for use during pregnancy.

ADVERSE EFFECTS: In rare cases, gastric and intestinal complaints may occur.

DRUG INTERACTIONS: None listed.

NOTE: This information was derived from the label of the manufacturer and consideration of additional safety information is advised. Please consult Brinker, 2001; McGuffin *et al.*, 1997, and the single herb monographs in this book for more information on the safety of each of the herbs listed in this multi-herb product. In some cases, potential toxicity may be reduced or otherwise altered through the combination of herbs into one product.

(Refer to table of Clinical Studies on next page.)

Clinical Studies on on Phytodolor®

Musculoskeletal Pain

Author/Year	Subject	Design	Duration	Dosage	Preparation	Results/Conclusion
Vajda, 1992	Rheumatoid arthritis	R, DB n=40	3 weeks	Phytodolor® (30 drops 3x/day) or 50 mg indomethacin 2x/day	Phytodolor®	Patients had relative risk reduction of 49% overall in all groups compared to placebo.
Bernhardt et al., 1991	Rheumatic diseases	R, DB, PC n=8	4 weeks	Phytodolor® (30 drops 3x/day), piroxicam or placebo	Phytodolor®, piroxicam, or placebo	Significant improvement in both actively treated groups with no observable difference.
Hawel, 1991	Osteoarthritis	R, DB n=240	3 weeks	Phytodolor® (30 drops 3x/day) or 25 mg diclofenac 3x/day	Phytodolor® or diclofenac	The authors noted equal therapeutic results in both groups, with less adverse effects in the Phytodolor® group (7.4% vs 14.2%).
Herzog et al., 1991	Rheumatic conditions, pain and joint function	R, DB n=432	4 weeks	Phytodolor® (30 drops 3x/day) or 25 mg diclofenac 3x/day	Phytodolor® or diclofenac	Both treatment groups showed improvement without a statistically significant difference. Patients taking Phytodolor® had better tolerance of the medication than the group taking diclofenac.
Bernhardt et al., 1990	Rheumatic diseases	R, DB, PC n = 47	4 weeks	Phytodolor® (60 drops 3x/day; or 30 drops or 15 drops 3x/daily)	Phytodolor® double strength, normal strength and half strength	Improvement noted in all active treatment groups without significant difference. All of the treatments reduced pain during movement, but chronic pain was alleviated only in the high dosage strength.
Baumann et al., 1989	Rheumatic conditions, pain, swelling, function	R, DB, MC n=108	2 weeks	Phytodolor® (30 drops 3x/day) or 25 mg diclofenac 3x/day	Phytodolor® or diclofenac	The authors concluded that the same clinical results were achieved with either Phytodolor® or diclofenac.
Huber, 1991	Rheumatic diseases	R,DB,PC n=40	3 weeks	Phytodolor® (30 drops 3x/day) or placebo	Phytodolor® or placebo	The study demonstrated a statistically significant improvement in symptoms (p<0.05) after one week, with prgressive improvement, in patients treated with Phytodolor® vs. placebo. No adverse effects were observed.
Hahn and Hubner-Steiner, 1988	Chronic epicondylitis	R, DB, PC n=45	4 weeks	Phytodolor® (30 drops 3x/day) or placebo	Phytodolor® or placebo	The study focused on pain and physical impairment outcomes and noted a significant differences in mobility (p<0.01) and pain due to movement (p<0.01) with the use of Phytodolor® vs. placebo.
Schreckenberger, 1988	Osteoarthritis	R, DB, PC n=45	4 weeks	Phytodolor® (30 drops 3x/day) or 25 mg diclofenac 3x/day or placebo	Phytodolor®, placebo, or diclofenac	The authors observed a significant difference (p<0.001) in pain and grip strength with both active treatments over placebo.

KEY: **C** – controlled, **CC** – case-control, **CH** – cohort, **CI** – confidence interval, **Cm** – comparison, **CO** – crossover, **CS** – cross-sectional, **DB** – double-blind, **E** – epidemiological, **LC** – longitudinal cohort, **MA** – meta-analysis, **MC** – multi-center, **n** – number of patients, **O** – open, **OB** – observational, **OL** – open label, **OR** – odds ratio, **P** – prospective, **PB** – patient-blind, **PC** – placebo-controlled, **PG** – parallel group, **PS** – pilot study, **R** – randomized, **RC** – reference-controlled, **RCS** – retrospective cross-sectional, **RS** - retrospective, **S** – surveillance, **SB** – single-blind, **SC** – single-center, **U** – uncontrolled, **UP** – unpublished, **VC** – vehicle-controlled.

Prostagutt® forte

MANUFACTURER: Dr. Willmar Schwabe GmbH, Karlsruhe, Germany. (Other brand names for this product, if any, may be found in the table on page 404.)

CONTENTS: WS®1473 is an ethanolic (90% w/w) extract containing a minium of 70% fatty acids and esters. 160 mg of saw palmetto (*Serenoa repens*) extract (WS® 1473), 10–14.3:1, and 120 mg of stinging nettle root (*Urtica dioica*) dry extract (WS® 1031), 8.3–12.5:1.

PRIMARY USES: Disturbances of micturition in case of benign enlargement of the prostate (prostatic hyperplasia stages I to II according to Alken).

DSHEA STRUCTURE-FUNCTION CLAIM: Promotes prostate health (Prostactive® Plus, Nature's Way).

DOSAGE: 2–160 mg capsules per day.

DURATION OF ADMINISTRATION: Duration of application is not limited in time.

ACTIONS: Inhibitory action on the enzymes 5α-reductase and aromatase which are both important for the androgen metabolism in the prostate. As concerns the aromatase inhibition, the combination of both extracts leads to an overadditive effect. Both extract have antiexudative-decongestive properties. The product increases the maximum urinary flow and improves micturition symptoms.

CONTRAINDICATIONS: None listed.

PREGNANCY AND LACTATION: Not applicable.

ADVERSE EFFECTS: In rare cases, mild gastric disorders may occur.

DRUG INTERACTIONS: None listed.

NOTE: This information was derived from the label of the manufacturer and consideration of additional safety information is advised. Please consult Brinker, 2001; McGuffin *et al.*, 1997, and the single herb monograph for saw palmetto in this book for more information on the safety of each of the herbs listed in this multi-herb product. In some cases, potential toxicity may be reduced or otherwise altered through the combination of herbs into one product.

Clinical Studies on Prostagutt® forte

Benign Prostatic Hyperplasia (BPH)

Author/Year	Subject	Design	Duration	Dosage	Preparation	Results/Conclusion
Sökeland, 2000 (Also published as Sökeland and Albrecht, 1997)	BPH (stages I and II)	R, RC, MC, DB, PG n=543	48 weeks	2 capsules per day	PRO 160/120 (Prostagutt® forte) or finasteride (Proscar®)	International-Prostate-Symptom-Score (I-PSS) value improved by a total of 4.8 points with the PRO 160/120. The study found equivalent efficacy between the 2 groups. The therapeutic outcome was unrelated to the prostate volume in either treatment group. Less adverse events, including diminished ejaculation volume, erectile dysfunction, and headache, were reported in the PRO 160/120 group. The study recommended that patients should receive finasteride only after the use of the combination for at least 3 months was unsuccessful.
Metzker et al., 1996	BPH (stages I and II)	DB, PC n=40	24 weeks, followed by 24 weeks single blind phase	2 capsules per day	PRO 160/120 (Prostagutt® forte)	The study concluded good efficacy and tolerance in the administration of PRO 160/120 for approximately 1 year of therapy. After 24 weeks, maximum urine volume per second by 3.3 ml/s had occurred with the combination compared to only a slight improvement of 0.55 ml/s with placebo. Subjective reports corresponding to the I-PSS found a highly significant (p<0.001) advantage with the combination vs. placebo.
Schneider et al., 1995	BPH (stages I and II)	O, MC, P, OB n=2,080	12 weeks	2 capsules per day	PRO 160/120 (Prostagutt® forte	Treatment with the combination was found to be an effective method to avoid surgery or not to make it necessary as soon. Physician and patient assessment confirmed the efficacy and tolerance of PRO 160/120. Side effects (mild gastrointestinal complaints) were observed in only 0.7% of patients.

KEY: **C** – controlled, **CC** – case-control, **CH** – cohort, **CI** – confidence interval, **Cm** – comparison, **CO** – crossover, **CS** – cross-sectional, **DB** – double-blind, **E** – epidemiological, **LC** – longitudinal cohort, **MA** – meta-analysis, **MC** – multi-center, **n** – number of patients, **O** – open, **OB** – observational, **OL** – open label, **OR** – odds ratio, **P** – prospective, **PB** – patient-blind, **PC** – placebo-controlled, **PG** – parallel group, **PS** – pilot study, **R** – randomized, **RC** – reference-controlled, **RCS** – retrospective cross-sectional, **RS** - retrospective, **S** – surveillance, **SB** – single-blind, **SC** – single-center, **U** – uncontrolled, **UP** – unpublished, **VC** – vehicle-controlled.

Sinupret®

MANUFACTURER: Bionorica AG; Neumarkt, Germany. (Other brand names for this product, if any, may be found in the table on page 404.)

CONTENTS: Gentian root (*Gentiana lutea*), primrose flowers with calyx (*Primula veris*), sorrel herb (*Rumex acetosa, R. crispus, R. obtusifolius*), elder flowers (*Sambucus nigra*), vervain herb (*Verbena officinalis*).

> *Tablets:* Dried powder of gentian 6 mg, primrose flowers 18 mg, common sorrel herb 18 mg, elder flowers 18 mg, vervain herb 18 mg.
>
> *Drops:* 29 g of aqueous-ethanolic extract (1:11) in the ratio of 1:3:3:3:3 (ethanol 53%).

PRIMARY USES: Sinusitis, acute or chronic bronchitis. Manufacturer's literature states, "Acute and chronic inflammation of the paranasal sinuses and of the respiratory tract, also as an additional measure in antibacterial therapy" (Anon., n.d.).

DSHEA STRUCTURE-FUNCTION CLAIM: N/A. Not available at this time. Product is scheduled to be available in the U.S. in May 2003.

DOSAGE: *Tablets:* Adults: 2 tablets 3 times daily; children of school age: 1 tablet 3 times daily. *Drops:* Adults: 50 drops 3 times daily; children of school age: 25 drops 3 times daily.

DURATION OF ADMINISTRATION: Manufacturer's literature says the preparation is indicated for long-term therapy (Anon., n.d.).

ACTIONS: Secretolytic, anti-inflammatory, anti-infective, immunostimulant, prevents bronchospasm. These actions are of clinical relevance in the established indications, with the primary therapeutic aims to normalize drainage and, especially in the case of sinusitis, to restore ventilation (Anon., n.d.).

CONTRAINDICATIONS: None listed.

PREGNANCY AND LACTATION: None listed for pregnancy. Neither the experience from several decades of use nor the known pharmacology and toxicology of the respective herbal ingredients suggest any evidence of risk associated with the use of this formula during pregnancy. A retrospective, multi-center study of Sinupret® use during all stages of pregnancy by 762 women did not reveal any evidence of adverse effects on the duration of the pregnancies nor on the children (Ismail *et al.*, 2001). In view of the documented relative safety during pregnancy and toxicological studies in animals, the manufacturer's literature provides a general statement, "Nevertheless, Sinupret® should be administered during pregnancy and lactation only after medical advice." (Anon., n.d.) No data was found on effects during lactation.

ADVERSE EFFECTS: The product is considered safe. Rare cases of gastric intolerance and isolated cases of allergic skin reactions (skin reddening, exanthema up to vesiculation) have been reported (Anon., n.d.). The incidence of ADR-reports (Adverse Drug Reaction) in clinical trials is less than 2% based on 2443 patients. The incidence of spontaneous ADR-reports in the period 1984–1999 is 0.000001%; based on approximately 100 million treated patients in 25 countries.

DRUG INTERACTIONS: None listed.

CLINICAL STUDIES: At least 4 controlled clinical trials have been conducted on the Sinupret® herbal combination, plus 1 comparative post-market surveillance study. Additional studies have been conducted on the individual ingredients. Only those studies conducted on the proprietary combination are listed in the table below.

EDITOR'S COMMENT: Sinupret® is the top-selling nonprescription medication in Germany; this includes sales for both herbal as well as conventional nonprescription medications.

NOTE: This information was derived from the label of the manufacturer and consideration of additional safety information is advised. Please consult Brinker, 2001; McGuffin *et al.*, 1997, and the single herb monographs in this book for more information on the safety of each of the herbs listed in this multi-herb product. In some cases, potential toxicity may be reduced or otherwise altered through the combination of herbs into one product.

Clinical Studies on on Sinupret®

Acute and Chronic Sinusitis or Bronchitis

Author/Year	Subject	Design	Duration	Dosage	Preparation	Results/Conclusion
Riechstein and Mann, 1999	Chronic sinusitis	R, PC, DB n=31	7 days	2 tablets 3/day; or 50 drops 3x/day	Sinupret® tablets & drops	Sinupret® group showed considerable improvement compared with placebo group on X-ray and ultrasound findings of paranasal sinuses. Complete recovery was seen in 12 of 16 Sinupret participants compared with 6 of 15 placebo participants.
Ernst et al., 1997	Acute bronchitis	Post-market surveillance n=3,187	10 days average	2 tablets, 3x daily; 25 drops to 50 drops 3x/day	Sinupret® tablets & drops	330 GPs and specialists; Sinupret® at least as effective as other expectorants.
Neubauer and März, 1994	Acute sinusitis	R,PC,DB n=160	14 days	2 tablets 3x/day	Sinupret® tablets	Therapy with antibiotics and decongestants improved in combination with Sinupret®.
Kraus and Schwender, 1992	Acute and chronic sinusitis	R, O, Cm n=134	14 days	2 tablets 3x/day	Sinupret® tablets	Study medication (Sinupret®) was as effective as the active control (volatile oil preparation).
Pinnow and Egentenmaier, 1992	Acute bronchitis	RC, SB n=158	14 days	2 tablets 3x/day	Sinupret® tablets and drops	Study medication (Sinupret®) was as effective as the active control (mucolytic agent).
Egetenmeier and März, 1991	Sinupret vs. ambroxol drops in acute bronchitis	C, DB n=80	14 days	100 drops 3x/day. (for the first 3 days); 50 drops 3x/day (for the rest of therapy)	Sinupret® drops	Study medication (Sinupret®) was found to be as effective as the active control (mucolytic agent).
Braum and März, 1990	Sinupret versus N-acetylcysteine for sinusitis	R, O, Cm n =160	21 days	2 tablets 3x/day	Sinupret® tablets vs. Fluimucil	Sinupret® was found to be as effective as the active control (mucolytic agent).

KEY: **C** – controlled, **CC** – case-control, **CH** – cohort, **CI** – confidence interval, **Cm** – comparison, **CO** – crossover, **CS** – cross-sectional, **DB** – double-blind, **E** – epidemiological, **LC** – longitudinal cohort, **MA** – meta-analysis, **MC** – multi-center, **n** – number of patients, **O** – open, **OB** – observational, **OL** – open label, **OR** – odds ratio, **P** – prospective, **PB** – patient-blind, **PC** – placebo-controlled, **PG** – parallel group, **PS** – pilot study, **R** – randomized, **RC** – reference-controlled, **RCS** – retrospective cross-sectional, **RS** - retrospective, **S** – surveillance, **SB** – single-blind, **SC** – single-center, **U** – uncontrolled, **UP** – unpublished, **VC** – vehicle-controlled.

REFERENCES

Alder D [BotanicLab]. Personal communication to M Blumenthal, Mar. 13, 2002.

Albrecht M, Berger W, Laux P, Schmidt U, Martin C. Psychopharmaceuticals and traffic safety: The influence of Euvegal® forte sugar-coated tablets on driving ability and combination effect with alcohol. *Z Allg Med* 1995;71:1215–25.

Ammer K, Melnizky P. Medicinal baths for treatment of generalized fibromyalgia [in German]. *Forsch Komplementarmed* 1999;6:80–5.

Anonymous. Sinupret® for sinusitis and inflammation of the respiratory tract. (manufacturer's booklet). Neumarkt, Germany: Bionorica Arzneimittel GmbH.

Anonymous. Various studies show Hochu-ekki-to® is effective in aiding recovery. *Kampo Today* 2001;4(2):1–3,6.

Arcangeli R. Pycnogenol in chronic venous insufficiency. *Fitoterapia* 2000;71(3):236–44.

Atal CK, Dubey RK, Singh J. Biochemical basis of enhanced drug bioavailability by piperine: evidence that piperine is a potent inhibitor of drug metabolism. *J Pharmacol Exp Ther* 1985;232(1):258–62.

Atal CK, Zutshi U, Rao PG. Scientific evidence on the role of Ayurvedic herbals on bioavailability of drugs. *J Ethnopharmacol* 1981;4(2):229–32.

Badmaev VV, Majeed M, Prakash L. Piperine derived from black pepper increases the plasma levels of coenzyme q10 following oral supplementation. *J Nutr Biochem* 2000;11(2):109–13.

Bahrman N, Zivy M, Damerval C, Baradat P. Organisation of the variability of abundant proteins in seven geographical origins of maritime pine (*Pinus pinaster* Ait.). *Theoretical & Applied Genetics* 1994;88(3–4):407–11.

Bano G, Raina RK, Zutshi U, Bedi KL, Johri RK, Sharma SC. Effect of piperine on bioavailability and pharmacokinetics of propranolol and theophylline in healthy volunteers. *Eur J Clin Pharmacol* 1991;41(6):615–7.

Baumann D, Focke G, Kornosoff G. Phytodolor® bei patienten mit aktivierter gonarthrosse, koxanthrose bzw. Schulter-Arm-Syndrom. Multizentrische randomisierte doppelblindstudie versus Diclofenac-Natrium. Steigerwald, Gmbh. Interner Forschungsbericht 1989.

Bensoussan A, Talley NJ, Hing M, et al. Treatment of irritable bowel syndrome with Chinese herbal medicine. *JAMA* 1998;280(18):1585–9.

Bernhardt M, Keimel A, Belucci G, Spasojevic P. Doppelblinde, randomisierte vergleich von Phytodolor® N und placebo sowie offener vergleich zu felden 20 tabs bei stationaren kurpatienten mit arthrotischen GelenkverSnderungen [in German]. Unpublished trial, Steigerwald, Germany, 1990.

Bernhardt M, Keimel A, Belucci G, Spasojevic P. Doppelblinde, randomisierte vergleichsstudie von Phytodol® N und placebo sowie offener vergleich zu felden 20 tabs bei stationaren kurpatienten mit arthrotischen GelenkverSnderungen [in German]. Unpublished trial, Steigerwald, Germany, 1991.

Blazsó G, Gábor M, Rohdewald P. Anti-inflammatory activities of procyanidin-containing extracts from *Pinus pinaster* Ait. after oral and cutaneous application. *Pharmazie* 1997;52(5):380–2.

Blazsó G, Gábor M, Sibbel R, Rohdewald P. Anti-inflammatory and superoxide radical scavenging activities of procyanidin-containing extracts from the bark of *Pinus pinaster* Sol. and its fractions. *Pharm Pharmacol Lett* 1994;3:217–20.

Blazsó G, Gaspar R, Gábor M, Rüve H-J, Rohdewald P. ACE inhibition and hypotensive effect of procyanidins containing extract from the bark of *Pinus pinaster* Sol. *Pharm Pharmacol Lett* 1996;6(1):8–11.

Blazsó G, Rohdewald P, Sibbel R, Gábor M. Anti-inflammatory activities of procyanidin-containing extracts from *Pinus pinaster* Sol. In: Antus S, Gábor M, Vetschera K, editors. *Proceedings of the International Bioflavonoid Symposium*; 1995 July 16–19; Vienna, Austria; 1995. p. 231–8.

Blumenthal M. Herb sales down 15% in mainstream market. *HerbalGram* 2001;51:69.

Blumenthal M, Busse WR, Goldberg A, Gruenwald J, Hall T, Riggins CW, Rister RS editors. Klein S, Rister RS (trans.). *The Complete German Commission E Monographs—Therapeutic Guide to Herbal Medicines*. Austin (TX): American Botanical Council; Boston (MA): Integrative Medicine Communication; 1998.

Bos R, Hendriks H, Scheffer J, Woerdenbag H. Cytotoxic potential of valerian constituents and valerian tinctures. *Phytomedicine* 1998;5:219–25.

Braeckow R, Eickstedt K, Kuhne U. Effects of chlorpromazine and valtratum on ethanol anesthesia and ethanol blood level. *Arzneimittelforschung* 1972;22:1977–80.

Braum D, März R. Randomised, open comparative study of sinupret versus n-acetyl-cysteine in cases of sinusitis. Bundeswehrkrankenhaus (military hospital), Giessen. 1990.

Brinker F. *Herb Contraindications and Drug Interactions*, 3d ed. Sandy (OR): Eclectic Institute;2001.

Buz'Zard AR, Peng Q, Lau BH. Kyolic® and Pycnogenol® increase human growth hormone secretion in genetically-engineered keratinocytes. *Growth Horm & IGF Res* 2002;12(1):34–40.

California State Dept. Human Services, Food and Drug Branch. State health director warns consumers about prescription drugs in herbal products. Feb 7, 2002.

Available from URL: http://www.dhs.ca.gov.

Chan T. An assessment of the delayed effects associated with valerian overdose [letter]. *Int J Clin Pharmacol Ther* 1998;36:569.

Chan T, Tang C, Critchley J. Poisoning due to an over-the-counter hypnotic sleep-Qik (hyoscine, cyproheptadine, valerian). *Postgrad Med J* 1995;71:227–8.

Chandler RF, Freeman L, Hooper SN. Herbal remedies of the maritime Indians. *J Ethnopharmacology* 1979;1(1):49–68.

Chauhan BL, Kulkarni RD. Liv.52 in alcoholic liver diseases: a profile of an herbal remedy. *Eur J Clin Pharmacol* 1991;40(2):189–91.

Cheshier JE, Ardestani-Kaboudanian S, Liang B, Araghiniknam M, Chung S, Lane L, et al. Immuno-modulation by Pycnogenol in retrovirus-infected or ethanol-fed mice. *Life Sci* 1996;58(5):87–96.

Crates E. Pycnogenol– barking up the right tree. *Funct Foods & Nutraceuticals* 2000;3(13):16–7.

Dharmananda S. The nature of ginseng: traditional use, modern research, and the question of dosage. *HerbalGram* 2002;54:34–51.

Dietary Supplement Health and Education Act of 1994 (DSHEA), Public Law 103-417, 21 USC § 3419.

Doucet M, Durand-Cagniart MO, Tanger-Rubin M. The value of FLAVAN for functional symptoms and the prevention of venous insufficiency. *Act Méd Int* 1987;4(59):2–4.

Drabaek H, Mehlsen J, Himmelstrup H, Winther K. A botanical compound, Padma® 28, increases walking distance in stable intermittent claudication. *Angiology* 1993;44(11):863–7.

Dressing H, Köhler S, Müller WE. Improvement of sleep quality with a high-dose valerian/lemon balm preparation: a placebo-controlled double-blind study. *Psychopharma* 1996;3:123–30.

Dressing H, Riemann D, Löw H, et al. Insomnia: are valerian/balm combinations of equal value to bezodiazepine? *Therapiewoche, 42* 1992 Mar;12:726–736.

DSHEA. See: Dietary Supplement Health and Education Act of 1994.

Dutkeiwicz T, Samochowiec L, Wójcicki J. Padma 28® modifies immunological functions in experimental atherosclerosis in rabbits. *Archivum Immunologiae et Therapia Experimentalis* 1992;40:291–5.

Egetenmaier J, März R. Double-blind study of Sinupret drops versus ambroxol drops in acute uncomplicated (tracheo-) bronchitis. 1991.

Elstner E, Kleber E. Radical scavenger properties of leucocyanidine. Proceedings of the 3rd International Symposium on Flavonoids in Biology & Medicine. 1989 Nov 13–17; Singapore, China; 1989.

Ernst E, März RW, Seider C. Acute bronchitis—benefits of Sinupret® [in German]. *Fortschritte der Medizin* 1997;115(11):52–3.

ESCOP. See: European Scientific Cooperative on Phytotherapy.

European Scientific Cooperative on Phytotherapy (ESCOP). *Valeriana radix. Monographs on the medicinal uses of plants*. Exeter: ESCOP;1997.

FAC. See: Food Advisory Committee.

Fallarino M. Tibetan medical paintings: illustrations to the blue beryl treatis of sangye gyamtso (1653–1705). *HerbalGram* 1994;31:38–44.

FDA. See: Food and Drug Administration.

Feine-Haake G. A new therapy for venous diseases with 3,3' 4,4' 5,7-hexadihydro-flavan. *Allgemeinmedizin* 1975;51:839.

Fishman RHB. Antioxidants and phytotherapy. *Lancet* 1994 Nov 12;344:1356.

Fitzpatrick DF, Bing B, Rohdewald P. Endothelium-dependent vascular effects of Pycnogenol. *J Cardiovasc Pharmacol* 1998;32(4):509–15.

Food Advisory Committee (FAC). French maritime pine bark extract. *Food for Thought* 1999;Autumn:2–3.

Food and Drug Administration (FDA). 65 FR 1000–1050. Jan 6, 2000. Regulations on statements made for dietary supplements concerning the effect of the product on the structure or function of the body. [Docket No. 98N–0044] 21 CFR Part 101–93..

Forth H, Beuscher N. Influence of Esberitox® on the frequency of the common cold [in German]. *Zeutschrift für Allgemeinmedizin* 1981;57:2272–5.

Foster S. *American Herbal Products Association: Herbs of Commerce*. Austin (TX): American Herbal Products Association; 2001.

Freise J, Köhler S. Peppermint oil-caraway oil fixed combination in non-ulcer dyspepsia—comparison of the effects of enteric preparations [in German]. *Pharmazie* 1999;54(3):210–5.

Fussel A, Wolf A, Brattström A. Effect of a fixed valerian-hop extract combination (Ze 9109) on sleep polygraphy in patients with non-organic insomnia: a pilot study. *Eur J Med Res* 2000;5:385–90.

Gábor M, Engi E, Sonkodi S. The influence of water soluble flavonoid derivates on capillary resistance in hypertonic rats [in German]. *Phlebologie* 1993;(22):178–82.

Gerhard U, Linnenbrink N, Georghiadou C, Hobi V. Vigilance-decreasing effects of 2 plant-derived sedatives. *Schweiz Rundsch Med Prax* 1996;85(15):473–81.

Gieldanowski J. Padma 28® modifies immunological functions in experimental atherosclerosis in rabbits. *Arch Immunol Ther Exp* 1992;40:291–5.

Ginsburg I, Sadovnik M, Sallon S, et al. PADMA-28, a traditional Tibetan herbal preparation inhibits the respiratory burst in human neutrophils, the killing of epithelial cells by mixtures of oxidants and pro-inflammatory agonists and peroxidation of lipids. *Inflammopharmacology* 1999;7(1):47–62.

Gulati OP. Pycnogenol® in venous disorders [review]. *Euro Bull Drug Res* 1999;7(2):8–13.

Guochang Z. Ultraviolet radiation-induced oxidative stress in cultured human skin fibroblasts and antioxidant protection [dissertation]. In: *Biological Research Reports from the University of Jyväskylä 33:1–86.* Jyväskylä, Finland: University of Jyväskylä; 1993.

Hahn S, Hubner-Steiner U. Behandlung schmerzhafter rheumatischer erkrankungen mit Phytodolar N im verglerch zur placebo- und Ammuno-Behandhung. *Rheuma Schmerz und Entznndung* 1988;8:55–8.

Hawel R. Phytodolor® vs. Diclofenac bei rheumatischen erkrankungen. Steigerwald, Gmbh. *Interner Forschungsbericht* 1991.

Health Canada. *Drug Product Database (DPD).* Ottawa, Ontario: Health Canada Therapeutic Products Programme (TPP); 2001.

Health Protection Branch. Pycnogenol®. In: *HPB Status Manual.* Ottawa, Ontario: Health Protection Branch; 1993. p. 158.

Hendriks H, Bos R, Allersma D, Malingre T, Koster A. Pharmacological screening of valerenal and some other components of essential oil of *Valeriana officinalis.* *Planta Med* 1981;42:62–8.

Henneicke-von Zepelin H, Hentschel C, Schnitker J, Kohnen R, Kohler G, Wustenberg P. Efficacy and safety of a fixed combination phytomedicine in the treatment of the common cold (acute viral respiratory tract infection): results of a randomised, double blind, placebo controlled, multicentre study. *Curr Med Res Opin* 1999;15(3):214–27.

Herzog U, Fitzek J, Franek H. Phytodolor® N versus Diclofenac Wirksamkeit und VertSglichkeit. Steigerwald, Gmbh. *Interner Forschungsbericht* 1991.

Hiller K. Neuropharmacological studies on ethanol extracts of *Valeriana officinalis* L: behavioral and anticonvulsant properties. *Phytother Res* 1996;10:145–51.

Hosseini S, Lee J, Sepulveda RT, Rohdewald P, Watson RR. A randomized, double-blind, placebo-controlled, prospective, 16 week crossover study to determine the role of Pycnogenol® in modifying blood pressure in mildly hypertensive patients. *Nutr Res* 2001a;21:12(9):1251-1260.

Hosseini S, Pishnamazi S, Sadrzadeh SMH, Farid F, Farid R, Watson RR. Pycnogenol® in the management of asthma. *Medicinal Food* 2001b;4(4):201–8.

HPB. See: Health Protection Branch.

Hsu, H-Y, et al. *Oriental Materia Medica: A Concise Guide.* Long Beach, Calif: Oriental Healing Arts Institute, 1986. http://www.tsumura.co.jp/english/kthp/4-2-01.htm#6

Huber B. Therapy of degenerative rheumatic diseases. Need for additional analgesic medication with Phytodolor N [in German]. *Fortschr Med* 1991;109;11:248–50.

Huynh HT, Teel RW. Selective induction of apoptosis in human mammary cancer cells (MCF-7) by Pycnogenol. *Anticancer Res* 2000;20(4):2417–20.

Igarashi T, Gonoi T, Hanada M, Sato H, et al. Study on effect of Hochu-ekki-to® (TJ-41) on anorexia, fatigue and malaise, and Kampo diagnosis of Hochu-ekki-to®. *Therapeutic Research* 1995;15(11):4526–30.

Ismail CH, Scharfetter K, Becker MKF, Marz RW. Sinupret® in pregnancy, submitted to *Archives of Gynecology and Obstetrics,* 2001.

Israelsen LD, Blumenthal M. FDA issues final rules for structure/function claims for dietary supplements under DSHEA. *HerbalGram* 2000;48:32–8.

Jankowski S, Jankowski A, Zielinska S, Walczuk M, Brzosko WJ. Influence of Padma 28® on the spontaneous bactericidal activity of blood serum in children suffering from recurrent infections of the respiratory tract. *Phytother Res* 1991;5:120–3.

Japan Kampo-Medicine Manufacturers Association. 1998 Sales Volume of Top Ten Kampo Formulations. *Kampo Today* 2001;4(2):2.

Kammerer E, Brattst öm A, Herberg K-W. Effects of a hop-valerian combination on fitness and driving safety. *Der Bay Int* 1996;16(3):32–6.

Kapoor LD. *Handbook of Ayurvedic Medicinal Plants.* Boca Raton (FL): CRC Press; 1990.

Karibe H. The effect of Japanese herbal medicine on MRSA carriers in neurosurgery. *Neurol Surg* 1997;25(10):893–7.

Khajuria A, Zutshi U, Bedi KL. Permeability characteristics of piperine on oral absorption — an active alkaloid from peppers and a bioavailability enhancer. *Indian J Exp Biol* 1998;36(1):46–50.

Khangkar LD. Lectures on Tibetan Medicine, 1986 Library of Tibetan Works and Archives, Dharamsala.

Kobayashi MS, Han D, Packer L. Antioxidants and herbal extracts protect HT4-neuronal cells against glutamate-induced cytoxicity. *Free Rad Res* 2000;32(2):115–24.

Kohama T, Suzuki N. The treatment of gynecological disorders with Pycnogenol®. *Euro Bull Drug Res* 1999;7(9):30–2.

Kraus P, Schwender W. Randomized, open comparative study with Sinupret® sugar-coated tablets vs. Gelomyrtol® F. conducted at the German Army Hospital in Amberg [abstract]. 4th National and 1st International Congress on Phytotherapy;

1992 Sep 10-13; Munich, Germany.

Kuratsune H, et al. Effect of Kampo medicine, "Hochu-ekki-to®", on chronic fatigue syndrome. *Clinic and Res* 1997;74:1837–45.

Lad V, Frawley D. *The Yoga of Herbs: An Ayurvedic Guide to Herbal Medicine.* Santa Fe (NM): Lotus Press; 1986.

Lataster MJ, Brattström A. The treatment of patients with sleep disorders: efficacy of tolerance of valerian-hop tablets. *Notabene Medici* 1996;4:182–5.

Leatherwood PD, Chauffard F, Heck E, Munoz-Box R. Aqueous extract of valerian root (*Valerianan officinalis* L.) improves sleep quality in man. *Pharmacol Biochem Behav* 1982;17(1):65–71.

Leuschner J, Mueller J, Rudmann M. Characterization of the central nervous depressant activity of a commercially available valerian root extract [in German]. *Arzneimittelfforschung* 1993;43:638–41.

Liu FJ, Zhang YX, Lau BHS. Pycnogenol® enhances immune and haemopoietic functions in senescence-accelerated mice. *Cell Mol Life Sci* 1998;54(10):1168–72.

Liu FJ, Zhang Y, Lau BHS. Pycnogenol® improves learning impairment and memory deficit in senescense-accelerated mice. *J Anti-Aging Med* 1999;2:349–55.

Madisch A, Heydenreich CJ, Wieland V, et al. Treatment of functional dyspepsia with a fixed peppermint oil and caraway oil combination preparation as compared to cisapride. A multicenter, reference-controlled double-blind equivalence study. *Arzen* 1999;49(11):925–32.

Magnard G, Franck JP, Dorne PA. Use of tetrahydroxy flavan-diol in ophthalmology especially in chronic retinopathy (40 cases) [in French]. *Lyon Medical* 1970;223(4):259–63.

Marks L, Hess D, Dorey F, et al. Tissue effects of saw palmetto and finasteride: use of biopsy cores for in situ quantification of prostatic androgens. *Urol* 2001;57(3):999–1005.

Marks L, Partin A, Epstein J, et al. Effects of a saw palmetto herbal blend in men with symptomatic benign prostatic hyperplasia. *Jour of Urol* 2000 May;163:1451–1456.

Matzner Y, Sallon S. The effect of Padma 28®, a traditional Tibetan herbal preparation, on human neutrophil function. *J Clin. Lab Immunol* 1995;46:13–23.

McGuffin M, Hobbs C, Upton R, Goldberg A. *American Herbal Product Association's Botanical Safety Handbook.* Boca Raton (FL): CRC Press;1997.

Medical Products Agency (MPA). *Naturläkemedel* (Authorised Natural Remedies). Uppsala, Sweden: Medical Products Agency; 2001.

Mehlsen J, Drabaek H, Peterson JR, Winther K. Der effekt einer tibetischen krautermischung (Padma 28®) auf die gehstrecke bei stabiler claudicatio intermittens. *Forsc Komplementarmed* 1995;2:240–5. (See also: *Angiology* 1993;44:863–7.)

Melchart D, Linde K, Worku F, Bauer R, Wagner H. Immunomodulation with Echinacea—a systematic review of controlled clinical trials. *Phytomed* 1994;1:245–254.

Mendal JN, Roy BK. Hepatitis, chronic active hepatitis and cirrhosis of the liver. *Probe* 1983;4:217.

Metzker H, Kieser M, Hölscher U. Efficacy of a combined Sabal-Urtica preparation in the treatment of benign prostatic hyperplasia (BPH): A double-blind, placebo-controlled, long-term study. *Urologe* 1996;36:292–300.

Micklefield GH, Greving I, May B. Effects of peppermint oil and caraway oil on gastroduodenal motility. *Phytother Res* 2000;14:20–3.

Miller L. Herbal medicinals: selected clinical considerations focusing on known or potential drug-herb interactions. *Arch Intern Med* 1998;158:2200–11.

Moerman D. *Native American Ethnobotany.* Portland (OR): Timber Press; 1998.

Moeslinger T, Friedl R, Volf I, Brunner M, Koller E, Spieckermann PG. Inhibition of inducible nitric oxide synthesis by the herbal preparation Padma 28® in macrophage cell line. *Can J Physiol* 2000:81:861–6.

Morazzoni P, Bombardelli E. *Valeriana officinalis*: traditional use and recent evaluation of activity. *Fitoterapia* 1995;66:99–112.

Mori K, Saito Y, Tominaga K. Utility of Hochu-ekki-to® in general malaise accompanying lung cancer chemotherapy. *Biotherapy* 1992;6(4):624–7.

MPA. See: Medical Products Agency.

Nefyodov LI, Doroshenko YM, Karavay NL, Brzosko WJ. Effect of Padma 28® on impaired amino acid metabolism induced by liver inflammatory pathology. *Herba Polonica* 2000;XLVI(4):340–5.

Nelson AB, Lau BHS, Ide N, Rong Y. Pycnogenol® inhibits macrophage oxidative burst, lipoprotein oxidation and hydroxyl radical-induced DNA damage. *Drug Development and Industrial Pharmacy* 1998;24(2):139–44.

Neubauer N, März RW. Placebo-controlled, randomized double-blind clinical trial with Sinupret® sugar-coated tablets on the basis of a therapy with antibiotics and decongestant nasal drops in acute sinusitis. *Phytomedicine* 1994;1(3):177–81.

Niwa M, et al. Effect of Hochu-ekki-to® (TJ-41) on immune function. *Progress in Medicine* 1996;16:1506–8.

ORG-MARG Private Limited. Syndicated retail audit conducted on the Indian Pharma industry. Operations Research Group (ORG) and Marketing & Research Group (MARG) (ORG-MARG Private Limited); 2001,

Ozaki, Y, Ma, JP. Inhibitory effects of tetramethylpyrazine and ferulic acid on spontaneous movement of rat uterus in situ. *Chem Pharm Bull* (Tokyo) 1990;38(6):1620–3.

Packer L, Rimbach G, Virgili F. Antioxidant activity and biologic properties of a procyanidin-rich extract from pine (*Pinus maritima*) bark, Pycnogenol. *Free Rad Biol & Med* 1999;27(5–6):704–24.

Padma Advertisement. *Alternative Therapies* 2000 Sept;6(5):45.

Patney NL, Kumar A. Preliminary Report on the Role of Liv. 52® – An Ayurvedic drug in Serum B hepatitis (Australian Antigen Positive) cases. *Probe* 1978;2:132.

Petrassi C, Mastromarino A, Spartera C. Pycnogenol in chronic venous insufficiency. *Phytomedicine* 2000;7(5):383–8.

Pinnow R, Egentenmaier J. Controlled clinical trials in achute (tracheo-) bronchitis: Sinupret® sugar-coated tablets vs. Mucret, Sinupret® drops vs. Mucosolvan drops in uncomplicated acute (tracheo-) bronchitis. Abstract presented at the 4th National and 1st International Congress on Phytomedicine, Munich, 1992.

Pütter M, Grotemeyer KH, Würthwein G, Araghi-Niknam M, Watson RR, Hosseini S, et al. Inhibition of smoking-induced platelet aggregation by aspirin and pycnogenol. *Thrombosis Res* 1999;95(4):155–61.

Queißer-Luft A., Ismail Ch. Safety of an herbal combination preparation in pregnancy—an example for using active detection systems for malformations, abstracts 3rd International Congress on Phytomedicine. 2000;7(2):12.

Reitz, HD. Immunomodulation with phytotherapeutic agents: a scientific study on the example of Esberitox® [in German]. *Notebene medici* 1990;20:362–6.

Riechstein A, Mann W. Treatment of chronic rhino-sinusitis with Sinupret®: a double-blind prospective clinical trial. *Schweizerische Zeitschrift fur Ganzheits Medizin* 1999;11(6):280–3.

Rihn B, Saliou C, Bottin MC, Keith G, Packer L. From ancient remedies to modern therapeutics: pine bark uses in skin disorders revisited. *Phytotherapy Res* 2001;15(1):76–8.

Rohdewald P. Pycnogenol® In: Rice-Evans CA, Packer L, editors. *Flavonoids in Health and Disease*. New York (NY): Marcel Dekker, Inc.; 1998. p. 405–19.

Rohdewald P. A review of the French maritime pine bark extract (Pycnogenol), a herbal medication with a diverse clinical pharmacology. *Int J Clin Pharm Ther* 2002;40(4):158–68.

Roseff SJ, Gulati R. Improvement of sperm quality by Pycnogenol®. *Euro Bull Drug Res* 1999;7(2):33–6.

Ruppanner H, Schaefer U, editors. Kräuterpfarrer Künzle AG Pygenol. In: *Codex 2000/01 — Die Schweizer Arzneimittel in einem Griff*. Basel, Switzerland: Documed AG; 2000. p. 459.

Rüve HJ. Identifizierung und Quantifizierung phenolischer Inhaltsstoffe sowi pharmakologisch-biochemische Untersuchungen eines Extraktes aus der Rind der Meereskiefer *Pinus pinaster* Ait. [doctoral thesis]. Münster, Germany:1996.

Sakamoto T, Mitani Y, Nakajima K. Psychotropic effects of Japanese valerian root extract. *Chem & Pharm Bull* 1992;40:758–61.

Saliou C, Rimbach G, Moini H, McLaughlin L, Hosseini S, Lee J, et al. Solar ultraviolet-induced erythema in human skin and nuclear factor-kappa-B-dependent gene expression in keratinocytes are modulated by a French maritime pine bark extract. *Free Radic Biol Med* 2001;30(2):154–60.

Sallon S, Beer G, Rosenfeld J, Anner H, Volcoff D, Ginsburg G, Paltiel O, Berlatzky Y. The efficacy of Padma 28®, a herbal preparation, in the treatment of intermittent claudication: a controlled double-blind pilot study with objective assessment of chronic occlusive arterial disease patients. *J Vasc Invest* 1998;4(3):129–36.

Sama SK, Krishnamurthy L, Ramachandran K, Krishnan L. Efficacy of Liv.52 in acute viral hepatitis: a double-blind study. *Indian Journal of Medical Research* 1976;5:738.

Samochowiec J, Palacz A, Bobnis W, Lisiecka B. Oscillating potentials of the electroretinogram in the evaluation of the effects of Padma 28® on lipid metabolism and vascular changes in humans. *Phytotherapy Research* 1992;6:200–4.

Samochowiec L, Wojcicki J. Effect of Padma 28® on lipid endoperoxides formation. *Herba Polonica* 1987;33(3):219–22.

Samochowiec L, Wojcicki J, Kosmider K, et al. Clinical test of the effectiveness of Padma 28® in the treatment of patients with chronic arterial occlusion. *Herba Polonica* 1987;33(1):29–41.

Saur E, Rotival N, Lambrot C, Trichet P. Maritime pine dieback on the West Coast of France: Growth response to sodium chloride of 3 geographic races in various edaphic conditions. *Ann des Sci Forestieres* (Paris) 1993;50(4):389–99.

Saxena S, Garg AK, Jain A. A study of Liv.52 therapy in Infective hepatitis in children. *Current Medical Practice* 1980;5:194.

Schilcher H. Personal communication to M. Blumenthal, Dec. 30, 1997.

Schilcher H. *Phytotherapy in Pediatrics: Handbook for Physicians and Pharmacists*, 2nd ed. Stuttgart: Medpharm Scientific Publishers;1997.

Schmidtke I, Schoop W. Hydrostatic oedema and the effect of medicinal products [in German]. *Swiss Med* 1984;6(4a):67–9.

Schmidtke I, Schoop W. Pycnogenol—stasis oedma and its medical treatment [in German]. *Z Ganzheits Med* 1995;3:114–5.

Schmitz M, Jackel M. [Comparative study for assessing quality of life of patients with exogenous sleep disorders (temporary sleep onset and sleep interruption disorders) treated with a hops-valerian preparation and a benzodiazepine drug]. *Wien Med Wochenschr* 1998;148(13):291–8.

Schneider HJ, Honold E, Masuhr Th. Treatment of benign prostatic hyperplasia: Results of a surveillance study in the practices of urological specialists using a combined plant-based preparation (Sabal extract WS 1473 and Urtica extract WS 1031). *Fortschr Med* 1995;113(3):37–40.

Schrader R, Nachbur M, Mahler F. Die Wirkung des tibetischen krauterpraparates Padma 28® auf die claudicatio intermittens. *Schweiz Med Wschr* 1985;115.

Schreckenberger F. Die behandlung von epicondylitiden mit Phytodolor®. *Österreichische Zeitschrift fur Allgemeinmedizin* 1988;42:1638–44.

Singh KK, Singh YK, Sinha SK, Sharma V, Mishra BN. Observatory treatment of infectious hepatitis with Ayurvedic drug - Liv.52. *Ind Med J* 1977;5:69.

Sirnelli-Walter L, Wiel-Masson D. Therapeutic evaluation of leucocyanidol (FLA-VAN) in venous insufficiency in medical gynaecological consultation [in French]. *Artéres et Veines* 1988;7.

Smulski HS, Wójcicki J. Placebo-controlled, double-blind trial to determine the efficacy of the Tibetan plant preparation Padma 28® for intermittent claudication. *Alternative Therapies* 1995 July;1(3). Reprinted from: Smulski HS, Wsojcici J. Plazebokontrollierte doppelblindstudie zur wirkung des tibetanischen krauterpraparates Padma 28® auf die claudicatio intermittens. *Forsch Komplementarmed* 1994;1.

Sökeland J, Albrecht J. A combination of Sabal and Urtica extracts vs. Finasteride in BPH (Stage I and II acc. To Alken): a comparison of therapeutic efficacy in a one-year double blind study. *Urologe* 1997;36:327–33.

Spadea L, Balestrazzi E. Treatment of vascular retinopathies with Pycnogenol®. *Phytotherapy Res* 2001;15(3):219–23.

Stefanescu M, Matache C, Onu A, Tanaseanu S, Dragomir C, Constantinescu I, et al. Pycnogenol efficacy in the treatment of systemic lupus erythematosus patients. *Phytother Res* 2001;15(8):698–704.

Suter M, Richter C. Anti- and pro-oxidative properties of PADMA 28®, a Tibetan herbal formulation. *Redox Report* 2000;5(1):17–22.

United States Congress (USC). Dietary Supplement Health and Education Act of 1994, Pub. l. No. 103–417 (1994).

USC. See: United States Congress.

Vonderheid-Guth B, Todorova A, Brattstöm A, Dimpfel W. Pharmacodynamic effects of valerian and hops extract combination (Ze 9109) on the quantitative-topographical EEG in healthy volunteers. *Eur J Med Res* 2000;5:139–44.

Vorberg G. For colds, stimulate the nonspecific immune system. *Arztl Prax* 1984;35(6):97–8.

Wang T, Duanjun T, Yusheng Z, Guankai G, Xue G, Hu L. The effect of Pycnogenol® on the microcirculation, platelet function and ischaemic myocardium in patients with coronary artery diseases. *Eur Bull Drug Res* 1999;7:19–25.

Watson RR. Reduction of cardiovascular disease risk factors by French maritime pine bark extracts. *CVR&R* 1999 June;326–9.

Wei ZH, Peng QL, Lau BHS. Pycnogenol enhances endothelial cell antioxidant defence. *Redox Report* 1997;3(4):219– 24.

WHO. See: World Health Organization.

Winther K, Kharazmi A, Himmelstrup H, Drabaek H, Mehlson J. Padma 28®, a botanical compound, decreased the oxidative burst response of monocytes and improves fibrinolysis in patients with stable intermittent claudication. *Fibrinolysis* 1994;8(Suppl 2):47–9.

Wójcicki J, Gonet B, Samochowiec L, Gnacin'ska K, Juz'wiak S. Effect of Padma 28® on ascorbate system in rats receiving a high fat diet. *Phytother Res* 1989b;3:54–6.

Wójcicki J, Samochowiec L.Controlled double-blind study of Padma 28® in Angina Pectoris. *Herba Pol* 1986;32:107–14.

Wójcicki J, Samochowiec L, Ceglecka M, Juzyszyn Z, Tustanowski S, Kadtubowska D, Juz'wiak S. Effect of Padma 28® on experimental hyperlipidaemia and atherosclerosis induced by high-fat diet in rabbits. *Phytother Res* 1988;2:119–23.

Wójcicki J, Samochowiec L, Kadlubowska D. Inhibition of ethanol-induced changes in rats by Padma 28®. *Acta Physiol Pol* 1989a;40:387–92.

World Health Organization (WHO). *WHO Monographs on Selected Medicinal Plants*, vol. 1. Geneva: WHO, 1999.

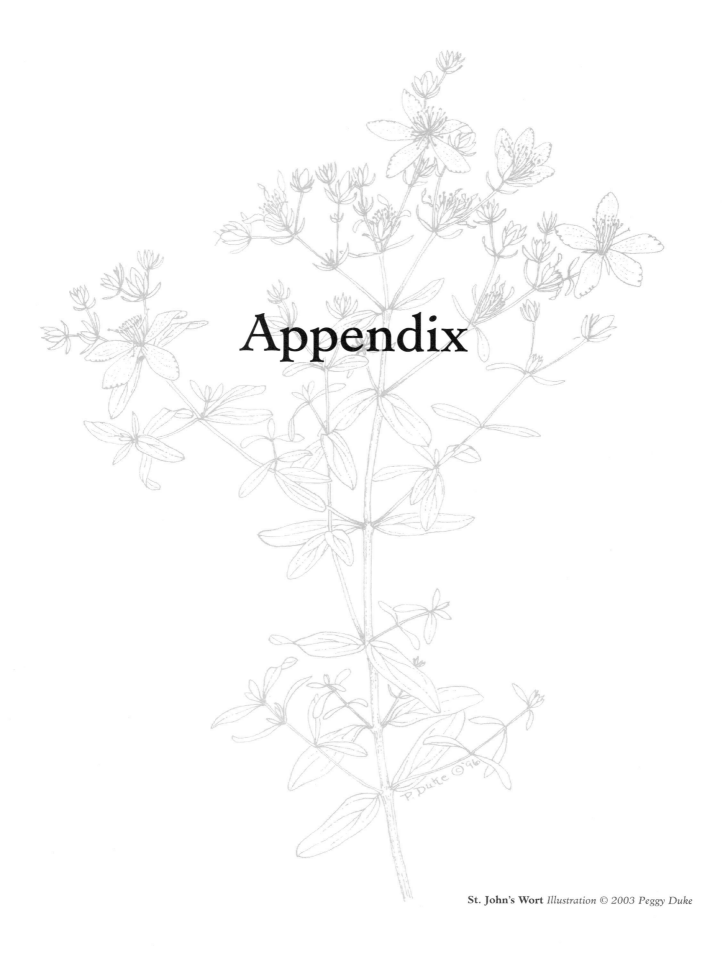

Appendix

St. John's Wort *Illustration © 2003 Peggy Duke*

REVIEWERS

The people listed below have had the opportunity to review one or more of the monographs during the editorial process. ABC is deeply grateful for each person's contribution of time and expertise in helping to review and offer editorial input in the preparation of this book.

Ronald Ackerman, M.D.

Harunobu Amagase, Ph.D.
Director of Research and Development
Wakunaga of America Co., Ltd.

Lenore Arab, Ph.D.*
Professor of Nutrition and Epidemiology
University of North Carolina, School of
Public Health

Dennis Awang, Ph.D., F.C.I.C. *
President
MediPlant Consulting Services

Bruce Barrett, M.D., Ph.D.
University of Wisconsin Medical School

Rudolf Bauer, Ph.D.
Professor
Heinrich Heine University, Düsseldorf

James Beck
JLB, Inc.

Paul Bergner
Editor/Herbalist
Medical Herbalism

Joseph M. Betz, Ph.D.
Director, Dietary Supplements Methods
and Reference Materials Program
Office of Dietary Supplements
National Institutes of Health

John Beutler, Ph.D. *
Molecular Targets Drug Discovery
Program
Laboratory of Natural Products
National Cancer Institute

Normann Boblitz, M.D.
Physician for Internal Medicine
Hanover

Donald Brown, N.D.
Director
Natural Product Research Consultants

Werner Busse, Ph.D.
Head of Regulatory & Scientific Affairs
W. Schwabe & Co.

John Cardellina, Ph.D.
Former Vice-President Botanical Science
Council for Responsible Nutrition

Hyla Cass, M.D.
Assistant Clinical Professor of Psychiatry
UCLA School of Medicine
President
Vitamin Relief USA, Vitamins for the
Homeless

John Cassady

Mary Chavez, Pharm.D. *
Professor of Pharmacy Practice
Midwestern University, College of
Pharmacy

Jerry Cott, Ph.D. *
Pharmacologist
Center for Drug Evaluation
Food and Drug Administration

Don Counts, M.D.
Physician
Seton Hospital

Edward Croom
Scientific and Regulatory Affairs
Manager
Indena U.S.A. Inc.

Jim Crowell, Ph.D.
Chief, Chemopreventative Agent
Development Research Group
Division of Cancer Prevention, NIH

Subhuti Dharmananda, Ph.D.
Director
Institute for Traditional Medicine

Edzard Ernst, M.D., Ph.D.
Director, Department of
Complementary Medicine
University of Exeter

Udo Erasmus, Ph.D.
Independent Researcher, Author,
Educator

W. Hardy Eshbaugh, Ph.D.
Professor Emeritus, Department of
Botany
Miami University

Norman R. Farnsworth, Ph.D.
Research Professor of Pharmacognosy
Senior University Scholar
College of Pharmacy, University of
Illinois at Chicago

Alan Feldstein
Chairman
Ephedra Committee of the American
Herbal Products Association

Steven Foster
Consultant, Author, Photographer
Steven Foster Group, Inc.

Jean Fourcroy, M.D., Ph.D., MPH
Consultant in Regulatory Issues

Michael Friede, Ph.D.
Head of Division of Gynecology and
Central Nervous System
Schaper-Bruemmer

Gary Friedman
Co–owner/Manager
Cosmopolitan Trading

Claus Gehringer, Dr. rer. nat.
President and CEO
Abkit, Inc.

Norman C. Gillis, Ph.D.†
Professor Emeritus
Department of Anesthesiology and
Pharmacology, Yale University School of
Medicine

Frank Greenway, M.D.
Medical Director, Professor
Pennington Biomedical Research Center
School of Medicine, Louisiana State
University

Om Gulati, Ph.D.
Director Scientific & Regulatory Affairs
Horphag Research Management

Robert Gutman, Ph.D.
Adjunct Research Scientist
Department of Pharmaceutics and
Biological Sciences
College of Pharmacy, University of
Georgia

Bill Haggerty, Ph.D.

Mary Hardy, M.D.
Medical Director
Cedars Sinai Integrative Medicine
Program

David Heber, M.D., Ph.D.
Director, Professor of Medicine and
Public Health
UCLA Center for Human Nutrition
David Geffen School of Medicine at
UCLA

Curt Hendrix
Chief Science Officer
Natural Science Corporation of America

Christopher Hobbs, LAc, AHG
Herbalist

David Horrobin, M.D., Ph.D.
Executive Chairman and Research
Director
Laxdale Ltd.

Peter Houghton, Ph.D.
Professor in Pharmacognosy
King's College

Gary Huber, M.D.

David Illingworth
Former President and Chief Executive
Officer
Lichtwer Pharma U.S., Inc.

Loren Israelsen
President
LDI Group

Thomas James, M.D.*

James Joseph, Ph.D.

Richard L. Kingston, Ph.D. *
Vice President & Sr. Clinical
Toxicologist
PROSAR International Poison Center
Associate Professor
Department of Experimental and
Clinical Pharmacology
University of Minnesota, College of
Pharmacy

Uwe Koetter, Ph.D.
Director, New Products Research
GlaxoSmithKline Consumer Healthcare

Rick Kulow
President
Bioriginal Food & Science Corp.

Thomas Kurt, M.D., MPH *
Clinical Professor
Department of Internal Medicine
University of Texas, Southwestern
Medical School

Larry Lawson, Ph.D.
Research Director
Plant Bioactives Research Institute

Marge Leahy, Ph.D.
Sr. Manager, Health and Nutrition
Ocean Spray Cranberries, Inc.

Albert Y. Leung, Ph.D.
President
Phyto-Technologies, Inc.

Eckehard Liske, Ph.D.
Professor and International Medical
Support and PR Division
Schaper & Brümmer GmbH & CO.
KG

Tieraona Lowdog, M.D. *
Physician
Integrative Medicine Education
Associates

Gail B. Mahady, Ph.D.
Assistant Professor
Departments of Pharmacy Practice,
Medicinal Chemistry and
Pharmacognosy
UIC/NIH Center for Botanical Dietary
Supplements Research
University of Illinois at Chicago

Leonard S. Marks, M.D.
Associate Clinical Professor, UCLA
Founder and Medical Director
Urological Sciences Research Foundation

Robin Marles, Ph.D.
Assoc. Prof. of Botany
Brandon University

Arja Miettinen-Baumann, Ph.D.
International Division
Lichtwer Pharma AG

Mark Miller, Ph.D.
Director/Professor
Pediatric Research Division
Albany Medical College

David Morrison
Scientific Affairs Director
Pharmaton Natural Health Products

Alister D. Muir, Ph.D.
Research Scientist
Agriculture and Agri-Food Canada-
Saskatoon Research Centre

Michael Murray, N.D.
Author

Cheryl Myers
Director of Product Development
Enzymatic Therapy

David J. Newman, D.Phil.
Natural Products Branch
Development Therapeutics Program
Division of Cancer Treatment and
Diagnosis, National Cancer Institute

Piergiorgio Pietta, Ph.D.
Professor
ITB-National Council of Research-
Segrate (Milano)

Ronald Pero
President/Professor Cell and Molecular
Biology
CampaMed, LLC

Gilbert Ramirez, R.Ph.
Associate Professor
Center for Leadership Studies
Our Lady of the Lake University

Peter Rohdewald, Ph.D.
Professor Emeritus
Institute for Pharmaceutical Chemistry
Westfälische Wilhelms-Universität
Münster

Megan Rooney
Technical Support
Indena U.S.A. Inc.

A. Wes Siegner, Jr., Esq.
Partner
Hyman, Phelps & McNamara, P.C.

Victor Sierpina, M.D.
Associate Professor
University of Texas Medical Branch at
Galveston

Reviewers

Yadhu N. Singh, Ph.D.
Professor
College of Pharmacy
South Dakota State University

Fabio Soldati, Ph.D.
Head of Research and Development
Pharmaton SA CH-6934 Bioggio

Marilyn Speedie, Ph.D.
Dean and Professor
College of Pharmacy
University of Minnesota

Meir Tenne, D.Sc.
General Manager
Kinarot - Technological Institute

Varro E. Tyler, Ph.D. ScD * †
Professor Emeritus, Pharmacognosy
Purdue University

Roy Upton
Executive Director
American Herbal Pharmacopoeia

Graham West
VP/Managing Director, Ingredient
Technology Group
Ocean Spray International, Inc.

Qun Yi Zheng, Ph.D.
Executive Vice President and Director of
Science and Technology
Pure World Botanicals, Inc.

Susan Zick, N.D., MPH
Research Investigator
Department of Family Medicine
Co-Investigator
Complementary and Alternative
Research Center
University of Michigan

* ABC-CRN Expert Panel
† Deceased

GENERAL REFERENCES

Development of the information in this book was initially based on the following authoritative general references. Additional references were drawn from toxicological and pharmacological studies and clinical trials obtained from HerbClip™ and the resource library of the American Botanical Council, Medline, Napralert and other databases. While by no means exhaustive, the list of references below constitutes a comprehensive array of many of the most authoritative texts in the current herbal medicine literature.

Arzneimittel—Kompendium der Schweiz. Basel, Switzerland: Documed AG; 2001.

Blumenthal M, Busse WR, Goldberg A, Gruenwald J, Hall T, Riggins CW, Rister RS, editors. Klein S, Rister RS, translators. *The Complete German Commission E Monographs—Therapeutic Guide to Herbal Medicines*. Austin (TX): American Botanical Council; Boston: Integrative Medicine Communication; 1998.

Blumenthal M, Goldberg A, Brinckmann J, editors. *Herbal Medicine: Expanded Commission E Monographs*. Newton (MA): Integrative Medicine Communications; 2000.

Bradley PR, editor. *British Herbal Compendium*, vol. 1. Dorset, England: British Herbal Medicine Association; 1992.

Bratman S, Kroll D. *Clinical Evaluation of Medicinal Herbs and Other Therapeutic Natural Products*. Roseville (CA): Prima Health; 1999.

Brinker F. *Herb Contraindications and Drug Interactions*. 3rd ed. Sandy (OR): Eclectic Medical Publications; 2001.

British Herbal Pharmacopoeia. Exeter, U.K.: British Herbal Medicine Association; 1996.

Bruneton J. *Pharmacognosy, Phytochemistry, Medicinal Plants*. 2nd ed. Paris: Lavoisier Publishing; 1999.

DeSmet P, Keller K, Hänsel R, Chandler RF, editors. *Adverse Effects of Herbal Drugs*, vol. 1. Berlin: Springs-Verlag; 1992.

DeSmet P, Keller K, Hänsel R, Chandler RF, editors. *Adverse Effects of Herbal Drugs*, vol. 2. Berlin: Springs-Verlag; 1993.

Deutsches Arzneibuch. Stuttgart, Germany: Deutscher Apotheker Verlag; 1999.

European Scientific Cooperative on Phytotherapy. *Monographs on the Medicinal Uses of Plant Drugs*. Exeter, U.K.: ESCOP; various years.

European Pharmacopoeia (3rd edition 1997, Supplement 2001). Strasbourg, France: Council of Europe; 2001.

Leung AY, Foster S. *Encyclopedia of Common Natural Ingredients Used in Food, Drugs, and Cosmetics*. 2nd ed. New York: John Wiley & Sons, Inc.; 1996.

McGuffin M, Hobbs C, Upton R, Goldberg A, editors. *American Herbal Products Association's Botanical Safety Handbook*. Boca Raton (FL): CRC Press; 1997.

Newall C, Anderson L, Phillipson J. *Herbal Medicines, A Guide for Health-Care Professionals*. London, U.K.: The Pharmaceutical Press; 1996.

Pizzorno JE, Murray MT, editors. *Textbook of Natural Medicine*. Vol. 1, 2nd ed. New York; Churchill Livingston; 1999.

Robbers JE, Tyler VE. *Tyler's Herbs of Choice: The Therapeutic Use of Phytomedicinals*. New York: Haworth Herbal Press; 1999.

Rotblatt M, Ziment I. *Evidence-Based Herbal Medicine*. Philadelphia: Hanley & Belfus; 2001.

Schultz V, Hänsel R, Tyler V. *Rational Phytotherapy: A Physicians' Guide to Herbal Medicine*. 4th ed. New York: Springer-Verlag; 2001.

United States Pharmacopeia, 25th revision; National Formulary, 20th ed. Rockville (MD): United States Pharmacopeial Convention, Inc.; 2002.

Upton R, editor. *American Herbal Pharmacopoeia and Therapeutic Compendium*. Santa Cruz (CA):AHP; various monographs.

Wagner, H, editor. *Immunomodulatory Agents from Plants*. Basel: Birkhäuser Verlag; 1999.

World Health Organization. *WHO Monographs on Selected Medicinal Plants*, vol. 1. Geneva, Switzerland: World Health Organization; 1999.

Commercial Products Used in Clinical Studies Listed in Single Herb Monographs

(in alphabetical order by herb)

(See table on pages 405-408 for contact information.)

Herb	Products Used in Clinical Studies (Manufacturer)	Other Names (Manufacturer/Distributor)
Bilberry	**Difrarel 100™** (Laboratories Chibret c/o Societe Anonyme Corporation) (Product no longer available)	
	Myrtocyan® (extract used in retail products) (Indena S.p.A.)	**MirtoSelect™** (U.S.: Indena USA Inc.) **Tegens™** (Synthelabo-Pharma SA of France)
	Tegens™ (Synthelabo-Pharma SA of France)	**MirtoSelect™** (U.S.: Indena USA Inc.) **Myrtocyan®** (extract used in retail products) (Indena S.p.A.)
Black Cohosh	**Remifemin® tablet** (Schaper & Brümmer GmbH & Co. KG)	**Remifemin® Menopause** (U.S.: GlaxoSmithKline)
	Remifemin® drops (Schaper & Brümmer GmbH & Co. KG) (Product no longer available)	
Cat's Claw	**C-MED 100®** (Campamed, LLC)	**C-MED 100®** (U.S.: AF Nutraceutical Group, Inc.)
	Krallendorn® Capsules (Immodal Pharmaka GmbH)	**Saventaro®** (U.S.: Enzymatic Therapy)
	Krallendorn® Drops (Immodal Pharmaka GmbH)	
	Krallendorn® Ointment (Immodal Pharmaka GmbH)	
	Krallendorn® Spray (Immodal Pharmaka GmbH)	
	Krallendorn® Tea (Immodal Pharmaka GmbH)	
Cayenne	**Axsain®** (GenDerm Corporation) (Product no longer available)	
	Capsig® (Schering-Plough) (Product no longer available)	
	Chili powder (no brand) (KNP Trading Pte Ltd)	
	Saemaul Kongjang 1 (Source company not found)	
	Zostrix®-HP (GenDerm Corporation)	
Chamomile	**Diarrhoesan®** (Dr. Loges & Co. GmbH)	
	Kamillosan® Creme (VIATRIS GmbH & Co. KG)	**CAMOCARE®** (U.S.: ABKIT, INC.)
	Kamillosan® Konzentrat (VIATRIS GmbH & Co. KG)	
	Kamillosan® Liquidum (VIATRIS GmbH & Co. KG)	
	Kneipp® Kamillen-Konzentrat (Kneipp-Werke)	
Chaste Tree	**Agnolyt® Capsules** (Madaus AG) (Product no longer available)	
	Agnolyt® Solution (Madaus AG)	
	Alyt® Solution (Ciba-Geigy AG) (Unable to verify source company and availability)	
	BNO 1095 Capsules (Bionorica AG) (Product not distributed)	
	Femicur® N Kapseln (Schaper & Brümmer GmbH & Co. KG)	
	Mastodynon® (Bionorica AG)	
	Premens® Ze440 (Zeller AG)	GNC's Women's Cycle (U.S.: GNC)
	Strotan® Kapseln (Strathmann AG & Co.)	
Cranberry	**Azo-Cranberry®** Capsules (PolyMedica Corp.)	
	Ocean Spray® Cranberry Juice Cocktail (Ocean Spray Cranberries Inc.)	
	Solaray® CranActin® (Nutraceutical Corporation)	

Commercial Products Used in Clinical Studies Listed in Single Herb Monographs (cont.)

(in alphabetical order by herb)

(See table on pages 405-408 for contact information.)

Herb	Products Used in Clinical Studies (Manufacturer)	Other Names (Manufacturer/Distributor)
Echinacea	**Echinacea Plus®** (Traditional Medicinals®, Inc.)	
	Echinacin® (Madaus AG)	**EchinaGuard®** (U.S.: Nature's Way Products, Inc.)
	Echinaforce® (Bioforce AG)	**Echinaforce®** (U.S.: Bioforce USA)
	EchinaGuard® (U.S.: Nature's Way Products, Inc.)	**Echinacin®** (Madaus AG)
	Esberitox® (prior to 1985) (Schaper & Brümmer GmbH & Co. KG)	
	Esberitox®-N[1] (1985 formulation based on Esberitox®) (Schaper & Brümmer GmbH & Co. KG)	
	Esberitox®-N[2] (1990 formulation based on Esberitox®) (Schaper & Brümmer GmbH & Co. KG)	**Esberitox®** (US: Enzymatic Therapy, Inc.)
	Resistan® (TRUW Arzneimittel Vertriebs GmbH) (Reformulation is in process)	
Eleuthero	**Elagen®** (Eladon Ltd.)	**Eleugetic®** (new name)
	Eleukokk® (Pharma-Inter-Med) (Product no longer available)	
	Maxim-L® (Omega Nutripharm)	
	Medexport (Source company not found)	
	Taigutan® (Dr. Mewes Heilmittel GmbH) (Unable to verify source company)	
Ephedra	**DietMax®** (NaturalMax Co./Kal Inc., Div. Nutraceutical Corporation)	
	Escalation™ (Enzymatic Therapy)	
	Excel (Excel Corporation) (no information available)	
	Metabolife 356® (Metabolife International)	
	Solaray® Ephedra (Nutraceutical Corporation)	
	Up Your Gas (National Health Products)	
Evening Primrose Oil	**Efamast® 500 mg EPO** (Scotia Pharmaceuticals Ltd.)	
	Efamol® 500 mg EPO (Scotia Pharmaceuticals Ltd.)	
	Efamol® Marine 500 mg (Scotia Pharmaceuticals Ltd.)	
	Epogam® 500 mg EPO (Scotia Pharmaceuticals Ltd.)	
	Quest Vitamins (Quest Vitamins)	
	Scotia Cream (Scotia Pharmaceuticals Ltd.)	
Feverfew	No branded products in monograph	
Flax	**Alena™** (ENRECO, Inc.)	
Garlic	**AGE™** (Wakunaga of America Co., Ltd.)	**Aged Garlic Extract™** (extract used in Kyolic® product line)
	Hofel's® Garlic Pearles One-A-Day (Seven Seas Ltd., division of Merck Group)	
	Kwai® forte 300 mg LI 111 (Lichtwer Pharma AG)	Kwai HeartFit™ Garlic (U.S.: ABKIT, INC.)
	Kwai®N LI 111 (Lichtwer Pharma AG)	Kwai® Garlic Supplement (U.S.: ABKIT, INC.)
	Kyolic® Liquid (Wakunaga of America Co., Ltd.)	
	Kyolic® Reserve (Wakunaga of America Co., Ltd.)	
	Kyolic® Super Formula 100 (Wakunaga of America Co., Ltd.)	
	Kyolic® Super Formula 101 (Wakunaga of America Co., Ltd.)	
	Kyolic® Super Formula 102 (Wakunaga of America Co., Ltd.)	
	Kyolic® Super Formula 103 (Wakunaga of America Co., Ltd.)	

Commercial Products Used in Clinical Studies Listed in Single Herb Monographs (cont.)

(in alphabetical order by herb)

(See table on pages 405-408 for contact information.)

Herb	Products Used in Clinical Studies (Manufacturer)	Other Names (Manufacturer/Distributor)
Garlic (cont)	**Kyolic® Super Formula 104** (Wakunaga of America Co., Ltd.)	
	Kyolic® Super Formula 105 (Wakunaga of America Co., Ltd.)	
	Kyolic® Super Formula 106 (Wakunaga of America Co., Ltd.)	
	Pure-Gar® Garlic Powder A-2000 (Essentially Pure Ingredients™)	
	Pure-Gar® Garlic Powder A-5000 (Essentially Pure Ingredients™)	
	Pure-Gar® Garlic Powder A-8000 (Essentially Pure Ingredients™)	
	Pure-Gar® Garlic Powder A-10000 (Essentially Pure Ingredients™)	
	Sapec® (Lichtwer Pharma AG)	
	Tegra® (Hermes Fabrick Pharma)	
Ginger	**Blackmores custom powdered ginger capsules** (Blackmores Ltd.)	
	EV. Ext® 33 (extract used in retail products) (Ferrosan A/S)	
	EV. Ext® 77 (extract used in retail products) (Ferrosan A/S)	**FlexAgility™** (U.S.: Enzymatic Therapy) **Zinaxin™** (Ferrosan A/S) **Zincosamine™** (U.S.: FreeLife International LLC)
	Martindale powdered ginger capsules (Martindale Pharmaceuticals Pty. Ltd.)	
	Zintona® (Dalidar Pharma c/o Bio-Dar Ltd.)	
Ginkgo	**Bio-Biloba®** (Pharma Nord ApS)	
	Concentrated Ginkgo leaf liquid (Quidao Fengyi Biotechnology Limited)	
	EGb-761 (extract used in retail products) (Dr. Willmar Schwabe Pharmaceuticals)	**Ginkgold®** (U.S.: Nature's Way Products, Inc.) **Ginkoba®** (Pharmaton Natural Health Products) **Rökan®** (Spitzner GmbH) **Tanakan®** (Beaufour-Ipsen) **Tebonin® forte** (Dr. Willmar Schwabe Pharmaceuticals)
	Geriaforce® (Bioforce AG)	
	Ginkgold® (Nature's Way Products, Inc.)	**EGb-761** (extract used in retail products) (Dr. Willmar Schwabe Pharmaceuticals)
	Kaveri® (Lichtwer Pharma AG)	**LI-1370** (extract used in retail products) (Lichtwer Pharma AG)
	LI-1370 (extract used in retail products) (Lichtwer Pharma AG)	**Ginkai®** (U.S.: ABKIT, INC.) **Ginkyo®** (Lichtwer Pharma AG) **Kaveri®** (Lichtwer Pharma AG) **Symphona®** (Lichtwer Pharma AG)
	Rökan® (Spitzner GmbH)	**EGb-761** (extract used in retail products) (Dr. Willmar Schwabe Pharmaceuticals)
	Tanakan® (Beaufour-Ipsen)	**EGb-761** (extract used in retail products) (Dr. Willmar Schwabe Pharmaceuticals)
	Tebonin® forte (Dr. Willmar Schwabe Pharmaceuticals)	**EGb-761** (extract used in retail products) (Dr. Willmar Schwabe Pharmaceuticals)
Ginseng, American	**Chai-Na-Ta®** (Cha-Na-Ta Corp.)	**CNT2000™** (Cha-Na-Ta Corp.)

Commercial Products Used in Clinical Studies Listed in Single Herb Monographs (cont.)

(in alphabetical order by herb)

(See table on pages 405-408 for contact information.)

Herb	Products Used in Clinical Studies (Manufacturer)	Other Names (Manufacturer/Distributor)
Ginseng, Asian	**Dansk Droge Ginseng tablets** (Dansk Droge A/S)	
	G115® (extract used in retail products) (Pharmaton Natural Health Products)	**Ginsana®** (Pharmaton Natural Health Products)
	Gerimax® Ginseng extract (Dansk Droge A/S)	
	Ginsana® G115 capsules (Pharmaton Natural Health Products, Division of Boehringer-Ingelheim Pharmaceuticals, Inc.)	**G115®** (extract used in retail products) (Pharmaton Natural Health Products)
	Pharmaton® capsules (Pharmaton Natural Health Products)	
	PKC 167/79 (investigational product only, not available) (Pharmaton S.A.)	
Goldenseal	No branded product in monograph	
Hawthorn	**Crataegutt® Dragées** (Dr. Willmar Schwabe Pharmaceuticals)	
	Crataegutt® forte Kapseln (Dr. Willmar Schwabe Pharmaceuticals)	**Crataegus Special Extract WS1442** (Dr. Willmar Schwabe Pharmaceuticals) **HeartCare™** (U.S.: Nature's Way Products, Inc.)
	Crataegutt® novo Filmtabletten (Dr. Willmar Schwabe Pharmaceuticals)	
	Crataegus Special Extract WS1442 (Dr. Willmar Schwabe Pharmaceuticals)	**Crataegutt® forte** (Dr. Willmar Schwabe Pharmaceuticals)
	Faros® 300 Dragées (Lichtwer Pharma AG)	
	Faros® LI 132 Dragées (Lichtwer Pharma AG)	
Horse Chestnut	**Aesculaforce® Venen-Gel** (Bioforce AG)	
	Aesculaforce® Venen-Tabletten (Bioforce AG)	**Aesculaforce®** (U.S.: Bioforce AG)
	Reparil® Dragées (Madaus AG)	
	Venoplant® retard S (Dr. Willmar Schwabe Pharmaceuticals)	
	Venostasin® Retardkapsel (Klinge Pharma GmbH)	**Venostat®** (U.S.: Pharmaton Natural Health Products)
Kava	**GITLY Kava extract** (Source company not found)	
	KavaPure® (PureWorld Botanicals Inc.)	
	Kavatrol® (Natrol Inc.)	
	Kavosporal® (Polcopharma F Polley & Co.)	
	Laitan® (Dr. Willmar Schwabe Pharmaceuticals)	**WS 1490** (extract used in retail products) (Dr. Willmar Schwabe Pharmaceuticals)
	Laitan® 100 (Dr. Willmar Schwabe Pharmaceuticals)	**WS 1490** (extract used in retail products) (Dr. Willmar Schwabe Pharmaceuticals)
	WS 1490 (extract used in retail products) (Dr. Willmar Schwabe Pharmaceuticals)	**Laitan®** (Dr. Willmar Schwabe Pharmaceuticals) **Laitan® 100** (Dr. Willmar Schwab Pharmaceuticals)
Licorice	**Caved-S®** (Tillots Pharma AG) (Product no longer available)	
	Saila Licorice Root Tablets (Saila S.p.A.)	
	Stronger Neo Minophagen-C (SNMC) (Minophagen Pharmaceutical Co.) (Product no longer available)	

Commercial Products Used in Clinical Studies Listed in Single Herb Monographs (cont.)

(in alphabetical order by herb)

(See table on pages 405-408 for contact information.)

Herb	Products Used in Clinical Studies (Manufacturer)	Other Names (Manufacturer/Distributor) Herb
Milk Thistle	**IdB 1016 Silipide** (Indena S.p.A.)	**Siliphos®** (U.S.: Indena USA Inc.)
	Legalon® 35 Dragées (Madaus AG)	
	Legalon® 70 (Madaus AG)	
	Legalon® 140 (Madaus AG)	**Thisilyn®** (U.S.: Nature's Way Products, Inc.)
Peppermint	**Colpermin®** (Tillots Pharma AG)	
	Enteroplant® (Dr. Willmar Schwabe Pharmaceuticals)	
	Euminz® (Lichtwer Pharma AG)	
	Peppermint Oil B.P (Source company not found)	
Saw Palmetto	**IDS 89** (extract used in retail products) (Strathmann AG & Co.)	**Strogen® 160 mg caps** (Strathmann AG & Co.) **Strogen® forte** (Strathmann AG & Co.) **Strogen® S** (Strathmann AG & Co.) **Strogen® UN** (Strathmann AG & Co.)
	LG 166/S (Laboratori Guidotti S.p.A.)	
	Nutrilite® Saw Palmetto with Nettle Root (Nutrilite®)	
	Permixon® (Pierre Fabre Médicament)	
	PRO 160/120® (Dr. Willmar Schwabe Pharmaceuticals)	**Prostagutt® forte** (Dr. Willmar Schwabe Pharmaceuticals)
	Prostagutt® (Dr. Willmar Schwabe Pharmaceuticals)	**WS 1473** (Dr. Willmar Schwabe Pharmaceuticals) **ProstActive™** (U.S.: Nature's Way Products, Inc.)
	Prostagutt® forte (Dr. Willmar Schwabe Pharmaceuticals)	**PRO 160/120®** (Dr. Willmar Schwabe Pharmaceuticals) **ProstActive Plus™** (U.S.: Nature's Way Products, Inc.)
	Prostaserene® (Therabel Research)	**SabalSelect™** (U.S.: Indena USA, Inc.)
	Solaray® Saw palmetto (Nutraceutical Corporation)	
	Strogen® forte (Strathmann AG & Co.)	**IDS 89** (extract used in retail products) (Strathmann AG & Co.)
	Strogen® S (Strathmann AG & Co.)	**IDS 89** (extract used in retail products) (Strathmann AG & Co.)
	Talso® (Sanofi Synthelabo GmbH)	**SG 291** (Indena S.p.A.) **SabalSelect™** (U.S.: Indena USA, Inc.)
St. John's wort	**Hyperiforce®** (Bioforce AG)	
	Jarsin® 300 (Lichtwer Pharma AG)	
	Kira® (Lichtwer Pharma AG)	**Kira®** (U.S.: ABKIT, INC.)
	LI 160 (extract used in retail products) (Lichtwer Pharma AG)	**Jarsin® 300** (Lichtwer Pharma AG) **Kira®** (Lichtwer Pharma AG / U.S.: ABKIT, INC.)
	Remotiv® (Bayer Vital GmbH & Co.)	**Ze 117** (extract used in retail products) (Zeller AG)
	STEI 300 (Steiner Arzneimittel)	
	WS 5570 (extract used in retail products) (Dr. Willmar Schwabe Pharmaceuticals)	

Commercial Products Used in Clinical Studies Listed in Single Herb Monographs (cont.)

(in alphabetical order by herb)

(See table on pages 405-408 for contact information.)

Herb	Products Used in Clinical Studies (Manufacturer)	Other Names (Manufacturer/Distributor)
St. John's wort (cont)	**WS 5572** (extract used in retail products) (Dr. Willmar Schwabe Pharmaceuticals)	**Neuroplant®** (Dr. Willmar Schwabe Pharmaceuticals) **Perika®** (Nature's Way Products, Inc.)
	WS 5573 (extract used in retail products) (Dr. Willmar Schwabe Pharmaceuticals)	
	Ze 117 (extract used in retail products) (Zeller AG)	**Remotiv®** (Bayer Vital GmbH & Co.)
Tea Leaf	**Arkocaps/Phytotrim®** (Arkopharma Laboratories)	
	Exolise® (Arkopharma Laboratories)	
	Lipton® Brisk Tea (Unilever Bestfoods North America)	
	Lipton® Green Tea (Unilever Bestfoods North America)	
	Twinings® Darjeeling Tea (Twinings London)	
Valerian	**Alluna™ Sleep** (U.S.: GlaxoSmithKline)	**Ze91019** (extract used in retail products) (GlaxoSmithKline)
	Euphytose® (Roche Nicholas SA)	
	Euvegal® forte (Dr. Willmar Schwabe Pharmaceuticals)	**Valerian Nighttime™** (U.S.: Nature's Way Products, Inc.)
	Harmonicum Much® (Prof. Dr. Much AG) (Unable to verify source company)	
	Hova® (Gebro Pharma GmbH)	
	Ivel® (Germany: Kanoldt Arzneimittel GmbH)	**Ze91019** (extract used in retail products) (Zeller AG)
	LI 156 (extract used in retail products) (Lichtwer Pharma AG)	**Sedonium®** (Lichtwer Pharma AG / U.S.: ABKIT, INC.)
	Nature's Way® Valerian root capsules (Nature's Way Products, Inc.)	
	Novo-Baldriparan® (Novo-Nordisk A/S)	
	ReDormin® (Switzerland: Zeller AG)	**Ze91019** (extract used in retail products) (Zeller AG)
	Sedariston® Konzetrat (Steiner Arzneimittel)	
	Sedonium® (Lichtwer Pharma AG / U.S.: ABKIT, INC.)	**LI 156** (extract used in retail products) (Lichtwer Pharma AG)
	Songha Night® (Pharmaton Natural Health Products)	
	Valdisperte® (Solvay Arzneimittel) (Unable to verify availability)	
	Valdisperte® forte (Solvay Arzneimittel)	
	Valerina Natt® (Pharbio Medical Suerigie c/o Cederroth International AB)	
	Valmane® (Lyssia GmbH c/o Solvay Arzneimittel) (Unable to verify availability)	
	Valverde® (Ciba-Geigy AG) (Product no longer available)	
	Ze91019 (extract used in retail products) (Zeller AG)	**Alluna™ Sleep** (U.S.: GlaxoSmithKline) **Ivel®** (Germany: Kanoldt Arzneimittel GmbH) **ReDormin®** (Switzerland: Zeller AG)

Commercial Products Used in Clinical Studies Listed in Proprietary Herbal Product Monographs (in alphabetical order by product name)

Proprietary Product (Manufacturer*)	Ingredients†	Other Names (Manufacturer/Distributor*)
Alluna™ Sleep (GlaxoSmithKline)	*Valeriana officinalis, Humulus lupulus*	Ivel® (Germany: Kanoldt Arzeneimittel GmbH) ReDormin® (Switzerland: Zeller AG) Ze 91019 (Zeller AG: extract used in retail products)
Esberitox® (Schaper & Brümmer GmbH & Co. KG) (pre-1985 formulation)	*Echinacea angustifolia* root, *Echinacea purpurea* root, *Thuja occidentalis* herb, *Baptisia tinctoria* root, additional homeopathic dilutions of herbs	Not marketed in the U.S.
Esberitox®N[1] (Schaper & Brümmer GmbH & Co. KG) (1985 formulation)	*Echinacea angustifolia* root, *Echinacea purpurea* root, *Thuja occidentalis* herb, *Baptistia tinctoria* root	Not marketed in the U.S.
Esberitox®N[2] (Schaper & Brümmer GmbH & Co. KG)	*Echinacea pallida* root, *Echinacea purpurea*, *Thuja occidentailis, Baptistia tinctoria* root	Esberitox® (U.S. Distributor: Enzymatic Therapy, Inc.)
Euvegal® forte (Dr. Willmar Schwabe Pharmaceuticals)	*Valeriana officinalis, Melissa officinalis*	Valerian Nighttime™ (U.S. Distributor: Nature's Way Products, Inc.)
Hochu-ekki-to® (Tsumura & Company)	*Astragalus membranaceus, Panax ginseng, Atractylodes lancea, Angelica sinensis, Bupleurum chinense, Zyzyphus jujuba, Citrus unshiu* peel, *Cimicifuga biternata, Zingiber officinale*	Not marketed in the U.S.
Hova® (Gebro Pharma GmbH)	*Valeriana officinalis, Humulus lupulus*	Not marketed in the U.S.
Liv.52® (Himalaya Drug Company)	*Capparis spinosa, Cichorium intybus,* Ferric oxide Calx., *Solanum nigrum, Terminalia arjuna, Cassia occidentalis, Achillea millefolium, Tamarix gallica* (specially processed in a base of *Eclipta prostrata, E. alba*)	LiverCare® (U.S. Distributor: Himalaya USA)
Mastodynon® (Bionorica AG)	10 g (10.8 ml) Mastodynon® drops contain as active ingredients 2.0 g *Vitex agnus-castus* ø, 1.0 g *Caulophyllum thalictroides* (HAB 34) Dil. D4 (HAB 1; V.3a), 1.0 g Cyclamen Dil. D4, 1.0 g Ignatia Dil. D6, 2.0 g Iris Dil. D2, 1.0 g *Lilium tigrinum* Dil. D3. Mastodynon® drops contain ethanol 53% *v/v*	Not marketed in the U.S.
Nutrilite® Saw Palmetto with Nettle Root (Nutrilite®)	*Serenoa repens, Urtica dioica* root, *Cucurbita pepo,* Lemon bioflavonoid concentrate, natural β-carotene concentrate	
Padma Basic® (PADMA AG)	*Saussurea lappa, Azadirachta indica, Cetraria islandica, Terminalia chebula, Elettaria cardamomum, Pterocarpus santalinus,* additional herbs	(U.S. Distributor: Econugenics)
Padma 28® (PADMA AG)	*Saussurea lappa, Azadirachta indica, Cetraria islandica, Terminalia chebula, Elettaria cardamomum, Pterocapus santalinus, Aconitum napellus,* additional herbs	Not marketed in the U.S.
Phytodolor® (Steigerwald)	*Fraxinus excelsior, Populus tremula, Solidago virgaurea*	Not marketed in the U.S.
Prostagutt® forte (Dr. Willmar Schwabe Pharmaceuticals)	*Serenoa repens, Urtica dioica* root	ProstActive Plus™ (U.S. Distributor: Nature'sWay Products, Inc.)
Pycnogenol® (Horphag Research)	French Maritime Pine Bark Extract (*Pinus pinaster* subsp. *Atlantica*)	(U.S. Distributor: Natural Health Science)
Sinupret® (Bionorica AG)	*Gentiana lutea, Primula veris, Rumex acetosa, R. crispus, R. obtusifolius, Sambucus nigra, Verbena officinalis*	(U.S. Distributor: Mountain Home Nutritionals)

* See pages 405-408 for contact information.
† Based on product label.

COMPANY CONTACT INFORMATION
FOR COMMERCIAL PRODUCTS USED IN CLINICAL STUDIES
(in alphabetical order by company name)

ABKIT, INC.: 207 East 94th Street, New York, NY 10128, U.S.A. / Tel: 800-226-6227 / Fax: 212-860-8323 / E-mail: info@abkit.com / Website: www.abkit.com (U.S. Distributor for Lichtwer Pharma AG and ASTA Medica AG)

AF Nutraceutical Group, Inc.: 786 Stonington Rd., Stonington, CT 06378, U.S.A. / Tel: 973-267-6691 / Fax: 973-267-6693 / Email: info@afnutra.com / Website: www.afnutra.com (U.S. Distributor for Campamed, LLC)

Arkopharma Laboratories: BP 28-06511, Carros Cedex, France / Tel: +33-49-32-91-128 / E-mail: info@arkopharma.com
U.S. DISTRIBUTOR: Health from the Sun, 19A Crosby Dr. #300, Bedford, MA 01730, U.S.A. / Tel: 781-276-0505 / Fax: 781-276-7335 / E-mail: seyrig@arkopharma-us.com

Bayer Vital GmbH & Co. KG: Consumer Care, Wesler Strasse 5-7, 51149 Köln, Germany / Tel: +49-01-30-82-6301 / Website: www.bayer-ag.de

Beaufour-Ipsen: Paris, France / Tel: +33 (0) 1 44 30 42 15 / Fax: +33 (0) 1 44 30 42 04 / Email: contact.web@beaufour-ipsen.com / Website: www.beaufour-ipsen.com

Bioforce AG: CH-9325 Roggwil TG, Switzerland / Tel: +41 71 454 61 61 / Fax: +41 71 454 61 62 / Email: info@bioforce.ch / Website: www.bioforce.com
U.S. DISTRIBUTOR: Bioforce USA / 1869 Route 9H, Suite #1, Hudson, New York 12534, U.S.A. / Tel: 1-800-641-7555 / Fax: 1-888-798-7555 / E-mail: Info@BioforceUSA.com / Website: www.bioforceusa.com

Bionorica AG: International Division, P.O. Box 1851, D-92308 Neumarkt, Germany / Tel: +49-91-81-2319-0 / Fax: +49-91-81-2312-65 / E-mail: international@bionorica.de / Website: www.bionorica.de
U.S. DISTRIBUTOR: Mountain Home Nutritionals, P.O. Box 1400, Ranson, WV 25438, U.S.A. / Tel: 800-888-1415 / Fax: 800-525-5562 (a subsidiary of Phillips International, Inc.)

Blackmores Ltd.: 23 Roseberry Street, Balgowlah, NSW 2093, Australia / Tel: +61-29-95-1011-1 / Fax: +61-29-94-9195-4 / Website: www.blackmores.com

Boehringer-Ingelheim: P.O. Box 368, Ridgefield, CT 06877, U.S.A. / Tel: 800-243-0127 / Website: www.us.boehringer-ingelheim.com

Campamed, LLC: 437 Madison Avenue, New York, NY 10022, U.S.A. / Tel: 212-616-6814 / Fax: 212-838-8918
U.S. DISTRIBUTOR: AF Nutraceutical Group, Inc., 786 Stonington Rd., Stonington, CT 06378, U.S.A. / Tel: 973-267-6691 / Fax: 973-267-6693 / Email: info@afnutra.com / Website: www.afnutra.com

Chai-Na-Ta Corp.: 5965 205A Street, Langley, BC V3A 8C4, Canada / Tel: 800-406-7668 / Fax: 623-553-8891 / Website: www.chainata.com

Ciba-Geigy AG: Novartis Consumer Health AG, Route de l'Entraz, CH 1260 Nyon 1, Switzerland / Website: www.consumer-health.novartis.com (a division of Novartis Consumer Health AG)

Dalidar Pharma: BioDar Ltd., Yavne Technology Park, P.O. Box 344, Yavne 81103, Israel / Tel: +972-08-942-0930 / Fax: +972-08-942-0928 / E-mail: dalidar@dalidar.com / Website: www.dalidar.com

Dansk Droga A/S: Industrigrenen 10, 2635, Ishoj, Copenhagen, Denmark / Tel: +43-56-5656 / Fax: +43-56-5600

Dr. Loges & Co. GmbH: Postfach 1262, Schützenstrasse 5, 21423 Winsen, Germany / Tel: +49-041-71-7070 / Fax: +49-041-71-7071-00 / E-mail: info@loges.com

Dr. Mewes Heilmittel GmbH: PF 1325, 56194 Höhr-Grenzhausen, Germany / Tel: +49-02-62-49-4529-0/ Fax: +49-02-62-49-4529-1 / Website: www.paesel.lorei.de

Dr. Willmar Schwabe Pharmaceuticals: International Division, Willmar Schwabe Str. 4, D-76227, Karlsruhe, Germany / Tel: +49-721-4005 ext. 294 / Email: melville-eaves@schwabe.de / Website: www.schwabepharma.com

Econugenics Inc.: 2208 Northpoint Parkway, Santa Rosa, CA 95407, U.S.A. / Tel: 800-308-5518 / Fax: 707-526-7689 / Website: www.padmabasic.com (U.S. Distributor for PADMA AG)

Efamol Nutraceuticals Inc.: 23 Dry Dock Ave., Boston, MA 02210, U.S.A. / Website: http://fox.nstn.ca/~scotlib/index.html

Eladon Ltd.: 63 High Street, Bangor, Gwynedd, LL57 1NR, U.K. / Tel: +44-01-24-83-7005-9 / Website: www.elagen.com

ENRECO, Inc.: P.O. Box 186, Newton, WI 53063, U.S.A. / Tel: 800-962-9536/ Fax: 920-926-4224 / E-mail: info@enreco.com / Website: www.enreco.com

Enzymatic Therapy, Inc.: 825 Challenger Drive, Green Bay, WI 54311, U.S.A. / Tel: 920-469-1313 / Website: www.enzy.com (U.S. Distributor for Ferrosan A/S, Immodal Pharmaka GmbH, Shaper & Brümmer Gmbh & Co. KG, and Steigerwald)

Essentially Pure Ingredients™: 21411 Prairie Street, Chatsworth, CA 91311, U.S.A. / Tel: 818-739-6046 / Website: www.essentiallypure.com

Excel Corporation: Contact information not available

Ferrosan A/S: Sydmarken 5, 2860 Soeborg, Denmark / Tel: +45-3969-2111 / Fax: +45-3969-6518 / Website: www.ferrosan.com
U.S. DISTRIBUTOR: Enzymatic Therapy, Inc., 825 Challenger Drive, Green Bay, WI 54311, U.S.A. / Tel: 920-469-1313 / Website: www.enzy.com
U.S. DISTRIBUTOR: FreeLife International LLC: 333 Quarry Road, Milford, CT 06460 / Tel: 800-882-7240 / Fax: 203-882-7255 / E-mail: info@freelife.com / Website: www.freelife.com

FreeLife International LLC: 333 Quarry Road, Milford, CT 06460 / Tel: 800-882-7240 / Fax: 203-882-7255 / E-mail: info@freelife.com / Website: www.freelife.com (U.S. Distributor for Ferrosan A/S)

Gebro Pharma GmbH: A-6391 Fieberbrunn, Austria / Tel: +43-53-54-5300-0 / Fax: +43-53-54-5300-0 / E-mail: pharma@gebro.com / Website: www.gebro.com

GenDerm Corp.: 4343 East Camelback Road, Phoenix, AZ 85012, U.S.A.

GlaxoSmithKline: One Franklin Plaza, Philadelphia, PA 19102, U.S.A. / Tel: 888-825-5249 / Website: www.gsk.com (U.S. Distributor for Schaper & Brümmer GmbH & Co. KG)

GNC (General Nutrition Centers, Inc.): 300 Sixth Avenue, Pittsburg, PA 15222 U.S.A. / Tel: 888-462-2548 / Website: www.gnc.com (U.S. Distributor for Zeller Medical)

Health from the Sun: 19A Crosby Dr. #300, Bedford, MA 01730, U.S.A. / Tel: 781-276-0505 / Fax: 781-276-7335 / E-mail: seyrig@arkopharma-us.com (U.S. Distributor for Arkopharma)

Heilmittel: See: Dr. Mewes Heilmittel GmbH

Hermes Fabrick Pharma: Georg-Kalb-Str. 5-8, 82049 Grosshesselohe, Germany

Himalaya Drug Company: Makali, Bangalore 562 123, India / Tel: +91-80 371-4444 / Fax: +91-80-371-4468 / Website: www.himalayahealthcare.com / Email: write.to.us@himalaya.ac
U.S. DISTRIBUTOR: Himalaya USA, 10440 Westoffice Drive, Houston, Texas 77042, U.S.A. / Tel: 800-869-4640 / Fax: 800-577-6930 /Email: healthcare@himalayausa.com / Website: www.himalayausa.com

Himalaya USA: 10440 Westoffice Drive, Houston, Texas 77042, U.S.A. / Tel: 800-869-4640 / Fax: 800-577-6930 / Email: healthcare@himalayausa.com / Website: www.himalayausa.com (exclusive North American representative of The Himalaya Drug Company)

Horphag Research: P.O. Box 80, Avenue Louis-Casai 71, 1216 Cointrin, Geneva, Switzerland / Tel: +41-22-71-0262-6 / Fax: +41-22-71-0260-0 / Website: www.pycnogenol.com
U.S. DISTRIBUTOR: Natural Health Science, 225 Long Avenue, Building 15, Hillside, NJ 07205, U.S.A. / Tel: 877-369-9934 / Fax: 973-926-4719 / Email: victor@pycnogenol.com

Immodal Pharmaka GmbH: Bundesstrasse 44, 6111 Volders, Austria / Tel: +43-05-22-45-7678 / Fax: 43-05-22-45-7646
U.S. DISTRIBUTOR: Enzymatic Therapy, 825 Challenger Drive, Green Bay, WI 54311, U.S.A. / Tel: 800-783-2286

Indena S.p.A.: Viale Ortles 12, 20139 Milano, Italy / Tel: +39-02-57-4961 / Fax: +39-02-57-4046-20 / E-mail: indenami@tin.it
U.S. DISTRIBUTOR: Indena USA, 1001 Fourth Avenue Plaza, Suite 3714, Seattle, WA 98154, U.S.A. / Tel: 206-340-6140 / Fax: 206-340-0863 / E-mail: botanicals@indena.com / Website: www.indena.com

Inverni Della Beffa S.p.A.: Via Ripamonti 99 / 20141 Milano, Italy / Tel: +39-02-57-4961 / Fax: +39-02-57-4964-28

Kanoldt Arzneimittel GmbH: c/o Knoll AG, Knollstrasse 50, 67008 Ludwigshafen, Germany / Tel: +49-06-21-5890 / Fax: +49-06-21-5892-896 / E-mail: info@knoll.de / Website: www.knoll.de

Klinge Pharma GmbH: Postfach 80 10 63 / D-81610 Munich, Germany / Tel: +089 45 44 – 01 / Fax: +089 45 44 - 13 29 / Website: www.klinge.com, www.fujisawa.com (a division of Fujisawa Group)
U.S. DISTRIBUTOR: Pharmaton Natural Health Products, P.O. Box 368, Ridgefield, CT 06877, U.S.A. / Tel: 800-451-6688 / Fax: 203-798-5771 / Email: askpharmaton@rdg.boehringer-ingelheim.com / Website: www.pharmaton.com (a division of Boehringer Ingelheim Pharmaceuticals, Inc.)

Kneipp-Werke: 105-107 Stonehurst Court, Northvale, NJ 07647, U.S.A. / Tel: 201-750-0600 / Fax: 201-750-2070 / Website: www.kneipp.com

KNP Trading Pte Ltd: 50 Senoko Drive, Singapore 758232 / Tel: 65-257-6916 / Fax: 65-753-6916 / Website: www.knp-housebrand.com

Laboratories Chibret: c/o Societe Anonyme Corporation, 200 Boulevard Etienne-Clementel Clermont-Ferrand, Puy-de-Dome, France

Laboratori Guidotti S.p.A.: Via Trieste 40 56126, Pisa, Italy / Tel: +39-05-05-0521-1 / Fax: +39-05-04-0250 / E-mail: a.viti@giofil.it / Website: www.giofil.it

Lichtwer Pharma AG: Wallenroder Strasse 8-14, 13435 Berlin, Germany / Tel: +49-30-40-3700 / Fax: +49-30-40-3704-49 / Website: www.lichtwer.de
U.S. DISTRIBUTOR: ABKIT, Inc., 207 East 94th Street, New York, NY, U.S.A. 10128 / Tel: 800-226-6227 / Fax: 212-860-8323 / E-mail: info@abkit.com / Website: www.abkit.com

Loges: See: Dr. Loges & Co. GmbH

Lyssia GmbH: c/o Solvay Arzeneimittel GmbH, Hans-Bockler-Allee 20, Hanover 30173, Germany / Tel: +49-511-8-5724e+006 / Fax: 49-511-8-57312e+006 / Website: www.solvay.com

Madaus AG: Osterheimer Strasse 198, Köln, Germany / Tel: +49-22-18-9984-76 Fax: +49-22-18-9987-21 / E-mail: b.lindener@madaus.de

Martindale Pharmaceuticals Pty. Ltd.: Hubert Road, Brentwood, Essex, CM14 4LZ, U.K. / Tel: +444-01-27-72-6660-0 / Fax: +44-01-27-78-4897-6 / E-mail: mail@martindalepharma.co.uk / Website: www.martindalepharma.co.uk

Medexport: Contact information not available

Metabolife International, Inc.: 5070 Santa Fe Street, San Diego, CA 92109, U.S.A / Tel: 858-490-5222 / Website: www.metabolife.com

Mewes: See: Dr. Mewes Heilmittel GmbH

Minophagen Pharmaceutical Co.: No. 3 Tomizawa Bldg., 2-7 Yotsuya 3-chrome, Shinjuku, Tokyo 160, Japan / Tel: +81-3-3355-6561 / Fax: +81-3-3355-6565

Mountain Home Nutritionals: P.O. Box 1400, Ranson, WV 25438, U.S.A. / Tel: 800-888-1415 / Fax: 800-525-5562 (a subsidiary of Phillips International, Inc.) (U.S. Distributor for Bionorica AG)

National Health Products: 731 South Kirkman Road, Orlando, FL 32811, U.S.A. / Tel: 407-297-7671

Natrol Inc.: 21411 Prairie Street, Chatsworth, CA 91311, U.S.A. / Tel: 800-326-1520 / Website: www. natrol.com

Natural Health Science: 225 Long Avenue, Building 15, Hillside, NJ 07205, U.S.A. / Tel: 877-369-9934 / Fax: 973-926-4719 / Email: victor@pycnogenol.com (U.S. Distributor for Horphag Research)

Nature's Way Products, Inc.: 10 Mountain Spring Parkway, Springville, UT 84663, U.S.A. / Tel: 801-489-1500 / Website: www.naturesway.com (U.S. subsidiary of Dr. Willmar Schwabe Pharmaceuticals)

Novartis Consumer Health AG: Route de l'Etraz, CH 1260 Nyon 1, Switzerland / Website: www.consumer-health.novartis.com

Novo-Naordisk A/S: Novo Allé, 2880 Bagsvaerd, Denmark / Tel: +45-4444-8888 / Fax: +45-4449-0555 / Email: webmaster@novonordisk.com

Nutraceutical Corporation: 1400 Kearns Blvd., Park City, UT 84060, U.S.A. / Tel: 800-669-8877 / Website: www.nutraceutical.com

Nutrilite®: 5600 Beach Blvd., Buena Park, CA 90622, U.S.A. / Tel: 714-562-6200 / Website: www.nutrilite.com (a division of Access Business Group LLC)

Ocean Spray: One Ocean Spray Drive, Lakeville-Middleboro, MA 02349, U.S.A. / Tel: 800-662-3263 / Website: www.oceanspray.com

Omega Nutripharm: Contact information not available

PADMA AG: Wiesenstrasse 5, CH-8603 Schwerzenbach, Switzerland / Tel: +41 (0)1 887 00 00 / Email: mail@padma.ch / Website: www.padma.ch
U.S. DISTRIBUTOR: Econugenics Inc., 2208 Northpoint Parkway, Santa Rosa, CA 95407, U.S.A. / Tel: 800-308-5518 / Fax: 707-526-7689 / Website: www.padmabasic.com

Pharbio Medical International AB: c/o Cederroth International AB, Box 715, S-19427 Upperlands, Väsby, Sweden / Tel: +46-85-90-9630-0 / Fax: +46-85-90-9614-1 / Email: info@cedarroth.com / Website: www.pharbio.cedarroth.com

Pharmacia Corporation: Pharmacia Corporation, 100 Route 206 North, Peapack, NJ 07977, U.S.A. / Tel: 908-901-8000 / Fax: 908-901-8379 / Website: www.pharmacia.com

Pharma Nord ApS: Pharma Nord ApS, Sadelmagervej 30-32, DK-7100, Vejle, Denmark / Tel: +43-75-85-7400 / Fax: +43-75-85-7474 / Website: www.pharmanord.com
MAILORDER: Phama Nord U.K., Mailorder, Telford Court, Morpeth, UK-NE61 2DB, U.K. / Tel: +44-01-67-0519-989 / Fax: +44-01-67-0513-222

Pharma-Inter-Med GmbH: Am Born 19, 22765 Hamburg, Germany

Pharmaton Natural Health Products: P.O. Box 368, Ridgefield, CT 06877, U.S.A. / Tel: 800-451-6688 / Fax: 203-798-5771 / Email: askpharmaton@rdg.boehringer-ingelheim.com / Website: www.pharmaton.com (a U.S. division of Boehringer Ingelheim Pharmaceuticals Inc.)

Pharmaton S.A.: CH-6903, Lugano, Switzerland / Tel: +41-91-610-3111 (a division of Boehringer Ingelheim Pharmaceuticals Inc.)

Pierre Fabre Médicament: 45 Place Abel-Gance, 92654 Boulogne, France / Tel: +33-01-49-10-8000 / Fax: +33-01-49-10-9712 / Website: www.dermaweb.com

Polcopharam F. Polley & Co.: P.O. Box 100 Epping, NSW 1710, Australia / Tel: +61-02-98-7664 / Fax: +61-02-98-6822-6 / Email: sales@polcopharma.com / Website: http://polcopharma.com.au

Polymedia Corp.: 11 State Street, Woburn, MA, 01801, U.S.A. / Tel: 781-933-2020 / Website: www.polymedia.com

Prof. Dr. Much AG: Contact information not available

PureWorld Botanicals Inc.: 375 Huyler Street, South Hackensack, NJ 07606, U.S.A. / Tel: 201-440-5000 / Fax: 201-342-8000 / Website: www.pureworld.com

Quest Vitamins: 7080 River Road #129, Richmond, BC, V6X 1X5, Canada / Tel: 604-273-0611 / Email: thartz@van.boehringer-ingelheim.com / Website: www.questvitamins.com

COMPANY CONTACT INFORMATION

Quindao Fengyi Biotechnology Limited: Contact information not available

Roche Nicholas SA: 33 rue de l'Industrie, 74240 Gaillard, France / Tel: 33-04-50-87-7070

Saila S.p.A.: 83 Viale Garibladi, Silvi Marina, Teramo, Italy

Sanofi Synthelabo: 174 avenue de France, 75013 Paris, France / Tel: +33 1 53 77 4000 / Website: www.sanofi-synthelabo.fr
U.S. DISTRIBUTOR: Sanofi-Synthelabo, Inc., 90 Park Avenue, New York, NY, 10016, U.S.A. / Tel: 212-551-4000 / Website: www.sanofi-synthelabous.com

Schaper & Brümmer GmbH & Co. KG: Bahnhofstrasse 35, 38259 Salzgitter, Ringelheim, Germany / Tel: +49-5341-30-70 / Fax: +49-5341-30-71-24 / Email: info@schaperbruemmer.de / Website: www.schaper-bruemmer.com
U.S. DISTRIBUTOR: Enzymatic Therapy, Inc., 825 Challenger Drive, Green Bay, WI 54311, U.S.A. / Tel: 920-469-1313 / Website: www.enzy.com
U.S. DISTRIBUTOR: GlaxoSmithKline, One Franklin Plaza, Philadelphia, PA 19102, U.S.A. / Tel: 888-825-5249 / Website: www.gsk.com

Schering-Plough: 2000 Galloping Hill Road, Kenilworth, NJ 07033, U.S.A. / Tel: 908-298-4000 / Website: www.sch-plough.com

Schwabe: See: Dr. Willmar Schwabe Pharmaceuticals

Scotia Pharmaceuticals Ltd.: Scotia House, Sterling, Scotland, FK9 4TZ, U.K. / Website: http://fox.nstn.ca/~scotlib/index.html

Seven Seas Ltd.: Hedon Road, Marfleet, Hull, HU9 5NJ, U.K. / Tel: +44-1482-37-5234 / Fax: +44-1482-37-4345 / Email: info@hofels.com or info@Seven-Seas.ltd.uk / Website: www.hofels.com (a division of the Merck Group)

Sidroga GmbH: Mumpferfährstrasse 68, D-79713 Bad Säckingen, Germany / Tel: +49-07-761-93976-46 / Fax: +49-07-761-93976-48 / Email: vertrieb@sidroga.de / Website: www.sidroga.de

Solvay Arznemittel GmbH: Hans-Bockeler-Allee 20, Hannover, 30173, Germany / Tel: +49-511-8-5724e +006 / Fax: +49-511-8-57312e +006 / Website: www.solvay.com

Spitzner GmbH: Postfach 763, 76261 Ettlingen, Germany / Tel: +49 72 43 – 106 01 / Fax: +49 72 43 – 106 333 / Email: info@spitzner.de / Website: www.spitzner.de

Steigerwald: Havelstrasse 5, D-64295 Darmstadt, Germany / Tel: +49-06-15-13-3050 / Email: info@steigerwald.de

Steiner Arzneimittel: Postfash 450520, 12175 Berlin, Germany / Tel: +49-03-07-1094-0 / Fax: +49-03-07-1250-12 / Website: www.steinerarznei-berlin.de

Strathmann AG & Co.: Sellhopsweg 1, 22459 Hamburg, Germany / Tel: +49-401-55-9050 / Fax: +49-40-55-9051-00 /

Email: info@strathmann.de / Website: www.strathmann.de

Synthelabo-Pharma SA: 11, Rue de Veyrot, 1217 Meyrin, France / Tel: +33-02-29-89-0147 / Fax: +33-02-29-89-0188

Therabel Research: Egide Van Ophemstraat 110, 1180, Bruxellus, Belgium / Tel: +32-02-370-4611 / Fax: +32-02-370-4690

Tillots Pharma AG: Hauptstrasse 27, CH-4417 Zeifen, Switzerland / Tel: +41-61-935-2626 / Fax: +41-61-935-2625

Traditional Medicinals: 4515 Ross Road, Sebastopol, CA 95472, U.S.A. / Tel: 707-823-8911 / Fax: 800-886-4349 / Website: www.traditionalmedicinals.com

TRUW Arzneimittel Vertriebs GmbH: Ziethenstrasse 8, 33330 Gutersloh, Germany / Tel: +49-52-41-3007-40 / Website: www.truw.de

Tsumura & Co.: 12-7, Nibancho, Chiyoda-ku, Tokyo, 102-8422, Japan / Tel: +81-3-3221-5262 / Fax: +81-3-3221-0016 / Website: www.tsumura.co.jp/english
U.S. BRANCH: Tsumura & Co., 20910 Normandie Avenue, Unit C, Torrance, CA 90502, U.S.A / Tel: 310-618-6012 / Fax: 310-328-5805

Twinings: 216 The Strand, London, U.K. / Website: www.twinings.com

Unilever Bestfoods North America: 800 Sylvan Ave., Englewood Cliffs, NJ 07632, U.S.A. / Tel: 800-697-7887 / Tel: 888-LIPTON-T / Email: letters.liptontusa@unilever.com / Website: www.liptont.com

VIATRIS GmbH & Co. KG: Weismüllerstrasse, 45, D-60314 Frankfurt/Main, Germany / Tel: +49-69-4001 2811 / Fax: +49-69-4001 2951 / Email: info@viatris.com / Website: www.viatris.com (formerly ASTA Medica AG)
U.S. DISTRIBUTOR: ABKIT, INC., 207 East 94th Street, New York, NY 10128, U.S.A. / Tel: 800-226-6227 / Fax: 212-860-8323 / Email: info@abkit.com / Website: www.abkit.com

Wakunaga of America Co., Ltd.: 23501 Madero, Mission Viejo, CA 92691, U.S.A. / Tel: 800-421-2998 / Website: www.kyolic.com

Warner Lambert: Pfizer, Consumer Affairs, 182 Tabor Road, Morris Plains, NJ 07950, U.S.A. / Tel: 800-223-0182 / Website: www.prodhelp.com

Willmar Schwabe: See: Dr. Willmar Schwabe Pharmaceuticals

Zeller AG: Seeblickstrasse 4, CH-8590 Romanshorn 1, Switzerland / Website: www.zellerag.ch
U.S. DISTRIBUTOR: GNC (General Nutrition Centers, Inc.), 300 Sixth Avenue, Pittsburgh, PA 15222, U.S.A. / Tel: 888-462-2548 / Website: www.gnc.com

TOP-SELLING HERBAL SUPPLEMENTS IN FOOD, DRUG, AND MASS MARKET RETAIL OUTLETS*

(52 weeks ending October 13, 2002)

This table lists retail sales figures for the top selling herbal supplements in mainstream outlets as reported by Information Resources, Inc., a market research firm based in Chicago, IL. Since 1998, herb sales have been decreasing in the mainstream channel of trade, defined as grocery stores, drug stores, and mass market retail stores. These statistics do *not* include warehouse buying clubs or convenience stores. Also, these data do not reflect sales from some of the traditional avenues of herb sales, e.g., health and natural food stores, multi-level marketing companies, direct sales via mail order (and internet), or sales via alternative or conventional healthcare practitioners. The primary reason often given for the recent decline in herb sales is negative media coverage. While some negative articles on herb quality and safety issues are warranted, often the information in the media is distorted and focuses on myths and misconceptions rather than the realities of herb regulation and the clinically documented safety and benefits of herbs when used responsibly and as directed by label information and/or the advice of a healthcare practitioner.

Some top selling herbs that are discussed in this book are not specified in this table due to their use in forms other than supplements. For example, chamomile and peppermint are top selling herbs but are for the most part, sold as teas. Additional herbs that are included in this book but not listed in this table are: chaste tree, eleuthero, ephedra, goldenseal, and horse chestnut.

Herb	Retail Sales ($)	% Change From Previous Year	Herb	Retail Sales ($)	% Change From Previous Year
1. Ginkgo	36,033,352	-29.3	21. Feverfew	456,544	-39.4
2. Garlic	34,695,496	-5.2	22. Dong Quai Root	413,596	-38.1
3. Echinacea	34,220,452	-22.3	23. Hawthorn	392,625	-27.6
4. Soy	27,517,698	-0.7	24. Guarana	361,326	-7.0
5. Saw palmetto	23,251,898	-9.7	25. Elderberry	345,884	-9.1
6. Ginseng	23,145,712	-32.7	26. Cat's Claw	339,543	-42.5
7. St John's wort	16,678,024	-38.8	27. Cayenne	283,291	-41.8
8. Cranberry	11,555,961	11.8	28. Spirulina	262,739	-1.8
9. Black cohosh	10,712,645	22.8	29. Barley	182,394	65.2
10. Valerian	8,509,827	-35.4	30. Dandelion	181,094	-9.5
11. Milk thistle	7,633,630	9.7	31. Gotu Kola	125,525	-44.5
12. Evening primrose	5,935,047	-1.1	32. Eyebright	96,718	-50.5
13. Kava kava	5,599,405	-44.4	33. Licorice Root	86,083	-19.1
14. Bilberry	3,433,132	-4.8	34. Pau D'Arco	68,004	-6.7
15. Grape Seed	3,145,202	-27.4	35. Yucca	11,887	-46.5
16. Yohimbe	2,389,610	12.7	36. Multi-herbs†	7,642,161	21.6
17. Green tea	1,669,361	-8.2	37. A/O herbs‡	28,512,642	-11.0
18. Ginger	1,140,264	-10.0	**Total Herbs§**	**298,597,952**	**-17.2**
19. Pycnogenol®	1,033,570	-34.3	Flaxseed§§	12,435,227	49.2
20. Aloe Vera	542,260	6.3			

Source: Information Resources, Inc. (IRI), Chicago, IL. www.infores.com Used with permission.

* Supermarkets, drug stores, mass merchandisers (except Wal-Mart, which does not provide sales data to market research companies).
† Multi-herb = herb combinations containing more than one herb. (Based on total sales in this channel of trade, this listing would be 11th, but single herbs are listed first.)
‡ A/O herbs = all other herbs not listed above.
§ Sales for Total Herbs as listed in this report varies from the sum of the individual sales values due to rounding by IRi.
§§ Flaxseed is listed separately because IRI reports list it in the Non-Herbal Supplement category.

RECENT STUDIES

In consideration of the continuously developing nature of medical and scientific information, we have created this section to provide citations for several significant studies that, due to their release immediately prior to the printing of this book, were not included in the corresponding monographs. For further information regarding new research developments and breaking news in the industry, the reader is referred to ABC's website www.herbalgram.org.

ASIAN GINSENG

Coon JT, Ernst E. *Panax ginseng*: a systematic review of adverse effects and drug interactions. *Drug safety* 2002;25(5):323–44.

Hong B, Ji YH, Nam KY, Ahn TY. A double-blind crossover study evaluating the efficacy of Korean red ginseng in patients with erectile dysfunction: a preliminary report. *J Urol* 2002;168:2070–3.

BLACK COHOSH

Bodinet C, Freudenstein J. Influence of *Cimicifuga racemosa* on the proliferation of estrogen receptor-positive human breast cancer cells. *Breast Cancer Res Treat* 2002;76:1–10.

Borrelli F, Ernst E. *Cimicifuga racemosa*: A systematic review of its clinical efficacy. *Eur J Clin Pharmacol* 2002;58:235–41.

Freudstein J, Dasenbrock C, Nißlein T. Lack of promotion of estrogen-dependent mammary gland tumor in vivo by an isopropanolic *Cimicifuga racemosa* extract. *Cancer Res* 2002;62:3448–52.

Kennelly EJ, Baggett S, Nuntanakorn P, Ososki AL, Mori SA, Duke J, et al. Analysis of thirteen populations of black cohosh for formononetin. *Phytomedicine* 2002;9(5):461–7.

Kronenberg F, Fugh-Berman A. Complementary and alternative medicine for menopausal symptoms: a review of randomized, controlled trials. *Ann Intern Med* 2002;137(10):805–14.

Liske E, Hänggi W, Henneicke-Von Zepelin HH, Boblitz N, Wüstenberg P, Rahlfs VW. Physiological investigation of a unique extract of black cohosh (*Cimicifuga racemosa rhizoma*): a 6-month clinical study demonstrates no systemic estrogenic effect. *J Womens Health and Gend Based Med* 2002;11(2):163–74.

Zierau O, Bodinet C, Kolba S, Wulf M, Vollmer G. Antiestrogenic activities of *Cimicifuga racemosa* extracts. *J Steroid Biochem Mol Biol* 2002;80:125–30.

CAT'S CLAW

Pero RW, Giampapa V, Vojdani A. Comparison of a broad spectrum anti-aging nutritional supplement with and without the addition of DNA repair enhancing cat's claw extract. *J Antiaging Medicine* 2002;(5)2:[in press].

CRANBERRY

Leahy M, Speroni J, Starr M. Latest developments in cranberry health research. *Pharmaceutical Biology* 2002;4 Suppl:50–4.

Terris MK, Issa MM, Tacker JR. Dietary supplementation with cranberry concentrate tablets may increase the risk of nephrolithiasis. *Urology* 2001;57(1):26–9.

University of Bonn, Germany. Cranberries and blackcurrants combat kidney stones. *European J Clin Nutr* 2002;51(2):283–5.

ECHINACEA

Barrett BP, Brown RL, Locken K, Maberry R, Bobula JA, D'Alessio D. Treatment of the common cold with unrefined echinacea: a randomized, double-blind, placebo-controlled trial. *Ann Intern Med* 2002;137(12):939–46.

Turner, RB. Echinacea for the common cold: can alternative medicine be evidence-based medicine [editorial]. *Ann Intern Med* 2002;137(12):1001–2.

EPHEDRA

Bailes JE, Cantu RC, Day AL. The neurosurgeon in sport: awareness of the risks of heatstroke and dietary supplements. *Neurosurgery* 2002;51(2):283–5.

GINKGO

Birks J, Grimley EJ, Van Dongen M. *Ginkgo biloba* for cognitive impairment and dementia [Cochrane Review]. In: *The Cochrane Library*, Issue 4, 2002. Oxford. Update Software.

Evans JR. *Ginkgo biloba* extract for age-related macular degeneration [Cochrane Review]. In: *The Cochrane Library*, Issue 4, 2002. Oxford: Update Software.

Hackett P, Roach R. High-altitude illness. *New Engl J Med* 2001;345(2):107–14.

Maakestad K, Leadbetter G, Olson S, Hackett P. *Ginkgo biloba* reduces incidence and severity of acute mountain sickness [abstract]. In: Abstracts from the Wilderness Medical Society's annual scientific meeting. Cited in: *Wildrns and Envir Med* 2001;12:51.

Mix JA, Crews WD. A double-blind, placebo-controlled, randomized trial of *Ginkgo biloba* extract Egb 761® in a sample of cognitively intact older adults: neuropsychological findings. *Hum Psychopharmacol Clin Exp* 2002;17:267–77.

Morgenstern C, Biermann E. The efficacy of ginkgo special extract EGb 761 in patients with tinnitus. *Int J Clin Pharmacol Ther* 2002;40(5):188–97.

KAVA

Loew D. Kava kava extract: risks, benefits or a problem of society? [in German]. *Dtsch Apoth Ztg* 2002;142(9):64–74.

Matthews JM, Etheridge AS, Black SR. Inhibition of human cytochrome P450 activities by kava extract and kavalactones. *Drug Metab Dispos* 2002;30(11):1153–7.

MILK THISTLE

Piscitelli SC, Formentini E, Burstein AH, Alfaro R, Jagannatha S, Falloon J. Effect of milk thistle on the pharmacokinetics of Indinavir in healthy volunteers. *Pharmacotherapy* 2002;22(5):551–6.

MILK THISTLE (cont.)

Venkatarmanan R, Ramachandran V, Komoroski BJ, Zhang S, Sciff PL, Strom SC. Milk thistle, a herbal supplement, decreases the activity of CYP3A4 and uridine diphosphoglucuronosyl transferase in human hepatocyte cultures. *Drug Metab Dispos* 2000;28(11):1270–3.

PEPPERMINT

Nair B. Final report on the safety assessment of *Mentha piperita* (peppermint) oil, *Mentha piperita* (peppermint) leaf extract, *Mentha piperita* (peppermint) leaf, and *Mentha piperita* (peppermint) leaf water. *Int J Toxicol* 2001;20 Suppl 3:61–73.

PYCNOGENOL®

Hosseini S, Pishnamazi S, Sadrzadeh SMH, Farid F, Farid R, Watson RR. Pycnogenol® in the management of asthma. *Jour Med Food* 2001;4(4):201–9.

Kimbrough C, Chun M, dela Roca G, Lau BHS. Pycnogenol® chewing gum minimizes gingival bleeding and plaque formation. *Phytomedicine* 2002;9:410–13.

Natural Health Science. Significant increase in men's fertility possible with 90-day Pycnogenol® treatment, study shows [press release]. 2002 Sept 20.

Roseff SJ. Improvement in sperm quality and function with French maritime pine tree bark extract. *J Reprod Med* 2002;47(10):821–4.

ST. JOHN'S WORT

Lecrubier Y, Clerc G, Didi R, Kieser M. Efficacy of St. John's wort extract WS 5570 in major depression: a double-blind, placebo-controlled trial. *Am J Psychiatry* 2002;159(8):1361–6.

Van Gurp G, Meterissian GB, Haiek LN, McCusker J, Bellavance F. St. John's wort or sertraline?: randomized controlled trial in primary care. *Can Fam Physician* 2002;48:905–12.

ABBREVIATIONS AND SYMBOLS

μg	microgram
%	percent
5-FU	5 fluorouracil
AA	arachidonic acid
AAFC	Agriculture and Agri-Food Canada
AAMI	age associated memory impairment
ABTS	2,2'-azinobis[3-ethyl-benzthiazoline-6-sulfonic acid]
ADAS-Cog	Alzheimer's Disease Assessment Scale-Cognitive subscale
ADL	activities of daily living
AER	adverse event report
AG	American ginseng
AGE	aged garlic extract
AgNOR	silver-stained nucleolar organizer regions
AHPA	American Herbal Products Association
AHRQ	Agency for Healthcare Research and Quality
AIDS	acquired immunodeficiency syndrome
AKS	*Arzneimittel Kompendium der Schweig*
ALA	alpha linolenic acid
Al-P	alkaline-phosphatase
ALT	alanine aminotransferase
ANOVA	analysis of variance
AST	aspartate aminotransferase
AZT	zidovudine
b.i.d	two times daily
BHP	*British Herbal Pharmacopoeia*
BMD	bone mineral density
BMI	body mass index
BP	blood pressure
BP	*British Pharmacopoeia*
BP	*Burkholderia pseudomallei*
BPC	*British Pharmaceutical Codex*
BPH	benign prostatic hyperplasia
bpm	beats per minute
C	caffeine
C	catechin
C	controlled (study)
ca.	circa, approximately
CAEs	carboxy alkyl esters
CAERS	CFSAN Adverse Event Reporting System
CAM	complementary and alternative medicine
cAMP	cyclic AMP, used as second messenger in cell signaling
CC	case-control (study)
CCRUM	Central Council for Research in Unami Medicine

CE	conjugated estrogens
CFSAN	Center for Foods and Applied Nutrition
CGI	clinical global impression scale
CGIC	clinical global assessment of change
CGI-I	clinical global impression improvement scale
CGI-S	clinical global impression severity scale
CH	cohort (study)
CHD	coronary heart disease
CI	confidence interval
cm	centimeter
Cm	comparison (study)
CNS	central nervous system
CO	crossover (study)
COMT	catechol-o-methyl-transferase
COX-1	cyclo-oxygenase-1
COX-2	cyclo-oxygenase-2
CS	contrast sensitivity
CS	cross sectional (study)
CVI	chronic venous insufficiency
CYP	cytochrome P450
D6D	delta-6-desaturase
DAB	*Deutsches Arzneibuch*
DB	double-blind (study)
DB, PC	double-blind, placebo-controlled (study)
DBP	diastolic blood pressure
DC	discontinued
DCO	double cross-over
DGL	deglycyrrhized licorice
DGLA	dihomogamma-linolenic acid
DHA	docosahexaenoic acid
DHT	dihydrotestosterone
DIN	drug identification number
DNA	deoxyribonucleic acid
DOCI	drugs of current interest
DPD	drug product database
DPPH	α, α-diphenyl-β-picrylhydrazyl
D-S	von Zerssen depression severity scale
DSHEA	Dietary Supplement Health and Education Act of 1994
DSM	Diagnostic and Statistical Manual of mental disorders
E	ephedrine
E	epidemiological (study)
E	epinephrine
EC	epicatechin
EEG	electroencephalogram

EFA	essential fatty acid	HCV	hepatitis C virus
EGC	epigallocatechin	HDL	high-density lipoprotein
EGCG	epigallocatechin gallate	HDL-C	high-density lipoprotein cholesterol
EGF	epidermal growth factor	HIV	human immunodeficiency virus
EPA	eicosapentaenoic acid	HMO	health maintenance organization
EPO	evening primrose oil	HPB	Health Protection Branch
ER+	estrogen receptor positive	HPLC	high performance liquid chromatography
ERG	electroretinogram	HPUS	Homeopathic Pharmacopoeia of the United States
ERT	estrogen replacement therapy		
ESCOP	European Scientific Cooperative on Phytotherapy	HRT	hormone replacement therapy
et al.	and others	IBS	irritable bowel syndrome
FDA	Food and Drug Administration	IC	immune complex
fl.	fluid	ICD-09	International Classification of Disease, 9th revision
FRAP	ferric reducing ability of plasma	ICD–10	International Classification of Disease, 10th revision
FSH	follicle stimulating hormone		
g	gram	IFN	interferon
g/ml	grams/milliliter	Ig	immunoglobulin
GABA	gamma-aminobutyric acid	IKS	*Interkantonale Konstroll stelle*
GAO	General Accounting Office	IL	interleukin
GAP	good agricultural practices	IL-1	interleukin-1
GBE	*Ginkgo biloba* extract	IL-6	interleukin-6
GC	gallocatechin	INOS	inducible nitric oxide synthase
GCP	good clinical practices	IP	*Indian Pharmacopoeia*
GERRI	Geriatric Evaluation by Relative's Rating Instrument	IU	international unit
		IUD	intrauterine device
GGT	gamma glutamyl transpeptidase	IVHD	isovaleroxyhydroxydihydrovaltrate
GHP	*German Homeopathic Pharmacopoeia*	JAMA	Journal of American Medical Association
GI	gastrointestinal	JP	*Pharmacopoeia of Japan*
GLA	gamma-linolenic acid	JSHM	*Japanese Herbal Medical Codex*
GLC	ginkgo leaf concentrate	KMHW	Korean Ministry of Health and Welfare
GLP	good laboratory practices	KPI	Kupperman-menopause index
GLDH	glutamate-dehydrogenase	LA	linoleic acid
GMP	good manufacturing practices	LC	longitudinal cohort (study)
GOT	glutamate oxaloacetate transaminase	LDL	low-density lipoprotein
GPT	glutamic pyruvic transaminase	LDL-C	low-density lipoprotein cholesterol
GRAS	generally recognized as safe	LH	luteinizing hormone
GSL	*General Sale List*	LVEF	left ventricular ejection fraction; a measure of cardiac output
GST	glutathione-s-transferase		
γ-GTP	gamma-glutamyl transpeptidase	MA	meta-analysis (study)
GTS	ginseng total saponin	MALDI-TOF	Matrix Assisted Laser Desorption Ionization-Time of Flight
HAB	*Homeopathisches Arzneibuch*		
HAMA	Hamilton Anxiety Scale	MAO	monoamine oxidase
HAMD	Hamilton Depression Scale	MAOI	monoamine oxidase inhibitor
HbA1c	hemoglobin A1c	MC	multi-center (study)
HBsAg	hepatitis B surface antigen	mcg (ug)	microgram
HBV	hepatitis B virus	MDA	malondialdehyde
HCC	hepatocellular carcinoma	MDR1	one of the 2 multi-drug resistance

mg	milligram
MIC	minimum inhibitory concentration
mm	millimeter
MMC	migrating motor complex
MMDQ	Moos menstrual distress questionnaire
MMSE	mini mental status exam
MPA	Medical Products Agency
n	number of patients
n.d.	no date
NAT	N-acetyltransferase
NE	norepinephrine
NF-kB	nuclear factor-kappa B
NFUM	*National Formulary of Unani Medicine*
NIH	National Institutes of Health
NK	natural killer
NLT	no less than
NO	nitric oxide
NPH	Natural Health Product
NSAID	nonsteroidal anti-inflammatory drug
O	open (study)
OA	osteoarthritis
ÖAB	*Österreichisches Arzneibuch*
OB	Observational (study)
OCD	obsessive compulsive disorder
ODS	Office of Dietary Supplements
OL	open label (study)
OR	odds ratio
ORP	oxidation-reduction potential
OSC	organosulfur compound
OTC	over-the-counter
OWH	Office of Women's Health
oz.	ounces
P	prospective (study)
PAF	platelet activating factor
PB	patient-blind (study)
PC	placebo-controlled (study)
PC, CO	placebo-controlled, cross-over (study)
PCC	peppermint caraway capsule
PCNA	proliferation cell nuclear antigen
PEH	pseudoepithelia hyperplasia
PG	parallel group (study)
PGE 1	prostaglandin E1
PGE 2	prostaglandin E2
PGE 3	prostaglandin E3
Ph.Eur	*European Pharmacopoeia*
Ph.Fr.X	*French Pharmacopoeia*
Ph.Helv.	*Swiss Pharmacopoeia*

ph.Ital	*Italian Pharmacopoeia*
Ph.USSR X	*State Pharmacopoeia of the Union of the Soviet Socialist Republics*
PIIINP	aminoterminal propeptide
PMN	polymorphonuclear leukocytes
PMS	premenstrual syndrome
PMTS	premenstrual tension syndrome
POAs	pentacyclic oxindole alkaloids
POMS	profile of mood status
PPA	phenylpropanolamine
ppm	parts per million
PPRC	*Pharmacopoeia of the People's Republic of China*
PS	pilot study
PSA	prostate specific antigen
PsA	psoriatic arthritis
PWV	pulse wave velocity
q.d.	once daily
q.i.d	four times daily
QPEG	quantitative pharmaco-eletroencephalogram
R	randomized (study)
R, DB, PC	randomized, double-blind, placebo-controlled (study)
RA	rheumatoid arthritis
RC	reference-controlled (study)
RCS	retrospective cross-sectional (study)
RES	reticuloendothelial system
RGTS	red ginseng total saponins
RMR	resting metabolic rate
RR	relative ratio
RS	retrospective (study)
S	surveillance (study)
SAD	seasonal affective disorder
SB	single-blind (study)
SBP	sulphobromophthalein sodium dye
SBP	systolic blood pressure
SC	single-center (study)
SCAG	Sandoz Clinical Assessment–Geriatric scale
SEM	standard error of the mean
SHBG	sex hormone binding globulin
SJW	St. John's wort
SKT	Syndrom-Kurytest
SLE	systemic lupus erythematosus
SN/AEMS	Special Nutritionals/Adverse Event Monitoring System
SNMC	Stronger Neo-Minophagen C
SOD	superoxide dismutase
SP	saw palmetto

spp	species	URTI	upper respiratory tract infection
SSRI	selective serotonin reuptake inhibitor	USC	United States Congress
T-47D	breast cancer cell line	USDA	United States Department of Agriculture
t.i.d.	three times daily	USDOC	The United States Department of Commerce
TC	total cholesterol	USFWS	United States Fish and Wildlife Service
TCM	traditional Chinese medicine	USP	*United States Pharmacopeia*
TEWL	transepidermal water loss	USP-NF	*United States Pharmacopeia-National Formulary*
TG	triglycerides		
TGA	Therapeutic Goods Administration	USSR	Union of Soviet Socialist Republics
THM	traditional herbal medicine	UT	*Uncaria tomentosa*
TNFα	tumor necrosis factor alpha	UTI	urinary tract infection
TOAs	tetracyclic oxindole alkaloids	UV	ultraviolet
TPP	Therapeutic Products Program	*v/m*	volume/measure
TRH	thyroxine releasing hormone	*v/v*	volume/volume
ug or μg	microgram	VA	visual acuity
U	uncontrolled (study)	VAS	visual analog scale
UG	*Uncaria guianensis*	VC	vehicle-controlled (study)
U.K.	United Kingdom	*w/v*	weight/volume
U.S.	United States	*w/w*	weight/weight
UP	unpublished (study)	WAIS	Wechsler Adult Intelligence Scale
UPC	Unani Pharmacopoeia committee	WHO	World Health Organization
URI	upper respiratory infection	x	times

GLOSSARY

ACE inhibitor: see: angiotensin-converting enzyme inhibitor

acylated: acid radical incorporated into an organic compound

adaptogen: an agent that increases the nonspecific resistance of an organism to harmful influences, while generating a normalizing action on bodily systems

Addison's disease: hormonal disorder, resulting from diminished production of cortisol and/or aldosterone, that causes weight loss, muscle weakness, fatigue, low blood pressure, and sometimes darkening of the skin

adenocarcinoma: cancerous growth of glandular tissue originating from the intestines, uterus, and breast

adenoma: benign tumor of glandular tissue epithelium (outer skin layer)

adrenergic: relating to nerve endings that use norepinephrine as primary neurotransmitters

adulteration: addition of any substance to a product, with the intent to defraud

adynamia: lack of physical or emotional drive; loss of strength or weakness

alveolar: refering to the air-filled space in the lungs formed by sac-like dilations of the lung tissue

amenorrhea: absence of a woman's monthly cycle

analgesic: a pain relieving product or compound

anaphylactic shock: severe allergic reaction characterized by any combination of: shortness of breath, fainting, itching skin rash, swelling of the throat, and a sudden decline in blood pressure

angiogenesis: blood vessel growth

angiotensin-converting enzyme inhibitor: agent (i.e., Enalapril, Captropril) that reduces peripheral vascular resistance via blockage of the angiotensin converting enzyme that reduces myocardial oxygen consumption, thereby improving cardiac output, reducing left ventricular and vascular hypertrophy, and improving blood pressure

anticholinergic: chemical that diminishes the effect of acetylcholine in the nervous system

anticoagulant: chemical compound that prevents blood from clotting

antiemetic: agent that stops or alleviates nausea and vomiting

antihistamine: drug that blocks the effect of histamines thereby blocking an allergic reaction

antilithic: prevents or dissolves stones (e.g., kidney stones, gallstones)

antioxidant: group of substances that prevent oxidative cell damage by scavenging free radicals generated during metabolic processes

antiphlogistic: reduction of inflammation

anti-schistosomal: medicines or remedies that protect against human parasitic infection (Schistosoma or blood flukes)

antithrombotic: treatment that dissolves blood clots or prevents their formation

aphthous ulcers: commonly called canker sores, characterized by mouth lesions

apoptosis: natural programmed cell destruction and death which is an important component of lifecycle events ranging from menstruation to arresting tumor growth

arrhythmia: change in heart rhythm, often noted as an irregular heart beat

ascorbic acid: vitamin C

asthenia: condition characterized by muscle weakness or loss of energy caused by muscular or psychological disorders

astringent: agent that controls bleeding or secretion by causing tissues to contract or draw together

ataxia: uncoordinated movement of muscle groups caused by a nerve disease characterized by unsteady gait

atherosclerosis: hardening of the arteries caused by cholesterol-lipid-calcium deposits

Ayurvedic: ancient medical practice based on total mental, physical, and spiritual health, and includes eight branches: internal medicine, general surgery, head and neck, pediatrics, toxicology, fertility and conception, rejuvenation, and psychiatry

AZT: also called zidovudine, the most widely used antiviral drug in the treatment of HIV/AIDS patients

bacteriuria: condition where bacteria are found in the urine

barium enema: barium sulfate suspension used as an enema (introduction of a fluid into the rectum and colon) to increase visibility of an X-ray during a colon exam

bathmotropic: response to a stimulus that increases nervous and muscular irritability

blood-brain barrier: membranous blood vessel barrier that selectively controls the entry of substances into the brain tissue

borborygmi: normal rumbling and gurgling sounds in the abdomen caused by gasses passing through intestinal liquids

bradycardia: a slow heartbeat (defined as a heart rate that is less than 60 beats per minute)

brix: unit of measure showing the percentage of sugar contained in a solution

bromsulphalein test: liver function test using an injected dye and measuring its excretion from the liver and thus the general functioning of the liver (especially cirrhosis)

cardiac glycoside: plant-derived substance used in cases of heart failure that strengthen contractions and regulate the heartbeat

carminative: agent that expels gas from the intestines and relieves gas pain and bloating

cataplasm: a poultice or soft external application, often medicated

catarrh: nasal discharge as a result of a viral or bacterial infection

cholagogue: an agent that stimulates the flow of bile from the liver

cholangitis: acute infection of the biliary tract usually caused by an obstruction of the bile duct

cholecystitis: inflammation of the gallbladder

choleretic: an agent or drug that stimulates evacuation of bile from the liver

cholestatic: stoppage or suppression of bile from the liver

chronotropic: an agent that affects the rate of contraction of the heart

cicatrizing: to heal, forming a scar

climacteric: the syndrome of endocrine, somatic, and psychic changes occurring at the termination of the reproductive period in the female, or the accompanying the normal diminution of sexual activity in the male

cold expression: method of extracting essential oils from various botanicals, usually citrus fruits, by using cold water and pressure

colic: painful spasm in the abdomen, usually pertains to the colon

collagenosis: term used for a group of diseases of unknown origin which attack the connective tissue (usually skin)

compress: folded material (wet, dry, hot, or cold) applied firmly to a section of the body

conjunctivitis: inflammation of the membrane (conjunctiva) that covers the eye and lines the inner surface of the eyelid; commonly known as "pink eye"

convalescence: recovery time after an illness or operation

corpus cavernosum: the erectile tissue of a penis or tissue leading to the clitoris

corpus luteum: glandular tissue in the ovary that releases progesterone and estrogen after the onset of ovulation

counterirritant: an agent (e.g., mustard plaster) that is applied to the skin to create inflammation with the purpose of remedying a deeply underlying inflammatory condition

Crocq's disease: disorder characterized by poor circulation to the hands, and at times the feet, resulting in a cold, blue, and sweaty condition (also known as acrocyanosis)

cryoprecipitate: a blood product made from fresh frozen plasma containing a concentration of the cold insoluble portion of plasma

cryotherapy: use of cold temperature for therapeutic purposes

cyclooxygenase pathway: an enzyme system that metabolizes arachidonic acid (AA), an essential fatty acid, to create prostaglandins and thromboxanes

cyst: a usually abnormal growth made up of a thick-walled sac filled with any combination of fluid, gas, or solid materials

cytokine: soluble glycoproteins which are produced and released by cells of the immune system to regulate the immune response

cytological: relating to cell formation, anatomy, and function

decoction: a medicinal preparation made by steeping plants, usually the more dense parts, e.g., roots, barks, etc., in boiling water

demulcent: a therapeutic substance that soothes irritated tissue, particularly mucous membranes

dermabrasion: removal of skin imperfections (e.g., scars, wrinkles, tattoos) through a surgical procedure and/or other mechanical methods

dermatitis: skin inflammation characterized by redness and itching

Dermatosis: a general term referring to any skin disease

detumescence: reduction of swelling, usually refers to the reversal of erection of the genital organ

diabetes mellitus: chronic metabolic disease caused by a deficiency of insulin produced, or lack of response to insulin, resulting in increased blood sugar concentrations

diaphoretic: an agent that causes perspiration

diazepam: generic name for an antianxiety sedative used to treat a variety of anxiety-related disorders, commonly known as Valium®

digitalis: dried leaves of *Digitalis purpurea,* containing cardiac glycosides and used in treating heart disease

dimer: a single compound formed by the joining of two identical molecules

diuresis: increased elimination of urine

dromotropic: effect on the electric conduction of the heart tissue

dysentery: an inflammation of the intestine that causes painful diarrhea and stools containing blood and mucus

dysmenorrhea: painful menstruation

dyspepsia: term derived from "bad" (dys) "digestion" (pepsia) describing a condition of the upper part of the gastro-intestinal tract characterized by heartburn, nausea, and loss of appetite

dyspnea: breathlessness or shortness of breath on exertion

ecchymosis: skin discoloration caused by ruptured blood vessels leaking blood into the surrounding tissues (bruises)

eicosanoid: a product of arachidonic acid metabolism

embolism: blood vessel obstruction, usually refers to a blood clot

emmenagogue: an agent that promotes or aids mentrual flow

emulsion: stable mixture of two or more immiscible liquids, such as milk (oil dispersed in water)

encephalomyelitis: acute brain inflammation caused either by a viral infection or in response to an infection

endogenous: produced within a cell or organism

endometriosis: gynecologic condition where endometrial tissue is located outside of the uterus and may result in painful, irregular menstrual cycles, or infertility

endometrium: uterus lining

endothelium: single cell layer that lines the lumen of all blood vessels forming the interface between the blood and the vessel wall

enteric coating: special tablet or capsule coating that does not dissolve until mixed with fluids in the small intestine, resulting in the coated agent's delayed release into the patient's system

enteritis: inflammation of the mucosal lining of the small intestine

enterocystoplasty: a surgical procedure that augments the bladder, using a portion of the intestine, for patients suffering from bladder innervation problems (e.g., in spinal cord injury)

enterocyte: skin cell in the intestinal lining

epithelia/epithelium: a layer of cells forming the surface of mucous membranes and the top layer of the skin

ergogenic: increased work output, actual and potential

ergometric: pertaining to measuring the amount of work done

eructation: condition where gas is produced from the stomach resulting in hiccoughing or belching sounds

erythema: spotted skin and redness usually indicative of infection or inflammation

exanthema: skin eruptions (break-out) in conjunction with a viral disease such as measles

fermentation: chemical reaction where enzymes decompose a complex material into more simple substances

fibrinolysis: dissolution of vascular system clots

fibromyalgia: chronic condition that includes debilitating muscle pain and fatigue

fimbriae: a thread-like structure or fingerlike filament

flavonoid: a plant-based compound containing a carbon skeleton with two aromatic rings bridged by a three-carbon aliphatic chain. Flavonoids are essential in maintaining capillary walls and protecting against infection. One subgroup (anthocyanins) creates plant pigmentation.

fluidextract: a liquid with the ratio of 1:1 whereby each cubic centimeter (cc) or milliliter (mL) of the solution contains 1 g of the extracted substance

fomentation: the application of warm liquid or moist heat to the surface of the body to relieve pain

Fontaines stage category (Stage I-IV): demonstration of the extent of peripheral arterial occlusive disease (PAOD)

formononetin: an isoflavone that is thought to be partially responsible for an herb's estrogenic effect

fortification: strengthening the nutritional value of a food by adding substances such as vitamins

furunculosis: condition marked by boils caused by bacterial skin infections

galenicals: infusions, decoctions, and tinctures prepared from medicinal plants

Geriatric Evaluation by Relative's Rating Instrument (GERRI): a test which assesses daily living and social behavior

GERRI: See: Geriatric Evaluation by Relative's Rating Instrument

glossodynia: tongue pain, also called burning tongue syndrome

glucose challenge: assesses glucose (blood sugar) metabolism capabilities, also known as a glucose tolerance test

glycoside: a plant substance that, when hydrolyzed, forms a sugar along with a non-sugar substance

gruel: porridge made by boiling grains in water or milk

halothane: a general anesthetic made from fluorinated hydrocarbon that is inhaled

Hamilton rating scale (HAM-D): depression rating scale for clinical evaluations

Hamilton rating scale (HAM-A): anxiety rating scale for clinical evaluations

hematoma: localized swelling and discoloration within an organ or tissue resulting from a blood vessel break, a bruise

heparin: a polysaccharide that is used therapeutically to inhibit blood platelet coagulation by forming an antithrombin

histaminergic: a substance or reaction that relates to histamine receptors (allergens and allergic reactions)

histological: relating to the microscopic structure of plant and animal tissues

hyperemesis gravidarum: unusually excessive vomiting during pregnancy that, if not treated, can lead to dehydration, weight loss, and death

hypermenorrhea: menstruation that is excessive in duration or is abnormally heavy

hyperplasia: excessive growth of normal tissue

hyperprolactinemia: condition linked to infertility and marked by increased levels of the pituitary gland hormone, prolactin

hyphema: bleeding in the eye between the cornea and iris

hypotensive: relates to lowered blood pressure

hypoxia: condition where cell tissues are deprived of an adequate supply of oxygen

idiosyncratic: an abnormal susceptibility to some drug, protein, or other agent which is peculiar to the individual

in vitro: Latin phrase used to indicate a process taking place within an artificial environment such as a test tube

in vivo: Latin phrase referring to a process (e.g., a drug reaction) that occurs within a living body, usually an animal

infusion: tea made by steeping (soaking) herbs in hot or cold water

inotropic: affecting a cardiac muscle's force of contraction (contractility)

intermittent claudication: tightness or pain in the calf muscles that arises when walking and subsides with rest, and is a result of insufficient blood circulation

intracranial: inside the skull

intraperitoneal injection: an injection into the abdominal cavity

ischemia: blood supply to a specific area is temporarily reduced or cut-off

Kampo: ancient Japanese healing practice that uses herbal formulas and focuses on treating systemic imbalances, thereby healing physical and psychological ailments

kernicterus: abnormal condition in some infants born with jaundice where excessive amounts of the bile pigment, bilirubin, collect within and damage the brain

Kruskal-Wallis test: a non-parametric test, that compares 3 or more randomly sampled groups with the objective of finding out if, no matter how they are grouped, they will have the same median range

lassitude: feeling lethargic, lacking energy

leukocyte: a white blood cell

leukopenia: reduction in the white blood cell count, i.e., 5,000 or less

leukoplakia: condition where thick, white patches form on mucus membranes (e.g. tounge, genitalia), and can be pre-cancerous

leukorrhea: vaginal discharge consisting of mucous that is white or yellow in color

leukotriene: a product of the metabolism of arachidonic acid mediating almost every aspect of an inflammatory reaction (including asthma)

lichenoid: crust-like patches on the skin that have a similar appearance and texture to a type of alga that grows on trees and rocks

lignan: potential anti-cancer compound that is found naturally in human and animal bodily fluids, as well as from more advanced plants, can be lab-created

liniment: medicinal liquid that relieves pain and stiffness when used externally

lipooxygenase pathway: means of metabolizing fats to produce leukotrienes

log rank test: over a period of time, recording events in people's lives (survival functions) to create a table on which statistical comparisons can be made, also known as Mantel-Cox

lumbago: backache located in the middle or lower back

lysis: process where cells are destroyed

maceration: soaking a solid for a defined period of time in a liquid

macrophage: mononuclear cells, originating from bone marrow, that enter the blood stream and are capable of producing antigens and activating immune system responses

GLOSSARY

Mann-Whitney test: a non-parametric inferential statistical test to compare two randomly drawn, independent samples

mast cell: tissue cells responsible for producing the mediators (i.e., histamines) for allergic reactions (e.g., sneezing, welts)

mastalgia: breast pain or discomfort

mastodynia: breast pain or discomfort

materia medica: general term referring to the curative substances in medicinal remedies and the science that studies them

menorrhagia: heavy or prolonged menstrual bleeding

metastasis: the spreading of a disease resulting in secondary signs and symptoms in another part of the body, usually cancerous

micturition: act of urinating

mitogenic: induction of cell division or change

motropic: relating to or influencing muscle motions

mucilage: thick, sticky gel-like agent produced by some plants and used as a therapeutic salve or to mix substances that would normally be insoluble

mucositis: inflammation of a mucous membrane

muscarinic: a subtype of the parasympathetic acetylcholinergic (ACh) receptor system

musculotropic: an agent that impacts or is drawn to muscle tissues

mutagenic: an agent that induces changes in genes

myalgia: muscle aches or pains

myalgic encephalomyelitis: painful disease that is characterized by inflammation of the brain and spinal cord, flu-like symptoms, and loss of muscle strength

myocarditis: inflammation of the heart muscle

myocardium: center muscle layer of the heart wall

myocyte: cell that makes up muscle tissue

myoglobinuria: losing myoglobins, beneficial proteins in the muscles that provide and store oxygen, via urination as a result of muscle trauma

native dry extract: an extract, typically hydroalcoholic, of plant material from which the solvent has been evaporated to leave a solid residue

neurogenic: relating to or stemming from nerve tissue impulses

Neurodermatitis: scaly patches of skin resulting from an itch that is irritated when scratched

neuropathy: general term for a disease involving any aspect of the nervous system

neurovegetative: relating to the autonomic nervous system's supplying of nerve fibers to internal organs

NF-kB: See: nuclear factor kappa beta

nociceptor: outer layer nerve ending that responds to painful or harmful agents

nocturia: persistent and excessive need to urinate during regular sleeping hours; oftentimes increases in frequency with aging

non-parametric: type of inferential statistical analysis where no assumptions are applied regarding the defining properties of the selected populations, commonly used in studies spanning the lifespan of a population

norepinephrine: an effective blood vessel constrictor secreted by the adrenal gland

notalgia paresthetica: dermatological condition characterized by intense itching of the scapula region (the upper back)

Nuclear factor kappa beta: a redox-sensitive transcription factor that promotes the transcription of genes that promote cell replication and tissue growth

nulliparous: a woman who, by choice or medical difficulties, has never given birth to a living child

octamer: DNA strands that carry polymer chains consisting of 8 amino acids

oculomotor: relates to movements of the eye

ointment: solid dosage form for use on the skin for soothing, healing, therapeutic, or cosmetic purposes

oleoresin: a mixture of essential oils and resins extracted from plants

oligomenorrhea: menstruation that is sporadic or has an unusually light flow

orthostatic: caused or impacted by standing upright (e.g., change in blood pressure)

osteoarthritis: non-inflammatory destruction of joint tissue resulting in pain and movement limitation

osteogenic: relating to the development, growth, or repair of bone

osteoporosis: a condition in which bone mass is decreased causing increased fracture risk and healing time

PAOD: see: peripheral arterial occlusive disease

papillary: surface of a lesion resembling a fold, frond or villous projection

pappus: cup-like structure (calyx) of plants, such as on dandelions, that is made of fibers, leaves, or thorns

paresthesia: often related to nerve damage, an abnormal sensation of the skin that can include prickling, numbness, and burning

paste: thick, smooth mixture that, when dry, is stiff and can be used as an adhesive or applied to the skin for therapeutic purposes

peripheral arterial occlusive disease (PAOD): an arterial disease leading to progressively increased pain, exhaustion, and debility

peroxidation: process characterized by oxidation of fatty acids affecting the integrity of cell membranes which can be modulated by the presence of antioxidants

pia mater: one of three membranes surrounding the brain and spinal cord

pial: pertaining to pia mater

phagocytosis: process of a cell taking in and digesting particles such as other cells or bacteria

Pharmacovigilence: the ongoing process of identification and reporting of drug safety issues to provide early detection in order to minimize the impact and extent of adverse drug reactions

pheochromocytoma: adrenal gland tumor that causes excessive epinephrine and norepinephrine secretion and eventually leads to high blood pressure

phlebopathy: any vein-related disease

phytochemicals: plant derived chemicals

plaster: paste-like material that hardens when dried and is used to create a model of, or immobilize, a body part

plethysmography: measuring the size of body parts or limbs to determine blood supply

polypectomy: extracting a polyp, a precancerous growth, by means of surgery

post-phlebitis syndrome: chronic inflammation of the deep veins of the legs, which then damages the vein or causes blockages in the superficial veins

postprandial: period of time after consuming food

poultice: a thick paste applied to the skin for the purpose of alleviating pain, reducing inflammation, and promoting healing

procyanidin: type of flavonoid that includes proanthocyanidins and procyanidin oligomers (PCOs)

prolactin: a pituitary gland hormone that when combined with estrogen and progesterone, stimulates breast development and milk formation during pregnancy

prophylactic: a preventative agent or process

prophylaxis: application of preventative measures to reduce the incidence of disease

prostaglandin: metabolized from arachidonic acid (unsaturated animal fatty acid) and important in several physicolgical functions (e.g., vasoconstriction, smooth muscle stimulation)

prurigo (nodular): on-going skin condition characterized by the eruption of severely itchy, pale papules (welts)

pruritus: condition characterized by intensely itchy skin

psychometric: pertaining to the surveying of psychological parameters including behavior, emotions, and cognitive abilities

psychomotor: mind-muscle connection, coordination of physical activities with mental operations

psychovegetative: depressive, catatonic-like state where a person appears to unknowingly respond to certain stimuli and lacks corresponding cognitive neurological function

purpura: disorder marked by hemorrhage in the skin or mucous membranes resulting in purple spots

putrefactive: an agent (usually bacteria) that breaks down, or decomposes, organic substances with a resulting foul odor

pyelonephritis: inflammation, brought on by bacterial infection, of the kidneys and surrounding area

pyuria: urine containing an abnormally high level of pus and white blood cells leading to urine that has a cloudy appearance, indication of a possible renal disease

qi: Chinese term referring to the vital force, or energy, that is believed to be present in all things

Raynaud's disease: disorder marked by episodic vasoconstriction of digits (hands and toes) leading to abnormally cold hands and feet; affects women three to five times more frequently than men

retinopathy: pertaining to any retinal disease or disorder

rheumatism: any inflammatory condition of the joints, ligaments, bursae, or muscles characterized by limitation of movement, pain, and structural degeneration

rheumatoid arthritis: progressive disorder characterized by painful inflammation and destruction of the joints and eventually malformation and disability

rhinitis: condition caused by chronic inflammation of the nasal mucosa characterized by runny nose, itching, and sneezing

rhizome: underground stem that grows horizontally, sometimes stores starch

rhynchophylline: indole alkaloid found in some species of *Uncaria*

GLOSSARY

rubefacient: externally applied agent that causes the skin to become red

saccade: rapid, involuntary eye movement made when shifting focus from one point to another

saponin: plant agent that creates a foam when shaken with water

sarcoma: malignant tumor growing from connective tissue such as bone or muscle

seborrheic dermatitis: chronic, recurring scaly rash predominantly affecting the face, ears, eyebrows, and scalp

secretolytic: a substance that reduces secretions

selective serotonin reuptake inhibitor (SSRI): antidepressant drug that is used to increase the amount of serotonin, a mood balancing neurotransmitter and hormone (e.g., Prozac®, Zoloft®)

septicemia: condition characterized by the presence of bacteria circulating in the blood, often associated with severe disease and increased mortality

sesquiterpene: a plant-derived compound usually with 15 carbons formed from isoprene units

Sjorgen's syndrome: autoimmune disorder marked by dry eyes and mouth, and occasional enlargement of the salivary glands

SKT: see: Syndrome Kurz Test

solute: substance dissolved in a liquid to create a solution

solvent: liquid in which substances are dissolved in order to create a solution

somatic: any agent, system, or process that affects or is related to the physical body

spectrophotometry: a method of analysis in which ultraviolet light or electromagnetic radiation is passed through a solution and measured against the light spectrum

SSRI: see: selective serotonin reuptake inhibitor

struvite: type of crystal found in some kidney stones

sympathomimetic: an agent that mediates sympathetic nervous system reactions, particularly the effects of adrenaline (e.g., increased heartrate and sweating)

Syndrom-Kurztest (SKT): a short, simple test used for determining cognitive impairment, specifically regarding attention and memory, developed in Germany

tachyarrhythmia: rapid, irregular heart beat

tachycardia: heart palpitations exceeding 100 beats per minute in the average adult

tachyphylaxis: marked desensitization to certain drugs or toxins following repeated administration of small doses

teratogenic: pertaining to abnormal embryo development

thermogenic: heat producing

thrombocytopenia: blood disease marked by decreased platelet count

thrombosis: condition characterized by vascular system blood clots

thromboxane: a by-product of the arachidonic acid metabolism, that can cause blood clotting and vein blockage

thrombophlebitis: inflammation of a vein combined with formation of a blood clot (thrombus)

thrombus: a blood clot formed by the aggregation of platelets, fibrin, clotting factors, and cellular elements that obstructs a blood vessel or heart chamber

thyrotoxicosis: disease caused by overactive thyroid gland leading to dangerous overproduction of thyroid hormones

tincture: a therapeutic solution created by soaking an herb in alcohol to extract the pharmacologically active components of the herb

tinnitus: condition marked by a ringing or buzzing in the ears

tocopherol: compound having the biochemical actions of vitamin E

tonic: a medicinal agent that improves systemic functions or sense of well-being

tumescence: state of being or becoming swollen

uremia: disease marked by kidney dysfunction leading to an increase of nitrogen-type waste products (toxins) in the blood

urogenital: regarding the organs in the urinary and reproductive systems

urostomy: surgically created urinary tract opening with an attached bag to collect urine

urticaria: allergic reaction resulting in itchy welts or bumps

vasomotor: relating to the nerves that control constriction and dilation of blood vessels

vertigo: dizziness or lightheadedness that leads to the sensation of spinning or moving

viscid: thick or sticky liquid

vulnerary: remedy used to heal wounds

Post Test, Applications for Receiving Credit, and Evaluation Forms

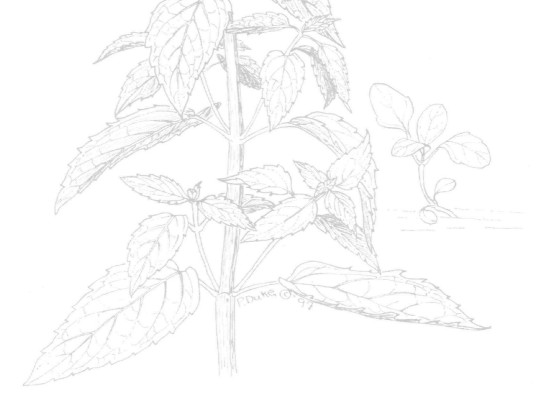

(This page intentionally left blank.)

POST TEST

1. **Which of these herbs can be used to treat menopausal symptoms such as hot flashes and irritability?**

    a. Ginkgo

    b. Black cohosh

    c. Chamomile

    d. Bilberry

2. **Which herb can be used to treat migraine headaches?**

    a. Licorice

    b. Horse chestnut

    c. Feverfew

    d. Milk thistle

3. **Which herb can be recommended to patients with chronic constipation who would benefit from more fiber in their diet?**

    a. Cat's claw

    b. Kava

    c. Flax

    d. Valerian

4. **Which herb is NOT used in the treatment of insomnia?**

    a. Chamomile

    b. Valerian

    c. Kava

    d. Echinacea

5. **Which of the following is NOT true about licorice?**

    a. The German Commission E contraindicates licorice in cholestatic liver disorders, liver cirrhosis, hypertension, hypokalemia, severe kidney insufficiency.

    b. Licorice root is not recommended during pregnancy.

    c. Because it is used as a flavoring agent in candies, its use is relatively safe, even in fairly large quantities.

    d. A particular type of licorice preparation is used in European phytotherapy for acute and chronic gastric/duodenal ulcers.

6. **Which herb is NOT used in the prevention or treatment of cardiovascular conditions?**

    a. Garlic

    b. Hawthorn

    c. Green tea

    d. St. John's wort

7. **Which herb is used to treat mild to moderate depression?**

    a. Hawthorn

    b. Chaste tree

    c. St. John's wort

    d. Black cohosh

8. **Regarding scientific research on garlic, which statement most accurately summarizes the *quantity of studies* conducted through at least the middle of 1996?**

    a. It is difficult to assess the volume of studies on garlic as there was no specific, standardized preparation used in all the studies.

    b. It is difficult to assess the volume of studies on garlic because garlic is also a food and the literature contains too many studies where garlic was employed merely as a flavoring agent.

    c. By 1996 there were 1,808 scientific studies (including chemical, pharmacological, clinical, and epidemiological) on garlic.

    d. It is difficult to count all the studies on garlic because garlic is so universally used that studies exist in too many languages to keep an accurate record.

9. **A sexually active young woman with recurrent urinary tract infections is wondering how to help prevent them. Which herb might she use?**

    a. Valerian

    b. Black cohosh

    c. Cranberry

    d. Flax

10. **A patient with HIV is taking the protease inhibitor Indinavir. Which herb do recent reports suggest may cause an herb-drug interaction?**

    a. Ginger

    b. Peppermint

    c. Milk thistle

    d. St. John's wort

11. **A colleague calls to ask if you have ever heard of an herb used for chronic venous insufficiency, backed by extensive clinical data. A patient is using this to treat the poor circulation in her lower legs. The herb she is taking is:**

    a. Horse chestnut

    b. American ginseng

    c. Cranberry

    d. Kava

12. **A female patient tells you she has had extreme fatigue, chronic colds all winter, and difficulty concentrating at work. Which herb might be recommended for these symptoms?**

    a. Evening primrose oil

    b. Chamomile

    c. Cat's claw

    d. Ginseng

13. **A patient's post surgical course was difficult and, due to severe depression, her physician has prescribed a monoamine oxidase (MAO) inhibitor. Which of the following herbs should she discontinue during MAO inhibitor therapy?**

    a. Horse chestnut

    b. Garlic

    c. Ephedra

    d. A and B

    e. A and C

14. **An older patient has been suffering from insomnia since moving to an assisted living situation and wants a natural sleep aid that is not known to interfere with the conventional drugs she is taking. What would you recommend?**

    a. Garlic

    b. Cayenne

    c. Valerian

    d. Ginseng

15. **A 13-year old suffers from repeated colds and ear infections. You could suggest that his mother boost his immune system with:**

    a. Saw palmetto

    b. Echinacea

    c. American ginseng

    d. A and B

    e. B and C

    f. All of the above

16. **Ginkgo reduces blood clotting time.**

    a. True

    b. False

17. **In general, patients with a history of liver disorders can safely use kava.**

    a. True

    b. False

18. **Kava is used to treat anxiety disorders.**

    a. True

    b. False

19. **Cayenne pepper is useful in the treatment of painful muscle spasms and neuralgias.**

    a. True

    b. False

20. **Hawthorn has been shown to be an effective treatment for NYHA Stages I and II in congestive heart failure.**

    a. True

    b. False

21. **Evening primrose oil can be used to treat cyclic breast pain.**

    a. True

    b. False

22. **Cat's claw can be used in the treatment of rheumatoid arthritis.**

    a. True

    b. False

23. **Green tea contains antioxidants.**

    a. True

    b. False

24. **Chaste tree is used to treat Premenstrual Syndrome.**

    a. True

    b. False

25. **The primary reason that goldenseal root is so popular in the U.S. market is the relatively large number of clinical studies conducted on this herb.**

    a. True

    b. False

26. **Pycnogenol® should be taken with meals to avoid possible gastric adverse effects.**

    a. True

    b. False

27. **A middle-aged man complains of increased fatigue and job stress and he also mentions that his libido has decreased over the last year. Which herb might help?**

    a. Eleuthero

    b. Bilberry

    c. Feverfew

    d. Chamomile

28. **A postpartum, healthy female comes to you after delivery of her second child, whom she is breast-feeding. The mother notes that the infant is irritable and not sleeping well. Which herb could she be taking that might be effecting the baby?**

    a. Chamomile

    b. Green tea

    c. Flax

    d. Evening primrose oil

29. **A man is having his gallbladder removed. Knowing that he takes large doses of herbal supplements daily, which of the following herbs is presumably safe for him to continue to take prior to and following surgery?**

    a. Garlic

    b. Ginger

    c. Ginkgo

    d. Peppermint

30. **A cancer patient asks if there are any herbs she can take to help with the nausea and vomiting caused by her chemotherapy. Which would you recommend?**

    a. Saw palmetto

    b. Hawthorn

    c. Cranberry

    d. Ginger

31. **A pregnant woman is suffering from severe morning sickness. Her husband has arranged for them to go on a sailing trip. She has a history of severe motion sickness and does NOT want to use Dramamine® (dimenhydrinate) because of the pregnancy. What would you recommend?**

    a. Cat's claw

    b. Saw palmetto

    c. Ginger

    d. EPO

32. **Which of the following best describes evening primrose oil?**

    a. Its trans-fatty acids can contribute to heart disease in chronic users.

    b. Its omega 6 fatty acids are precursors to anti-inflammatory prostanoids.

    c. In large clinical trials it has been proven useful for juvenile rheumatoid arthritis.

    d. Overdoses can cause joint pain and inflammation.

33. **Feverfew is commonly used to help prevent migraines. Which of the following is NOT a potential side effect of feverfew?**

    a. Oral ulceration

    b. Rebound headaches upon discontinuation

    c. Allergic reactions

    d. Tongue swelling

34. **Which of the following is a potential contraindication in the use of peppermint?**

    a. Allergy to the Compositae family of plants, such as ragweed

    b. Gastro-esophageal reflux disease

    c. Asthma

    d. Inflammatory bowel syndrome

35. **Which of the following could you reasonably suggest as a mild sedative?**

    a. Valerian

    b. Licorice

    c. Bilberry

    d. Echinacea

36. **Which of the following is NOT commonly used as a remedy for upset stomach?**

    a. Chamomile

    b. Peppermint

    c. Ginger

    d. Cranberry

37. An elderly woman comes in with agitation and insomnia. She tells you that she has been diagnosed with generalized anxiety disorder. What herb can you recommend?

    a.   Horse chestnut

    b.   Cayenne

    c.   Kava

    d.   Flax

38. An elderly man complains of urinary retention. After being diagnosed with benign prostatic hyperplasia (BPH), which herb is indicated?

    a.   Saw palmetto

    b.   Garlic

    c.   Green tea

    d.   Peppermint

39. A long-term psychiatric patient with a psychotropic medication history of several years comes to you with a question, "Are there any herbs that will protect my liver while I take these medications?" What would you recommend?

    a.   Valerian

    b.   Evening primrose oil

    c.   Milk thistle

    d.   Flax

40. Mrs. Green has been having trouble with psoriasis. Her niece gave her a cream containing capsaicin to relieve the itching. From what herb is capsaicin derived?

    a.   Cayenne

    b.   Garlic

    c.   Chamomile

    d.   Peppermint

41. Which herb is NOT used in therapeutic skin preparations?

    a.   Chamomile

    b.   Cayenne

    c.   Evening primrose oil

    d.   Cranberry

42. A patient with irritable bowel syndrome (IBS) wants to know if there have been any positive clinical studies on herbal supplements for the treatment of IBS. Your answer is yes, and the herb is:

    a.   Cranberry

    b.   Echinacea

    c.   Cat's claw

    d.   Peppermint oil in enteric-coated capsules

43. The recommended daily dose of ginkgo standardized dry extract in the treatment of dementia is:

    a.   90–130 mg

    b.   120–160 mg

    c.   120–240 mg

44. Which of the following would be considered a legal structure/function claim on an herbal dietary supplement label?

    a.   "Helps prevent heart disease"

    b.   "Helps support urinary tract health"

    c.   "Helps treat the common cold"

45. Herb product labels *must* specify:

    a.   Common name of the herb, as listed in *Herbs of Commerce*

    b.   Scientific name of the herb for herbs listed in *Herbs of Commerce*

    c.   Plant part used

    d.   A and C

46. Which of the following is NOT required on the labeling of an herbal product?

    a.   Serving size

    b.   A disclaimer

    c.   Expiration date

    d.   Amount of each individual herb if a combination product

47. **FDA published final rules for the labeling of herbs and other dietary supplements under the Dietary Supplemental Health and Education Act (DSHEA). These rules now allow labels on dietary supplements to:**

    a. Make therapeutic claims

    b. Claim to treat Alzheimer's disease and osteoporosis

    c. Make claims that do not directly relate to the treatment or prevention of a disease

    d. Claim to lower cholesterol and prevent cardiac arrhythmia

48. **Herbal and dietary supplement legislation regulates the industry in all of the following EXCEPT:**

    a. Required labeling elements

    b. Structure/function claim notices to FDA

    c. Good manufacturing practices

    d. Submission of pre-market safety data for old dietary ingredients

49. **The Federal Trade Commission (FTC) can stop an advertisement for herbs and dietary supplements making an inadequately substantiated claim.**

    a. True

    b. False

50. **In Germany, physicians often prescribe herbal medicines.**

    a. True

    b. False

CONTINUING EDUCATION FOR DIETITIANS/DIETETIC TECHNICIANS APPLICATION

To qualify for 12 CPE of CDR approved continuing education for Registered Dietitians, complete this original form (copies will not be accepted), the answer sheet, a check for $20, and mail to:

> Office of Continuing Education
> Southwest Texas State University
> 601 University Drive
> San Marcos, TX 78666-4616

Your certificate will be mailed to you at the address you have noted. Please allow 4-6 weeks for processing.

PERSONAL INFORMATION (PLEASE PRINT)

Title of Activity: ***ABC Clinical Guide to Herbs***   Date Completed: _____

Name: _____   Email: _____

Address: _____

City: _____   State: _____ Zip Code: _____

Lic. #: _____   Phone #: _____

Degree: ❑ Bachelors ❑ Master ❑ Ph.D.   Employed at: _____

ANSWER SHEET Fill in the circle next to the single best answer for each question.

1. a. O
   b. O
   c. O
   d. O
2. a. O
   b. O
   c. O
   d. O
3. a. O
   b. O
   c. O
   d. O
4. a. O
   b. O
   c. O
   d. O
5. a. O
   b. O
   c. O
   d. O
6. a. O
   b. O
   c. O
   d. O
7. a. O
   b. O
   c. O
   d. O
8. a. O
   b. O
   c. O
   d. O
9. a. O
   b. O
   c. O
   d. O
10. a. O
    b. O
    c. O
    d. O
11. a. O
    b. O
    c. O
    d. O
12. a. O
    b. O
    c. O
    d. O
13. a. O
    b. O
    c. O
    d. O
14. a. O
    b. O
    c. O
    d. O
15. a. O
    b. O
    c. O
    d. O
    e. O
    f. O
16. a. O
    b. O
17. a. O
    b. O
18. a. O
    b. O
    e. O
19. a. O
    b. O
20. a. O
    b. O
21. a. O
    b. O
22. a. O
    b. O
23. a. O
    b. O
24. a. O
    b. O
25. a. O
    b. O
26. a. O
    b. O
    b. O
    c. O
    d. O
27. a. O
    b. O
    c. O
    d. O
28. a. O
    b. O
    c. O
    d. O
29. a. O
    b. O
    c. O
    d. O
30. a. O
    b. O
    c. O
    d. O
31. a O
    b. O
    c. O
    d. O
32. a. O
    b. O
    c. O
    d. O
33. a. O
    b. O
    c. O
    d. O
34. a O
    b. O
    c. O
    d. O
35. a. O
    b. O
    c. O
    d. O
36. a. O
    b. O
    c. O
    d. O
37. a. O
    b. O
    c. O
    d. O
38. a. O
    b. O
    c. O
    d. O
39. a. O
    b. O
    c. O
    d. O
40. a. O
    b. O
    c. O
    d. O
41. a. O
    b. O
    c. O
    d. O
42. a. O
    b. O
    c. O
    d. O
43. a. O
    b. O
    c. O
44. a. O
    b. O
    c. O
45. a. O
    b. O
    c. O
    d. O
46. a. O
    b. O
    c. O
    d. O
47. a. O
    b. O
    c. O
    d. O
48. a. O
    b. O
    c. O
    d. O
49. a. O
    b. O
50. a. O
    b. O

ACTIVITY EVALUATION

SWT and the American Botanical Council would like to know how well this course met your professional and personal needs, and your degree of satisfaction with the program.

Please circle the number that best represents your opinion (select only one choice per question).

	Strongly Agree			Strongly Disagree
1. I was able to meet the learning objectives of this course. 1	2	3	4	5
2. The topic is relevant to the patients/clients I work with. 1	2	3	4	5

	Strongly Agree				Strongly Disagree
3. I increased my knowledge of the topic.	1	2	3	4	5
4. This was an effective method of learning.	1	2	3	4	5
5. I will be able to use what I have learned.	1	2	3	4	5

Comments or Suggestions:

POST-TEST

In order to receive continuing education credit for this program, you must complete all the post-test questions. Please attach your answer sheet to this form.

By signing below, you are acknowledging that the information given above is accurate based upon your participation in this program.

_____

Signature   Date

CHECKLIST

❏ I have enclosed the completed original application form.

❏ I have enclosed the completed answer sheet.

❏ I have enclosed a check for $20, payable to: Southwest Texas University.

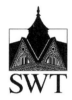

SWT

CONTINUING EDUCATION FOR NURSES AND ADVANCED PRACTICE NURSES
APPLICATION

To qualify for 10 contact hours of continuing education for Nurses and Advanced Practice Nurses, complete this original application form (copies with not be accepted), the answer sheet, include a check made payable to: Texas Nurses Association ($10 for members; $15 for non-members) and mail to:

Texas Nurses Association
7600 Burnet Road, Suite 440
Austin, TX 78757-1292

Your certificate will be mailed to you at the address you have noted. Please allow 4-6 weeks for processing.

PERSONAL INFORMATION (PLEASE PRINT)

Title of Activity: **ABC Clinical Guide to Herbs**   Date Completed: _____

Name: _____   Email: _____
(as it appears on the RN license)

Address: _____

City: _____   State: _____ Zip Code: _____

TNA Membership #: _____   Phone #: _____

Employed at: _____

ANSWER SHEET Fill in the circle next to the single best answer for each question.

1. a.O b.O c.O d.O	6. a.O b.O c.O d.O	11. a.O b.O c.O d.O	15. a.O b.O c.O d.O e.O f.O	21. a.O b.O	28. a.O b.O c.O d.O	33. a.O b.O c.O d.O	38. a.O b.O c.O d.O	43. a.O b.O c.O 44. a.O b.O c.O	48. a.O b.O c.O d.O
2. a.O b.O c.O d.O	7. a.O b.O c.O d.O	12. a.O b.O c.O d.O	16. a.O b.O	22. a.O b.O / 23. a.O b.O	29. a.O b.O c.O d.O	34. a.O b.O c.O d.O	39. a.O b.O c.O d.O	45. a.O b.O c.O d.O	49. a.O b.O / 50. a.O b.O
3. a.O b.O c.O d.O	8. a.O b.O c.O d.O	13. a.O b.O c.O d.O	17. a.O b.O	24. a.O b.O / 25. a.O b.O	30. a.O b.O c.O d.O	35. a.O b.O c.O d.O	40. a.O b.O c.O d.O	46. a.O b.O c.O d.O	
4. a.O b.O c.O d.O	9. a.O b.O c.O d.O	14. a.O b.O c.O d.O	18. a.O b.O / 19. a.O b.O	26. a.O b.O / 27. a.O b.O c.O d.O	31. a.O b.O c.O d.O	36. a.O b.O c.O d.O	41. a.O b.O c.O d.O	47. a.O b.O c.O d.O	
5. a.O b.O c.O d.O	10. a.O b.O c.O d.O		20. a.O b.O		32. a.O b.O c.O d.O	37. a.O b.O c.O d.O	42. a.O b.O c.O d.O		

ACTIVITY EVALUATION

The Texas Nurses Association and the American Botanical Council would like to know how well this course met your professional and personal needs and your degree of satisfaction with the program.

Please circle the number that best represents your opinion (select only one choice per question).

	Strongly Agree				Strongly Disagree
1. Rate your achievement of these objectives.					
a. I can identify the most popular medicinal herbs available to consumers in the U.S. market.	1	2	3	4	5

	Strongly Agree				Strongly Disagree
b. I can explain the common therapeutic indications of the leading herbs.	1	2	3	4	5
c. I can provide an overview of the clinical study research of the leading herbs.	1	2	3	4	5
d. I can identify potential drug interactions and side effects.	1	2	3	4	5
e. I can evaluate the safety issues and contraindications of the leading herbs.	1	2	3	4	5
f. I can interpret product labels for indications of clinical efficacy.	1	2	3	4	5
g. I can distinguish different brands on the marketplace which are backed by clinical research.	1	2	3	4	5
h. I can interpret the implications of government regulations on the clinical use of herbs.	1	2	3	4	5
2. The teaching/learning resource was effective.	1	2	3	4	5
3. The objectives were relevant to the following overall goals:	1	2	3	4	5

This activity emphasizes the importance of obtaining a detailed history of medication usage, over-the-counter herbs and pharmaceuticals, as well as prescriptive agents. It provides the nurse with clinical information on the effect of herbals and potential herb/drug interaction important for patient care and patient education. The nurse may utilize this information when encountering patients who take herbs.

	Very Good	Good	Fair	Poor
4. Overall I rate this learning activity.	1	2	3	4

Comments or Suggestions:

Post-Test

In order to receive continuing education credit for this program, you must complete all the post–test questions. Please attach your answer sheet to this form.

By signing below, you are acknowledging that the information given above is accurate based upon your participation in this program.

_____

Signature   Date

CHECKLIST

❏ I have enclosed the completed original application form.

❏ I have enclosed the completed answer sheet.

❏ I have enclosed a check payable to: Texas Nurses Association. Members of

Texas Nurses Association ($10)

Non-members ($15)

TNA
TEXAS NURSES ASSOCIATION

CONTINUING EDUCATION FOR PHARMACISTS
APPLICATION

To qualify for 1.2 CEU (12 credit hours) of ACPE accredited continuing pharmacy education for this program, complete this original application form (copies will not be accepted), the answer sheet, include a check for $7, and mail to:

Texas Pharmacy Association, CE Department
P.O. Box 14709
Austin, TX 78761–4709

Your certificate will be mailed to you at the address you have noted. Please allow 4-6 weeks for processing.

PERSONAL INFORMATION (PLEASE PRINT)

Title of Activity: **ABC Clinical Guide to Herbs**   Date Completed: _____

Name: _____   Email: _____

Address: _____

City: _____   State: _____ Zip Code: _____

Lic. #: _____   Phone #: _____   SS# _____

Degree: ❏ Bachelors ❏ Ph.D.   Employed at: _____

ANSWER SHEET Fill in the circle next to the single best answer for each question

1. a. O b. O c. O d. O	6. a. O b. O c. O d. O	11. a. O b. O c. O d. O	15. a. O b. O c. O d. O e. O f. O	21. a. O b. O	28. a. O b. O c. O d. O	33. a. O b. O c. O d. O	38. a. O b. O c. O d. O	43. a. O b. O c. O	48. a. O b. O c. O d. O
2. a. O b. O c. O d. O	7. a. O b. O c. O d. O	12. a. O b. O c. O d. O	16. a. O b. O	22. a. O b. O 23. a. O b. O	29. a. O b. O c. O d. O	34. a O b. O c. O d. O	39. a. O b. O c. O d. O	44. a. O b. O 45. a. O b. O	49. a. O b. O 50. a. O b. O
3. a. O b. O c. O d. O	8. a. O b. O c. O d. O	13. a. O b. O c. O d. O e. O	17. a. O b. O 18. a. O b. O	24. a. O b. O 25. a. O b. O 26. a. O b. O	30. a. O b. O c. O d. O	35. a. O b. O c. O d. O	40. a. O b. O c. O d. O	c. O d. O 46. a. O b. O	
4. a. O b. O c. O d. O	9. a. O b. O c. O d. O	14. a. O b. O c. O d. O	19. a. O b. O 20. a. O b. O	27. a. O b. O c. O d. O	31. a O b. O c. O d. O	36. a. O b. O c. O d. O	41. a. O b. O c. O d. O	c. O d. O 47. a. O b. O	
5. a. O b. O c. O d. O	10. a. O b. O c. O d. O				32. a. O b. O c. O d. O	37. a. O b. O c. O d. O	42. a. O b. O c. O d. O	c. O d. O	

ACTIVITY EVALUATION

The Texas Pharmacy Association and The American Botanical Council are interested in knowing your response to this type of CE program. Your input will help us in planning future programs to meet your needs and maintain high quality continuing pharmaceutical education. Please circle the number that best represents your opinion.

	Strongly Agree				Strongly Disagree
1. The program met the learning objectives.	1	2	3	4	5
2. The topic is relevant to my practice.	1	2	3	4	5

		Strongly Agree				Strongly Disagree
3.	The program increased my knowledge of the topic.	1	2	3	4	5
4.	The writer's approach to presenting the information was informative and easy to follow.	1	2	3	4	5
5.	This method of education was an effective method of learning.	1	2	3	4	5
6.	This program provided me with new information.	1	2	3	4	5
7.	I will be able to use what I have learned.	1	2	3	4	5

Comments or Suggestions:

Post-Test

By signing below, you are acknowledging that the information given above is accurate based upon your participation in this program.

_____

Signature   Date

The Texas Pharmacy Association is approved by the American Council on Pharmaceutical Education as a provider of continuing pharmaceutical education. A total of 1.2 CEU (12 contact hours) will be awarded to pharmacists for the successful completion of this program. The APCE Program number is 154–999–03–700–H01.

CHECKLIST

❏ I have enclosed the completed original application form.

❏ I have enclosed the completed answer sheet.

❏ I have enclosed a check for $7, payable to: Texas Pharmacy Association.

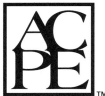

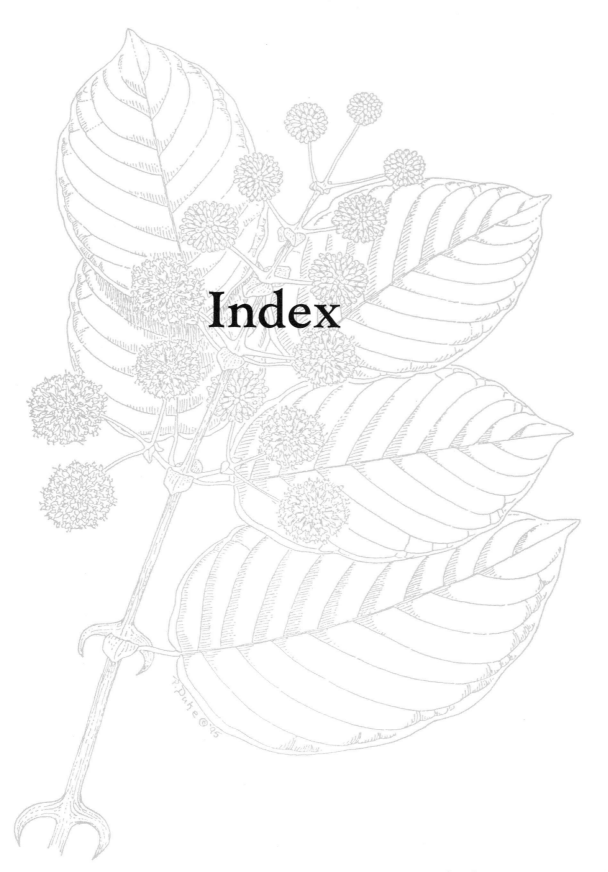

Index

INDEX

Bolded page numbers designate the herb chapter for the herb listed, or the monograph for the proprietary herbal product listed. For guidance on critical decision-making the reader is referred to the comprehensive information provided in the Monographs which are fully indexed. The Clinical Overview and Patient Information Sheet for each herb are indexed only under the scientific and common names for that herb because all material in these sections is discussed in further detail within the corresponding Monograph.

A

abdominal pain, 128, 139, 239, 264, 305, 373. *see also* gastrointestinal conditions

ABKIT, Inc., 405

abnormal sensations. *see* paresthesia

abrasions, 54, 57, 59, 90

absorption of drugs and nutrients, 147, 341, 367, 383

ABTS radicals, 29

Acanthopanax senticosus, **97–106**

Access Business Group, 382

Accreditation Council for Continuing Medical Education, xv, xvi

acetaldehyde, 380

acetaminophen, 162, 170, 308

acetazolamide, 116

acetyl salicylic acid. *see* aspirin

acetylacteol, 17

acetylcholinesterase inhibitors, 191

acetylcysteine, 389

acetylenic alcohols, 205

Achillea millefolium, 379

acne, 32, 64, 66, 67, 72, 381

Aconitum spp., 278, 383

Acquired Immune Deficiency Syndrome (AIDS). *see* HIV

Actaea racemosa, **13–22,** 410

actein, 17

activities of daily living (ADL), 189

activity levels influenced by eleuthero, 106

acute mountain sickness (AMS). *see* altitude sickness

adaptogens, 100, 101, 102, 105, 214, 215

ADAS-Cog score, 195

addiction potential, 113, 115

adenocarcinomas, mammary, 127

adenoma, prostatic, 114

adenomatous colorectal polyps, 161

adenosine, 157, 158, 231, 240

adeturone, 102

adhesions, bacterial, 77

adhesions, platelet, 168, 231. *see also* platelet aggregation

adipose tissue, 113, 115–116, 223

adrenoceptors, 239, 240, 313

adrenocorticotropic agents, 277

adverse effects, xviii, xxvii

abdominal pain, 128, 140

acne, 32, 66

allergic reactions/hypersensitivity, 44, 55, 56, 160, 326

alveolitis, 44

anaphylaxis, 55, 56, 90, 252

androgenization, 102

anxiety, 340

appetite reduction, 341

asthma, 160

bile obstruction, 264

bleeding/hemorrhage, 160, 190, 217, 326

breast tension/mastalgia, 66, 217

breath odor, 160

burning-mouth syndrome, 302

circulatory complaints, 18, 32

conjunctivitis, 55

constipation, 32, 115

contact sensitivity, oral, 302

dermatitis/skin reactions, 44, 55, 66, 69, 71, 139, 160, 252

diarrhea, 32, 78, 102, 140, 217, 295, 334

diuresis, 340

dizziness/vertigo, 18, 31, 190, 217

driving impairment, 356

dry mouth, 66

dyspepsia, 69, 140, 356

edema, 278

emesis/vomiting, 18, 31, 55, 115, 140

erectile/ejaculatory disturbances, 313, 317, 319

erythema, 326

erythrocytosis, 32

estrogen-like effects, 217

excitability, 356

fatigue, 66

flatulence, 140, 295

gastric reflux, 251

gastrointestinal complaints, 18, 22, 66, 71, 78, 190, 251, 295, 313, 317, 326, 332

giddiness, 115

hair loss, 66

hairy baby syndrome, 102

headaches, 18, 31, 66, 69, 71, 102, 115, 128, 190, 319, 340, 356

adverse effects (cont.)

heart irregularities, 66, 102, 115, 190, 278, 340

hepatitis, 264, 265

hepatotoxicity, 90, 264, 265

hyperaldosteronism, 278

hypertension, 115, 217, 278, 313, 340

hyphema, 190

hypokalemia, 278

ichthyosis, scaly, 264

icterus (jaundice), 264

impaired judgment, 356

impaired vision, 18

insomnia/sleep disturbances, 102, 115, 217, 334, 340, 356

irritability, 115, 217, 340

itching/pruritus, 66, 251

lichenoid reaction, 302

lip swelling, 139

liver dysfunction, 264, 265

loose stools, 128

lytic fever, 32

melioidosis, 264

menstrual disturbances, 66

morning sleepiness, 356

mucosal irritation, 44, 251, 340

mydriasis, 217

myoglobinuria, 278

nausea, 18, 31, 66, 69, 115, 128, 140, 251, 313

nephropathy/renal failure, 31, 252

nervousness/agitation, 66, 115, 217, 340

oral ulceration, 139, 302

photosensitization, 326

plasma cyclosporin reduction, 326

platelet aggregation inhibition, 32

potassium loss, 278

pulmonary edema, 278

respiratory arrest, 302

rhinitis, 160

sedative effects, 32

seizures, 115

skin odor, 160

sodium retention, 278

spinal epidural hematoma, 160

strokes, 115

tongue spasms, 302

tongue swelling, 139

tremors, 115, 340

urinary tract infections, 313, 317

adverse effects (cont.)

urination disturbances, 115

water retention, 278

weakness, 115

withdrawal symptoms, 356

adverse event reports (AERs), xviii, 111–112, 115, 262

Aegle marmelos, 383

aescin, 251

Aesculaforce®, 252, 255, 401

Aesculus hippocastanum, **247–258**

AF Nutraceutical Group, Inc., 33, 405

affective (emotional) disorders. *see also* anxiety; depression; mood; well-being/quality of life

agitation, 114, 115

anger, 70

approach-avoidance conflict, 355

bright light therapy, 333

daily stress, 270

dysphoria, 71, 205

emotional disturbances from dementia, 195

irritability, 16, 18, 70, 71, 215, 354

as adverse effect, 115, 217, 340

panicky states, 340

restlessness, 71, 114, 115, 263, 270, 354, 361, 376

as adverse effect, 340

seasonal affective disorder (SAD), 324, 327, 333

aflatoxin resistance, 216

Agathosma betulina, 76

aged garlic extract (AGE), 156, 162, 169, 170, 399

aging, 215, 224. *see also* elderly patients

agitation, 114, 115

Agnolyt®, 67, 69, 70, 71, 72, 398

agnuside, 64, 65

AHPA Safety Rating, xxviii

AIDS patients. *see* HIV patients

aji pepper, 42

ajoene, 157

akuammigine, 28

alanine aminotransferase (ALT), 264, 283, 289, 293, 294, 346, 378

albumin/globulin quotient, 294

alcohol

absorption, 380

abuse, 381

alcohol-induced disorders, 56, 216, 288, 290, 293, 294, 380

blood-alcohol levels, 217, 364

consumption, 265, 325

interactions, 326, 356, 364

alcohol (cont.)
  intoxication, 265
aldosteronism, 278, 279, 283, 377, 378
Alena™, 148, 152, 399
alkaline drugs, 341
alkaline elution, 36
alkaline phosphatase, 152, 380
alkamides, 89
allergic alveolitis, 44
allergies. *see* hypersensitivity
allicin, 157, 158, 161
alliin, 157, 161
alliinase, 157
Allium sativum, **153–170**
allspice, 383
Alluna™, 357, 363, **374,** 403
allyl methyl trisulfide, 157, 158
Aloe ferox, xx
aloe vera, 409
alpha-amylase activity, 339
alpha blockers, 313
alpha-linolenic acid (ALA), 146, 150, 151
alpha-reductase, 387
Alpinia galanga, 182
alprazolam, 265
Althaea officinalis, 276
altitude sickness, 101, 188, 191, 198. *see also* hypoxia
alveolar macrophages, 225
alveolitis, 44
Alyt®, 67, 70, 398
Alzheimer's disease, 188, 191, 195. *see also* memory
Amanita mushroom poisoning, 288, 289, 290, 295
ambroxol, 389
American Association of Poison Control Centers, xviii
American Botanical Council, vi, xiv, xvi
American Council on Pharmaceutical Education, xvi
American Dietetic Association, xvi
American ginseng, **201–209,** 216
American Herbal Products Association (AHPA), xix, 110, 116
American Medical Association, xv, 110
American Nurses Credentialing Center, xvi
aminoterminal propeptide, 222
aminotransferase levels, 290, 295
amiodarone, 90
amitriptyline, 326, 327, 332, 341
ammonia, fecal, 339, 349
ammonium chloride, 116

amoebicidal agents, 231
amoxicillin, 217
amyloid-β-protein toxicity, 370
anabolic steroids, 90
anaerobic threshold, 239, 244
analgesics, 42, 263, 301, 305, 308
anaphylaxis, 55, 56, 90, 252. *see also* hypersensitivity
androgens. *see* hormones
anemia, 157, 158, 215, 341
anesthetics, 263
Angelica acutiloba, 377
angina, 245, 375, 383, 384
angiogenesis, 339
angiotensin-converting enzyme (ACE), 44, 115, 370
angle-closure glaucoma, 115
animal protein drugs, 32
anise seed, 276
ankle circumference, 252, 255, 256
ankle edema, 244
ano-genital inflammations, 54
anorexia, 114, 116, 120, 293, 377, 378
anovulatory cycles, 65, 70, 151
antacids, 282, 302
Anthemis spp., 54, 56
anthocyanidins, 6
anthocyanins, 7, 77
anthocyanosides, 6, 7
anti-inflammatories
  berberine, 231
  bilberry, 7
  cat's claw, 26, 27, 28, 29, 30, 33
  cayenne, 49
  chamomile, 55
  cranberry combination, 76
  feverfew, 139
  flax, 147
  ginger, 175
  horse chestnut, 251
  licorice, 277
  milk thistle, 289
  Padma®28/Basic, 383, 384
  Phytodolor®, 385
  Pycnogenol®, 370
  saw palmetto, 313
  Sinupret®, 388
antibacterials
  Asian ginseng, 217, 225

antibacterials (cont.)

  berberine, 232, 234

  chamomile, 55

  cranberry, 76, 77, 82

  feverfew, 139

  garlic, 158

  ginger, 175

  goldenseal, 231

  Hochu-ekki-to®, 377

  peppermint, 301

  Sinupret®, 388

  St. John's wort, 325

antibiotic potentiation, 102

antibody production, 90

anticoagulants. *see also* thrombosis; warfarin

  interaction with Asian ginseng, 217

  interaction with cat's claw, 32

  interaction with feverfew, 140

  interaction with garlic, 159, 160

  interaction with ginkgo, 190

  interaction with goldenseal, 231

  interaction with horse chestnut, 252

  interaction with saw palmetto, 313

  interaction with St. John's wort, 326

antifungals, 157, 158, 175

antimetabolite drugs, 101

antioxidants

  American ginseng, 205

  bilberry, 7

  cat's claw, 26, 27, 29, 36

  cranberry, 77

  eleuthero, 101

  flax, 146

  garlic, 157, 158

  ginger, 175

  ginkgo, 189

  hawthorn, 240

  horse chestnut, 251

  licorice, 277, 279, 283

  milk thistle, 289

  Padma®28/Basic, 383

  Pycnogenol®, 370

  tea, 338, 339, 340, 346

antitumor. *see* tumor inhibitors

antivirals. *see also* herpes

  general, 301

antivirals (cont.)

  HIV (human immunodeficiency virus), 90, 206, 216, 223, 375

  influenza virus, 325

  polio virus, 77

  retrovirus, 27, 29, 38, 325

  rhinovirus, 30, 175

  vesicular stomatitis virus, 30

anxiety

  as adverse effect, 340

  anxiety disorder, 262

  anxiety-like conditions, 100

  and cerebral insufficiency, 191, 196

  in childbirth, 60

  as contraindication, 114, 340

  and insomnia, 100, 354, 362

  premenstrual, 71

  reduced symptoms, 245, 266, 270, 331, 333, 357, 361

  sedation, 354

anxiolytics, 55, 216, 263, 265, 266

aphrodisiacs, 215

aphthous ulcers, 276, 279, 282

apigenins, 54, 55, 301, 325

apoptosis, 27, 29, 146, 148, 152, 189, 313, 373

appetite, premenstrual, 71

appetite reduction, 215, 264, 295, 377

Aquilegiae vulgaris, 383

arabinogalactans, 89, 277

arabinose, 77, 89, 147, 312, 370

arabinoxylan, 89

arachidonic acid, 127, 162, 170, 231

Arctostaphylos uva-ursi, 76

arcurcumene, 174

arginine, 355

Arkocaps®, 341, 403

Arkopharma Laboratories, 341, 405

arnica hypersensitivity, 55, 90

aromatase, 387

arrest of descent, in childbirth, 133

arrhythmia. *see also* heart rate

  as adverse effect, 115

  animal studies, 277

  cardiac arrhythmia, 115

  cardiovascular antiarrhythmic action, 231

  drug interactions, 278

  effect of hawthorn, 244

  effect of valerian, 355

arrhythmia (cont.)
  proarrhythmic action, 231
  respiratory sinus arrhythmia (RSA), 271
  tachycardia, 66, 114, 115, 234, 278, 361
  ventricular arrhythmia, 231, 234, 278
Artemisia absinthium, 288
arteries. *see also* atherosclerosis; vascular conditions
  aortic stiffness, 157, 169
  arterial compliance, 150
  arterial pressure, 60, 150
  coronary artery, 182, 231, 240
  peripheral arterial occlusive disease (PAOD)
    and garlic, 156, 162, 170
    and ginkgo, 188, 189, 191, 192, 197
    and Padma®28, 383, 384
  radial artery pulse, 205
arteriosclerotic dementia, 196
arthritis. *see also* osteoarthritis
  chronic epicondylitis, 386
  general, 140, 148, 289
  psoriatic, 128, 132
  rheumatoid
    adjunct therapy, 27
    ineffective treatments, 140, 142, 148, 152
    morning stiffness, 28, 33, 37, 134
    pain reduction, 28, 33, 42, 45, 50
    potential treatment, 126, 146, 385, 386
    reduced inflammation, 49
articanin, 139
articular index, 134
arylamine N-acetyltransferase, 277
ascorbic acid, 43
ash, common, 385
Asian ginseng, 100, 204, **211–225,** 377, 410
aspartate aminotransferase (AST), 264, 289, 293, 294, 346, 378
aspen, 385
aspirin, 43, 44, 47, 113, 116, 140, 160, 190
ASTA Medica AG, 57
aster hypersensitivity, 55
asthenia/weakness
  as adverse effect, 115, 378
  from cerebrovascular insufficiency, 197
  debility, 100
  from diabetic neuropathy, 134
  functional asthenia, 100, 339
  menopausal, 223

asthenia/weakness (cont.)
  psychophysical, 224
  symptom of liver disease, 264, 293
  in TCM theory, 215
asthma. *see also* hypersensitivity; respiratory tract conditions
  as adverse effect, 160
  bronchial, 112, 276
  bronchial relaxation, 216, 341
  and ephedra, 110, 112
  and ginkgo, 191, 198
  and Pycnogenol®, 369, 370, 371, 373
  traditional Chinese medicine, 205, 276
Astragalus membranaceus, 377
astringents, xx, 7, 55, 56, 59, 76
ataxia, 30, 355
atherosclerosis
  aortic, 345
  atherogenesis, 146, 150
  atherogenic index, 339, 347
  general, 100, 175, 215, 370, 383
  plaque, 156, 158, 161, 169
  risk reduction, 146, 147, 153, 156, 157, 161, 338
  treatment, 162, 346
athletes, 91, 96, 102, 105, 112, 113, 218
athletic performance. *see also* exercise
  and American ginseng, 206, 209
  and Asian ginseng, 214, 218, 222, 223, 224
  and ephedra, 110, 111, 112, 113, 114
  physical fitness, 105, 223
atopic dermatitis, 126, 127, 128, 132, 133
Atractylodes lancea, 377
atrial fibrillation, chronic, 199
attention. *see* concentration
aucubin, 65
auditory disturbances, 102
auditory reaction time, 224
Australian Antigen Positive hepatitis, 380
autoimmune diseases, 31, 90, 91, 375. *see also* HIV
Axsain®, 45, 48, 49, 398
Ayurvedic medicine, 366, 367
Azadirachta indica, 383
azinobis ethyl benzthiazoline sulfonic acid (ABTS), 27
Azo-Cranberry®, 78, 81, 398

B
Bacillus spp., 158, 301
bacteria levels, fecal, 349

bacterial adherence, 77

bacterial clearance, 217, 225

bacteriostatic effects, 55, 114, 301

bacteriuria, 77, 78, 81, 82

baldrinal, 355

Ballota spp., 361

Baptisia tinctoria, 89, 92, 375

barbital metabolism, 101

barbiturates, 102, 265, 356

barium enemas, 300, 302, 305

barley, 409

barringtogenol, 251

bathmotropic effects, 239

Bayer Vital GmbH & Co., 328, 405

Beaufour-Ipsen, 405

behavior

    activities of daily living (ADL), 189

    activity levels, 106

    aggressiveness, 71, 355

    behavioral disturbances, 362

    fearful behaviors, 355

    obsessive-compulsive disorder, 324, 327, 334

    restless behaviors (*see under* nervous conditions)

    sleep behavior, 245

    social behavior, 195, 197

benefits of herbal products, xxi

Bengal quince, 383

benign prostatic hyperplasia, 115, 265, 312, 314, 317–319, 387

Benton Test of Visual Retention, 195

benzodiazepines, 265, 270, 354, 355, 356, 357, 363

benzoic acid, 370

benzopyrene binding, 127

benzoyl peroxide-induced tumors, 289

berberastine, 231

berberine, 230–232

beta-blocker drugs, 114, 115

beta-carotene, 382

bias against herbal medicine, xxv, 409

bifidobacteria levels, 349

bilberry, **3–12,** 409

bile. *see also* gallbladder

    cholagogic agents, 175, 232, 289, 301

    cholangitis, 294

    cholestatic liver disorders, 264, 277

    ducts, obstructions, 264, 302

    ducts, spasms, 300

bile (cont.)

    salts, 289

bilirubin, 231, 232, 289, 293, 294, 378, 380

bilobalide, 189, 190

binomial names, xix

Bio-Biloba®, 192, 199, 400

Bio-Quinone, 199

Bioforce AG, 91, 252, 328, 405

biological-protectives, 101

biomembrane damage, 158

Bionorica AG, 67, 381, 388, 405

bird pepper, 42

birth control pills. *see* contraceptives

bisabolane sesquiterpenes, 55

bisabolol, 60

bisaolene, 174

black cohosh, **13–22,** 409, 410

Blackmores, Ltd., 176, 181, 405

Blackmores ginger, 400

bladder, neurogenic, 78, 81

bladder, pediatric neuropathic, 78, 82

bladder cancer, 157, 158, 222

bladder outlet obstruction, 314, 319

bladder surgery, 82

bladder tonic, 76

bleeding. *see* hemorrhage/bleeding

bloating, 54, 70, 71, 128, 300, 306

blood. *see also* circulation; hemorrhage/bleeding; thrombosis

    bleeding time, 176, 182

    blood viscosity, 152

    clots (*see* thrombosis)

    ecchymoses, 372

    erythrocytes, 289, 373

    erythrocytosis, 32

    hematomas, 160, 250, 252, 258

    hemodynamic properties, 231

    hemoglobin, 222

    hyperemia, 43, 47

    hypoxia, 101, 188, 189, 191, 200

    ischemia, 169, 189, 231, 289, 339, 341, 345

    leukemia, 30, 31, 101

    leukocytes, 27, 28, 29, 33, 36, 37, 89, 223

    leukopenia, 29, 375

    plasma, 32

    plasma antioxidant activity, 338, 341, 345, 346

    plasma protein binding, 252

    serum microglobulin, 223

blood (cont.)
  serum protein carbonyl content, 150
blood alcohol levels, 217, 364
blood glucose/glycemia
  increased
    by ephedra, 113
  reduced
    by American ginseng, 205, 209, 217, 222
    by bilberry, 6
    by eleuthero, 101, 102
    by garlic, 157
    by milk thistle, 295
  and thermogenesis, 121
  unchanged
    by flax, 148, 152
    by garlic, 161, 168
blood pressure
  increased
    by chamomile, 60
    by ephedra, 115, 121
    by licorice, 283
    by tea, 345
  reduced
    by cat's claw, 29
    by ephedra, 112, 114, 120
    by garlic, 157, 161, 167
    by hawthorn, 244
    by Pycnogenol®, 373
    by valerian, 355
  unaffected by garlic, 169
blue cohosh hypersensitivity, 381
BNO-1095, 67, 69, 398
Boehringer-Ingelheim, 405
bone cancer, 127
bone formation, 152
bone loss/resorption, 17, 146, 148, 152. *see also* osteoporosis
bone marrow transplants, 31
bone mineral density, 349
bonnet pepper, 42
Borago officinalis, 128
borborygmi, 305
bornyl acetate, 65, 139
bornyl angelate, 139
botanical nomenclature, xix
bowel conditions
  anal prolapse, 377
  colonoscopy, 300

bowel conditions (cont.)
  colostomies, 300, 305
  constipation, 32, 115, 146, 371
  diverticulitis, 146
  fecal flora, 339, 341, 349
  fecal moisture, 339, 349
  hemorrhoids, 12, 44, 250, 377
  ileus (bowel obstruction), 147
  irritable bowel, 44, 146, 300, 302, 305–306
  light-colored stools, 264
  loose stools, 128
  pH, 339, 349
  polyps, colorectal, 161, 170, 306
bowel movements, 152, 306
brain cancer, 33, 37
brands of herbal products, xxiii, xxviii
breast cancer
  apoptosis, 370
  growth suppression, 17, 18, 30, 77, 127, 147, 206, 340
  recurrence reduction, 338, 347
  risk reduction, 146, 148, 151, 157
  unaffected, 222
breast swelling/tenderness, 12, 64, 66, 70, 71, 372. *see also under* pain
breath odor, 160
bromazepam, 266, 270
bromocriptine, 115, 131
bromsulphalein, 294, 295
bronchial asthma, 112, 276
bronchitis. *see also* respiratory tract conditions
  bacterial clearance, 217, 225
  and common cold, 94
  general treatment, 110, 276, 375, 388, 389
  and influenza, 105
  macrophage activity, 225
bronchoconstriction, 44, 139, 189
bronchodilation, 112, 113, 115, 216, 341
bronchospasms, 112, 388
brown adipose tissue (BAT), 113, 115–116
Brown's pepper, 42
BT-549 cells, 30
buchu leaf, 76
bufexamac, 59
Bupleurum falcatum, 377
burden of proof in herbal safety, xx
Burkholderia pseudomallei, 264
burning sensation, 49

burns, 324

butyrophenones, 290, 295

C

C-MED-100®, 33, 36, 398

C-peptide level, 189

caffeic acid, 89, 239, 301, 325, 355, 370

caffeine, 216, 240, 338, 339, 341

caffeine-ephedrine interaction, 111, 112, 113–114, 115–116, 120

caffeine-ginseng synergy, 217

caftaric acid, 89

calcium antagonists, 30

calcium excretion, urinary, 83

calcium mobilization, 313

calcium oxalate stones, 78

calendula, 383

calgranulin activity, 370

Camellia sinensis, 115, **335–349**

CAMOCARE®, 57, 398

Campamed, LLC, 32, 405

campesterol, 28, 30, 127, 147, 289

camphor, 139, 355, 357, 383

canadaline, 231

canadine, 231

cancer. *see* bladder cancer; bone cancer; brain cancer; breast cancer; cervical cancer; colorectal cancer; endometrial cancer; esophageal cancer; laryngeal cancer; liver cancer; lung cancer; oral cancer; ovarian cancer; pancreatic cancer; prostate cancer; renal cancer; skin cancer; stomach cancer

cancer prevention. *see* chemoprevention; tumor inhibitors

cancer treatment
    cancer therapy adjuncts, 27, 33, 37, 100, 191, 232
    chemotherapy side effects, 29, 54, 59, 158, 174, 183, 377
    extracorporeal chemotherapy (photopheresis), 183
    interaction with cat's claw, 32
    radiation therapy, 27, 29, 33, 37, 54, 59, 100, 158, 375

Candida spp., 158, 301, 325

candidiasis, 76, 88, 90, 91, 96, 162, 170

canin, 139

Cantox Health Sciences International (CHSI), 112

Cantox Toxicological Review, 113

caper stem bark, 76

capillary fragility, 6, 7, 12

capillary permeability, 7, 190, 251

Capparis spinosa, 379

capsaicin, 42, 43

capsaicinoids, 43

Capsicum spp., xx, **39–50**

Capsig®, 45, 50, 398

captopril, 244

carbamazepine clearance, 326, 334

carbohydrate oxidation, 43, 47

carboxy alkyl esters (CAEs), 26, 27, 28, 29, 32

carboxystrictosidine, 28

cardiac assessments
    cardiac index, 60, 231, 234
    cardiac muscle strength, 175
    cardiac output, 60, 245
    cardiac work tolerance, 239
    cardio-respiratory endurance, 204
    conductive dysfunction (ECGs), 334
    echocardiography, 241, 244
    electrocardiograms (ECGs), 245, 334
    heart function, 120
    pressure/rate product, 239, 244, 245
    radionuclide angio-cardiography, 245
    stroke index (stroke volume), 60, 231, 234
    ventricular ejection fraction, 231, 234, 238, 239, 244, 245

cardiac disorders. *see also* heart rate; vascular conditions
    angiocardiopathy, 215
    anxiety-related, 361
    atrial fibrillation, chronic, 199
    cardiac failure, 215, 230, 234, 238, 241, 244, 245
    cardiac insufficiency, 191, 200, 239, 241, 244, 245, 355
    cardiogenic shock, 215
    coronary disease, 114, 161, 169, 245, 338, 341, 346, 347
    flax as heart attack preventive, 148
    heart irregularities as adverse effect, 340
    myocardial infarction, 101, 115, 150, 161, 241, 338, 339, 341, 346
    myocarditis, 115
    nervous heart complaints, 238
    non-specific, 355
    NYHA Stages I, II, or III, 238, 239, 241, 244, 245
    pressure in cardiac region, 238
    and valerian, 355, 357

cardiac function. *see also* cardiac assessments; exercise
    bathmotropic effects, 239
    chronotropic effects, 30, 355
    dromotropic effects, 239
    inotropic effects, 30, 231, 239, 240, 355
    physical fitness, 105, 223
    stamina, 102, 105

cardiac glycosides, 115, 240

cardiotonics, 240

cardomom, 383

carminatives, 55, 301

carotenoids, 43

carvone, 301

caryophyllene, 65

cascara sagrada, xx

Cassia occidentalis, 379

Cassia senna, xx

casticin, 64, 65

catalase, 339, 370

cataracts, 6

catechin bioavailability, 349

catechins

    antioxidant activity, 345, 346

    bio-availability, 349

    component of bilberry, 7

    component of cat's claw, 28

    component of cranberry, 77

    component of St. John's wort, 325

    component of tea, 338, 339

    component of Pycnogenol, 369, 370

    and oxygen consumption, 115-116

    and phagocytosis, 30

catechol-O-methyl transferase, 116, 340

catecholamines, 44, 47, 209, 224

Catharanthus roseus, xvii

catheterization, cardiac, 57, 60

catheterization, urinary, 81

cat's claw, **23–38,** 409, 410

Caulophyllum thalictroides, 381

Caved-S®, 279, 282, 401

cayenne, **39–50,** 409

cayenne hypersensitivity, 44

CD4 cells, 27, 29, 33, 37, 38, 215, 223

CD8 cells, 37, 293

celandine, 264

cell proliferation, prostatic, 313

cell viability, 158. *see also* cytoprotectants

cellular defense, 105

cellular immune system, 101

Center for Foods and Applied Nutrition (CFSAN), xviii

central nervous system, 101, 190, 191, 199, 363

central nervous system depressants, 55, 265, 357

central nervous system stimulants, 113, 114, 325, 339

Cephaelis ipecacuanha, xx

cerebral conditions. *see* craniocerebral conditions

cervical cancer, 222

cervix, cytological smears, 223

Cetraria islandica, 383

CFSAN Adverse Event Reporting System (CAERS), xviii

Chai-Na-Ta®, 400

Chai-Na-Ta Corp., 206, 209, 405

chalcones, 263, 277

Chamaemelum nobile, 54, 56

chamazulene, 55, 59, 60

chamomile, 276, 409

chamomile, German, **51–60**

chamomile hypersensitivity, 90, 139

Chamomilla recutita, **51–60**

chaste tree, **61–72**

chaste tree hypersensitivity, 381

chebulic myrobalan, 383

chelation of metal ions, 205, 383

Chelidonium majus, 264

chemical standardization, xix

chemistry of herbs, xxvi

chemoprevention

    breast cancer, 340

    colon cancer, 347

    general, 7, 101, 162, 175, 277, 279

    liver cancer, 283

    oral cancer, 347

chemoprotection (against DMBA, urethane, aflatoxin), 216

childbirth. *see* pregnancy

children. *see also* infants

    bronchospasms, 112

    contraindicated, 31, 114, 139, 251, 302, 356, 377, 385

    coughs, 276

    dermatitis, 132

    diarrhea, 6, 54, 57, 60

    giardiasis, 234

    and herbal product storage, xxv

    infections, 76, 78, 81, 82, 383

    motion sickness, 179

chili pepper, 42

Chinese goldthread rhizome, 76

Chinese multi-herb products, 366

chlamydia, 231

Chlamydia trachomatis, 234

chlorogenic acid, 89, 231, 239, 301, 325, 355

chlorothiazide, 278

chlorpromazine, 355

chlorthalidone, 278

cholchicine, xvii

cholelithiasis. *see under* gallbladder

cholera, 231

cholesterol. *see* lipids

choline, 55, 325, 355

cholinesterase, 191, 301

Chondrodendron tomentosum, xvii

chronic fatigue syndrome, 100, 377

chronotropic effects, 30, 355

chrysanthemum hypersensitivity, 55, 90, 139

Chrysanthemum parthenium, **135–142**

chrysanthenyl acetate, 139

Ciba-Geigy AG, 67, 358, 405

cicatrizing activity, 90

cichoric acid, 89

Cichorium intybus, 379

cimetidine, 265, 282

Cimicifuga racemosa, **13–22,** 410

Cimicifuga simplex, 377

cimicifugoside, 17

cimigoside, 17

cimiracemosides, 17

cinchonain, 28, 30

cineole, 65, 301

cinnamic acid, 370

Cinnamomum camphora, 355, 383

circulation. *see also* vascular conditions
    capillaries, 6, 7, 12, 190, 251, 370
    cerebral circulation, 114, 189
    circulatory complaints, as adverse effects, 32
    coronary circulation, 239, 245, 355
    general, 206, 216, 218, 383
    impaired circulation, 18
    microcirculation, 6, 157, 169, 371, 373
    peripheral, 8, 157, 162, 170

cirrhosis, 232, 277, 290, 293, 294, 380

cisapride, 302, 307

citric acid, 77, 113

Citrus unshiu, 377

clary sage, 57, 60

clavulanic acid, 217

Clinical Global Impression (CGI) scale, 22, 71, 195, 307, 331, 332, 333, 334

Clinical Overview, xxix

clinical studies, xxviii

clobazam, 361

Clostridium spp., 158

clots, blood. *see* thrombosis

clotting time, 157, 160, 217

clove, 383

CNT2000™, 206, 400

co-dergocrine, 191

Cognex, 295

cognition. *see also* concentration; memory
    abstract thinking skills, 224
    alertness, 102, 223, 224, 325, 357, 364, 377
    Alzheimer's/dementia, 188, 189, 191, 195, 196
    amnesia, 205, 216
    cognitive impairment in elderly, 191, 195, 197
    cognitive/mental performance
        and American ginseng, 205, 209
        and Asian ginseng, 215, 224
        effects of alcohol, 265
        and eleuthero, 102, 106
        and flax, 147
        and ginkgo, 191, 192, 197
        and kava, 266, 271
        and peppermint, 308
        and Pycnogenol®, 370
        and St. John's wort, 325
        and valerian, 364
    cognitive restructuring, 114
    error-detection in proofreading, 205, 206, 209, 224
    errors of commision, 308
    figure connection test, 196
    impaired judgment, 356
    learning enhancement, 189, 195, 196
    mathematical performance, 197, 209
    psychometric performance, 364
    vigilance, 197, 308, 364
    word recognition tasks, 197

coitus frequency, 225

Cola nitida, 111, 116

Cola spp., 120, 361

Colchicum autumnale, xvii

cold exposure/hypothermia, 188, 198, 216, 355

cold limbs (TCM theory), 215

cold receptors, nasal, 301

cold sensations, neuropathic, 134

cold sores, 375

cold sweats, 180

colic, 276

collagen, 7, 139, 169, 231, 290

collagenosis, 90, 375

colorectal cancer
  diallyl disulfide as preventative, 158
  flax as preventative, 147
  garlic as preventative, 156, 157, 161, 162, 170
  2nd line treatment, 191, 199
  tea as preventative, 338, 340, 341, 347, 348
colostomies, 300, 305
Colpermin®, 302, 305, 306, 402
columbine, 383
combinations of herbs. *see* herbal combinations
Commission on Dietary Supplement Labels, xxi
common ash, 385
common colds. *see also* respiratory tract conditions
  nasal congestion, 112
  prevention, 223
  treatment, 54, 57, 60, 91, 94, 95, 156
complementary and alternative medicine (CAM), xxi–xxii
concentration (mental)
  and cerebral insufficiency, 188, 189, 191, 195, 196
  effects of eleuthero, 102, 106
  effects of ginseng, 224
  effects of peppermint, 308
  effects of St. John's wort, 325
  effects of valerian, 357, 364
  and fatigue, 100
  and premenstrual syndrome, 71
  prolonged attention, 308
conjunctivitis, allergic, 55
constipation, 32, 115, 146, 371
consumer use of herbal supplements, xvii, xxi
ConsumerLab.com, xvii
contraceptives, 8, 12, 26, 66, 326
contraindications, xxvii
contrast sensitivity, 100, 106
convalescence, 100
conventional drugs from plants, xvii
conventional medicine, xxi–xxiii
cooling effects, 55, 56, 59
cooling (TCM theory), 366
coordination, 224, 265
copper serum concentrations, 294
Coptis chinensis, 76, 230
CoQ10, 199
coronary artery, 182, 231, 240
coronary circulation, 239, 245, 355
corpus luteum abnormalities, 64, 66, 69, 70, 381
corticoid treatments, 278

corticosteroids, 90, 115, 258
cortisol, 96, 326, 333
corynantheine, 28, 30
corynoxeine, 28, 30
corypalmine, 231
coryza, acute, 112
costus, 383
coughs, 44, 114, 156, 205, 215, 276. *see also* respiratory tract conditions
Coumadin®, 159, 160, 170
cowslip, 276
cramps, menstrual, 370
cramps, muscular, 12, 250, 257, 370, 372, 383
cranberry, **73–83,** 409, 410
craniocerebral conditions
  brain activity, 189, 199
  brain cell protection, 370
  brain development, 147
  brain injuries, 308
  brain tumors, 37
  cerebral circulation, 114, 189
  cerebral cortex function, 205
  cerebral insufficiency, 188, 189, 191, 195, 196, 197
  cerebral ischemia, 189
  hypoxia, 101, 188, 189, 191, 200
  intracranial pressure, 250, 252, 258
  strokes, 115, 341
crataegolic acid, 239
Crataegus laevigata, **235–245**
Crataegus monogyna, **235–245**
Crataegus Special Extract WS-1442, 241, 244, 245, 401
Crataegus spp., 238, 355, 357, 361
Crataegutt®, 241, 245, 401
Crataeva nurvala, 76
creatinine, 147, 152
cryoprecipitates, 32
cryptococcal meningitis, 157
Cryptococcus spp., 157, 158
Cucurbita pepo, 382
cumaric acid, 370
cyanidin, 7, 77
cyanogenic glycosides, 147
cyclamen hypersensitivity, 381
cyclic AMP, 7, 158, 239-240
cyclic GMP synthesis, 216
cyclooxygenase (COX), 29, 30, 313
cyclosporine, 90, 326

cynarin, 89

cysteine sulfoxides, 157

cystic granular hyperplasia of endometrium, 70

cysticidal activity, 231

cytochrome P450, 56, 277, 326

cytokines, 29, 90, 152, 158

cytoprotectants, 27, 42, 127

cytotoxic lymphocytes, 289, 293

cytotoxicity, 29, 30, 90, 101, 105, 139, 158, 370

D

daily value (nutrients), xxiv

daisy hypersensitivity, 139

Dalidar Pharma, 176, 405

dammarane-type glycosides, 205

dammarane-type saponins, 215

danazol, 131

dandelion, 409

Dansk Droge A/S, 219, 405

Dansk Droge Ginseng, 219, 222, 401

Datura stramonium, xvii

daucosterol, 101

deafness, 188, 191, 199

deathcap mushroom poisoning, 289

deaths, 115

defecation. *see* bowel movements

delphinidin, 7

dementia, 188, 189, 191, 195, 196. *see also* memory

demulcents, xx, 276, 277

deodorants, 55

deoxyribose degradation, 27, 29

depolarization in ventricles, 334

depression

    antidepressant drugs, 190, 326, 327, 334

    antidepressant effects, 216, 324, 325, 355

    and cerebral insufficiency, 188, 196

    as contraindication, 114, 189, 264

    and dementia, 195

    depressive syndrome, 224

    menopausal, 16, 18, 22, 223, 270

    mild to moderate depression, 324, 325, 327, 331–333, 334

    premenstrual, 71

    severe depression, 191, 200, 327, 328, 331

depsides, 339

dermatological conditions. *see also* herpes; pruritus/itching

    abrasions, 54, 57, 59, 90

    acne, 32, 64, 66, 67, 72, 381

dermatological conditions (cont.)

    bacterial infections, 375

    bruises (*see* hematomas)

    cicatrizing activity, 90

    dermatitis

        atopic, 126, 127, 128, 132, 133

        in children, 126, 132

        chronic, 128, 132

        contact, 55, 56, 139, 160, 252

        neurodermatitis, 54, 59, 90

        seborrhoeic, 126

        ulcerative, 12

        zosteriform, 160

    dry skin, 132

    dyschromia, 12

    ecchymoses, 372

    eczema, 90, 128, 377

    epidermal thinning, 133

    erythema, 83, 132, 326, 333, 388

    exanthemas, 66, 381, 388

    hair loss, 66

    ichthyosis, 264

    inflammatory dermatoses, 54, 57, 59

    lichenoid reaction, 302

    melanin index, 333

    pemphigus, 160

    peristomial conditions, 83

    perspiration, 16, 17, 113, 361, 377

    psoriasis, 42, 45, 49, 370

    purpuras, 6

    rashes, 66, 69, 378

    rete ridge flattening, 133

    rubefacients, 43

    shingles (herpes zoster), 42

    skin cancer, 127, 175, 289

    skin lesions/ulcers, 43, 44, 49, 251

    skin metabolism stimulants, 55

    skin odor, 160

    skin reactions, non-specific, 71

    uremic skin symptoms, 126, 128, 132

    urticaria, 44, 55, 66, 160, 378

    vesiculation, 388

    wounds, 55, 88, 90, 251, 324

descriptions of herbs, xxvi

detoxifying enzymes, 339

detrusor pressure, 319

detumescence, early, 216

dexamethasone clearance, 115

diabetes. *see also* insulin

    as contraindication, 114, 277

    lactose- and gluten-free tablets, 383

    and liver disease, 288, 295

    nephropathy, 127

    neuropathy, 42, 43, 45, 48, 49, 128, 133, 134

    non-insulin dependent (type II), 152, 204, 205, 206, 209, 214, 218, 222

    retinopathy, 6, 11, 369

    streptozotocin-induced, 127

    traditional Chinese medicine, 215

    treatment, 7, 102

diallyl sulfides, 157, 158

diaphoretics, 113

diarrhea

    bacterial, 231, 234

    in cancer patients, 377

    in children, 6, 54, 57, 60

    in cholera patients, 231, 234

    dysentery, 102

    general, 230, 232

    in HIV patients, 162, 170

    symptomatic treatment, 338

diarrhea, as adverse effect

    Asian ginseng, 217

    cat's claw, 32

    cranberry, 78

    eleuthero, 102

    feverfew, 139, 140

    Hochu-ekki-to®, 377

    milk thistle, 295

    Pycnogenol®, 371

    St. John's wort, 334

Diarrhoesan®, 57, 60, 398

diastolic blood pressure reduction

    by garlic, 157, 161, 167, 168, 170

    by goldenseal, 231, 234

    by hawthorn, 244

    by Pycnogenol®, 373

diazepam, 22, 181, 355, 357, 361

diclofenac, 386

dietary fiber intake, 151

dietary/herbal supplements, xvii–xxi, xxiv, xxvii, 110–112, 115, 368, 409

Dietary Supplement Health and Education Act of 1994 (DSHEA), xvii, xx, xxi, 368

dietetic technicians, xvi, 431

dieticians, xvi, 431

DietMax®, 116, 120, 399

Difrarel™, 8, 11, 398

digitalis glycosides, 240, 278

Digitalis spp., xvii

digoxin, xvii, 102, 240, 326

dihomogammalinolenic acid (DGLA), 127

dilantin, 290

dimenhydrinate, 176, 179, 180

diosmetin, 301

diphenyl picrylhydrazyl (DPPH), 27, 29

dipyridamole, 341

disclaimers, xxiv, 368

disjunctive reaction time, 224

disorientation, 265

diuresis, 198, 338, 340. *see also* urodynamics

diuretics, 76, 113, 190, 278, 301, 313

dizziness, 114, 188, 191, 196, 197, 223, 265. *see also* vertigo

    as adverse effect, 31, 190, 217, 371

DMBA resistance, 216

DNA protection, 370

DNA repair, 27, 28, 29, 33, 36

DNA synthesis, 17

don quai, 409

donepezil, 191

dopamine, 65, 66, 115, 251, 252, 265, 325

dosages, xxvi

Dr. Loges & Co. GmbH, 57, 405

Dr. Mewes Heilmittel GmbH, 103, 405

Dr. Willmar Schwabe GmbH & Co., 192, 241, 253, 266, 303, 315, 357, 376, 387, 405

Dramamine®, 176

driving impairment, 356, 357, 364

dromotropic effects, 239

droperidol, 181

drug interactions. *see* herb-drug interactions

dry throat, 205

Duboisia spp., xvii

duration of administration, xxvi

dyschromia, 12

dysentery, 102

dyspepsia. *see also* gastrointestinal conditions

    as adverse effect, 69, 139, 356

    gastritis, acute, 44, 231, 301

    gastritis, general, 28, 33, 37, 146, 230

    non-ulcer, 300, 302, 307

    treatment, 54, 230, 276, 288

dysphoria, 71, 205

dyspnea/shortness of breath, 114, 215, 238, 239, 244, 245

dysuria, 313, 318, 339. *see also* urodynamics

E

eating disorders
    anorexia, 114, 116, 120, 293, 377, 378
    appetite reduction, 215, 264, 295, 377
    bulimia, 116

ecchymoses, 372

echinacea, **85–96,** 409, 410

Echinacea angustifolia, 88–90, 375

Echinacea pallida, 88–90, 375

Echinacea Plus®, 91, 94, 399

Echinacea purpurea, 88–90, 375

Echinacin®, 91, 95, 96, 105, 399

echinacoside, 89

Echinaforce®, 91, 94, 96, 399

EchinaGuard®, 91, 94, 399

econazole nitrate cream, 96

EcoNugenics, Inc., 383, 405

Ecstasy, 110

edema
    as adverse effect, 278
    ankle, 244
    cerebral, 189
    general, 251, 313, 339
    inflammations, 29
    nephritis, 112
    post-traumatic, 250
    postoperative, 250
    during pregnancy, 12
    pulmonary, 278
    with Raynaud's, 12
    vascular disorders, 12, 250, 255, 256, 257, 370, 372

Efamast®, 128, 131, 399

Efamol®, 128, 131, 132, 133, 134

Efamol Nutraceuticals Inc., 405

EGb-761, 192, 195, 196, 197, 198, 199, 200, 400

eicosanoid synthesis, 139, 182

ejaculation volume, 319

ejaculatory disturbances, 313, 317. *see also* reproduction

Eladon Ltd., 103, 405

Elagen®, 103, 105, 399

elder, 388

elderberry, 409

elderly patients, 77, 78, 82, 195–197, 224, 334, 377

Elettaria cardamomum, 383

Eleugetic®, 103, 399

Eleukokk®, 103, 105, 399

eleuthero, **97–106**

Eleutherococcus senticosus, **97–106,** 204, 218

eleutherosides, 101

embolisms. *see* thrombosis

emesis, 12, 55, 174, 175, 176, 305. *see also* vomiting

emetics, xx

emmenagogues, 18, 139

endometrial cancer, 161

endometrium, 17, 70, 369, 373

endoscopy, 306

endothelin, 205

energetics (TCM theory), 366

energy, 216, 224, 341, 345

English plantain, 383

ENRECO, Inc., 148, 405

enterobacteriaceae levels, fecal, 349

Enterococcus faecalis, 77

Enteroplant®, 303, 307, 402

Enzymatic Therapy, Inc., 117, 405

Ephedra sinica, xvii, **107–121,** 410

ephedrine, xvii, 110–112, 113

epicondylitis, chronic, 386

epidermal growth factor, 317

epilepsy, temporal lobe, 128

epileptic patients, 127, 128, 190. *see also* seizures

epinephrine, 47, 121, 169, 240

epithelial tissue, 29, 313, 314

Epogam®, 128, 132, 133

erectile dysfunction, 215, 216, 218, 225
    as adverse effect, 313, 319

ergogenic effects, 218, 222

ergogenic parameters, 102

ergogenic response, 209

ergometry, 209, 244, 245

ergospirometry, 244

eructation, 307

erysipelas, swine, 301

erythrocytes, 289, 373

erythrocytosis, 32

Esberitox®, 92, 94, 95, 96, **375,** 399

Escalation™, 117, 120, 399

Escherichia coli, 77, 231, 234, 301, 384

Escherichia spp., 158

escin, 251, 252

esculetin, 251, 252

esculin, 251

esophageal cancer, 215, 222, 338, 341, 348

esophageal reflux, 302

esophageal sphincter, 301

essential fatty acids (EFAs), 126, 127, 128, 132, 133, 134

Essential Nutrient Research Corp. (ENRECO), 148, 405

Essentially Pure Ingredients™, 162–163, 405

Essex cream, 49

estrogen receptor modulator, selective (SERM), 21

estrogen receptors, 18, 217, 277, 340

estrogenic effects, 17, 18, 21, 206, 217

estrogens, 17, 21, 65, 151, 152, 313. *see also* hormones

etoposide, xvii

eubacteria levels, fecal, 349

eudesmolides, 138, 139

Euminz®, 303, 308, 402

Euphytose®, 357, 361, 403

European goldenrod, 385

European multi-herb products, 366

Eurovita Extracts, 176, 182

Euvegal®, 357, 363, 364, 403

evening primrose, **123–134,** 409

EV.Ext-33, 400

EV.Ext-77, 400

evidence-based medicine, xxiii

Excel, 117, 399

Excel Corporation, 117

excess gas production, 54, 300

exercise
  aerobic, 105, 222
  and coronary disease, 241, 244, 245
  endurance, 101, 205, 209, 214, 218, 223, 384
  ephedra/caffeine effects, 114
  immunologic effects, 96

exhaustion, 12, 105, 209, 377. *see also* fatigue

Exolise®, 341, 345, 403

expectoration, 276, 277, 389

Expended Mental Control Test, 195

expiration dates, xxv

expiratory flow, 225

exudates, 251, 313

eyebright, 409

eyes. *see* ophthalmic conditions

eyewashes, 230, 232

F

factor XIII activity, 231

falcarindiol, 205

farnesene, 139

Faros®, 241, 244, 401

fat. *see* adipose tissue

fat composition of human milk, 127, 128, 134

fat intake, 151

fatigue
  as adverse effect, 66, 361
  and cardiovascular disorders, 238, 244, 255
  chronic, 100, 377
  and common colds, 95
  from exercise, 102, 105, 214
  general, 218, 222, 324, 327, 333
  premenstrual, 71
  prostration, 215

fatigue syndrome, chronic, 100, 377

fecal odor, colostomies, 300, 305

Femicur®, 67, 70, 398

fennel seed, 276

ferric-reducing ability, 345

Ferrosan A/S, 176, 406

fertility
  general, 215, 218
  during lactation, 66
  sperm quality, 147, 225, 369, 370
  trying to conceive, 69, 70, 381
  and valerian, 356

ferulic acid, 17, 325, 370

fever, 377

feverfew, **135–142,** 409

fibrinolysis, 43, 44, 48, 157, 383, 384

fibrocystic disease, 66

fibrocystic mastopathy, 381

fibrogenesis, 290, 295

fibroid cysts, 64

fibromyalgia, 42, 45, 50, 354

fibrosis, 295, 380

finasteride, 313, 314, 317, 318, 319

flatulence, 54, 140, 295, 305, 307

flatulent digestive pains, 300

flavone glycosides, 55

flavonoid intake, 347

flavonoids, 7, 28, 139, 189, 239

flavonol glycosides, 77

flavonolignans, 289

flax, **143–152**

flaxseed, 409

FlexAgility®, 400

flu. *see* respiratory tract conditions

flu vaccine response, 223

fluid retention, premenstrual, 71, 381

Fluimucil, 389

flunitrazepam, 364

fluocortin butyl ester, 59

fluorouracil (5-FU), 59, 191, 199

fluoxetine, 327, 331

fluphenazine precipitation, 341

Foeniculum vulgare, 276

follicle-stimulating hormone (FSH), 17, 18, 21, 65, 70, 314, 318. *see also* hormones

Food, Drug & Cosmetics Act, xx

Food and Drug Administration (FDA), xv, xix, xxiv, 110–112, 115, 368

forced expiratory volume, 225

formononetin, 17, 277

Formula One, 110

Fraxinus excelsior, 385

free radical scavengers, 7, 29, 30, 126, 189, 205, 277, 340, 370

FreeLife International LLC, 406

French maritime pine bark extract, **369–373**

frigidity, 215

fructosans, 89

G

G115®, 219, 401

GABA, 325, 355

galactose, 89, 147, 312

galactoside, 101

galacturonic acid, 147

galanga, 182

gallbladder. *see also* bile

cholecystectomy, 288, 295

cholecystitis, 232, 302

cholelithiasis, 175, 302

spasms, 300

gallic acid, 370

gamma-glutamyl transferase, 134

gamma-glutamyl transpeptidase (GGT), 289, 294

gamma-glutamylcysteines, 157

gamma-linolenic acid (GLA), 126, 127, 128, 132

ganglion blockage, 114

garlic, **153–170,** 409

garlic hypersensitivity, 159

gastric cancer. *see* stomach cancer

gastric complaints as adverse effect

black cohosh, 18, 22

chaste tree, 66, 69, 71, 78

feverfew, 139

ginkgo, 189

Hochu-ekki-to®, 378

horse chestnut, 251

Mastodynon®, 381

milk thistle, 295

Padma®28/Basic, 383

Phytodolor®, 385

Prostagutt®, 387

Pycnogenol®, 371

saw palmetto, 313, 317

St. John's wort, 326, 332

tea, 340–341

valerian, 356

gastrointestinal conditions. *see also* bowel conditions; dyspepsia

absorption of drugs and nutrients, 147, 341, 367, 383

achlorhydria, 302

activity of smooth muscles

migrating motor complex, 307

motility/spasms, 54, 175, 300, 301, 306, 355

relaxants, 301, 306, 307

spasms during barium enemas, 300, 302, 305

spastic colon syndrome, 306

stimulants, 43, 44, 302

bacteria adherence to epithelium, 77

carminatives, 55, 301

colon damage from laxative abuse, 146

colonoscopy, 300

digestive aids, 42, 64, 339

digestive system (TCM theory), 216

enteritis, 146

enterocolitis drug interaction, 102

enteropathy, 29

gastric emptying, 113, 251, 301

gastric function, 180, 302, 377

gastritis, acute, 44, 301

gastritis, general, 28, 33, 37, 146, 230

gastroesophageal reflux, 251, 302

gastrointestinal cancer, 339, 377 (*see also* colorectal cancer; stomach cancer)

gastroprotectants, 27, 29, 44, 47, 277, 289

gastroptosis, 377

ileus (bowel obstruction), 147

gastrointestinal conditions (cont.)
   inflammatory diseases, 54
   intestinal flora, 76, 160, 339, 341, 349
   mucosal irritation, 251, 340–341
   mucosal protection, 43, 44, 47, 127
   NSAID-induced gastric lesions, 134
   NSAID-induced gastritis, 27, 29
   pH in digestive tract, 339
   ulcers, duodenal
      and cayenne, 47
      and licorice, 276, 279, 282
   ulcers, gastric
      and Asian ginseng, 215
      and cat's claw, 26
      and cayenne, 42, 43, 44, 47
      and licorice, 276, 277, 279, 282
   ulcers as contraindication, 44, 114
Gebro Pharma GmbH, 357, 378, 406
Gefarnate, 282
GenDerm Corporation, 45, 406
General Accounting Office (GAO), 111
genetics
   DNA protection, 370
   DNA repair, 27, 28, 29, 33, 36
   DNA synthesis, 17
   genotoxins, 43
   mutagens
      antimutagenic effects, 27, 28, 29, 339
      chromosomal aberrations, 142
      photomutagenesis, 29
   sister chromatid exchanges, 142
Gentiana lutea, 388
geranial, 174
Geriaforce®, 192, 195, 400
geriatric clinical evaluation scale, 197
Gerimax®, 219, 224, 401
germacranolides, 139
germacrene, 139
German Commission E, xviii, xxi, 366
GERRI test, 195
giardiasis, 231, 234
giddiness as adverse effect, 115
ginger, **171–183,** 377, 409
gingerols, 174
Ginkai®, 400
Ginkgo biloba, **185–200,** 409, 410
ginkgo hypersensitivity, 189

Ginkgold®, 192, 195, 199, 400
ginkgolides, 189
Ginkoba® 400
Ginkyo®, 400
Ginsana® G115, 219, 222, 223, 224, 225, 401
ginseng, American, **201–209,** 216
ginseng, Asian, 100, 204, **211–225,** 377, 410
ginseng, Siberian, 100, 204
Ginseng Abuse Syndrome, 217
ginseng (non-specific), 409
ginsenosides, 204, 205, 215, 216, 218
GITLY Kava extract, 266, 270, 401
glaucoma, 114, 115, 116
GlaxoSmithKline, 19, 357, 374, 406
glomerulosclerosis, 147
glossodynia, 59
glucocorticoid drugs, 217
glucosamine, 89
glucosuria. *see* urinary glucose
glutamate, 370
glutamate-dehydrogenase (GLDH), 294
glutamic acid pyruvate transaminase (GPT), 264, 378
glutamine, 355
glutamyltransferase, 264
glutathione, 289, 293, 339, 370
glycans, 113
glycated hemoglobin, 222
glycemia. *see* blood glucose/glycemia
glycoproteins, 89
glycosaminoglycan hydrolases, 257
glycyrrhetic acid, 277
Glycyrrhiza spp., **273–283,** 276, 377, 383
glycyrrhizin, 277
GMP phosphodiesterase, 189
GNC (General Nutrition Centers), 406
GNC's Women's Cycle, 398
golden cinquefoil, 383
goldenrod, European, 385
goldenrod hypersensitivity, 56
goldenseal, 76, **227–234**
gonadal function, 279, 282
good agricultural practices (GAP), xix
good laboratory practices (GLP), xix
good manufacturing practices (GMP), xviii, xix, xx, xxiii
gotu kola, 409
granular layer absence, 133
granulocytes, 30, 38, 90

grape seed, 409

growth factor, 313

guaianolides, 138, 139

guanethidine, 115

guarana, 111, 116, 120, 409. *see also Paullinia* spp.

H

habanero pepper, 42

hairy baby syndrome, 102

halitosis, 160

haloperidol, 66, 341

halothane, 115

Hamamelis virginiana, xx

Hamilton Anxiety (HAMA) scale, 22, 270, 331, 361

Hamilton Depression (HAMD) scale, 331, 332, 333

hangover effects, 355, 362, 364

Harmonicum Much®, 357, 362, 403

hawthorn, **235–245,** 355, 357, 409

headaches. *see also* migraines

    cerebral insufficiency, 188, 191, 196, 197

    cluster, 42, 45, 50

    dysmenorrhea, 12

    general, 339

    high-altitude, 101

    menopausal, 17, 223

    premenstrual, 70, 71, 381

    severe, 114

    tension, 300, 301, 302, 308

headaches, as adverse effect

    black cohosh, 18

    cat's claw, 31

    chaste tree, 66, 69

    eleuthero, 102

    ephedra, 115

    evening primrose, 128

    ginkgo, 190

    Mastodynon®, 381

    Pycnogenol®, 371

    saw palmetto, 319

    tea, 340

    valerian, 356

Health from the Sun, 406

healthcare providers, xxi–xxiii

heart rate. *see also* arrhythmia

    baroreflex control of heart rate (BRC), 271

    cardiac arrhythmia, 115, 231

    and cat's claw, 29

heart rate (cont.)

    chronotropic effects, 30, 355

    and eleuthero, 105

    and ephedra, 112, 113, 121

    and exercise, 209

    and ginseng, 222

    and hawthorn, 239, 244, 245

    increased by imipramine, 334

    palpitations, 16, 18, 101, 115, 189, 238, 244, 245

    reduction, 29, 239, 244, 245, 355

    resting rate, 223

    and valerian, 355

heart tonics, 355

heart valves, mechanical, 199

heartbeat, rapid. *see* tachycardia

HeartCare™, 401

heartleaf sida, 383

heat (TCM theory), 205, 366

heaviness in legs, 250, 255, 370

Hedychium spicatum, 383

Heilmittel, 406

Helicobacter pylori, 77, 157, 158, 277

hellebore, 217

hematomas, 160, 250, 252, 258

hemiplegia, 377

hemoglobin, 222

hemorrhage/bleeding

    as adverse effect, 160, 170, 190

    bleeding disorders, 189

    breakthrough bleeding, 326

    postoperative, 6, 8, 12, 160

    retinal, 6, 11

    surgical, 6, 8, 12

    uterine, 67, 215

    vaginal, 217

hemorrhoids, 12, 44, 250, 372, 377

hepatic disorders. *see also* liver cancer

    alcoholic liver disease, 288, 290, 293, 294, 380

    cholangitic hepatopathies, 294

    cholestatic liver disorders, 264, 277

    chronic liver disease, 294

    cirrhosis, 232, 277, 290, 293, 294, 380

    as contraindication, 264–265, 302

    diabetes and liver disease, 288, 295

    hepatic failure, 276, 279, 283

    hepatotoxicity, 90, 205, 262, 264–265, 290, 295, 383

    jaundice, 231, 264

hepatic disorders (cont.)
  liver cell necrosis, 294
  liver dysfunction, 264, 265, 379
hepatitis
  alcoholic, 293
  Australian Antigen Positive, 380
  cholestatic, 264
  chronic, 276, 290, 294, 380
  drug-induced, 288
  infectious, 288, 380
  necrotizing, 264, 265
  non-specific, 215, 290
  viral, 133, 276, 290, 294
hepatocytes, 294, 326
hepatoprotective agents
  American ginseng, 205
  ephedra, 114
  licorice, 277
  Liv.52®, 379
  milk thistle, 289, 290, 294
  Padma®28, 383
  tea, 346
hepatoxicosis (in ruminants), 289
herb-drug interactions, xix, xxi, xxvii–xxviii
herbal combinations, 218, 366–368, 374–389, 409
Herbal Ecstacy, 110
herbal supplements. see dietary/herbal supplements
Herbs of Commerce, xix, xxiv
Hermes Fabrick Pharma, 163, 406
herpes
  genital, 91, 96, 162, 170
  simplex, 27, 33, 38, 90, 100, 102, 105, 301, 325
  simplex labialis, 375
  zoster (shingles), 42
heterocyclic amine activity, 339
hexobarbital metabolism, 101
high blood pressure. see hypertension
Himalaya Drug Company, 379, 406
hippocaesculin, 251
hippuric acid, 83
hirsuteine, 28, 30
hirsutine, 28, 30
histamines, 43, 49, 139
histidine decarboxylase, 114
HIV drugs, 26, 160, 215, 217
HIV (Human Immunodeficiency Virus), 90, 206, 216, 223, 375

HIV patients
  adjunct therapy, 27, 29, 33, 37, 38
  cautioned about cat's claw, 31
  CD4 T cell counts, 215
  and immunomodulators, 216
  natural killer cell activity, 162, 170
  saquinavir therapy, 160
  zidovudine (AZT) therapy, 26, 215, 217
Hochu-ekki-to®, 367, 377–378
Höfel's® Garlic Pearles, 162, 167, 399
holistic medicine, 367
homeostasis, 105
homocysteine, 157
hongshen, 215, 216
hops, 363, 364, 374, 378
hormones. see also estrogens; testosterone
  androgenization, 102
  androgens, 150, 313
  corpus luteum hormone, 65
  follicle-stimulating hormone (FSH), 17, 18, 21, 65, 70, 314, 318
  growth hormone, 333, 370
  hormone levels, 19, 151, 217
  hormone-like effects, 216
  hormone modulators, 65
  hormone therapy, 17, 18, 19, 21, 66
  luteinizing hormone (LH), 17, 18, 21, 65, 70, 314, 318
  peptide hormone drugs, 32
  progesterone, 64, 65, 66, 69, 70, 282
  progestin, 150
  prolactin, 17, 18, 21, 65, 66, 69, 225, 333
  sex hormone-binding globulin (SHBG), 17, 21
  thyroxin releasing hormone (TRH), 69
Horphag Research, 369, 406
horse chestnut, 247–258
horse chestnut seed extract (HCSE), 250
hot flashes, 16, 17, 21, 22, 128, 133, 263
Hova®, 357, 363, 364, 378, 403
Humulus lupulus, 354, 374, 378
hyaluronidase activity, 251
Hydergine®, 191
hydrastidine, 231
hydrastine, 231
Hydrastis canadensis, 76, 227–234
hydrochloric acid in gastric juice, 302
hydrochlorothiazide, 278
hydrocortisone, 59

hydrogen peroxide, 28, 29, 158

hydrooxyproline, 152

hydroxysteroid-dehydrogenase, 283

hyoscyamine, 305

hyperaldosteronism. *see* aldosteronism

hyperemesis gravidarum, 174, 176, 181

hyperemia, 43, 47

hyperforin, 324, 325, 326

hyperhidrosis, 377

hypericin, 324, 325

Hypericum perforatum, **321–334**, 357, 409, 411

Hyperiforce®, 328, 332, 402

hyperimmunoglobulin therapy, 32

hyperoside, 239, 325

hyperprolactinemia, 64, 66, 67, 69

hypersensitivity. *see also* anaphylaxis

    Asteraceae plants, 55, 56, 90, 139

    blue cohosh, 381

    Caulophyllum thalictroides, 381

    cayenne, 44

    chaste tree, 381

    composite flowers, 375

    cyclamens, 381

    echinacea, 375

    garlic, 159, 160

    ginkgo, 189

    hay fever, 112

    Hochu-ekki-to®, 377

    ignatia, 381

    irises, 381

    lilies, 381

    onions, 160

    ragweed, 55, 90, 139

    St. John's wort, 326

    tulips, 160

hypertension

    as adverse effect, 115, 116, 217, 278, 313, 340

    antihypertensives, 32, 44, 101, 115, 158, 161

    as contraindication, 102, 114, 216, 277

    drug interactions, 115

    and garlic, 156, 161, 168

    and hawthorn, 244

    portal, 293

    and Pycnogenol®, 369, 371, 373

    and valerian, 361

hypnotic effects, 265, 355

hypocorticoidism, 276

hypokalemia, 277, 278, 377, 378

hypotension, 357

hypotensive effects, 115, 355

hypothermia, 355

hypoxia, 101, 188, 189, 191, 200

hysterectomized patients, 18, 19

I

Ibuprofen, 182

ICD p24 antigen, 223

Iceland moss, 383

icterus. *see* jaundice

IdB 1016 Silipide, 291, 294, 402

IDS-89, 315, 317, 402

ignatia hypersensitivity, 381

IL-6 release, 96

ileum contractions, 301

Ilex paraguariensis, 111

imipramine, 327, 331, 332, 334, 341, 355

imminent health hazard, xx

Immodal Pharmaka GmbH, 33, 406

immune complex clearance, 277

immune function, 33, 36, 102, 105, 127, 231

immune support, 218

immunocompetent cells, 101, 105

immunoglobulin therapy, 32

immunologic effects of exercise, 96

immunomodulators

    Asian ginseng, 214, 216, 218, 223

    cat's claw, 26, 29–33, 36

    echinacea, 88, 89, 91

    eleuthero, 101, 102

    Esberitox®, 375

    evening primrose, 127

    garlic, 157, 159

    Hochu-ekki-to®, 377

    horse chestnut, 251

    Sinupret®, 388

immunoprotectants, 102

immunosuppression, 31, 90, 158

impaired concentration, premenstrual, 71

impotence, 215, 313, 317, 377. *see also* reproduction

Indena S.p.A., 8, 291, 406

India, traditional medicine, 366, 367

indigestion. *see* dyspepsia

indinavir clearance, 326

indole alkaloids, 28, 30

indomethacin, 386
inducible nitric oxide synthase (iNOS), 30, 206, 383
infants
    brain development, 147
    colic, 276
    contraindicated, 231, 302, 340
    dermatitis, 126
    formula fortification, 126
infections, acute phase, 102
inflammations
    bile duct, 294
    chronic, 26, 100, 127, 388
    gallbladder, 302
    gastrointestinal tract, 54
    mucosal, 6, 54, 56, 59, 300
    non-specific, 42, 114, 146, 147, 189
    respiratory, 388
    skin, 54, 57, 59, 90
    stomach, acute, 231
    throat, 54
influenza. *see* respiratory tract conditions
inotropic effects, 30, 231, 239, 240, 355
insomnia. *see also* sleep
    as adverse effect, 115, 217, 340, 356
    from anxiety/nervousness, 100, 354, 366
    as contraindication, 114
    general, 357, 362–364, 374, 378
    tradition Chinese medicine, 215
insulin
    dosage monitoring, 7, 206, 217
    insulin-like growth factor, 152
    interaction with herbs, 7, 32, 102, 157
    resistance, 295
    response to, 150, 161
    secretion, 148, 152, 189
    sensitivity, 161
intellectual functions, 197, 215. *see also* cognition
interactions. *see* herb-drug interactions
interferon gamma, 158
interleukin, 158, 325
intermittent claudication. *see* Peripheral Arterial Occlusive
    Disease (PAOD)
internal-heat (TCM theory), 205
International Olympic Committee, 113
International Prostate Symptom Score, 317, 318, 319
intractable pruritus, 42
intrauterine device side effects, 8, 12

inulin, 89
Inverni Della Beffa S.p.A., 406
invertose, 7
ipecac, xx
iridoids, 65, 355
iris hypersensitivity, 381
iron absorption, 341
irritability, 16, 18, 70, 71, 215, 354
    as adverse effect, 115, 217, 340
ischemia
    cardiac, 231, 339, 341, 345
    cerebral, 189
    ischemic mucosal injuries, 289
    juvenile ischemic attack, 169
isoajmalicin, 28
isoorientin, 65
itching. *see* pruritus/itching
IUD. *see* intrauterine device
Ivel®, 357, 363, 403

J

jalapeño peppers, 47
Japan, traditional medicine, 366, 367
Japanese ginseng, 218
Jarsin®, 327, 328, 334, 402
jaundice, 231, 264
jing (TCM theory), 216
joint mobility, 12, 49, 385
joint tenderness, 42
jujube, 377

K

kaempferol, 89, 189, 325
Kamillosan®, 57, 59, 398
Kampo medicine, 366, 367
kanamycin, 102
Kanoldt Arzneimittel GmbH, 357, 406
kava, **259–271,** 409, 410
kavain, 263
kavalactones, 262, 263, 264
KavaPure®, 266, 271, 401
Kavatrol®, 266, 270, 401
Kaveri®, 192, 195, 196, 400
Kavosporal®, 266, 271, 401
KB cells, 30
Kendrick battery test, 196
keratinocytes, 370

kernicterus, 231

ketoalkenes, 89

ketoalkynes, 89

ketoconazole, 90

kidney disorders. *see* renal/kidney disorders

kidney (TCM theory), 101

Kira®, 328, 333, 334, 402

Klebsiella spp., 158

Klinge Pharma GmbH, 406

Kneipp Kamillen-Konzentrat, 57, 60, 398

Kneipp-Werke®, 57, 406

knotweed, 383

KNP Trading Pte. Ltd., 45, 47, 406

kola nut. *see Cola* spp.

Krallendorn®, 28, 32, 33, 37, 38, 398

Kruskal-Wallis test, 305

Kupperman-Menopause Index (KPI), 19, 21, 22

Kwai®, 156, 162, 167, 168, 169, 170, 399

Kwai HeartFit™, 399

Kyolic®, 156, 162, 167, 168, 169, 170, 399, 400

L

L-glutamate uptake, 325

labdane diterpenoids, 65

labeling of herbal products, xx, xxi, xxiv, 368

labiate tannins, 301

labor. *see* pregnancy

Laboratoires Chibret, 8, 406

Laboratori Guidotti S.p.A., 314, 406

lactate levels, 47, 105, 209

lactation
    amenorrhea, 66
    in animals, 65
    beneficial herbs, 126, 147, 160
    as contraindication, 114, 139, 264, 326, 356, 376
    galactogogues, 66, 67
    insufficient, 64
    lactogenic response, 66

lactation contraindications, xxvii

lactic acid, 222

lactobacilli, 76, 81, 349

Laitan®, 266, 270, 271, 401

LAK cells, 158, 377

Lake Louise Self-report score, 198

lanoxin, xvii

laparoscopies, 181

laryngeal cancer, 161, 215, 222

lathosterol, 168

laxatives, xx, 147, 290. *see also* constipation

lectin, 293

Leeds anxiety questionnaire, 361

leg volume, 239, 250, 255, 256, 257, 372

Legalon®, 291, 293, 294, 295, 402

Leishmania donovani, 231

lemon balm, 276, 357, 363, 364, 376

lemon bioflavonoid, 314, 382

lettuce, 383

leucocyanidin, 325

leukemia, 30, 31, 101

leukocytes, 27, 28, 29, 33, 36, 37, 89, 223

leukopenia, 29

leukoplakia, 338, 347

leukosis, 90, 375

leukotrienes, 132, 373

levodopa, 265

levomenol, 59

LG-166/S, 314, 318, 402

LI-156, 357, 362, 364, 403

LI-160, 328, 331, 332, 333, 402

LI-1370, 192, 195, 196, 198, 400

libido, 216, 217, 225, 282, 313

lichenoid reaction, 302

Lichtwer Pharma AG, 162, 163, 192, 241, 303, 328, 357, 406

licorice, **273–283,** 377, 383, 409

light sensitivity, associated with migraines, 142

light therapy, 333

lignans, 146

lily hypersensitivity, 381

limonene, 65, 113, 301

linalool, 113

linamarin, 147

linoleic acid (LA), 127, 147, 289

linolenic acid, 251

Linum usitatissimum, **143–152**

linustatins, 147

lip swelling, 139

lipids
    apolipoproteins, 150, 167
    betalipoproteins, 384
    cholesterol, in milk thistle, 289
    cholesterol esters, 132
    cholesterol synthesis, 167, 168, 175
    HDL (high density lipoproteins) cholesterol
        levels raised, 120, 157, 168, 169, 216, 347

lipids (cont.)

HDL (high density lipoproteins) cholesterol (cont.)

levels unchanged, 150, 152, 167, 346, 349

hypercholesterolemia (lipidemia)

and flax, 146

and garlic, 156, 161, 167–169

and hawthorn, 240

and Padma®28/Basic, 383, 384

and tea, 339

hypocholesterolemia, 146, 346

LDL (low density lipoproteins) cholesterol

reduced by eleuthero, 100

reduced by ephedra, 120

reduced by flax, 146, 147, 148, 150, 152

reduced by garlic, 167, 168, 169

reduced by tea, 346, 347

lipid-lowering agents, 161, 240

lipopolysaccharides (LPS), 30, 205

liposterols in saw palmetto, 312

in maternal milk, 127, 128, 134

peroxidation, low density lipoproteins, 77, 157, 168, 282, 340, 341, 346

peroxidation, non-specific lipids, 7, 29, 105, 158, 189, 277, 345

peroxidation and liver damage, 290, 295

phospholipids, 133

total cholesterol (TC) reduced

by Asian ginseng, 216

by eleuthero, 100

by flax, 150, 152

by garlic, 157, 161, 167

by tea, 339, 346, 347, 349

triglycerides (triacylglycerol)

component of flax, 147

component of saw palmetto, 312

GLA levels in, 132

and hepatitis, 294

levels reduced

by Asian ginseng, 216

by eleuthero, 100

by ephedra, 120

by garlic, 157, 168, 169

by milk thistle, 289

by Padma®28, 384

by tea, 339, 347, 349

levels unchanged, 150, 152, 167, 346

lipoxygenase, 30, 313

Lipton® tea, 341, 346, 403

liquiritin, 277

lithiasis, 76, 77, 78, 83, 175, 302

Liv.52®, 367, **379–380**

liver cancer, 128, 134, 157, 158, 276, 283

liver enzymes, 264, 265, 378

liver function. *see also* hepatic disorders

compromised function, 290

hepatic metabolism of drugs, 44

indicators, 293

liver excretion function, 294

liver lecithin synthesis, 289

liver metabolic performance, 294

LiverCare®, 379

Loges, 406

lotaustralin, 147

lumbosacral pain (dysmenorrhea), 12

lung cancer, 147, 215, 222, 338, 340, 341, 348

lung function (TCM theory), 215, 216

lungs. *see* respiratory tract conditions

lupus, 148

lupus erythematosus, systemic (SLE), 31, 146, 152, 369, 371, 373

lupus nephritis, 146, 152

luteal phase of menstrual cycle, 71, 151

luteinizing hormone (LH), 17, 18, 21, 65, 70, 314, 318

luteolin, 55, 301

lyaloside, 28

lymphoblasts, 30

lymphocytes, 142

counts, as disease indicator, 94

and liver disease, 293

lymphocyte/neutrophil ratio, 28, 36

proliferation, 29, 30, 38, 90, 101, 223

and SLE, 373

SOD activity, 289, 293

subpopulations, 223

Lyssia GmbH, 358, 406

lytic fever, 32

M

macrophages, 29, 90, 158, 225

Madaus AG, 67, 91, 252, 291, 407

malic acid, 77, 113

malondialdehyde, 289, 293, 294, 295

malvidin, 7

mammary gland development, 340

mammary tumors. *see* breast cancer

Mann-Whitney test, 305

mannitol, 312

mannuronic acid, 147

maprotiline, 327, 332

marigold hypersensitivity, 55, 56, 90, 139

marker compounds, xxiii, 30

marshmallow root, 276

Martindale ginger, 400

Martindale Pharmaceuticals Pty. Ltd., 176, 181, 407

mastalgia, 64, 126, 128, 131, 217, 381

mastitis, 66

Mastodynon®, **381,** 398

mastopathy, fibrocystic, 381

maté, 111

Matricaria recutita, **51–60**

Matricaria spp., 54, 276

matricarin, 55

matricin, 55

Maxim-L®, 103, 105, 399

mechanisms of action, xxvii

Medexport, 103, 105, 399

medical education, xxi

MedWatch, xviii

melanin index, 333

melatonin, 139

melioidosis, 264

Melissa officinalis, 276, 354, 357, 376

memory

    and cerebral insufficiency, 191, 197

    in diabetics, 222

    general, 224, 325

    impairment, 188, 195, 196, 205

    performance, 215, 271

    selective, 100, 102, 106

    short-term, 189, 195, 196

    visual memory, 189, 195

meningitis, cryptococcal, 157

menopause

    adynamia, 223

    asthenia, 223

    depression, 16, 18, 22, 223, 270

    dizziness, 223

    general, 21–22, 67, 214, 271, 324, 327

    headaches, 17, 223

    heart palpitations, 16, 18

    hot flashes, 16, 17, 21, 22, 128, 133, 263, 372

    irritability, 16

menopause (cont.)

    mood disorder, 22

    motivation, 22

    nervousness, 16, 18, 22

    perimenopausal symptoms, 266

    psychological complaints, 18, 22, 334

    sleep disorders, 16, 18, 223

    tinnitus, 16, 18

    vertigo, 16, 17

    weariness, 22

menstrual cycle, luteal phase, 71, 151

menstrual cycle abnormalities. *see also* premenstrual syndrome (PMS)

    amenorrhea, 65, 66, 70, 381

    anovulatory cycles, 65, 70, 151

    cramps, 370, 373

    dysmenorrhea, 6, 8, 12, 16, 64

    menorrhagia, 70, 230

    oligomenorrhea, 70

    polymenorrhea, 12, 70

Mentha x *piperita,* 288, **297–308,** 409, 411

menthofuran, 301

menthol, 301

menthone, 301

menthyl acetate, 301

mesenchymal reaction, 294

Metabolife-356®, 117, 120, 399

Metabolife International, Inc., 117, 407

metabolism

    of drugs, 101, 326, 367

    energy, 216, 341, 345

    glucose, 355

    metabolic rate, 32, 44–45, 47

    and oxygen consumption, 120

metabolites

    antimetabolite drugs, 101

    estrogen metabolites, 151

metastasis, 146, 148, 151

meteorosensitivity, 357

methicillin-resistant microbes, 325, 377

methotrexate, 90

methyl jasmonate, 89

methyl propyl disulfide, 158

methyl xanthines, 115

methylephedrine, 113

methylgallic acid, 345

methysticin, 263

metoclopramide, 66, 176, 181

metolazone, 278

metronidazole, 234

Mewes, 407

micturition. *see* urodynamics

migraines, 138, 139, 140, 142, 381. *see also* headaches

migrating motor complex, 307

milk and tea, interaction, 339, 345, 346

milk composition, 127, 128, 134

milk crust, 126

milk thistle, **285–295,** 409, 410, 411

mineralocorticoid receptors, 283

Minophagen Pharmaceutical Co., 279, 407

MirtoSelect®, 8, 398

miscarriages, 64, 66

mitochondrial function, 277

mitraphylline, 28, 30

moclobemide, 115

monoamine oxidase (MAO) and ginkgo, 189

monoamine oxidase (MAO) inhibitors, 263, 325

    drug interaction, 44, 114, 115, 190, 217

monomycin, 102

monopreparations, 366

mood

    and aromatherapy, 57, 60

    and diabetes, 222

    in elderly, 189, 197

    menopausal, 22, 223

    mood-fatigue, 205, 206, 209, 224

    premenstrual, 70, 71

    sleep-related, 354, 357, 362

Moos Menstrual Distress Questionnaire (MMDQ), 71

motion sickness, 174, 176, 179, 180

Mountain Home Nutritionals, 407

mucilage, 55, 146, 147, 289

mucolytic effects, 301, 389

mucous membranes, 29, 43, 44, 54, 58, 59, 251, 300

multi-herb products. *see* herbal combinations

multiple sclerosis, 31, 90, 375

muscles. *see also* spasms

    calcium uptake in muscles, 175

    muscle strength, 175, 223, 378

    muscular contractions, 216, 301

    myalgia, 300, 324, 377

    myopathy, 377, 378

    neuromusculation, 147

    oxidative capacity of skeletal muscles, 216

muscles (cont.)

    relaxants, 7, 55, 263, 301, 306, 307, 308, 313

    smooth muscles, 231, 301, 307, 313, 355

mushroom poisoning, 288, 289, 290, 295

mutagenic urine, 142

mutagens

    antimutagenic effects, 27, 28, 29, 339

    chromosomal aberrations, 142

    photomutagenesis, 29

myalgia, 300, 324

Mycobacterium spp., 158

myoglobinuria, 278

myristic acid, 147

Myrtocyan®, 8, 11, 12, 398

N

naphthodianthrones, 325

narcotics toxicity, 288

Nardostachys jatamansii, 355

National Formulary, xvii

National Health Products, 117

National Institutes of Health (NIH), xxi

National Nutritional Foods Association (NNFA), 110

Natrol Inc., 266, 407

Natural Health Science, 407

natural killer (NK) cells

    activity stimulated, 90, 96, 158, 162, 170, 216, 377

    increased numbers, 101, 105, 223

NaturalMax Co., 116

Nature's Way Products, Inc., 192, 357, 376, 387, 407

Nature's Way® valerian, 357, 362, 403

naturopathic physicians, xvi, 435

nausea

    with dyspepsia, 174, 183, 307

    with liver disease, 264, 293, 295

    with migraines, 138, 140, 142

    postoperative, 174, 176, 181, 305

    prophylaxis, 181

nausea as adverse effect

    black cohosh, 18

    cat's claw, 31

    chaste tree, 66, 69

    ephedra, 115

    evening primrose, 128

    feverfew, 140

    Hochu-ekki-to®, 378

    horse chestnut, 251

nausea as adverse effect (cont.)
  Mastodynon®, 381
  saw palmetto, 313
neem, 383
negative bias toward herbal medicine, xxv, 409
nephropathy. *see* renal/kidney disorders
neral, 174
nervous conditions
  agitation, 66, 114, 115
  excitability, 356
  menopausal nervousness, 16, 18, 22
  nervous excitation, 115, 354
  nervousness as adverse effect, 115, 217, 340
  premenstrual nervousness, 71
  restless legs, 361
  restlessness, 114, 263, 270, 355, 361, 376
nervous system modulators
  drug interactions, 102, 127, 128, 190, 265, 326, 356
  physiogenic
    adrenocorticotropic agents, 277
    antispasmodics, 55, 190, 263, 295, 355
    CNS depressants, 55, 265, 357
    CNS stimulants, 113, 339, 340
    dopamine, 65, 66, 115, 251, 265, 325
    epinephrine, 47, 121, 169, 240
    muscle relaxants, 7, 55, 263, 301, 306, 307, 308, 313
    norepinephrine, 47, 116
    opioid analgesics, 305
    physical sedatives, 30, 32, 55, 64, 263, 301, 376
    serotonergic effects, 325
    sympathomimetic effects, 113, 115, 116
  psychotropic
    antidepressants, 190, 216, 324, 325, 326, 355
    antipsychotic drugs, 102
    anxiety reduction, 245, 266, 270, 331, 333, 357, 361
    anxiolytics, 55, 216, 263, 265, 266
    barbiturates, 102, 265, 356
    benzodiazepines, 265, 270, 354, 355, 356, 357, 363
    diazepam, 22, 181, 355, 357, 361
    hypnotic effects, 265, 355
    mental sedatives, 100, 101, 325, 354, 355, 357, 361, 364, 374, 378
    psychopharmacological drugs, 265, 290, 295
    relaxants, mental, 308
    selective serotonin reuptake inhibitors (SSRIs), 188, 190, 199, 327, 331
    sleep-promoting agents, 354, 374, 376, 378
    stimulant use, 216

nervous system modulators (cont.)
  psychotropic (cont.)
    withdrawal symptoms, 355, 356, 363
nettles, 314, 382, 387
neural function
  desensitization of sensory neurons, 43
  effects on afferent neurons, 49
  glutamate-induced neuronal death, 30
  nerve conduction, 127, 134
  nerve-damaging effects, 43
  neural irritants, 44
  neuromusculation, 147
  neuroprotection, 263
  neurotransmitters, 43, 147, 325
neuro-cardiac stability, 355
neurological conditions. *see also* neurosensory conditions
  diabetic neuropathy, 42, 49, 126, 128, 133, 134
  hemiplegia, 377
  meningitis, 157
  multiple sclerosis, 31, 90, 375
  neuralgia, 42, 43, 45, 48, 300
  neurodermatitis, 54, 59, 90
  neuropathic bladder, 78, 81, 82
  nonspecific neurological disorders, 56, 224
  notalgia paresthetica, 45, 50
  paralysis, 377, 378
  paresthesia, 12, 134, 255
  polyneuropathy, 45, 48
  surgical neuropathic pain, 48
Neuroplant®, 403
neurosensory conditions. *see also* pain; pruritus/itching; vision
  abnormal sensations (*see* paresthesia)
  algesimetric parameters, 308
  anesthetics, 263
  aromatherapy, 60
  auditory disturbances, 102
  auditory reaction time, 224
  bright light therapy, 333
  burning sensation, 49, 302
  cold/heat sensations, 134, 301
  deafness, 188, 191, 199
  disjunctive reaction time, 224
  light sensitivity, associated with migraines, 142
  meteorosensitivity (weather), 357
  noise sensitivity, associated with migraines, 142
  numbness, 134, 383
  olfactory stimulation, 57, 60, 308

neurosensory conditions (cont.)

paresthesia, 12, 45, 50, 134, 255

sensory-motor function, 224

sensory neuron desensitization, 43

signal detectability, 100, 106, 308

tinnitus, 16, 18, 188, 189, 191, 197, 198

tonometric (pressure) sensitivity, 258

trail making test, 196

vertigo, 16, 17, 18, 180, 188, 238

visual reaction time, 196, 224

neutrophils, 28, 36, 94, 101, 105, 139, 383

New York Heart Association (NYHA) classification, 238

Newcastle disease, 301

nicergoline, 191, 199

nicotine-induced striatal dopamine release, 216

night-blooming cereus, 355, 357

nighttime flushes, 133

nitric oxide generation, 216

nitrite production, 203

nitroglycerin tablets, 384

nitrosamine activity, 339

nitrosoproline formation, 339

nocturia, 244, 313, 314, 317, 318, 324

noise sensitivity, associated with migraines, 142

nomenclature, botanical, xix

nondisclosure of CAM therapy use, xxii–xxiii

nonsteroidal antiinflammatory drugs (NSAIDs), 27, 29, 36, 128, 132, 134

noradrenaline uptake, 325

norephedrine, 113

norepinephrine, 47, 116

notalgia paresthetica, 45, 50

Novartis Consumer Health AG, 407

Novo-Baldriparan, 358, 363, 403

Novo-Nordisk A/S, 358, 407

nuclear jaundice, 231

numbness, 134, 383

nurses, xvi, 437

nursing home patients, 82

nursing (infants). *see* lactation

Nutraceutical Corporation, 78, 116, 315, 407

Nutrilite®, 407

Nutrilite® Saw Palmetto with Nettle Root, 315, 318, **382**, 402

O

obesity, 112, 114, 341, 349

obsessive-compulsive disorder, 324, 327, 334

Ocean Spray® Cranberries, Inc., 78, 407

Ocean Spray® Cranberry, 398

odontalgia, 50

odors, 160, 305

Oenothera biennis, **123–134**

Office of Dietary Supplements (ODS), xxi

Office of Women's Health (OWH), 111

oleanane-type saponins, 215

oleanolic acid, 28, 205, 239

oleic acid, 127, 147, 289

oleoresin, 42, 174

olfactory stimulation, 57, 60, 308

oligoglycosides, 205

omega-3 fatty acids, 146, 150

Omega Nutripharm, 103, 407

omeprazole, 78

onions, sensitivity to, 160

ophthalmic conditions

allergic conjunctivitis, 55

cataracts, 6

conjunctival congestion, 234

corneoretinal resting potential, 200

day blindness, 6

dry eyes, 126

eye irritants, 44

glaucoma, 114, 115, 116

hyphema, 190

macular degeneration, 6, 192

mydriasis, 217

nystagmus, 180

ocular infections, 230, 231, 232, 234

ophthalmology, 106

pupillary reaction, 11, 234

retinal hemorrhage, 6, 11

retinal vascular disorder, 369, 370, 372

retinitis pigmentosa, 6

retinopathy, 6, 8, 11, 369, 371, 372

saccadic eye movements, 200

trachoma, 230, 231, 232, 234

opioid analgesics, 305

oral cancer, 347

oral conditions

aphthous ulcers, 276, 279, 282

burning-mouth syndrome, 302

cold sores, 375

contact sensitivity, 302

dry mouth, 66, 205

oral conditions (cont.)

dry throat, 205

glossodynia, 59

halitosis, 160

leukoplakia, 338, 347

lip swelling, 139

mucosal inflammation, 139, 300

odontalgia, 50

oral cancer, 347

sore throats, 95, 276

stomatitis, 56, 59, 276

throat inflammations, 54

tongue spasms, 302

tongue swelling, 139

ulceration, as adverse effect, 139, 302

Oregon Board of Naturopathic Examiners, xvi

organosulfur compounds (OSC), 157, 158

orphan nuclear receptor, 326

osteoarthritis

in hands, 49

joint tenderness, 42, 49, 50

in knee, 26, 27, 28, 32, 36, 182

pain from activity, 28, 32, 36, 182

pain reduction, 42, 45, 49, 50, 386

potential treatment, 26, 27, 174, 176

range of motion, 49

osteogenic sarcoma cells, 127

osteoporosis, 146, 152, 338, 341, 349

otitis, 105, 375

ovarian cancer, 30, 215, 222

ovarian dysfunction, 16, 21, 66, 151

ovariectomized patients, 18, 19

over-the-counter (OTC) drugs, xix, xx, xxvii, 42, 110, 113, 114

overviews of herbs, xxvi

Ovestin®, 21

oxalic acid, 113

oxazepam, 270, 271, 362

oxerutin, 255

oxidation-reduction potential, fecal, 349

oxidative metabolism of drugs, 326

oxidative stress, 150, 289

oxygen consumption. *see also* respiration

and American ginseng, 204, 206, 209

and Asian ginseng, 222, 223, 224, 225

and eleuthero, 105

and ephedra, 120

oxygen consumption (cont.)

and ephedra/caffeine, 115–116

and hawthorn, 244, 245

oxytocin, 116, 133

P

Padma®28/Padma® Basic, 367, **383–384**

Padma AG, 383, 407

pain

abdominal, 128, 139, 239, 264, 305, 373

algesimetric parameters, 308

analgesics, 42, 263, 301, 305, 308

anti-nociceptives, 139

breast, 64, 126, 128, 131, 217, 381

chest, 102, 238, 239

childbirth, 57, 60

chronic, 42

fibromyalgia, 42, 45, 50, 354

glossodynia, 59

leg, 250, 256, 370

muscle, 300, 324, 377

neuralgia, 42, 43, 45, 48, 300

postoperative, 42

pregnancy, 12

premenstrual, 71, 372

reduction, 43, 45, 50

sensitivity, 308

substance P, 43

palmitic acid, 127, 147, 251, 289

Panax ginseng, 100, 204, **211–225,** 377, 410

Panax japonicus, 218

Panax quinquefolius, **201–209,** 216

Panax vietnamensis, 218

panaxynol, 205

pancreatic β-cell function, 189

pancreatic cancer, 215, 222, 338, 341, 348

pansinusitis, 170

papaverine, 190, 240

paprika, 42

Paracetamol, 308

paralysis. *see* neurological conditions

parasites, 158, 175, 231, 234

paresthesia, 12, 45, 50, 134, 255

pargyline, 115

Parkinson symptoms, 265

parthenolide, 138, 139

Passiflora spp., 354, 361

patient counseling, xxii

Patient Information Sheet, xxix

pau d'arco, 409

Paullinia spp., 111, 116, 361

pelvic pain (dysmenorrhea), 12

pentacyclic oxindole alkaloids (POAs), 26, 27, 28, 29, 32, 33

pentobarbital, 355

peonidin, 7, 77

peppermint, 288, **297–308,** 409, 411

pepsin, 55

percent daily value, xxiv

performance enhancing agents. *see* athletic performance

Performance Status (PS) scale, 377

Perika®, 403

peripheral arterial occlusive disease (PAOD)
    and garlic, 156, 162, 170
    and ginkgo, 188, 189, 191, 192, 197
    and Padma®28, 383, 384

Periploca sepium, 102

permeability, capillary, 7, 190, 251

permeability, hepatocyte membrane, 294

permeability, vascular, 7, 11

Permixon®, 313, 314, 315, 317, 402

peroxynitrite, 29

perspiration, 16, 17, 113, 361, 377. *see also* hot flashes

Peruvian pepper, 42

petunidin, 7

pH, fecal, 339, 349

pH in digestive tract, 339

phagocytosis, 30, 89, 90, 101, 105, 139, 223

Pharbio Medical International AB, 407

Pharbio Medical Suerigie, 358

Pharma-Inter-Med GmbH, 103, 407

Pharma Nord A.p.S., 192, 407

Pharmacia Corporation, 407

pharmacists, xvi, 439

pharmacological actions, xxvii

Pharmaton Natural Health Products, 219, 222, 358, 407

phenelzine, 115, 217

phenolic acids, 339, 370

phenothiazines, 127, 128, 290, 295

phenylpropanolamine, 114

pheochromocytoma, 114

phlegm mixed with blood, 205

phlegm (TCM theory), 205

phloroglucinol, 325

phosphatase activity, 152

photodamage protection, 90

photopheresis, 183

phototoxicity, 325, 326, 333

physicians, xvi, 433

Physostigma venenosum, xvii

physostigmine, xvii

Phytodolor®, **385–386**

phytoestrogens, 151

phytohemagglutinin (PHA), 29, 36

Phytotrim®, 341, 403

Pierre Fabre Médicament, 315, 407

Pimenta dioica, 383

Pimpinella anisum, 276

pinene, 65, 139

Pinus pinaster, **369–373**

Piper methysticum, **259–271,** 409, 410

piquin, 42

piris, 42

piroxicam, 386

PKC-167/79, 219, 223, 401

Plantago arenaria, xx

Plantago lanceolata, 383

plantain, 383

plaque, atherosclerotic, 156, 158, 161, 162, 169

plasma. *see* blood

platelet aggregation
    and coronary disease, 182
    decreased, 7, 147, 150, 157, 174, 175
    and hypercholesterolemia, 169
    inhibited, 30, 32, 369, 370, 371, 373
    and juvenile ischemia, 168
    normalized, 370
    and PAOD, 170, 384
    unaffected, 176
    in vitro, 231

platelets
    antiplatelet agents, 7, 140, 160, 161, 190
    platelet activating factor (PAF), 139, 189
    platelet composition, 150
    platelet counts, 176, 182, 216
    platelet function, 156, 160, 161, 169

plethysmography, 198

pneumococcus vaccine, 27, 28, 33, 36

pneumonia. *see* respiratory tract conditions

Podophyllum peltatum, xvii

Polcopharma F. Polley & Co., 266, 407

polio virus, 77

pollakiuria, 318

polyacetylenes, 89, 215

polycyclic aromatic hydrocarbon activity, 339

Polygonum aviculare, 383

PolyMedica Corp., 78, 407

polymorphonuclear leukocytes, 223, 289

polypectomy, 306

polyphenols, 28, 338, 339, 346

polysaccharides, 101

polysomnography, 362, 363

Populus tremula, 385

portal hypertension, 293

postoperative bleeding. *see* hemorrhage/bleeding

postprandial glycemia, 204, 205, 206, 209

potassium levels, 278, 378

Potentilla aurea, 383

prednisolone, 217

pregnancy

    ability to conceive, 69, 70, 381

    arrest of descent, in childbirth, 133

    birth weights, 96, 133, 278, 282

    fetal development, 65, 96, 147

    fetal distress, 96

    fetotoxicity, 356

    gestation time, 133

    gestational safety, 91, 217

    hyperemesis gravidarum, 181

    labor, 57, 60, 128, 133

    miscarriages, 64

    morning sickness, 174

    phlebopathies, 12

    placenta expulsion, 64

    premature births, 278, 279, 282

    safety of echinacea, 96

    safety of ginseng, 217

    spontaneous abortions, 96

    teratogenicity, 102

pregnancy as contraindication

    chaste tree, 65–66

    ephedra, 114

    Euvegal®, 376

    feverfew, 139

    Hochu-ekki-to®, 378

    kava, 264

    licorice, 278

    Phytodolor®, 385

    Pycnogenol®, 371

pregnancy as contraindication (cont.)

    Sinupret®, 388

    St. John's wort, 326

    valerian, 356

pregnancy contraindications, xxvii

pregnane X receptor, 326

premature ejaculation, 225

PreMens® Ze440, 67, 70, 71, 398

premenstrual syndrome (PMS)

    and black cohosh, 16

    and chaste tree, 64, 66, 69–71

    and evening primrose, 126, 128, 131

    and Mastodynon®, 381

    and Pycnogenol®, 372

    and St. John's wort, 324, 327

premenstrual tension syndrome (PMTS) scale, 71

prescription drugs, xxvii

Presomen®, 21

Prevention magazine, xviii, xix

primroses, 388

Primula veris, 276, 388

Princeton Survey Research Associates, xviii, xix

PRO 160/120®, 314, 315, 319, 402

proanthocyanidins, 7, 77, 113, 325, 339

procarbazine, 115

procollagen, 222, 289, 293, 295

procyanidins, 28, 30, 239, 369, 370

product brands, xxiii, xxviii

Prof. Dr. Much AG, 357, 407

Profile of Mood States (POMS), 22

progesterone, 64, 65, 66, 69, 70, 282. *see also* hormones

prolactin, 17, 18, 21, 65, 66, 69, 225, 333. *see also* hormones; hyperprolactinemia

proliferation cell nuclear antigen (PCNA), 347

properties of herbs (TCM theory), 366

proprietary products, xxix, 366–392

Propulsid, 307

propylene sulfide, 158

Proscar, 314

ProstActive™, 387, 402

prostaglandins, 127, 132, 139, 251, 347

Prostagutt®, 315, 317, 319, **387,** 402

prostanoids, 127, 132

Prostaserene®, 315, 317, 402

prostate cancer

    as contraindication, 313, 314

    and flax, 146, 147, 148, 152

prostate cancer (cont.)
  and garlic, 158
  growth inhibition, 152, 158, 216, 289
  increased apoptosis, 146, 148, 152
  and milk thistle, 289
  risk reduction, 317
prostate enlargement, 114, 312. *see also* benign prostatic hyperplasia
prostate-specific antigen (PSA), 152, 314, 317
protease inhibitors, 326
proteinuria, 147
proteolytic activity of pepsin, 55
Proteus spp., 102, 158
prothrombin, 293, 326
protocatechic acid, 370
Prozac®, 327
prozacin, 313
pruritus/itching
  as adverse effect, 66, 251, 381
  psoriasis, 42, 49
  uremic skin conditions, 132
  varicosis, 257
  venous insufficiency, 12, 250, 255, 256, 372
pseudoephedrine, 110, 113, 114
pseudoepithelia hyperplasia (PEH), 83
pseudoginsenosides, 205, 216
Pseudomonas spp., 77, 231, 301
psoralen (8-MOP) therapy, 183
psoriasis, 42, 45, 49, 370
psoriatic arthritis, 128, 132
psychiatric conditions as contraindications, 114, 340
psychiatric/psychological conditions. *see* affective (emotional) disorders; behavior; cognition; neurosensory conditions; psychomotor conditions
psychological function testing, 60, 106, 195, 206, 218, 224
psychomotor conditions. *see also* spasms
  activity levels, 106
  ambulation, 355
  chronic fatigue syndrome, 100, 377
  coordination/ataxia, 30, 224, 265, 355
  driving impairment, 356, 357, 364
  motor restlessness, 115
  muscle relaxants, 7, 55, 263, 301, 306, 307, 308, 313, 325
  operating machinery, impairment, 357, 364
  paralysis, 377, 378
  psychomotor performance testing, 195, 206, 224
  seizures, 114, 115, 127, 128, 190, 326
  tremors, 115, 340

psychophysiological insomnia, 362
Psychotonin-M, 327
psyllium, xx
Pterocarpus santalinus, 383
pteropodine, 28, 30
pulegone, 301
pulse, 113, 115, 120, 215, 238, 244
pulse wave velocity, 162, 169
pumpkin seeds, 382
Pure-Gar®, 162–163, 167, 400
PureWorld Botanicals, Inc., 266
purpuras, 6
Pycnogenol®, **369–373,** 409, 411
pyrethrin, 139
pyridinoline, 17
pyrrolizidine alkaloids (PAs), 90
pyrrolketone, 355
pyuria, 77, 78, 82

Q
qi (TCM theory), 101, 205, 215, 216
quality of life. *see* well-being/quality of life
quercetin, 55, 89, 189, 239, 325
quercitrin, 325
Quest Vitamins, 128, 133, 399, 407
Quindao Fengyi Biotechnology Ltd., 192, 408
quinic acid, 77
quinoline alkaloids, 231
quinone reductase, 339
quinovic acid, 28, 30
quinovic glycosides, 28
quinqueginsin, 205, 206
quinquenosides, 205

R
racemoside, 17
radiation
  gamma, 101
  mucositis from, 54
  protectants, 101, 102, 216
  radiotherapy, 27, 29, 33, 37, 59, 100, 158, 375
  solar-simulated, 333
  ultraviolet (UV), 27, 29, 158
Radix ginseng, 214, 217
ragweed hypersensitivity, 55, 90, 139
rashes, 66, 69, 378
rational phytotherapy, xxiii

Rauvolfia serpentina, xvii
Raynaud's disease, 8, 12, 126
reaction time, 196, 224, 266, 270, 271, 357, 364
red pepper, 42
red saunders, 383
ReDormin®, 363, 403
reflux, gastroesophageal, 251, 302
regulation of herbal products, xix
regulatory status of herbs, xxviii
REM sleep, 271, 355, 362
Remifemin®, 16, 18, 19, 21, 22, 398
Remotiv®, 327, 328, 331, 402, 403
renal cancer, 158
renal/kidney disorders
    capillary fragility, 6
    as contraindication, 78, 231, 277, 340
    glomerulosclerosis, 147
    nephritis, 112, 146, 152
    nephrolithiasis, 76, 77, 78, 83
    nephropathy, 127, 252
    renal failure, 31, 114, 251, 252
    renal insufficiency, 78, 277
renshen, 215, 216
Reparil®, 252, 401
reproduction. *see also* fertility; hormones; menstrual cycle
    abnormalities; pregnancy
    aphrodisiacs, 215
    coitus frequency, 225
    contraceptives, 8, 12, 26, 66, 326
    corpus luteum abnormalities, 64, 66, 69, 70, 381
    ejaculation volume, 319
    ejaculatory disturbances, 225, 313, 317
    erectile function, 216, 225, 313, 319
    frigidity, 215
    gonadal function, 279, 283
    gynecological disorders, non-specific, 64
    impotence, general, 215, 377
    impotence as adverse effect, 313, 317
    libido, 216, 217, 225, 283, 313
    ovarian dysfunction, 16, 21, 66, 151
    sexual dysfunction as contraindication, 283
    sexual dysfunction from antidepressant use, 188, 190, 191,
    199
    sexuality, 334
    sperm quality, 147, 225, 369, 370
reserpine, xvii
reserpine-induced hypothermia, 355
Resistan®, 92, 95, 96, 399

respiration. *see also* oxygen consumption
    expiratory flow, 198, 225
    respiratory endurance, 205
    respiratory exchange ratio, 105, 222
    respiratory quotients, 47, 224, 345
respiratory sinus arrhythmia (RSA), 271
respiratory tract conditions. *see also* asthma; bronchitis; com-
    mon colds
    bronchoconstriction, 44, 139, 189
    bronchodilation, 112, 113, 115, 216, 341
    bronchospasms, 112, 388
    catarrh, 156, 205, 276, 300, 366
    chronic infections, 215, 225, 375, 383, 384
    chronic inflammations, 388
    decongestants, 389
    ergospirometry, 244
    flu-like symptoms, 94
    influenza, 90, 91, 100, 105, 325
    laryngeal cancer, 161, 215, 222
    laryngitis, 276
    lung cancer, 147, 215, 222, 338, 340, 341, 348
    nasal congestion, 112
    pharyngitis, 276, 375
    pneumonia, 105
    pulmonary complications during radiotherapy, 276, 279,
    283
    pulmonary edema, 278
    pulmonary function, 198, 215, 225, 370, 371, 373
    pulmonary tuberculosis, 44
    respiratory arrest, 302
    respiratory paralysis, 30
    rhinitis, 94, 95, 112, 156, 160
    rhinopathy, chronic, 42
    sinusitis, 105, 112, 170, 375, 388, 389
    upper respiratory tract infections (URTIs), 88, 91, 94–96,
    366
    ventilation, 204, 209, 388
restlessness
    as adverse effect, 115, 340
    as contraindication, 114
    premenstrual, 71
    restless legs, 361
    treatment with Euvegal®, 376
    treatment with kava, 263, 270
    treatment with valerian, 354, 361
rete ridge flattening, 133
reticuloendothelial system (RES) cells, 30
retinopathy. *see under* ophthalmic conditions

Rey Test, 195
reynosin, 139
rhamnetin, 55, 189
rhamnose, 147, 370
rhamnosides, 239
Rhamnus purshiana, xx
rheumatic disease, 386
rheumatic heart disease, 102
rheumatoid arthritis. *see under* arthritis
rhodopsin, 7
rhynchophylline, 28, 29, 30
Ribes nigrum, 128
rigidity (erectile), 216, 225
risk-benefit assessments, xxi
Ritchie Index, 33, 37
RNA polymerase, 158, 289
Roche Nicholas SA, 357, 408
Rökan®, 192, 196, 197, 198, 199, 400
rosmarinic acid, 301
rotundifuran, 65
rubefacients, 43
Rumex spp., 388
rupture of membranes, during childbirth, 133
rutin, 239, 325
rutoside, 89

S
S-allylcysteine (SAC), 157, 158, 161
S-allylmercaptocysteine (SAMC), 158, 159
Sabal serrulata, 312
SabalSelect™, 402
Saccade test, 196
Saccharomyces bayanus, 77
Saemaul Kongjang, 45, 47, 398
safety of ephedra, 110–112, 116, 120
safety of herbal products, xviii–xix, xxviii, 366
safety of kava, 262, 271
safety performance, 270
safety ratings, xxviii
Saila Licorice Root Tablets, 279, 283, 401
Saila S.p.A., 279, 408
salicin, 385
salicylate hypersensitivity, 385
salicylic acid, 17
Salmonella spp., 158, 384
Salvia sclarea, 57
Sambucus nigra, 388

Sanofi Synthelabo, 315, 408
santamarin, 139
Sapec®, 163, 167, 168, 400
sapogenins, 277
sapogenols, 251
saponins, 157
saquinavir, 160
Saussurea costus, 383
Saventaro®, 398
saw palmetto, **309–319,** 387, 409
SCAG questionnaire, 224
SCAG scale, 195, 197
scars. *see* cicatrizing activity
Schaper & Brümmer GmbH & Co., 19, 67, 92, 375, 408
Schering-Plough, 45, 408
schistosomes, 175
schizophrenic patients, 127
Schwabe, 408
scopolamine, xvii, 179, 205
Scotia Cream, 128, 133, 399
Scotia Pharmaceuticals Ltd., 128, 408
sea sickness, 179, 180
seasonal affective disorder (SAD), 324, 327, 333
secale alkaloid derivatives, 116
secoisolariciresinol diglucoside (SDG), 147
Secretary of Health and Human Services, xx
secretions
    antisecretory effects, 127
    secretolytic agents, 277, 301, 388
Sedariston®, 358, 361, 403
sedation as adverse effect, 32
sedative effects
    cat's claw, 30, 32
    chamomile, 55
    chaste tree, 64
    eleuthero, 100, 101
    kava, 263, 265
    peppermint, 301
    St. John's wort, 325
    valerian, 354, 355, 357, 361, 364
sedative-herb interactions, 102, 356
sedatives, 30, 55, 64, 100, 101, 102, 263, 265, 301, 325, 354, 355, 356, 357, 361, 364
    as adverse effect, 32
Sedonium®, 358, 362, 403
seizure disorders contraindicated, 114
seizure medication interactions, 127, 128, 190, 326

seizures as adverse effects, 115

selective estrogen receptor modulator (SERM), 21

selective serotonin reuptake inhibitors (SSRIs), 188, 190, 199, 327, 331

selegiline, 115

Selenicereus grandiflorus, 355, 357

Self-Assessment Depression scale, 22

Semliki Forest virus, 301

Senna alexandrina, xx

sensory conditions. *see* neurosensory conditions

Serenoa repens, **309–319,** 382, 387

Serenoa serrulata, **309–319**

serotonergic effects, 325

serotonin, 139, 325. *see also* selective serotonin reuptake inhibitors (SSRIs)

sertraline, 331

serving size, xxiv

sesquiphellandrene, 174

sesquiterpenes, 55, 139

Seven Seas Ltd., 162, 408

sexual dysfunction, 188, 190, 191, 199, 282, 313. *see also* reproduction

sexuality, 334

SG-291, 315, 402

Shigella spp., 102

shingles, 42

shogaols, 174

shortness of breath. *see* dyspnea/shortness of breath

Siberian ginseng, 100, 204, 218

sickle cell anemia, 157, 158

Sidroga GmbH, 408

signal detectability, 100, 106, 308

SIL-2R release, 96

Siliphos®, 291, 402

silver-stained nucleolar organizer regions (AgNOR), 347

silybin, 289

Silybum marianum, **285–295,** 409, 410

silychristin, 289

silydianin, 289

silymarin, 289, 290

Sinupret®, 366, **388–389**

sinusitis, 105, 112, 170, 375, 388

sister chromatid exchanges, 142

sitosterol, 28, 30, 127, 147, 251, 277, 289, 325, 355

Sjögren's syndrome, 126

SK-MEL cells, 30

SK-OV-3 cells, 30

skin cancer, 127, 289

skin disorders. *see* dermatological conditions

sleep. *see also* insomnia

  menopausal sleep disorders, 16, 18, 223

  morning sleepiness, 356

  nonpsychiatric sleep disorders, 357

  sleep behavior in cardiac patients, 245

  sleep disorders, non-specific, 263, 355

  sleep disorders as adverse effect, 102, 115, 217, 334, 340, 356

  sleep-promoting (soporific) agents, 354, 374, 376, 378

  sleep quality, 189, 266, 362, 363, 364

  somnolence, 265

sleep structure

  REM sleep, 271

  sleep latency, 271, 362, 363, 364

  sleep onset, 271, 333

  sleep time, 325

  slow wave sleep, 271, 362, 363

slippery elm, xx

Slone Survey, xviii, xix

smokers, 225, 364

sodium bicarbonate, 116

sodium nitrate, 240

sodium retention, 278

Solanum nigrum, 379

Solaray® CranActin®, 79, 81, 398

Solaray® ephedra, 117, 120, 399

Solaray® saw palmetto, 315, 319, 402

solid tumor growth, 339, 340

Solidago virgaurea, 385

soluble CD8 antigen, 223

Solvay Arzneimittel GmbH, 358, 408

Songha Night®, 358, 363, 403

sore throats, 95, 276

sorrel, 388

soy, 409

spasms

  anticonvulsants, 190, 263, 295, 355

  antispasmodics, 55, 263, 370

  during barium enema, 300, 302, 305

  bile ducts, 300

  bronchospasms, 112, 388

  during colonoscopy, 300

  gallbladder, 300

  gastrointestinal, 54, 300, 301, 355

  muscle cramps, 12, 250, 257, 370, 372, 383

  seizures, 114, 115, 326

spasms (cont.)

spastic colon syndrome, 306

susceptibility to, 340

tongue, 302

vasospasms, 190

Special Nutritionals/Adverse Event Monitoring System (SN/AEMS), xviii

speciophylline, 28

sperm counts, 225

sperm quality, 147, 225, 369, 370

spiked ginger lily, 383

spinal epidural hematoma, 160

spinasterol, 251

spirulina, 409

Spitzner GmbH, 192, 408

spleen function (TCM theory), 101, 215, 216

splenocytes, 29

squamous cell cancer, 338, 348

St. John's wort, **321–334**, 357, 409, 411

stable-plaque psoriasis, 128, 132

stamina, 102, 105

standardization of herbal products, xix, xxiii, xxiv

standardized common names, xxiv

Staphylococcus spp., 77, 158, 231, 301, 325, 377

statements of nutritional support, xx, xxiv, 368

stearic acid, 127, 147, 251

STEI-300, 328, 402

Steigerwald, 385, 408

Steiner Arzneimittel, 328, 358, 408

steroid-induced epidermal thinning, 133

steroid saponins, 157

steroidal drugs, 128

stigmasterol, 28, 30, 147, 251, 277, 289

stimulant use, 216

stomach cancer risk reduction

Asian ginseng, 215, 222

cayenne, 44, 47

garlic, 156, 157, 158, 161, 162, 170

tea, 339, 341, 348

storage of herbal products, xxv

Strathmann AG, 67, 315, 408

Streptococcus spp., 158, 231

stress, 101, 102, 105, 263

stress, daily, 270

stress, oxidative, 150, 289

stress, physical, 215

stress management, 305

stress reduction, 101

striatal dopamine release, 216

Strogen®, 315, 317, 402

strokes, 115, 341

stroma, prostatic, 313

Stronger Neo Minophagen-C, 279, 283, 401

Strotan®, 67, 69, 70, 398

structure/function claims, xxiv, 368

subcortical center stimulation, 205

subgingival microbiota, 77

substance P, 43

sulfacetamide, 234

sulfide, fecal, 339, 349

sulindac, 341

superoxide dismutase (SOD), 289, 293, 370

Supplement Facts panel, xx, xxiv

surgery, 160, 189

surgery, presurgical patients, 139, 189

surgery adjuvants, 33, 37

surgical bleeding, 6, 8, 12

surgical narcotics toxicity, 288, 295

sweating. *see* perspiration

sweet cravings, premenstrual, 71

swelling of soft tissue. *see* edema

swine erysipelas, 301

sympathomimetic effects of ephedra, 113, 115, 116

Symphona®, 400

Syndrom-Kurztest, 195

synergistic effects (TCM theory), 215

synovial fluid, 49

Synthelabo-Pharma SA, 8, 408

syringin, 101

systemic lupus erythematosus (SLE), 31, 146, 152, 369, 371, 373

systolic blood pressure reduction

by ephedra, 114

by garlic, 157, 161, 162, 167, 168

by hawthorn, 244

by Pycnogenol®, 373

by tea, 347

systremma, nocturnal, 250

Syzygium aromaticum, 383

T

T-cells, 95, 96, 101, 102, 105, 293

T4 cells, 38, 223

T8 cells, 38

T-cells, suppressor, 277

T-helper cells, 90

tabasco pepper, 42

tachycardia, 66, 114, 115, 234, 278, 361. *see also* heart rate

tachygastria, 180

tachyphylaxis, 113

tacrine, 295

Taigutan®, 103, 105, 399

Talso®, 315, 318, 402

Tamarisk gallica, 379

tamoxifen, 17, 18, 21, 128, 131, 341

tamsulosin, 313

Tanacetum parthenium, **135–142**

Tanakan®, 192, 196, 197, 198, 400

tannins, 7, 28, 139

taxifolin, 370

Taxol®, xvii

Taxus brevifolia, xvii

tea, black/green, 115, **335–349,** 409

Tebonin®, 192, 195, 197, 200, 400

Tegens®, 8, 11, 12, 398

Tegra®, 163, 167, 400

Tegretol®, 326

tension, 270, 361

tension in legs, 255, 256

terazosin, 265

Terminalia spp., 379, 383

terpene glycosides, 205

terpene lactones, 189

terpenes, 139

terpineol, 113

terpinyl acetate, 65

testosterone. *see also* hormones

    and Asian ginseng, 225

    and flax, 148, 152

    and licorice, 277, 282

    metabolism, 313

    and saw palmetto, 314, 317, 318

tetracyclic oxindole alkaloids (TOAs), 26, 27, 28, 29, 32

tetracycline, 234

tetrahydroalstonine, 28

tetrahydrocortisol, 283

Texas Medical Association, xiv, xv, xvi, 110

Texas Nurses Association, xvi

Texas Pharmacy Association, xvi

theaflavine, 339

thearubigins, 339

theobromine, 339

theophylline, 44, 115, 240, 326, 339, 341

Therabel Research, 315, 408

therapeutic claims, 368

Therapeutic Goods, xx

thermogenesis, 112, 113, 115, 121, 216, 339, 345

thiazide diuretics, 190, 278

thioacetamide damage, 289

thiopental, 355

thiosulfinates, 157, 158

thirst, 215

Thisilyn®, 402

thrombin, 48

thrombosis. *see also* anticoagulants; platelets

    antithrombotic effects, 48, 139, 157, 158, 161, 189, 263

    as contraindication, 251

    phlebothrombosis, 257

    thromboembolisms, 199, 251

    thrombophlebitis, 12, 257

    thrombus formation, 157, 231, 370

thromboxanes, 127, 158, 182, 231, 370, 373

Thuja occidentalis, 89, 92, 375

thymic extracts, intravenous, 32

thyroid disorders, 114, 116, 222, 340

thyrotoxicosis, 114

Tibetan medicine, 367

Tillots Pharma AG, 279, 302, 408

tinnitus, 16, 18, 188, 189, 191, 197, 198

tocopherol, 289

tongue spasms, 302

tongue swelling, 139

tonics, 214

tonometric sensitivity, 258

Toulouetes test, 224

Traditional Chinese Medicine (TCM), 101, 112, 204, 205, 215, 216, 366

Traditional Herbal Medicines (THMs), xx

Traditional Medicinals, Inc., 91, 408

traditional medicine systems, 366

trail making test, 196

tranquilizers, 101

transaminases, 294, 295

transcapillary filtration, 251, 257

transcription factor NF-kB, 30

transepidermal water loss, 132

transplant recipients, 31

transplant rejection, 190, 326

transplants, organ, 31, 190
tranylcypromine, 115
trauma, cranial, 250, 258
trazodone, 190, 225
tricyclic antidepressants, 327, 334
triglycerides. *see under* lipids
Trisequens®, 21
triterpene glycosides, 16, 17
TRUW Arzneimittel Vertriebs GmbH, 92, 408
Tsumura & Co., 377, 408
tuberculosis, 31, 44, 90, 375, 377
tubocurarine, xvii
tulips, sensitivity to, 160
tumescence (erectile), 216, 225
tumor inhibitors
    in animals, 43, 89, 127, 157, 158, 216, 289, 339–340
    cancer treatment adjuncts, 27, 33, 37, 100, 191, 232
    in humans, antiproliferation, 146, 147
    in humans, cancer prevention, 156, 161, 162, 170, 215, 218, 222, 338, 341, 348
    in vitro, 29, 77, 90, 127, 158, 175, 216, 251, 289
tumor necrosis factor (TNF), 29, 30, 31, 158, 277
Twinings, 342, 408
Twinings® tea, 342, 346, 403
tyramine levels, 232
tyrosine, 355

U
ulceration, 55
ulcers
    alcohol-induced, 56
    as contraindication, 114
    dermal, 251
    duodenal, 47, 276, 279, 282
    and *Helicobacter pylori,* 158
    leg ulcers, 250
    omeprazole treatment, 78
    oral, 139, 276, 279, 282, 302
    preventatives
        bilberry, 7
        cayenne, 42, 43, 44, 47
        chamomile, 55
        ephedra, 114
        evening primrose, 127
        ginger, 175
    treatment with Asian ginseng, 215
    treatment with cat's claw, 27, 28, 33, 37

ulcers (cont.)
    treatment with licorice, 279
Ulmus rubra, xx
Ultimate Xphoria, 110
ultraviolet (UV) light, 27, 29, 158, 370
uña de gato, 26
Uncaria guianensis, **23–38**
Uncaria rhynchophylla, 29, 30
Uncaria sinensis, 29, 30
Uncaria tomentosa, **23–38**
uncarine, 28
Unilever Bestfoods North America, 341, 342, 408
United States Pharmacopoeia, xvii
Up Your Gas, 117, 120, 399
upper respiratory tract infections (URTIs), 88, 91, 94–96, 366
urethane resistance, 216
uric acid, 32, 38, 78
urinary alkaloids, 231
urinary antisepsis, 76, 77
urinary bacteria, 77, 78, 81, 82
urinary catecholamines, 209, 224
urinary cortisol, 326
urinary estrogen metabolites, 151
urinary glucose, 6, 295
urinary methylgallic acid, 345
urinary nitrogen, 345
urinary norepinephrine, 345
urinary pathogens, 76, 77
urinary pH
    urinary acidification, 76, 81, 82, 83, 116
    urinary alkalizers, 116
urinary tract infections (UTIs), 76, 77, 78, 81, 82, 83
    as adverse effect, 313, 317
urine, brown, 264
urodynamics. *see also* bladder; prostate
    dysuria, 313, 318, 339
    micturition, 317, 318, 387
    nocturia, 244, 313, 314, 317, 318
    pollakiuria, 318
    residual urine, 114, 313, 317, 319
    urinary flow, 313, 314, 317, 318, 319, 382, 387
    urinary retention, 313, 318
    urination disturbances, 114, 115
uroepithelial cells, 77
urokinase inhibitors, 340
uronic acid, 312
urostomies, 83

ursolic acid, 28, 239
Urtica dioica, 382, 387
urticaria, 44, 55, 66, 160
uses, primary and potential, xxvi
uterine bleeding, 67, 215
uterine prolapse, 377
uterine stimulants, 18, 231
uterine tissue, 17, 18
uva ursi leaf, 76

V
vaccinia virus, 301
Vaccinium macrocarpon, **73–83,** 409, 410
Vaccinium myrtillus, **3–12**
vaginal conditions
    cervical cancer, 222
    cervix, cytological smears, 223
    vaginal bleeding, as adverse effect, 217
    vaginal cytology, 17, 18, 22, 223
    vaginal mucosa, 76
    vulvovaginal candidiasis, 76
Valdispert®, 355, 358, 361, 362, 403
valepotriates, 355, 356
valeranone, 355, 356
valerenic acid, 355, 356
Valerian Nighttime™, 403
Valeriana exaltata, 354
Valeriana officinalis, **351–364,** 374, 376, 378, 383, 409
Valerina Natt®, 358, 364, 403
Valmane®, 358, 361, 364, 403
valtrates, 355
Valverde®, 358, 364, 403
vanillic acid, 370
Varicella zoster, 27, 33, 38
varicosis, 6, 12, 127, 250, 257, 372
vascular conditions. *see also* arteries; circulation; veins
    capillary fragility, 6, 7, 12
    capillary permeability, 7, 190, 251
    capillary resistance, 370
    endothelium, 158
    peripheral vascular disorder, 6, 8, 12, 188, 191
    permeability, 7, 11, 231
    vascular resistance, 162, 169, 231, 234, 239
    vascular responses, 139
    vasoconstriction, 113, 251, 370
    vasodilation, 43, 77, 158, 216, 231, 240, 251, 341, 355
    vasomotor symptoms, 198, 223

vascular conditions (cont.)
    vasospasms, 190
vasopressin, 355
veins
    occlusions, 12
    thrombophlebitis, 12, 257
    varicosis, 6, 12, 127, 250, 257, 372
    venous disorders, non-specific, 252
    venous filling rate, 255
    venous insufficiencies, 6, 8, 12, 250, 255–257, 369, 370, 372
Venoplant®, 253, 255, 257, 258, 401
Venostasin®, 253, 255, 256, 257, 401
Venostat®, 401
ventilation, 204, 209, 388
ventricular cardiac myocytes, 240
ventricular ejection fraction, 231, 234, 238, 239, 244, 245
Veratrum nigrum, 217
verbascoside, 89
Verbena spp., 276, 388
vertigo, 16, 18, 180, 188, 238
vervain, 276, 388
vesicular stomatitis virus, 30
VIATRIS GmbH & Co. KG, 408
Vibrio cholerae, 231, 234
Vienna determination test, 196
Vietnamese ginseng, 218
vincristine, xvii
vinyldithiins, 157
vision
    altered, 263
    blindness, night/day, 6
    color discrimination speed, 100, 106
    color perception, 100, 106
    contrast sensitivity, 8, 11
    impairment, 18, 197, 370, 372
    infant development, 147
    night vision, 6, 8, 11
    spectral sensitivity, 100, 106
    visual reaction time, 196, 224
visual analog scale (VAS), 49, 50, 71, 307, 381
vital essence (TCM theory), 216
vitality, 27, 29, 33, 37, 38, 223
vitamin A, 314
vitamin B12, 78
vitamin E, 126
vitamin K, 341

Vitex agnus-castus, **61–72,** 381

vitexilactone, 65

vitexin rhamnosides, 239

vomiting
  as adverse effect, 18, 31, 115, 140
  antiemetics, 174, 175, 180
  associated with migraines, 138, 140, 142
  post-surgical, 181
  symptom of liver disease, 264

von Zerssen depression scale, 333

vulnerary activity, 90

W

Wakunaga of America Co., Ltd., 162, 408

walking distance, 170, 188, 192, 197, 225, 384

warfarin
  and Asian ginseng, 217
  and bilberry, 7
  and chamomile, 56
  and feverfew, 140
  and garlic, 159, 160, 162, 170
  and ginger, 175
  and ginkgo, 190, 191, 199
  and St. John's wort, 326
  and tea, 341

Warner Lambert, 408

water retention, 278

weakness. *see* asthenia/weakness

weariness, menopausal, 22

Wechsler-Bellevue test, 224

weight loss
  drug interactions, 115
  increased thermogenesis, 112, 113, 115
  studies, 116, 120, 121, 349
  and tea, 339, 341, 349

weight loss products, 110–112

well-being/quality of life
  and Asian ginseng, 215, 223, 224
  and eleuthero, 102, 106
  and garlic, 161, 167, 168
  and St. John's wort, 331, 332
  and valerian, 362, 363

West Nile virus, 301

white blood cells (WBC). *see* leukocytes

Willmar Schwabe. *see* Dr. Willmar Schwabe

wind (TCM theory), 205

witch hazel, xx

withdrawal symptoms, 355, 356, 363

work capacity, 100, 102, 244

wormwood, 288

wounds, 54, 55, 57, 59, 88, 90, 251, 324

WS-1031, 319

WS-1473, 315, 317, 319, 402

WS-1490, 266, 270, 271, 401

WS-5570, 328, 333, 402

WS-5572, 328, 332, 403

WS-5573, 328, 332, 403

X

xanthines, 115, 339

xanthones, 325

xylose, 147, 370

Y

Yale-Brown Obsessive-Compulsive Scale, 334

yangonin, 263

yarrow hypersensitivity, 55, 56, 90, 139

yin (TCM theory), 205

yohimbe, 409

yucca, 409

Z

Ze-117, 327, 328, 331, 332, 402, 403

Ze-91019, 358, 363, 403

Zeller Medical, 67, 328, 408

zidovudine (AZT), 26, 215, 217

Zinaxin®, 176, 400

zinc serum concentrations, 294

Zincosamine, 400

Zingiber officinale, **171–183,** 377

zingiberene, 174

Zintona®, 176, 179, 400

Zoloft®, 331

zosteriform dermatitis, 160

Zostrix®, 45, 48, 49, 50, 398

Zung self-rating depression scale, 331

zymozam, 384

Zyzyphus jujuba, 377